The Cleveland Clinic Intensive Review Of Pediatrics

THIRD EDITION

The Cleveland Clinic Intensive Review Of Pediatrics

THIRD EDITION

■ CAMILLE SABELLA, MD

Associate Professor of Pediatrics
Center for Pediatric Infectious Diseases
Cleveland Clinic Children's Hospital
Cleveland, Ohio

■ ROBERT J. CUNNINGHAM III, MD

Vice Chairman of Pediatrics
Section Head, Pediatric Nephrology and Hypertension
Ochsner Medical Center for Children
New Orleans, Louisianna

Wolters Kluwer | Lippincott Williams & Wilkins
Health

Philadelphia · Baltimore · New York · London
Buenos Aires · Hong Kong · Sydney · Tokyo

Acquisitions Editor: Sonya Seigafuse
Managing Editor: Kerry Barrett
Product Manager: Kevin Johnson/Nicole Walz
Senior Manufacturing Manager: Benjamin Rivera
Marketing Manager: Lisa Parry
Design Coordinator: Holly Reid McLaughlin
Production Service: Maryland Composition/ASI

Printed in The People's Republic of China

Library of Congress Cataloging-in-Publication Data

The Cleveland Clinic intensive review of pediatrics / [edited by] Camille Sabella, Robert J. Cunningham III. — 3rd ed.
   p. ; cm.
  Includes bibliographical references and index.
  ISBN 978-1-60547-137-2
  1. Pediatrics. I. Sabella, Camille. II. Cunningham, Robert J., III. III. Cleveland Clinic Foundation. IV. Title:
Intensive review of pediatrics.
  [DNLM: 1. Pediatrics. WS 200 C635 2009]
  RJ45.C593 2009
  618.92—dc22
                              2008052573

Care has been taken to confirm the accuracy of the information presented and to describe generally accepted practices. However, the authors, editors, and publisher are not responsible for errors or omissions or for any consequences from application of the information in this book and make no warranty, expressed or implied, with respect to the currency, completeness, or accuracy of the contents of the publication. Application of the information in a particular situation remains the professional responsibility of the practitioner.

   The authors, editors, and publisher have exerted every effort to ensure that drug selection and dosage set forth in this text are in accordance with current recommendations and practice at the time of publication. However, in view of ongoing research, changes in government regulations, and the constant flow of information relating to drug therapy and drug reactions, the reader is urged to check the package insert for each drug for any change in indications and dosage and for added warnings and precautions. This is particularly important when the recommended agent is a new or infrequently employed drug.

   Some drugs and medical devices presented in the publication have Food and Drug Administration (FDA) clearance for limited use in restricted research settings. It is the responsibility of the health care provider to ascertain the FDA status of each drug or device planned for use in their clinical practice.

To purchase additional copies of this book, call our customer service department at (800) 638-3030 or fax orders to (301) 223-2320. International customers should call (301) 223-2300.

Visit Lippincott Williams & Wilkins on the Internet: at LWW.com. Lippincott Williams & Wilkins customer service representatives are available from 8:30 am to 6 pm, EST.

10 9 8 7 6 5 4 3 2 1

To our wives—Paula and Mary Sue—for their love, support and understanding,

and our children—Carmen, Julia, Annmarie, *and* Patrick, Colin, Meghan, Brennan, Shannon, Conor, and Nina—who are our inspiration,

and our parents—Samira, Elie, Maripat, and in memory of Robert Cunningham—whose love and encouragement made this possible.

Contents

List of Contributors xi
Preface xiii

PART I: GENERAL PEDIATRICS 1

1 Pediatric Dermatology 1
   John B. Lampe

2 Immunizations 14
   Camille Sabella

3 Board Simulation: General Pediatrics 27
   Scott A. Francy

PART II: PEDIATRIC GASTROENTEROLOGY 37

4 Abdominal Pain 37
   Barbara Kaplan

5 Inflammatory Bowel Disease 46
   Robert Wyllie

6 Viral Hepatitis 53
   Marsha Kay

7 Foreign Bodies and Caustic Ingestions 62
   Marsha Kay and Robert Wyllie

8 Neonatal Jaundice and Liver Disease 70
   Vera F. Hupertz

9 Common Mucosal and Luminal Disorders 78
   Kadakkal R. Radhakrishnan

10 Board Simulation: Gastroenterology 82
   Lori Mahajan

PART III: PEDIATRIC NEPHROLOGY 88

11 Fluids and Electrolytes 88
   Robert J. Cunningham III

12 Proteinuria and Hematuria 94
   Robert J. Cunningham III

13 Hypertension, Obesity, Type II Diabetes Mellitus and Hyperlipidemia 102
   Robert J. Cunningham III

14 Board Simulation: Acid–Base and Complex Fluid and Electrolyte Problems 109
   Robert J. Cunningham III

15 Board Simulation: Nephrology 116
   Robert J. Cunningham III

PART IV: PEDIATRIC ENDOCRINOLOGY 123

16 Adrenal Disorders 123
   Anzar Haider

17 Thyroid Disease 129
   Douglas G. Rogers

18 Calcium and Phosphorus Metabolism 135
   Robert J. Cunningham III

19 Short Stature and Growth Hormone Therapy 141
   Douglas G. Rogers

20 Board Simulation: Endocrinology 147
   Elumalai Appachi

PART V: NEONATOLOGY 153

21 Respiratory Diseases of the Newborn 153
   Craig H. Raskind

22 Neonatal Sepsis and Congenital Infections 163
   Camille Sabella

23 Board Simulation: Neonatology 175
   Elumalai Appachi

PART VI: PEDIATRIC CARDIOLOGY 180

24 Recognition of Cardiovascular Disorders 180
   Daniel J. Murphy Jr.

25 Congenital Heart Disease 187
   Athar M. Qureshi

26 Acquired Heart Disease 194
    Daniel J. Murphy Jr.

27 Disorders of Cardiac Rate and Rhythm 200
    Richard Sterba

28 Board Simulation: Cardiology 208
    Daniel J. Murphy Jr.

PART VII: PEDIATRIC ALLERGY AND PULMONOLOGY 214

29 Allergic Disorders 214
    Alton L. Melton Jr.

30 Asthma 219
    Velma L. Paschall

31 Board Simulation: Airway and Pulmonary Disorders 233
    Samiya Razvi

32 Board Simulation: Allergy and Immunology 241
    Nicola M. Vogel

PART VIII: PEDIATRIC NEUROLOGY 247

33 Epilepsy and Anticonvulsant Therapy 247
    Deepak K. Lachhwani and Elaine Wyllie

34 Nonepileptic Paroxysmal Disorders in Children 258
    Ajay Gupta, Bruce H. Cohen, and Elaine Wyllie

35 Neurocutaneous Syndromes 266
    George E. Tiller

36 Neuromuscular Disorders: Muscular Dystrophies and Congenital Myopathies 274
    Neil R. Friedman

37 Board Simulation: Neurology 282
    Bruce H. Cohen

PART IX: DEVELOPMENTAL PEDIATRICS 292

38 Normal Child Growth and Development 292
    Mark H. Deis and Roberta E. Bauer

39 Developmental Disabilities 300
    Roberta E. Bauer and Mark H. Deis

40 Board Simulation: Development 315
    Roberta E. Bauer and Mark H. Deis

PART X: GENETIC AND METABOLIC DISORDERS 325

41 Chromosomal Abnormalities 325
    George E. Tiller

42 Dysmorphic Syndromes 331
    George E. Tiller

43 Inborn Errors of Metabolism 341
    George E. Tiller

PART XI: ADOLESCENT MEDICINE 350

44 Adolescent Development and Tanner Staging 350
    Ajuah Davis

45 Sexually Transmitted Diseases 357
    Ellen S. Rome

46 Amenorrhea 368
    Karen S. Vargo

PART XII: PEDIATRIC INFECTIOUS DISEASES AND IMMUNOLOGY 377

47 Inherited Immunodeficiency Disorders 377
    Alton L. Melton Jr.

48 Infectious Diseases, Part I 383
    Camille Sabella and Johanna Goldfarb

49 Infectious Diseases, Part II 398
    Camille Sabella and Johanna Goldfarb

50 Infectious Diseases, Part III 406
    Lara A. Danziger-Isakov and Camille Sabella

51 Board Simulation: Infectious Diseases 415
    Camille Sabella

PART XIII: PEDIATRIC RHEUMATOLOGY 430

52 Rheumatic Disorders 430
    Philip J. Hashkes

53 Board Simulation: Pediatric Rheumatology 444
    Steven Spalding

PART XIV: PEDIATRIC HEMATOLOGY-ONCOLOGY 448

54   **Anemia: An Approach to Evaluation 448**
Jawhar Rawwas and L. Kate Gowans

55   **Hemoglobinopathies 457**
David J. Slomiany and Michael Levien

56   **Clinical Signs and Prognostic Factors in Common Pediatric Malignancies 467**
Michael Levien and L. Kate Gowans

57   **Bleeding Disorders 480**
Gregory E. Plautz

58   **Board Simulation: Hematology-Oncology 486**
Michael Levien and L. Kate Gowans

PART XV: PEDIATRIC EMERGENCIES AND CRITICAL CARE 493

59   **Ingestions and Poisonings 493**
Steve Davis

60   **Musculoskeletal Emergencies 500**
Martin G. Hellman

61   **Pediatric Trauma 506**
Michelle Walsh

62   **Board Simulation: Pediatric Critical Care 512**
Michael McHugh

PART XVI: PEDIATRIC SURGERY 516

63   **Board Simulation: Common Problems in Pediatric Surgery 516**
Anthony Stallion

64   **Orthopaedics for the Pediatrician 525**
Thomas E. Kuivila

65   **Urology for the Pediatrician 535**
Jonathan H. Ross

66   **Ophthalmology Overview 543**
Elias I. Traboulsi

PART XVII: BOARD SIMULATION 549

67   **Board Simulation: Potpourri 549**
Elumalai Appachi

68   **Board Simulation: Potpourri 557**
Robert J. Cunningham III and Camille Sabella

Index 569

List of Contributors

ELUMALAI APPACHI, MD Department of Pediatric Critical Care Medicine, Cleveland Clinic Children's Hospital, Cleveland, Ohio

ROBERTA E. BAUER, MD Chair, Department of Behavioral and Developmental Pediatrics, Cleveland Clinic Children's Hospital, Cleveland, Ohio

BRUCE H. COHEN, MD Center for Pediatric Neurology, Neurology Institute, Cleveland Clinic Children's Hospital, Cleveland, Ohio

ROBERT J. CUNNINGHAM III, MD Vice Chairman of Pediatrics, Section Head, Pediatric Nephrology and Hypertension, Ochsner Medical Center for Children, New Orleans, Louisiana

LARA A. DANZIGER-ISAKOV, MD, MPH Assistant Professor of Pediatrics, Cleveland Clinic Lerner College of Medicine of Case Western Reserve University, Center for Pediatric Infectious Diseases, Cleveland Clinic Children's Hospital, Cleveland, Ohio

AJUAH DAVIS, MD Center for Pediatric Endocrinology, Cleveland Clinic Children's Hospital, Cleveland, Ohio

STEVE DAVIS, MD Chair, Department of Pediatric Critical Care Medicine, Cleveland Clinic Children's Hospital, Cleveland, Ohio

MARK H. DEIS, MD Pediatric Associates, PSC, Crestview Hills, Kentucky

SCOTT A. FRANCY, MD Pediatric Institute/Regional Medical Practice, Cleveland Clinic Children's Hospital, Lorain, Ohio

NEIL R. FRIEDMAN, MBChB Center for Pediatric Neurology, Neurology Institute, Cleveland Clinic Children's Hospital, Cleveland, Ohio

JOHANNA GOLDFARB, MD Professor of Pediatrics, Cleveland Clinic Lerner College of Medicine of Case Western Reserve University; Head, Center of Pediatric Infectious Diseases, Cleveland Clinic Children's Hospital, Cleveland, Ohio

L. KATE GOWANS, MD Clinical Assistant Professor of Pediatrics, Cleveland Clinic Lerner College of Medicine of Case Western Reserve University, Department of Pediatric Hematology/Oncology, Cleveland Clinic Children's Hospital, Cleveland, Ohio

AJAY GUPTA, MD Assistant Professor, Cleveland Clinic Lerner College of Medicine of Case Western Reserve University; Director, Tuberous Sclerosis Program, Center for Pediatric Epilepsy and Neurology, Cleveland Clinic Children's Hospital, Cleveland, Ohio

ANZAR HAIDER, MD Center for Pediatric Endocrinology, Cleveland Clinic Children's Hospital, Cleveland, Ohio

PHILIP J. HASHKES, MD, MSc Associate Professor of Medicine and Pediatrics, Department of Rheumatic Diseases, Cleveland Clinic Children's Hospital, Cleveland, Ohio

MARTIN G. HELLMAN, MD, FAAP, FACEP Clinical Assistant Professor of Pediatrics, University of Pittsburgh School of Medicine; Attending Physician, Department of Emergency Medicine, Children's Hospital of Pittsburgh, Pittsburgh, Pennsylvania

VERA F. HUPERTZ, MD Department of Pediatric Gastroenterology and Hepatology, Cleveland Clinic Children's Hospital, Cleveland, Ohio

BARBARA KAPLAN, MD Department of Pediatric Gastroenterology and Hepatology, Cleveland Clinic Children's Hospital, Cleveland, Ohio

MARSHA KAY, MD Director, Pediatric Endoscopy, Department of Pediatric Gastroenterology and Nutrition, Cleveland Clinic Children's Hospital, Cleveland, Ohio

THOMAS E. KUIVILA, MD Orthopedic and Rheumatology Institute, Cleveland Clinic Children's Hospital, Cleveland, Ohio

DEEPAK K. LACHHWANI, MB, BS, MD Center for Pediatric Epilepsy and Neurology, Cleveland Clinic Children's Hospital, Cleveland, Ohio

JOHN B. LAMPE, MD Pediatric Institute/Regional Medical Practice, Cleveland Clinic Children's Hospital, Solon, Ohio

MICHAEL LEVIEN, MD Department of Pediatric Hematology/Oncology, Cleveland Clinic Children's Hospital, Cleveland, Ohio

LORI MAHAJAN, MD   Department of Pediatric Gastroenterology and Nutrition, Cleveland Clinic Children's Hospital, Cleveland, Ohio

MICHAEL MCHUGH, MD   Department of Pediatric Critical Care Medicine, Cleveland Clinic Children's Hospital, Cleveland, Ohio

ALTON L. MELTON JR., MD   Head, Center for Pediatric Allergy and Immunology, Cleveland Clinic Children's Hospital, Cleveland, Ohio

DANIEL J. MURPHY JR., MD   Associate Professor of Pediatrics, Stanford University School of Medicine; Associate Director, Pediatric Cardiology Clinical Services, Lucile Packard Children's Hospital, Stanford, California

VELMA L. PASCHALL, MD   Center for Pediatric Allergy and Immunology, Cleveland Clinic Children's Hospital, Cleveland, Ohio

GREGORY E. PLAUTZ, MD   Associate Professor of Pediatrics, Cleveland Clinic Lerner College of Medicine of Case Western Reserve University; Chair, Department of Pediatric Hematology/Oncology, Cleveland Clinic Children's Hospital, Cleveland, Ohio

ATHAR M. QURESHI, MD   Department of Pediatric Cardiology, Cleveland Clinic Children's Hospital, Cleveland, Ohio

KADAKKAL R. RADHAKRISHNAN, MD (Peds), DCH, MRCP (UK), MRCPCH, FAAP   Professor of Pediatrics, Cleveland Clinic Lerner College of Medicine of Case Western Reserve University, Department of Pediatric Gastroenterology, Cleveland Clinic Children's Hospital, Cleveland, Ohio

CRAIG H. RASKIND, MD   Department of Neonatology, Cleveland Clinic Children's Hospital, Cleveland, Ohio

JAWHAR RAWWAS, MD   Staff Physician in Hematology and Oncology, Children's Hospitals and Clinic of Minnesota, Minneapolis, Minnesota

SAMIYA RAZVI, MD, MS   Center for Pediatric Pulmonology, Cleveland Clinic Children's Hospital,Cleveland, Ohio

DOUGLAS G. ROGERS, MD   Head, Center for Pediatric Endocrinology, Cleveland Clinic Children's Hospital, Cleveland, Ohio

ELLEN S. ROME, MD, MPH   Associate Professor of Pediatrics, Cleveland Clinic Lerner College of Medicine of Case Western Reserve University, Department of General Pediatrics, Cleveland Clinic Children's Hospital, Cleveland, Ohio

JONATHAN H. ROSS, MD   Associate Professor of Surgery, Cleveland Clinic Lerner College of Medicine of Case Western Reserve University, Department of Urology Glickman Urological and Kidney Institute, Cleveland Clinic Children's Hospital, Cleveland, Ohio

CAMILLE SABELLA, MD   Associate Professor of Pediatrics, Cleveland Clinic Lerner College of Medicine of Case Western Reserve University, Center for Pediatric Infectious Diseases, Cleveland Clinic Children's Hospital, Cleveland, Ohio

DAVID J. SLOMIANY, MD   Department of Pediatric Hematology/Oncology, Children's Hospital of Minnesota, St. Paul, Minnesota

STEVEN SPALDING, MD   Associate Staff, Department of Rheumatic and Immunologic Disease, Cleveland Clinic, Cleveland, Ohio

ANTHONY STALLION, MD   Department of Pediatric Surgery, Cleveland Clinic Children's Hospital, Cleveland, Ohio

RICHARD STERBA, MD   Department of Pediatric Cardiology, Cleveland Clinic Children's Hospital, Cleveland, Ohio

GEORGE E. TILLER, MD, PhD   Department of Genetics, Southern California Permanente Medical Group, Los Angeles, California

ELIAS I. TRABOULSI, MD   Professor of Ophthalmology, Cole Eye Institute, Cleveland Clinic Children's Hospital, Cleveland, Ohio

KAREN S. VARGO, MD   Pediatric Institute/Regional Medical Practice, Cleveland Clinic Children's Hospital, Independence, Ohio

NICOLA M. VOGEL, MD   Allergy Associates of New Hampshire, Portsmouth Regional Hospital, Portsmouth, NH

MICHELLE WALSH, MD   Attending Physician, Department of Emergency Services, Akron Children's Hospital, Akron, Ohio

ELAINE WYLLIE, MD   Director, Center for Pediatric Neurology, Cleveland Clinic Children's Hospital, Cleveland, Ohio

ROBERT WYLLIE, MD   Calabrese Chair of Pediatrics; Chairman, Pediatric Institute; Physician-in-Chief, Cleveland Clinic Children's Hospital, Department of Pediatric Gastroenterology, Cleveland Clinic Children's Hospital, Cleveland, Ohio

Preface

The *Cleveland Clinic Intensive Review of Pediatrics* represents a compilation of pediatric topics reviewed at the "Cleveland Clinic Annual Pediatric Board Review Symposium," which we have had the honor and privilege of directing over the 14 years. As is the intent of the symposium, the intent of the book is to provide relevant, factual material in a format conducive to board review and preparation. We envision this text as an excellent tool for those seeking primary board certification in pediatrics, as well as physicians seeking board re-certification.

Each chapter provides review questions to reinforce reader's perspective understanding of important concepts covered in the text. In addition to topic chapters, we have incorporated "board simulation" chapters, which contain questions dealing with a specific subspecialty, along with detailed rationales to the questions. This allows the reader to:

- evaluate their strengths and weaknesses
- review important concepts in an efficient manner
- gain experience with multiple choice questions

Because the mission of this book is to provide an intensive, factual review of topics essential for board preparation, it is important to realize that the material presented is not necessarily indicative of the frequency of problems encountered by a pediatrician or primary care provider. Controversial issues in diagnosis or management are rarely represented on board examinations, and you will not find much information on topics where controversy exists. For example, the management of otitis media is rarely addressed to any degree in the book, whereas noncontroversial factual topics, such as vitamin deficiencies and metabolic disorders, are amply reviewed.

This third edition contains several new "board simulation" chapters, including the topics of airway and pulmonary disorders, rheumatology, emergency medicine, and common pediatric surgical problems. In addition, there are new chapters on gastrointestinal mucosal disorders and infectious diseases.

We are indebted to the many contributors of this book for their expertise, commitment to excellence, and love of patient care. Their commitment to education has been an inspiration in our endeavor to synthesize the knowledge and wisdom that we have gained from them. They have helped make the Cleveland Clinic Annual Pediatric Board Review Symposium an important resource for physicians preparing for board examinations, as well as primary care physicians seeking to update their knowledge. We expect you will find this book an equally valuable resource as you prepare for board certification or re-certification.

The Cleveland Clinic Intensive Review Of Pediatrics

THIRD EDITION

Chapter 1

Pediatric Dermatology

John B. Lampe

Dermatologic disease and normal skin variants are common considerations in a pediatric practice, accounting for up to 10% to 15% of pediatric office visits. For the physician who is familiar with common skin conditions and the available treatment options, the management of these conditions can be an enjoyable part of clinical pediatrics.

COMMON TRANSIENT NEONATAL SKIN CONDITIONS

Several common neonatal rashes are easily distinguished on close observation. *Erythema toxicum (neonatorum)* is possibly the most frequently encountered rash (Fig. 1.1). Appearing within the first 3 to 5 days of life, it resolves spontaneously in 1 to 2 weeks. The individual lesions are characterized by a central, small "welt" or pustule on a broader erythematous base and can appear anywhere on the body. The fact that they are individual lesions makes it possible to differentiate them from the clustered microvesicles of herpes simplex (which also yields a positive direct fluorescent antibody stain when the base of the lesion is scraped) and the wider pustules of impetigo (which can be confirmed by a positive Gram stain for neutrophils and the presence of gram-positive cocci in clusters or chains). For unknown reasons, a Wright stain of a scraping of erythema toxicum reveals predominantly eosinophils. No treatment of this rash is necessary.

Miliaria ("prickly heat") is another rash that is relatively common in the first few weeks of life (Fig. 1.2). Caused by keratin plugging of eccrine (sweat) glands in the skin, miliaria presents as an eruption of microvesicular lesions on the face, neck, scalp, or diaper area. If the eccrine obstruction is relatively deep in the epidermis, sweat can leak out of the duct and cause an inflammatory response, in which case the lesion has a red base. Treatment consists of dressing the infant in light clothes and avoiding excessive humidity.

Milia are white or yellow micropapules that develop when the pilosebaceous unit is obstructed by keratin/sebaceous material. They are most commonly found clustered on the nose, cheeks, chin, or forehead, and they resolve without treatment within several months.

ECZEMATOUS RASHES

Eczematous rashes are among the most frequently encountered skin disorders in children from infancy through adolescence. The neonatal form of *seborrheic dermatitis* often appears during the first several months of life. It may present as "cradle cap" and then extend to other areas of the skin where sebaceous glands are dense: the forehead and eyebrows, behind the ears, the sides of the nose, the middle of the chest, and the umbilical, intertriginous, and perineal areas in infants (Fig. 1.3). A *lack of pruritus* is characteristic of seborrhea. The individual lesions are often well-circumscribed plaques with greasy, yellow-to-orange overlying scales.

The lesions of infantile seborrhea often resolve by 8 to 12 months of age, but they can recur in childhood and especially in adolescence (in association with a hormonally related, general increase in sebaceous activity in the skin). Some dermatologists have proposed an association of seborrhea with skin colonization by *Pityrosporum ovale*, although it is unclear whether this is a primary or secondary phenomenon. The treatment of seborrheic dermatitis in infants is often expedited by controlling the scalp seborrhea with an antiseborrheic shampoo. In persistent cases of scalp seborrhea, one may consider treatment with 2% ketoconazole (Nizoral) shampoo. Once the scalp lesions are controlled, any residual skin lesions that do not resolve spontaneously can be treated with a brief course of a mild (1% hydrocortisone) topical steroid cream.

If a seborrheic-like rash is quite persistent or severe or is accompanied by anemia, adenopathy, or hepatosplenomegaly, consideration of a more systemic illness, such as *histiocytosis*, is appropriate.

Atopic dermatitis is the most often encountered chronic skin condition in pediatric practice (Fig. 1.4). The clinical term *eczema*, which is often used to indicate this diagnosis,

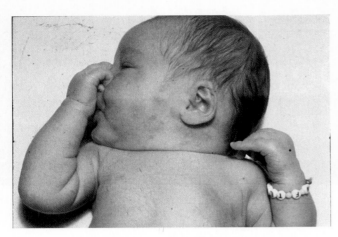

Figure 1.1   Erythema toxicum in a neonate. (See color insert.)

actually describes a clinical constellation of physical signs, including the following:

- Erythema
- Microvesicles (often confluent)
- Weeping and crusting
- Thickening (lichenification) of the involved skin as a result of chronic scratching

Atopic dermatitis represents an inherited predisposition of the skin to become excessively dry, to itch, and to display the noted features of eczema. Besides an underlying defect of stratum corneum barrier function, there is also altered T-cell expression with resultant local expression of inflammatory cytokines. The incidence in children is now estimated at 20%, and the condition is seen more often at times of the year (winter in temperate or cold climates) when the air is dry. *Atopic dermatitis often develops in conjunction with two other diagnoses of the so-called atopic triad—namely, asthma and allergic rhinitis (in the same patient or family members).*

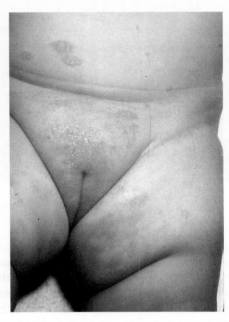

Figure 1.3   Seborrheic dermatitis in an infant. (See color insert.)

The pattern of distribution of atopic dermatitis often changes during the childhood years. Although it is often seen on the face in infants, it is found more often on extensor surfaces of the arms and legs in the first year of life, and in the more familiar sites of the antecubital and popliteal areas, front of ankles, neck, and face in older children and teenagers.

The treatment of atopic dermatitis strives to address the underlying physiologic events. Interrupting the "itch–scratch" cycle (e.g., with oral antihistamines or col-

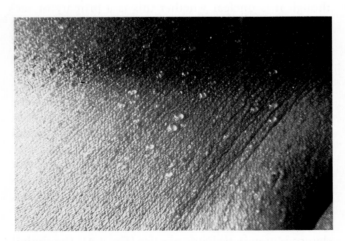

Figure 1.2   Microvesicular lesions representing miliaria. (See color insert.)

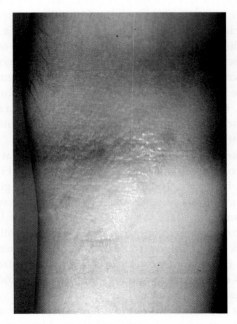

Figure 1.4   Atopic dermatitis in the antecubital fossa of an older child. (See color insert.)

loidal oatmeal baths) is important. The frequent and liberal use of unscented topical moisturizers to combat dry skin is helpful, especially immediately after a bath with tepid water and mild soap, if any. Newer, more expensive "physiologic moisturizers" are now available that attempt to replenish depleted intracellular lipids in the epidermis. Actively weeping patches can be partially relieved with wet compresses soaked in aluminum acetate solution (Domeboro, Burow; available over the counter as tablets or powder packets). Inflamed (red, scaly) lesions are usually treated with a topical steroid cream or ointment until the inflammation is controlled. (Ointments are more potent, with better penetration of lichenified lesions that are not on the face or on intertriginous, occluded areas of skin). Topical calcineurin inhibitors that block T-cell transcription upregulating inflammatory modulators, such as tacrolimus (Protopic) ointment and pimecrolimus (Elidel) cream, are effective in the treatment of moderate or refractory cases of atopic dermatitis. These agents are safe to use even on delicate skin such as on the face or neck. These calcineurin inhibitors, however, are currently recommended for children older than 2 years of age, and as second-line agents to be used if topical steroid therapy and moisturizers are ineffective. Finally, being alert to the presence of possible secondary infection (especially *Staphylococcus aureus*) and treating such infection with a course of an effective oral antibiotic or topical mupirocin (if the lesions are more localized) often leads to significant improvement.

Most easily recognized by its typical pattern of rashes, *contact dermatitis* is seen in patches, linear arrays, and unusual distributions (Fig. 1.5). Poison ivy (also oak or sumac), also known as *Rhus* dermatitis, is a paradigm for contact dermatitis. Lines and patches of textured ("orange peel") erythema soon develop on the skin that has come in contact with the oil of the plant leaves or stem. These rapidly become microvesicular rashes and can progress to larger blisters, which then open and weep. Contact dermatitis is typically pruritic. Treatment involves the following:

- Oral antihistamine to control itching
- Topical steroids (moderate potency)
- Consideration of oral steroids (prednisone or prednisolone for 1 week at a dosage of 1 to 2 mg/kg per day, with the dose tapered during the second week to prevent rebound of the rash) if the rash is extensive or involves the genitalia or skin around the eyes, potentially causing eyelid edema

Finally, *acrodermatitis enteropathica* can be considered in the same general category. This autosomal-recessive disorder causes zinc deficiency, and its clinical presentation is similar to that of nutritional zinc deficiency (as occurs in premature or chronically malnourished infants). In genetically susceptible infants who have been breast-fed, it often presents at the time of weaning, an observation that raises the possibility that a zinc-binding ligand in breast milk enhances zinc absorption up to the time of weaning. The associated rash is moist, erythematous, and papular, forming plaques on the skin around orifices (mouth, nose, ears, and perineum) and on the acral areas (hands and feet) (see Fig. 67.5). Associated systemic symptoms include a foul-smelling, frothy diarrhea; alopecia; irritability or apathy; and a generalized failure to thrive. Abnormal laboratory values include low levels of serum zinc and serum alkaline phosphatase (a zinc-dependent enzyme). Treatment is with zinc sulfate 5 mg/kg per day, which usually brings about a dramatic reversal of the symptoms and rash within several weeks.

PAPULOSQUAMOUS RASHES

Papulosquamous rashes are both raised ("papulo-") and covered with fine scaling ("-squamous"). *Pityriasis rosea* (Fig. 1.6) is a rash that may be seen every month or two in a pediatric practice, more commonly in teenagers and older children than in younger patients. The cause is unknown; it may be viral, although the condition is infrequently seen in more than one family member. The initial lesion is a "herald patch," a 2- to 4-cm scaly round or oval plaque with a raised border. A typical exanthem follows within 5 to 7 days, producing 2- to 10-mm ovoid, slightly raised plaques with central scaling in addition to smaller individual papules. The long axes of the smaller ovoid lesions are parallel to the crease lines of the skin, producing a "Christmas tree" pattern over the back if the rash is well developed. The rash lasts for 6 to 10 weeks and resolves without treatment. *Secondary syphilis sometimes mimics pityr-*

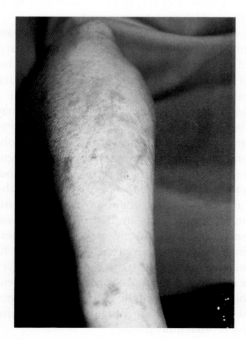

Figure 1.5 A child with contact dermatitis of the arm. (See color insert.)

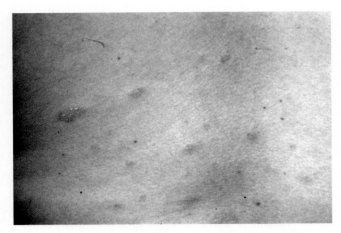

Figure 1.6 Papulosquamous lesions of pityriasis rosea. (See color insert.)

iasis rosea, but unlike pityriasis rosea, often includes lesions on the palms and soles.

Psoriasis (Fig. 1.7) is an unusual cause of scaly patches in children but must be kept in mind for the differential diagnosis, which includes tinea corporis, seborrhea, and pityriasis rosea. Psoriasis affects as many as 1% to 2% of adults, and approximately 35% of these instances present before the age of 20 years. Approximately 60% of pediatric patients have a first-degree relative with psoriasis. Sometimes precipitating factors can be uncovered, including trauma, cold, stress, and group A β-hemolytic streptococcal infection. One form of psoriasis, guttate psoriasis, can develop 2 to 4 weeks after a streptococcal infection,

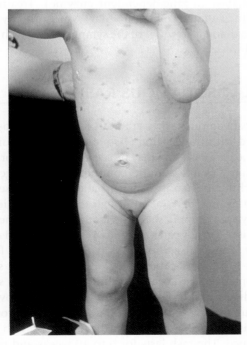

Figure 1.7 Scaly patches of psoriasis in a child. (See color insert.)

presenting with predominantly small, "drop-like" lesions. Psoriasiform lesions are red-based plaques with a fine, adherent silvery scale; their removal produces pinpoints of bleeding (Auspitz sign). The lesions are found on the knees, elbows, scrotum, and scalp. Nail pitting occurs in about half of clinical cases of psoriasis.

The treatment of psoriasis entails a minimal use of soap and the liberal use of thick emollients, keratolytics (with salicylic or lactic acid), and topical steroids of adequate potency to control inflamed lesions. Calcipotriene (a synthetic vitamin D_3 analog) topical cream or ointment has been an efficacious addition to therapy for teenagers and adults. Psoriasis is usually a chronic condition that is often difficult to treat and usually warrants consultation with a dermatologist who treats children.

VASCULAR MALFORMATIONS AND HEMANGIOMAS

Vascular malformations are hamartomas (anomalous morphogenesis) of mature endothelial cells that are present (but not always seen) at birth and enlarge with body growth. The blood flow through these lesions is either normal or slower than normal. Vascular malformations can affect the growth of underlying bone and soft tissue, causing asymmetric overgrowth (Klippel-Trenaunay syndrome). The most common vascular malformation is the "salmon patch" seen on the middle of the forehead, glabella, philtrum, or upper eyelids of about one third of newborns. This dull, reddish lesion becomes quite red when the infant cries, but the parents can be reassured that it will fade by 18 to 24 months of age, except if located on the nape of the neck, in which case it may persist.

Port wine stains are composed of mature, dilated dermal capillaries and are persistent. They range from light to dark red in color, and often deepen to a purplish hue with aging. If the distribution of the port wine stain includes the ophthalmic (upper eyelid to forehead) branch of the trigeminal nerve (see Fig. 35.8), the patient may have Sturge-Weber syndrome (estimated risk 8% to 29%). This syndrome includes ipsilateral leptomeningeal involvement and intracranial calcifications, which may be seen at the earliest with magnetic resonance imaging or computed tomography. Seizures develop in 60% to 90% of these patients, and about half of them have mental retardation. Concomitant eye findings in patients with this syndrome in whom the ophthalmic and maxillary branches of the trigeminal nerve are involved include glaucoma. It is recommended that port wine stains be treated with the pulsed tunable dye laser, emitted at a wavelength absorbed by hemoglobin in the vessels of the most superficial 1-mm layer of the skin. Multiple treatments are generally required, and the result is often quite good.

Hemangiomas can, by distinction, be considered benign neoplasms of endothelial cells, characterized by rapid

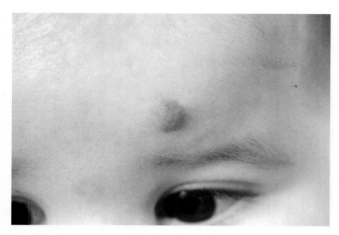

Figure 1.8   A superficial ("strawberry") hemangioma. (See color insert.)

blood flow and an increased density of mast cells within the lesion. They grow rapidly during infancy, then plateau and begin to involute by 18 to 24 months of age. *As a rough rule, approximately 50% of hemangiomas resolve by 5 years of age, 70% by 7 years, and 90% by 9 years.* The several different types of hemangiomas are classified by morphology. Superficial hemangiomas (formerly called "strawberry" hemangiomas) (**Fig. 1.8**) are well defined, raised, and light to deep red in color. Deeper ("cavernous") hemangiomas (**Fig. 1.9**) involve capillary growth into the dermis and subcutaneous tissue; therefore, they are often soft blue to red in color.

Hemangiomas occur in 10% to 12% of children, and at least 90% of them resolve without treatment. Exceptions to the watchful waiting approach are necessary if the growing hemangioma interferes with vision or obstructs the airway; in such cases, active intervention with steroids, interferon, or laser treatment (if superficial) is indicated. Midline lumbar or sacral hemangiomas may be associated with underlying spinal cord involvement and would warrant consideration of imaging of the cord. Hemangiomas involving the lip or breast tissue or those in a segmental pattern may also warrant more active therapy. A particular situation involving a *large "hemangioma," thrombocytopenia, and consumptive coagulopathy is the Kasabach-Merritt syndrome.* These lesions are actually not true hemangiomas, but rather tufted angiomas or kaposiform hemangioendotheliomas.

PIGMENTED AND HYPOPIGMENTED LESIONS

Several dermatologic conditions are associated with hyperpigmentation. Mongolian spots (dermal melanosis) (**Fig. 1.10**) are commonly observed in children of African-American, Asian, Hispanic, or Mediterranean descent. The dull, blue-black macule is found most commonly over the lower spine, but can be seen anywhere on the body, especially the shoulders and arms.

Incontinentia pigmenti is an x-linked dominant syndrome affecting the skin, central nervous system, eyes, and skeleton. (This condition is prenatally lethal in a male fetus.) The skin manifestations evolve in four phases. Inflammatory vesicles are first seen in neonates (**Fig. 1.11**) and evolve over several months to verrucous lesions. The lesions then develop into swirled, brown to gray patches and finally become hypopigmented.

Nevus sebaceous of Jadassohn (**Fig. 1.12**) is seen infrequently, but is important to recognize. Composed of sebaceous glands and rudimentary hair follicles, the lesion is initially a hairless, yellow-to-orange plaque that becomes

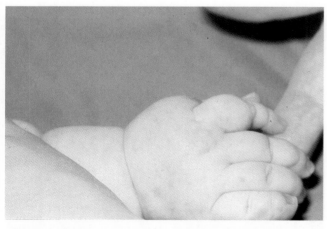

Figure 1.9   A deep or cavernous hemangioma. (See color insert.)

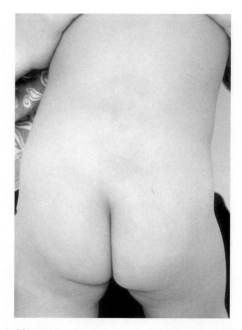

Figure 1.10   A blue-black colored macule, representing dermal melanosis (mongolian spot). (See color insert.)

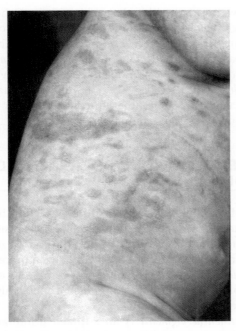

Figure 1.11 Inflammatory vesicular lesions in a neonate with incontinentia pigmenti. (See color insert.)

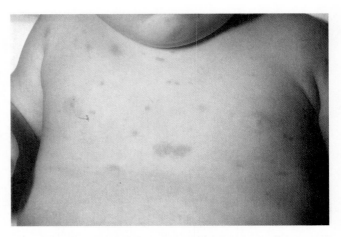

Figure 1.13 Urticaria pigmentosa on the trunk of an infant. (See color insert.)

darker and thicker during puberty. It is found usually on the scalp. Excision before puberty is advised to avoid the 10% to 15% risk for neoplastic transformation.

Urticaria pigmentosa (**Fig. 1.13**) is the most common example of the general diagnostic group of mastocytosis disorders, which have in common the pathologic accumulation of mast cells. Most of the urticaria pigmentosa cases present at 3 to 9 months of age, but the onset can certainly be later. Typically, patients have multiple reddish brown macules, papules, or nodules. The lesions urticate (welt) when rubbed firmly. This characteristic feature is the *Darier sign*. The lesions tend to be concentrated on the trunk more than on the extremities. Systemic involvement (of bone, liver, spleen, lymph nodes, or other tissues) can occur in up to 10% to 30% of children, primarily when the onset is after the age of 10 years. The prognosis for children in whom the onset is before 10 years of age is favorable. In this group, the condition usually remains cutaneous and often remits with time. Treatment consists of oral antihistamines as needed and the avoidance of food and medications that can cause mast cell degranulation (e.g., codeine, aspirin, opiates, procaine, radiographic contrast agents, alcohol, cheese, and certain spicy foods).

Nevi (nevocellular nevi) are classified according to the histologic depth at which the nevus cells are found. Nevus cells are thought to be derived from epidermal melanocytes and Schwann cells of the neural crest. Congenital melanocytic nevi (**Fig. 1.14**) are present at birth and carry a small risk for eventual malignant trans-

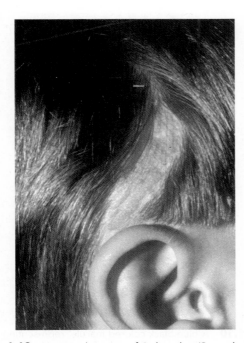

Figure 1.12 Nevus sebaceous of Jadassohn. (See color insert.)

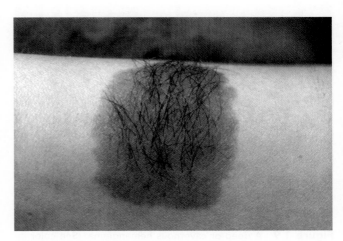

Figure 1.14 Congenital hairy nevus. (See color insert.)

formation: a 2% to 4% lifetime risk for small (<1.5 cm in diameter) congenital nevi, and a 6% to 7% risk for giant (>20 cm in diameter) congenital nevi.

Junctional nevi are characterized histologically by a location of the nevus cells at the dermal–epidermal junction and are sometimes the initial lesions of acquired nevi. They are brown to dark brown in color and flat, with a notable retention of skin crease lines across the lesion.

Intradermal nevi are characterized by nests of nevus cells in the dermis. They are flesh-colored to brown, slightly raised plaques that become more papillomatous and darker during adolescence.

Compound nevi exhibit nevus cells both at the dermal–epidermal junction and in the dermis. They are more commonly found in older children and adults. Morphologically, they are dome-shaped and range in color from light to dark brown or nearly black.

Malignant melanoma (**Fig. 1.15**), of course, is the skin malignancy for which clinicians are vigilant. The incidence of this cutaneous malignancy, which is more common in relatively lightly pigmented skin, has increased significantly during the past several decades, even in children and teenagers and the lifetime risk of melanoma is estimated to be 1 in 55. Worrisome signs of possible malignant transformation into melanoma include the following:

- Asymmetric shape
- Irregular borders
- Color changes (haphazard intermingling of black, blue, or red)
- Rapid growth
- Inflammation or ulceration

A final and interesting nevus to consider is the halo nevus. This lesion originates as a nevus (often compound or intradermal), and its periphery then becomes a depigmented halo. In about half of the cases, the central pigmented lesion resolves within several years. The rare incidence of a central melanoma has been reported.

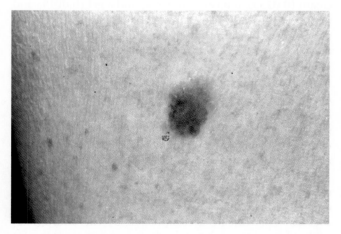

Figure 1.15 Malignant melanoma, characterized by asymmetry of shape, irregular borders, and diverse color. (See color insert.)

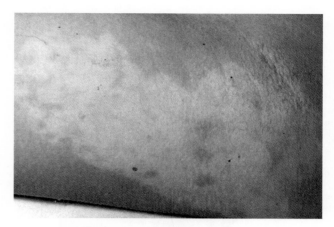

Figure 1.16 Vitiligo. (See color insert.)

Vitiligo (**Fig. 1.16**) is occasionally seen in pediatric practice. Thought to be an autoimmune disorder, it is caused by the destruction of melanocytes. Therefore, repigmentation is often not accomplished completely, if at all, although the chances of improvement are better in patients with more darkly pigmented skin. The likelihood of the coexistence of another autoimmune process (e.g., Graves or Hashimoto thyroid disease, Addison disease, myasthenia gravis) is 10% to 15%.

In approximately 50% of the cases of vitiligo, the onset is before the age of 20 years, and approximately 25% of patients have a positive family history of skin hypopigmentation disorder. Two types of vitiligo are seen clinically. A generalized type is often symmetric in distribution, involving the skin around the nose, mouth, umbilicus, or genitalia. This type is often progressive. The second type of vitiligo is segmental in distribution. It is usually linear, unilateral, and generally stabilizes after the first year of presentation.

The administration of sufficiently potent topical steroids early during the course of vitiligo can be helpful. Consultation with a dermatologist is helpful in all but the mildest nonprogressive cases. Treatment with topical psoralens plus ultraviolet A phototherapy may be considered in selected patients with vitiligo. Topical calcineurin inhibitors also have been employed, as well as narrow band UVB (311 nm) light therapy or the excimer laser for smaller lesions.

Neurofibromatosis (NF) is one of the several neurocutaneous syndromes associated with macules of variable pigmentation. Classified into eight distinct types, NF type 1 accounts for approximately 85% of cases, with an incidence of 1 in 4000 births. In NF type 1, *café au lait* macules (CALMs) appear during childhood, most often between birth and 2 years (see Fig. 35.1). The diagnostic criteria for NF type 1 in prepubertal children include the presence of at least six CALMs at least 0.5 cm in diameter and in postpubertal patients, more than 1.5 cm in diameter. Axillary freckling (Crowe sign) is found in up to half of the pa-

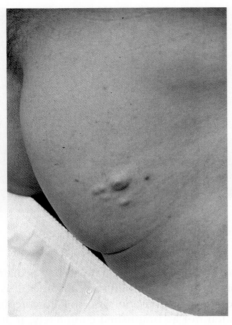

Figure 1.17 Neurofibroma in a child with neurofibromatosis (NF). (See color insert.)

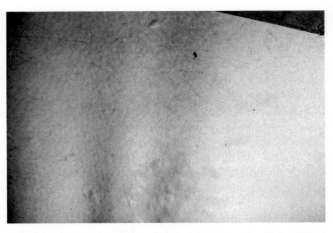

Figure 1.18 Shagreen patch in a child with tuberous sclerosis. (See color insert.)

tients. Other diagnostic criteria include the presence of two or more neurofibromas (of dermal or Schwann cell origin) (Fig. 1.17), often appearing at puberty, Lisch nodules (yellow-brown hamartomas on the iris seen on slit lamp examination), and neurologic manifestations (optic glioma, mental retardation, and seizures in approximately 10% of patients).

Tuberous sclerosis is also associated with skin pigmentary manifestations. Although an autosomal-dominant pattern of inheritance is cited, at least 50% of cases represent new mutations. DNA testing can now identify mutations in about 80% of cases. Hypopigmented macules ("ash leaf" pattern) are seen in 80% to 90% of cases, in addition to tiny, hypopigmented macules in a confetti-like pattern on the pretibial skin (see Fig. 35.5). Fifty percent of patients have five or less "ash leaf" macules, and 10% have only one (as do 1% of unaffected newborns). Other skin symptoms include Shagreen patches (connective tissue nevi with an orange peel texture, often evident over the lumbosacral spine) (Fig. 1.18), adenoma sebaceum (angiofibromas that are rounded, almost acneiform papules of the midface), and subungual fibromas. Systemic symptoms include seizures; cranial tubers (hamartomas); retinal phakomas; renal hamartomas; cardiac rhabdomyomas; and cystic, pulmonary, and osseous lesions.

ACNE

No dermatologic disorder is as ubiquitous in prepubertal children, adolescents, and young adults as acne, which is a disorder of the pilosebaceous unit precipitated by the hor-

monal milieu of puberty. Androgenic hormones cause an increase in sebaceous activity; therefore, more substrate is available for the lipolytic enzymes of *Propionibacterium acnes* bacteria dwelling in the skin to lyse into free fatty acids, so that an inflammatory response is generated. Altered keratinization of the follicular canal also leads to obstruction of the pilosebaceous unit, which is integral to the pathogenesis of the acne lesion.

The earliest lesion of acne is the microcomedo ("whitehead"), which progresses, if left untreated, to become an inflamed papule or pustule by dint of the processes noted in the preceding text. An open comedo ("blackhead") represents a dilated pilosebaceous orifice with melanized keratin debris visible within.

The treatment of acne seeks to address the physiologic causes. In early, noninflammatory acne with comedones, the objective of the treatment is to retard the development of closed microcomedones by attacking the excessive and abnormal desquamation of the follicular canal wall. Several topical treatments are applied to this effect, including topical tretinoin (Retin-A), which is available as a cream (0.025%, 0.05%, and 0.1%) and a gel (0.001% and 0.025%) for daily use. Topical adapalene (Differin), a naphthoic acid with retinoid activity, is also effective as a 0.1% gel or cream for daily use. Finally, topical 20% azelaic acid (Azelex), used twice daily, is an antibiotic with effects on keratinization. It also can be helpful in the treatment of cases of acne in which postinflammatory hyperpigmentation is troublesome. Tazarotene (Tazorac) gel or cream is a retinoid prodrug; used once daily for comedonal acne, it has a higher incidence of associated erythema or skin irritation.

In mild inflammatory acne, characterized by the development of scattered papules and pustules arising from microcomedones, the proliferation of *P. acnes* must be addressed. This can be accomplished by the addition of topical benzoyl peroxide (as a lotion, cream, or gel), also available in a combined cream with erythromycin

(Benzamycin) or clindamycin (BenzaClin or Duac). Other topical antibiotics that are useful include erythromycin, clindamycin, and azelaic acid.

Moderate inflammatory acne is marked by an increased density of papules and pustules, first on the face, then on the shoulders, upper back, and chest. An oral antibiotic is an appropriate addition to therapy at this point. Possible options include tetracycline, doxycycline, minocycline, and erythromycin.

Nodular cystic acne represents the most severe end of the acne spectrum. Patients have larger inflammatory papules; cystic lesions and often pitted scars can ensue. Oral *cis*-retinoic acid (Accutane) is frequently indicated and effective, reducing sebum production and altering keratinization. Up to 50% to 60% of the cases can remit with a single course. This medication has significant side effects, which must be closely monitored; the most significant of these is teratogenicity, which mandates contraception by two methods concurrently as well as following the prescribed program for monitoring toxicity and possible depressive symptoms.

VISUAL DIAGNOSIS OF SKIN MANIFESTATIONS OF KNOWN AGENTS

Viral Agents

■ *Varicella* (Fig. 1.19) is characterized by developing crops of initially erythematous papules that quickly develop into clear vesicles on a red base. The vesicular fluid becomes turbid, then white to yellow. The lesions subsequently dry and crust. Mucosal lesions are seen in the mouth and vagina, but not on the palms and soles (unlike the lesions of smallpox).

■ *Fifth disease (infection with human parvovirus B19)* is first evident as a macular erythematous blush on the cheeks. This is followed by a reticulated (lacy) erythematous

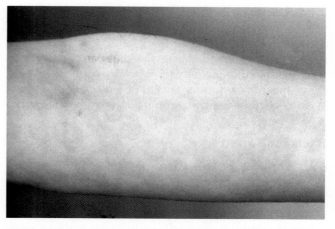

Figure 1.20 Lace-like reticular rash in a child with erythema infectiosum (fifth disease). (See color insert.)

rash (Fig. 1.20), most easily seen on the volar aspect of the arms and the anterolateral thighs. The rash can last for several weeks, during which time it can recur when the body temperature rises (e.g., during exercise or bathing).

■ *Herpes simplex virus* causes lesions that are typified as clusters of tiny vesicles, the fluid of which changes from clear to cloudy and then crusts. Recurrence of the lesion at the same (nerve distribution) site fairly confirms the diagnosis.

■ *Herpangina (infection with coxsackievirus, usually A16)* causes 1- to 2-mm ulcers on a red base in the posterior pharynx (on the pretonsillar pillars and adjacent palate). It can also cause concomitant intradermal blisters on the palms (Fig. 1.21) and soles, and vesicles on the buttocks. It usually shows strong seasonal predilection (end of summer).

■ *Molluscum contagiosum (a pox virus)* causes typical flesh-colored 1- to 2-mm dome-shaped papules with central umbilication over a central opaque "core" that some-

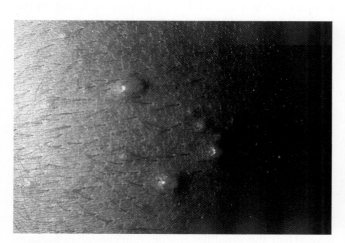

Figure 1.19 Vesicular lesion on an erythematous base, characteristic of varicella. (See color insert.)

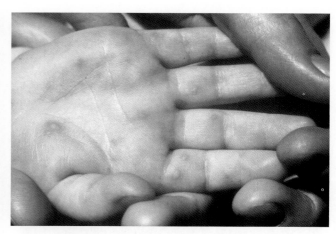

Figure 1.21 Intradermal blisters in a child with enterovirus infection. (See color insert.)

times can be seen through fair skin. Lesions can proliferate in patients with atopic dermatitis or an immunodeficiency.

■ *Warts (human papillomavirus).* More than 100 types of human papillomavirus cause a variety of wart lesions, ranging from common warts to filiform (columnar on a narrow base) and plantar (on the soles of the feet) warts.

Bacterial Agents

■ *Scarlet fever* is the rash that accompanies a group A β-hemolytic streptococcal infection. The fine erythematous confluent rash (described as having a "sandpapery" texture) appears first on the neck, in the axillae, and then over the groin. It dries and desquamates within a week to 10 days. This illness is also associated with circumoral pallor, *Pastia lines* (accentuated erythema of the crease lines in the antecubital fossae and axillae), and "strawberry tongue" (protrusion of red papillae through a white-coated surface of the dorsal tongue).

■ *Impetigo,* caused by staphylococcal or streptococcal bacteria, begins in a follicular pattern, with tiny pustules at hair follicle sites. These progress to blistered (bullous) or honey-crusted plaques that enlarge and spread to new sites without appropriate antibiotic treatment. Smaller lesions can be treated with the topical antibiotic mupirocin (Bactroban).

Fungal Agents

■ *Tinea corporis* is a superficial fungal infection of the skin. It causes an enlarging scaly plaque, often with some degree of central clearing and a raised scaly, papular, or even microvesicular border.

■ *Tinea versicolor* (Fig. 1.22) is a superficial fungal skin colonization by *Pityrosporum orbiculare* (also called *Malassezia furfur*). It causes hyperpigmented or hypopigmented plaques on the upper and middle areas of the

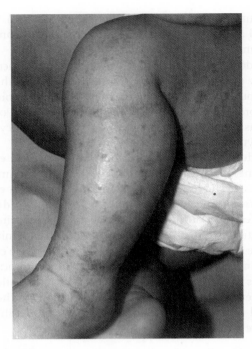

Figure 1.23 Pruritic erythematous papules and vesicles of scabies. (See color insert.)

back, the upper and sternal chest, and occasionally the face. It is seen most commonly in teenagers and young adults and is most evident in the summer months, when it causes an uneven tanning of the skin.

Mites

Scabies (Fig. 1.23) is caused by a microscopic mite, *Sarcoptes scabiei,* the pregnant female of which burrows into the epidermis to deposit its eggs. The skin lesions thereby created are erythematous papules, vesicles, or burrows. In infants and young children, the lesions are found on the arms, lower legs, feet (including the soles), and face. In older children and adults, the lesions are found on the finger webs, wrists, axillae, umbilical area, and groin. The rash is intensely pruritic, particularly at night, and easily spreads among family members. The diagnosis is confirmed by scraping an active lesion onto an oil droplet to search under the light microscope for the mite, its eggs, or fecal pellets. Scabies is safely treated by massaging 5% permethrin cream (Elimite) into the entire skin surface (including the head, palms, and soles in infants) and washing it off 8 hours later. Close family members should be treated concomitantly.

HAIR ABNORMALITIES

Several hair abnormalities are common enough in pediatric practice to warrant attention. *Trichotillomania* (Fig. 1.24) is self-inflicted pulling of the hair. Usually, the scalp hair is af-

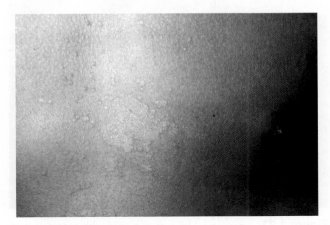

Figure 1.22 Hypopigmented, finely scaled plaques in a child with tinea versicolor. (See color insert.)

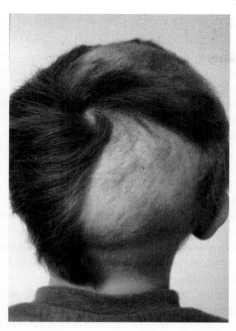

Figure 1.24 Patchy pattern of hair loss, consistent with trichotillomania. (See color insert.)

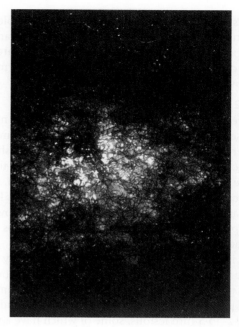

Figure 1.25 Tinea capitis in a child, causing an inflammatory loss of hair with crusting and pustule formation. (See color insert.)

fected, but eyelashes or eyebrows can also be lost. The clinical diagnosis is suspected on the basis of an unusual patchy pattern of hair loss, with an uneven pattern of hair regrowth. Trichotillomania can coexist with other compulsive behaviors, and treatment options include behavior modification or medication for severe cases (such as those used to treat obsessive-compulsive disorders).

Alopecia areata is diagnosed on the basis of the sudden appearance of sharply defined patches of hair loss; smooth areas of the scalp are left without scaling or inflammation. This process can progress for several weeks. If the hair loss is limited to several patches, regrowth usually occurs in 6 to 12 months. The condition is considered to be of autoimmune origin, and topical steroids of moderate to high potency are sometimes prescribed by dermatologists in more extensive or persistent cases.

Finally, *tinea capitis* (**Fig. 1.25**) is a quite common cause of inflammatory hair loss in children, more commonly seen in African-American patients. The involved areas of scalp can exhibit any degree of inflammation, from subtle scaling (easily confused with seborrhea) to crusting and pustule formation. Currently the most common cause in the United States is the endothrix (growing within the hair shaft and therefore not fluorescent under the Wood lamp) *Trichophyton tonsurans.* This fungus is easily grown in culture from a moistened swab rubbed vigorously over the affected scalp or from an opened pustule. The affected hairs break off at the skin surface, giving a "black dot" appearance to the scalp. Tinea capitis can be treated with oral griseofulvin (15–20 mg/kg per day given once daily with fatty food or beverage to enhance absorption) for a 6- to 8-week course. Use of a selenium sulfide–containing shampoo twice a

week can diminish spore carriage on the scalp and thereby decrease infectivity. In the unusual case of treatment failure with griseofulvin, an alternative antifungal, such as itraconazole or terbinafine, may be considered.

REVIEW EXERCISES

QUESTIONS

Case 1
You are asked by a nursery nurse during your morning rounds to check a 3-day-old newborn with a rash. The infant was delivered by cesarean section, has been feeding well, and has had normal vital signs. The rash you see on the infant is scattered on the trunk and consists of individual white, 1- to 2-mm papules on a blanchable erythematous base. Six to eight such lesions are evident.

1. Your diagnosis would likely be:
a) Milia
b) Impetigo
c) Herpes simplex virus infection
d) Erythema toxicum neonatorum

Answer
The answer is d. This is the classic description of erythema toxicum lesions. Milia are pinpoint white papules—usually over the nose, chin, or forehead of infants—that develop a little later. Impetigo lesions are more pustular or crusted and are often more clustered. Impetigo can be ruled out with a Gram stain if the diagnosis is in doubt. Herpes simplex virus generally causes

clusters of microvesicular lesions. If herpes simplex virus infection is suspected, a direct fluorescent antibody examination of the swabbed base of an unroofed lesion can be performed. A positive result confirms the diagnosis.

Case 2

An 8-year-old boy is brought to the office by his mother because of a spreading rash. She can recall no symptoms of fever or illness, and the boy denies that the rash is pruritic or bothersome. When questioned about the initial site and subsequent development of the rash, the boy recalls the appearance of a larger spot on his left lower abdomen several weeks ago. This was followed by the appearance of multiple lesions, mostly on his back and anterior trunk, but some on his extremities.

On inspection, you find a 2-cm-diameter scaly round plaque with a raised border at the noted initial spot. The rest of the rash consists of a combination of 1-mm individual papules intermingled with multiple, round to ovoid, 2- to 5-mm lesions, some of which have a superficial fine scale and most of which have a defined, raised edge.

2. Your initial thought of the *most* likely diagnosis is:
a) Contact dermatitis
b) Pityriasis rosea
c) Guttate psoriasis
d) Secondary syphilis

Answer
The answer is b.

3. Stepping back a bit, you notice that the long axes of the ovoid lesions are parallel with the skin crease lines, creating on the boy's back a pattern reminiscent of a fir tree. No rash is evident on the palms or soles. You are now confident in diagnosing:
a) Contact dermatitis
b) Pityriasis rosea
c) Guttate psoriasis
d) Secondary syphilis

Answer
The answer is b.

4. Based on this diagnosis, you advise the following treatment:
a) Mild topical steroid cream, expecting resolution within 5 to 7 days
b) Referral to a pediatric dermatologist to consider ultraviolet A phototherapy
c) Referral to a pediatric dermatologist for evaluation and possible biopsy
d) No treatment or topical emollients if the rash becomes pruritic, with the advice that the rash may persist for 6 to 8 weeks

Answer
The answer is d. The initial herald patch and the subsequent development of the characteristic ovoid, scaly lesions with defined edges are characteristic of pityriasis rosea, especially when the long axes of the ovoid lesions are aligned parallel to the skin crease lines and hence to each other (as seen on the back when the rash is more fully developed). The treatment is primarily reassurance that the rash is benign, although long-lasting, and that topical emollients may prove helpful if the patient experiences mild pruritus.

Case 3

A 3-year-old African-American boy is seen in your practice with a chief complaint of "bald spots." The child has been happy and playful. His father relates that the bald spots became evident at the child's most recent haircut 2 days ago.

The scalp examination reveals three areas of hair loss on the parieto-occipital scalp, ranging from 0.5 to 2.5 cm in diameter. The smaller two lesions are nearly devoid of hair, and five to ten black dots of broken hairs within hair follicles are seen. The larger patch of alopecia is reddened and a bit scaly, with several small pustules noted. When you check, you can palpate a 1 × 1.5-cm posterior cervical node over the adjacent neck area.

5. You are fairly confident that this represents:
a) Alopecia areata
b) Traction alopecia
c) Trichotillomania
d) Tinea capitis

Answer
The answer is d.

6. You advise the boy's father that:
a) You will obtain a fungal culture of the scalp.
b) The boy should be put on treatment once daily with 15 to 20 mg of oral griseofulvin/kg per day for 6 to 8 weeks, the medication to be taken with a fatty food or beverage.
c) The father should be aware that this condition is quite communicable by direct contact to siblings and playmates.
d) He should shampoo his son's hair twice a week with a selenium sulfide shampoo.

Answer
The answer is all of the above (*a–d*). Tinea capitis is clearly present in this case. The pattern of hair loss, notably with "black dots" representing broken, endothrix-weakened hairs, is well established. The erythema and scaling (signs of inflammation) and pustule formation in this case are also not unusual. The treatment advice given in question 6 is well considered and sound.

Case 4

The mother of a 6-year-old patient has called your office, worried about a spreading rash on her son's arms. He feels well except for complaining of pruritus. The rash started on his wrist 2 days ago, spread to his other forearm, and then to his cheek and the side of his neck. Embarrassed, when asked directly about other sites of rash, he confides that he has some rash on his penis as well, since this morning.

On examination, the original rash on his wrist is red and finely papular; with magnification by your otoscope it is actually noted to be microvesicular. The rash on his forearm is in a patchy distribution of plaques and linear arrays. The newest rash, on the penis, is red with a finely papular surface, in several lines.

7. To clarify the history, you ask further history about:
a) Recent travel
b) Camping or playing in the woods
c) Contact with siblings or playmates with similar rash
d) Fever or sore throat

Answer
The answer is b.

8. Clarifying the picture with the support of this added history, you diagnose:
a) Poison ivy (*Rhus* contact dermatitis)
b) Erythema infectiosum (Fifth disease)
c) Scarlet fever
d) Nickel dermatitis

Answer
The answer is a. Often a history of playing in the woods, or on the edge of a playground or yard where poison ivy might be found can be elicited as occurring in the preceding several days. It is also possible for the oil (urushiol) of the plant leaf or vine to be transmitted to the fur of a pet, which can cause a more diffused rash on the extremities. The rash itself is not contagious after the initial plant oil deposited on the skin is cleansed, but can be spread from the fingers (to face, neck, or genitals for instance) before the hands are washed, causing linear arrays of rash.

9. You advise treatment with:
a) Penicillin or amoxicillin
b) Lactic acid– or urea–containing emollient cream
c) Observation, with isolation until the rash has resolved
d) Topical steroid cream and oral antihistamine

Answer
The answer is d. If the oil of the plant can be washed off thoroughly with soap within several hours of exposure, the subsequent contact dermatitis might be lessened or even avoided. Once the rash is evident, treatment with a mild to moderate strength topical steroid cream can help lessen the pruritus (although it does not modify the several-week course of the rash), and a first- or second-generation oral antihistamine might help. If the rash is extensive, around the eyes or mouth where edema can be problematic, or over the genital skin, a several-week tapering course of oral steroid may be warranted.

SUGGESTED READINGS

1. Bittencourt FV, Marghoob AA, Kopf AW, et al. Large congenital melanocytic nevi and the risk for the development of malignant melanoma and neurocutaneous melanocytosis. *Pediatrics* 2000;106:736–741.
2. Drolet BA, Esterly NB, Frieden IJ. Hemangiomas in children. *NEJM* 1999;341:173–181.
3. Haggstrom AN, Drolet BA, Baselga A, et al. Prospective study of infantile hemangiomas: clinical characteristics predicting complication and treatment. *Pediatrics* 2006;118:882–888.
4. Hebert AA, Goller MM. Papulosquamous disorders in the pediatric patient. *Contemp Pediatr* 1996;13:69–88.
5. Huggins RH, Schwartz RA, Janniger CK. Childhood vitiligo. *Pediatric Derm* 2007;79:277–280.
6. Hurwitz S. *Clinical pediatric dermatology*, 2nd ed. Philadelphia: WB Saunders, 1993.
7. Mendenhall AK, Eichenfield LF. Back to basics: caring for the newborn's skin. *Contemp Pediatr* 2000;17:98–114.
8. Mulliken JB, Glowacki J. Hemangiomas and vascular malformations in infants and children: a classification based on endothelial characteristics. *Pediatr Reconstr Surg* 1982;69:412–420.
9. Schachner LA, Hansen RC. *Pediatric dermatology*, 2nd ed. New York: Churchill Livingstone, 1995.
10. Zaenglein AL, Thibautot DM. Expert committee recommendations for acne management. *Pediatrics* 2006;118:1188–1199.

Chapter 2

Immunizations

Camille Sabella

The goal of immunization is to prevent infectious diseases. In the United States, immunization programs have resulted in the elimination or significantly diminished incidence of many infectious diseases. The implementation of universal immunization against certain infections, such as measles, rubella, and infection with *Haemophilus influenzae* Type b (Hib), has resulted in a decrease of more than 99% in the prevalence of these infections.

Active immunization involves administering all or part of a microorganism or a modified product of such virulence to evoke an immunologic response. This response mimics the response to natural infection but poses little or no risk to the recipient. Active immunization can be accomplished with either live attenuated vaccines or killed (inactivated) vaccines. Vaccination with a live vaccine causes an active infection in the vaccinee but usually results in little or no adverse host reaction in an immunocompetent person. An immunocompromised person, however, may experience an adverse effect after vaccination with a live virus vaccine. The microorganisms in inactivated vaccines are incapable of replicating in the host and therefore do not pose a threat to an immunosuppressed host.

Passive immunization involves the administration of preformed antibody. This can be given for the following reasons:

- Prevention or amelioration of an infection in a susceptible host who has been exposed to the infection and is at high risk for its complications. A clinical example would be the administration of varicella-zoster immunoglobulin (Ig) to a susceptible immunocompromised host who has been exposed to varicella.
- Amelioration or provision of aid in suppressing the effect of the toxin when an infection is already present. A clinical example would be administration of tetanus Ig to treat a patient with tetanus.
- Replenishment of Ig in a person with deficient antibody synthesis because of a congenital or acquired B-cell defect. A clinical example would be administration of intravenous Ig monthly to a child with Bruton (X-linked) agammaglobulinemia.

GENERAL CONSIDERATIONS

In general, multiple vaccines can be administered simultaneously in a safe and effective manner. The immune response to one of the vaccines included in the routine immunization schedules generally does not interfere with the immune response to the others. A causal relationship between multiple immunizations and the development of immune system dysfunction has recently been *rejected* by an Institute of Medicine Safety Review Committee.

The recommended doses of vaccines are based on clinical trials and experience. Administering a reduced dose of a vaccine may result in a suboptimal immunogenic response to the vaccine. Therefore, reducing or dividing the dose of a vaccine is *not* recommended, even in premature or low-birth-weight infants.

The administration of parenteral *live virus vaccines* shortly before to several months after the administration of Ig products can result in diminished immunogenicity. This phenomenon has been documented for *measles vaccine* and theorized for *varicella vaccine*. The degree and duration of inhibition of the immune response vary with the dose and route of administration of the Ig product. If an Ig product has been administered within 14 days of the administration of measles, mumps, and rubella (MMR) or varicella vaccine, the vaccine should be readministered after a period deemed appropriate, depending on the dose and type of Ig given. If a child has received an Ig product and is due to receive an MMR or varicella vaccination, the vaccination should be deferred until an appropriate amount of time has elapsed. The intervals between the administration of select Ig products and the vaccination with measles and varicella vaccines recommended by the Committee on Infectious Diseases of the American Academy of Pediatrics are summarized in Table 2.1.

The National Childhood Vaccine Injury Act of 1986 requires health care professionals who administer routine vaccines to:

- Maintain permanent immunization records
- Report occurrences of specified adverse events to the Vaccine Adverse Event Reporting System (VAERS)

TABLE 2.1

RECOMMENDED TIME INTERVALS BETWEEN ADMINISTRATION OF AN IMMUNOGLOBULIN PRODUCT AND IMMUNIZATION WITH MEASLES OR VARICELLA VACCINES

Immunoglobulin Product/ Indication	Recommended Interval (Months)
Tetanus Ig	3
Ig for hepatitis A prophylaxis	3
Hepatitis B Ig	3
Varicella-zoster Ig	5
Intravenous Ig for replacement therapy	8
Intravenous Ig for Kawasaki syndrome	11

Ig, immunoglobulin.

CONTRAINDICATIONS TO VACCINATION

Contraindications to vaccination are discussed in the subsequent text in the sections on specific vaccines. In general, if an infant or child has an acute febrile illness, unless it is mild with only low-grade fever, immunizations should be deferred until recovery. An otherwise healthy child who is on antimicrobial therapy, has a mild diarrheal illness, or recently has been exposed to an infectious disease can be vaccinated. Likewise, an otherwise healthy child who has a pregnant, unimmunized, or immunodeficient household contact can be vaccinated. Breast-feeding, malnutrition, and a family history of seizures or adverse events after immunizations are *not* contraindications to immunizations.

Premature infants generally can be immunized at the usual chronologic age. The one possible *exception* concerns hepatitis B immunization in infants weighing *less than 2 kg*. These infants vaccinated with hepatitis B vaccine *at birth* have seroconversion rates after hepatitis B vaccination that are lower than those in term infants and in preterm infants vaccinated at a later date. However, medically stable preterm neonates appear to respond to hepatitis B vaccination as well as older infants. Thus the following recommendations apply for hepatitis B vaccination of infants weighing less than 2 kg.

If the mother is hepatitis B surface antigen (HBsAg)-*negative*:

■ Defer the first dose of hepatitis B vaccine until the infant is 30 days of age if medically stable or at hospital discharge if the infant is discharged before 30 days of chronologic age. The second and third doses of vaccine can then be administered at 1 to 2 months and 6 to 18 months of age, respectively.

If the mother is HBsAg-*positive*:

■ Administer the first dose of hepatitis B vaccine to the infant within 12 hours of birth, along with hepatitis B Ig.

■ Complete the immunization series with *three* subsequent doses of hepatitis B vaccine (do not count the first dose given as part of the immunization series), when the infant is 1 month, 2 to 3 months, and 6 to 7 months of age.

■ Test the infant for the presence of HBsAg and antibody to HBsAg (anti-HBs) at 9 to 18 months of age.

ACTIVE IMMUNIZATIONS ROUTINELY RECOMMENDED FOR ALL CHILDREN (Figs. 2.1 and 2.2)

Tetanus Vaccine

Tetanus vaccine is a killed toxin (toxoid) vaccine that is usually combined with diphtheria and acellular pertussis vaccine (DTaP and Tdap) or with diphtheria vaccine (DT or Td). Vaccination with a primary series and booster doses every 10 years is nearly 100% effective in preventing tetanus. Natural disease usually does not confer immunity to tetanus.

After the primary series is complete, booster doses should be given every 10 years. Booster doses should not be given more frequently than every 10 years except for tetanus postexposure wound prophylaxis (see subsequent text).

Adverse effects include extremely rare reports of severe anaphylactic reactions, Guillain-Barré syndrome, and brachial neuritis. *The only contraindication to tetanus vaccination is an immediate anaphylactic reaction to a previous dose of tetanus-containing vaccine.* In this rare circumstance, referral to an allergist and possible desensitization is warranted.

Tetanus Prophylaxis in Wound Management

For children who have received three or more doses of tetanus toxoid previously, tetanus vaccination is recommended if the time elapsed since the last dose of vaccine is 5 years (for contaminated wounds) or 10 years (for clean, minor wounds). For children who have received no or fewer than three doses of tetanus vaccine, this vaccine, along with *tetanus Ig*, should be administered for contaminated wounds, whereas only tetanus vaccine should be administered for clean, minor wounds. The choice of tetanus vaccine depends on the age of the child and whether pertussis vaccine is contraindicated:

■ For children younger than 7 years, DTaP is recommended unless pertussis vaccine is contraindicated, in which case DT should be given.

■ For children 7 to 10 years of age or older, adult-type diphtheria vaccine should be administered in combination with tetanus vaccine (Td).

■ For adolescents 11 to 18 years of age, Tdap should be administered instead of Td, unless they have received Tdap previously.

Diphtheria Vaccine

Diphtheria vaccine is a killed toxin (toxoid) vaccine given in combination with tetanus toxoid and acellular pertussis

Vaccine ▼ Age ►	Birth	1 month	2 months	4 months	6 months	12 months	15 months	18 months	19–23 months	2–3 years	4–6 years
Hepatitis B	HepB	HepB			HepB						
Rotavirus			Rota	Rota	Rota						
Diphtheria, Tetanus, Pertussis			DTaP	DTaP	DTaP		DTaP				DTaP
Haemophilus influenzae type b			Hib	Hib	*Hib*	Hib					
Pneumococcal			PCV	PCV	PCV	PCV				PPV	
Inactivated Poliovirus			IPV	IPV		IPV					IPV
Influenza					Influenza (Yearly)						
Measles, Mumps, Rubella						MMR					MMR
Varicella						Varicella					Varicella
Hepatitis A						HepA (2 doses)				HepA Series	
Meningococcal										MCV4	

Range of recommended ages

Certain high-risk groups

Figure 2.1   Recommended Immunization Schedule for Persons Aged 0–6 Years, United States, 2008. Adapted from the recommendations of the Advisory Committee on Immunization Practices (http://www.cdc.gov/vaccines/recs/acip), the American Academy of Pediatrics (http://www.aap.org), and the American Academy of Family Physicians (http://www.aafp.org).

vaccine (DTaP or Tdap) or with tetanus toxoid (DT or Td). DTaP and DT should be used for infants and children younger than 7 years, Td should be given to children 7 to 10 years of age, and Tdap used in adolescents 11 to 18 years of age. The dose of diphtheria toxoid in the Td and Tdap preparations are significantly lower than that in DTaP and DT and are therefore less reactogenic in older children and adults.

Immunization with diphtheria toxoid is effective in preventing infection and decreasing colonization by toxinogenic strains of *Corynebacterium diphtheriae*, as evidenced by the rarity of this disease in countries with high immunization rates.

Adverse reactions to diphtheria toxoid include mild local reactions, such as tenderness, swelling, and erythema. In children 7 years of age and older, the incidence of local

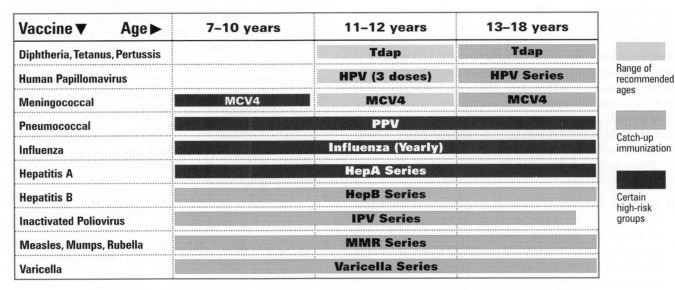

Figure 2.2   Recommended Immunization Schedule for Persons Aged 7–18 years, United States, 2008. Adapted from the recommendations of the Advisory Committee on Immunization Practices (http://www.cdc.gov/vaccines/recs/acip), the American Academy of Pediatrics (http://www.aap.org), and the American Academy of Family Physicians (http://www.aafp.org).

reactions to the standard diphtheria dose contained in DTaP and DT is higher; therefore, they should be immunized with Td or Tdap. Anaphylaxis is an extraordinarily rare event following diphtheria and tetanus vaccination.

The only contraindication to diphtheria vaccination is a history of an immediate severe or life-threatening event after a previous dose of diphtheria vaccine.

Pertussis Vaccines

Whole-cell vaccines containing inactivated *Bordetella pertussis* organisms have been replaced by acellular vaccines for routine immunization in the United States. Acellular vaccines contain one or more purified antigens of the bacteria and are combined with diphtheria and tetanus toxoids. Acellular vaccines cause fewer reactions than whole-cell vaccines.

The immunogenicity and efficacy of acellular vaccines are comparable with those of whole-cell vaccines. The efficacy of these vaccines in preventing pertussis following primary vaccination is between 70% and 85%.

Acellular pertussis vaccines are recommended for infants and children in the United States because they are associated with fewer adverse events, such as fever, irritability, and local reactions, than whole-cell vaccines. Pertussis vaccines are *not* currently indicated for children 7 to 10 years of age, although Tdap vaccines are now approved for use in adolescents 11 to 18 years of age.

Adverse events following pertussis vaccination include the following:

- Erythema, swelling, and pain at the injection site
- Fever, usually low-grade, very rarely to 40.5°C (104.9°F) or higher
- Anaphylaxis and allergic reactions
- Seizures, most of which are febrile seizures
- Hypotonic-hyporesponsive episodes
- Persistent, inconsolable crying
- Limb swelling

The incidence of systemic and local reactions is significantly less following acellular pertussis vaccination than following whole-cell vaccination. The seizures that follow the administration of pertussis vaccines are thought to be mostly febrile seizures and are not associated with long-term sequelae. Likewise, the hypotonic and prolonged episodes of crying do not appear to be associated with any sequelae. Limb swelling involving the entire thigh or upper arm, sometimes occurring with fever, erythema, and pain, has been reported to occur after *booster* doses of acellular pertussis vaccines. This condition resolves spontaneously and without sequelae.

Examination of occurrences of sudden infant death syndrome, brain damage, seizure disorder, and developmental delay following pertussis vaccination has *not* established a causal relationship.

Contraindications to pertussis vaccination include the following:

- Immediate anaphylactic reaction to a previous dose of the vaccine
- Severe encephalopathy occurring within 7 days after a previous dose of a vaccine that cannot be explained by another cause

Adverse events associated with pertussis vaccination, such as seizures within 3 days of after vaccination, inconsolable crying within 3 hours of vaccination, a hypotonic episode within 48 hours of vaccination, and fever to 40.5°C (104.9°F) or higher, are *not* considered true contraindications to further vaccination. However, in these situations, the benefits and risks should be carefully considered before vaccination.

The decision to administer pertussis vaccines to children with underlying neurologic disorders must be considered carefully and on an individual basis. In general, in children with *progressive,* unstable, or evolving neurologic disorders, including recent or uncontrolled seizures, pertussis vaccination should be deferred until the condition has been stabilized. Children with stable neurologic conditions or well-controlled seizure disorders may be immunized with DTaP. A family history of seizure disorder is not a contraindication to immunizing a child with pertussis vaccine.

Poliovirus Vaccines

Poliovirus vaccination, which began with the introduction of the inactivated poliovirus vaccine (IPV) in the 1950s, followed by the oral poliovirus vaccine (OPV) in the 1960s, has virtually eliminated paralytic poliomyelitis worldwide. The last indigenously acquired case of polio caused by wild-type poliovirus in the United States was in 1979; since that time, *the only cases of indigenous paralytic polio reported in the United States have been associated with OPV.*

Until 2000, OPV was used exclusively in the United States and around the world to control poliovirus. However, because of the risk for vaccine-associated paralytic poliomyelitis (VAPP) with OPV, *an all-IPV schedule is now recommended in the United States.* IPV is now the only polio vaccine available in the United States. OPV is still the only vaccine recommended in countries in which polio remains endemic.

Inactivated Poliovirus Vaccine
IPV, developed by Jonas Salk in the early 1950s, consists of formalin-inactivated noninfectious viral particles. The currently available vaccine is an enhanced formulation that contains higher concentrations of all three poliovirus serotypes and is highly immunogenic against all three. Nearly 100% of children have antibodies to all three

serotypes of poliovirus after two doses of IPV in the first year of life and a booster dose in the second year of life. Therefore, IPV is at least as immunogenic as OPV.

Because IPV is a killed virus vaccine, adverse events associated with vaccination are exceedingly rare. No risks of VAPP or of spread to immunocompromised persons are associated with IPV. Therefore, the vaccine can be administered to immunodeficient persons and their contacts. The only contraindication to IPV immunization is a severe allergic reaction to a previous dose or to streptomycin, polymyxin B, or neomycin, which the vaccine contains in trace amounts.

Oral Poliovirus Vaccine

OPV, developed by Albert Sabin and licensed for use in 1961, is a live attenuated virus vaccine containing all three poliovirus strains. The vaccine is highly immunogenic and provides durable protection that is probably life long. OPV induces mucosal immunity in the oropharynx and intestine and the virus is shed in the pharynx and feces for weeks after vaccination.

Because the virus is shed in the stool and saliva, it can be transmitted to close contacts and provide protection for those not previously immunized. OPV remains the vaccine of choice in many parts of the world and was the vaccine of choice for decades in the United States because of its:

- Low production cost
- Ease of administration and acceptance by patients
- Ability to transmit immunity to and protect unimmunized persons (herd immunity)
- Ability to induce intestinal immunity

The problem with OPV is its potential to cause paralytic disease in vaccine recipients and their contacts. The overall risk for VAPP, when both recipients and contacts are included, is 1/2.4 million doses. The risk is highest following the first dose (approximately 1/760,000 doses). The risk for VAPP is 3200- to 6800-fold higher in immunodeficient than in immunocompetent persons.

Licensed OPV is no longer available in the United States.

Measles Vaccine

The current measles vaccine is a live attenuated wholevirus vaccine grown in chicken embryo cell culture. Although monovalent measles vaccine is available, it is preferable to administer measles vaccine in combination with rubella and mumps vaccines (MMR vaccine).

Immunity to measles develops in approximately 95% of children following vaccination at 12 to 15 months of age. When children are given two doses of the vaccine separated by at least 4 weeks, immunity develops in more than 99%. Because of this 5% primary vaccine failure rate with one dose of the vaccine, a *two-dose schedule* is routinely recommended. Measles outbreaks in the United

States in the late 1980s and early 1990s were a direct result of poor immunization rates in preschool children. Since that time, the incidence of measles in the United States has fallen, and currently the incidence of measles in this country is at an all-time low. Although indigenous cases of measles are rare, imported cases from other countries continue to occur.

The seroconversion rates in infants younger than 1 year who are immunized with measles vaccine are significantly lower than those in children 1 year of age and older. This finding has been attributed to the presence of maternal passive antibody, although deficiencies in humoral immunity in the first year of life may contribute to the lack of immunogenicity of the vaccine. However, during an outbreak, the vaccine can be given as early as 6 months of age. Children immunized before their first birthday must be revaccinated at 12 to 15 months of age and then receive a third dose at least 1 month after the second dose.

Adverse Events

A fever of 39.4°C (102.9°F) or higher develops in approximately 5% to 15% of vaccinees approximately 7 to 12 days after vaccination. The seizures associated with these fevers are usually simple febrile seizures and are not associated with long-term sequelae. Transient rashes occur in 5% of vaccinees. A transient thrombocytopenia occurs rarely, and encephalitis or encephalopathy is estimated to be associated with fewer than one in 1 million doses administered. Several recent studies, as well as an Institute of Medicine Immunization Safety Review Committee report, have refuted a causal relationship between measles vaccine and autism.

The following individuals should *not* receive measles vaccine:

- Pregnant women
- Children who have had an anaphylactic reaction to a previous dose of measles vaccine
- Persons with immunocompromising conditions (except asymptomatic human immunodeficiency virus [HIV] infection; see subsequent text)

In addition, in children who have recently received Ig, measles vaccination should be delayed for a specified period on the basis of the Ig preparation and dose received (see Table 2.1).

Human Immunodeficiency Virus Infection and Measles Vaccine

Infants and children infected with HIV are at risk for severe complications of measles infection, such as severe pneumonia. Therefore, measles vaccine should be given to persons with *asymptomatic* HIV infection and those with symptomatic infection but *without* severe immunosuppression on the basis of $CD4^+$ T-lymphocyte counts and percentages. Individuals infected with HIV who have severe immunosuppression should *not* receive measles vaccine because of the risk for vaccine-related pneumonia.

Egg Allergies and Measles Vaccine

Measles vaccine is produced in chicken embryo cells but does *not* contain significant amounts of egg white cross-reacting proteins. Most children with a history of anaphylaxis to eggs have no untoward reaction to MMR vaccine. Furthermore, in children who are allergic to eggs, skin testing with measles vaccine is not predictive of immediate hypersensitivity reaction. Therefore, children with a history of egg allergy *can* be given MMR vaccine without prior skin testing.

Mumps Vaccine

Mumps vaccine is a live attenuated strain prepared in chicken embryo cell cultures. A monovalent vaccine is available, but a combination with measles and rubella vaccines (MMR vaccine) is preferred. The vaccine is highly immunogenic, and vaccine-induced immunity is long-lasting.

Adverse reactions to mumps vaccine are extremely rare. The recommendations and contraindications for mumps vaccination are as described in the preceding text for measles vaccination.

Rubella Vaccine

Rubella vaccine is a live attenuated vaccine grown in human diploid cell cultures and usually administered in combination with measles and mumps vaccines (MMR vaccine). Like measles and mumps vaccines, rubella vaccine is highly immunogenic and efficacious, and it provides long-term immunity. Special efforts should be made to immunize susceptible postpubertal persons because congenital rubella syndrome continues to be a problem in communities with low immunization rates.

Adverse events associated with rubella vaccine include mild lymphadenopathy, fever, and rash occurring 5 to 12 days after vaccination. Transient arthralgias and mild arthritis occur in 0.5% of vaccinated young children but are much more common in susceptible postpubertal women.

Like measles vaccine, rubella vaccine should not be given to pregnant women, persons with altered immunity (other than HIV infection; see preceding section on measles vaccine), and persons who have recently received Ig.

Haemophilus Influenzae Type b Vaccines

Vaccines against Hib were introduced in 1988. The first were polysaccharide vaccines that did not elicit an immune response in infants and children younger than 2 years. During the next few years, capsular polysaccharide vaccines were covalently linked (conjugated) to carrier proteins. These conjugate vaccines activate helper T cells and induce T-dependent (thymus-dependent) immunity, resulting in:

- Greatly enhanced quantitative responses, especially in infants
- Immunologic memory
- Reliance on IgG rather than IgM antibody

Currently, three single-antigen conjugate Hib vaccines and two combination vaccines that contain Hib are available in the United States. All are highly immunogenic in infants and children. Their efficacy is evidenced by the virtual elimination of invasive Hib disease in the United States since their introduction.

Hib vaccines are recommended for use in all infants, starting at 2 months of life. After the primary series, a booster dose is recommended at 12 to 15 months of life.

Adverse events associated with Hib vaccines are uncommon. Local reactions at the injection site occur, but these are usually mild and short-lived. Systemic reactions are rare.

Hepatitis B Vaccines

The hepatitis B vaccines currently available in the United States are produced by a recombinant DNA technology, in which common baker's yeast is genetically modified to synthesize HBsAg. Hepatitis B vaccines are 90% to 95% effective in preventing hepatitis B viral infection and clinical hepatitis in children and adults. Although antibody levels may wane over time and become undetectable, long-term studies indicate that the memory response remains intact for at least 15 years.

Routine immunization against hepatitis B is recommended for *all infants, children, and adolescents.* In addition, all persons at high risk for hepatitis B viral infection should be immunized (**Table 2.2**). *Routine immunization of all infants is the most effective method to prevent the transmission of hepatitis B viral infection and eventually eliminate it.* In addition, special efforts should be taken to vaccinate all children before they reach adolescence.

Postexposure immunoprophylaxis is the most effective method to prevent the vertical transmission of hepatitis B virus. Recommendations are based on the hepatitis B status of the pregnant mother. The management of infants born to HBsAg-*positive* mothers includes the following:

- Administration of hepatitis B Ig within 12 hours of birth
- Administration of hepatitis B vaccine within 12 hours of birth at a different site
- Administration of a second dose of hepatitis B vaccine at 1 to 2 months of life
- Administration of a third dose of hepatitis B vaccine at 6 months of life
- Testing of infants for HBsAg and anti-HBs at 9 to 15 months of age

TABLE 2.2

PERSONS AT HIGH RISK FOR HEPATITIS B VIRUS INFECTION

Alaskan native and Asian-Pacific islander children
Children born to first-generation immigrants from HBV-
   endemic areas
Sexually active heterosexual adolescents and adults
Household contacts and sexual partners of individuals with
   chronic HBV infection
Healthcare professionals
Residents and staff of institutions for individuals with
   developmental disabilities
Patients undergoing hemodialysis
Adoptees and their household contacts from countries in which
   HBV infection is endemic
Inmates in juvenile detention and other correctional facilities
Patients with bleeding disorders who receive clotting factor
   concentrates
Long-term international travelers to areas in which HBV
   infection is endemic

HBV, hepatitis B virus.

The management of infants born to mothers not tested during pregnancy should include the following:

- Administration of hepatitis B vaccine to the infant within 12 hours of birth
- Testing of the mother for HBsAg status as soon as possible after childbirth
    - *If* the mother is found to be HBsAg-*positive*, administer hepatitis B Ig to the infant as soon as possible but before 7 days of birth and complete the hepatitis B vaccine series at 6 months of age

For infants born to HBsAg-*negative* mothers, hepatitis B vaccine should be given according to the following schedule:

- Dose 1: birth (before discharge)
- Dose 2: between 1 and 2 months of age
- Dose 3: between 6 and 18 months of age

Adverse reactions to hepatitis B vaccine include local pain and low-grade fever. Anaphylaxis appears to be a very rare event. A causal relationship between hepatitis B vaccine and Guillain-Barré syndrome or demyelinating diseases of the central nervous system has *not* been found.

Varicella Vaccine

Varicella vaccine is a live attenuated vaccine derived from the wild Oka strain and contains trace amounts of gelatin and neomycin. The vaccine was licensed in the United States in 1995 for healthy persons 12 months of age and older who are susceptible to varicella.

When one dose of vaccine is given to healthy susceptible children, an immune response develops in more than

95%. The seroconversion rate in children older than 13 years and in adults is approximately 80% after one dose of vaccine and approximately 99% after two doses. The vaccine is 95% effective in preventing moderate or severe disease and approximately 70% to 85% effective in preventing mild varicella. Varicella in vaccinated individuals is significantly milder than in unvaccinated individuals, with a lower rate of fever, significantly fewer vesicular lesions, and more rapid recovery. Studies in Japan and the United States have documented long-term (10–20 years) immunity after vaccination with varicella vaccine.

Varicella vaccine is recommended as part of the routine childhood immunization schedule. All children 12 months of age and older who do not have a history of varicella should be vaccinated with one dose of varicella vaccine unless the vaccine is contraindicated (see subsequent text). A second dose of varicella vaccine for all children, given at 4 to 6 years of age, has been recommended recently to decrease the risk of breakthrough infection. Susceptible adolescents 13 years of age and older should receive two doses of the vaccine 4 to 8 weeks apart.

Adverse Effects

Discomfort develops at the injection site in approximately 20% of vaccinees. Six to ten percent of immunized children develop a localized or generalized rash, which usually consists of two to five maculopapular or vesicular lesions, occurring 5 to 26 days after immunization. Transmission of vaccine strain virus to susceptible contacts occurs very rarely and only if a vaccine-associated rash develops in the vaccinee. Therefore, *contacts of immunocompromised persons can be vaccinated with varicella vaccine.*

The administration of varicella vaccine is contraindicated in:

- Pregnant women
- Immunocompromised persons, including children with T-lymphocyte immunodeficiencies, malignancies, and those receiving high doses of systemic corticosteroids (≥ 2 mg/kg per day or ≥ 20 mg/day of prednisone)
- Children who have had anaphylactic reactions to gelatin or neomycin
- Children who have recently received an Ig, as for measles vaccine (see Table 2.1)
- Persons with intercurrent illness, defined as moderate or severe, with or without fever

Children with only impaired humoral immunity *may* be immunized with varicella vaccine. Varicella vaccine should be *considered* for asymptomatic children infected by HIV who do not have evidence of immunosuppression (CD4$^+$ T-lymphocyte percentage of 25% or greater).

Pneumococcal Vaccines

Two vaccines against *Streptococcus pneumoniae* are currently available: a 23-valent polysaccharide vaccine (PS23) and a

7-valent conjugate vaccine (PCV7). As with the Hib vaccines, a conjugate pneumococcal vaccine was developed to provide protection against pneumococcal disease in infants and children younger than 2 years, the age group at highest risk for invasive pneumococcal disease. This conjugate vaccine was licensed in the United States in 2000.

PCV7 comprises seven capsular pneumococcal serotypes that are responsible for approximately 85% of cases of invasive disease and 65% to 70% of cases of otitis media in the United States. This vaccine is immunogenic and highly effective in the prevention of invasive pneumococcal disease when given to infants, starting at 2 months of age, as has been evidenced by a significant decrease in invasive pneumococcal infections in children and adults in this country since the licensure of this vaccine. Additionally, in infants and children immunized with this vaccine, the incidence of otitis media is mildly reduced, whereas the incidence of recurrent otitis media and nasopharyngeal carriage are modestly reduced.

PCV7 is indicated for all infants, starting at 2 months of age. Four doses of vaccine are administered before the age of 15 months. The vaccine is also recommended for children 24 to 59 months of age who are at high risk for invasive pneumococcal disease (Table 2.3) if they have not received their series of four injections before 24 months of age.

Adverse effects following vaccination with PCV7 are mild and include low-grade fever and local reactions.

The PS23 vaccine is not immunogenic in children younger than 2 years. This vaccine is recommended for children older than 2 years who are at high risk for invasive pneumococcal disease (see Table 2.3). For children who have completed their PCV7 vaccination before the age of 2 years, PS23 can be given to high-risk children at 24 months of age to provide broader pneumococcal coverage against serotypes not contained in PCV7. A second dose of PS23 is recommended for these children 3 to 5 years after the first dose. Adverse effects of PS23 include mild local reactions and, very rarely, fever and severe local reactions.

TABLE 2.3

RISK FACTORS FOR INVASIVE PNEUMOCOCCAL DISEASE IN CHILDREN

Sickle cell disease
Asplenia
Human immunodeficiency virus infection
Congenital immunodeficiencies
Cochlear implants
Cerebrospinal fluid leaks
Chronic illnesses, including the following:
   Chronic cardiac disease
   Renal failure and nephrotic syndrome
   Chronic pulmonary disease (including asthma treated with
     corticosteroids)
   Diabetes mellitus
   Immunosuppressive therapy

Influenza Vaccine

Inactivated influenza vaccines are produced in embryonated eggs and are composed of subvirion vaccine or purified surface antigen vaccine containing strains of influenza A and B. They are revised periodically according to the anticipated prevalent circulating influenza strains. All vaccines contain residual egg proteins.

The efficacy of inactivated influenza vaccine in healthy children is estimated to be approximately 70%. The duration of protection is brief; therefore, annual vaccination is required. The efficacy has not been evaluated in infants younger than 6 months; consequently, it is not indicated for infants younger than 6 months of age. Two doses of vaccine, given 1 month apart, are required in children younger than 9 years who have not been previously immunized. Once children have been primed by immunization, the administration of one dose of vaccine annually results in a brisk immune response.

A *live attenuated, cold-adapted influenza vaccine* is approved for use in healthy children and adults 2 to 49 years old. This live trivalent vaccine is administered intranasally, induces high antibody responses in vaccinees, and is more than 90% protective against culture-proven cases. This vaccine is indicated only for vaccination of *healthy* individuals 2 to 49 years old.

Annual influenza vaccination is now recommended for *all infants and children 6 months of age and older*. This is especially critical for children with:

- Chronic pulmonary diseases or asthma
- Hemodynamically significant cardiac disease
- Immunocompromising conditions, including HIV infection
- Hemoglobinopathies, including sickle cell anemia
- Chronic renal and metabolic disease
- Diseases for which long-term aspirin therapy is required

In addition, annual influenza vaccination is recommended for persons who are in close contact with high-risk patients. Pregnant women who will be in their second or third trimester during the influenza season should be vaccinated.

Adverse Effects

Fever and local reactions are rare following vaccination of children with inactivated vaccine. Approximately 10% of adolescents experience local reactions following vaccination. Influenza vaccination is *not* associated with an increased risk for Guillain-Barré syndrome in infants, children, and adolescents.

Adverse effects of the *live* attenuated influenza vaccine include runny nose, sneezing, and nasal congestion. This vaccine is generally *not* indicated for:

- Persons with asthma or reactive airway disease
- Persons with immunodeficiencies or chronic illness

In addition, live virus vaccinees should avoid contact with severely immunocompromised individuals for at least 21 days after vaccination with this live vaccine.

Contraindications

Children experiencing severe anaphylactic reactions to eggs or chickens generally should *not* receive any influenza vaccination.

In addition the live attenuated vaccine is *contraindicated* in:

- Children receiving salicylates
- Individuals with Guillain-Barré syndrome

Hepatitis A Vaccine

The currently available hepatitis A vaccines are formalin-inactivated, approved for persons 12 months of age and older, and given according to a two-dose schedule.

The seroconversion rate in children vaccinated with two doses of hepatitis A vaccine approaches 100%. The efficacy of the vaccine in preventing clinical hepatitis A, based on controlled, randomized trials performed in the United States and Thailand, is 95% to 100%. The duration of protection with hepatitis A vaccine is not known, but kinetic models estimate that protective antibody concentrations will persist for at least 20 years.

Hepatitis A vaccine is routinely recommended for:

- *All* children at 1 year of age; children who are not immunized by 2 years of age can be immunized at subsequent visits
- Travelers to areas in which hepatitis A is endemic
- Patients with chronic liver disease, including those awaiting or who have undergone liver transplantation
- Homosexual and bisexual men
- Users of injection and illicit drugs
- Persons working with hepatitis A virus in a research laboratory
- Persons with clotting factor disorders
- Children 2 to 18 years of age living in states and communities in which the average annual rate of hepatitis A is at least twice the national average (≥20 cases/100,000 population)

In addition, routine hepatitis A vaccination should be *considered* for persons in states and communities in which the average annual rate of hepatitis A is between the national average and twice the national average (10–20 cases/100,000 population).

Currently, routine immunization with hepatitis A vaccine is *not* routinely recommended for the children and staff in day care centers, hospital personnel, or food handlers. However, hepatitis A vaccination can be considered in child care centers with ongoing or recurrent outbreaks. Traditionally, Ig, given within 14 days of exposure to hepatitis A, is recommended for postexposure prophylaxis, such as in the setting of household, sexual, perinatal, or child care exposure to hepatitis A. However, recent data indicate that hepatitis A vaccination is as effective as immunoglobulin for postexposure prophylaxis.

Adverse reactions to hepatitis A vaccine are mild. Local reactions are most common. No serious effects have been documented. The only contraindication to vaccination is a known hypersensitivity reaction to a vaccine component, such as alum or phenoxyethanol.

Meningococcal Vaccine

Two vaccines are currently available against infections caused by *Neisseria meningitidis:* the traditional polysaccharide vaccine (MPSV4) and a polysaccharide conjugate vaccine (MCV4). The MPSV4 vaccine is a quadrivalent purified capsular vaccine. Serogroups A C, Y, and W135 are contained in the vaccine. Serogroup B is not represented in the currently available polysaccharide vaccine. Like other polysaccharide vaccines, the meningococcal vaccine is not immunogenic in children younger than 2 years, although the group A component is immunogenic in infants 3 months of age and older and has been used to control outbreaks in infants.

The MCV4 vaccine is a quadrivalent polysaccharide *conjugate* meningococcal vaccine, whose immune response relies on T-cell rather than B-cell immunity. Like the polysaccharide vaccine, this vaccine does not provide protection against serogroup B. Currently the conjugate vaccine is approved for children 2 years of age and older.

MCV4 vaccine is now recommended routinely for:

- *All* adolescents at the 11- to 12-year health care visit
- All adolescents at high school entry or 15 years of age, whichever comes first, and if not previously immunized with MCV4
- Entering college students who plan to live in dormitories, if not previously immunized with MCV4

Meningococcal vaccination is also indicated for individuals 2 years of age and older at high risk for meningococcal disease, including the following:

- Children with functional and anatomic asplenia
- Children with terminal complement or properdin deficiencies
- Travelers to countries in which disease is hyperendemic or epidemic
- Military recruits
- Patients with HIV infection

Meningococcal vaccines are safe, with only mild local reactions reported following administration.

Human Papillomavirus Vaccine

Anogenital HPV infection is the most prevalent sexually transmitted infection in the United States. Although subclinical and transient infection is common, persistent infection with this virus account for the majority of cervical cancer and precancerous lesions in the female genital tract. Most adolescents acquire this infection soon after the initiation of sexual activity. HPV serotypes 16 and 18 are responsible for the majority of cases of cervical cancer, and serotypes 6 and 11 are account for the majority of genital warts.

The currently available HPV vaccine is a quadrivalent, bioengineered vaccine, providing protection against serotypes 6, 11, 16, and 18. It has been shown to be safe and immunogenic. It is currently approved for females 9 to 26 years of age and is recommended for routine immunization of adolescents at 11 to 12 years of age, in a 3 dose series given at 2 and 6 months.

The vaccine should not be given to pregnant women, or to individuals with a moderate to severe febrile illness. The vaccine also can cause syncopal episodes in adolescent females after injections. The only contraindication to HPV vaccine is a severe hypersensitivity reaction to a previous dose or component of the vaccine.

Vaccines to Be Used in Special Circumstances

Rabies Vaccines

Three rabies vaccines are licensed in the United States, all of which consist of inactivated whole-virus preparations:

- Human diploid cell vaccine
- Rabies vaccine adsorbed
- Purified chick embryo cell vaccine

The decision to provide postexposure prophylaxis depends on the type of exposure, offending animal, nature of the attack, and risk for rabies associated with each species of animal in the locality in which the attack occurred. Local health departments should be consulted to help in decision making.

In the United States, *bats, raccoons, foxes,* and *skunks* are more likely to be rabid than other animals; therefore, persons who have been bitten by these animals require postexposure prophylaxis unless the geographic area is known to be free of rabies or until the animal is proved to be free of rabies by immunofluorescent testing. In addition to bites from these animals, seemingly insignificant exposure to bats has resulted in human infection. Therefore, postexposure prophylaxis is indicated when a bat has been physically present, and a bite, scratch, or contamination of mucous membranes cannot reliably be excluded, unless prompt testing of the bat has ruled out rabies infection.

Dogs, cats, and ferrets that have bitten a human should be observed by a veterinarian for 10 days. If they are proved or suspected to be rabid, immediate postexposure prophylaxis should be administered.

Persons who have been bitten by rodents, rabbits, hares, and livestock almost never require antirabies vaccination. These cases should be considered individually in consultation with local public health officials.

Postexposure prophylaxis requires the following:

- Local wound care
- Administration of rabies Ig unless the person who has been bitten has previously received pre-exposure prophylaxis with rabies vaccine or has had an adequate antirabies titer after previous immunization
- Administration of rabies vaccine

Local wound care involves the prompt, thorough local treatment of all wounds and an assessment of the need for tetanus prophylaxis. Rabies Ig should be administered concomitantly with the first dose of rabies vaccine. As much of the dose of rabies Ig as possible is given locally to infiltrate the wound, with the remainder of the dose given intramuscularly. Any of the three available rabies vaccines can be administered for postexposure prophylaxis, but the same product should be used for all five doses. The vaccine is administered intramuscularly on the first day of therapy, with repeated doses given on days 3, 7, 14, and 28.

Pre-exposure prophylaxis (three-dose series) with rabies vaccine is indicated for persons in high-risk groups, such as veterinarians, animal handlers, certain laboratory workers, and persons moving to an area in which canine rabies is common.

In children, adverse events following rabies vaccination are uncommon. Local reactions occur in approximately 20% of adult vaccinees, and mild systemic reactions are reported in 10% to 20%. Serum sickness–like reactions have been reported in adults receiving booster doses of human diploid cell vaccine for pre-exposure prophylaxis but are rare following primary vaccination and vaccination with the other rabies vaccines.

REVIEW EXERCISES

QUESTIONS

1. An 8-year-old boy who has had no previous immunizations sustains a puncture wound to the foot. Which of the following regimens should you administer to the child for postexposure prophylaxis against tetanus?
a) DTaP vaccine
b) Td vaccine
c) DTaP vaccine and tetanus Ig
d) Td vaccine and tetanus Ig
e) Tetanus Ig

Answer

The answer is d. Puncture wounds, burns, and frostbite, in addition to wounds contaminated with dirt, soil, feces, and saliva, should be considered "contaminated" wounds. Therefore, for a child who has received no previous vaccinations or fewer than three doses against tetanus, tetanus Ig must be given in addition to tetanus vaccine. The choice of tetanus vaccine depends on whether pertussis vaccine also should be given. Because pertussis vaccination is currently not indicated in children 7 to 11 years of age, this child should receive tetanus vaccine in the form of Td, which contains a lower dose of diphtheria toxoid and therefore is less reactogenic in older children and adults.

2. Which of the following is a *true* statement about acellular pertussis vaccination?
a) In comparison with whole-cell vaccines, acellular pertussis vaccines have superior efficacy.
b) Acellular vaccines are less reactogenic than whole-cell vaccines.
c) Immunocompromised children should not be vaccinated with acellular pertussis vaccines.
d) Both *a* and *b*

Answer
The answer is b. The major advantage of the acellular pertussis vaccines over the whole-cell vaccines is that they are associated with a significantly decreased rate of local and systemic adverse effects. The two types of vaccines are comparable in immunogenicity and efficacy. Because acellular pertussis vaccines are composed of purified antigens of *Bordetella pertussis,* they are not contraindicated in immunocompromised children.

3. Which of the following statements is an absolute contraindication to pertussis vaccination?
a) Fever to 41°C (105.8°F) following a previous dose of the vaccine
b) A hypotonic episode within 48 hours of a previous dose of the vaccine
c) Inconsolable crying for 3 hours following a previous dose of the vaccine
d) Severe unexplained encephalopathy following a previous dose of the vaccine
e) All of the above

Answer
The answer is d. Absolute contraindications to pertussis vaccinations include an immediate anaphylactic reaction and encephalopathy occurring within 7 days of the vaccine. The encephalopathy is defined as a major, severe, acute alteration of consciousness or seizures, which persists for more than a few hours without recovery within 24 hours and is not explained by another cause. High fever to or above 40.5°C (104.9°F), collapse or shock-like state, and inconsolable crying following vaccination, although once considered contraindications, are now considered *precautions* because they have not been proved to cause permanent sequelae. In these circumstances, the decision to vaccinate with pertussis vaccine should be considered carefully and should be based on the clinical assessment of the earlier adverse event, the likelihood of pertussis exposure in the community, and the overall benefits and risks of the vaccine.

4. Which of the following is a *true* statement about poliovirus vaccination?
a) IPV is less immunogenic than OPV.
b) VAPP is a risk of OPV immunization.
c) VAPP has been described following the administration of IPV.
d) Both *a* and *b*

Answer
The answer is b. The immunogenicity of IPV against all three serotypes of poliovirus is comparable with that of OPV. VAPP is a risk only of OPV, not of IPV vaccination. IPV is a formalin-inactivated vaccine and not capable of causing poliomyelitis. The risk for VAPP is the major reason why an all-IPV schedule against poliomyelitis is currently recommended in the United States. Since 1979, the only cases of indigenous poliomyelitis in the United States have been caused by the administration of OPV.

5. Who among the following can be vaccinated with MMR vaccine?
a) A 12-month-old boy with advanced HIV infection and a CD4$^+$ percentage of 10%
b) An 18-year-old college student who is pregnant
c) A 12-month-old child with a history of anaphylaxis after egg ingestion
d) A 15-month-old girl who had Kawasaki disease at the age of 12 months and received intravenous Ig therapy

Answer
The answer is c. Measles vaccine contains only a small amount of egg white cross-reacting proteins, and most children with a history of anaphylaxis after egg ingestion have no untoward reaction to MMR vaccination. In contrast, influenza vaccine contains a significant amount of egg white cross-reacting proteins. Children who have asymptomatic HIV infection or are symptomatic but without severe immunosuppression can be vaccinated with MMR vaccine. However, children with advanced HIV infection and those with a low percentage of CD4$^+$ T lymphocytes (<15%) should not receive MMR vaccine because of the risk for vaccine-associated pneumonia. Pregnancy is a contraindication to MMR vaccination because of the theoretic risk for fetal infection from a live virus vaccine. In children who have received intravenous Ig therapy for Kawasaki disease, MMR and varicella vaccination should be deferred for 11 months after receipt of the intravenous Ig. The Ig interferes with the immune response to these live virus vaccines.

6. An infant born to a mother whose HBsAg status at birth is unknown should receive:
a) A first dose of hepatitis B vaccine some time within the first 2 months of life
b) Hepatitis B vaccine within 12 hours of birth; the infant can then also be given hepatitis B Ig within

7 days of birth if the mother is found to be HBsAg-positive

c) Hepatitis B Ig and a first dose of hepatitis B vaccine between 3 and 6 months of life

d) Hepatitis B vaccine and hepatitis B Ig within the first 12 hours of life

Answer

The answer is b. The management of the infant and mother in situations in which the mother's hepatitis B status at birth is not known is as follows: The infant should be given hepatitis B vaccine at birth (within 12 hours). Mothers should undergo hepatitis B testing as soon as possible after delivery. If the mother is found to be HBsAg-positive, the infant should then be given hepatitis B Ig as soon as possible, but before 7 days of age. This recommendation is based on the fact that the hepatitis B vaccine when given at birth is highly effective in preventing perinatal transmission in term infants. The added benefits of coadministering hepatitis B Ig in these situations is low and does not justify routine use of hepatitis B Ig when the mother's status is unknown, until/unless the mother is proved to be HBsAg-positive.

7. Varicella vaccination is contraindicated in which of the following persons?

a) A 12-month-old child whose mother is taking chemotherapy for lymphoma

b) An 18-month-old child whose mother is pregnant

c) A 12-month-old child with newly diagnosed acute lymphoblastic leukemia who is undergoing induction chemotherapy

d) A 13-year-old healthy boy with no history of varicella

Answer

The answer is c. Varicella vaccine is a live attenuated virus vaccine. Therefore, immunocompromised persons, including those with malignancies, should not receive varicella vaccine. The vaccine is recommended as part of the routine childhood immunization schedule, and all children 12 months of age and older who are susceptible should be vaccinated. Because transmission of the virus from a vaccine recipient to a susceptible person occurs very rarely, *contacts* of immunocompromised persons and pregnant women can be vaccinated with varicella vaccine.

8. Hepatitis A vaccine is indicated in each of the following persons, *except:*

a) A 4-month-old boy with biliary atresia

b) A 3-year-old girl traveling with her family to Central America

c) A 2-year-old girl with chronic hepatitis B infection

d) An adolescent engaging in high-risk behavior

Answer

The answer is a. Hepatitis A vaccine is not recommended for children younger than 12 months of age. Therefore, a 4-month-old child with biliary atresia

should not receive the vaccine. Children with chronic liver disease, including those with chronic hepatitis B and hepatitis C infection who are 12 months of age and older, should be vaccinated. Travelers to areas in which hepatitis A is endemic and all adolescents should be vaccinated with hepatitis A vaccine. Hepatitis A is endemic in all countries except Western Europe and Scandinavia, Australia, Canada, Japan, and New Zealand.

9. Which of the following is a *true* statement about pneumococcal vaccination?

a) 7-Valent conjugate vaccine is indicated for all children 2 years of age and older.

b) 23-Valent polysaccharide vaccine is not immunogenic in children younger than 2 years.

c) Children with congenital immunodeficiencies should receive polysaccharide pneumococcal vaccination rather than conjugate vaccine.

d) Polysaccharide pneumococcal vaccine is associated with significant adverse reactions, as compared with conjugate vaccine.

Answer

The answer is b. 23-Valent polysaccharide pneumococcal vaccine, like other polysaccharide vaccines, elicits T-cell independent responses, which results in weak and variable immune responses with minimal T-cell influence. Therefore, there is restricted IgG subclass response, no memory cells formation, and no booster effect with these vaccines. The result is that these vaccines are poorly immunogenic in children younger than 2 years. Protein conjugation of the polysaccharide vaccine allows a T-cell–dependent response, which depends on IgG1 and IgG3 responses (rather than IgG2 and IgG4, which are formed earlier in life). Therefore, these conjugate vaccines are immunogenic in infants. The 7-valent pneumococcal conjugate vaccine is currently indicated for all infants, starting at 2 months of life. Neither the polysaccharide nor the conjugate pneumococcal vaccines are live virus vaccines and therefore not contraindicated for persons with altered immunity. Both vaccines have excellent safety profiles and cause only mild adverse events following vaccination.

10. Influenza vaccine is indicated for each of the following patients *except:*

a) A 2-year-old boy with asthma

b) A 5-year-old girl with juvenile rheumatoid arthritis who is taking long-term aspirin therapy

c) A 4-month-old boy with congenital heart disease

d) A 2-year-old girl with HIV infection

e) A 6-year-old heart transplant recipient

Answer

The answer is c. Inactivated influenza vaccine is a subvirion or purified-antigen vaccine, which is revised periodically according to the anticipated prevalent circulating influenza strains. Influenza vaccine is indicated for all infants and children 6 months of age and older. Special attention should be paid to giving inactivated vaccine to infants and children with chronic pulmonary, cardiac, renal, or metabolic diseases; immunocompromising conditions, including HIV infection; hemoglobinopathies; and diseases for which long-term aspirin therapy is required. The efficacy of the vaccine has not been evaluated in infants younger than 6 months. A cold-adapted, trivalent live attenuated influenza vaccine is available and approved for use in *healthy* individuals 2 to 49 years of age.

SUGGESTED READINGS

1. American Academy of Pediatrics. Immunization in special clinical circumstances. In: Pickering LK, Baker CJ, Long SS, McMillan JA, eds. *Red book: 2006 Report of the Committee on Infectious Diseases*, 27th ed. Elk Grove Village, IL: American Academy of Pediatrics, 2006:67–103.
2. American Academy of Pediatrics. Measles. In: Pickering LK, Baker CJ, Long SS, McMillan JA, eds. *Red book: 2006 Report of the Committee on Infectious Diseases*, 27th ed. Elk Grove Village, IL: American Academy of Pediatrics, 2006:441–452.
3. American Academy of Pediatrics. Pertussis. In: Pickering LK, Baker CJ, Long SS, McMillan JA, eds. *Red book: 2006 Report of the Committee on Infectious Diseases*, 27th ed. Elk Grove Village, IL: American Academy of Pediatrics, 2006:498–520.
4. American Academy of Pediatrics. Policy statement: recommendations for the prevention of pneumococcal infections, including the use of pneumococcal conjugate vaccine (Prevnar), pneumococcal polysaccharide vaccine, and antibiotic prophylaxis. *Pediatrics* 2000; 106:362–366.
5. Arvin AM. Live attenuated varicella vaccine. *Pediatr Ann* 1997;26: 384–388.
6. Barlow WE, Davis RL, Glasser JW, et al. The risk of seizures after receipt of whole-cell pertussis or measles, mumps, and rubella vaccine. *NEJM* 2001;345:656–661.
7. Bisgard KM, Wenger JD. Recommendations for the use of *Haemophilus influenzae* type b vaccines among children in the United States. *Pediatr Ann* 1997;26:361–365.
8. Centers for Disease Control and Prevention. Poliomyelitis prevention in the United States: updated recommendations of the Advisory Committee on Immunization Practices. *MMWR Morb Mortal Wkly Rep* 2000;49:RR-5.
9. Centers for Disease Control and Prevention. Recommended childhood immunization schedule—United States 2002. *MMWR Morb Mortal Wkly Rep* 2002;51:31–33.
10. Gans HA, Arvin AM, Galinus J, et al. Deficiency of the humoral immune response to measles vaccine in infants immunized at age 6 months. *JAMA* 1998;280:527–532.
11. Giebink GS. The prevention of pneumococcal disease in children. *NEJM* 2001;345:1177–1183.
12. Lieberman JM. Varicella vaccine: what have we learned? *Contemp Pediatr* 2001;18:50–60.
13. Margolis HS, Coleman PJ, Brown RE, et al. Prevention of hepatitis B virus transmission by immunization. *JAMA* 1995;274: 1201–1208.
14. Markowitz LE, Dunne EF, Saraiya M, et al. Quadrivalent human papillomavirus vaccine: recommendations of the Advisory Committee on Immunization Practices (ACIP). *MMWR Recomm Rep.* 2007; 56(RR-2):1–24. Available at: http://www.cdc.gov/mmwr/preview/mmwrhtml/rr56e312a1.htm

Chapter 3

BOARD SIMULATION: General Pediatrics

Scott A. Francy

QUESTIONS

1. Of the following, the *least* likely cause of death in a child between the ages of 2 and 18 years is:
a. Suicide
b. Homicide
c. Motor vehicle accident
d. Cancer
e. Drowning

Answer
The answer is d.

2. The parents of a 4-year-old boy are concerned because during the past 2 weeks he has been waking up in the middle of the night. The boy awakens in a frightened, confused, and disoriented state. He appears flushed and is sweating profusely during the episodes. The child returns to sleep in a few minutes and has no recollection of the event the next morning. There is a 3-week-old infant at home. What is the *most* likely cause of this child's sleep disturbance?
a. Night terror
b. Nightmare
c. Separation anxiety
d. Depression
e. Sibling rivalry

Answer
The answer is a. This boy is most likely experiencing *night terrors*, which occur in 1% to 4% of children. Night terrors are more common in boys than in girls, and the incidence is highest in preschool-age children. The disturbance commonly occurs during non–rapid eye movement sleep; a history of fright, confusion, and disorientation, along with intense autonomic signs, is characteristic. Sleepwalking may accompany the episodes, which usually last a few minutes. Typically, the child does not become lucid before the end of the episode and has no recollec-

tion of the event the next morning. The episodes frequently are related to a specific precipitating stressful event, such as the birth of a sibling. The events are self-limited. Management involves an understanding of the precipitating factors, reassurance, and support.

Unlike night terrors, *nightmares*:

- Are more common in girls than in boys
- Occur during rapid eye movement sleep
- Are not confined to children in their preschool years

In addition, a person who has had a nightmare awakens, quickly becomes lucid, and often remembers the content of the dream.

Separation anxiety and depression can cause sleep disturbances but are not commonly associated with episodes of fright and confusion. Sibling rivalry is rarely manifested as a sleep disturbance.

3. An 8-year-old boy who has a lifelong history of thumb sucking continues to suck his thumb. The *best* advice to the family would be to:
a. Recommend behavior modification with the use of positive reinforcement.
b. Reassure them that the problem will resolve spontaneously.
c. Insert an occlusive dental appliance.
d. Have the child undergo psychological testing.
e. Constantly remind the child to stop thumb sucking.

Answer
The answer is a. Thumb sucking, although normal in infancy, should never be considered normal after the age of 5 years or after the permanent teeth have begun to erupt. Potential complications in the older child include malocclusion and flaring of the incisors. The management of thumb sucking in the older child is controversial, although most experts recommend behavior modification with positive reinforcement as the most appropriate form

of therapy. Occlusive dental appliances are generally not recommended, and psychological testing is not warranted unless other abnormal behaviors are present.

4. A 5-year-old boy whom you are seeing for the first time has enuresis. The *best* initial intervention for this child is to:
a. Tell the parents to wake the child each evening when they go to sleep to let the child void in the toilet.
b. Use negative reinforcement techniques each morning after he has wet the bed.
c. Obtain a urinalysis.
d. Use conditioning devices.
e. Obtain urine and serum electrolytes.

Answer
The answer is c. Enuresis (bed wetting) is a common problem encountered by pediatricians. Persistent (primary) enuresis, in which the child has never been dry at night, accounts for 75% of cases and is often the result of inappropriate or inadequate toilet training. In the regressive type of enuresis, the child has been dry for 1 year and then begins to wet the bed. This type is often the result of a stressful or traumatic event in the child's life. In both types of enuresis, an organic cause is rarely found. A thorough physical examination and urinalysis are indicated to rule out conditions such as urinary tract infection and diabetes mellitus. Modifying behavior with positive reinforcement, avoiding liquids at bedtime, and making older children launder their own clothing and bed sheets have been suggested as methods of management. Punishment and negative reinforcement should be avoided. Conditioning devices such as alarms should be reserved for recurrent and refractory cases. Drug therapy with desmopressin acetate should be used with caution as side effects can include hyponatremia, seizures, and volume overload. FDA ALERT [12/4/2007]: "FDA has requested the manufacturers update the prescribing information for desmopressin to include important new information about severe hyponatremia and seizures. Certain patients taking desmopressin are at risk for developing severe hyponatremia that can result in seizures and death. Children treated with desmopressin *intranasal* formulations for primary nocturnal enuresis (PNE) are particularly susceptible to severe hyponatremia and seizures. As such, desmopressin *intranasal* formulations are no longer indicated for the treatment of primary nocturnal enuresis and should not be used in hyponatremic patients or patients with a history of hyponatremia. PNE treatment with desmopressin *tablets* should be interrupted during acute illnesses that may lead to fluid and/or electrolyte imbalance. *All* desmopressin formulations should be used cautiously in patients at risk for water intoxication with hyponatremia."

5. A previously healthy 7-year-old girl presents with patchy scaling of the scalp and hair loss. Potassium hydroxide staining of the scalp and hair reveal branching fungal hyphae. Which of the following is a *true* statement concerning the treatment of this child's condition?
a. Routine monitoring with liver function tests will be required during the course of treatment.
b. Adjunctive antibacterial therapy will likely be required.
c. Topical antifungal agents should be used as first-line therapy.
d. Treatment with systemic antifungal therapy for 6 to 8 weeks will likely be required to eradicate the infection.

Answer
The answer is d. Fungal infection of the scalp (tinea capitis) can present in the form of:

■ Patchy scaliness with hair loss
■ Discrete areas of hair loss and broken hairs
■ Discrete pustules without hair loss
■ Boggy inflammatory masses surrounded by pustules (kerion)

In the United States, *Trichophyton tonsurans* is the most common etiologic agent. Fungal hyphae or spores can often be seen when scaly areas or hair is examined with a potassium hydroxide preparation, or when material from the affected area is plated onto appropriate fungal media and incubated for 2 to 3 weeks. Because *T. tonsurans* does not produce fluorescence, an examination under ultraviolet light (Wood lamp) is not a reliable diagnostic tool.

Systemic therapy with an oral antifungal agent is required for the effective treatment of tinea capitis. Topical agents cannot penetrate the hair and therefore are not effective. Griseofulvin remains the preferred agent based on its long history of success and proven safety record. The drug should be administered with a lipid-containing meal to enhance absorption, which may be erratic. Because the drug is fungistatic, a prolonged course of therapy (6–8 weeks or longer) is required, and therapy should be continued for at least 2 weeks after clinical resolution. Adverse side effects associated with griseofulvin include nausea, headaches, rash, and rarely leukopenia and elevated transaminases. Routine monitoring with liver function tests is not indicated in healthy children receiving griseofulvin for the treatment of tinea capitis. Selenium sulfide shampoos may be used with oral antifungal agents to reduce fungal shedding. Corticosteroids may be used as adjunctive therapy for the treatment of kerion. Antibiotics are not indicated for tinea capitis or kerion.

6. An adolescent boy presents with a skin eruption consisting of approximately 5- to 7-mm salmon-pink macular lesions with scaly plaques at the center. The lesions are found on the trunk in a symmetric, bilateral pattern. The hands and feet are spared. On further examination, you note a 2 × 3-cm oval-shaped scaly plaque on his chest. Of the following, the *most* likely diagnosis is:

a. Syphilis
b. Pityriasis rosea
c. Tinea corporis
d. Erythema multiforme

Answer

The answer is b. The description of this eruption is most consistent with pityriasis rosea, a self-limited disorder commonly affecting healthy children and adolescents. The incidence of pityriasis rosea is highest in adolescents and is slightly higher in girls than in boys. The cause remains unknown, but a viral infection is suspected. Although atypical cases are not uncommon, the classic form begins with a *herald patch*, a solitary, oval, pink scaly lesion usually found on the trunk. Several days after the appearance of the herald patch, a secondary eruption develops in which small crops of macules with a scaly center appear in a fir tree pattern. The eruption usually spares the face, feet, and hands. Pruritus is not uncommon. The diagnosis can usually be made clinically, although atypical cases may be difficult to diagnose. The differential diagnosis of pityriasis should include:

- Secondary syphilis
- Tinea corporis
- Erythema multiforme
- Drug eruptions
- Guttate psoriasis

Secondary syphilis more typically involves the palms and soles; erythema multiforme does not typically appear in a symmetric fir tree pattern; tinea corporis may be confused with the herald patch but rarely results in the eruption of crops of lesions. Drug eruptions most typically manifest as morbilliform rashes, urticaria, or as a "fixed" demarcated, erythematous lesions. None of these lesions are usually associated with any scaling as described in the question.

The herald patch is lacking in guttate psoriasis. The scale in psoriasis is usually thick and diffuse.

7. A 4-year-old girl presents with sporadic vaginal irritation. She has no history of fever, urinary urgency or frequency, and examination reveals a mildly hyperemic vulva bilaterally with a fetid odor. No discharge is noted. The *most* appropriate initial step in the management of this child would be to:

a. Refer the child for a sexual abuse workup.
b. Obtain a vaginal culture for group A streptococci.
c. Give instructions regarding proper hygiene and bowel and bladder habits.
d. Recommend a trial of an antistaphylococcal antibiotic.

Answer

The answer is c. This child presents with nonspecific vulvovaginitis, which in young girls is most often caused by poor perineal hygiene, which results in contamination of the vaginal area with stool flora. Irritation also may be caused by soaps, shampoos, bubble baths, detergents, and tight clothing. The clinical features include intermittent signs of vaginal irritation, including erythema and a fetid odor. The most important concepts in the management of this common problem include reassuring the child and her family and stressing the importance of proper perineal hygiene. This includes having the child take sitz baths and removing potential irritants. Close follow-up is prudent because recurrent or refractory symptomatology would warrant investigation for sexual abuse.

Children with group A streptococcal vulvovaginitis present with an acute, progressive, painful rash that often involves the perianal area. Purulent drainage is also common.

8. The parents of an otherwise healthy 14-month-old child are concerned because the child is not yet walking by himself. He is able to pull to stand and cruise and has a six-word vocabulary. The next *most* appropriate step in the care of this child is:

a. Neurology consultation
b. Physical and speech therapy
c. Reassurance and a follow-up evaluation in 2 months
d. Muscle biopsy
e. Serum and urine analysis for amino acids and urine analysis for organic acids

Answer

The answer is c. The average age to attain the ability to walk alone is 12 to 13 months, and most children are walking by 15 months. This 14-month-old child is able to pull to stand and cruise. His language skills are slightly advanced for his age. Given the choices, it is most appropriate to reassure the parents and re-evaluate the child's development in 2 months.

9. A 12-year-old female soccer player comes to your office with complaints of anterior knee pain. It seems to hurt most with activity, especially jumping and kicking a ball. She does not recall any trauma. With normal ambulation, she does not experience pain or instability. The *most* likely cause of her symptoms is:

a. Anterior cruciate ligament strain
b. Patellar dislocation
c. Distal quadriceps tear
d. Osgood-Schlatter disease
e. Shin splint

Answer

The answer is d. *Osgood-Schlatter disease*, or *tibial tubercle apophysitis*, is the most likely cause of her pain. This condition most commonly occurs between 10 and 15 years of age. The examination is usually positive for swelling, prominence, and tenderness of the tubercle. Symptoms may be present for 6 to 24 months. Treatment consists of attempting to identify training errors, to decrease the frequency and intensity of exercise; stretching of the hamstrings and quadriceps; and applying ice postactivity. "Shin splint" pain does not occur at the knee.

10. A 2-month-old term infant is not "sleeping through the night." You tell the exhausted parents that most (70%–80%) infants sleep through the night (uninterrupted sleep for 6–8 hours) by:
a. 2 months
b. 4 to 6 months
c. 7 to 9 months
d. 12 months

Answer
The answer is b. By 4 to 6 months of age total sleep requirements are 14 to 16 hours per day. Seventy to eighty percent of infants sleep for a 6- to 8-hour period by 4 to 6 months of age.

11. An 18-month-old child should typically be able to:
a. Stand on one foot
b. Jump off the floor with both feet
c. Walk up the stairs alternating feet forward
d. Walk backward

Answer
The answer is d. The skills mentioned in the question and the average age when they are attained are as follows:

- Stand on one foot: 23 months (16–30 months)
- Jump off floor with both feet: 23 months (18–30 months)
- Walk up the stairs alternating feet forward: 30 months (23–33 months)
- Walking backward: 15 months (11–20 months)

12. A 4-year-old child should be able to perform all of the following *except*:
a. Copy a circle
b. Pedal a tricycle
c. Hop on one foot
d. Skip

Answer
The answer is d. Children aged 3 to 4 years should be able to copy a circle, pedal a tricycle, and hop on one foot. A typical 5-year-old child should be able to skip.

13. The parents of a healthy 14-month-old girl are concerned because she bangs her head as she transitions to sleep. She does not bang her head at other times. Appropriate action by the pediatrician would include:
a. Refer the patient for psychological testing, specifically autism.

b. Assure the parents that this typically resolves by age 4 years.
c. Begin a trial of diazepam at times of head banging.
d. Discuss the increased risk of mental retardation or brain injury in children who bang their heads.
e. Inform the parents that this should have resolved by 12 months.

Answer
The answer is b. Head banging is a sleep–wake transition disorder. Head banging and body rocking are very common. They occur in approximately 60% of 9 to 12 month olds, 20% of 2 year olds, and usually resolve in the remainder by 4 years. A typical session usually lasts less than 15 minutes. It is usually not a sign of central nervous system injury, headache, ear pathology, neglect, abuse, or other pathology.

14. A 16-year-old wrestler has been encouraged by several individuals at his gym to take anabolic steroids. He is considering it as he hopes to get a college scholarship. He asks about the potential negative side effects. All of the following are known potential side effects of anabolic steroids *except*:
a. Testicular atrophy
b. Late epiphyseal closure
c. Aggressive behavior
d. Elevated blood pressure
e. Elevated liver enzymes

Answer
The answer is b. Potential adverse effects of anabolic steroids include:

- Psychological: Emotional instability, aggression, depression, altered libido
- Dermatologic: Increased acne, male-patterned baldness
- Musculoskeletal: Early epiphyseal closure, increased risk of muscle/tendon injuries
- Cardiovascular: Elevated blood pressure, increased low-density lipoprotein (LDL) cholesterol
- Hepatic: Elevated liver enzymes and bilirubin levels
- Genitourinary: Testicular atrophy, clitoral hypertrophy, oligospermia

15. An 18-year-old basketball player injures his knee during a game. He remembers someone falling on the outside of his knee as he was pivoting on his foot that was planted on the ground. His knee examination 18 hours after the injury shows a large effusion. The *most* likely diagnosis is:
a. Patellar tendon rupture
b. Anterior cruciate ligament injury
c. Ruptured popliteal (Baker) cyst
d. Patellofemoral tracking syndrome

Answer
The answer is b. Given the mechanism of the injury and the development of a large effusion, an intrasubstance

anterior cruciate ligament injury is the best answer. This injury occurs after skeletal maturity. Before skeletal maturity, the same mechanism may result in a tibial eminence avulsion fracture.

Joint effusion in the first 24 hours is a result of hemarthrosis. This same injury mechanism may result in a tear of the medial collateral ligament. Initial treatment involves rest, ice application, compression, and elevation. Most often, surgical stabilization of the ligament is necessary.

16. A 17-year-old male basketball player (height 50th percentile) is being seen in July for a preparticipation sports physical. His blood pressure is 140/88. This elevated blood pressure is confirmed on subsequent visits. You discuss hypertension with the patient. All of the following points are correct *except*:
a. He should adopt healthy lifestyle habits, such as avoiding anabolic steroids, drugs of abuse, and high sodium intake.
b. He should avoid active sports such as football and basketball, and choose a more sedentary sport such as weight lifting.
c. He should have his blood pressure monitored regularly, every 1–2 months.
d. If cardiovascular disease coexists, the type and severity of this disease should impact your decision regarding sports participation.

Answer
The answer is b. His blood pressure falls into the category of "significant hypertension" for his age.

According to the American Academy of Pediatrics (AAP), "the presence of significant hypertension in the absence of target organ damage or concomitant heart disease should not limit a person's eligibility for competitive athletics." The AAP states, "those with significant essential (unexplained) hypertension should avoid weight and power lifting, body building, and strength training. Those with secondary hypertension (hypertension caused by a previously identified disease) or severe essential hypertension need evaluation."

17. A 4-year-old boy presents to your office with a history of dog bite on the forearm, which occurred approximately 18 hours ago. Examination reveals a small 7-mm laceration as well as adjacent apparent puncture wounds. His mother states the area is much more swollen, red, and warm than just 6 hours ago. She has noted some drainage from the wound. The following statements about dog bites are true, *except*:
a. Dog bites are less likely to become infected than cat bites.
b. The erythema and swelling noted likely represent infection and not just local tissue trauma.
c. Cephalexin is the best initial antibiotic of choice because of its good coverage against Staphylococcal and Streptococcal organisms.

d. After copious irrigation, some facial lacerations as a result of dog bites may be closed primarily in the first 6 hours after the bite.

Answer
The answer is c. Approximately 5% to 15% of dog bites become infected and 25% to 50% of cat bites become infected. Copious irrigation is an important part of the initial management. It is important to be aware of the tetanus status of the patient and evaluate the risk of rabies. Some facial wounds may be appropriate for suturing. Crush injuries, animal bites, and puncture wounds have the greatest rate of infection. Organisms likely to cause infection are *Staphylococcus aureus*, *Pasteurella* species, Streptococci, *Corynebacterium* species, *Eikenella* species, *Capnocytophaga* species, and anaerobes. Other organisms may also cause infection. Amoxicillin–Clavulanate has excellent activity against these organisms and therefore is the preferred oral first-line agent for treating animal bites. Cephalexin, a first generation cephalosporin, does not have activity against *Pasteurella* or anaerobic bacteria and therefore is not the first-line agent for treating animal bites.

18. A breast-fed 6½-month-old child (born at 38 weeks of gestation, weight of 2600 g) is thought to have vitamin D–deficient rickets. His examination findings would most likely include all of the following, *except*:
a. Poor growth
b. Costochondral beading (rosary)
c. Bowlegs
d. Softening of the skull (craniotabes)
e. Widening of the epiphyses

Answer
The answer is c. *Vitamin D–deficient rickets* is characterized by a failure of mineralization of growing bone, secondary to a lack of calcium and phosphorus salts. Vitamin D deficiency may occur in breast-fed infants who are dark-skinned or unexposed to sunlight. Skeletal manifestations may be present as early as the first few months of life, especially in low-birth-weight infants.

Craniotabes, a thinning of the outer table of the skull, may be detected by a "ping-pong" ball sensation when pressure is exerted over the parietal or occipital bones. Epiphyseal widening or enlargement may be seen, especially at the wrist or ankles. Bending or bowing of the shafts of the fibula, tibia, or femur is exacerbated only by *weight bearing*, so that bowlegs are unlikely in this 6-month-old child. Another early manifestation may be enlargement of the costochondral junctions, also known as the *rachitic rosary*.

19. A 1-week-old infant who is on an appropriate amount of formula feedings has excessive vomiting and episodes of choking and exhibits abnormal head posturing following feedings. You suspect gastroesophageal reflux. Which one of the following is a *true* statement concerning gastroesophageal reflux?

a. Without therapy, most children continue to have symptoms into their school-age years.
b. Sandifer syndrome is a complication.
c. Histamine$_2$ receptor blockers are used to increase gastric emptying.
d. Older children with reflux have a better long-term prognosis than infants.
e. It has no role in reactive airways disease.

Answer
The answer is b. Episodes of physiologic *gastroesophageal reflux* occur in healthy infants and children. However, reflux may produce pathologic effects. In abnormal situations, an increased frequency of reflux and amount of refluxate potentially lead to esophagitis. Symptoms of abnormal reflux include irritability, feeding problems, interrupted sleep, poor weight gain, episodes of choking, and respiratory symptoms, which may include reactive airway disease, laryngospasm, and apnea. Sandifer syndrome consists of gastroesophageal reflux disease, iron deficiency anemia, vomiting, head tilting, arching, irritability, and rumination. Eighty-five percent of infants with pathologic reflux present in the first week of life. Older children may present with substernal burning. Sixty percent of infants with reflux are free of symptoms by the age of 2 years, whereas older children in whom gastroesophageal reflux disease is diagnosed have a more chronic course. Treatment options for infants with pathologic reflux include proper positioning (prone or seated completely upright), dietary changes (thickening feeds, small and frequent feedings), medical therapy (prokinetic agents, acid-reducing agents, mucosa-protecting agents), and surgery (fundoplication). Specifically, histamine$_2$ receptor blockers are used to treat or prevent esophagitis but do not increase gastric emptying.

20. A 2-week-old breast-fed infant presents with persistent jaundice, vomiting, lethargy, and irritability. The examination reveals poor weight gain, jaundice, and hepatomegaly. The infant's mother reports episodes of hypoglycemia in the nursery. You suspect galactosemia. Which of the following clinical features is *not* typically associated with classic galactosemia?

a. Hepatomegaly
b. Cataracts
c. Seizures
d. Presence of urine-reducing substances
e. Choanal atresia

Answer
The answer is e. Classic *galactosemia* is caused by a deficiency of galactose-1-phosphate uridyltransferase, which results in the accumulation of galactose-1-phosphate in

infants ingesting lactose (glucose and galactose). The accumulation leads to parenchymal injury in the kidneys, liver, and brain. Clinical manifestations include jaundice, vomiting, hepatomegaly, seizures, lethargy, hypoglycemia, lethargy, failure to thrive, and cataracts. When the condition is not diagnosed in the neonatal period, an ongoing intake of lactose may lead to irreversible liver (cirrhosis) and brain (mental retardation) damage. Patients with galactosemia are at an increased risk for neonatal *Escherichia coli* sepsis. Specific enzyme assays confirm the diagnosis. Treatment centers on the elimination of lactose from the diet.

21. A 2-year-old girl with failure to thrive is referred to you for further evaluation. At the interview, you elicit a history of bulky/fatty stools. The *most* likely cause of these symptoms is:

a. Hypothyroidism
b. Celiac disease
c. Renal tubular acidosis
d. Cystic fibrosis
e. Carbohydrate malabsorption

Answer
The answer is d. Although all the diseases listed may manifest as failure to thrive, the additional history of steatorrhea and wheezing makes cystic fibrosis the most likely diagnosis.

Gastrointestinal manifestations of cystic fibrosis include the following:

- Intestinal manifestations:
  - Meconium ileus in the newborn: intestinal obstruction secondary to a thick and viscid meconium mass
  - Distal intestinal obstructive syndrome: colicky abdominal pain, distension, and a palpable mass (inspissated stool causing partial obstruction)
  - Rectal prolapse
  - Fat-soluble vitamin deficiency: vitamins A, D, E, and K
- Hepatobiliary manifestations:
  - Prolonged neonatal cholestasis in 5% to 10% of cases
  - Cirrhosis in approximately 10% of patients older than 25 years
  - Cholelithiasis and cholecystitis in young adult patients
- Pancreatic manifestations:
  - Exocrine pancreatic insufficiency in 80% to 90% of patients with cystic fibrosis

22. A 12-year-old girl, with a history of a resolving upper respiratory infection and fever, now presents with emesis, confusion, and lethargy. She is without fever presently. She was treated for respiratory tract infection with rest, fluids, and aspirin. The serum electrolytes and glucose levels are normal. You suspect that the patient has Reye syndrome. The medical student working with you asks which laboratory result best predicts

whether a patient will progress to coma. You inform her that it is the:
a. Blood ammonia level
b. Blood urea nitrogen level
c. Complete blood cell count
d. Sedimentation rate
e. Serum albumin level

Answer

The answer is a. *Reye syndrome* is thought to be a disorder of mitochondrial function. Although the exact cause is unknown, a viral syndrome with *influenza* or *varicella* may be noted before the onset of symptoms. Studies have suggested a link between the use of aspirin during influenza or varicella infection and the development of Reye syndrome, which involves acute encephalopathy and fatty degeneration of the liver.

Classic Reye syndrome follows a stereotypic, biphasic course. A prodromal, febrile illness that is beginning to resolve is followed by the abrupt onset of vomiting and mental status changes that may progress to seizures, coma, and death. The neurologic examination is nonfocal. Aminotransferase levels are elevated, and the prothrombin time is increased. Patients in whom the serum ammonia level is increased threefold or more, are more likely to progress to coma.

23. A 7-month-old infant on parenteral feeding is transferred to your hospital. During the examination, you note perioral and perianal scaling and erythema. This *most* likely is a manifestation of a deficiency of:
a. Vitamin D
b. Zinc
c. Vitamin A
d. Selenium
e. Copper

Answer

The answer is b. *Zinc* is an essential cofactor for hundreds of enzymes. It plays a role in fat, protein, carbohydrate, and nucleic acid metabolism. Zinc is found in meats, grains, and nuts. A deficiency may result from poor dietary intake, malabsorption, or increased excretion. Zinc deficiency manifests as perioral and facial dermatitis, alopecia, angular stomatitis, poor wound healing, diarrhea, impaired taste sensation, or failure to thrive.

Acrodermatitis enteropathica (see Fig. 67.5) is an autosomal-recessive disorder in which insufficient zinc is absorbed from the diet as a consequence of a reduced transport of zinc across the small intestinal mucosa.

24. A 4-week-old boy is brought to the emergency department with a history of several episodes of projectile nonbilious emesis during the past 2 to 3 days. The laboratory results are as follows:
Na = 139 mmol/L
K = 3.4 mmol/L
Cl = 94 mmol/L
CO^2 = 34 mmol/L
The *most* likely diagnosis is:
a. Congenital adrenal hyperplasia
b. Milk protein allergy
c. Pyloric stenosis
d. Gastroesophageal reflux disease

Answer

The answer is c. *Pyloric stenosis* is caused by muscular hypertrophy of the circular muscle of the pyloric canal. It is more common in male and first-born infants. An increased incidence is noted in the siblings and future offspring of affected children. Pyloric stenosis manifests as nonbilious vomiting that is usually progressive. Prolonged vomiting may lead to dehydration and weight loss. Laboratory results may reveal a hypochloremic metabolic alkalosis and hypokalemia.

Congenital adrenal hyperplasia may present with salt-wasting crisis and vomiting, failure to gain weight, and potential cardiovascular collapse. Ninety percent of cases of congenital adrenal hyperplasia are caused by a deficiency of 21-hydroxylase. Seventy-five percent of cases of 21-hydroxylase deficiency are of the salt-wasting form. Laboratory results may reveal a metabolic acidosis, hyperkalemia, and increased urine sodium level with or without hypoglycemia.

25. What percentage of newborns will pass a meconium stool within the first 48 hours of life?
a. 50% to 60%
b. 60% to 70%
c. 70% to 80%
d. 80% to 90%
e. 90% to 100%

Answer

The answer is e. A stool is passed by 94% to 99% of newborns during the first 48 hours of life. In *Hirschsprung disease,* ganglion cells are lacking in an affected area of the bowel. The abnormal innervation extends proximally from the rectum for a variable distance. The transition to normal bowel is most commonly at the rectosigmoid area. The diagnosis is made by 1 month of age in 50% of patients with Hirschsprung disease, and by 1 year in approximately 80%. Symptoms include abdominal distension, vomiting, and constipation. Neonates more frequently present with vomiting, whereas older infants and children usually present with constipation. Hirschsprung disease is not typically characterized by significant encopresis. The diagnosis is made by anorectal manometry, barium enema, or rectal biopsy. An association between trisomy 21 and Hirschsprung disease has been noted.

26. A 15-year-old patient who underwent resection of the terminal ileum 2 years ago comes to see you after being "lost to follow-up." He is complaining of a loss of coordination. Deficiency of which vitamin is *most* likely causing this symptom?

a. Vitamin A
b. Vitamin D
c. Vitamin C
d. Vitamin K
e. Vitamin B_{12}

Answer

The answer is e. Resection of the terminal ileum is associated with deficiencies of:

- *Vitamin A:* night blindness, xerophthalmia, follicular hyperkeratosis, poor growth
- *Vitamin D:* frontal bossing, beading of the rib cage, bowing of the shafts of the legs, widening of the epiphyses
- *Vitamin E (membrane antioxidant):* hemolytic anemia (decrease in red cell half-life), progressive neurologic disorders (e.g., loss of deep tendon reflexes, loss of coordination, weakness)
- *Vitamin K:* bleeding diathesis, petechiae, purpura, ecchymoses
- *Vitamin B_{12}:* glossitis, cheilosis, megaloblastic anemia, peripheral neuropathy

27. A 12-month-old boy is being discharged from the hospital after undergoing successful radiologic reduction of an intussusception. His parents ask about the likelihood of a recurrent episode. You tell them that the risk is closest to:

a. 10%
b. 25%
c. 40%
d. 55%

Answer

The answer is a. *Intussusception* is a common cause of bowel obstruction in children younger than 2 years. Intussusception is the invagination of one segment of bowel into another. Involvement of the mesentery of the proximal segment results in venous and lymphatic congestion. In children younger than 2 years, 80% to 90% of cases are idiopathic, with no identifiable lead point. Lead points are more common in older children. Examples of lead points are polyps, duplication cysts, lymphomas, hematomas associated with Henoch-Schönlein purpura, hypertrophic Peyer patches, Meckel diverticula, and hemangiomas. Ileocolic intussusceptions account for approximately 90% of the cases.

The clinical presentation is usually characterized by the sudden onset of intermittent episodes of abdominal colic that often result in inconsolable crying. Between the initial attacks, the child may very well be asymptomatic. Bilious emesis usually develops. With time, the child may become listless or lethargic. The examination may reveal a sausage-shaped abdominal mass in the right upper quadrant and emptiness in the right lower

quadrant. Microscopic blood in the stools or *"currant jelly"* stools may be seen.

Diagnosis and therapy are aided by ultrasonography or air enema with fluoroscopy. A surgical consultation should be obtained before any type of radiologic, diagnostic, or therapeutic procedures are undertaken. Children with evidence of free intraperitoneal air, peritoneal irritation, and prolonged symptoms are surgical candidates.

The risk for recurrence after successful nonsurgical reduction is approximately 10%.

28. A mother brings in her 3-week-old term infant after noting blood and mucus in the baby's stool four times in the 36 hours before the visit. The stool otherwise is "seedy and not hard." The child's physical examination findings were normal at his 2-week visit. The infant is drinking 2 to 3 oz of a cow's milk–based formula every 2 to 3 hours. The mother has noted increased irritability during the last few days. The examination findings today are normal except for an obvious small amount of gross blood with stool in the diaper. The *most* likely explanation is:

a. Food allergy–associated colitis
b. Inflammatory bowel disease
c. Necrotizing enterocolitis
d. Intussusception

Answer

The answer is a. The most likely cause of the infant's symptoms is *cow's milk protein allergy.* Enterocolitis may develop in an infant days to weeks after the initial ingestion of cow's milk protein. Patients usually present within the first 2 to 3 months of life with symptoms of colic, bloody stools, and diarrhea. Other symptoms may include vomiting, eczema, and poor feeding. In most cases, weight gain has been normal. Small bowel mucosal injury may lead to carbohydrate malabsorption.

Between 30% to 50% of infants with cow's milk protein allergy are also intolerant of soy protein. Most infants with protein allergy respond to a casein hydrolysate– or amino acid–containing formula. After withdrawal of the offending protein, most infants' symptoms resolve within a few days. Suspected cow's milk protein allergy in a breast-fed infant should be treated by removing milk protein from the mother's diet.

In 50% to 60% of infants with protein allergy, tolerance develops by 12 months, and more than 80% tolerate cow's milk protein by 3 or 4 years of age.

Necrotizing enterocolitis usually would be suspected in an ill-appearing preterm infant. Inflammatory bowel disease would be extremely unusual at this age. Intussusception would be less likely than cow's milk protein allergy given this clinical scenario.

29. During your evening shift in the emergency department, you are asked to see a 7-month-old male infant with a 2- to 3-day history of several episodes of vomiting and diarrhea. The mother describes him as awake but moderately irritable. On examination, he is alert but irritable, with dry mucous membranes, a sunken fontanelle, slightly sunken eyes, tachycardia, and a 2- to 3-second capillary refill. His serum sodium level is 140 mEq/L. You estimate his percentage dehydration to be:

a. <1%
b. 1% to 4%
c. 5% to 10%
d. 11% to 20%

Answer

The answer is c. The clinical features described in this case correlate with an isotonic *dehydration* of 5% to 10%. An infant with less than 5% dehydration may present only with thirst and restlessness. An infant with more than 10% to 15% dehydration may appear lethargic or obtunded, have cool extremities, a capillary refill longer than 3 seconds, very dry mucous membranes, poor skin elasticity, tachycardia, and very sunken eyes.

30. A 7-year-old boy presents to your office with a several-day history of perianal itching. The patient's mother followed instructions from the triage nurse and noticed a "white worm or something" in her son's perianal region at night. You diagnose *Enterobius vermicularis* infection. The treatment of choice would be:

a. Trimethoprim/sulfamethoxazole
b. Amoxicillin
c. Erythromycin
d. Pyrantel pamoate
e. Mebendazole

Answer

The answer is e. *E. vermicularis* (pinworm) infection is common in preschool and school-age children (5%–10%). Fecal–oral transmission is the most important route. Eggs are ingested and they hatch in the duodenum. Adult pinworms mature in the cecum. Female worms migrate to the anus and deposit their eggs in the perianal region. Itching leads to autoinfection and possible transmission to others.

The diagnosis can be made by directly observing the perianal region at night or by applying transparent adhesive tape to the perianal skin and looking for eggs. Of the treatment choices listed only mebendazole and pyrantel pamoate have activity against Enterobius vermicularis. Mebendazole has greater than 95% efficacy. Pyrantel pamoate has an efficacy of approximately 90%. It can lead to adverse reactions including anorexia, nausea, vomiting, abdominal cramps, and diarrhea, and is also associated with neurotoxic effects and transient increases in hepatic enzymes. Mebendazole is the drug of choice as pyrantel pamoate is associated with more side effects and lower efficacy.

31. You are asked to see a 5-day-old boy because of poor feeding, abdominal distension, and the acute onset of bilious emesis. This term infant is the product of an uncomplicated vaginal delivery and had Apgar scores of 9 at 1 minute and 9 at 5 minutes. In the nursery, he fed "okay, not great" and passed meconium within a few hours after birth. He has had a few more stools at home since discharge on the second day. The examination is significant for abdominal distension and tenderness. The *most* likely condition causing this clinical picture is:

a. Hirschsprung disease
b. Gastroesophageal reflux disease
c. Pyloric stenosis
d. Midgut volvulus
e. Meconium ileus

Answer

The answer is d. In the case described, an acute onset of bilious emesis in combination with a history of normal passage of meconium in the first 24 hours of life makes *midgut volvulus* the best choice.

During fetal development, the midgut rotates 270 degrees in a counterclockwise direction. The superior mesenteric artery serves as an axis for this rotation. Abnormalities of fixation and rotation predispose the midgut to volvulus, which occurs most often in the newborn period but can develop later in life. A volvulus can obstruct the intestinal blood supply, causing ischemia and infarction. Signs and symptoms of midgut volvulus include the acute onset of bilious emesis, abdominal distension and pain, and the passage of blood or mucus per rectum. The initial management of the infant described in the question would include placement of a nasogastric tube, the administration of intravenous fluids and parenteral antibiotics, and surgical consultation/intervention.

The passage of meconium in the first 24 hours of life makes Hirschsprung disease and meconium ileus poor choices. The presence of bilious emesis and the remainder of the scenario as presented make reflux disease and pyloric stenosis unlikely.

32. A 5-year-old boy and his 7-year-old brother have had 2 days of fever and multiple episodes of vomiting and diarrhea. The 5-year-old has been healthy, specifically without any history of abdominal pain, before the last 2 days. During the last 48 hours, he has been given two correct doses of acetaminophen. The patient is brought in because he has been vomiting "clear stuff," but now his mother has noted possible bloody vomit. His examination is unremarkable except for vague abdominal pain with palpation. He proceeds to have a timely episode of hematemesis in your office. The *most* likely cause of this patient's hematemesis is:

a. Peptic ulcer disease
b. Esophageal varices
c. Münchhausen syndrome by proxy
d. Crohn disease
e. Mallory-Weiss tear

Answer

The answer is e. The most likely cause of this patient's hematemesis is a *Mallory-Weiss tear* complicating a course of gastroenteritis. A Mallory-Weiss tear is an esophageal or gastric mucosal lesion that occurs in response to forceful retching and vomiting. It is usually a self-limited condition. The patient's age, lack of previous symptoms or problems, and current history of an acute illness make the other choices offered less likely.

33. Regarding concussions, choose the following statement that is false:

a. The majority of concussive episodes in young athletes are not reported
b. Multiple concussions can result in cumulative brain damage
c. There should be loss of consciousness for there to be a diagnosis of concussion
d. Close observation of the athlete is of critical importance after a head injury

Answer

The answer is c. Concussion is a complex pathophysiologic process affecting the brain, induced by traumatic biomechanical forces. Signs and symptoms may include alterations in consciousness, confusion, amnesia, visual and hearing impairment, irritability and mood changes, difficulties with balance, headache, lethargy, insomnia, memory impairment, nausea, and vomiting. Loss of consciousness does *not* have to occur to make the diagnosis of concussion. Guidelines for return to activity are somewhat controversial. Physical and cognitive rest are important. There should be a sequential, functional progression of increasing activity as symptoms clear. Symptoms should not return with exertion. Neuropsychological testing may be needed in some cases. Postconcussive syndrome involves residual symptoms from a concussion including headache, dizziness, irritability, and difficulty concentrating; these symptoms can occur after any concussion, regardless of severity.

SUGGESTED READINGS

1. American Academy of Pediatrics. Committee on sports medicine and fitness: athletic participation by children and adolescents who have systemic hypertension. *Pediatrics* 1997;99(4):637–638.
2. Hartley AH. Pityriasis rosea. *Pediatr Rev* 1999;20:266–270.
3. Howard BJ, Wong J. Sleep disorders. *Pediatr Rev* 2001;22:327–341.
4. Lawless MR, McElderry DH. Nocturnal enuresis: current concepts. *Pediatr Rev* 2001;22:399–407.
5. MacMillan JA, DeAngelis CD, Feigin RD, Warshaw JB, eds. *Oski's pediatrics: principles and practice.* Philadelphia: Lippincott Williams & Wilkins, 2006.
6. McCrory P, Johnston K, Meeuwisse W, et al. Summary and agreement statement of the 2nd International Conference on Concussion in Sport, Prague 2004. *Br J Sports Med* 2005;39:196–204.
7. Roy CC, Silverman A, Alagille D, et al., eds. *Pediatric clinical gastroenterology.* St. Louis: Mosby-Year Book, 1995.
8. Rudolph AM, Hoffman JIE, Rudolph CD, et al., eds. *Rudolph's pediatrics.* McGraw-Hill, 2003.
9. Stein DH. Tineas: superficial dermatophyte infections. *Pediatr Rev* 1998;19:368–372.
10. U.S. Food and Drug Administration Center For Drug Evaluation and Research. http://www.fda.gov/CDER/DRUG/InfoSheets/HCP/desmopressinHCP.htm
11. Walker WA, Durie PR, Hamilton JR, et al., eds. *Pediatric gastrointestinal disease: pathophysiology, diagnosis, management.* Hamilton, Ontario: BC Decker, 2000.
12. Wyllie R, Hyams JS, eds. *Pediatric gastrointestinal and liver disease.* Philadelphia: WB Saunders, 2005.

Chapter 4

Abdominal Pain

Barbara Kaplan

Chronic abdominal pain is one of the most common problems encountered in pediatric practice. Abdominal pain occurs in an estimated 10% to 15% of school-age children and is responsible for multiple office visits and school absences. The causes of pain considered in the evaluation of these children are extensive. However, they can be divided into two general groups:

- Functional pain
- Pain caused by an identifiable organic disorder

In large reported series evaluating children with symptoms of chronic abdominal pain, organic causes of pain are found in 10% to 30%, whereas 70% to 90% experience pain that can be categorized as functional.

The evaluation of children with chronic abdominal pain should include a detailed history to elicit characteristics of pain, including, severity, timing and location, precipitating and alleviating factors, appetite, dietary intake, and stool history. Particular attention should be focused on the identification of "red flags" noted on history or physical examination which would trigger a search for an organic cause. These include:

- Age <5 years
- Dysphagia
- Persistent vomiting
- Persistent right upper quadrant or right lower quadrant pain
- Gastrointestinal blood loss
- Nocturnal diarrhea
- Pain that awakens child from sleep
- Arthritis
- Hepatomegaly or splenomegaly
- Perianal disease
- Involuntary weight loss
- Deceleration in linear growth
- Delayed puberty
- Unexplained fever
- FH of celiac disease, inflammatory bowel disease or peptic ulcer disease

FUNCTIONAL ABDOMINAL PAIN

The term *functional abdominal pain* is used to describe chronic or recurrent abdominal pain in children for which there is no structural, inflammatory, infectious, or metabolic cause. Functional abdominal pain in young children was first described by Apley 50 years ago, in a group of children who presented with a vague, nonspecific abdominal pain that lasted for more than 3 months and for which no organic cause could be identified. He labeled this symptom complex as *recurrent abdominal pain of childhood*. As varying patterns of functional abdominal pain in children have become recognized, functional abdominal pain in children, a broadly defined entity, has been subdivided into three, more specifically defined patterns:

- Functional dyspepsia: abdominal pain associated with dyspepsia and localized to the upper abdomen
- Irritable bowel syndrome: abdominal pain associated with an altered stool pattern
- Childhood functional abdominal pain: episodes of isolated, vague, nonspecific abdominal pain that does not meet the criteria for other types of functional abdominal pain

The pathophysiology of this heterogeneous group of disorders is not entirely clear. However, it is important to recognize that the pain experienced by the affected children is genuine and is not simply an excuse to avoid specific activities. Proposed pathogenetic mechanisms of symptoms in patients with functional abdominal pain implicate a dysregulation of the enteric nervous system, the "gut brain." It is theorized that individuals with functional abdominal pain exhibit a pattern of visceral hyperalgesia, a decreased threshold for pain related to biochemical changes in the afferent neurons of the enteric and central nervous systems. The development of visceral hyperalgesia may be triggered by different mucosal inflammatory processes including infection, allergy, or primary inflammation resulting in sensitization. This leads to the development of abnormal bowel reactivity to normal physiologic stimuli associated with eating, luminal distension, inflammation, or psychological stress.

Functional Dyspepsia

Functional dyspepsia is defined as persistent or recurrent abdominal pain localized to the upper abdomen occurring once per week for at least 2 months. As in all functional disorders there is no inflammatory, anatomic, metabolic, or neoplastic process that explains the child's symptoms. Epigastric or midabdominal discomfort or burning occurs in the absence of associated gastrointestinal inflammation, gastroesophageal reflux, or structural abnormalities. Other dyspeptic symptoms may include nausea, bloating, regurgitation, heartburn, belching, anorexia, early satiety, and upper abdominal fullness. These symptoms may be similar to those reported by patients with acid peptic disease, lactose intolerance, and gallbladder or pancreatic disease. Patients with functional dyspepsia also may have an irritable bowel component to their pain, with lower abdominal cramping and alteration in stool frequency or consistency. The evaluation of these patients can include a complete blood cell count, comprehensive metabolic profile, determination of the sedimentation rate, measurement of amylase and lipase levels, and stool examination for ova and parasites. In selected cases, an abdominal ultrasonography, upper gastrointestinal series with small bowel follow-through, or upper gastrointestinal endoscopy with biopsy should be performed to exclude anatomic abnormalities and evaluate for the presence of significant mucosal inflammation or infection. The controversy regarding the significance of *Helicobacter pylori* infection and its treatment in patients with dyspepsia is ongoing. As for all patients with functional abdominal pain, education and reassurance are the most important components of treatment. Avoidance of aggravating foods and medications such as nonsteroidal anti-inflammatory medications is recommended. In patients with functional dyspepsia, stress reduction and an empiric trial of a histamine$_2$ (H$_2$) receptor antagonists or proton pump inhibitors may decrease symptoms.

Irritable Bowel Syndrome

Individuals with irritable bowel syndrome experience pain that occurs at least once a week for at least 2 months. Pain is typically described as cramping in nature and is associated with an altered stool pattern. Patients with irritable bowel syndrome report at least two of the following three symptoms:

- Relief from pain with defecation
- Onset associated with a change in stool frequency
- Onset associated with a change in stool form

Irritable bowel syndrome afflicts 10% to 20% of adolescents and adults. Patients with irritable bowel syn-

drome typically experience abdominal pain in the periumbilical region or lower abdomen. Patients can have diarrhea, constipation, or both. Patients may also have such symptoms as fecal urgency, straining during a bowel movement, a sensation of incomplete stool evacuation, relief from pain with the passage of stools, the passage of mucus, and increased flatulence or bloating. The symptoms of irritable bowel syndrome may be similar to those described by patients with inflammatory bowel disease, parasitic infections, or lactose intolerance, all of which should be considered in the evaluation. Screening should include a complete blood cell count, measurement of the sedimentation rate, examination of the stool for occult blood as well as ova and parasites, and a lactose breath test. For patients with intractable symptoms or symptoms suggestive of inflammatory bowel disease, a colonoscopy may be indicated to detect evidence of mucosal inflammation. Once the diagnosis of irritable bowel syndrome has been made, the treatment is focused on education, reassurance, and the identification of possible psychosocial triggers. Studies evaluating the treatment of children with irritable bowel syndrome support the benefits of cognitive behavioral therapy, high-fiber diets, and peppermint oil. Other medications prescribed include antidiarrheals, anticholinergics, tricyclic antidepressants, and selective serotonin reuptake inhibitors.

Childhood Functional Abdominal Pain

Children with childhood functional abdominal pain experience episodic or continuous abdominal pain once per week for at least 2 months. The children categorized as having childhood functional abdominal pain do not meet the specific criteria for functional dyspepsia or irritable bowel syndrome. The pain described by these children is typically nonspecific, vaguely localized, often to the periumbilical area, and of variable severity. The abdominal pain onset of pain is gradual, with a clustering of episodes of pain that can last for weeks to months, occurring daily or several times per week. No consistent, temporal relationship to activity or meals is reported. The pain typically does not awaken children from sleep but can interfere with their daily functioning. These children may also experience other somatic symptoms, including nausea, headache, fatigue, and difficulty sleeping. Psychological stressors or "triggers" that precipitate symptoms may be identified and an associated family history of other chronic pain syndromes also may be elicited. However, it is important to recognize that a history of anxiety, depression, behavioral problems, and negative life events do not differentiate children with functional pain from those with an organic cause for their symptoms.

The physical examination findings and the results of laboratory studies in children with childhood functional abdominal pain are normal. In that functional abdominal lacks a specific diagnostic marker, the evaluation in these children may be variable, depending on the presence or absence of "red flags," duration and severity of pain, impact on daily life, and the level of concern. The laboratory evaluation of these patients may include a complete blood cell count, comprehensive metabolic profile, determination of the sedimentation rate, measurement of amylase and lipase levels, urinalysis, urine culture, examination of the stool for occult blood as well as ova and parasites, and lactose breath test. Abdominal and pelvic ultrasounds as a screening test in the absence of "red flags" have little diagnostic yield.

The diagnosis of childhood functional abdominal pain as well as other types of functional pain, is a positive diagnosis, not simply a reflection of an inability to "correctly" identify an underlying organic problem. Acknowledgment that the pain is real and not fabricated is particularly important in helping the patient and family. Treatment includes reassurance, and a discussion of visceral hypersensitivity, and the interaction of the enteric nervous system in children with functional abdominal pain. Identifying triggers, discussing the relationship between stress and symptoms, and limiting pain-induced disability are all beneficial. Cognitive behavioral therapy, relaxation techniques, and self-hypnosis have been shown to be effective in the treatment of children with functional abdominal pain. Medications also may be utilized selectively in the treatment of individual patients.

ABDOMINAL PAIN WITH AN ORGANIC CAUSE

The list of potential organic causes of abdominal pain in children is extensive (Table 4.1). Pain may be caused by disease in the gastrointestinal tract, liver, gallbladder, pancreas, or genitourinary system and also may be a consequence of metabolic, hematologic, or musculoskeletal disorders. Organic causes of abdominal pain can be further categorized as relatively common, less common, and rare.

Common Causes of Abdominal Pain

Common causes of abdominal pain include the following:

- Gastroesophageal reflux
- Peptic ulcer disease
- Carbohydrate intolerance
- Intestinal parasites
- Constipation

Gastroesophageal Reflux
Gastroesophageal reflux is defined as the regurgitation of the gastric contents into the esophagus or oropharynx. Symptoms of gastroesophageal reflux include epigastric and periumbilical abdominal pain, chest pain, heartburn, chronic regurgitation, dysphagia, odynophagia, and in-

TABLE 4.1
ORGANIC CAUSES OF ABDOMINAL PAIN IN CHILDREN

Gastrointestinal
  Gastroesophageal reflux
  Peptic ulcer disease
  Carbohydrate intolerance
  Constipation
  Celiac disease
  Intussusception
  Parasitic disease
  Inflammatory bowel disease
Hepatobiliary/pancreatic
  Cholelithiasis
  Cholecystitis
  Choledochal cyst
  Pancreatitis
Genitourinary
  Pyelonephritis/cystitis
  Nephrolithiasis
  Ureteropelvic junction obstruction
  Mittelschmerz
  Pelvic inflammatory disease
  Endometriosis
  Ovarian cyst
  Fitz-Hugh and Curtis syndrome
Metabolic/hematologic/miscellaneous
  Acute intermittent porphyria
  Diabetes mellitus
  Lead poisoning
  Sickle cell disease
  Familial Mediterranean fever
  Angioneurotic edema
  Henoch-Schönlein purpura
  Musculoskeletal
  Trauma
  Hernia

creased belching. Respiratory symptoms attributed to gastroesophageal reflux include wheezing, nocturnal cough, and hoarseness. Symptoms result from the retrograde flow of the gastric contents into the esophagus with or without the development of esophageal inflammation. Transient relaxation of the lower esophageal sphincter that is not associated with normal esophageal peristaltic propagation with swallowing is thought to be one of the primary factors responsible for reflux in infants and children. Factors related to the development of symptoms and esophageal injury in patients with gastroesophageal reflux include the frequency of reflux events, esophageal clearance mechanisms, esophageal motility, esophageal mucosal barrier function, gastric acidity, gastric emptying, airway reactivity, and visceral hypersensitivity. The evaluation of children for gastroesophageal reflux depends on the individual patient's symptoms and may include an upper gastrointestinal series, upper gastrointestinal endoscopy, esophageal pH and impedance monitoring, and a gastric-emptying study. Treatment includes dietary modifications, maintaining an upright position after meals, and the administration of antacids, H_2 receptor antagonists, proton pump inhibitors, cytoprotective agents, and prokinetic medications.

Gastritis and Peptic Ulcer Disease

Gastritis and peptic ulcer disease occur in children either as the result of primary mucosal injury, or secondary to underlying disease or exposure to gastric irritants. Primary inflammation is most commonly caused by infection with the organism *H. pylori*, a gram-negative spiral flagellated bacterium first linked with peptic ulcer disease in adult patients in 1982. *H. pylori* infection has since been associated with peptic ulcer disease and chronic nodular gastritis in children. *H. pylori* has also been reported in 20% of children with gastric ulcers and 90% of children with duodenal ulcers. The diagnosis of *H. pylori* infection is made most accurately by endoscopy, mucosal gastric biopsy, and the histologic identification of bacteria adherent to the gastric mucosa. *H. pylori* serum immunoglobulin G titers are of limited value in detecting infection; in that the sensitivity and specificity of these tests in children are variable. A ^{13}C-urease breath test and *H. pylori* stool antigen screening offer noninvasive methods to detect bacterial gastric colonization and confirm successful eradication following treatment.

Gastritis and ulcers also can be caused by exposure to gastric irritants, such as nonsteroidal anti-inflammatory medications, aspirin, and alcohol. Other conditions associated with gastric inflammation that may result in inflammation or the formation of ulcers include eosinophilic gastroenteritis, hypertrophic gastritis, and Crohn disease. Systemic conditions associated with increased acid production have been implicated as secondary causes of peptic ulcer disease in children. These include:

- Zollinger-Ellison syndrome
- Systemic mastocytosis
- Renal failure
- Hyperparathyroidism
- Shock
- Burns
- Sepsis

The symptoms of children with acid peptic disease vary. Younger children may have nonspecific and vague abdominal pain, a poor appetite, belching, early satiety, and nausea and vomiting. Older children more often experience the classic symptoms of acid peptic disease, such as postprandial epigastric burning, nausea, and vomiting. The medications used to treat acid peptic disease include H_2 receptor antagonists, proton pump inhibitors, and cytoprotective agents. H_2 receptor antagonists decrease fluid and acid secretion by acting as selective competitive agonists to the action of histamine on H_2 receptors. Proton pump inhibitors irreversibly inhibit H^+/K^+-adenosine triphosphatase, blocking gastric acid production by the parietal cell. Sucralfate, sucrose octasulfate, and polyaluminum hydroxide complex bind to the injured gastric mucosa and are cytoprotective. For the treatment of *H. pylori* infection, triple therapy regimens are recommended with a proton pump inhibitor in combination with two of three antibiotics: amoxicillin, clarithromycin, and metronidazole.

Carbohydrate Intolerance

Carbohydrate malabsorption occurs as a result of an inability to digest and absorb specific dietary sugars. When carbohydrates are not absorbed in the small intestine, they create an osmotic load that stimulates peristalsis and intraluminal fluid production. The result is a flow of the increased output of intestinal fluid in the form of diarrhea. Unabsorbed sugar may be excreted in the stool or fermented by colonic bacteria into hydrogen, methane, carbon dioxide, and short-chain fatty acids. These byproducts are responsible for the development of the symptoms of abdominal pain, flatulence, borborygmus, abdominal distension, and diarrhea. Patients with carbohydrate malabsorption pass acidic stools with a pH of less than 5.7, and depending on the type of malabsorbed carbohydrate, reducing substances may be present in the stools.

The most common type of carbohydrate intolerance is dietary lactose intolerance. It is caused by a decrease or absence of mucosal lactase enzyme activity. Lactase is an intestinal enzyme complex found within the brush border of the small intestinal villi. Lactase hydrolyzes lactose, a nonabsorbable polysaccharide, into two absorbable monosaccharides: glucose and galactose. The three types of lactase deficiency are congenital lactase deficiency, adult-type hypolactasia, and acquired lactase deficiency. Congenital lactase deficiency is associated with a complete absence of mucosal lactase activity; it is very rare and a cause of infantile diarrhea. Primary adult-type hypolactasia is the most common type of lactose intolerance and develops as a genetically determined partial loss of intestinal lactase activity. The prevalence of adult-type lactase deficiency varies worldwide; it is highest among Asian populations, Native Americans, and African Americans, and is lowest in persons of northern European origin. Symptoms typically develop during adolescence or early adulthood. Acquired lactase deficiency can develop at any age, with a loss of mucosal lactase activity occurring as a result of mucosal injury secondary to an acute infection or inflammation. This transient deficiency, associated with typical symptoms of lactose intolerance, resolves within weeks to months, with a restoration of normal lactase activity. The diagnosis of lactose intolerance can be made by means of a noninvasive lactose hydrogen breath test. The criterion for a positive result is a rise in the breath hydrogen ion excretion of more than 20 ppm over baseline following administration of an oral lactose load. In addition, stool evaluation, with findings of an acidic stool pH and the presence of reducing substances, are suggestive of lactose malabsorption. The mucosal lactase activity also be can assayed from small intestinal mucosal biopsy specimens to confirm the diagnosis of lactase deficiency. The treatment of lactose intolerance includes the elimination or limitation of dietary lactose intake and the administration of oral supplemental lactase enzyme.

The ingestion of excessive amounts of other nonabsorbable or incompletely absorbed sugars, including sorbitol and fructose, can also cause abdominal pain and bloating. These products are commonly found in fruits, fruit juices, and artificially sweetened foods.

Intestinal Parasites

Parasitic infections can be a cause of nonspecific abdominal pain in children. Children with parasitic infections may be asymptomatic or have symptoms of abdominal pain, diarrhea, malabsorption, and weight loss. The symptom onset may be acute or more chronic.

Giardia lamblia is the most common cause of intestinal protozoan infection in the United States. *Giardia* organisms are transmitted by the fecal–oral route from person to person or from contaminated water or food. Natural reservoirs for this parasite are humans, dogs, and beavers. Persons at greatest risk are children in day care, residents of long-term care facilities, campers exposed to contaminated water, and travelers to areas of endemicity. Infection develops following ingestion of the infective cyst form of the parasite. Within the gastrointestinal tract, the *Giardia* cyst excysts in the proximal small intestine into a binucleate flagellated parasite that adheres to the mucosal surface. Parasitic infection impairs absorption, thereby causing symptoms. *Giardia* infection is diagnosed by direct examination of the stool or the detection of *Giardia* antigen in stool samples. Treatment with metronidazole or nitazoxanide is recommended in symptomatic patients. Asymptomatic patients, in most cases, do not require treatment.

Cryptosporidium parvum is a spore-forming coccidian protozoan transmitted by contact with infected animals or humans or by exposure to contaminated water. *Cryptosporidium* has been reported as a cause of outbreaks of diarrhea in child care centers, waterborne epidemics, and traveler's diarrhea. Natural reservoirs are domestic cattle and wild animals. In immunocompetent persons, the infection is self-limited; it may be asymptomatic or cause gastrointestinal symptoms, including cramping, abdominal pain, vomiting, and diarrhea. In immunocompromised persons, *Cryptosporidium* has been recognized as a more significant pathogen that causes chronic, protracted watery diarrhea. *Cryptosporidium* infection is diagnosed by direct examination of the stool or the detection of *Cryptosporidium* antigen in stool samples. A 3-day course of nitazoxanide is effective in the treatment of immune competent children with diarrhea caused by this infection.

Blastocystis hominis and *Dientamoeba fragilis*, other intestinal protozoans, also have been implicated as possible etiologic agents of abdominal pain. These parasites have been frequently identified in the stools of asymptomatic individuals and there continues to be debate as to whether or not these parasites are true pathogens or commensal organisms. The diagnosis is made by direct examination of the stool. Indications for treatment are not established.

Constipation

Constipation is one of the most common causes of abdominal pain in children. This problem accounts for 3% of general pediatric outpatient visits and 25% of pediatric gastroenterology visits. Constipation is defined as a delay or difficulty in defecation lasting for 2 weeks or longer. Most cases of constipation in children are functional. Functional constipation may be situational, secondary to toilet phobia, avoidance of school bathrooms, or excessive parental intervention; it may be constitutional, resulting from colonic inertia or a genetic predisposition; or it may be secondary to stool dryness and reduced stool volume in children on low-fiber diets or with a limited fluid intake. It is important to consider organic causes of constipation in the evaluation of these patients. Included in this category are anatomic malformations, anal stenosis, imperforate anus, anterior displacement of the anal opening and pelvic mass, metabolic disorders, hypothyroidism, hypokalemia, hypercalcemia, malabsorption, celiac disease, cystic fibrosis, and gluten enteropathy. Constipation also may be caused by medications, or develop as a component of a generalized systemic or localized myopathic or neuropathic condition, or result from a specific intestinal nerve or muscle abnormality, as in Hirschsprung disease. Constipation is treated with many different therapeutic regimens. Dietary modification with an increase in fluid and fiber intake, behavioral modification, and medications are the primary therapies recommended for these children. Medications that may be beneficial in the treatment of constipation include osmotic agents, bulk-forming agents, lubricants, and less often stimulant laxatives.

Less Common Causes of Abdominal Pain

Less common causes of abdominal pain are as follows:

- Inflammatory bowel disease (Crohn disease)
- Intussusception
- Cholelithiasis
- Pancreatitis
- Celiac disease
- Nephrolithiasis
- Sickle cell disease
- Mittelschmerz

Crohn Disease

Crohn disease (also see Chapter 5) is a form of chronic inflammatory bowel disease that can involve the entire gastrointestinal tract, from the mouth to the anus. The inflammation is transmural, involving all layers of the intestinal wall, including the mesentery and lymph nodes. The inflammation may be continuous, or the disease may manifest as skip lesions. Inflammation is limited to the terminal ileum in 40% of cases, the small intestine and colon in 50%, and the colon in 10%. Symptoms in patients with Crohn disease vary depending on the distribution of the disease and severity of inflammation. Symptoms include abdominal pain, nausea, anorexia, vomiting, diarrhea, rectal bleeding, and extraintestinal manifestations of fever, weight loss, fatigue, rash, perianal discomfort, joint pain, and delay in sexual maturation or linear growth. Patients with isolated ileal disease may present with only right lower quadrant pain. A mass in the right lower quadrant or findings of perianal disease, fistulae, fissures, and skin tags are suggestive of Crohn disease. The diagnosis of Crohn disease is suspected based on the history, physical examination findings, and laboratory values suggesting a chronic inflammatory process. These laboratory values include an elevated sedimentation rate, thrombocytosis, a decreased serum albumin level, and iron deficiency anemia. In patients with Crohn disease involving the small intestine, an upper gastrointestinal series with small bowel follow-through demonstrates mucosal ulcerations, nodular thickening of folds, luminal narrowing, bowel wall separation, and sinus tracts and fistulae in any area of the small intestine. Terminal ileal involvement is most common. Upper gastrointestinal endoscopy and colonoscopy with biopsy are important in establishing the diagnosis of Crohn disease. These are also helpful in distinguishing changes attributed to Crohn disease from other causes of mucosal thickening, such as infection with *Mycobacterium tuberculosis* or *Yersinia*, eosinophilic gastroenteritis, polyarteritis nodosa, intestinal ischemia, and lymphoma. In patients with Crohn disease, the findings at colonoscopy include patchy nonspecific inflammation, mucosal ulcerations, nodularity, and strictures. Intubation of the ileocecal valve with examination and biopsy of the distal ileum can be important in establishing the diagnosis of Crohn disease. On biopsy, noncaseating granuloma is the most characteristic histologic feature of Crohn disease; however, granulomas are found in only 30% to 40% of patients. Other histologic features include a patchy transmural enterocolitis with an infiltrate of lymphocytes, plasma cells, and histiocytes in addition to lymphoid aggregates, goblet cell depletion, and crypt abscesses. The treatment of patients with Crohn disease is individualized, and specific therapy is recommended based on the severity and distribution of the disease. Therapy most frequently incorporates nutritional support, anti-inflammatory and immunomodulatory medications, and more recently the addition of newer biologic therapies. Surgery is indicated in select patients in whom significant complications develop, including obstruction, abscess, and fistulae, and in patients with severe disease that does not respond to medical therapy.

Intussusception
Intussusception is the most common cause of intestinal obstruction in children between the ages of 3 months and 6 years. Intussusception is the telescoping of a proximal segment of the bowel into a distal segment. This can occur anywhere in the intestine, but most commonly intussusceptions are ileocolic. Most (70%–90%) cases of intussusception are idiopathic. A seasonal peak—occurring in the spring and fall, corresponding to the peak season for gastroenteritis and suggesting that distal ileal mesenteric lymph node enlargements and Peyer patches hypertrophy secondary to an intercurrent infection—may serve as a lead point for an intussusception. Other lead points known to cause intussusception include intestinal polyps, hemangioma, Meckel diverticulum, lymphoma, round worm infestation with *Ascaris lumbricoides*, and swallowed foreign bodies. Intussusception may follow an episode of Henoch-Schönlein purpura and can occur in patients with cystic fibrosis, in which inspissated stool serves as the lead point. Symptoms of intussusception include the sudden onset of severe colicky pain, vomiting, fever, lethargy, and the passage of "currant jelly" stool. *A sausage-shaped abdominal mass, typically in the right upper quadrant, is palpable in two thirds of patients.* The diagnosis can be confirmed with ultrasonography, or the intussusception can be demonstrated and reduced with an air contrast enema or hydrostatic barium enema.

Cholelithiasis
Gallstones in children and adolescents are a cause of recurrent colicky abdominal pain localized to the right upper quadrant. Other symptoms are nausea, vomiting, and fatty food intolerance. Jaundice may be the only symptom of gallstones in infants. In younger children with gallstones, an associated underlying predisposing condition is typically present; this is most frequently hemolytic disease, predominantly sickle cell disease and hereditary spherocytosis. Other conditions associated with gallstones are obesity, hyperlipidemia, pregnancy, cystic fibrosis, the prolonged use of total parenteral nutrition, ileal disease or previous ileal resection, and the use of specific medications, including furosemide, ceftriaxone, and oral contraceptives. On the basis of their composition, gallstones are determined to be either pigmented stones or cholesterol stones. Black stones are the most common type of pigmented stones and are found in younger children and patients who have underlying hemolytic disease or are receiving long-term parenteral nutrition. Cholesterol stones are more frequent in adolescents. Gallstones are best identified with ultrasonography because cholesterol stones and some pigmented stones are radiolucent and not apparent on standard abdominal x-ray films. Complications of gallstones in children include cholecystitis, cholangitis, and pancreatitis.

Pancreatitis
Acute and chronic forms of pancreatitis have become increasingly recognized as significant causes of abdominal pain in children. Symptoms in patients with pancreatitis

include pain localized to the epigastric region or right upper quadrant with radiation to the back, nausea, vomiting, dehydration, and in some cases low-grade fever. Patients may be more comfortable in the antalgic position, with their hips and knees flexed and sitting forward. The list of causes of acute and chronic pancreatitis is extensive and includes trauma, infectious or metabolic disorders, structural or inflammatory disease of the pancreas or biliary tree, exposure to specific medications or toxins, and other underlying systemic inflammatory or vasculitic conditions that may affect the pancreas. Pancreatitis is associated with the use of specific antibiotics, anticonvulsants, diuretics, chemotherapy agents, and consumption of alcohol. Pancreatitis is also associated with hypercalcemia, hyperlipidemia (types I, IV, and V), cystic fibrosis, gallstones, choledochal cyst, systemic lupus erythematosus, Crohn disease, Kawasaki disease, hemolytic uremic syndrome, and shock. Inherited forms of pancreatitis, occur secondary to abnormalities in the serine protease 1 gene (PRSS1), the gene encoding cationic trypsinogen, mutations in serine protease inhibitor Kazal type 1(SPINK1 gene) a pancreatic trypsin inhibitor and with CFTR mutations. The diagnosis of acute pancreatitis is established by demonstrating a rise in the serum amylase and lipase levels. The rise in amylase may be helpful but is nonspecific because it may be elevated in patients with other medical conditions, such as parotitis, intestinal injury, tubo-ovarian disease, renal failure, and macroamylasemia. The rise in lipase elevation greater than three times the upper limit of normal is more specific; the serum lipase may remain elevated longer than the serum amylase. Pancreatitis can be suspected on a radiographic examination of the abdomen, with findings of a sentinel loop or a colon cutoff sign. In children, ultrasonography is most helpful in evaluating patients for evidence of anatomic abnormalities, obstruction of the pancreatic or bile ducts, and pancreatic inflammation. CT and magnetic resonance cholangiopancreatography (MRCP) also may be utilized in the evaluation of selected patients.

Celiac disease

Celiac disease (see Chapter 9) is an autoimmune disorder that develops as a consequence of an immune-mediated intestinal response to dietary gluten protein. Celiac disease previously was felt to be relatively uncommon; however, with the availability of more specific diagnostic tests, celiac disease has become increasingly recognized. The prevalence of celiac disease is estimated to be 0.5% to 1% of the population in the United States. Infants and young children with celiac disease can exhibit more classic symptoms of chronic diarrhea, malabsorption, and failure to thrive. Children and adolescents with celiac disease, however, may present with more subtle symptoms of abdominal pain, diarrhea, vomiting, anorexia, constipation, or extraintestinal manifestations that would include failure to thrive, short stature, iron deficiency anemia, elevated liver function studies, or dermatitis herpetiformis. The most common serologic screening tests for celiac disease are serum endomysial IgA antibodies and anti-tissue transglutaminase IgA antibodies. Overall the sensitivity for these tests is greater than 90%. The diagnosis is confirmed with a small bowel biopsy demonstrating histologic features of celiac disease, including prominent intraepithelial lymphocytes and partial to total villous atrophy. Celiac disease is treated with lifelong adherence to a gluten-free diet, excluding foods containing wheat, rye, barley, and oats.

Uncommon Causes of Abdominal Pain

- Choledochal cyst
- Acute intermittent porphyria
- Familial Mediterranean fever
- Obstruction of the ureteropelvic junction
- Endometriosis
- Henoch-Schönlein purpura
- Lead poisoning
- Angioneurotic edema
- Tumors/lymphoma

Choledochal Cyst

A choledochal cyst is a cystic dilatation of all or a portion of the intrahepatic or extrahepatic biliary tree. The most common type, type I, found in 70% of patients, is dilatation of the common bile duct. The classic presenting triad of symptoms in children with a choledochal cyst includes:

- Jaundice
- Abdominal pain
- Abdominal mass

Patients rarely present with all three symptoms together. In 50% of patients with choledochal cysts, the cysts are diagnosed in the newborn period. Choledochal cysts occur four times more frequently in girls than in boys. The diagnosis, when suspected, is confirmed by ultrasonography. The treatment of choledochal cysts is surgical, with complete resection of the cyst because of the potential for adenocarcinoma to arise from the cyst or its remnant after incomplete or partial resection.

Acute Intermittent Porphyria

Acute intermittent porphyria is an inherited disorder of heme biosynthesis. It is the most common of the acute porphyrias and is characterized by a deficiency of the enzyme porphobilinogen deaminase. The condition is inherited in an autosomal-dominant fashion. Clinical symptoms develop in only 10% to 15% of gene carriers. The disorder is expressed most often after puberty, and occurs more frequently in women. Characteristic symptoms are the acute onset of severe abdominal pain, nausea, and vomiting that may be accompanied by neurologic and psychiatric symptoms, including muscle weakness, confusion, hallucinations, and seizures. The attacks are triggered by stress or exposure to exogenous precipitating factors, such as fasting, smoking, alcohol, and a variety of medications. In women, premenstrual attacks are common. The frequency and severity of attacks vary. Acute intermittent porphyria is diagnosed during an acute attack by detecting elevated urinary excretion of aminolevulinic acid and porphobilinogen. Attacks are prevented by the avoidance of precipitants. Oral and intravenous glucose and heme arginate are the mainstays of therapy.

Familial Mediterranean Fever

Familial Mediterranean fever (FMF) is an inherited autosomal-recessive disorder characterized by recurrent acute attacks of *fever* and *polyserositis*. Nonsense or missense mutations on the MEFV gene cause FMF. The MEFV gene regulates the production of pyrin, a protein present in white blood cells, thought to activate the biosynthesis of chemotactic factor inactivators. When pyrin is absent, inactivators are not produced, resulting in the exaggerated inflammatory response seen in patients with FMF. The manifestations of this disease are fever, one or more symptoms of peritonitis (including abdominal pain), arthritis/arthralgia (most commonly in the larger joints), pleuritis, and various skin lesions. It occurs primarily in ethnic groups of Mediterranean origin, Arabs, Armenians, Sephardic Jews, and less commonly Turks, Greeks, Hispanics, and Italians. Symptoms begin in the first decade of life in 50% of patients. The frequency of attacks varies, and acute attacks last 2 to 3 days. The attacks begin with a high fever, which may rise to 40°C (104°F) and can be associated with chills. Ninety percent of patients experience abdominal pain during the attacks. The pain is diffuse and may be severe enough to mimic that of acute abdomen. During acute attacks, the sedimentation rate and levels of acute phase reactants, such as C-reactive protein, plasma fibrinogen, and serum haptoglobin, are elevated. The diagnosis of FMF is made based on clinical criteria and/or genetic testing. Colchicine greatly decreases the frequency, length, and severity of attacks and prevents the long-term complication of renal dysfunction secondary to amyloidosis.

Henoch-Schönlein Purpura

Henoch-Schönlein purpura is a systemic vasculitis involving the blood vessels of the skin, gastrointestinal tract, kidneys, and joints. The cause is unknown. Clinical observation, however, suggests that an infection or medication triggers an immune response that leads to the deposition of immunoglobulin A immune complex in blood vessel walls. Henoch-Schönlein purpura mainly affects children between the ages of 3 and 10 years, with a peak incidence between the ages of 4 and 5 years. Boys are affected more frequently than girls. A seasonal variation is noted, with a peak incidence between November and January. In two thirds of affected patients, an upper respiratory infection precedes the onset of symptoms by 1 to 3 weeks. The gastrointestinal system is involved in two thirds of patients with Henoch-Schönlein purpura, and in 14% to 36% of patients, the gastrointestinal symptoms precede the appearance of the typical purpuric rash. Gastrointestinal symptoms may include colicky abdominal pain, vomiting, and bloody diarrhea or melena. Petechiae and a red non-blanching macular rash symmetrically involving the extensor surfaces of the arms and legs and the buttocks, with sparing of the trunk, develop in 95% to 100% of patients. Renal involvement is noted in 20% to 50% of patients. Glomerulonephritis with hematuria and mild to moderate proteinuria and hypertension develop in patients with Henoch-Schönlein purpura. Patients with mild renal involvement are at low risk for the development of residual renal disease. The most common gastrointestinal complication is intussusception. More unusual complications of Henoch-Schönlein purpura are bowel ischemia, perforation, acute appendicitis, massive gastrointestinal hemorrhage, pancreatitis, hydrops of the gallbladder, and pseudomembranous colitis. The diagnosis is based on the clinical features with supportive laboratory findings of leukocytosis, an elevated sedimentation rate, hematuria, proteinuria, and guaiac-positive stools. The treatment of Henoch-Schönlein purpura is primarily supportive, with careful monitoring for the development of renal and gastrointestinal complications. Corticosteroids can alleviate the arthralgias and gastrointestinal symptoms, but they do not influence the long-term outcome of renal disease. Patients with Henoch-Schönlein purpura may relapse in up to 40% of cases.

Obstruction of the Ureteropelvic Junction

The ureteropelvic junction is the most common site of obstruction in the upper urinary tract in children. The condition is most often congenital and may be secondary to an intrinsic ureteral stenosis or external compression. It can appear at any age and may be detected on routine prenatal ultrasonography. Newborns most often present with an abdominal mass. Older children typically present with acute episodes of severe unilateral colicky abdominal pain that radiates to the flank and is often associated with nausea and vomiting. The symptoms can last for several hours, and then spontaneously resolve. The diagnosis is suspected based on the history and is usually confirmed by ultrasonography. The treatment is surgical intervention to relieve the obstruction.

REVIEW EXERCISES

QUESTIONS

1. Of the following, which is *not* a typical feature of functional abdominal pain in children?
a) Lasts longer than 2 months
b) Begins before the age of 5 years
c) Interrupts normal daily activities
d) Is often severe and diffusely localized

Answer

The answer is b. The onset of pain in children before the age of 5 years requires a more in-depth evaluation for an organic cause of pain. Other "red flags" in the history that suggest an organic cause of pain in children are pain that causes awakening from sleep, an acute onset of the pain, and localization of the pain away from the periumbilical region.

2. The *most* appropriate form of initial therapy for an 11-year-old girl in whom functional abdominal pain was recently diagnosed is:
a) Antispasmodic medications
b) A lactose-free diet
c) Education, reassurance, and limitation of pain-induced disability
d) Antidepressants

Answer

The answer is c. The initial therapeutic intervention that is most effective in children with functional abdominal pain consists of education, reassurance, and an explanation of the pathophysiologic factors contributing to the development of pain. Identifying triggers and limiting pain-induced disability can be helpful. Medications and dietary modifications can be considered in selected patients but are not used as initial therapy.

3. The *most* common cause of intestinal protozoan infection is:
a) *G. lamblia*
b) *C. parvum*
c) *D. fragilis*
d) *B. hominis*

Answer

The answer is a. *G. lamblia* is the most common cause of intestinal protozoan infection. Many children with giardiasis are asymptomatic. Symptomatic children may experience abdominal pain, bloating, diarrhea, and weight loss.

4. An 11-month-old boy is brought to the emergency department with an acute onset of intermittent colicky abdominal pain, vomiting, lethargy, and "currant jelly" stools. Which of the following is the *most* likely diagnosis?
a) Acute appendicitis
b) Obstruction of the ureteropelvic junction
c) Intussusception
d) Choledochal cyst

Answer

The answer is c. All the choices are possible causes of abdominal pain in a child of this age. The characteristic features of intussusception are a sudden onset of severe intermittent colicky abdominal pain and vomiting, followed by the development of lethargy and the passage of "currant jelly" stools. A sausage-shaped abdominal mass may be palpable in the right upper quadrant.

5. Risk factors for the development of gallstones include the following, *except*:
a) Peptic ulcer disease
b) Obesity
c) Hemolytic disease
d) Cystic fibrosis

Answer

The answer is a. Risk factors for the development of gallstones in children and adolescents are hemolytic disease, hyperlipidemia, obesity, pregnancy, cystic fibrosis, prolonged total parenteral nutrition, ileal disease, ileal resection, and the use of several medications, including furosemide, ceftriaxone, and oral contraceptives.

6. A 13-year-old girl is seen for evaluation with a 3-month history of diffuse abdominal pain, fever, weight loss, joint pain, and intermittent rectal bleeding. The *most* likely diagnosis is:
a) Lactose intolerance
b) Crohn disease
c) Meckel diverticulum
d) Irritable bowel syndrome

Answer

The answer is b. The most common presenting clinical features in children with Crohn disease are abdominal pain, diarrhea, weight loss, and growth retardation. Some patients have nausea and vomiting, perianal disease, rectal bleeding, fever, and arthralgia. Patients with irritable bowel syndrome or lactose intolerance may have diarrhea and abdominal pain but not rectal bleeding or guaiac-positive stools. The most common presentation of a Meckel diverticulum is painless rectal bleeding. Meckel diverticulum can also cause partial or complete intestinal obstruction.

SUGGESTED READINGS

1. Apley J, Narsh N. Recurrent abdominal pain: a field survey of 1,000 school children. *Arch Dis Child* 1958;33:165–170.
2. Boyle J. Recurrent abdominal pain: an update. *Pediatr Rev* 1997;18:310–320.
3. Collins B, Thomas D. Chronic abdominal pain. *Pedaitr Rev* 2007;28:323–331.
4. DiLorenzo C, Colletti RB, Lehmann HP, et al. Chronic abdominal pain in children: a technical report of the American Academy of Pediatrics and the North American Society for Pediatric Gastroenterology, Hepatology and Nutrition. *J Pediatr Gastroenterol Nutr* 2005;40:249–261.
5. DiLorenzo C, Colletti RB, Lehmann HP, et al. Chronic abdominal pain in children: a clinical report of the American Academy of Pediatrics and the North American Society for Pediatric Gastroenterology, Hepatology and Nutrition. *J Pediatr Gastroenterol Nutr* 2005;40:245–248.
6. Drossman DA. The functional gastrointestinal disorders and the Rome III process. *Gastroenterology* 2006;130:1377–1390.
7. Hyams J. Irritable bowel syndrome, functional dyspepsia and functional abdominal pain syndrome. *Adolesc Med Clin* 2004;15:1–15.
8. Zeiter D, Hyams J. Clinical aspects of recurrent abdominal pain. *Pediatr Rev* 2001;30:17–21.

Chapter 5

Inflammatory Bowel Disease

Robert Wyllie

Inflammatory bowel disease (IBD) is a general term referring to two chronic conditions of the gastrointestinal tract: Crohn disease (CD) and ulcerative colitis (UC). Although the clinical spectrum of symptoms may be similar in both diseases, the clinical differentiation of CD from UC has important therapeutic implications.

EPIDEMIOLOGY OF INFLAMMATORY BOWEL DISEASE

Forty-five hundred children are diagnosed with IBD every year, and there are approximately 1 million people in the United States who have either CD or UC. The peak incidence is between 15 and 25 years of age, and 25% of the newly diagnosed cases occur in the childhood and adolescent age group. In the pediatric age group CD is more common than UC, accounting for 60% versus 20% to 30%. Approximately 10% to 20% of the children diagnosed with IBD can not definitively be classified as having CD or UC and are placed in a category called Indeterminate Colitis.

CROHN DISEASE

CD may involve any portion of the gastrointestinal tract from the mouth to the anus, but it most often affects the terminal ileum. The terminal ileum and colon are involved in approximately 50% of patients, and 40% have isolated small bowel disease. In patients with small bowel disease, the inflammation is localized in the terminal ileum in 50%, and 50% have multifocal involvement of the small bowel. In 10% of patients, disease is isolated to the large bowel, with no involvement of the small bowel. The inflammation is usually patchy, and ulcerations are interspersed with normal mucosa. Grossly, the bowel wall is thickened by chronic inflammation and edema; as a result, the bowel lumen may

be narrowed and adjacent loops of bowel may be displaced. The mesentery may be thickened and edematous. Fat migrates over the serosal surface of the bowel, creating a characteristic appearance of "fat wrapping." Microscopically, the diagnostic lesion is a granuloma, but granulomas can be identified in only 25% of the mucosal endoscopic biopsy specimens of the large bowel and only 40% of surgically resected specimens. Endoscopically, the appearance of the mucosa may be one of superficial ulcerations overlying lymphoid follicles or of large, linear ("bear claw") ulcers. A cobblestone appearance may result when linear ulcerations isolate blocks of regenerating mucosa.

The initial inflammatory lesion typically evolves into stricturing (fibrostenotic) or penetrating (fistulizing) disease. Fistulae arise when transmural inflammation erodes into adjacent structures. The most common site of fistula formation is an adjacent loop of bowel, but fistulae may occur anywhere, including the perineum, abdominal wall, bladder, or vagina. An ulcer may also erode the bowel wall and end blindly in a localized inflammatory mass, or phlegmon. Stricturing disease occurs when circumferential inflammation results, and fibrosis restricts the size of the intestinal lumen and limits the flow of contents through the intestine.

A general increase in incidence was documented between 1950 and 2000. In approximately 60% pediatric patients with CD, the diagnosis is made between the ages of 16 and 20 years, and in 30% between 11 and 15 years. Only 10% of patients present between 6 and 10 years of age. CD is more common in the white and Jewish populations. Girls are 20% more likely to develop CD than boys. The frequency of CD is higher in certain disorders, including:

- Turner syndrome
- Glycogen storage disease type 1B
- Cystic fibrosis
- Pachydermoperiostosis
- Hermansky-Pudlak syndrome

ULCERATIVE COLITIS

The inflammation of UC is limited to the large bowel. Classically, the inflammation is continuous from the distal to the proximal bowel. At the time of the initial diagnosis in children, approximately two thirds have disease involving the total colon. Disease is limited to the rectum in 15%, and to the left side of the colon in 25%. Occasionally in children, the rectum is spared at the time of the initial diagnosis, but continuous inflammation usually develops during the course of the disease. Of the children who initially have left-sided inflammation or inflammation limited to the rectum, 75% progress to total colonic disease within 10 years.

The endoscopic changes in UC consist of mucosal erythema and edema that produce a granular appearance. In severe disease, deep ulceration and sloughing of the mucosa may be seen. The typical histologic findings are uninterrupted inflammation of the crypts with crypt abscesses and chronic inflammatory cells.

The onset of symptoms is typically between the ages of 16 and 20 years, with symptoms developing in approximately one third of children between the ages of 11 and 15 years. Symptoms appear within the first decade of life in approximately 10% of cases, but UC is uncommon before the age of 6 years.

The epidemiology of UC is similar to that of CD. UC is more common in whites than in individuals of color and is identified more often in the Jewish population. Boys are slightly more likely to develop UC than girls. IBD is more common in the northern United States, and the incidence is higher in urban areas than in rural settings.

ETIOLOGIC CONSIDERATIONS

A variety of studies have investigated the relationship of IBD to nutritional, infectious, and psychologic abnormalities. The incidence of CD is higher in persons with diets high in sugar and lower in those with a higher intake of fluids, fruits, vitamin C, and magnesium. Diets rich in vegetables and potassium also have been associated with a lower risk for development of the disease. Smoking increases the relative risk for CD and decreases the risk for UC. A variety of infectious organisms have been implicated in the pathophysiology of IBD. Measles infection early in life has been associated with a higher risk for CD. Investigation into the possible role of *Mycobacterium paratuberculosis* has yielded conflicting results, but more recent DNA hybridization studies suggest it is not associated with the development of IBD. Abnormalities in intestinal mucus have been demonstrated to enhance the inflammatory process and are associated with IBD. No specific emotional factors have been associated with the development of IBD. A genetic predisposition to IBD is suggested by a predisposition to the development of IBD in certain ethnic

groups and an increased incidence among the family members of initially identified persons. Twin studies demonstrate a high concordance rate for CD among monozygotic twins, approximately 40%, and a concordance rate among dizygotic twins of 10%. Less dramatic increases in concordance rates are seen in UC (10% for monozygotic twins and 3% for dizygotic twins). The incidence of both CD and UC is increased in the first-degree and more distant relatives of initially identified persons. Overall, 10% to 20% of patients with IBD report having a relative with IBD. After an index case has been identified, the likelihood that CD will develop in a sibling is 5% to 10% over a lifetime. The lifetime risk that CD will develop in the offspring of a parent with CD is similar, approximately 10%. In families in which both parents have CD, the risk may be as high as 50%. Familial statistics for UC tend to follow the same patterns but with less dramatic associations. Overall, IBD is found five to ten times more frequently in the relatives of individuals with CD or UC than in control families. In families with IBD, disease is generally diagnosed at a younger age, tends to involve the small bowel, and Jewish ethnicity is relatively common. The lack of an increased risk in adopted siblings and spouses makes an environmental influence unlikely.

NOD2/CARD15 mutations have been identified and associated with CD. Three variations of the gene were found to be associated with CD but not UC. The pathophysiology of how mutations in the NOD2 gene suggest the mutations are associated with a decreased ability of the immune system to respond to bacterial products suggesting CD may be related to a defective host response to normal intestinal flora. Recently genome wide association studies have identified several other areas that also are related to the development of IBD. Defects in the IL23R gene region have been associated with both UC and CD.

SYMPTOMS

The various presenting features of CD and UC are listed in Table 5.1. *Rectal bleeding is more common in UC, whereas*

TABLE 5.1

PRESENTING FEATURES OF CROHN DISEASE AND ULCERATIVE COLITIS IN CHILDHOOD

	Crohn Disease	Ulcerative Colitis
Abdominal pain	++++	++++
Diarrhea	++	+++
Weight loss	++++	++
Fever	++	+
Rectal bleeding	++	++++
Arthritis	+	+
Perianal fissures/fistulae	++	–
Growth failure	+++	+

weight loss and growth failure are more common in CD. The typical presentation of UC is bloody diarrhea. Occasional patients in whom inflammation is limited to the rectum may present with formed stools that are coated with blood and mucus. Most children also have cramping abdominal pain that is relieved by the passage of stool. Bowel movements are typically more frequent in the mornings, when patients may experience rectal spasm associated with muscular irritability. The muscular spasm creates the sensation that stool is within the rectal vault, and patients may be in and out of the bathroom until the spasm subsides.

Children with CD most often have abdominal pain in the right lower quadrant secondary to ileal inflammation. The pain is not necessarily associated with meals or defecation. If the upper gastrointestinal tract (gastroduodenal region) is involved, they may experience epigastric pain simulating that associated with peptic ulcer disease. Diarrhea occurs in approximately half of the patients with CD. Blood is more likely to be present in the stools of patients with disease of the distal colon. Many children with CD have oral aphthous ulcers. They usually persist for a

longer period than lesions associated with viral inflammation. Perianal inflammation is present in 25% or more of children with CD. The most common findings are rectal fissures and surrounding tags. The finding of significant perianal disease or inflammation of the small bowel distinguishes CD from UC.

Growth failure is a hallmark of CD, although it may also occur in UC. Typically, serial measurements of growth demonstrate weight and height decreases that may precede other signs and symptoms of disease (Fig. 5.1). A deceleration in growth velocity is seen in up to 90% of patients. Growth failure is secondary to inadequate caloric intake in most children. Fever is more common in CD than in UC. It is usually of low grade and may occasionally occur without other gastrointestinal symptoms. Arthritis is more common in CD than in UC and may precede the development of bowel symptoms by months or years (see Table 5.1). A typical form of joint involvement is a unilateral migratory arthritis of the large joints of the lower extremities. The joints may be erythematous or swollen, but the arthritis is not usually associated with joint destruction. Joint

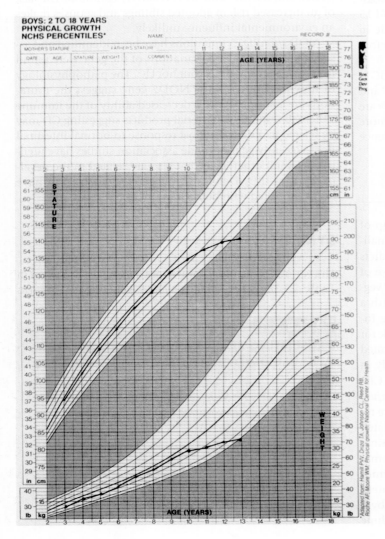

Figure 5.1 Typical growth chart of a patient with Crohn disease.

inflammation usually parallels the activity of the underlying bowel disease. Ankylosing spondylitis occurs in 2% to 6% of patients with IBD and is independent of the bowel disease. Clubbing is typically found in CD and is the result of hypertrophic osteoarthropathy.

The most common cutaneous manifestations are erythema nodosum and pyoderma gangrenosum, which occur in 1% to 4% of patients with IBD (Table 5.2). Other, less common skin conditions include polyarteritis nodosa and epidermolysis bullosa. Ocular complications are uncommon, occurring in fewer than 10% of patients. Episcleritis produces painless red eyes with no changes in vision. Iritis and uveitis are typically painful and may affect vision. Subcapsular cataracts are typically associated with the use of corticosteroids.

Patients with IBD may have symptoms related to their hypercoagulable state. Elevated levels of fibrinogen, factor V, and factor VIII, and depressed levels of antithrombin III may be associated with pathologic clotting. Manifestations include deep vein thrombosis, pulmonary emboli, and neurovascular complications. Patients with CD are susceptible to the development of calcium oxalate and uric acid stones, which may occur in up to 5% of cases.

Hepatobiliary complications are rare in children, but occasional children with primary sclerosing cholangitis and UC have been identified. Children are typically asymptomatic at the time of diagnosis, but the diagnosis is made when persistently abnormal results of liver function studies are noted. Autoimmune hepatitis occasionally has been identified in children with IBD. Gastrointestinal complications include massive hemorrhage that occurs in 1% to 3% of patients with IBD. Major hemorrhagic events are typically preceded by a "herald bleed" that may alert the clinician to an impending problem. Intestinal obstruction is usually partial and associated with CD. Colonic strictures are more typical of patients with UC. In patients with UC, a toxic dilation of the colon may lead to spontaneous perforation. So-called toxic megacolon usually occurs in patients with severe UC and may be precipitated by the use of agents that slow down intestinal transit.

DIAGNOSIS

The diagnosis of IBD is suggested by a compatible history and appropriate physical findings. Serial measurements of growth and calculation of the growth velocity are particularly useful adjuncts to the usual physical examination. Routine laboratory studies include a complete blood cell count, comprehensive metabolic profile, and determination of the sedimentation rate. Anemia is common, found in 70% of patients. Hypoalbuminemia and thrombocytosis are found in 60% of patients. Occult blood is present in the stool of 35% of patients. The sedimentation rate may be elevated in up to 80% of patients. Bacterial and parasitic infections must be ruled out by appropriate fecal testing.

Commercial antibody tests have been used to assist in the diagnosis of IBD. Tests to detect perinuclear antineutrophil cytoplasmic antibody (pANCA) and *anti–Saccharomyces cerevisiae* antibody (ASCA) are commercially available and may aid in identifying children with IBD and in distinguishing CD from UC. The presence of ASCA is significantly associated with CD of the small bowel. Approximately 70% of children with UC involving the entire colon test positive for pANCA. The result of antibody testing is less likely to be positive in those with UC limited to the left side of the colon. A recent analysis found the combination of anemia and elevated sedimentation rate was as effective as the newer serologic testing in predicting IBD in children.

The diagnosis of CD and UC is typically established by a combined radiologic and endoscopic evaluation. In 80% to 90% of children with CD, abnormalities are demonstrated on an upper gastrointestinal series and small bowel followthrough. The involved small bowel is typically nodular, and adjacent bowel loops are displaced. Some patients have strictures of the small bowel with dilatation of the proximal segments. Computed tomography is useful in identifying abscesses and demonstrating edema of the bowel wall (Fig. 5.2).

Endoscopy allows direct observation of the mucosa with histologic sampling. If the rectosigmoid area is visually and histologically normal, UC is unlikely. Segmental involvement, ileal disease, or the identification of granulomas on biopsy specimens establishes a diagnosis of CD. Tissue that appears normal macroscopically may demonstrate significant histologic abnormalities. Capsule endoscopy of the small bowel is a new technique that has a higher yield than barium examination in identifying patients with small bowel CD. Barium enema examinations are usually not useful in establishing a diagnosis of CD or UC.

TABLE 5.2

COMPARISON OF EXTRAINTESTINAL MANIFESTATIONS OF CROHN DISEASE AND ULCERATIVE COLITIS IN CHILDREN

	Crohn Disease (%)	Ulcerative Colitis (%)
Joints	10	15
Eyes	0.2	1–2
Skin	5–15	2–5
Liver	1–2	1–2
Fistulae	15	0
Renal disease/calculi	5	1–5

Adapted from Hamilton JR, Bruce GA, Abdourhaman M, et al. Inflammatory bowel disease in children and adolescents. *Adv Pediatr* 1979;26:311–341; Grand RJ, Ramakrishna J, Calenda KA. Inflammatory bowel disease in the pediatric patient. *Gastroenterol Clin North Am* 1995;24:613–632; Michener WM, Whelan G, Greenstreet RL, et al. Comparison of the clinical features of Crohn's disease and ulcerative colitis with onset in childhood or adolescence. *Cleve Clin Q* 1982;49:13–16.

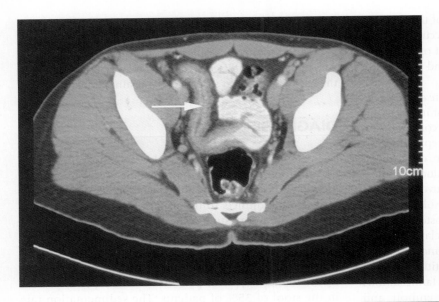

Figure 5.2 Abdominal computed tomogram demonstrating thickened terminal ileum (*arrow*) in a patient with Crohn disease.

TREATMENT

The goal of the treatment of IBD in childhood is to establish and maintain remission while allowing normal growth and preserving quality of life. Although remission is maintained, it is important to minimize therapy-related complications. The therapy utilized for establishing remission usually depends on the severity and extent of bowel involvement (Table 5.3). Therapy for mild IBD usually involves the use of 5-aminosalicylic acid (5-ASA) agents, which can be given topically by suppository or enema in limited colonic disease or orally for more extensive disease. A combination of oral and topical agents is more effective in left-sided colonic disease that has not responded to the administration of single agents. For children who have more severe disease or are not responding to 5-ASA therapy, steroids are typically added. Intravenous steroids are utilized for patients who have severe disease or are not responding to 5-ASA medications and oral steroids.

The formulation of aminosalicylates allows some leeway as to which product is selected for an individual patient. 5-ASA conjugates are available as sulfasalazine (Azulfidine), olsalazine (Dipentum), balsalazide (Colazal), and MMX mesalamine or Lialda. Sulfasalazine is composed of sulfapyridine and 5-ASA. The 5-ASA is liberated in the colon after being metabolized by colonic bacteria. Olsalazine consists of two 5-ASA molecules linked by a diazo bond. After bacterial degradation, the 5-ASA is liberated in the colon. Unfortunately, olsalazine causes diarrhea as a side effect, so its use is limited.

Mesalamine preparations are pure 5-ASA coated either with ethylcellulose as a timed-release capsule (Pentasa) or with acrylic resin as a tablet that dissolves at a pH of 7 or higher (Asacol). The newest formulation, Lialda, can be given as a single daily dose and may improve compliance among teenagers. An oral mesalamine preparation is the

TABLE 5.3

THERAPY FOR INFLAMMATORY BOWEL DISEASE IN CHILDREN AND ADOLESCENTS

Mild disease—5-ASA
Topical for distal colonic disease
   Suppositories (disease limited to the rectum)
   Enemas (disease confined to the distal colon)
Combination of topical 5-ASA and one of the oral products
Oral for disease limited to the colon
   Left colon disease
   Balsalazide
   Pancolonic disease
   Sulfasalazine
   Olsalazine
   Mesalamine (Pentasa, Asacol)
Oral for more extensive colonic disease or a combination of large and small bowel disease
   Mesalamine
   pH release: Asacol
   Timed release: Pentasa
Moderate disease—5-ASA as above plus consideration of the following:
Glucocorticoids
   Topical for distal colon disease
   Oral
Antibiotics
   Metronidazole
   Ciprofloxacin
Immune modulators
   Azathioprine
   6-Mercaptopurine
   Methotrexate
Severe disease—additive therapy for severe disease
Glucocorticoids
   Intravenous
Crohn disease
   Infliximab
Ulcerative colitis
   Cyclosporine
   Tacrolimus

5-ASA, 5-aminosalicylic acid.

preferred 5-ASA product in the treatment of small bowel and proximal large bowel disease. Mesalamine suppositories are used to treat proctitis, and enemas are useful in treating disease extending to the splenic flexure.

Sulfasalazine and the newer mesalamine preparations exhibit a dose–response relationship, but the toxicity of the carrier drug (sulfapyridine) in sulfasalazine limits the dose. A dose–response relationship of oral mesalamine is evident in dosages of up to 4.8 g/day, and side effects are fewer than with sulfasalazine. Common side effects of sulfasalazine include headache, nausea, and vomiting. Less common side effects include allergic reactions, pancreatitis, hepatotoxicity, interstitial nephritis, and hemolytic anemia. 5-ASA products are generally used to achieve remission in mild disease and maintain remission after treatment of the active phase of the disease.

Glucocorticoids are very effective in establishing remission in moderate and severe disease but are not effective in maintaining remission. Prednisone is usually given orally at first and then intravenously if oral treatment fails. Budesonide is a recently available coated formulation of oral steroid that delivers active drug to the terminal ileum and proximal large bowel. It is currently used for CD of the distal ileum and right colon.

Toxicity is a major concern with the use of glucocorticoids. Cosmetic side effects of concern to teenagers include exacerbation of facial acne and hair growth. Facial puffiness, weight gain, and striae are also bothersome side effects. Medical concerns include growth failure, cataracts, glaucoma, osteoporosis, myopathy, hypertension, and depression. Budesonide causes significantly fewer side effects because most of the drug is inactivated following the first pass through the liver.

Glucocorticoids have not been effective in the treatment of perianal disease or the maintenance of remission in IBD. These limitations, coupled with the side effects of steroid therapy, have led to the development of a variety of alternate therapies. The most frequently used medications are immune modulators, including azathioprine and 6-mercaptopurine. Azathioprine and 6-mercaptopurine are used to induce and maintain remission in CD and UC. Their onset of action is after 3 to 4 months, and therefore they are usually used as steroid-sparing medications in patients who require the frequent administration of glucocorticoids. Complications of therapy with 6-mercaptopurine and azathioprine include bone marrow suppression, pancreatitis, leukopenia, and liver toxicity. Laboratory measurement of the active metabolites 6-thioguanine (6-TG) and 6-methyl-mercaptopurine (6-MMP) has led to dose adjustments, which may be helpful in preventing side effects, and the use of drug doses that are more likely to maintain remission. The have been recent reports about the use of azathioprine in combination with remicade resulting in hepatosplenic T-cell lymphoma in teenagers.

Methotrexate is also useful in the management of IBD, particularly in patients with joint symptoms. Methotrexate can be given orally or intramuscularly. The usual onset of action is after 3 to 4 weeks. Side effects include marrow suppression and hepatotoxicity. Methotrexate, azathioprine, and 6-mercaptopurine may be associated with fetal deformities. An increased risk of lymphoma risk when methotrexate and remicade are used in combination has not been reported.

Nutritional therapy is more effective in CD than in UC. The use of polymeric or elemental diets as the sole source of nutrition has been associated with remission rates similar to those achieved with glucocorticoids in CD in small series of pediatric patients. In addition, dietary therapy has led to increases in body weight and growth velocity. However, because of nutritional fatigue and an inability to sustain the diet, compliance has been poor in most cases. Once the dietary therapy is stopped, the relapse rate is higher than it is after the withdrawal of steroids.

Other treatments include antibiotics, particularly metronidazole, ciprofloxacin, and more recently rifaximin. All inhibit the growth of anaerobic bacteria, but it is not clear whether their antibacterial activity is responsible for the improvement in patients with IBD. The administration of both antibiotics together may be associated with greater clinical improvement than the administration of either one in IBD.

One of the newest forms of therapy for IBD is monoclonal antibodies to tumor necrosis factor (TNF), particularly in CD. Infliximab is a monoclonal antibody to TNF. It is administered intravenously, and most patients respond within days to weeks after administration. Infliximab has been successfully used to close fistulas and induce remission. In patients who lose their tolerance to infliximab, humanized TNF inhibitors (adalimumab and centrolizumab) have been used with reported success, although limited information is available in children.

Approximately half of the patients with CD have traditionally required surgery. Surgery is typically performed to treat strictures, although in the past it was more commonly performed for the treatment of fistulae and failure of medical therapy to induce remission. Strictureplasty is a bowel-sparing operation that has effectively relieved obstruction in adults and children without a loss of mucosal surface area. Surgery in CD is invariably associated with eventual relapse and is not curative. Relapse occurs less often if immune modulators are started as a chemoprophylactic agent in the postoperative period. Advances in medical therapy should be associated with a reduced requirement for surgery in the future.

In patients with UC, removal of the colon "cures" the disease. The most common procedures are ileorectal anastomosis and ileal pouch-anal anastomosis. Ileorectal anastomosis is associated with frequent bowel movements, which are reduced with pouch surgery. "Pouchitis" is inflammation of the surgically created pouch and is associated with diarrhea and abdominal pain. Pouchitis usually responds to antibiotics and tends to occur less frequently with time.

REVIEW EXERCISES

QUESTIONS

1. Which of the following is the *most* important clue in differentiating UC from CD?
a) Joint symptoms
b) Disease limited to the large bowel
c) Small bowel disease
d) Kidney stone

Answer
The answer is c. UC affects only the colon, whereas CD may affect the small bowel, colon, or both. Extraintestinal manifestations are frequent in both UC and CD.

2. Which of the following is *more* common in CD?
a) Perianal disease
b) Onset during the teen years
c) Growth failure
d) Both *a* and *c*
e) None of the above

Answer
The answer is d. Both UC and CD may present with growth failure during the teen years. Growth failure and perianal disease are both more common in CD.

3. Initial therapy for mild IBD typically includes all of the following, *except:*
a) Cyclosporine
b) Mesalamine
c) Sulfasalazine
d) Olsalazine
e) 5-ASA suppositories

Answer
The answer is a. Cyclosporine is typically limited to patients with refractory UC. A variety of 5-ASA medications can be used, depending on the location and extent of disease.

4. The *best* choice of ASA product for the treatment of small bowel disease is:
a) Balsalazide
b) Olsalazine
c) Sulfapyridine
d) 5-ASA enemas
e) Timed-release mesalamine

Answer
The answer is e. The most appropriate choice for the treatment of small bowel disease would be either pH-dependent or timed-release mesalamine. The other 5-ASA dimers are best used for isolated disease of the large bowel.

5. The most common side effects of azathioprine include all of the following, *except:*
a) Pancreatitis
b) Bone marrow suppression
c) Liver toxicity
d) Cardiomyopathy

Answer
The answer is d. Pancreatitis occurs in approximately 5% of children started on azathioprine. Bone marrow toxicity may be either an acute or a chronic side effect. Liver function abnormalities usually develop after prolonged therapy.

6. The most common etiology of growth failure in children with CD is:
a) Excessive utilization of calories
b) Decreased caloric intake
c) Loss of protein through bowel inflammation
d) Bacterial overgrowth

Answer
The answer is b. Although any of the above may occur in children with CD and growth failure, the cause of growth problems is typically inadequate caloric intake. Increased caloric intake in children with CD may result in clinical improvement.

SUGGESTED READINGS

1. Bernstein CN, Wajda A, Svenson LW, et al. The epidemiology of inflammatory bowel disease in Canada: a population-based study. *Am J Gastroenterol* 2007;102:1749–57. quiz 1748, 1758.
2. Biancone L, Calabrese E, Petruzziello C, et al. Treatment with biologic therapies and the risk of cancer in patients with IBD. *Nat Clin Pract Gastroenterol Hepatol* 2007;4:78–91.
3. Bousvaros A, Antonioli DA, Colletti RB, et al. Differentiating ulcerative colitis from crohn disease in children and young adults: report of a working group of the North American Society for Pediatric Gastroenterology, Hepatology, and Nutrition and The Crohn's and Colitis Foundation of America. *J Pediatr Gastroenterol Nutr* 2007; 45:3–14.
4. de'Angelis GL, Fornaroli F, de'Angelis N, et al. Wireless capsule endoscopy for pediatric small-bowel diseases. *Aliment Pharmacol Ther* 2007;25:941–947.
5. Kozuch PL, Hanauer SB. General principles and pharmacology of biologics in inflammatory bowel disease. *Gastroenterol Clin North Am.* 2006;35:757–773.
6. Mack DR, Langton C, Markowitz J, et al. Laboratory values for children with newly diagnosed inflammatory bowel disease. *Paediatr Drugs.* 2006;8:279–302.
7. Mackey AC, Green L, Liang LC, et al. Hepatosplenic T cell lymphoma associated with infliximab use in young patients treated for inflammatory bowel disease. *J Pediatr Gastroenterol Nutr* 2007;44: 653–674.
8. Ooi CY, Bohane TD, Lee D, et al. Thiopurine metabolite monitoring in paediatric inflammatory bowel disease. *Acta Paediatr* 2007;96:128–130.
9. Rufo PA, Bousvaros A. Current therapy of inflammatory bowel disease in children. *J Pediatr Gastroenterol Nutr* 2007;44:265–267.
10. Rufo PA, Bousvaros A. Current therapy of inflammatory bowel disease in children. *Paediatr Drugs* 2006;8:279–302.
11. Sabery N, Bass D. Use of serologic markers as a screening tool in inflammatory bowel disease compared with elevated erythrocyte sedimentation rate and anemia. *Pediatrics* 2007;119: 1113–1119.

Chapter 6

Viral Hepatitis

Marsha Kay

Although a number of recent developments have increased our understanding of the causes and consequences of viral hepatitis, the various agents responsible for viral hepatitis have been present for several thousand years. Epidemic jaundice associated with fever, anorexia, malaise, and fatigue was described by Hippocrates more than 2000 years ago. From the 1940s through the 1960s hepatitis A and hepatitis B were differentiated as separate clinical entities. In 1970 Dane et al. identified the viral particle responsible for hepatitis B infection. Feinstone identified the hepatitis A virus (HAV) in 1972, and in 1989 an immunoassay was developed to detect antibodies to hepatitis C virus (HCV). In 1994 the hepatitis C viral particle was identified by immunoelectron microscopic study in Japan. In 1993 research tests became available to detect the antibody to hepatitis E, although the virus was first described in 1983. Although investigators became aware of hepatitis E in the 1980–1990s, the agent was retrospectively identified as having caused a large epidemic of viral hepatitis in India in 1955 and a second major outbreak there in 1980, with a high fatality rate among pregnant women. Research is ongoing to identify "new hepatitis viruses" to join the list of currently recognized viruses, which include the agents responsible for hepatitis A, B, C, D, E, F, G, and GB infection.

According to recent data from the U.S Centers for Disease Control and Prevention (CDC), the annual incidence of new cases of hepatitis A and B viral infection in the United States is decreasing. The most dramatic decreases have been in the pediatric population as a result of pediatric vaccination strategies for both hepatitis A and B. After a decline in the incidence of acute hepatitis C infection in the 1990s, since 2003 the rates have plateaued, with a slight increase in the reported cases in 2006, the most recent year for which data are available. The prevalence of each type of hepatitis in the United States varies by patient age. In adults, hepatitis B is the most common, accounting for approximately 50% of cases, followed by hepatitis A (30%) and hepatitis C (20%); hepatitis D and hepatitis E account for less than 1% of the cases. The relative prevalence and recognition of hepatitis C are anticipated to increase in the coming years and because of the

high likelihood of developing chronic infection, this entity will likely be the most prevalent form of hepatitis in adults in the United States. In children, hepatitis A is the most common form in the United States (50%) and hepatitis B the second most common (30%), with hepatitis C accounting for approximately 20% of the cases. With the significant decrease in the rates of hepatitis A and B infection in pediatric patients, the relative prevalence of hepatitis C infection will likely increase, and it is anticipated that hepatitis C will become the most prevalent form of hepatitis in children and adolescents in the United States. The relative increase in the importance of HCV infection is the consequence of two factors: effective vaccination strategies for hepatitis A and hepatitis B, which have decreased the rates of hepatitis A and hepatitis B infection in children, young adults and their contacts, and the high rate of chronic infection following hepatitis C infection. Hepatitis D and hepatitis E account for less than 1% of the cases of pediatric viral hepatitis in the United States, and as in adults, hepatitis E occurs almost exclusively in patients who have traveled to areas in which the infection is endemic.

HEPATITIS A

Hepatitis A is a RNA virus in the family Picornaviridae. Infection with HAV results in acute illness only. Most infected patients are asymptomatic. Hepatitis A occurs most frequently in developing countries, in which the prevalence may reach 100% and most individuals have been infected by the age of 5 years. Approximately 30% of adults in the United States have had hepatitis A infection. It is estimated that only one fifth of individuals with hepatitis A undergo diagnostic testing, the results of which by law must be reported to the CDC. For example, 29,000 cases were reported in the United States in 1990, but 130,000 to 150,000 cases of hepatitis A were estimated to have occurred that year. CDC data in 2006 the most recent year available indicate a significant decrease in reported HAV cases in the United States (3579 cases reported, estimated 15,000 acute clinical cases, and 32,000 new infections) with similar rates now in all age groups (0.7–1.4 cases/100,000 population). This is the result of availability of HAV vaccine starting in 1995, with the largest comparative decreases in the rates of infection during childhood. The mean incubation period for hepatitis A virus is 28 days, with a range of 15 to 50 days. Patients are contagious up to 14 days before the development of symptoms and for 1 week after jaundice appears (Fig. 6.1). The primary route of transmission is fecal–oral, but transmission from contaminated shellfish and rare percutaneous and transfusion-associated transmission also occurs. The diagnosis is established by the presence of elevated levels of anti-HAV immunoglobulin M (IgM), which can be detected at 5 weeks following exposure, at the time when clinical symptoms have appeared. This antibody typically persists for 3 to 4 months. Anti-HAV IgG, which can usually be detected 4 months after exposure, may persist for years. *Children with hepatitis A, especially those younger than 3 years, are usually asymptomatic.* If they do have symptoms, they are similar to those of a viral upper respiratory tract infection. The frequency of clinical symptoms is higher in adolescents and adults, and their symptoms, including nausea, vomiting, diarrhea, fatigue, dark-colored urine, and anorexia, may be more severe. The fraction of individuals hospitalized with acute HAV infection increases with increasing age with a 22% rate in children less than age 5 and a rate of 52% in persons ≥60 years of age. Fulminant hepatic failure from hepatitis A is uncommon, but can be fatal, with approximately 100 cases per year in the United States (0.3% death rate). A long-term carrier state does not exist.

Two methods are available to prevent hepatitis A infection:

■ Passive immunoprophylaxis
■ Active immunization

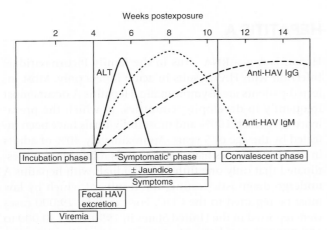

Weeks postexposure

Figure 6.1 Hepatitis A infection: development of immunoglobulin G (IgG) antibody to hepatitis A virus (HAV) anti-HAV (IgG) indicates immunity to infection. ALT, alanine aminotransferase. (Adapted from Nowicki MJ, Balistreri WF. Hepatitis A to E: building up the alphabet. *Contemp Pediatr* 1992;9:118–128, with permission.)

Before 1995, hepatitis A Ig was the only form of prophylaxis available and was administered before travel to areas of endemicity or following acute exposure. Areas in which hepatitis A is endemic include Mexico, the Caribbean, South America, Central America, Africa, and Asia (not including Japan). This type of passively acquired immunity lasts 12 weeks or less, and Ig must be readministered in cases of ongoing exposure. Hepatitis A Ig is also indicated for:

■ Acute exposure, if given within 14 days after exposure to household members or intimate contacts of individuals with acute hepatitis A
■ Outbreaks in day care or custodial settings
■ Common source outbreaks

Two hepatitis A vaccines are now available. Immunization is now routinely recommended for all children 12 months of age or older regardless of state of residence. Coadministration of HAV vaccine with other immunizations is not associated with impairment of vaccine induced immunity. In addition to all children, vaccination is recommended for travelers and high-risk populations, which include American Indians, Alaskans, illicit drug users, laboratory workers, handlers of primate animals, and individuals with chronic liver disease, patients with clotting factor disorders, and men who have sex with men. A booster dose is required for both hepatitis A vaccines. Vaccination is being evaluated for postexposure prophylaxis, especially in areas of a confined outbreak. In this setting both vaccine or hepatitis A immunoglobulin are highly efficacious and are associated with a reduction of the rate of acute hepatitis A infection to ≤5% of exposed contacts.

HEPATITIS B

Hepatitis B virus (HBV) is a DNA virus in the family Hepadnaviridae with a mean incubation period of 120 days (range, 45–160 days). Currently there are 8 genotypes (A-H) and two subtypes (Aa/Ae, Ba/Bj). It is extremely common worldwide, with more than 300 million carriers. Areas in which hepatitis B is highly endemic include China, sub-Saharan Africa, Southeast Asia, the Mediterranean basin, and Alaska (among the Eskimo population). In Asia, the hepatitis B surface antigen (HBsAg) carrier rate is 5% to 20% of the general population. The annual rate of HBV infection in the United States is estimated to be about 50,000 cases, which has decreased by more than 60% from the 1990s and represents approximately 20% of the mean number of new infections in the 1980s. Overall in the United States, approximately 0.5% to 0.7% of the population are long-term carriers (approximately 1.25 million individuals), with 4.9% of the population having been infected with Hepatitis B at some point in their lifetime. The mortality rate is 1.4%. *The major risk factor for HBV infection in children is having a mother who is positive for HBsAg, especially if the mother is also positive for hepatitis B early antigen (HBeAg)*. Without immunoprophylaxis, rates of transmission from mother to infant may approach 90%, and up to 30% to 90% of these children remain long-term carriers until at least 30 years of age. Children adopted from areas of endemicity are another population at risk in the United States. Currently the majority of new childhood infections in the United States excluding perinatal infections are found in immigrant children themselves, children born to infected immigrant women, and children who acquire HBV horizontally within these households or enclaves. Children also can acquire HBV infection intravenously from drugs and blood products, following tattooing and piercing, in the course of institutionalized care (especially when the incidence of biting is high), and through high-risk sexual behaviors.

Hepatitis B Serology

HBsAg is acquired by almost all infected individuals. Detection is coincident with symptom onset and increased values of serum liver chemistries. It is typically detectable 45 days following infection, and levels may decrease before symptoms resolve (Fig. 6.2). Persistence of this antigen for 6 months or longer indicates a long-term carrier state (Fig. 6.3). HBeAg, a low-molecular-weight soluble protein associated with the viral core, is a marker of infectivity. Anti-HBc is antibody to hepatitis B core antigen (HBcAg). HBcAg is not detectable by commercial testing. Initially, anti-HBc is an IgM antibody and subsequently an IgG antibody. Levels increase shortly after symptom onset and the appearance of HBsAg, and anti-HBc typically persists for many years. Its presence indicates acute, resolved, or chronic infection, but anti-HBc is not detected following immunization. The development of anti-HBe indicates a reduced risk for transmission of HBV, but not immunity. *The development of antibody to HBsAg (anti-HBs) indicates immunity, and anti-HBs is acquired after effective immunization or the resolution of*

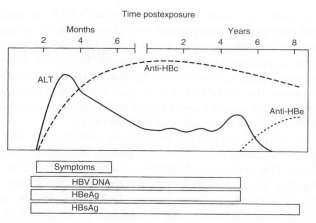

Figure 6.3 Chronic hepatitis B infection: note persistence of hepatitis B surface antigen (HBsAg). The development of antibody to hepatitis B early antigen (anti-HBe) indicates reduction of infectivity, but not resolution of the infection. ALT, alanine aminotransferase. (Adapted from Nowicki MJ, Balistreri WF. Hepatitis A to E: building up the alphabet. *Contemp Pediatr* 1992;9(11):118–128, with permission.)

infection. HBV DNA is found in the viral core and is currently the best measure for viral replication. Rarely, patients may be positive for both HBsAg and anti-HBs. This finding likely represents the development of immunity to vaccine virus in a patient who was already a long-term carrier of wild-type virus and is associated with chronic disease.

Clinical symptoms are more frequent with HBV infection than with HAV infection, and fulminant hepatitis develops in a higher proportion of patients. Symptoms of infection include anorexia, malaise, nausea, vomiting, and abdominal pain. *Chronic disease develops in approximately 10% of adults, 50% of older children who are infected and in 90% of infants who acquire the infection vertically.* The high rate of perinatal acquisition reflects the large viral inoculum in maternal blood during birth and in maternal secretions after birth, and the infant's immune tolerance to the virus. Factors associated with immune tolerance to HBV infection and therefore with chronic infection include downregulation of the expression of immune recognition signals on the surface of infected hepatocytes, viral antigenic variation, suppressing the immune response by inducing tolerance, exhausting viral specific cytotoxic T lymphocytes, and interfering with cytokine function. In children with chronic HBV infection, who had acquired the infection vertically, transaminase levels are characteristically normal or minimally elevated, usually up to 100 international unit (IU)/L, with simultaneously high levels of viral replication. In older children who acquire the infection horizontally, the pattern of transaminase elevation may be more similar to that of adults. *Chronic HBV infection can result in chronic hepatitis, liver necrosis, cirrhosis, and hepatocellular carcinoma (HCC).* The risk for HCC in an individual with chronic HBV infection can be 200 to 500 times greater than that of an unaffected patient, and the risk correlates with the duration of

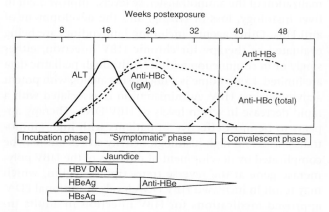

Figure 6.2 Acute hepatitis B infection: development of antibody to hepatitis B surface antigen (anti-HBs) indicates immunity to infection. ALT, alanine aminotransferase. (Adapted from Nowicki MJ, Balistreri WF. Hepatitis A to E: building up the alphabet. *Contemp Pediatr* 1992;9(11):118–128, with permission.)

infection. In Taiwan, 80% of children with HCC are anti-HBe seropositive and patients with chronic HBsAg carriage have a 25% lifetime risk of developing HCC, with highest rates in patients who are HBeAg positive. Hepatitis C infection also significantly increases the risk for HCC in pediatric patients. The rate of HCC has decreased by 75% in children between the ages of 6 and 14 years in Taiwan after universal HBV vaccination was initiated there in 1984.

Effective strategies are available to prevent HBV infection, including vaccination and passive immunoprophylaxis. The two types of HBV vaccine are plasma-derived vaccine and recombinant vaccine; recombinant vaccine is used primarily because plasma-derived vaccine is no longer manufactured in the United States. Hepatitis B immunoglobulin (HBIg) is used in conjunction with the vaccine. When HBIg and HBV vaccines are administered at birth and an appropriate vaccination schedule is followed, perinatal HBV infection is prevented in more than 90% of infants, whereas the efficacy rate is 75% to 80% when either HBV vaccine or HBIg is given alone. HBV vaccination and the administration of HBIg are indicated for:

- Neonates with an HBsAg-positive mother
- Intimate contacts of a patient with acute HBV infection
- HBsAg-negative individuals who sustain an HBsAg-positive needlestick injury

Universal hepatitis B vaccination is recommended for all infants at birth by the American Academy of Pediatrics. All children and adolescents who have not been immunized against HBV should begin the series as soon as possible. In addition to the groups listed in the preceding text, HBV vaccination is recommended for intimate or household contacts of a patient with chronic HBV infection, ethnic populations at high risk of HBV infection, all injection drug users, sexually active individuals with more than one partner per 6-month period or a history of a sexually transmitted disease, sexually active homosexual men, health care personnel, residents and staff of institutions for developmentally disabled individuals, patients undergoing hemodialysis, patients with bleeding disorders who require clotting factor concentrates, travelers to areas in which HBV infection is endemic, and inmates of juvenile detention or correctional facilities.

Once chronic infection is established, the rate of spontaneous seroconversion and development of anti-HBs is low; however, seroconversion from HBeAg-positive to anti-HBe-positive may occur and this indicates a less contagious state. Clearance of HBeAg and development of anti-HBe may be preceded by an acute increase in serum aminotransferase levels. Because of the long-term risks associated with chronic hepatitis B infection, we recommend that patients with chronic infection be evaluated to determine whether they are candidates for antiviral therapy. The goals of the therapy are to remove the stimulus to ongoing inflammation by eliminating the virus, thereby interrupting the progression to fibrosis and cir-

rhosis and decreasing the risk for the development of HCC. Interferon α (IFN-α), a naturally occurring protein produced by B lymphocytes and monocytes, is currently the mainstay of therapy. The synthetic form of IFN-α is produced by recombinant DNA techniques with the use of *Escherichia coli*. IFN-α acts by inducing protein synthesis within the recipient's cells, and the proteins affect various stages of the viral replication cycle. IFN-α interrupts translation of the viral genome into virus-specified proteins, and as a result of its immunoregulatory actions, major histocompatibility complex (MHC) antigen expression, macrophage activation, cytokine induction, and regulation of T-cell activity are altered. IFN-α is given by subcutaneous injection, typically three times a week, with the dosage based on body weight and the duration of therapy, which ranges from 6 to 12 months. Pegylated forms of interferon with a longer half-life, which therefore require injection only once a week, are currently undergoing evaluation. Children with chronic HBV infection with the following characteristics are more likely to respond to antiviral therapy:

- Increased levels of serum transaminases
- Low levels of HBV DNA
- Horizontally acquired disease
- Younger patient age
- Infection of short duration
- Negativity for anti-human immunodeficiency virus (HIV)
- Active liver histology

The transaminases of children on therapy may flare before a response is noted. While receiving this medication, patients may have flu-like symptoms, which are usually more severe at the initiation of therapy. Patients must be monitored for side effects of the medication, which can include hematologic and cardiac disturbances, weight loss, the development of antithyroid antibodies, and psychiatric problems. A positive response to therapy consists of normalization of the aminotransferase levels, improvement in liver histology, loss of HBsAg, and the development of anti-HBs. Other agents, including lamivudine, are being evaluated as therapy for chronic HBV infection, either singly or in conjunction with IFN, although pediatric data are limited. Lamivudine is a nucleoside analog with potent activity against HBV. Administration is associated with a rapid decrease in serum levels of HBV DNA. Therapy appears to be most effective in patients with high aminotransferases and high histologic activity scores but may be complicated by development of mutants of the HBV polymerase gene at the reverse transcriptase region, which may result in increased HBV DNA levels. Additional FDA-approved medications for HBV infection in adults include Adefovir dipivoxil, an oral nucleotide analog, and Entecavir, an oral guanosine nucleoside analog. Adefovir dipivoxil is currently undergoing evaluation in a multicenter pediatric trial. Cirrhosis secondary to HBV infection is currently an indication for liver transplantation. The recurrence rate in allografts is very high, often because of autoinfection from other sites. Currently, a variety of prophylaxis and treatment strategies at the time of transplantation are being studied to reduce the recurrence rate of HBV infection in grafts.

HEPATITIS DELTA

Hepatitis delta virus (HDV) is a defective RNA virus that *requires the machinery of HBV for replication.* It consists of an RNA genome and a delta protein antigen (HDAg), both of which are coated with HBsAg. The prevalence of this virus is increased in developing countries and the Mediterranean basin, including southern Italy, Eastern Europe, South America, Africa, and the Middle East. HDV infection is often transmitted by intrafamilial or intimate contact, and in developed countries transmission is usually percutaneous. Two types of infection can occur. In coinfection, an individual acquires HBV and HDV infections at the same time. Perinatal coinfection is rare. Superinfection occurs when a long-term HBV carrier becomes infected with HDV, and it may be the cause of an acute deterioration in the status of an otherwise stable carrier of HBV. The diagnosis is established by measuring anti-HDV IgG (commercially available) or anti-HDV IgM, HDAg, or HDV RNA (research-based) (**Figs. 6.4 and 6.5**). The incubation period for coinfection is similar to that for HBV infection. The incubation period for superinfection is 2 to 8 weeks. Coinfection typically results in acute hepatitis, which is fulminant in 5% of patients. Superinfection can result in chronic or fulminant hepatitis. HDV is directly hepatotoxic, and infection accelerates the progression to cirrhosis in comparison with HBV infection alone, carries a higher risk for the development of HCC, and is associated with a higher mortality rate. HDV infection is prevented by effective HBV vaccination. The therapy for

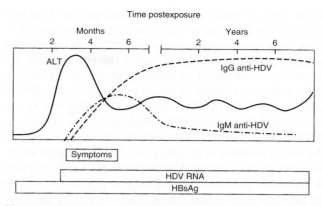

Figure 6.5 Chronic hepatitis delta and hepatitis B infection: note persistence of hepatitis B surface antigen (HBsAg) and hepatitis delta virus RNA. ALT, alanine aminotransferase. (Adapted from Nowicki MJ, Balistreri WF. The C's, D's, and E's of viral hepatitis. *Contemp Pediatr* 1992;9(12):23–42, with permission.)

chronic infection is similar to that for chronic HBV infection, although the response rate to therapy with IFN-α is reduced. Clearance of HDV infection requires clearance of HBV infection.

HEPATITIS C

HCV is a single-stranded RNA virus that accounted for approximately 90% of cases of post-transfusion or non-A and -B hepatitis, before the tests to screen for HCV antibody became available in 1990. This virus is transmitted primarily by parenteral routes and replicates preferentially in hepatocytes. The incubation period is wide, ranging from 2 to 52 weeks. The HCV particle was identified in 1994 by immunoelectron microscopy in Japan. It is an enveloped 9.5-kb virus with significant genomic heterogeneity resulting from frequently occurring mutations. There are nine major genotypes and at least 90 subtypes. The prevalence of the different genotypes varies by geographical region and genotypes are associated with differential response rates to antiviral therapy. Genotype 1, the most common type in the United States, is associated with a decreased response rate to antiviral therapy. HCV is now classified in the Hepacivirus family.

The seroprevalence of hepatitis C infection in the general population in the United States is 1.6% to 1.8%. Lowest prevalence rates worldwide are in the United Kingdom and Scandinavian countries, where the rate is 0.01% to 0.1%. Countries with high prevalence rates include the Mediterranean countries, Brazil, the Middle East, and the Indian subcontinent, with rates between 1% and 5%. The seroprevalence rate in the United States is 0.2% in children up to 12 years of age and 0.4% in children who are 12 to 19 years old. By contrast, the prevalence rate in pediatric patients is more than 14% in Cameroon. More than 4 million individuals are infected

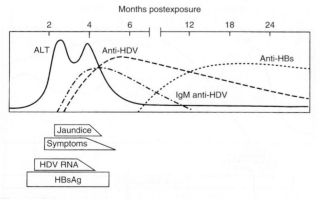

Figure 6.4 Resolution of acute hepatitis delta and acute hepatitis B infection: development of antibody to hepatitis B surface antigen (anti-HBs) indicates immunity to infection. ALT, alanine aminotransferase. (Adapted from Nowicki MJ, Balistreri WF. The C's, D's, and E's of viral hepatitis. *Contemp Pediatr* 1992;9(12): 23–42, with permission.)

in the United States, and it is estimated that worldwide at least 175 million individuals are positive for anti-HCV. Risk factors for transmission in adults include intravenous drug use, snorting of drugs, blood transfusion, and administration of blood products, dialysis, needlestick injury, and occupational or sexual exposure. Up to 40% of adults with HCV infection lack an identified risk factor. Risk factors for acquisition in children include the preceding factors and perinatal acquisition. *The rate of maternal to infant transmission is thought to be 4% to 6%, with an increased risk for transmission when the mother is coinfected with HIV or has high titers of HCV at the time of delivery.* The rate of perinatal transmission in infants born to HIV and HCV coinfected mothers is approximately 20%. Children who acquire the infection perinatally may have a high rate of chronic disease because of immune tolerance, although longitudinal studies are required to determine the exact risk. Although there are no significant differences in perinatal transmission rates between infants delivered vaginally versus those born by cesarean section, prolonged rupture of membranes for more than 6 hours is an independent risk factor for HCV transmission. Other pediatric patients at risk include recipients of blood products, especially before 1990, such as hemophiliacs, survivors of leukemia or other childhood malignancies, and children who have undergone cardiac surgery. Children with a higher number of transfusions have a higher prevalence rate. Viral sequences are detected by polymerase chain reaction, and antibodies are detected by enzyme-linked immunoadsorbent assay (ELISA) or recombinant immunoblot assay (RIBA), the preferred test. Patients who received blood or serum products before the year 1990, when screening became available, should be considered at risk for this infection. Infection acquired from the intravenous administration of Ig after 1990 has been reported.

Approximately 10% to 30% of patients with acute HCV infection develop jaundice, 10% to 20% have nonspecific symptoms, and the majority are asymptomatic. The symptoms of HCV infection include fatigue, abdominal pain, anorexia, weight loss, and malaise. In a fraction of patients, the course of acute HCV may be more fulminant than that of HAV or HBV infection (Fig. 6.6). HCV infection may be associated with aplastic anemia or agranulocytosis. The mortality rate of patients with infection is approximately 1% to 2%. *Chronic disease is thought to develop in approximately 80% of infected patients, although the range is from 50% to 80%, depending on the series.* Most patients with chronic HCV infection are identified as part of a workup for elevated transaminase levels. Approximately 70% of patients with chronic HCV have symptoms that are nonspecific. Chronic infection is characterized by fluctuating aminotransferase levels, which in some cases may be persistently normal despite positivity for HCV RNA (Fig. 6.7). Cirrhosis ultimately develops in 50% of chronically infected patients. Therefore, cirrhosis develops in 25% to 40% of infected patients.

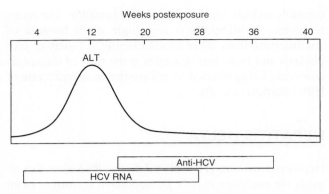

Figure 6.6 Acute hepatitis C virus (HCV) infection. Sustained normalization of serum aminotransferase levels and persistent negativity for HCV RNA suggests resolution of infection. Note that antibody to HCV (anti-HCV) may persist even with resolution of infection. ALT, alanine aminotransferase. (Adapted from Nowicki MJ, Balistreri WF. The C's, D's, and E's of viral hepatitis. *Contemp Pediatr* 1992;9(12):23–42, with permission.)

Hepatitis C is one of the major risk factors for the development of HCC. The annual incidence of developing HCC in chronic HCV patients with cirrhosis is 3% to 4%. Serial ultrasound screening and regular measurement of serum α-fetoprotein levels are used to detect the development of HCC, which in some cases is unsuspected preoperatively and is diagnosed in the explanted liver at the time of transplantation. In Japan, 60% to 80% of patients with HCC are positive for hepatitis C. Cirrhosis secondary to HCV infection is currently the number one indication for liver transplantation in adults in the United States. It is estimated that 8000 to 10,000 people die annually in the United States as a result of chronic liver disease caused by HCV infection. Higher morbidity and mortality rates are predicted in the future because of the prolonged period between infection and development of clinical disease.

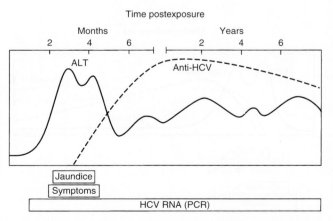

Figure 6.7 Chronic hepatitis C virus (HCV) infection. Fluctuation of aminotransferase levels is characteristic. Persistent positivity for HCV RNA may occur in chronic infection. ALT, alanine aminotransferase. (Adapted from Nowicki MJ, Balistreri WF. The C's, D's, and E's of viral hepatitis. *Contemp Pediatr* 1992;9(12):23–42, with permission.)

Currently, no vaccine is available to prevent HCV infection. The frequency of aminotransferase normalization in untreated adults ranges from 0% to 4%; the rate is 3% to 10% in untreated children with 1 to 6 years of follow-up. The rate of spontaneous HCV RNA clearance is not known. Therapy for chronic HCV infection includes IFN-α. Addition of polyethylene glycol to the interferon (pegylated interferon) increases the medication half-life, decreases the incidence of flu-like symptoms, and is associated with a higher sustained viral response rate compared with standard interferon. Coadministration of interferon and the oral nucleoside analog ribavirin is now the FDA approved treatment regimen for children aged ≥ 3 with chronic HCV infection. Ribavirin coadministration is associated with an increased long-term viral clearance rate. Hemolysis is a potential complication of combination therapy. The response to IFN varies based on a number of host factors. The best response typically occurs in patients who have low levels of HCV RNA, increased levels of aminotransferases, minimal inflammation on liver biopsy and no cirrhosis, and in those who are negative for anti-HIV. Certain viral genotypes, which vary by country, such as genotypes 2 and 3, are associated with an improved response to therapy. Horizontal acquisition, short duration of infection, and younger patient age may increase the likelihood of a response. Patients with normal aminotransferase levels despite positivity for HCV RNA are currently not considered candidates for therapy because of their poor response rate. Criteria for a response to antiviral therapy include persistent loss of HCV RNA, persistent normalization of the aminotransferase levels, and improved findings on liver biopsy. Patients remain positive for anti-HCV, which is not a protective antibody. Recent reports suggest that treatment of acute hepatitis C infection within 8 to 12 weeks of exposure with pegylated interferon may be associated with significantly higher sustained virologic response rates compared with patients treated for established disease.

HEPATITIS E

Hepatitis E virus (HEV) is an enteric and epidemic form of non-A, -B, and -C hepatitis. It is a single-stranded RNA virus that belongs to the unassigned genus Hepatitis E–like viruses. Research-based tests are available to detect anti-HEV and HEV RNA by PCR. Areas of high prevalence include the Indian subcontinent, Middle East, Southeast and Central Asia, North Africa, West Africa, South Africa, and Mexico. Most patients infected in the industrialized areas have traveled to the endemic areas. HEV-infected patients are typically older than those infected with hepatitis A, with a peak incidence between 15 and 34 years of age. The incubation period is 2 to 9 weeks, with a mean of 45 days. Transmission is fecal–oral, often by fecal contamination of drinking water, although sporadic food-borne cases have

been reported in nonendemic areas. The onset of symptoms is abrupt. *The mortality rate is 0% to 2%, except in pregnant women, in whom the mortality rate in the third trimester may be up to 20%.* Infection also may be a risk factor for premature delivery. In developing countries such as India and Nepal, HEV may account for more than 50% of cases of acute hepatic failure. Acute HEV infection may also be associated with fulminant hepatitis or liver decompensation in patients with chronic HBV infection. No chronic form exists, and no method of prevention is known except for hygienic practices. HEV vaccines are in the initial development stage.

OTHER HEPATITIS VIRUSES AND CAUSES OF HEPATITIS IN PEDIATRIC PATIENTS

At least three other causes of viral hepatitis have been identified. Hepatitis F virus, an enteric agent identified in 1994, is a double-stranded DNA virus that has been transmitted experimentally to primates. Hepatitis G virus (HGV) is an RNA virus of the Flaviviridae family, similar to HCV although it has not yet been isolated. It has a worldwide distribution, is transmitted parenterally, and may be present within the accepted blood donor pool in the United States and abroad (rate 1.5%–1.7%). Infection can result in acute and chronic hepatitis and can occur following blood transfusion or community acquisition. Infected blood donors are not typically identified by elevated aminotransferase levels. The incidence of HGV infection is up to 17% following transfusion of infected blood with a higher risk of acquisition with multiple transfusions. Nontransfusion-associated transmission may occur by percutaneous, transplant, injection, hemodialysis, mother to infant, and sexual transmission routes. The long-term consequences of infection are currently unknown. HGV can coinfect with HBV and HCV, which occurs most commonly in injection drug users. HGV RNA can be identified by research tests; commercial testing is not currently available.

Hepatitis GB virus is structurally similar to HGV. It is known to have caused hepatitis as early as the 1960s, although the responsible virus has only recently been identified. This agent is thought to cause chronic hepatitis, and specialized research testing is required for its identification.

Cytomegalovirus and Epstein-Barr virus infections can present as acute hepatitis in pediatric patients. Other less common causes of viral hepatitis in children include human parvovirus B19, herpes simplex virus, echovirus, and adenovirus infections. Other causes of hepatitis in pediatric patients include medications and toxins (e.g., alcohol, anticonvulsants, acetaminophen, isoniazid, propylthiouracil, sulfonamides, poisoning by *Amanita phalloides*), and metabolic causes (e.g., Wilson disease, α_1-antitrypsin deficiency, autoimmune disease, inflammatory bowel disease). These are discussed elsewhere in this book.

REVIEW EXERCISES

QUESTIONS

1. The *most* common form of viral hepatitis in children in the United States is:
a) Hepatitis A
b) Hepatitis B
c) Hepatitis C
d) Hepatitis D
e) Hepatitis E

Answer

The answer is a. Hepatitis A is the most common form of viral hepatitis in children in the United States. With increasing vaccination, the frequency of hepatitis A may decrease in childhood. Infection with other hepatitis viruses, such as HCV, for which no vaccine is available, may become increasingly common in children in the United States.

2. All of the following are true of hepatitis B, *except:*
a) HBV is a DNA virus with a mean incubation period of 120 days.
b) A smaller viral inoculum is required for HBV infection than for HIV infection.
c) The parenteral and perinatal routes are important in the transmission of HBV infection.
d) Positivity for HBeAg indicates a long-term carrier state.
e) Chronic infection is associated with an increased risk for HCC.

Answer

The answer is d. Positivity for HBsAg for >6 months indicates a long-term carrier state. Positivity for HBeAg is associated with an increased risk for transmitting the infection but is not specific for chronic carriage of the virus.

3. Which of the following are *true* of hepatitis C infection?
a) Patients may be asymptomatic.
b) No long-term carrier state exists.
c) Detection may be delayed because of a delay in antibody formation.
d) Transmission is primarily by the fecal–oral route.
e) Both *a* and *c*
f) Both *b* and *d*

Answer

The answer is e. Chronic infection develops in approximately 50% to 80% of patients infected with HCV. This rate is much higher than that in adults infected with HBV, for example. Although all the routes of infection are not known, HCV is thought to be transmitted primarily by contact with infected blood or body fluids rather than by the fecal–oral route.

4. Which of the following statements are *true* for children?
a) Approximately 90% of infants of mothers with chronic hepatitis B infection acquire the infection at birth, even if vaccine and Ig are administered within the first 48 hours after birth.
b) The risk for maternal to infant transmission of HCV is increased in mothers who are coinfected with HIV or who have a high viral load of HCV at the time of delivery.
c) Currently, no effective treatment is available for chronic HBV infection in children.
d) Hepatitis E infection is acquired primarily by parenteral exposure.
e) Both *b* and *d*

Answer

The answer is b. Approximately 90% of infants of mothers with chronic hepatitis B infection are prevented from acquiring the disease if they receive Ig and vaccine, which work synergistically, at the time of birth or within 48 hours. Chronic HBV infection in children can be treated with IFN-α. This medication is most effective in patients who acquired the infection horizontally and have a low viral load. Hepatitis E is thought to be transmitted by the fecal–oral route.

5. Which of the following is *true* of hepatitis E infection?
a) It is endemic in the United States.
b) Infection is associated with a high long-term carrier rate.
c) Detection of HBeAg in blood indicates acute infection.
d) Infection in pregnant women is associated with a high case fatality rate.
e) This is a new agent; the first cases of infection were reported in the mid-1990s.

Answer

The answer is d. Hepatitis E infection in pregnant women is associated with a high case fatality rate. To date, infection in the United States has been reported primarily in patients who have traveled to areas of endemicity and then returned to the United States. HBeAg positivity is a marker for hepatitis B infection, not hepatitis E infection. Although the agent responsible for hepatitis E infection has only recently been identified, outbreaks of this type of infection have occurred for more than 50 years.

6. Which of the following are *true* regarding hepatitis C infection?
a) Chronic infection is associated with an increased rate of HCC (hepatocellular carcinoma).
b) Chronic infection is associated with an increased rate of hepatoblastoma.
c) Anti-HCV is a protective antibody; development coincides with resolution of disease.

d) Most patients are symptomatic at the time of infection.

e) Chronic hepatitis B infection confers an increased risk for the development of chronic hepatitis C infection.

Answer

The answer is a. As in hepatitis B, chronic hepatitis C infection is associated with a 200- to 500-fold increased risk for the development of HCC. Anti-HCV is not a protective antibody. Most patients are asymptomatic at the time of infection and are not aware that they are long-term carriers. Although HBV and HCV infection commonly occur in the same individuals because of common risk factors, HBV infection does not predispose to the development of HCV infection.

7. All of the following are true regarding the treatment of chronic HBV and HCV infections, *except*:

a) Ribavirin increases the risk for hemolysis.

b) Psychiatric disturbances are a relative contraindication to IFN therapy.

c) Therapy is successful over the long term in more than 80% of treated patients.

d) New forms of IFN are being developed in an attempt to provide steadier serum concentrations.

e) Patients with chronic HCV infection and normal aminotransferase levels respond poorly to current treatment regimens.

Answer

The answer is c. Currently, the best long-term viral clearance rates following therapy for chronic HBV or HCV infection are in the range of 20% to 50%. These relatively disappointing rates have prompted use of combination therapy or enhanced forms of IFN, such as pegylated IFN, in an effort to improve sustained response rates by decreasing the development of escape mutants and providing more consistent concentrations of medication in serum.

8. Since the availability of hepatitis A vaccination starting in 1995, the most recent CDC data (2006) indicates a decrease in the reported HAV cases in the United States.

a) True

b) False

Answer

The answer is a. True. CDC Data in 2006 indicates a significant decrease in reported HAV cases in the United States. This trend has been linked to the availability of HAV vaccine starting in 1995.

SUGGESTED READINGS

1. American Academy of Pediatrics. Hepatitis. In: Pickering LK, ed. *2006 Red book: report of the committee on infectious diseases*, 27th ed. Elk Grove Village, IL: American Academy of Pediatrics, 2006: 326–361.
2. Arora NK, Das MK, Mathur P, et al. Hepatitis C in childhood. *Int Semin Pediatr Gastroenterol Nutr* 2004;12(4):3–9.
3. Chang MH. New insights in Hepatitis B virus infection. *Int Semin Pediatr Gastroenterol Nutr* 2004;12(4):9–14.
4. Committee on Infectious Diseases American Academy of Pediatrics. Hepatitis A vaccine recommendations. *Pediatrics* 2007; 120:189–199.
5. Elisofon SA, Jonas MM. Hepatitis B and C in children: current treatment and future strategies. *Clin Liv Dis* 2006;10:133–148.
6. Jacobson KR, Murray K, Zellos A, et al. An analysis of published trials of interferon monotherapy in children with chronic hepatitis C. *J Pediatr Gastroenterol Nutr* 2002;34(1):52–58.
7. Jonas MM. Treatment of chronic Hepatitis B in children. *J Pediatr Gastroenterol Nutr* 2006;43(1):S56–60.
8. Leach CT. Hepatitis A in the United States. *Pediatr Infect Dis J* 2004;23(6):551–552.
9. Nowicki MJ, Balistreri WF. Hepatitis A to E: building up the alphabet. *Contemp Pediatr* 1992;9(11):118–128.
10. Nowicki MJ, Balistreri WF. The C's, D's, and E's of viral hepatitis. *Contemp Pediatr* 1992;9(12):23–42.
11. Rustgi VK. The epidemiology of hepatitis C infection in the United States. *J Gastroenterol* 2007;42:513–521.
12. Victor JC, Monto AS, Surdina TY, et al. Hepatitis A Vaccine versus immune globulin for postexposure prophylaxis. *NEJM* 2007;357: 1685–1694.
13. Wasley A, Grydtal S, Gallagher K. Surveillance for acute viral hepatitis United States 2006 *MMWR* 2008;57(SSO2):1–24.

Chapter 7

Foreign Bodies and Caustic Ingestions

Marsha Kay and Robert Wyllie

FOREIGN BODIES

In the first recorded case of an ingestion of a foreign body, Frederick Wilheim, later known as Frederick the Great, swallowed a shoe buckle at the age of 5 years, which apparently passed without incident. In 1937, Jackson and Jackson reported 3266 esophageal and airway foreign body ingestions. These authors coined the phrase, "Advancing points perforate and trailing points do not," subsequently referred to as *Jackson's axiom*. In addition, their writings formed the basis of the U.S. Consumer Product Safety Commission small parts regulation, which bans toys and other articles intended for use by children ≤ age 3 that represent a hazard for choking, swallowing, and inhaling based on size criteria (≤2.25 × 1.25 in. [≤5.7 × 3.2 cm]). In 1966, Bigler reported extracting an esophageal foreign body with the use of a Foley catheter, and in 1972, Morissey reported the first case in which a foreign body was extracted endoscopically. By 1978, three reports of the endoscopic removal of foreign bodies in a total of 16 patients had been published, by Ament, van Thiel, and Bendig. Starting in the 1980s, a number of large series of endoscopic or radiologic retrieval of foreign bodies were reported.

Epidemiology

The type and incidence of foreign bodies ingested and reported vary by geographic region and the specialty of the authors. One of the largest reports published in the last two decades was by Nandi and Ong, who reported 2934 foreign body ingestions in China in the *British Journal of Medicine*. Eighty-four percent of the foreign bodies ingested in their series were fish bones, which were usually lodged in the esophagus. Three hundred and forty-three children were included in the series. Ingestions of fish bones were reported in 146 of the children, but coin ingestion was the second most common type of ingestion in children, accounting for 134 cases in the same series. In the United States, coin ingestion is the most common type of foreign body ingested during childhood. The exact incidence of foreign body ingestion in the United States is unknown, but data from the American Association of Poison Control Centers suggests that in 2004 alone there were more than 109,000 cases of foreign body ingestion by children and adolescents. Data from Sweden's National Health Service indicate an incidence of foreign body ingestion of 122/million population per year. Approximately 1500 deaths in patients of all ages are caused annually in the United States by foreign body ingestion.

Approximately 80% of cases of foreign body ingestion occur in children, predominantly between the ages of 6 and 36 months, with coins being the objects most often ingested. In adults, the most common unintentional ingestions that become lodged are meat and fish bones. Intentional ingestions occur primarily in psychiatrically impaired individuals and prisoners. Individuals under the influence of alcohol may unintentionally swallow objects because their perception is impaired. Foreign body ingestions by gang members as part of initiation practices are becoming more frequent. A significant number of foreign body ingestions do not come to medical attention, and the objects pass without incident. It is estimated that 80% to 90% of foreign bodies ingested that come to medical attention pass spontaneously. For 10% to 20%, endoscopic removal is required, and surgery is ultimately required for 1% or fewer. Perforation of the intestinal tract, the most serious sequela of foreign body ingestion, occurs in less than 1% of cases. The higher rates reported in some series are primarily related to the subspecialty of the authors reporting the data. For example, the perforation rate would be anticipated to be higher in series reported by thoracic surgeons than in a series of all patients presenting to an emergency room for evaluation. Sharp objects are associated with a higher perforation rate than dull objects. Approximately 75% of perforations occur at the appendix or near the ileocecal valve. Foreign body entrapment and subsequent perforation are also more likely to occur in the region of a congenital malformation, such as a Meckel diverticulum, or at a site of prior surgery.

The largest number of foreign bodies ingested by a single individual was 2533, reported by Chalk et al. in 1928. The woman, who had melancholia, was sent to a sewing room for therapy, where she ingested an assortment of pins, needles, and bobbins. Remarkably, the objects passed uneventfully, and the patient survived. In 1987, Henderson et al. reported a case of ingestion of 500 straight pins, which resulted in the patient's death within 2 months as a consequence of multiple intestinal perforations. High number foreign body ingestions continue to be reported in the psychiatrically impaired, who may "save their treasure" by ingesting a variety of objects and who typically present with abdominal pain, distension, obstruction, and anemia, and require surgical removal of the foreign bodies, which may weigh several kilograms. One of the most remarkable reports of foreign body ingestion was by Yamamoto et al. in 1985, who reported the endoscopic removal of a chopstick from the duodenum of a 71-year-old man who had ingested the object 60 years earlier.

Esophageal Foreign Bodies

Clinical and Radiographic Features

Ninety percent of children have a history of ingestion or are observed to ingest an object. Approximately 90% of foreign bodies ingested in children are radiopaque. It is appropriate to obtain an x-ray film in every case of foreign body ingestion of an opaque object because objects may be lodged in the esophagus even in asymptomatic patients.

The most common site of foreign body obstruction in the gastrointestinal tract in children is the esophagus. Approximately 60% to 70% of foreign bodies that become entrapped in the esophagus are located in the proximal esophagus at the region of the cricopharyngeus. The second most common site is just above the lower esophageal sphincter, with approximately 20% of obstructions occurring in the mid-esophagus.

Coins are the foreign bodies most frequently ingested by children in the United States. The anteroposterior view on an x-ray film will demonstrate the coin *en face*, whereas the lateral view will show the edge of the coin (Fig. 7.1). This pattern is the opposite of the radiographic appearance of a coin lodged in the trachea. Coins lodged in the esophagus most frequently appear *en face* on the anteroposterior view, but the appearance of the lateral edge of a coin lodged in the esophagus on the anteroposterior view has also been reported.

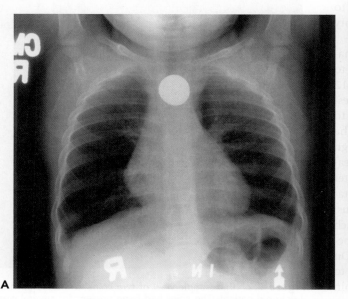
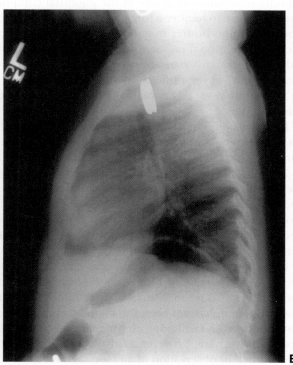

Figure 7.1 Anteroposterior (**A**) and lateral (**B**) chest x-ray film of an 11-month-old infant with a 3-month history of stridor, wheezing, and persistent cough. Two coins were found in the proximal esophagus and are best demonstrated on the lateral film. Tracheal narrowing as a result of edema also was noted.

Symptoms

The symptoms of foreign body obstruction vary according to the patient's age and the nature of the foreign body. Symptoms in young children are nonspecific and can include choking, drooling, and poor feeding. Some children modify their diet to compensate for a partial obstruction—for example, consuming only liquids. Older children and teenagers report dysphagia and substernal chest pain. On occasion, the only symptoms of an esophageal foreign body are respiratory. These include wheezing, stridor, impaired speech, and recurrent infection. The foreign body may be noted incidentally on an x-ray film obtained to evaluate suspected pneumonia or reactive airway disease. The cause of the stridor is edema secondary to foreign body obstruction with subsequent impingement on the trachea. Rarely a patient with an esophageal foreign body may present with massive hematemesis as their initial presentation. This is caused by erosion of the foreign body into the aorta. Unfortunately, identification of the foreign body as the underlying cause of the hematemesis is usually at autopsy, as the hematemesis is typically life threatening, and these patients often can not be resuscitated.

Management

If patients are symptomatic (i.e., unable to swallow their secretions or experiencing respiratory difficulty), emergency endoscopy is indicated to remove the foreign body. Aspiration pneumonia is one of the potential complications of failure to remove a foreign body. In some centers, smooth foreign bodies may be removed by an experienced interventional radiologist with catheters. This procedure is potentially dangerous because the foreign body can "flip out" as the catheter is withdrawn and come to lie flat on the vocal cords, causing immediate respiratory compromise.

If patients are symptomatic (i.e., experiencing dysphagia or a "feeling that something is there") but are able to handle their secretions, endoscopy can be deferred for 12 to 24 hours to allow for an appropriate period of preanesthetic fasting; an x-ray film should be obtained prior to endoscopy to verify that the foreign body is still in the esophagus. This management strategy is true for foreign bodies such as coins but does not apply to esophageal batteries, which are an exception and are discussed later in the chapter. Objects such as coins can pass spontaneously, especially coins located in the distal esophagus. Spontaneous passage may occur in up to one third of such cases. Glucagon has not been shown to be effective in pediatric patients in facilitating esophageal coin passage. On a cost per case basis, however, admission of the patient to the hospital for observation of an esophageal located coin with endoscopy reserved for coins that fail to pass within 16 hours has been shown to be less cost effective than earlier endoscopic removal.

Gastric and Small Intestinal Foreign Bodies

Most foreign bodies that reach the stomach pass uneventfully through the remainder of the gastrointestinal tract within 4 to 6 days. Patients are instructed to consume a regular diet. The use of prokinetic agents such as metoclopramide is not indicated to increase the speed of passage. Parents should monitor the stools of their children to detect passage of the foreign body. Metal detectors have been used by a few for this purpose. If a patient is asymptomatic and the foreign body has not been noted in the stool, we generally recommend waiting for 3 weeks before obtaining an x-ray film to localize a known gastric foreign body. We generally wait an additional 3 weeks after obtaining the x-ray film if the patient remains asymptomatic, and obtain a second film 6 weeks after the ingestion. If the object is still in the stomach, we recommend endoscopic removal at that time. We have anecdotally noted that in cases of ingestion of multiple coins, gastric passage may be delayed as the coins appear to adhere to each other and endoscopic removal may be required (Fig. 7.2). No toxicity has been reported from retention of modern zinc containing "copper" pennies following the change in composition of the penny in 1982 to a zinc-predominant coin. Toxicity studies were carried out prior to the release of the various Euro coins with regard to the potential of zinc toxicity following ingestion. These coins have a lower zinc content than the American penny, and to date no cases of zinc intoxication following ingestion have been identified.

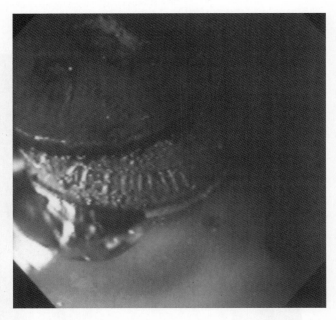

Figure 7.2 Endoscopic view of two coins in the stomach of a 4-year-old patient. The coins had been present for several weeks without passage. Alligator forceps are used to remove the coins. Note erosion of the penny from prolonged contact with gastric acid. (See color insert.)

Potential problem sites downstream for foreign bodies include the pylorus, the fixed curves of the C loop of the duodenum, and the ileocecal valve. The duodenal C loop poses a problem because of its fixed retroperitoneal location. Objects that require endoscopic removal from the stomach and proximal small intestine can be placed into two categories, those that require removal because of their size and those that require removal because of their composition and physical characteristics.

Objects in the stomach of an adult patient that are longer than 10 cm cannot negotiate the duodenal C loop and therefore should be removed endoscopically at the time of identification. Successful negotiation of the duodenum by a toothbrush has never been reported. An ovoid object with a length of more than 5 cm or a thickness of more than 2 cm is unlikely to pass the pylorus in an adult and should be removed. Appropriate size modifications are required to make recommendations in younger patients. Patients with a congenital malformation, such as a duodenal web, an annular pancreas, or a surgical anastomosis may not be able to pass objects significantly smaller than the sizes indicated above. The size of an object may be magnified on x-ray films, and therefore some estimation is required, or measurement of a similar object can be used if the identity of the ingested object is known.

Management of Specific Ingested Foreign Bodies

Impacted Meat

Impacted meat is the most common foreign body causing obstruction in adolescents and adults. Up to 95% of adult patients who experience a meat impaction have underlying esophageal pathology, and the rate is also high in adolescents. Conditions that predispose patients to esophageal meat impaction include esophageal strictures or narrowing from a variety of etiologies including acid peptic disease, post-caustic ingestion, and postoperatively, esophageal motility disorders, and eosinophilic esophagitis. This condition, which is increasingly recognized in children and adults, results in a characteristic ringed esophageal appearance.

For patients who are symptomatic and unable to handle their secretions, immediate endoscopy is required to relieve the obstruction and prevent the potential complication of aspiration. Patients who are symptomatic but able to handle their secretions require endoscopy within 12 hours. Contrast radiography is contraindicated because of the potential for aspirating the contrast in addition to the impacted food. The use of meat tenderizers is also contraindicated because these agents have been associated with esophageal perforation and hypernatremia.

Batteries

The largest series of battery ingestions was reported by Litovitz et al. in 1992. This series, comprised of data from a national registry, reported 2382 ingestions in 2320 patients. Almost all the reported ingestions were button batteries. In that series, only 62 cylindric batteries were ingested. Hearing aids were the most common source of button batteries, representing more than 40% of the reported cases. In a third of these cases, the hearing aid was the child's own. In this series, only 10% of the patients were symptomatic, and only two children sustained residual injury—in both cases esophageal strictures that required dilation. The battery transit time in the gastrointestinal tract was less than 24 hours in 23% of cases, less than 48 hours in 61% of cases, and less than 96 hours in 86% of cases. The transit time was longer than 1 week in only 4.5% of the cases.

Complications of retained esophageal batteries are serious and occur frequently. Symptoms correlate poorly with clinical outcome and serious complications may occur in asymptomatic patients. The same report details the outcome of 25 patients reported with a battery lodged in the esophagus, five patients ingested a small battery with a diameter between 8 and 11 mm, and the battery passed spontaneously into the stomach. However, 10 of the 25 patients experienced major complications. These included esophageal perforation, development of a tracheoesophageal fistula, esophageal stricture, and death. Of the ten patients with a major complication, eight had swallowed a large battery (20–23 mm in diameter) and two had swallowed a small battery. Nine of the 25 patients who had a battery lodged in the esophagus were asymptomatic. Esophageal perforation following the ingestion of a battery has been reported within 6 hours after ingestion, and development of esophageal stenosis has been reported after a battery was lodged for 10 hours. The early development of complications following ingestion of a battery is probably a consequence of the nature of the battery, the caustic material contained within it (sodium or potassium hydroxide), and perhaps from the discharge of current.

An x-ray film should be obtained *immediately* following the ingestion of any battery. If the battery is lodged in the esophagus, emergency endoscopy to remove it is indicated to avoid the aforementioned complications, even if the patient is asymptomatic. If the battery is located in the stomach and the patient is asymptomatic, the patient can be observed. If significant symptoms develop while the battery is in the stomach, endoscopic retrieval is indicated. If the battery is larger than 15 mm in an adult-size patient and does not pass the pylorus within 48 hours after ingestion, endoscopic retrieval should be considered because such batteries tend not to pass. This situation represents fewer than 3% of ingestions. Gastric ulceration following the ingestion of a battery has been reported. Mercury poisoning is a theoretical concern following the ingestion of a button battery but this has not been reported in more than 500 patients; in some patients elevated mercury levels have been reported without clinical sequelae. One patient who experienced elevation of serum lithium levels but was asymptomatic was reported following gastric retention of a lithium battery for >96 hours; levels returned to normal within 24 hours of endoscopic removal.

Sharp and Pointed Foreign Bodies

These objects represent a relatively small fraction of foreign bodies ingested by pediatric patients. Common objects ingested include toothpicks, nails, needles, glass, and safety pins. The use of diapers with plastic tabs has decreased the frequency of safety pin ingestions in the United States, although cultural practices in some countries where items are pinned to infants' clothing result in an increased rate of safety pin ingestion in those countries and communities. The risk of perforation increases significantly when a sharp object is ingested, increasing from 1% to between 15% and 35%, depending on the number of objects ingested and their contact time within the gastrointestinal tract. Straight pins are the exception and usually pass uneventfully following Jackson's axiom, with the blunt head passing first through the digestive tract. The ingestion of a large number of straight pins, however, is associated with a higher rate of intestinal perforation and gastric impaction of a single straight pin has been reported. Glass ingestion represents a challenging foreign body to diagnose radiologically if the history is unclear as glass is not radiopaque and is therefore may be hard to localize prior to endoscopy.

The endoscopic removal of sharp objects other than straight pins should be considered, depending on their size and location. In some cases, an overtube is employed, although an increased risk for esophageal perforation is associated with its use. Other protective devices such as a latex foreign body hood, can be employed to reduce the risk of complications related to sharp foreign object removal. Ingestion of sharp objects is particularly common with intentional ingestions in the prison populations or in the psychiatrically impaired, and is associated with a very high rate of complications in these settings.

Magnets

Ingestion of magnets is increasingly being reported in pediatric patients. This is because of their ubiquitous nature and the perception that they are benign objects. Magnets are being increasingly utilized in children's toys, jewelry, and common household objects. In 2008, magnets were identified by the Consumer Product Safety Review as #1 of the top five hidden home hazards. Since 2005 one death and more than 86 pediatric injuries have been reported related to magnet ingestion. At least two major toy manufacturers have issued voluntary recalls of toys with magnets since 2006. Although ingestion of one magnet is generally benign if located in the stomach or distally, ingestion of more than one magnet is extremely hazardous, as they are able to attract each other and can result in fistulization, obstruction, and perforation. Therefore, x-ray evaluation and early endoscopic removal of multiple magnets is indicated if they are located within reach of the endoscope.

Cocaine and Other Drugs

The phenomenon of cocaine ingestion is known as "body bagger" or "body packer" syndrome. In the past it was uncommon in children, occurring primarily in older adolescents and young adults. However, because of increased scrutiny by U.S. Customs and border patrol agents, younger children are now being enlisted to act as "mules." In an attempt to smuggle cocaine, an individual ingests several condoms, each usually filled with 3 to 5 g of cocaine. Other drugs smuggled in this manner include heroin, amphetamines, and ecstasy. Because the rupture of just one condom with the absorption of 1 to 3 g of cocaine is fatal, endoscopic retrieval of the condoms is contraindicated. In patients who are asymptomatic, observation for passage of the condoms is the only treatment recommended. Symptomatic patients require stabilization, and the administration of activated charcoal has been reported. Some patients have undergone surgery to remove the condoms if numerous bags are present in the gastrointestinal tract.

CAUSTIC INGESTIONS

Epidemiology

It is estimated that more than 1.3 million nonpharmaceutical toxic exposures occur annually in the United States. In more than 90% of cases, the exposure is to a single substance and a similar percentage of exposures occur in the home. Caustic ingestions occur most frequently in children younger than 6 years, with the majority of cases occurring in children between 12 and 48 months of age. Children generally have to be ambulatory, with access to cabinets or areas where cleaning products are stored. Although they account for 51% of ingestions, children under age 6 account for only 2.3% of fatalities resulting from caustic ingestions (fatality rate of 0.0022%) primarily because of the accidental nature of their ingestions.

More than 50% of ingestions in teenagers or adults occur as part of a suicide attempt. In 2004 the most recent year for which data is available, there were 1183 fatalities resulting from caustic ingestions in the United States. Fifty-six percent of fatalities in that year occurred in patients between 20 and 49 years of age. Eighty-eight percent of adolescent deaths and 80% of adult deaths caused by caustics were a result of an intentional ingestion (adult fatality rate 0.12%). The significantly increased case fatality rate in adolescents and adults compared with pediatric patients is primarily the result of the different outcomes associated with an intentional ingestion of a high volume and high concentration caustic vs. a typically lower volume unintentional ingestion of a caustic of varying concentrations.

Household bleach accounts for 30% to 40% of caustic ingestions, laundry detergents for 20%, and acids and alkalis from various cleaners (oven, toilet, tile, and drain) for

50%. Although laws have been enacted in the United States to reduce the concentration of various household agents, farm and industrial chemicals represent a dangerous source of caustic ingestions and use of "nonoriginal" containers increases the risk of accidental ingestion substantially. Abroad, legislation to reduce the concentrations of various household caustics may not be in place; therefore, injury following unintentional ingestion may be more severe. Caustic agents can be subclassified into strong alkalis, strong acids, weak alkalis, and weak acids.

Mechanism of Injury

Injury following ingestion is dependent on both the concentration and the pH of an agent. The ingestion of a strong alkali results in liquefaction necrosis, which is associated with deep penetration and perforation, usually in the esophagus, but sometimes also in the stomach. Alkalis are usually odorless and tasteless, resulting in consumption of a large volume. Alkalis with a pH between 9 and 11, including many household detergents, rarely cause serious injury. Ingestion of even small quantities of an alkali with a pH >11 may cause severe burns and ingestion of a substance with a pH >12.5 will cause injury regardless of the concentration. Specific examples of strong alkali are sodium hydroxides (lye products, drain cleaner, oven cleaner, and dishwashing detergents) and sodium phosphates (dishwashing detergents and laundry detergents). Granular forms of detergents are associated with a higher rate of injury than liquid forms and are often not perceived by families to represent a potential caustic.

Acid ingestions represent approximately 15% of ingestions in children. Ingestion of a strong acid results in coagulation necrosis, which limits the extent of penetration (Fig. 7.3). Their low viscosity and specific gravity result in rapid transit to the stomach, and gastric injury is more common than esophageal injury, especially in the prepyloric area. However, their bitter taste and development of pain with ingestion may result in lower volumes of ingestion. Gastric injury following ingestion may result in gastric outlet obstruction or perforation. Specific strong acids include sulfuric acid (drain cleaner), hydrochloric acid (toilet bowl cleaner), sodium bisulfate (toilet bowl cleaner), hydrofluoric acid (metal cleaner, photography products), phosphoric acid, and sodium hypochlorite, which has a low concentration in bleach (relatively nontoxic) and a very high concentration in swimming pool and tile cleaners and is associated with a high rate of toxicity.

Clinical Manifestations

Multiple studies have demonstrated that the presence or absence of symptoms does not predict the likelihood that an ingestion has occurred or correlate with the severity of

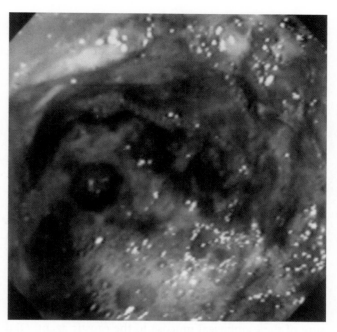

Figure 7.3 The endoscopic appearance of the stomach following an intentional caustic ingestion of a strong acid in a teenager. Note the *black* appearance of the rugal folds representing coagulative necrosis. The patient later went on to develop gastric outlet obstruction. (See color insert.)

injury to the gastrointestinal tract. In a review of 378 pediatric ingestions by Gaudreault et al., 12% of asymptomatic children had severe esophageal burns, whereas 82% of symptomatic children had no esophageal burns. The presence or absence of oral lesions is also a poor indicator of esophageal injury. In a recent Turkish series of 473 pediatric caustic ingestions, primarily of alkaline agents, 240/389 (61%) patients without oral cavity burns had esophageal lesions found at endoscopy. In that series 80% of patients had an esophageal injury and 17% of patients had gastric injury. The most common symptoms following a caustic ingestion are dysphagia, drooling, retrosternal pain, abdominal pain, and vomiting. Although minor symptoms do not rule out the presence of relevant injury, an increased number of symptoms correlates with a greater likelihood of significant injury. Symptoms involving the airway are less common, although dyspnea is associated with a high risk of significant gastrointestinal injury.

Management

For patients with a questionable history of ingestion, who are asymptomatic and have no oral burns, we recommend observation and intake of liquids. If dysphagia—which can occur anytime between 2 and 6 weeks following ingestion—subsequently develops, we perform upper gastrointestinal roentgenography to rule out an esophageal stricture. In patients with a questionable history of ingestion, esophageal burns, if present, are most often minor, liquids generally are tolerated, and no other specific therapy is required. Patients with a history of ingesting household bleach rarely require therapy, and observation is usually the only treatment required unless they become symptomatic. If patients have a strong history of ingestion, have oral burns, or are symptomatic, we recommend an endoscopic evaluation within 24 hours to evaluate the extent of injury to the esophagus and stomach. Endoscopic evaluation is rarely indicated in patients with ingestion of "no lye" hair relaxer. Despite a very high pH of 12 or more, injury is usually limited to the face or oral mucosa. Endoscopy is required in all cases of intentional ingestion, even if the patient is asymptomatic, because there is a higher likelihood of oropharyngeal sparing resulting from rapid swallowing of the caustic and the presence or absence of oral burns or symptoms in this setting is a poor indicator of the extent of oral of gastric injury.

The administration of ipecac is contraindicated following a caustic ingestion because of potential re-exposure of the esophageal mucosa to the caustic agent. Oral dilution or neutralizing agents are also contraindicated because they may result in vomiting, with further esophageal injury. Nasogastric tubes should not be placed blindly because of the risk for esophageal perforation if severe esophageal ulceration is present. Nasogastric tubes are sometimes placed in patients with severe circumferential burns as a stent to keep the esophagus open when the development of strictures is anticipated. Corticosteroid administration is controversial and is usually confined to patients with symptoms involving the airway. The concomitant administration of broad-spectrum antibiotics is required if corticosteroids are initiated.

Esophageal injury is graded at the time of endoscopy to direct the therapy. The likelihood of complications correlates with the degree of injury. Grade 1 injury, seen in 80% of patients who have injury, consists of edema and erythema. Patients can be fed normally and discharged home. Grade 2 esophageal injury consists of linear ulcerations and necrotic tissue with whitish plaques. Patients with Grade 2 injury require intravenous nutrition but generally do well on long-term follow-up. Grade 2 lesions rarely progress to esophageal stenosis. Grade 3 esophageal injury is characterized by circumferential injury, which may be transmural with mucosal sloughing. Patients require intravenous nutrition, strictures often develop, and esophageal stenting may be required. Such patients require long-term follow-up, may have to undergo repeated endoscopic procedures and dilations, may require surgery, and are at increased long-term risk for esophageal carcinoma. Patients with evidence of Grade 4 injury (perforation at endoscopy, or evident by x-ray or at the time of surgery) have a very poor prognosis and high case fatality rate caused by systemic complications. If perforation is suspected, endoscopy is contraindicated and initial management is surgical.

Long-Term Complications

The development of esophageal strictures is the major complication following caustic ingestion. In 80% of the patients in whom strictures ultimately develop, the strictures develop within 8 weeks after the ingestion. Strictures may develop as early as 3 weeks following ingestion. Other complications include dysphagia, esophageal motility abnormalities, gastric outlet obstruction, and pancreatic and bowel injury. Esophageal carcinoma (both adenocarcinoma and squamous cell carcinoma) is a late but serious complication of severe caustic injury. The incidence following caustic ingestion ranges from 2% to 30%, depending on the series, with the carcinoma developing one to three decades after the ingestion. The incidence is 1000 times the expected occurrence rate in patients of a similar age. Cancer is most commonly at the site of the tracheal bifurcation, an area of anatomic narrowing, and may be related to increased exposure to the caustic at this site. Dysplasia screening is recommended for patients following a severe caustic ingestion to allow for the early detection of precancerous changes. Esophageal bypass surgery does not prevent the development of esophageal cancer following a caustic ingestion.

REVIEW EXERCISES

QUESTIONS

1. All foreign bodies in the esophagus require immediate removal.
a) True
b) False

Answer
The answer is b. Coins in an asymptomatic patient do not require immediate removal, especially if located in the region of the lower esophageal sphincter. Follow-up x-ray films can be obtained within 24 hours. In up to one third of cases, the coin will have passed into the stomach. All esophageal batteries require immediate endoscopic removal. All esophageal-lodged foreign bodies should be removed within 24 hours following ingestion.

2. Which of the following statements is *true* regarding esophageal meat impactions?
a) The obstruction should be confirmed with barium contrast studies.
b) The administration of meat tenderizers is indicated.
c) Immediate endoscopy (within 2 hours) is indicated in patients who are able to handle their secretions.
d) Obstruction may indicate underlying esophageal pathology.
e) All of the above

Answer
The answer is d. If patients are able to handle their secretions, endoscopy is recommended within 12 hours, but immediate endoscopy is not required. The administration of meat tenderizer is contraindicated because this

may result in esophageal perforation and hypernatremia. Esophageal pathology is present in most children and adults with esophageal meat impaction.

3. Button batteries should be removed when:
a) They remain in the stomach for 24 hours.
b) They are lodged in the esophagus.
c) Whenever they are ingested.
d) Both *a* and *b*
e) None of the above

Answer
The answer is b. Button batteries should be removed when they lodge in the esophagus because of the risk for perforation, which can occur as early as 6 hours following ingestion. Button batteries in the stomach are likely to pass without sequelae. Batteries larger than 20 mm that remain in the stomach for more than 48 hours generally require endoscopic removal.

4. Which of the following is *true* regarding caustic ingestions?
a) Bleach ingestions are usually associated with esophageal injury.
b) Esophageal injury is always associated with oral injury.
c) The risk for esophageal carcinoma is increased following caustic ingestion.
d) All of the above
e) None of the above

Answer
The answer is c. The rate of esophageal cancer in patients 20 to 30 years after a severe caustic injury is significantly higher than that in their peers. Screening for dysplasia is indicated to detect precancerous changes in these at-risk patients. The ingestion of household bleach does not usually result in significant injury. The presence or absence of oral burns does not predict the likelihood or severity of esophageal injury.

5. Which of the following statements are *true*?
a) Cocaine-filled condoms ingested by body baggers should be endoscopically removed to minimize their potential toxicity.
b) In 80% to 90% of cases of foreign body ingestion, endoscopy is ultimately required for evaluation or therapy.
c) The presence or absence of symptoms with swallowing is the best discriminating factor for determining an esophageal or gastric location of an ingested coin.
d) The administration of ipecac to induce vomiting is contraindicated following a caustic ingestion.
e) Coins are the most common foreign body causing obstruction in adults in the United States.

Answer
The answer is d. The administration of ipecac is contraindicated following a caustic ingestion because of the

potential to re-injure the esophagus when the caustic agent is vomited. Cocaine-filled condoms should not be endoscopically removed because they may rupture. It is estimated that 80% to 90% of foreign bodies ingested pass spontaneously and never require endoscopic removal. The presence or absence of symptoms does not predict an esophageal location of an ingested coin. An x-ray film should be obtained to locate the position of the coin. The most common foreign body causing obstruction in adolescents and adults is impacted food, usually meat.

6. What is Jackson's axiom?
a) All button batteries should be endoscopically removed.
b) Advancing points perforate and trailing points do not.
c) Trailing points perforate and advancing points do not.
d) Objects in the stomach larger than 10 cm cannot negotiate the C loop of the duodenum.

Answer
The answer is b.

7. Regarding alkaline ingestions, which of the following are *true*?
a) They are generally odorless and tasteless, resulting in a larger volume ingestion.
b) Endoscopy is required following ingestion of alkaline hair relaxer with a pH of 12 or more.
c) Injury is dependent on both the concentration and the pH of the product.
d) Common agents include toilet bowl cleaner and swimming pool cleaner.
e) *a* and *c*
f) *a*, *c*, and *d*

Answer
The answer is e (*a* and *c*). Because injury is usually limited to the face and oral mucosa, endoscopy is rarely indicated following ingestion of alkali hair relaxer. Toilet bowl cleaners (hydrochloric acid and sodium bisulfate) and swimming pool cleaners (sodium hypochlorite) are usually strong acids.

8. A 3-year-old boy swallows three round magnets, each <1 cm in diameter. He is asymptomatic. An x-ray is obtained localizing all three magnets to the stomach. On the basis of currently available data the best approach would be to "watch and wait" for passage of the magnets.
a) True
b) False

Answer
The answer is b, False. A watch and wait approach would be appropriate if only one magnet was ingested, if it was located in the stomach or distally and the patient was asymptomatic. However, the presence of multiple magnets warrants early intervention if possible, as some of the magnets may pass into the small bowel or colon, whereas others may remain in the stomach and attraction between the magnets may result in the development of a perforation or an entero-enteric fistula.

SUGGESTED READINGS

1. Betalli P, Falchetti D, Giuliani S, et al. Caustic ingestion in children: is endoscopy always indicated? The results of an Italian multicenter observational study *Gastrointest Endosc* 2008;68:434–439.
2. Dogan Y, Erkan T, Cokugras FC, et al. Caustic gastroesophageal lesions in childhood: an analysis of 473 cases. *Clin Pediatr* 2006; 45:435–438.
3. Eisen GM, Barron TH, Dominitz JA, et al. American Society for Gastrointestinal Endoscopy guideline for the management of ingested foreign bodies. *Gastrointest Endosc* 2002;55(7):802–806.
4. Fox VL, Nurko S, Furuta GT. Eosinophilic esophagitis: it's not just kid's stuff. *Gastrointest Endosc* 2002;56(2):260–270.
5. Kay M., Wyllie R. Foreign bodies and bezoars. In Liacouras CA, Piccoli DA, eds. *Pediatric Gastroenterology: the Requisites in Pediatrics*, 1st ed. Philadelphia: Elsevier, 2008;64–73.
6. Kay M, Wyllie R. Caustic ingestions and the role of endoscopy. *J Pediatr Gastroenterol Nutr* 2001;32:8–10.
7. Kay M, Wyllie R. Techniques of foreign body removal in infants and children. *Tech Gastrointest Endosc* 2002;4(4):188–195.
8. Litovitz T, Schmitz BF. Ingestion of cylindrical and button batteries: an analysis of 2,382 cases. *Pediatrics* 1992;89:747–757.
9. Liu S, de Blacam C, Lim FY, et al. Magnetic foreign body ingestions leading to duodenocolic fistula. *J Pediatr Gastroenterol Nutr* 2005;41:670–672.
10. Traub SJ, Kohn GL, Hoffamn RS, et al. Pediatric "body packing." *Arch Pediatr Adolesc Med* 2003;157(2):174–177.
11. Waltzman ML, Baskin M, Wypij D, et al. A randomized clinical trial of the management of esophageal coins in children. *Pediatrics* 2005;116:614–619.
12. Watson WA, Litovitz TL, Rodgers GC Jr, et al. 2004 Annual Report of the American Association of Poison Control Centers Toxic Exposure Surveillance System. *Am J Emerg Med* 2005;23(5): 589–666.

Chapter 8

Neonatal Jaundice and Liver Disease

Vera F. Hupertz

Neonatal jaundice is most often first seen by the parents of the patient. Yellowness of the skin and sclerae start at the head and progress in a caudal direction. A number of conditions, both benign and not so benign, can be responsible and are described in the subsequent text. A careful history and physical examination will narrow the differential diagnosis.

INDIRECT (UNCONJUGATED) HYPERBILIRUBINEMIA

Etiology and Pathophysiology

Bilirubin is formed by the destruction of both erythropoietic heme and nonerythropoietic heme. Erythropoietic heme, derived from the destruction of red blood cells, accounts for 85% of the total bilirubin. Nonerythropoietic heme is derived from the breakdown of proteins such as myoglobin, catalase, tryptophan pyrrolase, and cytochromes. The breakdown of heme is catalyzed by heme oxygenase in the presence of cytochrome P-450. Heme oxygenase is produced in greater amounts during times of stress, such as fasting. Bilirubin is conjugated in the microsomes of the smooth endoplasmic reticulum to two molecules of glucuronide. Glucuronide is made by uridine diphosphate glucose (UDPG) dehydrogenase. Conjugated (direct) bilirubin is then excreted into the bile and subsequently into the intestines, where bacteria transform it into urobilinogen.

In both physiologic jaundice and breast milk jaundice, the level of indirect (unconjugated) bilirubin is elevated.

This fraction of bilirubin is not measured, so its value is obtained by subtracting the value for direct bilirubin from the value for total bilirubin. The value for direct bilirubin is normal in all cases of physiologic and breast milk jaundice. Physiologic jaundice is thought to be caused by delayed conjugation and increased turnover of hemoglobin, in addition to an immature secretory system within the liver (biliary tract) and an immature excretory system outside the liver (intestines). The exact cause of breast milk jaundice is unknown. The elevated levels of 5β-pregnane-3α, 20β-diol, or nonesterified long-chain fatty acids found in some maternal breast milk, in addition to glucuronidase, may interfere with the glucuronidation of bilirubin.

Hemolytic anemia leads to indirect hyperbilirubinemia because the production of heme-activated heme oxygenase leads to an increase in bilirubin. In addition, conjugation is slower in infants because of their low levels of UDPG dehydrogenase. Hemolytic anemia has been associated with blood group incompatibilities, hereditary hemolytic syndromes, and neonatal infections of bacterial or viral origin.

Genetic enzyme defects are responsible for syndromes such as Crigler-Najjar syndrome types I and II and Gilbert syndrome. Both types of Crigler-Najjar syndrome are caused by an absence of uridine diphosphate (UDP) glucuronosyltransferase; the inheritance is autosomal recessive. Gilbert syndrome is caused by a deficiency of UDP glucuronosyltransferase; the inheritance is autosomal dominant with incomplete penetrance.

Clinical Presentation

All infants with the disorders described in the preceding text appear jaundiced to varying degrees. Infants with physiologic jaundice or breast milk jaundice appear healthy, without signs of lethargy or organomegaly. The timing and degree of jaundice and a history of breast-feeding can often differentiate the two. The urine is normal in color because the unconjugated bilirubin is not water soluble. The stool does not become acholic in color because excretion of conjugated bilirubin occurs. Jaundice rarely appears during the first 36 hours of life. The bilirubin levels often peak by day 4 to 6 of life, with maximum levels of 6 to 12 mg/dL in physiologic jaundice. In breast milk jaundice, the peak bilirubin level can be as high as 20 mg/dL and usually appears by day 5 to 6 of life. Jaundice associated with hemolytic anemia appears within the first 36 hours of life and may be associated with hydrops fetalis or hepatosplenomegaly.

Crigler-Najjar syndrome is associated with an early rapid rise in bilirubin that if left untreated results in neurologic devastation (kernicterus). The urine color is pale. In addition, because conjugated bilirubin is not excreted, the stools are clay-colored. A therapeutic trial of phenobarbital causes the bilirubin level to drop in patients with type II Crigler-Najjar syndrome but not in those with type I.

In patients with *Gilbert syndrome*, the bilirubin levels rise to a point of clinical detection during physiologic stress, such as fasting and intercurrent illness. Gilbert syndrome is more common in boys, with a male-to-female ratio of 2:1 to 7:1.

Red flags for neonatal unconjugated hyperbilirubinemia are as follows:

- Jaundice in the first 36 hours of life
- Total bilirubin level above 12 mg/dL
- Persistent hyperbilirubinemia after 12 days of life in full-term infants or after 15 days in preterm infants
- Elevated level of conjugated bilirubin (>1.5 mg/dL or >15% of total bilirubin)

Diagnosis

If an infant is jaundiced beyond 2 weeks of age, the total and direct bilirubin levels should be measured. If the direct component is <15% of the total and the total bilirubin is elevated, indirect hyperbilirubinemia is diagnosed. A positive Coombs test result identifies a problem with isoimmunization that can be associated with:

- Rh incompatibility
- ABO incompatibility
- Kell incompatibility

If the Coombs test result is negative, then other causes should be sought (Table 8.1).

TABLE 8.1

CAUSES OF COOMBS-NEGATIVE HYPERBILIRUBINEMIA

Causes	Underlying Disease
Extravasated blood	Cephalohematoma, ecchymoses, petechiae, hemorrhage, swallowed blood
Metabolic errors	Crigler-Najjar syndrome (types I, II, III) Gilbert syndrome Lucy-Driscoll syndrome
Hormonal	Hypothyroidism Hypopituitarism Anencephaly Infants of diabetic mothers
Drugs	Antibiotics (sulfonamides, ceftriaxone) Chuen-lin (Chinese herb)
Red blood cell abnormalities	Spherocytosis Elliptocytosis Stomatocytosis
Hemoglobinopathies	Sickle cell disease Hemoglobin C disease
Disseminated intravascular coagulation	Sepsis
Enzyme deficiencies	Prematurity
Twin–twin transfusion	
Maternal–infant transfusion Intrauterine hypoxia	

Treatment and Complications

The goal of treatment is to avoid the most serious complication of indirect hyperbilirubinemia, kernicterus. Various treatments include phototherapy, exchange transfusion, enzyme induction, alteration of breast-feeding, and interruption of the enterohepatic circulation. In breast milk jaundice, withholding breast-feeding for 1 to 3 days should result in a reduction of the total bilirubin level >50%. Phototherapy changes the course of indirect hyperbilirubinemia by converting the insoluble form of bilirubin to a water-soluble, nontoxic form, lumirubin that can be excreted in the urine.

The treatment of Crigler-Najjar type II disease is phenobarbital, which may lower the bilirubin to acceptable levels. In both types I and II, long-term phototherapy may be required. If phototherapy is not applied consistently in type I disease, kernicterus may develop. Liver transplantation is an accepted and recommended therapy for type I disease because of the high level of associated morbidity and quality-of-life issues related to daily night-time phototherapy.

Prognosis

The prognosis for patients with uncomplicated physiologic jaundice, breast milk jaundice, and Gilbert syndrome are excellent, with no long-term sequelae. If kernicterus develops, the infant will have severe mental and motor retardation. If liver transplantation is performed for Crigler-Najjar type I disease, the chance of a normal life expectancy is better than 85%, and further phototherapy is not needed. However, these patients will require long-term immunosuppression.

NEONATAL CHOLESTASIS

Etiology

Cholestatic liver disease in infants has numerous causes. The overall incidence is approximately 1 in 2500 live births. *The two most common causes of neonatal cholestasis are neonatal hepatitis (idiopathic) and biliary atresia.* Other causes, in decreasing frequency, are listed in Table 8.2.

The intrahepatic cholestatic syndromes include diseases such as *Alagille syndrome, Byler disease* (PFIC1), and other *bile acid defect syndromes* (e.g., bile salt export pump [BSEP] deficiency, multidrug resistance [MDR]3 deficiency, and 3β-hydroxysteroid dehydrogenase [3β-HSD]). Endocrine and metabolic defects that are associated with cholestasis include:

- Thyroid disease (hyperthyroidism or hypothyroidism)
- Panhypopituitarism
- Cystic fibrosis
- Mitochondrial cytopathies
- Tyrosinemia
- Galactosemia

TABLE 8.2

CAUSES AND FREQUENCY OF NEONATAL CHOLESTASIS

Disease	Estimated Frequency
Idiopathic neonatal hepatitis	1:8000
Extrahepatic biliary atresia	1:14,000
a-j-Antitrypsin deficiency	1:40,000
Intrahepatic cholestasis syndrome	1:70,000
Bacterial sepsis	1:100,000
Hepatitis secondary to congenital infection	1:100,000
Endocrine/metabolic causes	1:100,000

- Hereditary fructosemia
- Glycogen storage disease type 4
- Niemann-Pick disease types B and C
- Gaucher disease
- Neonatal hemochromatosis
- Wilson disease
- Citrin deficiency
- Organic acidemias

Pathophysiology

Idiopathic neonatal hepatitis can occur in either a sporadic or a familial form. Cholestasis develops in the central zones within hepatocytes and canaliculi, but rarely in the bile ducts. Prominent giant cell transformation and extramedullary hematopoiesis are characteristic. No steatosis is noted on liver biopsy specimens.

Extrahepatic biliary atresia is a progressive, sclerosing, inflammatory process that can affect any portion of the extrahepatic biliary tree. Segmental or complete obliteration of the ductular lumen leads to rapid progression to end-stage liver disease. The two types of presentation are related to the underlying cause of the disease. The fetal form is possibly caused by an unknown gene mutation because laterality anomalies are often associated. The perinatal form (most common) is probably secondary to an insult, such as a viral infection.

Abnormalities typically associated with extrahepatic biliary atresia include:

- Polysplenia or asplenia
- Cardiovascular defects
- Abdominal situs inversus
- Intestinal malrotation
- Portal vein anomalies
- Hepatic artery anomalies

α_1-*Antitrypsin deficiency* is inherited as an autosomal-recessive condition. Liver disease associated with α_1-antitrypsin deficiency occurs in patients with the PiZZ phenotype, although on rare occasions it may be associated with

PiZS and PiZ null. Liver damage is thought to be caused by the accumulation of an abnormal α_1-antitrypsin gene product within the hepatocytes. Histologically, the liver biopsy reveals giant cells, extramedullary hematopoiesis, hepatocellular cholestasis and plugs in the canaliculi, periodic acid-Schiff-positive and diastase-resistant eosinophilic globules.

Two types of bile duct paucity syndromes are associated with neonatal cholestasis: Alagille syndrome (arteriohepatic dysplasia) and nonsyndromic bile duct paucity syndrome. On microscopy, the two appear identical and can be differentiated only by the associated abnormalities seen in patients with Alagille syndrome. Under the light microscope, both diseases are characterized by a paucity of bile ducts (<0.5 ducts/portal triad). As a result, bile cannot be adequately drained from the liver.

Abnormalities associated with Alagille syndrome include:

■ Ophthalmic: Posterior embryotoxon
■ Cardiac: Pulmonic stenosis, tetralogy of Fallot, others
■ Skeletal: Butterfly vertebrae, foreshortened finger, stunted growth
■ Renal: Interstitial nephritis, glomerular disease
■ Facial: Prominent forehead, hypertelorism, flattened malar eminence, pointed chin
■ Other: Developmental delay or mental retardation (possibly nutrition-related)

Two major causes of liver disease in patients with metabolic disorders are as follows:

■ Accumulation of gene products within the liver cells (e.g., α_1-antitrypsin deficiency, glycogen storage disease)
■ Inappropriate metabolism of products leading to the production of toxic metabolites (e.g., bile acid defects)

These processes can result in the development of hypoglycemia, lactic acidosis, bile stasis, or hyperammonemia.

Clinical Presentation

Most infants and children who have cholestatic disorders present with jaundice. In infants, jaundice may not be noticed until the serum bilirubin level reaches approximately 7 mg/dL, but in older children, jaundice is more quickly noticed at a bilirubin level of 2 to 3 mg/dL. Jaundice beyond 12 days of age in a full-term infant or beyond 15 days of age in a premature infant is unusual and requires further evaluation. Pruritus is also a hallmark symptom of cholestasis, although infants may not be affected. Other clinical symptoms that occur with varying frequencies include failure to thrive, vomiting, poor eating, lethargy, and sleep disturbances. These are seen commonly in children with tyrosinemia and galactosemia, other metabolic diseases, and also in cases of sepsis. Prematurity is often associated with neonatal hepatitis, whereas most children with biliary atresia are full-term. Patients who have extrahepatic biliary atresia are generally born with an appropriate weight for their gestational age.

A low birth weight is more often associated with intrahepatic cholestasis, as in Alagille syndrome and congenital infections. The stools may be acholic, the color of pale clay, and the urine is darkened by the direct hyperbilirubin, which is water soluble.

On physical examination, the patient may appear jaundiced. With causes of jaundice such as biliary atresia and Alagille syndrome, the patient appears well. An ill appearance is more common in patients with infection (e.g., sepsis) or an inborn error of metabolism. A congenital infection may be associated with a low birth weight, microcephaly, and chorioretinitis. Congenital heart disease may be associated with extrahepatic biliary atresia and syndromic bile duct paucity (Alagille syndrome). The facial features characteristic of Alagille syndrome may become more prominent with age. Dysmorphic features are also not uncommon with various chromosomal defects. Polysplenia, which sometimes accompanies biliary atresia, may be associated with a midline liver. Hepatomegaly is common, and the liver is often almost rock hard in advanced disease due to cirrhosis. Hepatomegaly is also seen in glycogen storage disease types I, III, IV, VI, and VIII (Table 8.3). It may be accompanied by varying degrees of hypoglycemia and hypotonia. If a cystic mass is palpable, ultrasonography may

TABLE 8.3

GLYCOGEN STORAGE DISEASES ASSOCIATED WITH LIVER FINDINGS

Type	Diagnostic Tests	Findings
GSD I (von Gierke disease, glucose-6-phosphatase deficiency	DNA testing, liver biopsy with enzyme assay	Hepatomegaly, ketotic hypoglycemia
GSD III (Debrancher deficiency)	Fibroblast or liver enzyme assay	Hepatomegaly, ketotic hypoglycemia
GSD IV (Brancher deficiency)	Fibroblast, muscle, or liver biopsy	Hepatomegaly, cirrhosis
GSD VI (Hers disease, liver phosphorylase deficiency)	Liver biopsy and enzyme assay	Hepatomegaly, hypoglycemia
GSD VIII (phosphorylase b kinase deficiency)	Liver and muscle biopsy	Hepatomegaly, hypoglycemia, fatigue

GSD, glycogen storage diseases.

confirm the diagnosis of choledochal cyst. Splenomegaly is frequently seen in congenital infection and advanced liver disease. Signs of severe liver failure in excess of that expected for the degree of cholestasis are associated with metabolic diseases such as neonatal iron storage disease (neonatal hemochromatosis) and tyrosinemia. Purpura, bleeding, ascites, and edema can develop rapidly, with massive hepatocyte necrosis.

Diagnosis

The diagnostic tests that should be performed first are listed in Table 8.4. These help establish the diagnosis of cholestasis and the degree of dysfunction. Tests should be requested after thoughtful consideration of the amount of blood volume that can be safely removed from the infant within a short period of time. The illnesses most likely to become rapidly life-threatening or for which a specific treatment is available should be evaluated first.

While the initial evaluation is being completed, further diagnostic workup should include ultrasonography of the liver and biliary system. Abdominal ultrasonography can gauge the size and texture of the liver and assess the gallbladder, which is often absent or small in extra-

hepatic biliary atresia. It can also detect a choledochal cyst, ascites, splenomegaly, or other intra-abdominal abnormalities. Specific laboratory tests should be performed to define specific disorders: α_1-antitrypsin phenotyping, immunoglobulin M (IgM) antibodies to toxoplasmosis, rubella, cytomegalovirus, and herpes simplex (TORCH) infections, cultures and smears of vesicular lesions for herpesvirus, and urine culture for cytomegalovirus. Serologies can be obtained for parvovirus B19 and human herpesvirus 6. Metabolic studies of the serum and urine and screening of the urine for organic acids should be performed to detect metabolic disease. Hepatobiliary scanning with hepatic dimethyliminodiacetic acid (HIDA) or disopropyliminodiacetic acid (DISIDA) provides information about hepatic uptake and the excretory ability of the liver. Failure of excretion is suggestive of biliary atresia but may also occur in other diseases in which the cholestasis is caused by such severe hepatocellular damage that the cells cannot excrete the radionuclide. Delayed uptake by the liver indicates hepatocellular dysfunction, as in advanced cases of biliary atresia and neonatal or other forms of hepatitis. Excretion of radionuclide makes biliary atresia less likely, but since the disease is progressive, a hepatobiliary scan performed too early may be falsely reassuring. The scan should be repeated if any concern remains.

If the hepatobiliary scan indicates excretory failure, a liver biopsy should be performed. It can often rule out biliary atresia or identify other causes of hepatobiliary disease, such as α_1-antitrypsin deficiency and neonatal hepatitis. If findings consistent with biliary atresia are identified, open cholangiography should be performed by an experienced pediatric surgeon who is prepared to carry out a portoenterostomy (Kasai procedure) under the same anesthesia if the external biliary system cannot be identified.

Treatment

The treatment of cholestasis should be aimed at the underlying disease process. In addition, complications of cholestasis, such as deficiencies of fat-soluble vitamins and pruritus, must be treated. Extrahepatic biliary atresia is currently treated with a portoenterostomy to allow bile flow to the intestinal lumen. Fat-soluble vitamin supplementation is essential if the patient remains cholestatic (Table 8.5).

Pruritus can be treated with conservative measures, such as oatmeal baths, emollients, antihistamines, and rifampin (10 mg/kg per day). In some cases, severe pruritus is a compelling reason for liver transplantation. Xanthomas can be very disfiguring and can be treated with bile salt resin binders, such as cholestyramine. Some children with cholestasis respond to therapy with bile salts, such as ursodeoxycholic acid. This particular bile salt can improve

---

TABLE 8.4

FIRST-LINE DIAGNOSTIC STUDIES FOR NEONATAL CHOLESTASIS

History and Physical Examination	Pregnancy
	Family history
	Neonatal course
	Stool color
	Extrahepatic abnormalities
	Organomegaly
	Signs of hepatic dysfunction
Fractionated bilirubin	Total bilirubin and direct bilirubin (abnormal if direct bilirubin >15% of total)
Liver injury tests	ALT
	AST
	Alkaline phosphatase
	GGTP
Liver function tests	Prothrombin time
	Partial thromboplastin time
	Albumin
	Glucose
	Cholesterol
	Ammonia
Hematology	Complete blood cell count with differential, platelets
Evaluation for infection	Bacterial cultures of blood, urine, and ascitic fluid (if present)

ALT, alanine aminotransferase; AST, aspartate aminotransferase; GGTP, γ-glutamyl transpeptidase.

TABLE 8.5

FAT-SOLUBLE VITAMIN SUPPLEMENTATION

Vitamin	Deficiency	Treatment	Toxicity
Vitamin A	Corneal damage	5000–25,000 U/day	Hepatotoxicity Pseudotumor cerebri Dermatitis
Vitamin D	Rickets Hypocalcemia	800–4000 U/day	Hypercalcemia Arrhythmia Lethargy Nephrocalcinosis
Vitamin E	Ataxia Peripheral neuropathy Ophthalmoplegia	TPGS 15–25 U/kg per day, or α-Tocopherol 25–200 I U/kg per day	Hyperosmolarity secondary to PEG in TPGS if patient in renal failure
Vitamin K	Coagulopathy	2.5 mg twice weekly to 5 mg/day	Clotting diathesis

PEG, polyethylene glycol; TPGS, tocopheryl polyethylene glycol succinate.

bile flow by increasing the fluidity of the bile through the stimulation of biliary bicarbonate secretion, and it may also affect the local immune system of the biliary tree. Poor growth requires the delivery of extra calories and possibly the placement of a nasogastric tube or semipermanent gastrostomy tube. Immunizations should be given without delay, including both the hepatitis A and B vaccines. Repeated bouts of cholangitis can further damage the liver of patients who have undergone a portoenterostomy and must be treated quickly and adequately with broad-spectrum antibiotics that achieve good concentrations within the liver, such as piperacillin/tazobactam and gentamicin. It may be necessary to treat ascites by fluid restriction and diuretics. Encephalopathy can be treated with lactulose or neomycin, or both.

Specific metabolic diseases, such as tyrosinemia, may require specific dietary restrictions, and the input of a metabolic specialist is necessary. If the disease process progresses, liver transplantation should be considered, not only to cure the underlying disease but also to improve the patient's quality of life that can be affected by poor growth, xanthomas, pruritus, and lethargy.

Prognosis

The prognosis of infants with biliary atresia is markedly improved by early referral to a subspecialist. The chance of success is 86% if surgery is performed before 8 weeks of age, but drops to 36% if surgery is performed later than that. Reasons for late referral include inadequate medical follow-up, ignoring jaundice until the patient fails to thrive, a mild fall in the serum bilirubin level, misdiagnosis of breast milk jaundice, pigmented stools, left-sided liver, a nondiagnostic result of early biopsy, and inade-

quate surgical experience. Cholangitis causes further damage to the liver. The prognosis also depends on the experience of the pediatric surgeon. Better outcomes have been achieved in centers that perform several portoenterostomies each year. Developmental delay may be caused by vitamin deficiencies and parental/social anxieties. Children should be encouraged to participate in all the age-appropriate activities that they can perform safely.

In 15% of patients with α_1-antitrypsin deficiency, liver disease develops by 20 years of age. If the liver disease presents in the neonatal period, micronodular cirrhosis develops in 50% of the cases. The mortality of patients with Alagille syndrome is 17% to 25%, caused either by liver disease or cardiac complications. Survival after transplantation is 75% because of the presence of other complicating disorders, such as heart disease. The prognosis of patients with idiopathic neonatal hepatitis depends on whether it is the sporadic or familial type of neonatal hepatitis. Prognosis percentages for the sporadic form of the disease are as follows:

- Recovery, 74%
- Chronic liver disease, 7%
- Death, 19%

For the familial form of the disease, they are as follows:

- Recovery, 22%
- Chronic liver disease, 15%
- Death, 63%

The life expectancy of infants with cholestasis has improved markedly from what it was 20 to 30 years ago. The correction of vitamin deficiencies, symptomatic treatment of pruritus, and liver transplantation have markedly improved the outcome of these children.

REVIEW EXERCISES

QUESTIONS

Case

A full-term male infant born to a gravida I, para I 32-year-old mother with no prenatal risk factors weighed 5 lb at birth. He was noted to be jaundiced at 24 hours of age, with a total bilirubin level of 4.5 mg/dL. He was discharged home with a recommendation for close follow-up. The patient was lost to follow-up until the 2-week-old visit and was seen to be gaining weight appropriately on maternal breast milk. On physical examination, the baby was noted to be alert but jaundiced.

1. What is the next appropriate step?
a) Reassure the mother that everything is okay.
b) Reassure the mother but obtain a total bilirubin level.
c) Reassure the mother but obtain a total and direct bilirubin level.
d) Stop breast-feeding.

Answer

The answer is c. Although it is most likely that the bilirubin is almost entirely indirect, measurement of the direct bilirubin is important in ruling out liver disease. Jaundice at 2 weeks of age is abnormal, although the infant may appear well. The mother can be reassured about the physical examination findings, but should be informed about the higher probability of a physiologic process. The total bilirubin level is important, but does not rule out underlying liver disease. Breast-feeding may be stopped for a short time to see whether the bilirubin level drops, but only if the direct bilirubin level is normal.

2. The total bilirubin was 7.0 mg/dL, and the direct bilirubin was 1.1 mg/dL. What would be the next step?
a) Perform a blood smear for hemolysis.
b) Perform liver function tests.
c) Have the patient undergo ultrasonography of the liver.
d) Have the mother give the infant glycerin suppositories.

Answer

The answer is b. Direct hyperbilirubinemia is always abnormal. The serum hepatocellular enzymes (alanine aminotransferase and aspartate aminotransferase), biliary enzymes (alkaline phosphatase), and serum electrolytes should be evaluated. Although hemolysis can cause an elevated bilirubin level, it does not cause direct hyperbilirubinemia (direct bilirubin ≥15% of total bilirubin). Ultrasonography will be necessary, but not as a first priority. It will help to rule out or confirm the presence of an obstructive lesion, such as a choledochal cyst or mass. It is not helpful in diagnosing biliary atresia. Although it is important to increase biliary excretion, the degree of the patient's hyperbilirubinemia at this point is such that excessive therapy is not required.

3. The results of laboratory tests showed that the alanine aminotransferase and aspartate aminotransferase levels were more than twice the upper limit of normal and that the alkaline phosphatase level was thrice the upper limit of normal. All the following should be evaluated, *except:*
a) Sweat chloride
b) TORCH IgG titers
c) Serum thyroid levels
d) Hepatitis viral antibodies

Answer

The answer is b. Although it is important to evaluate for the various TORCH infections, the serum levels of IgG at this age are most likely of maternal origin. It is more appropriate to check the serum IgM levels. Cystic fibrosis is a metabolic cause of cholestasis and should be considered as part of the workup. The cholestasis is most likely secondary to an increased viscosity of the bile. Hypothyroidism and hyperthyroidism are associated with hyperbilirubinemia. In many states, serum thyroid tests are part of the neonatal state screening process, and the results can be easily reviewed. If these are unavailable for some reason, the tests should be performed. Antihepatitis A IgM, hepatitis B surface antigen (HBsAg), antihepatitis B core antigen IgM, and hepatitis C viral antibodies should be measured. It is necessary to measure antihepatitis A IgM to rule out an acute infection, whereas IgG may represent the mother's antibody status. In the United States, all neonates are immunized against hepatitis B at birth, but serologic testing should be performed if the status is unclear. Hepatitis C viral antibodies may be the patient's own or of maternal origin. If the result of the antibody test is positive, further testing for hepatitis C viral RNA by polymerase chain reaction is indicated.

4. The results of the workup for this child were negative, showing no signs of metabolic or infectious disease. Ultrasonography showed no evidence of biliary obstruction. The extrahepatic bile ducts and gallbladder were not visualized, but the baby had just finished a bottle. An HIDA scan was performed and showed no excretion of radionuclide into the intestines in 24 hours. What is the next step?
a) Consult a pediatric surgeon to perform biliary surgery.
b) Perform a liver biopsy.
c) Stop breast-feeding.
d) Wait and see.

Answer

The answer is b. With an abnormal HIDA scan, the next step is to perform a liver biopsy to look for portal tract expansion and bile duct proliferation, consistent with extrahepatic obstruction. A percutaneous liver biopsy can be performed relatively safely if the patient's coagulation status and platelets are normal or correctable.

Otherwise, an open laparotomy may be required. Without a pathologic finding consistent with biliary atresia, it would be premature to have a surgeon perform a portoenterostomy. Nonetheless, maintaining a line of communication with the surgeon is important because time is of the essence. If the surgeon is notified that a child who may have biliary atresia is being evaluated, the surgeon's schedule can be arranged so that surgery can be performed as quickly as possible. It is sometimes recommended that breast-feeding be stopped so that a formula high in medium-chain triglycerides (the absorption of which does not require bile) can be provided, but discontinuation is not mandatory so long as the child can absorb an adequate number of calories and continue to gain and grow. There is some concern that formulas excessively high in medium-chain triglycerides may lead to a deficiency of essential fatty acids (essential fatty acids are long-chain triglycerides). Watching and waiting are not appropriate because infants do best after a portoenterostomy when they undergo surgery early.

5. The baby underwent a portoenterostomy and began passing green stools, and his jaundice markedly improved. What would be the *most* appropriate thing to tell the family?
a) The vitamins in his formula should be more than adequate.
b) The liver may continue to be inflamed, even with initial excretion, so close follow-up will be necessary.
c) Immunizations should be withheld because of the patient's liver disease.
d) Poor growth and developmental delay are expected outcomes.

Answer
The answer is b. Because of the nature of the disease itself, which is a progressive inflammatory process, and because of complications, such as repeated bouts of cholangitis, the liver damage continues, and liver transplantation may become necessary in the future. If the cholestasis continued, then the infant should be given supplementary fat-soluble vitamins (vitamins A, D, E, and K). Supplementation is often in excess of the recommended daily allowance to compensate for poor absorption. Patients with liver disease should receive all necessary immunizations, especially the hepatitis A and B vaccines. Vaccination is especially important if liver transplantation becomes necessary because the administration of live vaccines is not currently recommended after liver transplantation. With close monitoring, growth can be supported through additional caloric intake, either with a concentrated formula or even nasogastric feeding. Developmental delay is unlikely to occur, especially if the nutritional status and fat-soluble vitamin supplementation of the infant are closely monitored.

6. The parents of this baby are interested in having more children and request information about the risk to future progeny. Your *best* answer would be that:
a) The inheritance of this disease is autosomal dominant, so their risk of having another affected baby is one in two.
b) The inheritance of this disease is autosomal recessive, so their risk of having another affected baby is one in four.
c) The disease is passed on by maternal infection, so the best protection is for the mother to avoid all sick contacts.
d) The disease is not hereditary, so the risk to future infants is the same as that in the general population.

Answer
The answer is d. No specific inheritance patterns are associated with extrahepatic biliary atresia, which is thought to be caused either by an unidentified infectious agent or an insult *in utero* that affects ductal plate formation. The inheritance of Gilbert disease is autosomal dominant with incomplete penetrance. Liver diseases with autosomal-recessive inheritance include α_1-antitrypsin deficiency and Crigler-Najjar syndrome types I and II. Although data are available to support a possible infectious etiology (newer animal models), no specific organisms have been identified, nor have any maternal risk factors. Telling the mother to avoid all sick contacts would make her unduly anxious and would probably have an untoward effect on her pregnancy.

SUGGESTED READINGS

1. Chardot C, Carton M, Spire-Bendelac N, et al. Is the Kasai operation still indicated in children older than 3 months diagnosed with biliary atresia? *J Pediatr* 2001;138:224–228.
2. Chuang JH, Lin JN. Biliary atresia at the dawn of a new century [Review]. *Chang Gung Med J* 2001;24:217–228.
3. Kaufman SS, Murray ND, Wood RP, et al. Nutritional support for the infant with extrahepatic biliary atresia [Review]. *J Pediatr* 1987;110:679–686.
4. Mieli-Vergani G, Vergani D. Immunological liver diseases in children [Review]. *Semin Liver Dis* 1998;18:271–279.
5. Migliazza L, Lopez SM, Murcia J, et al. Long-term survival expectancy after liver transplantation in children. *J Pediatr Surg* 2000;35:5–7.
6. Poupon R, Chazouilleres O, Poupon RE. Chronic cholestatic diseases [Review]. *J Hepatol* 2000;32:129–140.
7. Shneider BL. Genetic cholestasis syndromes. *J Pediatr Gastroenterol Nutr* 1999;28:124–131.
8. Shneider B, Cronin J, van Marter L, et al. A prospective analysis of cholestasis in infants supported with extracorporeal membrane oxygenation. *J Pediatr Gastroenterol Nutr* 1991;13:285–289.
9. Sokol RJ, Treem WR. Mitochondria and childhood liver diseases. *J Pediatr Gastroenterol Nutr* 1999;28:4–16.
10. Volpert D, White F, Finegold MJ, et al. Outcome of early hepatic portoenterostomy for biliary atresia. *J Pediatr Gastroenterol Nutr* 2001;32:265–269.

Chapter 9

Common Mucosal and Luminal Disorders

Kadakkal R. Radhakrishnan

CELIAC DISEASE

Celiac disease, also called gluten-sensitive enteropathy, is a permanent intestinal intolerance to dietary wheat protein gliadin and related proteins. This disorder occurs only in genetically susceptible individuals.

Epidemiology

In the United States, the incidence of celiac disease using persistent IgA transglutaminase positivity is 1 per 104 individuals and 1 per 105 individuals when IgA anti-endomysial antibodies are used to detect this disorder. In Sweden, the incidence ranges from 1 per 77 individuals to 1 per 285 individuals. In Finland the incidence of biopsy proven celiac disease is 1 per 99 individuals. Celiac disease is generally uncommon in Asia and Africa, although the highest incidence of celiac disease by serological methods was reported in sub-Saharan Africa at 1 per 60 individuals.

Pathogenesis

The pathogenesis of celiac disease is thought to be dependent on three components (Fig. 9.1):

- Genetic susceptibility (HLA DQ-2 and DQ-8 are seen in over 90% of individuals with celiac disease, but these same genes are also present in 30% of whites who do not have celiac disease).
- Exposure to incriminating proteins, especially gliadin
- T-cell–mediated inflammatory response in the small bowel, causing inflammation and mucosal change in genetically susceptible individuals

Dietary Factors

The three main cereals that are implicated in celiac disease fall under the tribe Triticeae. They include:

- Wheat (Gliadin)
- Barley (Hordein)
- Rye (Secalin)

Oats, which are considered part of the Avenae tribe, rarely activates celiac disease, playing a role in a small fraction of patients. All these proteins are structurally similar, with the last 33 amino acids being resistant to digestion. This amino acid sequence is believed to be the inflammation-stimulating sequence.

Clinical Manifestations

The *classic* manifestations of celiac disease include:

- Failure to thrive
- Loose stools and/or diarrhea

However, a *more common* presentation of celiac disease is an *asymptomatic* patient who is incidentally identified by serologic screening. Refractory iron deficiency in *adults* is a common manifestation of celiac disease. *Uncommon* presentations of celiac disease include constipation, osteoporosis, fat-soluble vitamin deficiency, elevation in transaminases, depression, and dermatitis herpetiformis.

Diagnosis

Definitive diagnosis is established by endoscopy and small bowel biopsy in the appropriate clinical setting. Changes in the small bowel include subtotal to total villous atrophy and increased round cell infiltration.

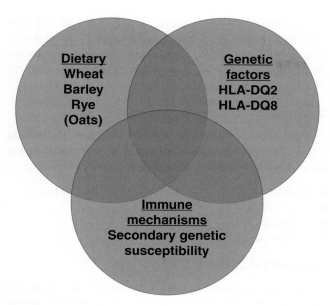

Figure 9.1 Schematic showing the relationship between the three components thought to be important in the pathogenesis of celiac disease.

Serologic methods of diagnosis include:

- Tissue transglutaminase (TTG) IgA: sensitivity >90% and specificity >95%
- Anti-endomysial antibody IgA: sensitivity >95% and specificity >98%
- Gliadin IgG and IgA antibodies: relatively high false positivity rate (low specificity)

Measurement of total IgA levels is recommended when screening for celiac disease, given the high incidence of IgA deficiency in the general population.

It is important to remember other entities that cause villous atrophy, including:

- Severe Crohn disease
- Cell-mediated, congenital, and acquired immune deficiency states
- Radiation enteritis
- Severe cow milk protein allergy
- *Giardia* infection

Treatment

The definitive treatment for celiac disease is complete and lifelong institution of a gluten-free diet. Patients are advised not to share cooking utensils to avoid the risk of contamination. Follow-up serologic studies of endomysial antibody are recommended, preferably every 6 months, to evaluate the response to diet and compliance. Oats may be reintroduced after 6 months of a strict gluten-free diet. Patient with celiac disease should have a complete blood count and metabolic

panels an annual basis, and bone densities should be performed every 2 to 3 years after the age of 10 years.

Celiac disease is associated with other disorders, including:

- Type 1 diabetes (7% of patients have celiac disease)
- Down syndrome (up to 7% have celiac disease)
- Hypothyroidism (20% of patients with celiac disease may have hypothyroidism)
- T-cell lymphoma of the gut (relative risk is 3 in patients with celiac disease)

CYSTIC FIBROSIS AND GASTROINTESTINAL SYSTEM

Cystic fibrosis (CF) is the most common genetic disease affecting the pancreas. The prevalence of CF is 1 per 2500 whites, 1 per 15,000 African Americans, and 1 per 100,000 Asians.

Pathogenesis

CF is caused by mutations affecting the cystic fibrosis transmembrane regulator (CFTR) gene. Over 1400 mutations have been reported in the CFTR gene but only 10 of these cause 90% of the disease. Homozygous delta 508 is the most common mutation, and this accounts for 70% of the disease. Ninety-nine percent of children with homozygous delta 508 mutations have pancreatic insufficiency by 1 year of age. Seventy percent of compound delta 508 mutations have pancreatic insufficiency by one year of age.

Pancreatic Insufficiency

Patients with untreated CF often have greasy stools because of fat malabsorption. Severe malabsorption may lead to failure to thrive and hypoalbuminemia. Fat-soluble vitamin deficiencies and their consequences in CF include:

- Vitamin E: Hemolysis and ataxia
- Vitamin K: Coagulopathy
- Vitamin A: Night blindness, xerosis of cornea, and conjunctiva

Patients may compensate for malabsorption with an increased intake of protein and carbohydrates and fat. However, patient with CF commonly decompensate when oral intake decreases as a result of intercurrent infections.

Other Gastrointestinal Manifestations

Meconium ileus is seen in 10% to 20% of neonates with CF who present with symptoms of malabsorption. Older children with CF present with features caused by distal intestinal obstruction syndrome. Gastroesophageal reflux disease (GERD) and gastric acid hypersecretion are fairly common, and are seen in up to 40% of patients. Rectal prolapse is a well-recognized presentation of CF. Fibrosing colonopathy is an iatrogenic complication of CF, occurring from lipase supplementation of more than 20,000 IU/kg.

Cystic Fibrosis–Related Liver Disease

Hepatic steatosis is the most common liver abnormality in CF patients, manifesting in approximately 60% of patients. Neonatal cholestasis is seen in 5% of patients, whereas neonatal jaundice and late onset hemorrhagic disease are well recognized. Focal biliary cirrhosis, often occurring without specific clinical findings, occurs in 10% of patients with CF at 3 months of age and the incidence increases to 70% in young adults. Multilobular biliary cirrhosis occurs in 5% of CF patients and this may evolves into portal hypertension.

Evaluation for Patients with Cystic Fibrosis

The gastrointestinal evaluation of patients with suspected and proven CF includes:

- Sweat chloride and mutation analysis
- 72 fecal fat estimation (and yearly)
- Fat-soluble estimation (and yearly)
- Ultrasonography of the abdomen (and yearly)
- Nutritional evaluation (every 6 months)

Management of Gastrointestinal Issues

All patients with CF require close clinical follow-up. It is important to assure an adequate intake of calories for these patients. Energy intake should be about 120% RDA with 40% as long chain fatty acid. It is recommended that protein intake be maintained at 100% RDA. Enzyme supplementation should be close to 5000 to 10,000/kg for lipase. Fat-soluble vitamin supplementation (vitamins A, D, E, K) should be five to ten times the RDA for fat-soluble vitamins.

LACTOSE INTOLERANCE

Lactose intolerance is the prototype entity for malabsorption resulting from lack of brush border enzymes. Lactose intolerance is caused by deficiency or inactivity of lactase/phlorizin enzyme. Almost all Asians and Native Americans, 80% of African Americans and 30% to 50% of whites are lactose intolerant. Primary lactose intolerance is rare; common manifestations include gas, bloating, and diarrhea. Women are generally more symptomatic than men. Also, symptoms become more evident as people become older.

Diagnosis of Lactose Intolerance

The diagnosis of lactose intolerance is made with a breath test using lactose. The dose of lactose in this test is 50 g, which is equivalent to 4 cups of milk. Patients blow into

the machine every 15 minutes. A rise in breath H2 over 20 PPM is diagnostic of lactose intolerance. This test is positive in 90% of patients with lactose intolerance. Patients are advised to fast for 6 hours before test and to take no antibiotics within 10 days of the test.

Secondary Lactose Intolerance

Primary hypolactasia should never be diagnosed before 5 years of age. Children less than 5 years of age likely have secondary lactose intolerance, which may be caused by:

- Rotavirus gastroenteritis or other postinfective states
- Celiac disease
- Crohn disease
- Immune deficiency

Congenital Lactose Deficiency

Congenital lactose deficiency is exceedingly rare. Breast-fed neonates with this entity present in the newborn period with profuse diarrhea. Stool reducing substances are positive. This disorder is most common in Scandinavia. The diagnosis is made by eliminating lactose from the diet.

EOSINOPHILIC DISORDERS OF THE GASTROINTESTINAL SYSTEM

Eosinophils, which are present in the gastrointestinal tract in utero, normally reside in the gastrointestinal tract. Eosinophils may have a role in gastrointestinal development, and are believed to play an important role in host defense against parasitic infections. They serve as antigen-presenting cells to T cells.

Eosinophilic Esophagitis

Primary eosinophilic esophagitis (EE) may be an atopic, nonatopic, or familial disorder (10%). Most cases are believed to represent an adverse response to a dietary antigen. EE can also occur as a part of the spectrum of eosinophilic gastroenteritis.

The precise incidence of EE is not known, although it occurs in approximately 3.5% of children with GERD and 7% of children with esophagitis. In addition, EE is present in 20% of patients with dysphagia and 50% of those with unexplained dysphagia. Seventy to ninety-five percent of children unresponsive to proton-pump inhibitors may have EE. There is a marked male predominance.

The clinical features of EE include dysphagia, vomiting, and pain (chest, epigastric, and/or abdominal pain). Food impaction is a common presentation. Endoscopic findings in EE include furrows, vertical lines, and corrugation. Rings may be seen in the esophagus that look like tracheal mucosa. Adherent whitish plaques that are eosinophil-laden abscesses are frequently in patients with EG. Rarely, strictures may be seen. A response to dietary therapy of specific antigen avoidance supports the diagnosis of atopic EE.

Eosinophilic Gastroenteritis

Eosinophilic gastroenteritis (EG) is a term designated to refer to eosinophilic inflammation of the stomach and small intestine, although the designation of eosinophilic gastrointestinal disorders (EGID) refers to a broad spectrum of eosinophilic inflammation of one or more gastrointestinal sites, including esophagitis, gastritis, enteritis, and colitis. A history of allergic disorders is common in patients who have primary EG, although secondary causes, especially parasitic infections, can cause eosinophilic inflammation.

The clinical features of EG may include:

■ Failure to thrive
■ Abdominal pain
■ Irritability
■ Gastric dysmotility
■ Nausea, vomiting, and diarrhea
■ Dysphagia
■ Microcytic anemia
■ Protein-losing enteropathy

The initial work up for EG includes a full history and physical examination, serum IgE level, and erythrocyte sedimentation rate. Skin testing and radioallergosorbent test (RAST) for common food antigens may be considered in selected patients. A search for parasitic infections should be undertaken. Finally, esophagogastroduodenoscopy and colonoscopy may be performed in selected cases.

■ Swallowed fluticasone or budesonide for mild to moderate EE patients
■ Short courses (2–3 weeks) of systemic steroids for EGE and severe EE (strictures or not responding to fluticasone or budesonide)
■ Trial of elemental diet and dietary elimination in selected patients with EE and EGE
■ IL-5 antibody (Mepolizumab) for patients with very severe disease and not responding to above treatment options

REVIEW EXERCISES

QUESTIONS

1. A 19-month-old white girl has dropped weight from the 50th percentile to the 5th percentile since 10 months of age. Her appetite is decreased, she has become more irritable, and she is having three to four loose stools per day. Her physical examination is remarkable for a protuberant abdomen and loose folds of skin in her arms and thighs. A complete white count shows a microcytic, hypochromic anemia, normal erythrocyte sedimentation rate, C-reactive protein, and complete metabolic panel. Urinalysis and stool Hemoccult is negative. What is the most likely diagnosis?
a) Cow milk protein allergy
b) Celiac disease
c) Ulcerative colitis
d) Immune deficiency
e) Ascariasis
f) All of the above

Answer
The answer is b. Celiac disease is one of the most common causes of failure to thrive in the Western world, second only to low nutritional intake. The symptoms start after gluten-containing weaning foods are introduced into the child's diet. The presentation of the child in this scenario is very classical for celiac disease. Ulcerative colitis is less likely given the age and lack of blood in stool. It is unusual for cow milk protein allergy to persist past 12 months of age. It is generally unusual for a cellular immune deficiency to manifest at this age, and Ascariasis rarely presents in this manner.

2. A 2-month-old male infant presents with irritability for less than 1 day, and later develops a generalized seizure. Treatment is started for sepsis, and a computed tomography of the head is done that shows a right-sided parietal lobe hemorrhage. The patient required surgery on day 3 of life for meconium ileus. The patient had a mild conjugated hyperbilirubinemia (4.8/2.7); AST- 202 ALT 313 PT- 39sec PTT 42 sec. What is the most helpful test in confirming the diagnosis: What simple test can you order to make the diagnosis?
a) Factor V assay
b) HIDA scan
c) Sweat chloride
d) Ultrasound of abdomen
e) Stool 72-hour fat estimation

Answer
The answer is c. Cystic fibrosis is a recognized cause of late onset hemorrhagic disease of the newborn. In this patient, the history of meconium ileus is a clue to the diagnosis. Five percent of all patients with CF have cholestatic jaundice at birth.

3. During teaching rounds you come across a patient with Rotavirus diarrhea. The patient continues to have diarrhea for 10 days after the onset. You tell the residents that the diarrhea is secondary to malabsorption due to loss of cells lining the villi. One smart resident asks you how long it would take for the average intestinal cell to turn over? The best answer is:
a) 1 day
b) 2 to 3 weeks
c) 3 to 5 days
d) 1 to 2 months
e) 8 to 10 days

Answer
The answer is c.

4. A 14-year old white male has been having trouble with swallowing for 2 years. Today, he is having difficulty handling his secretions after eating a steak. He claims that "It is stuck." He previously had a similar event a year ago. He is otherwise healthy except for mild seasonal allergy. He denies a history of "heartburn."

The most likely diagnosis is:
a) Congenital anomaly of the esophagus
b) Mediastinal mass
c) Mitral stenosis
d) Eosinophilic esophagitis
e) GERD with stricture
f) Functional

Answer

The answer is d. The history of food impaction is a classic presentation of Eosinophilic gastroenteritis.

SUGGESTED READINGS

1. Khan S, Orenstein SR. Eosinophilic gastroenteritis. *Gastroenterol Clin North Am* 2008;37:333–348.
2. National Institutes of Health Consensus Development Conference Statement on Celiac Disease, June 28–30, 2004. *Gastroenterology* 2005;128(4 Suppl 1):S1–9.
3. Putnam PE. Eosinophilic esophagitis in children: clinical manifestations. *Gastroenterol Clin North Am* 2008;37:369–381.
4. Wyllie R, Hyams J, eds. *Pediatric Gastroenterology and Liver disease.* Philadelphia: Saunders, 2006.

Chapter 10

BOARD SIMULATION:
Gastroenterology

Lori Mahajan

QUESTIONS

1. Name the *most* likely hematologic abnormality that would result from feeding an infant exclusively with goat's milk.
a) Thrombocytosis
b) Iron deficiency anemia
c) Folate deficiency anemia
d) Vitamin B_{12} deficiency anemia
e) Neutropenia

Answer

The answer is c. Although similar to cow's milk in composition, goat's milk is very low in folic acid. Infants fed with goat's milk exclusively are susceptible to megaloblastic anemia resulting from folate deficiency.

2. A strict vegetarian diet (excluding eggs and dairy products) for a young child is likely to lead to a deficiency of:
a) Vitamin B_1
b) Vitamin B_{12}
c) Vitamin C
d) Vitamin D
e) Vitamin E

Answer

The answer is b. Vegetarians who consume eggs are known as ovo-vegetarians; those who consume dairy products are called lactovegetarians; and those who consume both are known as lacto-ovo-vegetarians. Vegetarians who consume neither eggs nor dairy products are called vegans. This diet contains almost no vitamin B_{12}; therefore, vegans are at high risk for developing a deficiency state. Nursing vegan mothers must be given supplemental vitamin B_{12} to prevent the development of methylmalonic acidemia in their infants. (Adenosylcobalamin, a metabolite of vitamin B_{12}, serves as a coenzyme in the metabolism of methyl-malonic acid. Deficiency of vitamin B_{12} can, therefore, lead to methylmalonic acidemia characterized by keto-sis, acidosis, anemia, neutropenia, thrombocytopenia, hyperammonemia, coma, and death.)

3. A 3-year-old boy status post-Kasai procedure for bil-iary atresia at age 12 weeks presents with a 1-month course of increasing irritability, pruritus, and clumsiness. Records indicate that he has not gained weight over the past 6 months. On examination, the patient has a wide-based gait, enlargement of both his liver and spleen, and diminished deep tendon reflexes in all the extremities. Which nutrient deficiency *most* likely accounts for these complaints and physical findings?
a) Vitamin A
b) Vitamin B_{12}
c) Vitamin D
d) Vitamin E
e) Zinc

Answer
The answer is d. Vitamin E (α-tocopherol) is a fat-soluble antioxidant that is present in milk and in a wide variety of foods. Supplementation is necessary in only select conditions such as in preterm infants who demon-strate poor absorption and in clinical conditions leading to fat malabsorption (biliary atresia, cystic fibrosis, pan-creatic insufficiency, short bowel syndrome). Clinical manifestations of vitamin E deficiency include progres-sive neurologic degeneration such as cerebellar ataxia, peripheral neuropathy, posterior column abnormalities with loss of deep tendon reflexes, and weakness.

4. A full-term newborn develops bilious emesis shortly after delivery. The pregnancy was complicated by poly-hydramnios. Physical features are suggestive of trisomy 21. On examination, the newborn's abdomen is soft and nondistended. What is the *most* likely diagnosis?
a) Pyloric stenosis
b) Midgut volvulus
c) Hirschsprung disease
d) Ileal duplication
e) Duodenal atresia

Answer
The answer is e. Bilious emesis without abdominal dis-tention is the most typical presentation of congenital duodenal obstruction. The relative incidence of various forms of congenital duodenal obstruction is duodenal atresia in 42%, annular pancreas in 33%, and duodenal diaphragm in 23% of neonates. Down syndrome is present in up to 30% of infants with duodenal atresia. Polyhydramnios occurs in approximately 50% of

pregnancies in which there is congenital duodenal ob-struction. This occurs because high intestinal obstruction prevents the normal absorption of amniotic fluid in the distal small intestine. The radiographic finding of a markedly distended stomach and first portion of the duodenum without air in the bowel distal to this is known as the *double-bubble sign* and is pathognomonic of duodenal atresia (see Fig. 63.3).

Pyloric stenosis is typically not present at birth, but presents between 3 weeks and 5 months of age. Emesis with this condition is nonbilious, as the obstruction is proximal to the second portion of the duodenum, where bile enters the lumen of the gut. A midgut volvu-lus is also not typically present at birth. This should al-ways be considered in the differential diagnosis of any infant that initially does well for several days to several months of life and subsequently develops bilious eme-sis. Hirschsprung disease may present with bilious eme-sis; however, the patient's abdomen would be markedly distended because of the distal location of the obstruc-tion. For the same reason, the presentation is not con-sistent with ileal duplication; as such a distal obstruc-tion would result in significant abdominal distension. The ileum is the most common location for GI duplica-tion cysts. The presentation is typically in childhood or adulthood.

5. An exclusively breast-fed 2-week-old male infant is brought to the emergency room with bilious emesis and abdominal distention. His parents report that he had been somewhat irritable with decreased oral intake for the preceding 12 hours. In addition, he has not stooled today, but previously had been stooling normally. Which of the following is *most* likely the diagnosis?
a) Midgut volvulus
b) Hirschsprung disease
c) Sepsis
d) Milk protein allergy
e) Viral gastroenteritis

Answer
The answer is a. Intestinal malrotation is a congenital anomaly occurring in approximately 1 in 500 live births. It results from failure of the normal 270-degree counter-clockwise rotation of the midgut around the superior mesenteric artery during fetal development. Symptoms may be intermittent and chronic or acute and cata-strophic. Approximately 50% of infants with this condi-tion will develop symptoms in the first month, whereas 90% become symptomatic within the first year of life. Vomiting is the most common presenting sign and is bilious in over 80% of patients. The diagnostic test of choice is an upper GI series. Because intestinal malrota-tion with midgut volvulus can rapidly lead to irreversible intestinal ischemia and death, every individual in whom this anomaly is clinically suspected should have an im-mediate upper GI study.

6. A term newborn develops bilious emesis and abdominal distension on the first day of life. No meconium passage has yet occurred. Pregnancy was complicated by maternal insulin-dependent diabetes mellitus. On examination, the newborn's abdomen is markedly distended, but nontender. Rectal examination is normal. What is the *most* likely diagnosis?
a) Intestinal malrotation with volvulus
b) Hypoplastic left colon syndrome
c) Meconium ileus
d) Jejunal atresia
e) Hirschsprung disease

Answer
The answer is b. Infants born to mothers with insulin-dependent diabetes mellitus are at up to an eightfold increased risk of congenital malformation as compared with infants born to mothers without this condition. Associated GI malformations include a small or hypoplastic left colon syndrome, also referred to as functional immaturity of the colon. In addition, there is an increased incidence of duodenal and anorectal atresia.

7. An otherwise healthy 6-day-old white female infant is brought to your office for evaluation of blood in the stool. She was delivered at home without complication and has been exclusively breast-fed. She has not been examined previously by a physician. On examination, she has what appear to be areas of ecchymosis over the buttocks and lower extremities. She is mildly tachycardic and her stool is grossly bloody. Physical examination is otherwise normal. Of the following, what is the *most* likely diagnosis?
a) Sepsis
b) *Salmonella* infection
c) Hemorrhagic disease of the newborn
d) Physical abuse
e) Colonic polyposis

Answer
The answer is c. A moderate decrease in serum levels of factors II, VII, IX, and X normally occurs in all newborns by 72 hours following delivery. This deficiency of vitamin K–dependent factors is secondary to lack of free vitamin K in the mother as well as breast milk (a poor source of vitamin K) and absence of bacterial intestinal flora normally responsible for production of vitamin K. Maternal medications, including anticonvulsants (phenobarbital, phenytoin) and antituberculous medications (isoniazid [INH] and rifampin) have been identified as risk factors for hemorrhagic disease of the newborn. Administration of 1 mg of natural oil-soluble vitamin K (phylloquinone) intramuscularly to the newborn at the time of delivery prevents the fall in vitamin K–dependent factors in full-term infants. In the clinical scenario, the delivery at home implies that no prophylactic vitamin K was administered. This was followed by the development of classic hemorrhagic disease of the

newborn. Sites of hemorrhage with this condition include the GI tract and the intracranial, circumcision, cutaneous, and injection sites.

8. A 14-year-old girl presents with an 8-month history of intermittent low-grade fevers and right lower quadrant pain. Her appetite has been decreasing, as pain worsens with eating. Her weight and height have decreased from the 50th percentile to below the 10th percentile for her age over the past 2 years and her parents are concerned that she has developed an eating disorder. On examination, the patient has mild right lower quadrant pain and fullness. No peritoneal signs are present. Her stool is Hemoccult positive. Of the following, the *most* appropriate initial diagnostic test would be:
a) Abdominal computed tomography (CT) scan to rule out a perforated appendix
b) Barium enema
c) Upper gastrointestinal (GI) series with small bowel follow-through
d) Abdominal ultrasonography
e) Stool culture

Answer
The answer is c. In the clinical scenario presented, there are several "red flags" that suggest an organic disease process rather than an eating disorder in this teenaged girl with significant weight loss. Intermittent low-grade fevers and pain localizing to the right lower quadrant region in an adolescent with growth failure are highly suggestive of inflammatory bowel disease, specifically Crohn disease. Fullness in the right lower quadrant on examination, in addition to Hemoccult positive stool, is also suggestive of this diagnosis. The presentation of Crohn disease may be insidious and complaints of diarrhea and visible blood in the stool are often not present. The only symptoms may be that of growth failure or extraintestinal manifestations such as arthralgia/arthritis, rashes (erythema nodosum, pyoderma gangrenosum), uveitis, oral aphthous ulcers, anemia, and osteopenia.

In Crohn disease, inflammation can involve any region of the GI tract from the mouth to the anus. Of the diagnostic tests listed, an upper GI series with small bowel follow-through is the most appropriate initial diagnostic test for the evaluation of possible Crohn disease. For further evaluation, this study would likely be followed by upper and lower endoscopy and possibly wireless capsule endoscopy for direct visualization of the small intestinal mucosa.

In the absence of peritoneal signs, an abdominal CT scan is not currently indicated and would expose the patient to unnecessary radiation. A barium enema would not provide adequate visualization of the terminal ileum (which is the area of interest) and would put the patient through significant discomfort. An abdominal ultrasonography may show bowel wall thickening, but it is not a routinely ordered study for the evaluation of the bowel when inflammatory bowel disease is suspected. Its diagnostic value is very operator-dependent. A stool culture would also have a low yield given the chronicity of symptoms.

9. A 2-year-old boy is brought to the emergency room following painless passage of a large maroon-colored stool. The patient is mildly tachycardic on examination with heme-positive and tarry stool in the rectal vault. His hemoglobin level is 6.8 gm/dL. Of the following, what is the *most* likely diagnosis?
a) Inflammatory bowel disease
b) Peptic ulcer disease
c) Colonic polyp
d) Meckel diverticulum
e) Bleeding diathesis

Answer

The answer is d. Meckel diverticula represent the most common congenital GI anomaly, occurring in 1% to 4% of all infants. The diverticulum represents a remnant of the omphalomesenteric or vitelline duct. It is typically located on the antimesenteric border of the distal small bowel, usually within 50 cm of the ileocecal valve. Pathology related to a Meckel diverticulum occurs more commonly in men. In symptomatic cases, 80% of the diverticula contain ectopic tissue. In most of these cases, the tissue is gastric, with pancreatic tissue being the second most common finding. The most common presentation is painless rectal bleeding caused by acid production by the gastric mucosal parietal cells with development of a marginal ulcer at the junction of the gastric and ileal mucosa. A Meckel diverticulum may also act as a lead point for an intussusception.

As in this clinical scenario, when bleeding occurs from a Meckel diverticulum, the stool is typically maroon or brick colored. Bleeding can lead to significant anemia, but is often self-limited because of contraction of the splanchnic vessels as the patient becomes hypovolemic. The most sensitive diagnostic test, known as a Meckel scan, permits visualization of the diverticulum following intravenous infusion of technetium-99m pertechnetate. The mucous-secreting cells of the ectopic gastric mucosa take up pertechnetate, allowing visualization of the diverticulum. The sensitivity of the scan can be enhanced by administering histamine (H_2) receptor blockers prior to the study.

Inflammatory bowel disease and peptic ulcer disease typically have a more insidious presentation and are associated with abdominal pain. Although a juvenile polyp is certainly a possibility in this age range, bleeding is more often bright red colored, as the polyp is colonic (more distal) in location. An isolated GI bleed would be an exceedingly rare presentation for a bleeding disorder in a 2 year old.

10. A 20-month-old infant is brought to your office with a 3-month history of one to four loose, nonbloody stools per day. The mother is concerned because she frequently sees undigested food particles in the stool. History is negative for recurrent fevers, abdominal pain, weight loss, or nocturnal symptoms. Growth and development have been normal. Examination, including rectal examination, is normal. What is the *most* likely diagnosis?
a) Chronic nonspecific diarrhea
b) Inflammatory bowel disease
c) Lactose intolerance
d) Giardiasis
e) Cow milk protein–allergy

Answer

The answer is a. Chronic nonspecific diarrhea (toddler's diarrhea) is the most likely diagnosis in this patient given the normal growth and development. (Failure to thrive would be expected with inflammatory bowel disease or untreated cow milk protein–allergy at this age.) Lactose intolerance is more commonly seen in school-aged children. Giardiasis also would be expected to result in abdominal pain, weight loss, and nocturnal symptoms.

Chronic nonspecific diarrhea is the most common cause of chronic diarrhea in infancy and typically has its onset after the first year of age. This condition may last until 40 months of age. The presence of vegetable matter such as peas or corn in the stool is normal and consistent with poor chewing instead of a malabsorption syndrome. The diarrhea is secondary to ingestion of juices high in fructose and sorbitol as well as "colonic fluid-overload." Stooling typically occurs during the day and not overnight. Limitation of juices and overall fluid intake between meals as well as increasing dietary fat often leads to resolution of this pattern.

11. In the United States, what is the *most* common cause of rectal prolapse?
a) Chronic diarrhea
b) Chronic constipation
c) Malnutrition
d) Anorectal malformations
e) Parasitic infestation

Answer

The answer is b. Rectal prolapse refers to the exteriorization of rectal tissue through the anus. When visualized, the tissue protruding is usually rectal and not a polyp or other tissue. Causes of rectal prolapse include:

- Chronic constipation
- Acute or chronic diarrhea
- Pertussis
- Ehlers-Danlos syndrome
- Cystic fibrosis

Of the causes listed, the most common in the United States is chronic constipation.

12. A 3-month-old female infant is brought to your office for evaluation of constipation. She has been passing small, hard stools every 4 to 5 days and the mother is concerned with the infant's fussiness and straining prior to and during stooling. The patient passed meconium within the first few hours of life. Newborn screening was normal. Her current diet consists of 900 mL/day of cow milk–based formula. Physical examination, including rectal examination, is normal. Of the following, which is the *most* appropriate nutritional recommendation?
a) Change to soy formula
b) Change to formula with a lower iron content (1.5 mg/L)
c) Begin rice cereal
d) Change to elemental formula
e) Give pear or apple juice in addition to the current formula

Answer
The answer is e. The most appropriate nutritional recommendation is the addition of pasteurized pear or apple juice. These juices in particular contain increased amounts of sorbitol and fructose, which act as natural osmotic laxatives. Soy formula and rice cereal may exacerbate the condition, leading to increased difficulty with stooling. Lower iron content formulas have no place in infant nutrition and should be avoided. The iron content of standard infant formulas do not lead to constipation. Although most elemental formulas would lead to increased stooling, these formulas are only indicated for cow milk protein–allergic and soy protein–allergic infants. They are significantly more expensive and could represent an unnecessary financial burden for the family in this clinical scenario.

13. A 15-year-old girl is followed up in your office for recurrent headaches for which you had prescribed ibuprofen. The patient returns with severe epigastric pain and melenic stool. The gastroenterologist performs upper endoscopy and finds a large gastric ulcer. What is the *most* likely mechanism by which the ibuprofen caused the ulcer?
a) Decreased pepsinogen production
b) Increased gastrin production
c) Stimulation of *Helicobacter pylori* overgrowth
d) Inhibition of prostaglandin synthesis
e) Gastric mast cell degranulation with histamine release

Answer
The answer is d. Nonsteroidal anti-inflammatory medications are a common cause of gastritis and peptic ulcer disease. These medications can lead to damage of the GI mucosa through the inhibition of prostaglandin synthesis, thereby inhibiting mucous secretion and mucosal bicarbonate.

14. A 16-year-old boy comes to your office complaining of bilateral breast enlargement since you prescribed medication for his gastroesophageal reflux 6 months earlier. Which medication prescribed by you for reflux could have resulted in this complaint?
a) Omeprazole (Prilosec)
b) Lansoprazole (Prevacid)
c) Metoclopramide (Reglan)
d) Ranitidine (Zantac)
e) Famotidine (Pepcid)

Answer
The answer is c. Metoclopramide, a dopamine antagonist, raises lower esophageal sphincter pressure and improves gastric emptying. It is commonly used in the treatment of gastroesophageal reflux disease and gastroparesis. Potential side effects mandate caution in use. Metoclopramide crosses the blood–brain barrier and may produce central nervous system side effects including irritability, sedation, and extrapyramidal side effects such as torticollis. These side effects are transient or reversible with diphenhydramine in almost all cases. Irreversible changes such as tardive dyskinesia have, however, occurred. Dopamine receptor antagonism may also promote hyperprolactinemia, leading to impotence, galactorrhea, gynecomastia, or amenorrhea. These side effects are usually reversed when the medication is discontinued.

15. A 16-year-old girl presents with a several-year history of intermittent scleral icterus. She notices that the whites of her eyes become yellow most often during or after cold or flu-like illnesses. Occasionally, this also happens during periods of stress or menstruation. Otherwise, she is healthy and on no medications. Physical examination is completely normal. Laboratory evaluation is as follows:

Indirect bilirubin = 4 mg/dL

Direct bilirubin = 0.3 mg/dL

Aminotransferase and albumin levels and coagulation studies are all normal. Of the following, which is the *most* likely diagnosis?
a) Gilbert syndrome
b) Epstein-Barr virus infection
c) Chronic viral hepatitis
d) Hepatitis A
e) Rotor syndrome

Answer
The answer is a. Gilbert syndrome is an inherited cause of recurrent, mild, unconjugated hyperbilirubinemia. The condition typically manifests after puberty with mild jaundice during periods of fasting, stress, menstruation, or concomitant illness. The syndrome results from abnormal expression of the enzyme UDP-glucuronosyltransferase. There are no associated negative implications for health or longevity. Some patients may complain of symptoms

ranging from occasional fatigue to abdominal pain. No therapy is indicated.

16. Vitamin B_{12} deficiency is most likely to occur in a child following which of the following surgical procedures?

a) Gastrojejunostomy
b) Resection of jejunum
c) Resection of ileum
d) Colectomy
e) Colostomy

Answer

The answer is c. Vitamin B_{12} receptors are restricted to the ileum and there is no adaptation of absorption of this vitamin following ileal resection. Vitamin B_{12} malabsorption is almost invariably present following resection of more than 100 cm of the terminal ileum.

17. A 2-year-old boy has just swallowed a nickel. Physical examination reveals a quiet child in no distress. Which of the following is the *most* appropriate first step in managing this patient?

a) Administer glucagon intramuscularly.
b) Administer papain.
c) Admit for observation.
d) Complete plain radiographs of the chest and abdomen.
e) Perform emergency endoscopy.

Answer

The answer is d. Coins represent the most frequently ingested foreign body in children. The first and most appropriate step in the management of children with suspected foreign body ingestion is prompt radiographic evaluation to determine the number and location of the coin(s) ingested. If located in the esophagus, the face view of the coin should be seen on an anteroposterior view and the edge on the lateral view. The opposite is true for coins in the trachea. (The edge of the coin is seen on the anteroposterior view and the lateral view shows the face of the coin.)

18. A 3-year-old is brought to your office after swallowing a penny. The x-ray reveals the coin to be in the stomach. What is the next *most* appropriate step in management?

a) Give the child an emetic.
b) Perform gastric lavage.
c) Admit the patient for observation for signs of intestinal obstruction.
d) Discharge the patient and advise the mother to examine stools for the coin.
e) Refer the patient to a gastroenterologist for endoscopic removal of the penny.

Answer

The answer is d. As a general rule, if a coin makes it spontaneously into the stomach, it is expected to make it through the rest of the GI tract. Once it is determined that the coin is in the stomach, the parents should be instructed to examine the patient's stools for passage of the coin. Endoscopic removal of the coin can be delayed for up to 4 weeks unless symptoms of gastric outlet obstruction (emesis, abdominal pain) occur. If after 4 weeks, the parents have not confirmed passage of the coin in the stool, another radiograph should be taken prior to endoscopic removal to confirm the presence and location of the coin.

19. A 3-year-old girl is found crying and drooling in front of an open container of oven cleaner. The bottle was previously full, but is now half empty. On examination in the emergency room, she has blisters and ulceration of her lips and buccal mucosa. Initial management should include which of the following?

a) Induction of emesis to decrease the amount of caustic agent in the GI tract
b) Administration of milk or another neutralizing agent
c) Gastric lavage
d) Intravenous fluids, nothing to eat by mouth, and admission to the hospital

Answer

The answer is d. The clinical scenario presented is consistent with a potentially significant ingestion of a strong alkali. Emesis should not be induced because of the risk of increasing the injury to the esophagus through re-exposure as well as the risk of aspiration. Administration of milk or another neutralizing agent is also contraindicated as this may induce emesis or result in a harmful exothermic reaction with thermal injury to the GI tract. Gastric lavage is also contraindicated, as passage of a nasogastric/orogastric tube would likely induce emesis.

Following a caustic ingestion the symptomatic child should be administered intravenous fluid therapy, admitted to the hospital, and given nothing by mouth until endoscopic evaluation of upper GI tract damage can be made. Endoscopic evaluation should be performed 12 to 24 hours after the ingestion. If it is performed too early, damage may be underestimated.

SUGGESTED READINGS

1. Kay M. Wyllie R. Pediatric foreign bodies and their management. *Curr Gastroenterol Rpt* 2005;7(3):212–218.
2. Kliegman RM, Behrman RE, Jenson HB, et al., eds. *Nelson textbook of pediatrics*, 18th ed. Philadelphia: Saunders, 2007.
3. Walker WA, Kleinman, Mieli-Vergani, et al., eds. *Walker's Pediatric Gastrointestinal Disease: Pathophysiology, Diagnosis, Management*, 5th ed. New York: McGraw-Hill, 2008.
4. Wyllie R, Hyams J, eds. *Pediatric Gastrointestinal and Liver Disease: Pathophysiology, Diagnosis, Management*, 3rd ed. Philadelphia: Saunders, 2005.

Chapter 11

Fluids and Electrolytes

Robert J. Cunningham III

The appropriate fluid and electrolyte therapy involves the understanding of a few basic principles that can be applied systematically to calculate the requirements for an individual patient. The maintenance requirements for water are based on the studies of the energy expenditures of hospitalized children performed by Holliday and Segar. In these studies, the average energy expenditure was measured as a function of body weight. The requirement for water was then calculated by assuming that the child was consuming 2 g of protein/kg per day. A second assumption was that the products of protein metabolism were to be excreted in urine that was neither concentrated nor diluted—that is, urine with a specific gravity of 1.008 to 1.015. Given these two assumptions, the water requirement is then 1 mL/calorie expended. A simplified graph of the data on energy expenditure described in the original work of Holliday and Segar is shown in **Figure 11.1**. By breaking the continuous line into three segments, it is possible to approximate the daily fluid requirements. They are as follows:

- 100 mL/kg for the first 10 kg of body weight
- 50 mL/kg for the second 10 kg of body weight
- 20 mL/kg for each kg above 20 kg (at least until 80 kg is reached)

This is a simple method of estimating maintenance water requirements. The daily electrolyte requirements are summarized in **Table 11.1**.

The fluid and electrolyte requirements of a 40-kg child are outlined in **Tables 11.2** and **11.3** Note that in 0.2% normal saline (NS) solution, the concentration of NaCl is 34 mEq/L, and if 20 mEq of KCl is added to each liter of fluid, then a correct calculation of the water requirements automatically gives the correct complement of Na, K, and Cl. This is why commercially available solutions contain 0.2% NS—because they provide adequate concentrations of electrolytes if the patient has no deficits, is stable, and requires intravenous (IV) fluids only to maintain homeostasis.

A situation that the pediatrician encounters more commonly is when the patient arrives with a history of diarrhea and dehydration and requires not only maintenance IV fluids, but also replenishment of a fluid and electrolyte deficit that has resulted from vomiting and diarrhea. Physical findings that help in estimating the severity of the deficit are shown in **Figure 11.2**.

Note that Figure 11.2 gives an estimation of the percentage of dehydration. To translate this into how much "fluid" the patient has lost, multiply the percentage loss with the body weight in kilograms. The result is the fluid deficit in liters. For example, if you evaluate a 1-year-old child who appears dehydrated, and the best estimate from the physical finding appears to be that he is 10% dehydrated and weighs 10 kg, then 0.10 (10%) × 10 kg = 1 kg (or 1 L) of fluid deficit. Remember, 1 L or 1000 mL of water weighs 1 kg!

When a fluid prescription is calculated for an individual patient, the task should involve answering three questions:

- What is the deficit?
- What is the maintenance fluid requirement?
- What is the estimate of ongoing losses over the next 24 hours?

If this approach is applied consistently, fluid and electrolyte calculations will cease to be perplexing and can become routine. The major source of error when the approach is utilized is the estimation of ongoing losses. This is always a guess, and although (it is hoped) a thoughtful one, like any projection into the future, it is subject to error. Therefore, when a patient is treated with a fluid regimen and the response is not the expected one, always check to determine if a source of continuing fluid loss is present that which you did not anticipate. Or conversely, did you anticipate fluid losses that are not present?

Another calculation that is frequently utilized on board exams is that of free water deficit or free water excess. In order to solve this in a given patient, you need to know the patients weight (in kg) and the serum Na in mEq/L. Then there are 2 assumptions that are made (**Table 11.4**):

- The volume of distribution of Na is the extracellular fluid volume and is calculated by taking 0.6 (l/kg) × weight (kg) = volume of distribution of Na (in liters).
- The number of Na ions will stay constant; the change in concentration will be the result of adding or subtracting water.

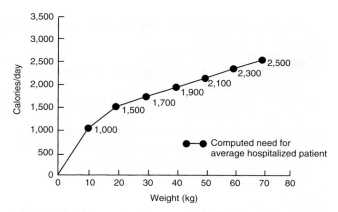

Figure 11.1 Energy requirement as a function of body weight. This calculation allows an estimation of fluid requirements and works out to 1 mL of fluid for each calorie expended. (Modified from Holliday MA, Segar WF. The maintenance need for water in parenteral fluid therapy. *Pediatrics* 1957;19:825.)

% Wt. loss	Sensorium	Mucous membranes	Skin turgor	Eyes	Vital signs	Urine output
3–5	Normal	Normal/dry	Normal/ decreased	Normal	Normal	Normal
6–10	Lethargic	Dry	Decreased	Decreased	Pulse up Respiration rate normal/up	Decreased
10–15	Semicoma	Parched	Marked decrease	Very decreased	Pulse up Respiration rate up BP up/down	Decreased
>15	Coma	Parched	Cold/dry	Very decreased	Pulse weak Respiration rate up BP up/down	Absent

Figure 11.2 Clinical signs as a function of the degree of dehydration. As pointed out in the text, these signs depend on the intravascular and extracellular fluid volumes. BP, blood pressure.

TABLE 11.1

MAINTENANCE ELECTROLYTE REQUIREMENTS

Easiest way to remember is 1 . . . 2 . . . 3
1. mEq of potassium/kg/day
2. mEq of sodium/kg/day
3. mEq of chloride/kg/day

TABLE 11.2

MAINTENANCE CALCULATIONS FOR A 40-KG CHILD: FLUIDS

Water requirement
100 mL/kg/24 hour × 10 kg = 1000 mL *plus*
50 mL/kg/24 hour × 10 kg = 500 mL *plus*
20 mL/kg/24 hour × 20 kg = 400 mL
Total water requirement = 1900 mL

TABLE 11.3

MAINTENANCE CALCULATIONS FOR A 40-KG CHILD: ELECTROLYTES

Severity of deficit
K = 1 mEq/kg/24 hour × 40 kg = 40 mEq
Na = 2 mEq/kg/24 hour × 40 kg = 80 mEq
Cl = 3 mEq/kg/24 hour × 40 kg = 120 mEq
Therefore, 2 L of 0.2% NS plus 20 mEq of KCl/L will approximate the requirements.
0.2% NaCl provides 34 mEq of Na/L.
Addition of 5% dextrose is recommended.

NS, normal saline.

TABLE 11.4

CALCULATION OF FREE WATER DEFICIT OR FREE WATER EXCESS

V_{Dist} L = 0.6 × body weight in kg × 1 L/kg
V_{Dist} L × Na_{Serum} mEq/L = # of Na in mEq
# of mEq of Na/$V_{New\ Dist}$ L = 140 mEq/L
# of mEq of Na /140 mEq/L = $V_{New\ Dist}$ L
Deficit or excess = $V_{New\ Dist}$ L − V_{Dist} L

In the review exercises, three cases are presented for which you are asked to estimate fluid deficits and calculate replacement regimens.

REVIEW EXERCISES

QUESTIONS

Case 1

A 1-year-old boy is brought to you with vomiting and diarrhea of 4 days' duration. Initially, the mother gave him an oral electrolyte maintenance solution (Pedialyte) every 3 to 4 hours, but the baby has been vomiting all feeds for the last 24 hours. The mother does not know when he last urinated.

The infant appeared sleepy and responded only disinterestedly when blood was drawn.

- Temperature, 38°C (100°F); pulse, 142/minute; respiratory rate, 32/minute; weight, 10 kg.
- Skin turgor was decreased with obvious tenting. Nail beds were pink with prompt capillary refill. Orbits were "squishy."

1. The estimated degree of dehydration is:
a) 3.5%
b) 5%
c) 10%
d) 15%

Answer

The answer is c. My estimation of the degree of dehydration is 10%. The skin turgor is decreased with obvious tenting, which suggests 5% to 10% dehydration. The patient is listless and responds only when blood is drawn; this also suggests a level of dehydration of approximately 10%. The fact that capillary refill is present and no comment is made that the extremities are cold or that the pulse is not higher or thready goes against 15% dehydration.

2. Calculate the fluid requirements for the next 24 hours assuming his diarrhea persists and he loses an additional 400 mL of fluids during the next 24 hours.
a) 1200 mL
b) 1600 mL
c) 2100 mL
d) 2400 mL

Answer

The answer is d. My calculations are shown in the following:

- Deficit: 10 kg × 10% = 1 kg = 1000 mL*
- Maintenance: 10 kg × 100 mL/kg = 1000 mL
- Losses ongoing (an estimate) = 400 mL
- Total = 2400 mL

3. Which of the following would represent the *best* choice for the initial fluid orders?
a) D_5W (5% dextrose in water)/0.2% NS to run at 100 mL/hour. Add 20 mEq of KCl/L after urination
b) D_5W/0.45% NS to run at 150 mL/hour for the next 8 hours. Add 20 mEq of KCl/L after urination
c) D_5W/0.45% NS to run at 150 mL/hour for the next 8 hours
d) 9% NS to run at 150 mL/hour for the next 8 hours

Answer

The answer is b. A good general approach is to replenish half of the estimated need for 24 hours in the first 8 hours. This helps to eliminate the deficit more quickly. One choice that was not given and would be a very reasonable one would be to restore the circulating blood volume quickly by first giving a bolus of 0.9% NS at 20 mL/kg over 20 minutes or as quickly as the IV line will run. At levels of dehydration that compromise circulating blood volume, the first goal is to normalize the intravascular volume and then proceed with normal fluid resuscitation. I do not include the bolus fluid in my calculations and would give fluids as described in choice *b* following the 0.9% NS.

*1 kg = 1000 mL of fluid

4. Which of the following is *most* helpful in assessing the adequacy of the therapy?
a) Normalization of electrolytes
b) Patient's level of alertness, skin turgor, pulse rate, and blood urea nitrogen (BUN)
c) Presence of diarrhea, resumption of urine output, and decrease in irritability
d) Normal creatinine clearance, decrease in the white blood cell count and hemoglobin levels to normal values, which were increased secondary to hemoconcentration

Answer

The answer is b. The best way to assess fluid balance is by repeatedly examining the patient. Laboratory values are of little benefit in the ongoing evaluation of fluid therapy.

The second case is a slight variation of the first one, but with important implications for fluid therapy.

Case 2

An 8-month-old infant is brought to the emergency department with a history of fever, diarrhea for 96 hours, and vomiting for the past 24 hours. Beginning 4 days ago, fever and profuse diarrhea developed. He was switched to an oral electrolyte maintenance solution (Pedialyte) but was getting no nutrition, so he was given boiled skim milk for the next 48 hours. Yesterday, he became irritable and began vomiting all feeds.

The physical examination reveals a very irritable infant with a high-pitched scream when disturbed. Temperature, 38°C (100°F); pulse, 130/minute; blood pressure, 80/45 mm Hg. His fontanelle is flat but not sunken, his eyeballs feel normal, and his skin has an odd "silly putty" or doughy feel.

5. The estimated degree of dehydration is:
a) 3.5%
b) 5%
c) 10%
d) 15%

Answer

The answer is c.

6. What would you predict the serum sodium to be in this patient at presentation?
a) 125 mEq/L
b) 135 mEq/L
c) 145 mEq/L
d) 155 mEq/L

The following electrolyte values were obtained:

- Na = 156 mEq/L
- K = 5.4 mEq/L
- Cl = 123 mEq/L
- HCO_3 = 17 mEq/L

- BUN = 36 mg/dL
- Creatinine = 1.2 mg/dL
- Glucose = 126 mg/dL

Calculate the serum osmolarity.

The formula for calculating the serum osmolarity is shown below along with the calculations for this patient.

- $(2 \times [Na]) + 10 + ([BUN]/3) + ([Glucose]/18)$
- $(2 \times 156) + 10 + (36/3) + (126/18) = 341$ mOsm/L.
  In most cases, a reasonable estimate of osmolarity can be obtained by multiplying the value for the serum sodium by 2 and adding 10. The glucose and BUN do not add much to the calculation when the levels are in the normal range. Obviously, if one or the other is elevated, then it may make a significant contribution to the serum osmolarity.

Answer

The answer is d. Although this patient does not appear as "volume-contracted" as the first one, there is a critical difference between them. The second patient was given boiled skim milk as a fluid replacement solution. Boiling the milk removes the water and thereby makes it solute-rich. It is being used to replace losses secondary to diarrhea, in which the losses are more water than solute. Because a low-solute loss is being replaced with a very high-solute solution, the patient is at high risk for hypernatremia. Patients with hypertonic dehydration do not present the same clinical picture as those with the more routine forms of dehydration that we are accustomed to evaluating. If you look at Figure 10.2, the signs of dehydration are the result of intravascular and extracellular fluid contraction. If we administer hypertonic solutions into the extracellular space, the solute serves to draw fluid from the intracellular space to the intravascular and extracellular compartments. Hence, the dehydration in hypertonic states is an intracellular phenomenon, and the extracellular fluid volume is reasonably maintained. The hints that this patient was hypertonic, aside from the history of being given boiled skim milk, are the high-pitched scream and extreme irritability. The other characteristic is the "silly putty" or doughy feel to the skin, a characteristic of patients with hypertonic dehydration. These clues should alert you to the fact that the patient may be hypertonic and therefore more dehydrated than he first appears.

7. Calculate the fluid requirements for the next 24 hours, assuming another 400 mL of diarrhea.
- a) 2000 mL
- b) 2400 mL
- c) 3000 mL
- d) 3500 mL

Answer

The answer is b. The answer, as in the first case, is 2400 mL. The percentage of dehydration, maintenance fluid requirement, and ongoing losses are all identical to those of the first patient.

8. What is the optimal fluid regimen?
- a) $D_5W/0.45\%$ NS to run at 150 mL/hour for 8 hours and at 100 mL/hour for the next 16 hours: Add 20 mEq of KCl/L after patient urinates
- b) $D_5W/0.9\%$ NS plus 20 mEq of KCl/L to run at 150 mL/hour for 8 hours and at 75 mL/hour thereafter
- c) $D_5W/0.3\%$ NS plus 20 mEq of KCl/L to run at 70 mL/hour for 48 hours
- d) Run fluids as outlined in choice b and introduce oral feeds ad libitum at 24 hours.

Answer

The answer is c. This is where the second case differs significantly from the first. The method used to derive this answer was to calculate the maintenance for the second 24 hours (1000 mL), add it to the requirements for the first 24 hours (2400 mL), and divide the resultant sum by 48 hours so that the dehydration would be corrected slowly. Why should we tarry with this one? The reason is that hypernatremia has developed in the patient during a period of 4 days, and the normal response of the brain is to generate "idiogenic" osmoles from amino acids (lysine). This response serves to keep the intracranial osmolarity identical to that of the serum, so that as the dehydration progresses, the brain cells are protected from severe dehydration. Only a vascular barrier is present between the circulating blood and brain cells. If idiogenic osmoles were not formed, intracellular dehydration of the brain cells would be severe and life- threatening. It takes 48 hours for these osmoles to develop, and it also takes time for them to be metabolized as the osmolarity returns to normal. If fluids were administered quickly, the serum osmolarity would drop suddenly, a net movement of water from the circulation into the brain would occur, and the result would be the development of cerebral edema, seizures, and possibly death. Hence, in patients who are severely hypernatremic, correction should proceed at a rate slow enough to give the brain cells time to metabolize the idiogenic osmoles. In this way, sudden intracranial shifts of fluid are prevented!

Please note that the preceding discussion refers to patients in whom hypernatremia develops during days, not hours. In a patient who has diabetes insipidus and in whom the serum sodium level rises from 140 mEq/L in the morning to 168 mEq/L in the evening, the sodium level may be corrected quickly; idiogenic osmoles have not developed because the process takes time. A good general rule for the correction of hypernatremia or hyponatremia is not to attempt to correct the abnormalities at a rate different from the rate at which the abnormalities were established.

After the first 18 hours of therapy, the following electrolyte values were obtained:

- Na = 152 mEq/L
- K = 5.4 mEq/L
- Cl = 115 mEq/L
- HCO_3 = 22 mEq/L
- BUN = 27 mg/dL
- Creatinine = 0.8 mg/dL
- Glucose = 378 mg/dL

9. Your next step in the treatment should be:
a) Give 1 U of regular insulin/kg subcutaneously.
b) Give 0.1 U/kg every hour IV until the blood sugar level is <200 mg/dL.
c) Remove dextrose from the IV fluids.
d) Continue current treatment and give insulin only if the blood sugar level is >500 mg/dL.

Answer
The answer is c. The best answer is to remove dextrose from the IV solutions. Again, a sudden drop in osmolarity is to be avoided; therefore, the blood glucose should not drop suddenly either. Hyperglycemia is a frequent complication of hypernatremic dehydration, and blood glucose levels should be followed up carefully.

After 30 hours of treatment, the following electrolyte values were obtained:

- Na = 148 mEq/L
- K = 5.4 mEq/L
- Cl = 112 mEq/L
- HCO_3 = 25 mEq/L
- BUN = 23 mg/dL
- Creatinine = 0.7 mg/dL
- Glucose = 150 mg/dL

10. Fifteen minutes later, the patient has a seizure. The *most* likely cause is:
a) Hypocalcemia
b) Hypoglycemia
c) Pyridoxine deficiency
d) Intracranial hemorrhage

Answer
The answer is a. The answer is hypocalcemia. This, too, is a complication of hypernatremic dehydration. Serum calcium determinations should be followed up closely and calcium supplements given if hypocalcemia is developing.

11. Calculate the free water deficit. It is:
a) 6 L
b) 6.68 L
c) 680 mL
d) 340 mL

Answer
The answer is c. Please see Table 11.4

Volume of distribution is 10 kg × 0.6 = 6 L
6 L × 156 mEq/L = 936 meq of Na
963 mEq Na/140 mEq/L = $V_{New\ Dist}$ L or 6.68 L
Deficit = 6.68 L − 6.0 L = 680 mL
Therefore, free water deficit = 680 mL

Summary of Hypernatremic Dehydration
Hypernatremic dehydration occurs when hypotonic fluid is lost (e.g., diarrhea) and replaced with a hypertonic fluid. A source of hypertonic fluid can nearly always be identified, and boiled skim milk is an old, grandmother's remedy. When hypertonic dehydration is suspected, initiate fluid resuscitation slowly, obtain the electrolyte determinations as quickly as possible, and if the serum sodium is high, tailor the fluid resuscitation scheme over 48 hours. Watch for both hyperglycemia and hypocalcemia. The critical variable is the time taken to correct the deficit, not the type of fluids that you choose to administer. If you correct too quickly with a more hypertonic fluid (e.g., 0.9% NS), the kidneys will excrete the additional sodium and conserve water, and the correction of the serum osmolarity will proceed at nearly the same rate as if you had corrected with pure water. The only way to limit the rate of fall of the serum sodium is to change the time frame over which you are making the correction.

Case 3
A 10-year-old developmentally delayed white girl was well until 4 days before admission, when she developed low-grade fever. Because she did not appear to be very ill, these symptoms were treated only with aspirin. Her oral intake of fluids was well maintained until 2 days before admission, when it decreased significantly, and she subsequently began to refuse fluids. On the day before admission, her intake remained poor, and she passed green, watery stools. Approximately 12 hours before admission, her temperature spiked to 41°C (105°F), and an erythematous rash erupted on her face, trunk, and upper extremities. Close questioning revealed that she had apparently not voided in the last 2 days.

Physical examination revealed a semicomatose child with a generalized rash. Her weight was 44 kg (surface area, 1.15 m²); blood pressure, 70/50 supine and 50/0 sitting; pulse, 200/minute; respirations, 32/minute. Her mucous membranes were parched, and her peripheral extremities were cold and moderately cyanotic. She had a whitish tonsillar exudate and a beefy red tongue.

12. The estimated degree of dehydration is:
a) 3.5%
b) 5%
c) 10%
d) 15%

Answer

The answer is d. This patient is 15% dehydrated and in shock. Her blood pressure is down to 70/50 mm Hg, her pulse is 200/minute, and she has poorly perfused extremities, evidenced by the fact that they are both cold and cyanotic.

13. The first step in therapy should be which of the following?

a) $D_5W/0.45\%$ NS to run at 490 mL/hour for 8 hours

b) $D_5W/0.45\%$ NS plus 20 mEq of KCl/L to run at 490 mL/hour

c) 0.9% NS, 900 mL to run over 20 minutes followed by $D_5W/0.45\%$ NS plus 20 mEq of KCl to run at 500 mL/hour

d) 0.9% NS, 900 mL to run over 30 minutes followed by $D_5W/0.45\%$ NS to run at 500 mL/hour: Add 20 mEq of KCl/L when the patient has urinated twice

e) 0.9% NS, 900 mL to run over 20 minutes followed by $D_5W/0.45\%$ NS to run at a rate of 200 mL/hour for 24 hours: Add 20 mEq of KCl/L when the patient has urinated twice

Answer

The answer is d. The infusion of 0.9% NS may have to be repeated more than once to re-establish the circulating vascular volume. You would want to see improved perfusion, and evidence of this would be an increase in the blood pressure, a lower pulse rate, and warmer extremities. A rate of 500 mL/hour seems high, but as shown from the calculations below, it will replace approximately half of the deficit in 8 hours.

Approach to the fluid calculations:

- Deficit (0.15 × 44 kg) = 6600 mL
- Maintenance = 1980 mL/day
    = 8580 mL/24 hour

Assuming *no* ongoing losses, if intravascular volume is depleted, give 20 mL of 0.9% NS/kg over 20 minutes. In most cases, you should calculate the total fluids for 1 day, and then give half of the total in the first 8 hours.

After you have initiated therapy, the following laboratory values that were sent *stat* are given to you:

- Na = 145 mEq/L
- K = 3.3 mEq/L
- Cl = 110 mEq/L
- HCO_3 = 10 mEq/L
- BUN = 96 mg/dL
- Creatinine = 6.7 mg/dL
- Hemoglobin = 15.8 g/dL
- Hematocrit = 50%

14. Your next step is to:

a) Decrease the rate of fluid administration to insensible loss, remove KCl from the IV fluids, and give 1 mEq of $NaHCO_3$/kg.

b) Obtain a urinalysis and a urine specimen for measurement of the sodium and creatinine.

c) Decrease the IV fluid rate to two thirds of maintenance and correct the acidosis with a solution of $D_5W/0.33\%$ NS plus 50 mEq of $NaHCO_3$/L.

d) Order renal ultrasonography and a urine culture and continue current IV administration of fluids.

Answer

The answer is b. Do not assume a patient is in renal failure until hydration is normal and evidence of renal insufficiency is still present. Volume contraction and severe dehydration can cause severe laboratory abnormalities. Choices *a* and *c* both assume that this patient is in renal failure; and even if this proves to be the case, she needs adequate circulating volume. She should be back to a normal state of hydration before the IV fluid administration is decreased. Choice *d* is less likely than choice *b* to help you determine whether this patient is in acute renal failure.

Urinalysis shows the following values:

- Specific gravity = 1.027
- Protein = 1+
- Ketones = 3+
- pH = 5.0
- Na = 4 mEq/L
- Creatinine = 450 mg/L

15. The data are *most* consistent with which of the following:

a) Chronic renal failure

b) Acute renal failure

c) Glomerulonephritis

d) Acute dehydration

Answer

The answer is d. The fractional excretion of sodium is <1%, which indicates that the renal tubules are continuing to conserve sodium, and therefore volume, in the face of dehydration. This is the desired response. Were the urine sodium elevated, it would mean that the kidneys were no longer capable of conserving sodium, and this would be a consequence of tubular damage. In general, when you see a urine sodium level of <10 mEq/L, you can assume that the kidneys are conserving sodium well.

The method of calculating the fractional excretion of sodium is as follows:

- $FE_{Na} = ([U_{Na} \times PCr]/[UC_r \times P_{Na}]) \times 100 = ([4 \text{ mEq/L} \times 6.7 \text{ mg/dL}]/[450 \text{ mg/dL} \times 145 \text{mEq/L}]) \times 100 = 0.0004 \times 100 = 0.04\%$
- Fractional excretion of sodium (FE_{Na}) <1% indicates dehydration.
- FE_{Na} >1% indicates acute renal insufficiency.

Comment

The preceding scenario is a real one, and I chose it to demonstrate that even if a patient has severe abnormalities and a very high creatinine level, this approach must be followed. The patient in this example received 8 L of IV fluids over 24 hours, and her serum creatinine was 1.2 mg/dL with a BUN of 35 mg/dL on the day after the IV fluids had been administered. And yes, she did have streptococcal pharyngitis! Her pharynx was very inflamed, and the pain was sufficiently intense that she did not take in any oral fluids for 2 to 3 days before she was seen. She was given penicillin for this condition in addition to the IV hydration.

SUGGESTED READINGS

1. Finberg L. Hypernatremic (hypertonic) dehydration in infants. *N Engl J Med* 1973;289:196.
2. Finberg L, Kravath R, Fleischman A. *Water and electrolytes in pediatrics.* Philadelphia: Saunders, 1982.
3. Friedman AL. Pediatric hydration therapy: historical review and a new approach. *Kidney Int* 2005;67:380–388.
4. Holliday MA, Segar WF. The maintenance need for water in parenteral fluid therapy. *Pediatrics* 1957;19:825.
5. Mathew OP, Jones AS, James E, et al. Neonatal renal failure: usefulness of diagnostic indices. *Pediatrics* 1980;65:57–60.
6. Roberts KB. Fluid and electrolytes: parenteral fluid therapy. *Pediatr Rev* 2001;22:380–386.

Chapter 12

Proteinuria and Hematuria

Robert J. Cunningham III

This chapter discusses the evaluation of the child or adolescent with proteinuria or hematuria. Because proteinuria is more likely than hematuria to indicate significant renal disease, the focus is first on the major causes and evaluation of proteinuria, after which the etiology and workup of hematuria are considered.

PROTEINURIA AND NEPHROTIC SYNDROME

The most severe form of proteinuria is the nephrotic syndrome, which is characterized by:

■ Proteinuria (>40 mg/m^2 per hour)
■ Elevated serum cholesterol
■ Evidence of edema

To understand the approach to patients with lesser degrees of proteinuria, one must first understand the rationale for the evaluation of patients with nephrotic syndrome. In 10% of patients, the condition is secondary to a systemic disease and the three diseases that are commonly seen in the pediatric age group are Henoch-Schönlein purpura, systemic lupus erythematosus, and hemolytic uremic syndrome. In the other 90% of the cases, the nephrotic syndrome represents a primary kidney disease and the three most common histologic causes of primary nephrotic syndrome in children, as shown in Table 12.1 are:

■ Minimal-change disease
■ Focal segmental glomerulosclerosis (FSGS)
■ Membranoproliferative glomerulonephritis (MPGN)

TABLE 12.1

HISTOLOGY OF UNSELECTED PATIENTS WITH NEPHROTIC SYNDROME

Histology	No.	%
Minimal-change disease	398	76.4
Focal sclerosis	45	8.6
Membranoproliferative glomerulonephritis	39	7.5
Mesangial proliferative glomerulonephritis	12	2.3
Proliferative glomerulonephritis	12	2.3
Membranous glomerulonephritis	8	1.5
Other	7	1.4
Total	521	100.0

The data in Table 12.1 are derived from the International Study of Kidney Disease in Children, a cooperative study performed during the 1960s and 1970s in a large number of centers in the United States, Canada, Europe, and Japan. The data represent the histologic diagnoses of all patients between 1 and 17 years of age who presented with nephrotic syndrome. They remain relevant today, although the incidence of FSGS may be increasing relative to that of minimal-change disease. A patient younger than 1 year diagnosed with nephrotic syndrome should be referred directly to a pediatric nephrologist because the child may have congenital nephrotic syndrome, a life-threatening illness that is discussed in the subsequent text.

The clinical characteristics of patients with the three major types of nephrotic syndrome are summarized in Table 12.2.

Minimal-Change Disease

Patients with minimal-change disease are characteristically of preschool age. Boys are more frequently affected; the male-to-female ratio is 6:4. Of these children, 23% have hematuria and 18% have hypertension. In most cases, the hematuria is microscopic. The cholesterol values are severely elevated, usually in the range of 300 to 500 mg/dL; serum cholesterol levels <250 mg/dL are unusual. The serum creatinine values may be elevated, although the elevations are usually mild. *The hallmark of minimal-change disease is that this form of nephrotic syndrome responds to daily prednisone therapy with total clearing of the proteinuria.* Furthermore, 90% of the patients with minimal-change disease who will respond to prednisone therapy do so within 4 weeks.

Once a patient has responded to daily prednisone therapy, the standard is to continue prednisone on alternate days for 4 weeks, then discontinue the steroid therapy. Unfortunately, relapse in minimal-change disease is the rule rather than the exception. Patients who have responded to prednisone therapy with total clearing of the proteinuria can be divided into three subgroups according to their course:

- Thirty-nine percent never have a relapse and never require another course of prednisone therapy.
- Nineteen percent have relapses at infrequent intervals (fewer than two in a 6-month period).
- Forty-two percent have more frequent relapses (more than two in a 6-month period).

The first group poses little difficulty. Patients in the second group can be treated with daily prednisone therapy. Most pediatric nephrologists continue the daily therapy for 3 to 4 days after the proteinuria has cleared, after which alternate-day prednisone therapy is given for 2 to 3 weeks. For patients who relapse only one to three times each year, the prednisone exposure is acceptable, and side effects are minimal. Patients in the third group are difficult to manage. Because neither the side effects of steroid therapy nor the edema associated with nephrosis is acceptable, a number of alternative therapies are utilized. Cyclophosphamide or chlorambucil alone without other therapy offers a 70% chance of a 2.5- to 3-year remission. Likewise, daily cyclosporine therapy can be given instead of prednisone and

TABLE 12.2

NEPHROTIC SYNDROME: CLINICAL CHARACTERISTICS AT DIAGNOSIS

Characteristic	Minimal-Change Disease (%)	FSGS (%)	MPGN (%)
Age <6 years	79.6	50.0	2.6
Female sex	39.9	30.6	64.1
Hypertension (>98th percentile)	13.5	33.3	27.0
Hematuria	23.0	48.0	48.0
Low C3 level	1.5	3.7	74.0
Cholesterol <250 mg/dL	5.4	8.6	19.4
Increased creatinine	32.5	40.6	50.0
Response to prednisone	93.0	7.0	0

C3, third component of complement; FSGS, focal segmental glomerulosclerosis; MPGN, membranoproliferative glomerulonephritis.

may maintain patients with minimal-change disease in remission. The advantages of these therapies must be weighed against their side effects.

The side effects of cyclophosphamide include:

■ Hair loss
■ Leukopenia
■ Hemorrhagic cystitis
■ Sterility in male patients while they are taking the drug and possibly for 5 to 10 years following therapy
■ Risk for neoplasia, although cases of cancer following the use of cyclophosphamide to treat nephrotic syndrome have not been reported

The side effects of chlorambucil include:

■ Leukopenia
■ Sterility in male patients, probably similar to that associated with cyclophosphamide
■ Risk for neoplasia, with reported cases of lymphoma following the use of chlorambucil to treat nephrotic syndrome

The side effects of cyclosporine include:

■ Gingival hyperplasia
■ Hypertension
■ Renal insufficiency
■ Headache
■ Tremors

The lymphomas associated with chlorambucil therapy for frequently relapsing nephrotic syndrome occurred in patients who had received a total dose of chlorambucil >14 mg/kg. The dosage currently administered is 0.01 mg/kg per day for 8 weeks, making a total dose of 8.4 mg/kg. No tumors have been reported since the standard therapy was lowered to this total dose.

The choice of agent depends on the patient's ability to tolerate side effects. Most youngsters would rather not take cyclophosphamide because of the hair loss, but this is a temporary phenomenon, and the hair does grow back.

The long-term prognosis of patients with minimal-change disease is excellent. In most cases, the disease remits and the proteinuria and edema resolve.

Two important complications of this disease are worthy of note:

■ Primary peritonitis
■ Vascular thromboses or pulmonary emboli

Patients in whom nephrotic syndrome recurs and ascites develops are susceptible to primary peritonitis. The most common organisms causing this are *Streptococcus pneumoniae* and *Escherichia coli*. This diagnosis must be excluded in any patient with nephrotic syndrome who is receiving steroid therapy and who presents with abdominal pain, with or without fever.

Vascular thromboses or pulmonary emboli may develop in patients with active nephrotic syndrome, who are in a hypercoagulable state. These entities must be considered in patients with nephrotic syndrome who present with pain in an extremity, a change in the color of an extremity, or a sudden onset of chest pain.

When the proteinuria does not clear totally after 4 weeks of daily steroid therapy, other diagnoses and renal biopsy must be considered. The continuation of daily prednisone therapy in such cases exposes patients to the side effects of steroid therapy without much hope of benefit, so that they simultaneously experience the worst of the disease and the worst of the treatment.

Focal Segmental Glomerulosclerosis

The most likely diagnosis in young patients who meet the criteria for minimal-change disease but fail to respond to prednisone therapy is FSGS. The clinical characteristics of patients with this histologic diagnosis are shown in Table 12.2. It is difficult to distinguish between FSGS and minimal-change disease on the basis of a patient's clinical signs and symptoms at presentation. A large percentage of patients with FSGS have hematuria (33%) and hypertension (48%). As in minimal-change disease, the serum cholesterol is severely elevated in FSGS, and the creatinine level may also be elevated. *The only consistent feature that distinguishes patients with FSGS is that their proteinuria persists despite prednisone therapy.* Only 7% of patients with FSGS respond initially to prednisone therapy. The prognosis for patients with FSGS is poor, with 50% to 70% progressing to chronic renal failure during a 5- to 10-year time frame. Although a number of treatment options are available, including high-dose cyclosporine and high-dose intravenous methylprednisolone, the success rates with these options do not exceed 50% to 60%.

Unfortunately, FSGS is increasing in importance because the incidence is rising, particularly in the adolescent and young adult African-American population. A study done in Houston, Texas, examined the incidence of FSGS in renal biopsies prior to 1990 and compared it with those done from 1990 to 1998. The percentage of biopsies that showed FSGS increased from 23% to 47% over this time frame. In children older than 8 years, the incidence of FSGS doubled from 33% to 67%. The incidence of FSGS in adults is also increasing, especially in young African-American men; the reasons for this sudden increase in this specific population are not clear.

Additionally, this disease recurs in a transplanted kidney in approximately 30% of patients who have undergone transplantation.

Membranoproliferative Glomerulonephritis

The clinical features of MPGN differ significantly from those of both minimal-change disease and FSGS. MPGN is more common in girls and children who are 8 years of age or older. Hematuria and hypertension are common, and the *level of the third component of complement (C3) is depressed* in 75% of the cases at the initial presentation. If it is suspected that MPGN is the cause of nephrotic syndrome, a renal biopsy should be performed before therapy is initiated. Daily steroid therapy can exacerbate hypertension, and numerous anecdotal reports have appeared of the development of malignant hypertension in patients with MPGN treated with high-dose prednisone. Patients with MPGN are often treated with a low dose of prednisone on alternate days for years. Despite therapy, renal insufficiency develops in 10% to 40% of patients.

Congenital Nephrotic Syndrome

Congenital nephrotic syndrome should be considered in any infant who presents with proteinuria and edema in the first year of life. This disease is inherited (in an autosomal-recessive pattern) and the highest frequency is in the Finnish population. Congenital nephrotic syndrome is associated with the following:

- Maternal history of oligohydramnios during pregnancy
- High concentration of α-fetoprotein in the amniotic fluid
- Very large placenta at birth

Most patients are edematous in the first week of life, and all are edematous by 3 months of age. Renal biopsy in these patients shows diffuse mesangial sclerosis. The prognosis is dismal, and without aggressive therapy, most children die of sepsis in the first year of life, most commonly caused by *E. coli.* Patients generally die before renal failure develops. Because the urinary losses of protein are massive, resulting in protein malnutrition and an immune deficiency, the therapeutic approach involves stemming the protein losses with either unilateral or bilateral nephrectomy. Peritoneal dialysis and daily infusions of albumin have been used to maintain these infants until they have

grown sufficiently to undergo successful renal transplantation. If patients grow well enough to receive a kidney transplant, the success rate is high, and the disease does not recur in the new kidney.

Evaluation of Proteinuria

The question frequently confronting the pediatrician is how to evaluate a patient when proteinuria is discovered on routine urinalysis. An approach to patients with this finding is outlined in the algorithm in **Figure 12.1.** The first rule is that proteinuria is not significant unless it is *persistent and present in both the supine and standing positions.* Therefore, when eight urine specimens are tested and protein is found in only five, the patient does not require further evaluation. When no protein is found in specimens obtained in the supine position, the patient probably has *postural proteinuria,* a benign entity. If you examine the algorithm, you will note that the second urine specimen obtained is a first morning specimen, to measure urine filtration in the supine position while the patient was sleeping. If this specimen is negative for protein, the extent of the evaluation is reduced, and the patient is spared the inconvenience of performing an orthostatic proteinuria test, outlined in **Table 12.3.**

If the protein in the urine is both persistent and nonpostural, the age of the patient dictates how to proceed. Children younger than 7 years can be followed up clinically and treated only if the proteinuria worsens or edema develops. It is wise to check the serum protein levels; if the albumin level is reduced, treatment with prednisone is warranted.

The difficult decision is if a trial of prednisone is given to an asymptomatic patient and the proteinuria does not clear. Then, the logical next step is to perform a renal biopsy but if the patient has no edema, has normal renal function and if proteinuria persists, one may defer the

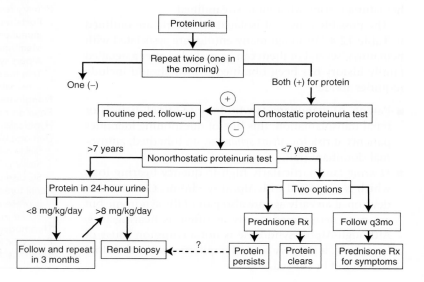

Figure 12.1 Algorithm for the evaluation of proteinuria.

TABLE 12.3

TEST FOR ORTHOSTATIC PROTEINURIA

1. Have patient void before bedtime between 9:00 and 10:00 p.m. and save specimen in a labeled container.
2. Patient should then go to bed and lie flat. At midnight, patient should void into a container (while in bed). Again, put the urine specimen in a container and label it.
3. Patient should void again between 5:00 and 6:00 a.m. (remaining in bed and flat). Again, place specimen in labeled container. Repeat procedure between 7:00 and 7:30 a.m. (patient still in bed, still lying flat).
4. Patient may then rise. Obtain another urine specimen between 9:00 and 9:30 a.m. The specimen may be obtained in the standing or sitting position. Place the specimen in a labeled container. Patients should bring urine sample with them to the next clinic visit (all five specimens in separate containers).

A result is positive when the 5:00 a.m. and 7:00 a.m. specimens are negative for protein. This finding is indicative of *postural proteinuria,* for which the prognosis is excellent.

biopsy and follow. This is the reason for the dashed line and "?" leading to biopsy in the algorithm. Remember, in children of this age, the most likely diagnosis is minimal-change disease.

In children older than 7 years, the serum albumin level and total protein concentrations should be determined. In addition, a 24-hour urine specimen should be obtained for protein level determination. In the algorithm, renal biopsy is recommended if the protein level is >800 mg/m². This is not a firm rule; if the patient is asymptomatic, another option is to repeat the 24-hour urine test in 4 to 6 weeks. If the proteinuria is diminishing, following-up the patient clinically and repeating the 24-hour urine test at monthly intervals is acceptable. Obviously, if the proteinuria is increasing, then a renal biopsy is more urgently required.

HEMATURIA

Isolated hematuria is much less worrisome than proteinuria to the pediatric nephrologist. If a patient presents with both hematuria and proteinuria, the evaluation should follow the proteinuria algorithm. The evaluation of isolated hematuria is somewhat more streamlined.

The possible causes of isolated hematuria are outlined in Table 12.4. Although many entities are associated with hematuria, several of them can be excluded after a detailed family history has been obtained, which should include inquiries about:

- Parents or grandparents who have required dialysis or renal transplantation; this line of questioning identifies patients at risk for *Alport syndrome,* an inherited, autosomal-dominant trait.
- *Hearing loss,* particularly high-frequency hearing loss, which is associated with Alport syndrome. *Cataracts* that develop at an early age are also part of the syndrome but are not encountered nearly as often as hearing loss. Although Alport syndrome is not a common cause of hematuria, it has very serious implications and therefore should not be missed.

- A family history of benign hematuria, which may point to *thin basement membrane disease.*
- A family history of nephrolithiasis, which may suggest the presence of *hypercalciuria,* a very common cause of hematuria; 80% of patients with hypercalciuria have a family history of nephrolithiasis.
- A history of *sickle cell trait,* which is a very common cause of hematuria, both gross and microscopic, in the African-American population. The incidence of hematuria is higher in individuals with sickle cell trait than in those with homozygous sickle cell disease.

TABLE 12.4

CAUSES OF HEMATURIA

Glomerular causes
Secondary to systemic diseases
  Systemic lupus erythematosus
  Henoch-Schönlein purpura
  Hemolytic uremic syndrome
  Subacute bacterial endocarditis
  Shunt nephritis (seen in patients with a ventriculoatrial shunt)
Primary renal diseases
  Poststreptococcal glomerulonephritis
  Immunoglobulin A nephropathy
  Membranoproliferative glomerulonephritis
  Alport syndrome
  Thin basement membrane disease (benign familial recurrent hematuria)
Nonglomerular causes
Renal stones
Hypercalciuria
Hemoglobinopathies
  Sickle cell trait
  Sickle cell disease (less commonly than trait)
  SC disease
Renal tumors (a rare cause in children unless a palpable tumor is present)
Vascular malformations
Thrombocytopenia
Polycystic kidneys
Tuberous sclerosis with angiomyolipomas

TABLE 12.5

RECOMMENDED STUDIES FOR PATIENTS WITH HEMATURIA

Urinalysis
Determination of serum electrolytes and creatinine, and blood urea levels
Complete blood cell count
Urinary calcium/creatinine ratio
Sickle cell screening in selected patients
Renal ultrasonography in patients with gross hematuria or associated abdominal pain
Urine culture in selected patients or those with pyuria or leukocyte esterase found on urinalysis

After a detailed history has been taken and a physical examination performed, certain studies should be carried out for patients with isolated hematuria. These are listed in Table 12.5.

In addition to hypercalciuria and sickle cell trait, two other entities are common causes of hematuria and worthy of special mention:

- Immunoglobulin A (IgA) nephropathy
- Poststreptococcal glomerulonephritis

Immunoglobulin A Nephropathy

Few historical features are specific for IgA nephropathy; the diagnosis can be made with certainty only by renal biopsy. A historical feature that may *suggest* the diagnosis is that the hematuria associated with IgA nephropathy often increases markedly during minor viral or upper respiratory infections. In many cases, the hematuria is microscopic, but it may become gross when the patient has a minor illness. Of patients with IgA nephropathy, 80% to 90% have a benign course. In the remaining 10% to 15% of patients, who are at risk for the development of chronic renal disease, proteinuria is either present at the time of diagnosis or develops with time. Therefore, it is not necessary to pursue a renal biopsy when patients are first evaluated with isolated hematuria; if persistent proteinuria develops subsequently, then a more exhaustive investigation, including a renal biopsy, may be necessary. One entity that should be included here is Henoch-Schönlein, or anaphylactoid purpura. This disease is associated with hematuria that may persist for 1 to 2 years after other signs of the disease have dissipated. The reason for including this syndrome with IgA nephropathy is that the *histologic findings on renal biopsy material from patients with Henoch-Schönlein purpura are identical to those seen in IgA nephropathy.* The clinical course and prognosis for the two entities are very similar; children at risk for the development of chronic renal failure in association with Henoch-Schönlein purpura have persistent proteinuria, as do children at risk for the development of renal failure in association with IgA nephropathy.

Poststreptococcal Glomerulonephritis

Poststreptococcal glomerulonephritis is another common cause of hematuria in children and adolescents. This disease follows group A streptococcal infection, most commonly pharyngitis in the northern United States and impetigo in the southern United States, and is recognized 10 to 14 days following the infection. The disease is *not* prevented by timely antibiotic treatment of the streptococcal infection. *The hallmarks of poststreptococcal glomerulonephritis are hematuria, hypertension, and edema.*

A *low level of C3* is seen at the time of diagnosis and may persist for 6 weeks. Hence, if hematuria develops in a patient following a streptococcal infection, it is worthwhile to obtain a C3 level. Many cases of poststreptococcal glomerulonephritis are subclinical, and patients manifest few symptoms; therefore, medical attention is not sought during the "acute" phase of the disease. The hematuria that is associated with poststreptococcal glomerulonephritis may persist for 12 to 18 months, although the C3 level has returned to normal and no evidence of the disease is present. Therefore, the incidence of poststreptococcal glomerulonephritis is likely to be underestimated. In a 6-year survey of Galveston County school-aged children, the incidence of hematuria found on urinalysis increased two- to threefold in the year following an epidemic of impetigo. This finding gives further credence to the contention that subclinical poststreptococcal glomerulonephritis is a very common cause of hematuria.

Other Causes of Hematuria

Although *urinary tract infection* may cause hematuria, isolated hematuria is rare. The urinalysis will be positive not only for hemoglobin but also for leukocyte esterase. Urine cultures should be obtained when the diagnosis is suspected. In general, isolated hematuria should not be attributed to a symptomatic urinary tract infection without a concomitant search for other causes.

The role of imaging studies in the evaluation of persistent microhematuria is controversial, whereas imaging studies are recommended for patients with gross hematuria. Congenital lesions with associated hydronephrosis may cause intermittent gross hematuria. Other entities that may be diagnosed with renal ultrasonography include renal stones, cysts, and tumors.

Cancer is a rare cause of hematuria in children. Children with Wilms tumor often have hematuria when the abdominal mass is palpable on physical examination. *This tumor rarely presents with hematuria;* the abdominal mass is noted first.

Although parents are often worried about the possibility of cancer, they are reluctant to vocalize their concerns. Therefore, the pediatrician should address the family's fears and explain that hematuria is unlikely to be a sign of cancer.

REVIEW EXERCISES

QUESTIONS

1. A 10-year-old patient who presents with a history of intermittent gross hematuria and 1+ proteinuria that is more pronounced during an upper respiratory infection is likely to have which of the following findings?
a) Low C3 level
b) Calcium oxalate crystals on urinalysis
c) Urine with a specific gravity of 1.020 and a pH of 5.0, and a red blood cell cast on microscopic examination
d) Evidence of hemolytic anemia with anisocytosis and poikilocytosis and very few platelets demonstrated on a smear

Answer
The answer is c. The fact that the patient has hematuria *and* mild proteinuria indicates that this is likely a glomerular lesion. The history of constant hematuria that is markedly increased even with mild upper respiratory infection is most characteristic of IgA nephropathy. In this disease, the C3 level is normal, and there is no association with hemolytic anemia.

2–6. Match the following diseases with the clinical description that most closely fits:
a) Minimal-change nephrotic syndrome
b) FSGS
c) MPGN
d) Membranous glomerulonephritis
e) Poststreptococcal glomerulonephritis

2. A 4-year-old boy presented 1 month ago with swelling, ascites, and a cholesterol level of 648 mg/dL. After treatment with prednisone (2 mg/kg per day) for 1 month, he continues to have 4+ proteinuria but less swelling. (He has also been taking 2 mg of furosemide/kg per day.)

Answer
The answer is b. Minimal-change disease is the most likely diagnosis in a 4-year-old boy. However, because he failed to respond to a 4-week course of prednisone therapy, the most likely diagnosis becomes FSGS.

3. A 4-year-old boy presented 1 month ago with swelling, ascites, and a cholesterol level of 648 mg/dL. After treatment with prednisone (2 mg/kg per day) for 1 month, his proteinuria has cleared. However, every time his prednisone dose is tapered to alternate-day therapy, the proteinuria returns.

Answer
The answer is a. However, this patient falls into the "frequent relapse" group.

4. A 4-year-old boy with a history of otitis media 10 days ago now presents with gross hematuria and increased blood pressure (130/94 mm Hg).

Answer
The answer is e. The clues that poststreptococcal glomerulonephritis is the most likely diagnosis in this patient are prior infection, hypertension, and a urinalysis showing hematuria (with no mention of proteinuria, which may or may not be present).

5. A 7-year-old girl who was adopted from China has episodic gross hematuria and persistent microscopic hematuria.

Answer
The answer is d. This is the trickiest of the questions. Membranous glomerulonephritis is very rare in childhood. When it is present, you must think of infectious causes, such as hepatitis B (membranous glomerulonephritis is seen in chronic carriers of hepatitis B). When membranous glomerulonephritis is diagnosed in an infant, congenital syphilis must be considered. The clue in this question is that the child was adopted from China, where the incidence of hepatitis B infection and chronic hepatitis B carriage is high.

6. A 13-year-old girl presented with swelling of her lower extremities, a mildly elevated blood pressure of 134/92 mm Hg, and 3+ protein and 2+ hemoglobin on urinalysis. Blood test result shows a serum creatinine level of 1.4 mg/dL and a cholesterol level of 249 mg/dL.

Answer
The answer is c. This adolescent has nephrotic syndrome and exhibits the clinical characteristics of the disease. She has hematuria, hypertension, and a serum cholesterol level that is nearly normal.

7. Which of the patients listed earlier (questions 2–6) are likely to have a low C3 level?

Answer
The answers are 4 and 6. Three diseases associated with a low C3 level are as follows:

- Poststreptococcal glomerulonephritis
- MPGN
- Systemic lupus erythematosus

8. A 7-year-old girl is sent to you for an evaluation of dysuria and frequency. She has had four prior urinary tract infections, all of which were diagnosed when she complained of dysuria and frequency and was found to have blood in her urine. During her last two episodes, the urine cultures were negative. (No cultures were obtained during the first two episodes.) Urinalysis shows 15 to 20 red blood cells and is negative for protein. What single question regarding the family history will you ask, and what single laboratory study will you do if the family history is positive?

Answer
The answer is that you should look for a *family history of renal stones*, and the important laboratory study is a

urinary ratio of calcium to creatinine or a 24-hour urine for calcium. Hypercalciuria is one of the more frequent causes of renal stones and may also cause dysuria and frequency.

9. The following are all complications of nephrotic syndrome, *except*:

a) *E. coli* peritonitis
b) Pulmonary embolus
c) Thrombosis of an extremity
d) *Haemophilus influenzae* peritonitis
e) Kwashiorkor

Answer

The answer is d. The two most common organisms causing peritonitis are *S. pneumoniae* and *E. coli*. Thrombosis is also a known complication, and in a patient with unremitting nephrotic syndrome, protein malnutrition may develop (as in congenital nephrotic syndrome). *H. influenzae* is a very rare cause of peritonitis in these patients.

10. Which of the following statements are true regarding congenital nephrotic syndrome? (You may choose more than one answer.)

a) The prognosis is dismal, with death often occurring within the first year.
b) It can be inherited as an autosomal-recessive trait.
c) It is associated with an abnormally large placenta.
d) It is associated with polyhydramnios.
e) Major causes of death are early renal failure and hyperkalemia.

Answer

The answer is that all are true with the exception of *e*. The major cause of death is sepsis and infection. Most patients die of other causes before the onset of renal failure.

SUGGESTED READINGS

1. Arbeitsgemeinschaft Für Pädiatrische Nephrologie. Effect of cytotoxic drugs in frequently relapsing nephrotic syndrome with and without steroid dependence. *N Engl J Med* 1982;306:451–453.
2. Bonilla-Felix M, Parra C, Dajani T, et al. Changing patterns in the histopathology of idiopathic nephrotic syndrome in children. *Kidney Int* 1999;55:1885–1890.
3. Brouhard BH. Hematuria. In: Kliegman R, Nieder ML, Super DM, eds. *Practical strategies in pediatric diagnosis and therapy.* Philadelphia: Saunders, 1996:424–433.
4. Cunningham RJ. Proteinuria. In: Kliegman R, Nieder ML, Super DM, eds. *Practical strategies in pediatric diagnosis and therapy.* Philadelphia: Saunders, 1996:415–424.
5. Dodge WF, West EF, Smith EH, et al. Proteinuria and hematuria in schoolchildren: epidemiology and early natural history. *J Pediatr* 1976;88:327.
6. Gorensek MJ, Lebel MH, Nelson JD. Peritonitis in children with nephrotic syndrome. *Pediatrics* 1988;81:849–856.
7. Report of the International Study of Kidney Disease in Children. Nephrotic syndrome in children: prediction of histopathology from clinical and laboratory characteristics at the time of diagnosis. *Kidney Int* 1978;13:159–165.
8. Report of the International Study of Kidney Disease in Children. Minimal-change nephrotic syndrome in children: deaths during the first 5 to 15 years' observation. *Pediatrics* 1984;73:497–501.

Chapter 13

Hypertension, Obesity, Type II Diabetes Mellitus, and Hyperlipidemia

Robert J. Cunningham III

INTRODUCTION

Assessment of a patient's risk for cardiovascular disease had traditionally required an evaluation of the following factors:

- Is there a family history of myocardial infarction (MI) or cerebrovascular accident (CVA) in relatives at an age of <55 years?
- Does the patient smoke and if so, how many cigarettes per day?
- Is the patient hypertensive?
- Does the patient have an abnormal lipid profile?
- Is the patient obese?
- Does the patient have diabetes mellitus? (In adults this is more often type II.)
- Does the patient exercise on a regular basis?

These assessments have been the purview of the internist or family practitioners who care for patients who are older and have exhibited a number of these risks. Unfortunately, these factors are now present in the pediatric population with an increasing frequency so that the pediatrician now needs to evaluate and address them. This changing paradigm forms the basis of this chapter.

EPIDEMIOLOGY

Hypertension has become an increasingly common problem over the past 20 years and the incidence has been rising at an alarming rate. Fixler et al. studied children in the Dallas school system in the 1970s and found that 8% of them had a blood pressure reading above the 95th percentile for age when a single reading was taken. However, fewer than 2% of children had three such readings when these were obtained at separate visits. In contrast, studies done in 2002 showed that the incidence of hypertension when blood pressures were taken in children on three separate visits had risen to 9.5%.

The incidence of obesity and of type 2 diabetes mellitus has also risen dramatically and parallels the rise in childhood hypertension. The increase in obesity and type 2 diabetes mellitus is most striking in adolescent boys; in particular, Hispanic and African-American adolescents are at highest risk for obesity (Table 13.1). There is also a direct correlation between the increased incidence of obesity and Type II diabetes mellitus. In the adult population, metabolic syndrome is a recognized entity and includes three of the following five elements:

- Obesity
- Hypertension
- Insulin resistance
- Hyperlipidemia
- Hyperglycemia

This syndrome is associated with a very high risk of cardiovascular and cerebrovascular disease. The alarming phenomena in pediatrics is that 28% to 30% of boys who are overweight (>95 percentile) will have three or more of the elements of metabolic syndrome. This indicates that they are at a much higher risk of early myocardial infarction or

TABLE 13.1

DIFFERENCES IN INCIDENCE OF OBESITY AMONG ETHNIC GROUPS IN THE UNITED STATES BETWEEN 1988–1994 AND 1999–2000

	% Overweight	
Period	1988–1994	1999–2000
Ethnic group	Boys 12–19 yr	
Non-Hispanic whites	12	14
Non-Hispanic blacks	11	20
Mexican Americans	14	28
	Girls 12–19 yr	
Non-Hispanic whites	9	13
Non-Hispanic blacks	16	27
Mexican Americans	14	19

Adapted from: Ogden CL, Flegtal KM, et al. Prevalence and trends in overweight among US children and adolescents, 1999–2000. *JAMA* 2002;288:1728–1732.

cerebrovascular accident than were prior generations who did not demonstrate these criteria until middle age.

HYPERTENSION

Definitions

Blood pressure nomograms are similar to growth charts for infants and children (Table 13.2). Children whose blood pressure falls between the 90th and 95th percentiles have *borderline* hypertension, and those whose blood pressure is consistently between the 95th and 99th percentiles have *significant* hypertension. Children whose blood pressure is higher than the 99th percentile for age are considered to have *severe* hypertension.

The study by Fixler et al. illuminated two points regarding the diagnosis of hypertension in children. First, the blood pressure may be labile, and therefore repeated measurements are required before any evaluation or treatment is considered. Within a single visit, the blood pressure may vary markedly, and efforts should be made to document pressures on at least three visits before an investigation into possible causes is initiated.

A second important consideration, especially in older or larger children, is to make sure that the blood pressure cuff covers at least two thirds of the upper arm. The use of a cuff that is smaller than recommended, a particularly common occurrence in athletic or obese adolescents, will result in a falsely elevated pressure.

Etiology

Once the cuff size has been determined to be appropriate and the blood pressure is seen to be consistently elevated, the evaluation and treatment outlined in the algorithm shown in Figure 13.1 can be applied.

Patients whose blood pressure is above the 99th percentile for age are candidates for a more thorough evaluation. The higher the pressure, the more urgent it is to evaluate, and the more likely it is that a cause of the hypertension will be identified.

TABLE 13.2

CLASSIFICATION OF HYPERTENSION IN THE YOUNG BY AGE GROUP

	High Normal Hypertension 90th–95th Percentile (mm Hg)	Significant Hypertension 95th–99th Percentile (mm Hg)	Severe Hypertension >99th Percentile (mm Hg)
Newborns			
(7 days)		SBP 96–105	SBP ≥106
(8–30 days)		SBP 104–109	SBP ≥110
Infants (≤2 years)	SBP 104–111	SBP 112–117	SBP ≥118
	DBP 70–74	DBP 76–81	DBP ≥82
Children (3–5 years)	SBP 108–115	SBP 116–123	SBP ≥124
	DBP 70–75	DBP 76–83	DBP ≥84
Children (6–9 years)	SBP 114–121	SBP 122–129	SBP ≥130
	DBP 74–77	DBP 78–85	DBP ≥86
Children (10–12 years)	SBP 122–125	SBP 126–133	SBP ≥134
	DBP 78–81	DBP 82–89	DBP ≥90
Children (13–15 years)	SBP 130–135	SBP 136–143	SBP ≥144
	DBP 80–85	DBP 86–91	DBP ≥92
Adolescents (16–18 years)	SBP 136–141	SBP 142–149	SBP ≥150
	DBP 84–91	DBP 92–97	DBP ≥98

DBP, diastolic blood pressure; SBP, systolic blood pressure.
Adapted from *Report of the Second Task Force on Blood Pressure in Children*—1987. U.S. Department of Health and Human Services, Public Health Service, National Institutes of Health. January 1987.

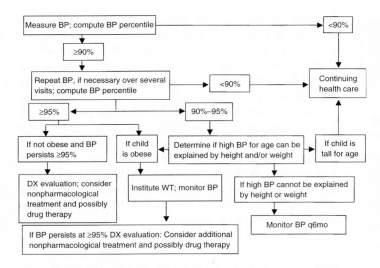

Figure 13.1 Algorithm giving an outline of the evaluation and treatment of hypertension. DX, diagnostic evaluation; WT, weight control. (Reprinted from National Heart, Lung, and Blood Institute. Task Force on Blood Pressure Control in Children. *Report of the Second Task Force on Blood Pressure Control in Children—1987*. U.S. Department of Health and Human Services, Public Health Service, National Institutes of Health, 1987:1–32.)

The causes of hypertension by age are listed in **Table 13.3**. Note that renal disease and coarctation of the aorta are prominent in the *younger* age groups.

Historical points that help determine the cause of hypertension include a detailed family history and evidence of renal parenchymal disease (e.g., a history of urinary tract infections or abnormal findings on prenatal ultrasonography). Inquiries should also be made to determine whether the patient has episodes of sweating, flushing, and palpitations, which are symptomatic of a pheochromocytoma. Without such symptoms, it is unlikely that a tumor will be found. If they are present, it is essential to obtain 24-hour urine studies for vanillylmandelic acid to detect catecholamine excess.

Two lesions that should be considered during the physical examination are:

- Coarctation of the aorta
- Renal artery stenosis

Evidence of coarctation of the aorta includes the absence of a femoral pulse and a lag between the time the brachial or radial pulse is felt with one hand and the femoral pulse with the other. Another clue that coarctation is present is a lower blood pressure reading in the leg than in the arm. Under normal circumstances, the blood pressure reading in the leg is higher than that in the arm.

The most common cause of severe hypertension in childhood is renal artery stenosis. An abdominal or flank bruit leads one to suspect a renal artery stenosis. The origin of the bruit is turbulent blood flow at the site of the stricture, akin to the flow of water through a hose. Imagine a kink in the hose—the resulting noise is like the bruit heard in a narrowed renal artery.

Diagnostic Evaluation

Initial laboratory studies recommended for a child with hypertension include:

- Urinalysis
- Measurement of serum electrolytes
- Measurement of serum creatinine
- Fasting lipography—lipogram
- Echocardiography
- Renal ultrasonography (with Doppler flow studies if possible)
- Other studies suggested by historical points or physical examination findings

TABLE 13.3

COMMON CAUSES OF HYPERTENSION IN CHILDHOOD

Ages 1–6	Ages 6–12	Ages 12–18
Renal parenchymal disease	Renal parenchymal disease	Essential hypertension
Renovascular disease	Renovascular disease	Iatrogenic
Coarctation of the aorta	Essential hypertension	Renal parenchymal disease
Endocrine causes[a]	Coarctation of the aorta	Renovascular disease[a]
Iatrogenic[a]	Endocrine causes[a]	Endocrine causes[a]
Essential hypertension[a]	Iatrogenic[a]	Coarctation of the aorta[a]

[a]Less common.

The purpose of most of these studies is apparent. An echocardiogram should be obtained to search for evidence of either septal or left ventricular hypertrophy. A lipogram detects lipid abnormalities that would predispose the patient to atherosclerosis. If a patient has both hypertension and lipid abnormalities, both conditions require treatment.

Management and Treatment

When an underlying cause of hypertension is found, it is of paramount importance to correct it. In most cases, however, a cause is not found. In these situations, the next step depends on the degree of hypertension and the effectiveness of nonpharmacologic therapy.

Children with borderline hypertension should be followed up clinically. If they are overweight, dietary counseling regarding weight loss is recommended. Patients with significant hypertension (95th–99th percentile) should be counseled regarding both weight loss and salt restriction. Children who remain hypertensive despite these measures or, as is common, fail to lose weight are candidates for antihypertensive medication. Few drugs are approved for the treatment of hypertension in children. Those that might be used as initial therapy are shown in Table 13.4, including the following:

- Diuretics
- Angiotensin-converting enzyme (ACE) inhibitors (contraindicated in pregnancy!)
- Calcium channel blockers
- β-Blockers

The mechanisms of action and side effects of each class of drugs are also shown in Table 13.4. Drugs that are used less frequently appear in Table 13.5. The adverse effects of these medications determine the tolerability and ultimately the success of the treatment regimen. Angiotensin receptor blockers are beginning to be used in children only recently and their side effects are similar to those outlined for the ACE inhibitors with the exception that there is a very low incidence of cough.

TYPE II DIABETES

Type II diabetes mellitus is a disease that is related to both to a genetic predisposition and the presence of obesity. The genetic tendency is inherited as an autosomal dominant

---

TABLE 13.4

DRUGS APPROVED FOR THE TREATMENT OF HYPERTENSION IN CHILDREN: INITIAL THERAPY

Drug Class	Examples	Action	Use	Common Side Effects
Diuretics	■ Thiazide ■ Loop (furosemide)	■ Increase salt and water excretion	■ Decrease salt retention ■ Decrease volume component of blood pressure	■ Hypokalemia ■ Alkalosis ■ Volume depletion
Angiotensin-converting enzyme inhibitors	■ Captopril ■ Enalapril ■ Lisinopril	■ Prevent conversion of angiotensin I to angiotensin II, thereby decreasing vasoconstriction and salt retention	■ Oral ■ Persistent hypertension, Hyperreninemia ■ Diabetes mellitus	■ Cough ■ Increased serum K^+ with impaired renal function ■ Decreased renal function with decreased renal function (one kidney with renal artery stenosis)
Calcium channel blockers	■ Nifedipine ■ Amlodipine ■ Diltiazem ■ Verapamil	■ Decrease vascular smooth-muscle calcium concentration ■ Decrease peripheral resistance ■ Decrease heart rate, myocardial contractility	■ Oral/sublingual ■ Acute lowering of blood pressure (nifedipine) ■ Long-term control of blood pressure	■ Edema ■ Constipation
β-Blockers	■ Atenolol (Inderal)	■ Peripheral β-receptor blockade ■ Decrease heart rate	■ Persistent hypertension ■ Usually oral; can be IV	■ Bradycardia ■ Exacerbation of asthma ■ Impotence ■ Unrecognized hypoglycemia

IV, intravenous.

TABLE 13.5

DRUGS APPROVED FOR THE TREATMENT OF HYPERTENSION IN CHILDREN: LESS FREQUENTLY USED

Drug Class	Examples	Use	Action	Common Side Effects
α-Blockers	■ Prazosin	■ Peripheral α-receptor	■ Persistent blockade ■ Oral only	■ Dizziness ■ Headaches ■ Hypertension
Combination α/β-blockers	■ Labetalol	■ α/β-Blockers; less blockage than single agents	■ Oral or IV ■ Persistent or acute hypertension	■ Decreased heart rate ■ Impotence
Peripheral vasodilator	■ Hydralazine ■ Diazoxide ■ Minoxidil ■ Sodium nitroprusside	■ Direct peripheral vasodilatation	■ Immediate lowering of blood pressure ■ Oral or IV	■ Sodium retention drug-specific ■ Hydralazine: lupus-like syndrome ■ Minoxidil: hirsutism
Central α stimulation	■ Clonidine	■ Decreased sympathetic outflow from CNS	■ Oral ■ Persistent hypertension	■ Rebound hypertension if stopped acutely ■ Sleepiness ■ First-dose effect

CNS, central nervous system; IV, intravenous.

trait and the hallmark of this disease is insulin insensitivity. The first clinical sign of this in an individual patient is often the presence of *acanthosis nigrans*. This hallmark finding is an increase in pigmentation and a "roughness" of the skin particularly over the back of the neck and in the axillary region. When pointed out to a parent, the response is often that they have been exasperated because the assumption was that the patient was not washing his or her neck. This should be searched for in any patient who is obese and particularly in patients in whom there is a history of diabetes in either parent. The darkening of the skin is the result of hyperinsulinemia. If this is found on physical examination, laboratory evaluation to determine if the patient has Type II diabetes mellitus should include a glucose tolerance test with insulin levels. Often, the fasting insulin levels will be elevated so a fasting insulin and glucose level may be done as a screen. Patients with early type II diabetes often are not hyperglycemic and therefore, fasting blood sugar determinations and glucose tolerance tests without insulin levels are of little value.

The treatment of choice is to *encourage weight loss!* Patients who successfully lose weight and achieve a weight compatible with their percentile for height may lose the acanthosis nigrans; even a small weight loss of 3% to 5% may help restore normal insulin sensitivity. It is not within the scope of this chapter to outline plans for successful weight loss but there are three components that are almost universally agreed upon. First, all sugared soft drinks must be eliminated from the diet; second, the patient must increase the baseline of physical activity and third, the rules for the child need to apply to the parents as well. For those patients with documented hyperinsulinemia, *metformin* may be prescribed. This is a biguanide compound that serves both to increase hepatic release of glucose and increase peripheral sensitivity to insulin so that it more effectively moves glucose into fat and muscle cells. There is some evidence that improving insulin sensitivity will also promote weight loss. The major side effects with this drug are stomach upset, which is common, and *lactic acidosis*, which is not common, but is a potentially lethal adverse effect.

HYPERLIPIDEMIA

The importance of hyperlipidemia in the pediatric population has recently undergone reexamination and recommendations have suggested a more aggressive approach to therapy. Previously, the American Academy of Pediatrics had considered a total serum cholesterol of 200 mg/dL or lower acceptable but, as the evidence that even lower levels of total cholesterol are associated with an increased risk of cardiovascular disease in the adult population, the pediatric standards are changing as well. For those patients who are overweight, weight loss, a diet with no more than 7% of calories from saturated fats and total intake of cholesterol that is less than 200 mg/day and increased exercise is the first line of therapy. It is now recommended that pharmacologic intervention be considered for children with a LDL concentration of >190 mg/dL (160 mg/dL if there is a family history of early heart disease or two other risk factors are present). The agents available for the treatment of hyperlipidemia, with the exception of the HMA Co-reductase inhibitors, are, in general, not well tolerated by pediatric patients. As a result, these are being utilized with increasing frequency for the treatment of hyperlipidemia in children who are as young as 8 years of age.

These drugs lower cholesterol by 30% to 50% and they lower the endogenous synthesis of cholesterol and upregulate LDL receptors, which results in an increased clearance of LDL from the circulation.

The major adverse effects include an increase in liver enzymes. Thus, when a patient is to begin one of these agents, it is imperative to obtain liver function studies prior to initiation and within 1 to 2 months after therapy is initiated. Rhabdomyolysis is also seen, albeit infrequently, and patients need to be told that if they experience muscle soreness or fatigue after therapy has been instituted, they need to be seen, at which time a creatine phosphokinase (CPK) levels need to be checked and, if they are elevated, the drug need to be discontinued. These agents are *contraindicated* in pregnancy and any female who is of childbearing age needs to be warned about this!

REVIEW EXERCISES

QUESTIONS

1. A 16-year-old boy with a 13-year history of insulin-dependent diabetes mellitus is referred to you for syncopal/seizure episodes. These occur three to four times per week, last several minutes, and are relieved by the administration of glucose. The blood sugar level during the episodes has been documented to be <50 mg/dL. The patient is unable tell that his blood sugar is low, as he could in the past.

He has had hypertension and is currently taking propranolol (Inderal), chlorothiazide (Diuril), a potassium supplement, and amlodipine besylate (Norvasc) for blood pressure control.

His physical examination findings are unremarkable; his blood pressure is 115/75 mm Hg, and laboratory studies show a value for hemoglobin A_{1C} of 6.1% (normal, 3%–6%). You recommend:
a) Discontinuing the Norvasc
b) Insulin pump therapy
c) Discontinuing the Diuril
d) Adding an ACE inhibitor
e) Discontinuing the Inderal

Answer
The answer is e. Inderal is contraindicated in patients with diabetes mellitus because it prevents the symptoms of hypoglycemia. The patient is unaware that hypoglycemia is developing and therefore cannot intervene. Seizures occur when the sugar level becomes too low and the level of glucose in the brain plummets.

2. A 16-year-old boy is brought to your office for a routine examination. He has had insulin-dependent diabetes for 13 years. He has been well but admits to nocturia and polyuria. His last hemoglobin A_{1C} measurement was 13.2%.

Physical examination shows a blood pressure of 142/92 mm Hg. The remainder of the examination is unremarkable. Laboratory data show:

- Hemoglobin A_{1C} = 14.1%
- Urinalysis
- Specific gravity = 1.035
- pH = 6.0
- Blood, negative
- Sugar >1000 mg/dL
- Ketones, trace
- Protein = 1+

The best class of drug to control his blood pressure would be:
a) Calcium channel blocker
b) β-Blocker
c) Peripheral vasodilator
d) ACE inhibitor
e) Diuretic

Answer
The answer is d. This patient should be taking an ACE inhibitor. These are the drugs of choice for a patient with hypertension and diabetes mellitus because the evidence is compelling that ACE inhibitors slow the progression of diabetic nephropathy. The fact that this patient has both hypertension and proteinuria implies that an element of diabetic nephropathy may be present.

3. You are asked to see a hypertensive infant in the intensive care nursery. He was born at 28 weeks after a complicated pregnancy. He is 3 weeks old and had been doing well until several days ago, when the systolic pressure readings in his umbilical artery catheter increased to 110 mm Hg.

His physical examination is unremarkable. An umbilical artery catheter and oral endotracheal tube are in place.

The *most* likely cause of his hypertension is:
a) Stimulation of the renin–angiotensin system
b) Increased epinephrine concentration
c) Renal immaturity
d) Increased cortisol production
e) Congenital hypothyroidism

Answer
The answer is a. The most likely cause is a thrombus secondary to the umbilical artery catheter. It may be a very small clot affecting only a peripheral branch of the renal artery, and results of studies may be normal. Although these patients often require medical treatment, the blood pressure is usually normal by 1 year of age, even without medications.

4. A 15-year-old girl is brought to your office for a follow-up visit for hypertension. Her hypertension is secondary to chronic renal scarring from pyelonephritis. Her current medication is 25 mg of captopril three times a day. She is adhering to a low-sodium diet. She has no complaints and has been well.

Her blood pressure is 135/72 mm Hg. The remainder of her physical examination is normal.

Laboratory studies reveal:

- Hemoglobin =13.5 g/dL
- Na = 137 mEq/L
- K = 6.5 mEq/L
- Cl = 102 mEq/L
- HCO_3 = 19 mEq/L
- Blood urea nitrogen = 43 mg/dL
- Creatinine = 3.1 mg/dL

The *most* likely explanation for the hyperkalemia is:
a) Decreased urine output
b) Metabolic acidosis
c) Decreased aldosterone production
d) Increased potassium intake
e) Decreased cortisol production

Answer

The answer is c. The production of aldosterone is decreased because the ACE inhibitor inhibits the production of angiotensin II. Without angiotensin II stimulation, aldosterone secretion is diminished. Given the patient's

serum creatinine level of 3.1 mg/dL, it is apparent that the glomerular filtration rate is low. As the filtration rate falls, the excretion of K^+ becomes increasingly dependent on the tubular action of aldosterone stimulating Na^+/K^+ exchange.

SUGGESTED READINGS

1. Daniels SR, Greer FR, and the Committee on Nutrition. Lipid screening and cardiovascular health in childhood. *Pediatrics* 2008;122:198–208.
2. Kay JD, Sinaiko AR, Daniels SR. Pediatric hypertension. *Am Heart J* 2001;142:422–432.
3. National Heart, Lung, and Blood Institute. Report of the second task force on blood pressure control in children—1987. *Pediatrics* 1987;79:1–24.
4. National Heart, Lung, and Blood Institute. Task force on blood pressure control in children. *Report of the second task force on blood pressure control in children—1987*. US Department of Health and Human Services, Public Health Service, National Institutes of Health, 1987:1–32.
5. Norwood VF. Hypertension. *Pediatr Rev* 2002;23:197–209.
6. Ogden CL, Flegtal KM, et al. Prevalence and trends in overweight among US children and adolescents, 1999–2000. *JAMA* 2002;288:1728–1732.
7. Sorof JM, Lai D, Turner J, et al. Overweight, ethnicity, and the prevalence of hypertension in school-aged children. *Pediatrics* 2004;113:475–482.
8. Vogt B, Davis ID. Treatment of hypertension in pediatric nephrology. In: Avner ED, Harmon WE, Niaudet P, eds. *Pediatric nephrology.* Philadelphia: Lippincott Williams & Wilkins, 2004:1199–1220.

Chapter 14

BOARD SIMULATION: Acid–Base and Complex Fluid and Electrolyte Problems

Robert J. Cunningham III

In this chapter, a board simulation format is utilized to review acid–base physiology and transmit an approach that will allow you to tackle more complex fluid problems. A number of cases are presented with relevant questions. The correct answers and the logic used to arrive at each answer appear following each question.

QUESTIONS

Case 1

A 6-year-old boy is being evaluated for short stature. His physical examination findings are normal, except that his height is below the fifth percentile. His height was in the fifth percentile when he was 3 years old and has slowly fallen off the curve to just below the fifth percentile. His weight is proportional to his height.

His urinalysis is normal, with a urinary pH of 6.5. No protein, blood, or white blood cells are noted. His electrolyte values are as follows:

- $Na = 141$ mEq/L
- $K = 3.9$ mEq/L
- $Cl = 110$ mEq/L
- $HCO_3 = 19$ mEq/L

1. The data are *most* consistent with which of the following?
a. Chronic renal failure
b. Diabetic ketoacidosis
c. Urea cycle defect with acidosis
d. Renal tubular acidosis (RTA)

Answer

The answer is d. When you are confronted with a patient with evidence of acidosis, the first step is to calculate the anion gap, as shown:

$$Na - (Cl + HCO_3) = 141 - (110 + 19) = 12$$

A normal value for the anion gap is from 8 to 16. Acidosis with a *normal* anion gap can be caused by:

- Renal loss of bicarbonate
- RTA
- Carbonic anhydrase inhibitors
- Posthypocapnia
- Gastrointestinal loss of bicarbonate
- Diarrheal stool
- Ileostomy drainage, digestive fistulae
- Ileal conduits
- Administration of cation exchange resins
- Administration of acid
- Arginine chloride, hydrochloric acid
- Parenteral nutrition
- Dilution acidosis

The origin of the anion gap is that under normal circumstances, the Na^+ ions are balanced by the sum of the Cl and HCO_3 ions, in addition to other anions not accounted for in the equation. The anion gap of 8 to 16 accounts for these ions, which include PO_4, albumin, and other protein molecules that carry a negative charge. There is no net charge because the numbers of positively and negatively charged molecules in the circulation are equal.

A normal value for the anion gap is 8 to 16, so that the gap in this example is well within the normal range. All causes of a normal anion gap acidosis represent situations of either a direct loss of bicarbonate or an addition of acid to the body fluids. In nearly all cases, you are directed to the kidney or gastrointestinal tract, the two organs with the capacity to eliminate bicarbonate. Situations of active addition of H^+ to the blood are special. The one most often encountered in practice is the patient who is dependent on total parenteral nutrition. In this scenario, no additional anion is present in the circulation. The mechanism for the development of acidosis is loss of bicarbonate; and with each loss of a bicarbonate ion, a cation (e.g., Na^+) is lost simultaneously. In this way, electrical neutrality is maintained, and a normal anion gap is preserved.

In the earlier example, assume that you are considering the diagnosis of RTA and that you obtained a first morning urine sample along with a blood gas. The results are shown in the subsequent text:

Urinalysis	Blood Gas
pH = 6.0	pH = 7.34
Specific gravity = 1.025	HCO_3 = 18 mEq/L
Glucose, negative	P_{CO_2} = 32 mm Hg
Protein, negative	
Hemoglobin, negative	

2. These results effectively:
a. Confirm a diagnosis of type I (distal) RTA
b. Confirm a diagnosis of type II (proximal) RTA
c. Exclude RTA as a cause of acidosis
d. Establish acidemia without identifying a specific defect

Answer

The answer is d. You have now established that the patient has acidemia; the bicarbonate is low, the pH is low, and a compensatory low P_{CO_2} is present. How do you know that this is a metabolic acidosis and not a compensatory response to a respiratory alkalosis? The answer is that the pH is <7.40, and overcompensation never occurs.

After the administration of ammonium chloride, an acid, the following results were obtained:

Urinalysis	Blood Gas
pH = 6.0	pH = 7.29
Specific gravity = 1.014	HCO_3 = 14 mEq/L
	P_{CO_2} = 32 mm Hg

3. The diagnosis is consistent with:
a. Type I distal RTA
b. Type II proximal RTA

Answer

The answer is a. This patient has received an acid load, and even in the face of severe acidosis, the urine has a pH of 6.0. This finding indicates a distal tubular defect and an inability to excrete acid. The normal response to the acid load would be to excrete enough H^+ to drive the urine pH to a value of 5.5 or lower. Hence, a pH of 6.0 indicates that the distal tubule function is inadequate. If the patient had a type II (proximal) RTA, with a bicarbonate level of 15 mEq/L, the proximal tubule would reabsorb all the bicarbonate presented to it. As shown in **Figure 14.1**, the pH of the fluid entering the distal tubule would be 7.0, and with the addition of acid

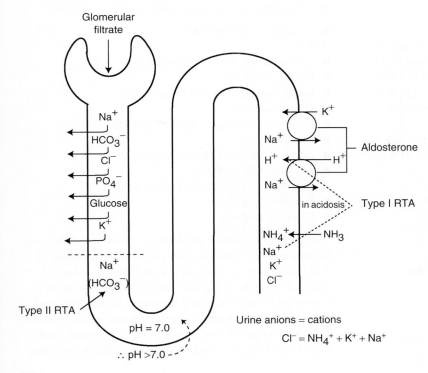

Figure 14.1 The glomerular filtrate. In the proximal tubule, represented by the section above the *dotted line*, bicarbonate is reabsorbed back into the circulation. This is also the area where K^+, Cl, PO_4 glucose, and amino acids are reabsorbed. In normal circumstances, the pH of the fluid exiting the proximal tubule is 7.0. In type II renal tubular acidosis (RTA), the proximal tubule fails to reabsorb all the bicarbonate and HCO_3 escapes, so that the pH of the exiting fluid is >7.0. In type I RTA, acid transport in the distal tubule fails. This is depicted by the *dotted line*, which indicates that the transport system is not functional for H^+. During acidosis, NH_3 is secreted and "captures" the H^+ ion and this is excreted in the urine. The major anion is Chloride and this equals the sum of the $NH_4^+ + K^+ + Na^+$ ions. Hence urinary $(K^+ + Na^+) - Cl^-$ will be negative in acidosis with normal distal tubular secretion of H^+ ion but in type I RTA, $(K^+ + Na^+) - Cl^-$ will be positive neutral or + because of the lack of NH_4^+ in the urine.

by distal tubular cells, the pH would fall to at least 5.5, if not lower.

4. Further history that would increase your suspicion of RTA would include:
a. Father with a history of polycystic disease
b. Mother with a history of renal stones
c. Father with a history of anemia
d. Sibling who is also in the fifth percentile for height

Answer
The answer is b. In an individual with a chronic inability to excrete an acid load, H^+ is buffered in the bone. For every 2 H^+ ion that is buffered in the bone, one Ca^{2+} ion is released and must be excreted. As a result, hypercalciuria develops and predisposes the patient to the formation of renal stones. When renal stones develop in an adult, RTA must be considered as a predisposing cause.

5. If this child is begun on therapy with sodium bicarbonate or sodium citrate, what is the major side effect to be avoided?
a. Hypokalemia
b. Metabolic alkalosis
c. Volume overload
d. Hypernatremia

Answer
The answer is a. Hypokalemia develops in patients with RTA and is exacerbated by treatment with base solutions containing sodium but not potassium. The reason is that the patient is acidotic, and the aldosterone level is elevated in an attempt to increase H^+ excretion. K^+ is excreted by the same mechanism; K^+ ions are excreted in the distal tubule in exchange for Na^+ ions. When a patient is treated with sodium solutions, the result is decreased sodium reabsorption in the proximal tubule and enhanced delivery of Na^+ to the distal tubule. With a high aldosterone level and an increase in the amount of substrate available for exchange, potassium excretion is enhanced and hypokalemia results. This process is illustrated in **Figure 14.2**.

Case 2
A 6-year-old boy is brought to the emergency department in respiratory distress. His breathing rate is 44/minute, and his respirations are deep. The physical examination shows that he is moving air extremely well and has no rales, wheezes, or rhonchi. Blood pressure is 130/70 mm Hg, pulse 90/minute, temperature 37.4°C (99.32°F), and weight 25 kg. He had a viral illness 7 to 10 days ago with diarrhea but seemed to be doing well with a good appetite. Initial blood gas and electrolytes determination shows:

- pH = 7.25
- P_{CO_2} = 20 mm Hg
- Na = 128 mEq/L
- K = 5.1mEq/L

Prior to treatment with sodium bicarbonate
Blood–brain barrier

Blood	CSF
pH = 7.02 (normal = 7.40)	pH = 7.27 (normal = 7.25–7.32)
$[HCO_3^-]$ = 5 mEq/L	$[HCO_3^-]$ = 9 mEq/L
P_{CO_2} = 20 mm Hg	P_{CO_2} = 20 mm Hg

$$pH = pK + \log \frac{[HCO_3^-]}{(P_{CO_2})0.03}$$
$$= pK + \log \frac{[9]}{0.03(20)}$$

After infusion of bicarbonate

Blood	CSF
pH = 7.37	pH = 7.07
$[HCO_3^-]$ = 18 mEq/L	$[HCO_3^-]$ = 9 mEq/L
P_{CO_2} = 32 mm Hg	P_{CO_2} = 32 mm Hg

$$pH = pK + \log \frac{[9]}{0.03(32)}$$

Figure 14.2 Acid–base balance in the blood and cerebrospinal fluid (CSF) of a patient such as the one described in case 4. When the blood pH was 7.02, the serum bicarbonate was only 5 mEq/L, and the P_{CO_2} was 20 mm Hg. Active transport of bicarbonate and rapid diffusion of carbon dioxide into the CSF take place. After treatment with intravenous bicarbonate, the blood pH is corrected, and the bicarbonate level rises to 18 mEq/L. With this improvement, compensatory hyperventilation slows and the P_{CO_2} rises rapidly. This carbon dioxide also diffuses freely into the CSF. Bicarbonate is not transported quickly. At the bottom of each CSF panel, the Henderson-Hasselbalch equation shows that the pH of the CSF actually fell with treatment because the P_{CO_2} rose whereas the bicarbonate level remained constant. Hence, the numerator remained the same, the denominator increased, and the CSF acidosis actually worsened.

- HCO_3 = 5 mEq/L
- Cl = 98 mEq/L

6. This clinical presentation is consistent with all of the following *except*:
a. Acute renal insufficiency (uremia)
b. Salicylate intoxication
c. Diarrhea
d. Diabetic ketoacidosis

Answer
The answer is c. Diarrhea would result in a nongap acidosis. The gap here is $128 - (98 + 5)$, or 25. This is an elevated anion gap and therefore is not consistent with a gastrointestinal loss of bicarbonate. In cases of gap acidosis, the mnemonic *MUDPILES* is helpful. The causes of gap acidosis are outlined in **Table 14.1**.

Hence, the clinical scenario in this case would be consistent with uremia, diabetic ketoacidosis, or salicylate intoxication.

The blood glucose was reported to be 473 mg/dL. The following therapy was instituted in the emergency department:

- Four fluids were begun: 0.45% normal saline (NS) + KCl of 30 mEq/L running at 125 mL/hour.

TABLE 14.1

CAUSES OF GAP ACIDOSIS

M	Methanol intoxication
U	Uremia
D	Diabetic ketoacidosis
P	Paraldehyde intoxication
I	Inborn errors of metabolism (or isoniazid intoxication)
L	Lactic acidosis
E	Ethylene glycol (antifreeze) intoxication
S	Salicylate intoxication

- Sodium bicarbonate (2 mEq/kg) was given IV over 5 minutes to correct the acidosis.
- Insulin (0.2 U/kg) was administered IV for the first hour, and then the rate was adjusted to 0.1 U/kg per hour.

7. When he arrived at the pediatric ward, he was comatose and unresponsive. The likely cause is:

a. Hypoglycemia
b. Hypokalemia
c. Worsening central nervous system acidosis
d. Progressive dehydration
e. Hypercapnia

Answer

The answer is c. Worsening central nervous system acidosis. The pH of the cerebrospinal fluid (CSF) is maintained by the active transport of bicarbonate across the blood–brain barrier. As shown in Figure 14.2, the CSF pH is normally slightly lower than the serum pH (usually 7.25–7.30), whereas the pH of the arterial blood is stable at approximately 7.40. However, the CSF pH is maintained during the development of arterial acidosis by an active transport of bicarbonate. Before the patient received any bicarbonate, the CSF bicarbonate level was 9 mEq/L, and that of the plasma was 5 mEq/L.

Following the infusion, the arterial bicarbonate level increases but that of the CSF does not because bicarbonate enters the CSF by active transport, a process that takes time. The P_{CO_2} rises quickly as the respiratory drive is blunted because the arterial acidosis has improved. Carbon dioxide diffuses very rapidly into the CSF. As a result, the denominator of the Henderson-Hasselbalch equation increases without a concomitant increase in the numerator. The net result is a rapid fall in the CSF pH (shown in the lower part of Fig. 14.2).

For this reason, it is unwise to correct rapidly a systemic acidosis that has evolved over a matter of days. If bicarbonate is to be administered, it should be infused over several hours, with time allowed for the active transport of bicarbonate across the blood–brain barrier at a rate similar to that at which the systemic acidosis is corrected.

Case 3

A 3-year-old child is brought to the emergency department with rapid respiration and decreasing responsive-

ness. He has not been ill and was playing in the back yard of his grandmother's house this morning, but when he came in for his nap, he was found to be lethargic and breathing rapidly.

Physical examination reveals a respiratory rate of 44/minute and a blood pressure of 100/60 mm Hg. He is semicomatose but has no signs of trauma, and no focal neurologic signs are noted.

- Na = 141 mmol/L
- K = 4.8 mmol/L
- Cl = 101 mmol/L
- HCO_3 = 9 mmol/L
- Blood urea nitrogen (BUN) = 14 mg/dL
- Creatinine = 0.9 mg/dL
- Glucose = 115 mg/dL
- Bilirubin = 0.9 mg/dL
- Transaminases, normal
- Prothrombin time = 12 seconds

8. The data are *most* consistent with:

a. RTA
b. Ammonium chloride ingestion
c. Diabetic ketoacidosis
d. Salicylate intoxication
e. Reye syndrome

Answer

The answer is d. Choices *a* and *b* would result in a non-gap acidosis, and the gap value in this case is 21. Choice *c* is ruled out by a normal blood glucose level, and choice *e* is unlikely because the patient has no history of a preceding illness and the prothrombin time and transaminase levels are normal.

9. Studies that would help establish the diagnosis include:

a. Urinalysis
b. Serum protein electrophoresis
c. Blood ammonia level
d. Salicylate level

Answer

The answer is d. The most likely diagnosis is salicylate intoxication. A hint is that the child was at his grandmother's house, a place less likely to be childproof and where aspirin is probably available. A urinalysis would not be helpful. There is no reason to suspect that the serum proteins are abnormal, and if Reye syndrome were more likely, then a blood ammonia level would be helpful.

10. Treatment modalities that increase the excretion of salicylates include all the following *except*:

a. Intravenous (IV) hydration and alkalinization of the urine
b. Hemodialysis
c. Peritoneal dialysis
d. Administration of mannitol

Answer

The answer is d. Aspirin is an acid substance, and excretion of the acid is facilitated when the urine is alkalinized. Both hemodialysis and peritoneal dialysis increase the rate of salicylate removal, but of the two, hemodialysis is much more efficient and preferred for serious intoxication. Treatment with mannitol increases the urine flow but does not enhance the tubular secretion of salicylate and therefore does not facilitate its removal.

Case 4

KF is a 14-month-old white girl presenting with failure to thrive. She weighed 2.9 kg at birth with Apgar scores of 9 and 9 at 1 and 5 minutes, respectively. Her growth was along the 10th percentile for the first 6 months of life, but subsequently, it fell below the fifth percentile. She has been hospitalized three times with complaints of tachypnea, and the results of numerous HCO_3 determinations have ranged from 18 to 20 mEq/L.

The physical examination reveals a small blond girl with normal findings. Her height and weight are below the fifth percentile; the head circumference is at the 50th percentile.

Her electrolyte values are as follows:

- Na = 140 mEq/L
- Cl = 109 mEq/L
- HCO_3 = 18 mEq/L
- K = 4.9 mEq/L

Her blood gas measurement shows:

- pH = 7.34
- P_{CO_2} = 34 mm Hg
- HCO_3 = 19 mEq/L

11. Reasonable next steps include:
a. Obtaining a first morning urine for pH
b. Checking the serum creatinine level
c. Simultaneously measuring the serum pH and urine pH after an ammonium chloride load
d. Obtaining a 24-hour urine for amino acids and phosphorus

Answer

The answer is a. The first morning urine is the one most likely to have a low pH, and that in itself may eliminate type I RTA as a possibility. The anion gap is 13, which is normal; therefore, measuring the serum creatinine level will not be helpful because this is a nongap acidosis. Obtaining a serum pH and a urine pH following an acid load may not be necessary if the pH of the first morning urine is <5.5. A 24-hour urine might be helpful if you established that the defect was a proximal tubular one (i.e., type II RTA). You would then be looking for more generalized evidence of proximal tubular dysfunction, or Fanconi syndrome, in which a generalized failure of proximal tubular reabsorption leads to elimination of bicarbonate, glucose, phosphorus, and amino acids. All

these are reabsorbed primarily by the proximal tubule (Fig. 14.1).

12. A first morning urine shows a pH of 5.0 with a urine Na of 70 mEq/L, K of 27 mEq/L and a urine Cl of 120 mEq/L. These values:
a. Rule out the diagnosis of RTA
b. Rule out the diagnosis of distal RTA (type I)
c. Both
d. Neither

Answer

The answer is b. The fact that the urine pH is <5.5 establishes that the patient's urine can be acidified and rules out the possibility of type I RTA. In addition, the urine electrolytes show that there is H^+ secretion into the urine. The urine $(Na^+ + K^+) - Cl^-$ is −23 and the unmeasured cation is likely NH_4^+. This indicates that the distal tubule is secreting hydrogen ion in response to acidosis, thereby ruling out type I RTA. She may still have a bicarbonate leak. If the serum bicarbonate is low enough that all the bicarbonate presented to the proximal tubule is reabsorbed, then the urine pH can be this low, and the patient can still have a type II RTA.

13. If a plasma pH, obtained at the same time that the first morning urine was collected, showed a pH of 7.38 with a bicarbonate level of 25 mEq/L, this would:
a. Rule out the diagnosis of RTA
b. Rule out the diagnosis of distal RTA (type I)
c. Both
d. Neither

Answer

The answer is c. If, however, the bicarbonate level is 25 mEq/L and the pH is 7.38 at the time that the urine is collected, then you have established that the patient is capable of reabsorbing bicarbonate normally and has neither type I nor type II RTA.

In this case, the bicarbonate was 17 mEq/L at the time the urine pH was obtained and when the patient was given an IV infusion of sodium bicarbonate, the urine pH "jumped" to 8.0 when the serum bicarbonate reached 19 mEq/L. Hence, the patient was leaking bicarbonate indicating a low renal threshold for bicarbonate reabsorption and this is consistent with type II (proximal) RTA.

Case 5

A 3-month-old boy is seen in your office for recurrent vomiting during the past 10 days. The mother states that the vomiting has become progressively more forceful and occurs with every feeding. You have the mother give him a bottle in the office and observe peristaltic waves cross his abdomen followed by projectile vomiting.

The physical examination reveals a lethargic infant with a weight of 7.2 kg, pulse of 120, blood pressure of 80/40 mm Hg, and respiratory rate of 16/minute. His skin turgor is poor, and he has a weak cry.

14. Which of the following serum electrolyte/blood gas patterns do you suspect will *most* likely be found?
a. Na = 137, K = 4.6, Cl = 110, HCO_3 = 22
b. Na = 134, K = 4.6, Cl = 105, HCO_3 = 23
c. Na = 132, K = 3.2, Cl = 90, HCO_3 = 35
d. Na = 132, K = 3.2, Cl = 100, HCO_3 = 32

Answer

The answer is c. This is obviously a clinical description of a patient with pyloric stenosis, so that you would expect to see an *alkalosis*. Therefore, choices *a* and *b* are incorrect. Why is *d* not correct? Note that the anion gap in choice *d* would be 0. That is impossible, so the choice is c.

15. Which of the following would provide the *best* approach to IV therapy?
a. D_5W (5% dextrose in water)/0.2% NS + KCl of 20 mEq/L to run at 30 mL/hour
b. D_5W/0.45% NS + KCl of 20 mEq/L to run at 30 mL/hour
c. D_5W/0.9% NS to run at 90 mL/hour for 8 hours, then add KCl of 20 mEq/L and run at 60 mL/hour for the next 16 hours
d. D_5W/0.9% NS + KCl of 30 mEq/L to run at 90 mL/hour for 8 hours and at 50 mL/hour for the next 16 hours

Answer

The answer is d. This patient is close to being 10% dehydrated and requires 1,520 mL of fluids over the next 24 hours. Both *c* and *d* give approximately one-half that amount in the first 8 hours, but *d* gives more K^+ and more Cl. The correction of alkalosis requires volume replacement and adequate chloride replenishment. In simple terms, the kidney always preserves volume, and preservation of volume takes precedence over normal chemical balance. Sodium is reabsorbed in the proximal tubule, and to maintain volume, it is reabsorbed avidly. For every Na^+ ion that is reabsorbed, an accompanying anion is needed. If the numbers of chloride ions available to accompany the sodium ions are inadequate, then sodium takes its second choice to the dance, a bicarbonate ion, even if too many are there already. It was shown that metabolic alkalosis persists indefinitely until chloride balance is restored, in an experiment performed on volunteer medical students. Nasogastric tubes were placed and the stomach contents were drained for 48 hours. The expected alkalosis developed, and the nasogastric tubes were removed. The alkalosis persisted for as long as 15 days when the subjects were maintained on a diet low in sodium chloride.

Case 6

TW is a 6-year-old girl brought to you because the parents suspect that she has diabetes mellitus. She has begun to urinate frequently, has lost weight during the last 6 months, and has not been growing at the same rate as her friends during the last year. Her appetite has not changed appreciably, although the parents think that she may be eating less because she is drinking too much water, which is her preferred drink.

She is the product of a normal pregnancy and delivery and has developed normally. She is in the first grade and doing well. The family has a history of adult-onset diabetes (type 2); both grandmothers are being treated for diabetes with diet and oral hypoglycemic agents.

The physical examination reveals a healthy girl who is at the fifth percentile for height and who interrupts the examination twice to get a drink of water.

16. This case is *most* consistent with:
a. Renal insufficiency
b. Diabetes mellitus
c. Diabetes insipidus
d. Hypothyroidism

Answer

The answer is c. Diabetes mellitus is unlikely because the patient's appetite has not increased. Chronic renal failure is associated with an inability to concentrate urine and a loss of appetite, so this is also a possibility. The girl's thirst seems exaggerated; she could not even get through the examination without drinking water twice. Hypothyroidism can also result in a dilute urine, but again, the degree of her thirst would negate this, and she probably would have gained weight if she were hypothyroid.

17. The electrolyte levels are measured along with the blood glucose and creatinine levels. The results are as follows:

Na = 151 mEq/L
K = 4.9 mEq/L
Cl = 110 mEq/L
HCO_3 = 27 mEq/L
Creatinine = 0.7 mg/dL
BUN = 12 mg/dL
Glucose = 96 mg/dL

The serum osmolarity can be approximated from these data. It is approximately:
a. 270 mOsm/kg
b. 290 mOsm/kg
c. 300 mOsm/kg
d. 315 mOsm/kg

Answer

The answer is d. The osmolarity is calculated with the formula $(2 \times [Na]) + 10 + (Glucose/18) + (BUN/3)$.

18. The next step in the evaluation is to:
a. Determine the urine osmolarity and serum osmolarity simultaneously.
b. Have the patient come into office first thing in the morning to perform these studies but allow her no oral fluids after midnight.

c. Administer intranasal desmopressin acetate (DD-AVP) and repeat the electrolyte determination.
d. Admit the patient to the hospital and perform water deprivation under controlled conditions.

Answer

The answer is a. If the urine osmolarity is less than the serum osmolarity, which is clearly elevated, then the diagnosis of diabetes insipidus is established. Having the patient come in for a morning visit after being deprived of fluid overnight is *dangerous*. If diabetes insipidus is genuinely suspected, then any deprivation of water must be carried out under very controlled circumstances and halted after 7% of the body weight has been lost. Administering DDAVP immediately assumes a diagnosis of central diabetes insipidus. Option *d* is reasonable and may also be considered, but hospitalization is required.

19. If the patient's urine does not become concentrated following water deprivation, the next step would be to:
a. Administer DDAVP.
b. Place the patient on a high-protein diet and repeat the study in a week.
c. Obtain a computed tomogram of the pituitary fossa.
d. Continue to deprive her of fluids until she has lost 10% of her body weight.

Answer

The answer is that both *a* and *c* are correct. If a patient's urine fails to become concentrated even with water deprivation, administration of DDAVP is the second part of the test. However, nephrogenic diabetes insipidus is rare, even more so in girls, and is usually evident shortly after birth. Central diabetes insipidus is more common, and a pituitary tumor is one of the most common causes of this entity. A search for the cause of diabetes insipidus should be undertaken.

Case 7

JT is a 12-year-old, 50-kg boy admitted from the emergency department, where he underwent therapy for a depressed skull fracture sustained when he fell from a tree while trying to retrieve his cat. He has multiple bruises but no other fractures. Findings on the chest roentgenogram and urinalysis are normal. He was begun on IV fluids ($D_5W/0.3\%$ NS + KCl of 20 mEq/L) at a maintenance rate.

However, 12 hours after admission, the electrolyte values reveal hyponatremia:

- Na = 127 mEq/L
- K = 4.9 mEq/L
- Cl = 97 mEq/L
- HCO_3 = 22 mEq/L
- Creatinine = 0.4 mg/dL
- BUN = 9 mg/dL

20. Hyponetremia is *most* likely the result of:
a. Water intoxication

b. Inappropriate secretion of antidiuretic hormone (SIADH)
c. Diabetes insipidus
d. Inadequate sodium replacement

Answer

The answer is b. SIADH is not uncommon following head trauma. The serum osmolarity in this patient is 270 mOsm/kg, and in diabetes insipidus it would be low, not high. With normal renal function, the kidney conserves sodium, and therefore inadequate replacement is not reasonable. In fact, whenever you see hyponatremia, your first thought should not be, "Why is there too little sodium?" but rather, "Why is there too much water?" Hyponatremia is usually a dilution phenomenon, not one of inadequate salt intake. Water intoxication does not appear reasonable when you examine the fluids that this patient has received during the past 12 hours. There is no reason to assume that he was water intoxicated before his fall.

21. What should be the initial treatment?
a. Restrict fluids to insensible loss.
b. Change IV fluids to $D_5W/0.9\%$ NS + KCl of 20 mEq/L and keep the rate at maintenance.
c. Change IV fluids to $D_5W/0.9\%$ NS + KCl of 20 mEq/L and cut the rate to two thirds of maintenance.
d. Administer 2 mg of furosemide/kg and give back sodium IV following the diuresis as 3% NaCl.

Answer

The answer is a. The first step in the treatment of SIADH is fluid restriction to insensible losses (approximately 400 mL/m^2 per day). The kidney is excreting Na$^+$ normally but is preserving water excessively under the influence of antidiuretic hormone (ADH). Therefore, options *b* and *c* will not solve the problem, and the Na$^+$ concentration will most likely continue to fall if either of these strategies is used. Option *d* is too drastic and generally reserved for very refractory cases of SIADH or for patients at risk for seizures.

22. Calculate the free water excess. It is:
a. 30 L
b. 27.2 L
c. 2.8 L
d. 1.4 L

Answer

The answer is c.
See Table 11.4.

Volume of distribution is 50 kg × 0.6 = 30 L
30 L × 127 mEq/L = 3810 mEq of Na
3810 mEq Na/140 mEq/L = $V_{New Dist}$ L or 27.2 L
Excess = L 27.2 L − 30 L = −2.8 L
Therefore free water excess = 2.8 L

The new volume of distribution is 2.8 L less than the current volume of distribution, hence the negative number

SUGGESTED READINGS

1. Adrogue HJ, Wesson DE. *Acid-base.* Houston: Libra and Gemini Publications, 1991.
2. Arief AI, de Fronzo RA. *Fluid electrolyte and acid-base disorders.* New York: Churchill Livingstone, 1985.
3. Chan JCM, Gill JR Jr. *Kidney electrolyte disorders.* New York: Churchill Livingstone, 1990.
4. Finberg L, Kravath R, Fleischman A. *Water and electrolytes in pediatrics.* Philadelphia: Saunders, 1982.
5. Gluck SL. Acid-base. *Lancet* 1998;352:474–479.
6. Roth KS, Chan JCM. Renal tubular acidosis: a new look at an old problem. *Clin Pediatr* 2001;40:533–543.

Chapter 15

BOARD SIMULATION: Nephrology

Robert J. Cunningham III

This chapter utilizes a board simulation format to review general principles in pediatric nephrology. A number of cases are presented, each followed by an explanation of the correct answer and the logic used to arrive at that particular solution.

QUESTIONS

1. A 3-year-old, previously healthy, white girl presents for a routine physical examination and is found to have a blood pressure (BP) of 164/93 mm Hg. Upon obtaining further history and physical examination, the parents state that she has been increasingly irritable recently. Eight *café au lait* lesions measuring >3 cm × 2 cm are noted. Of the following, which is the *most* likely etiology of the hypertension?
a. Coarctation of the thoracic aorta
b. Renal artery stenosis
c. Urinary tract infection
d. Renal dysplasia

Answer
The answer is b. The patient's history and physical examination are consistent with a diagnosis of *neurofibromatosis* (von Recklinghausen disease). The diagnosis of neurofibromatosis is made on the basis of the history

and physical examination findings of at least two of the following:

- Six or more *café au lait* macules of greatest diameter >5 mm in prepubertal and >15 mm in postpubertal individuals
- Two or more neurofibromas of any type or one plexiform neurofibroma
- Freckling in the axillary or inguinal regions
- Optic glioma
- Two or more Lisch nodules (iris hamartomas)
- A distinctive bony lesion such as sphenoid dysplasia or thinning of the long bone cortex with or without pseudoarthrosis
- A first-degree relative (parent, sibling, or child) with neurofibromatosis

Hypertension in these patients is usually secondary to *renal artery stenosis*, which can occur because of extrinsic compression of the renal artery, vascular neurofibroma formation, or aneurysmal dilation; and can occur at any age. Coarctation of the abdominal aorta may be associated with neurofibromatosis as well as other conditions such as tuberous sclerosis, William syndrome, or other vasculitic disorders. However, coarctation of the thoracic aorta is not a typical finding of neurofibromatosis, but can occur in other conditions such as Turner syndrome. Additionally, pheochromocytomas have been associated with neurofibromatosis but this is seen much more frequently in adults, whereas pediatric patients with neurofibromatosis more commonly have renal artery stenosis. Urinary tract infections generally do not cause hypertension. Renal dysplasia may be associated with hypertension; however, the presenting signs are usually those of failure to thrive.

2. A 4-year-old white boy presents with a 5-day history of generalized edema, which began approximately 1 week after an upper respiratory infection. On physical examination, you find an alert, interactive child, who is noted to have periorbital edema, and ascites. Urinalysis reveals a specific gravity of 1.020, pH 7.0, 4+ proteinuria, and is otherwise unremarkable. Serum cholesterol level was found to be 648 mg/dL, albumin 2.3 g/dL, C3 of 68 mg/dL, C4 of 128 mg/dL, and serum creatinine 0.3 mg/dL. What is the next appropriate step in the management of this child?
a. Perform a renal biopsy.
b. Begin therapy with amoxicillin.
c. Begin therapy with oral prednisone.
d. Admit the patient for intravenous fluids.

Answer
The answer is c. This patient presents with nephrotic syndrome as defined by edema, hypoalbuminemia, and proteinuria. The most common etiology in children is *minimal change disease,* which has a peak incidence in preschool children. Boys are more affected than girls in this age group. Clinical presentation includes generalized edema, often preceded by an infection. Laboratory evaluation will reveal proteinuria, hypoalbuminemia, and hypercholesterolemia. A hypercoagulable state because of derangement in anticoagulant proteins also occurs. In nephrotic syndrome caused by minimal change disease, the serum complement levels are normal.

Management of newly diagnosed nephrotic syndrome clinically consistent with minimal change disease demographically involves a trial of oral prednisone therapy. To induce initial remission, a dosage of 60 mg/m² per day is prescribed with a maximum dose of 80 mg/day. Although 80% of patients will respond within the first 2 weeks of therapy, a 4- to 6-week trial is given before the patient is declared steroid resistant. If the patient is found to be steroid resistant, a renal biopsy should be performed to determine a diagnosis and therapy altered on the basis of the diagnosis.

Although nephrotic patients are at higher risk of developing infections, especially due to *Streptococcus pneumoniae,* prophylactic antibiotics are not recommended at this time. These patients should, however, be immunized using the polyvalent pneumococcal vaccines. Patients with nephrotic syndrome have total body

volume overload resulting from interstitial edema as a result of the hypoalbuminemia. Treatment with intravenous fluids may result in further third spacing and worsening of the nephrotic state. If the patient exhibits signs of intravascular volume depletion, replacement using colloid replacement solution (i.e., albumin infusion therapy) should be considered.

3. The obstetrician calls you because of a concern that one of his patients is carrying a baby with polycystic kidney disease, which has been discovered on prenatal fetal ultrasonography at 28 weeks gestation. The ultrasonography shows numerous huge cysts in the left kidney and a large right kidney with no obvious cysts. Your *best* recommendation would be to:
a. Have a discussion regarding therapeutic abortion.
b. Have a discussion with the mother regarding the fact that this infant will most likely have severe respiratory difficulty immediately after birth and if he survives will most likely go into renal failure shortly after birth.
c. Advise the mother that this most likely represents autosomal-dominant polycystic disease and that she and her husband should have renal ultrasonography to rule out this possibility.
d. Advise that a renal ultrasonography be repeated shortly after birth and that you think the baby will most likely do well.

Answer
The answer is d. This patient presents with unilateral cystic disease. The diagnosis is consistent with a multicystic dysplastic kidney. The dysplastic kidney consists of a group of cysts with a small amount of connective tissue present without the presence of identifiable renal parenchyma. Cystic dysplasia may result from congenital obstructive abnormalities. The contralateral kidney may be enlarged to compensate for the multicystic dysplastic kidney; however, the parenchyma should appear and function normally. With time, the dysplastic kidney involutes and its function deteriorates. The management includes postnatal renal ultrasonography to confirm the diagnosis. Approximately 40% of patients have contralateral vesicoureteral reflux; therefore, a voiding cystourethrogram may be warranted. These patients should be followed up with ultrasound monitoring. The affected kidney need not be removed unless recurrent urinary tract infections or hypertension develop.

Autosomal-dominant polycystic kidney disease (ADPKD) and autosomal-recessive polycystic kidney disease (ARPKD) are genetic defects that cause cyst formation within the kidneys without dysplasia. The defect causes bilateral renal involvement. The management and prognoses vary depending upon clinical features.

4. An 18-month-old girl presents to your office with dysuria and fever. Urinalysis shows 3+ leukocyte esterase and microscopic examination reveals too numerous to count white blood cells (WBCs) and numerous bacteria. You diagnose a urinary tract infection and treat with trimethoprim-sulfamethoxazole for 10 days and the symptoms resolve. She has had one other urinary tract infection, so you obtain an ultrasonography, which is normal, and a voiding cystourethrogram, which shows left-sided grade III reflux. There is no reflux on the right side. The *most* appropriate course of action now is to:

a. Refer the patient to a urologist for ureteral reimplantation.
b. Begin prophylactic antibiotic therapy once daily.
c. Hospitalize the patient and treat with intravenous antibiotics.
d. No further evaluation or intervention is warranted.

Answer
The answer is b. On the basis of the American Academy of Pediatrics guidelines, all the children between 2 months and 2 years of age presenting with a first-time febrile urinary tract infection should undergo a screening renal ultrasonography and voiding cystourethrogram to evaluate for the presence of vesicoureteral reflux.

Recurrent urinary tract infections in the presence of vesicoureteral reflux may lead to renal scarring and eventually chronic renal failure, and as such, should be avoided. In the presence of reflux, children should be placed on once-daily prophylactic antibiotics, preferable at bedtime. Acceptable antibiotic choices include trimethoprim-sulfamethoxazole, nitrofurantoin, or amoxicillin. Quarterly urine cultures should be performed routinely, as well as during times of urinary infection symptoms or unexplained fevers. Annual cystograms should be performed. After the first voiding cystourethrogram, reevaluations can be performed using radionucleotide cystograms to decrease the risk of radiation exposure.

No absolute data define the resolution rates based on grade; however, large retrospective studies show that grades I to III of reflux often resolve. Of those cases of reflux that resolve, approximately 80% resolve within 5 years of diagnosis. Furthermore, approximately 80% of all cases of grades I to II reflux resolve spontaneously, as compared with 60% of those with grade III reflux, and 40% of those with grade IV reflux. Surgical intervention should be considered in children who have breakthrough infections, have high-grade reflux (IV or V) and evidence of renal scars, or children older than 6 year of age with persistent high-grade reflux.

5. You are called to see a 5-day-old male infant in the emergency room for generalized edema. After examination of the child, your presumed diagnosis is congenital nephrotic syndrome of the Finnish type. All of the following are true regarding congenital nephrotic syndrome *except:*

a. It is associated with an abnormally large placenta and oligohydramnios.
b. It is associated with hypothyroidism.
c. It should be managed with aggressive nutrition therapy.
d. Corticosteroids are the mainstay of pharmacotherapy.

Answer
The answer is d. Congenital nephrotic syndrome is an inherited disorder involving a defect in chromosome 19, NPHS1, which encodes for nephrin. This defect causes a disruption of the glomerular capillary filter. The result is loss of protein in the urine, initially albuminuria; however, because of the severity of proteinuria, losses of immunoglobulin, antithrombin III, vitamin D-binding protein, and thyroid-binding globulin occur. These children are often born prematurely, are below the fifth percentile for weight (with normal birth lengths), and the placenta is enlarged (comprising at least 25% of the birth weight). Approximately 90% of these children present with generalized edema within the first week of life. Progressive protein loss results in malnutrition, hypothyroidism, a markedly increased susceptibility to infections, and hypercoagulable state. *Progressive renal failure also occurs, with most patients requiring dialysis or renal transplantation within the first decade of life.* Because of a kwashiorkor state, these patients require aggressive nutrition therapy to achieve normal growth and development. Because of high protein losses, these patients often require daily albumin infusion therapy. In many cases, medical or surgical nephrectomy may be indicated to decrease the degree of proteinuria. Supplementation with thyroxine is required, often from birth, with adjustments for growth. The major cause of early death is sepsis. Most patients who survive for the first 12 months undergo renal transplantation. The major barrier is to overcome the nutritional deficiencies and achieve a dry weight that allows for a renal transplant to be performed. Many of the patients who have had transplantation have undergone unilateral or bilateral nephrectomies in order to limit protein losses and allow for more normal growth. Recurrent disease in the transplant has been reported but is a rare phenomenon.

6. You are asked to see a patient in the pediatric intensive care unit with a falling urine output following an automobile accident during which the patient developed a renal hematoma and a liver laceration for which he underwent an exploratory laparotomy. His serum creatinine is 2.4 mg/dL, his serum Na is 137 mEq/L, his urinary Na is 9 mEq/L, and his urinary creatinine is 278 mg/dL. This is consistent with which of the following diagnoses?
a. Acute tubular necrosis
b. Intravascular volume depletion
c. Renal compression syndrome
d. Underlying glomerular disease

Answer
The answer is b. This patient has acute renal failure, which can be clinically from either prerenal or renal

etiology. The fractional excretion of sodium (FENa), calculated as:

$$\frac{U_{Na} \times P_{Cr}}{P_{Na} \times U_{Cr}} \times 100$$

can help differentiate prerenal etiologies from renal etiologies of acute renal failure. In this equation, the U_{Na} is the urine sodium, P_{Cr} is plasma creatinine, P_{Na} is plasma sodium, and U_{Cr} is the urine creatinine, all measured on random urine and blood samples. These values should be obtained when the patient is not taking diuretics. In the setting of an acute renal failure, a FENa >2.5% is indicative of a renal cause, whereas an FENa of <1% is indicative of a prerenal cause. In this patient, the FENa is indeed <1%. Management should include determination of the prerenal cause (i.e., intravascular volume depletion, poor cardiac output, reduced renal perfusion) and appropriate intervention should be implemented. In most cases, if the urinary Na is <10 mEq/L, the kidney is avidly conserving Na and the FENa is going to be <1%.

7. A 15-year-old teenage boy presents to your office for a routine physical examination after football practice. You find him to be healthy, and at the 95th percentile for height and 75th percentile for weight. He is an active young man who plays football and basketball. Vital signs are normal as is the physical examination. A routine urine dipstick test in the office reveals 2+ proteinuria. The appropriate next step in evaluation of the proteinuria is:
a. Obtain three first morning voids.
b. Obtain a 24-hour urine collection.
c. Perform a renal biopsy.
d. Initiate treatment with an angiotensin converting enzyme inhibitor.

Answer
The answer is a. Proteinuria may be a transient finding in the urine and is influenced by many factors. False-positive tests may occur with an alkaline urine or gross hematuria. Transient proteinuria may occur with exercise, fever, intrinsic cardiac disease, and so on. Orthostatic proteinuria is a transient proteinuria that has been associated with urine samples taken later during the day and is typically found in tall, athletic, adolescent boys. To differentiate orthostatic proteinuria, three first morning void samples can be obtained and checked for protein. Because this urine is produced overnight, while the patient is supine, protein should not be present in the first morning void sample.

If protein is present in all of the first morning voids, then a 24-hour urine collection should be obtained to quantify the degree of proteinuria. Additionally, laboratory evaluation, including a renal function panel, complete blood count, and C3 and C4 levels, should be obtained. If proteinuria is greater than 8 mg/kg per day, then a renal biopsy should be performed to determine

its etiology. Angiotensin converting *enzyme* inhibitors and/or angiotensin receptor blockers are recommended to decrease the glomerular filtration pressure, thereby decreasing proteinuria and preserving renal function.

8. A 5-year-old girl presents with a 2-day history of gross hematuria and slight facial edema. She had a sore throat 2 weeks ago for which she was seen in an emergency care center. According to the mother, the rapid group A streptococcal test was positive and the patient was treated with penicillin intramuscularly. Vital signs show a temperature of 37.7°C (99.86°F), heart rate (HR) 90 beats/minute, respiratory rate (RR) 18, and BP 118/86 mm Hg. Her physical examination is significant only for slight periorbital edema and ascites. The single *most* appropriate laboratory test that you should obtain is:
a. Antistreptolysin O (ASO) titer
b. C3 level
c. Antinuclear antibody (ANA)
d. Renal ultrasonography

Answer
The answer is b. The most likely diagnosis is poststreptococcal glomerulonephritis (PSGN), of which the hallmark laboratory abnormality is a depressed C3 level. PSGN is the most common cause of glomerulonephritis in children and affects preschool and elementary school students. Boys are affected more frequently than girls. The serum C3 levels are depressed initially, but should normalize within 8 to 12 weeks after presentation. If this does not occur, then systemic lupus erythematosus or membranoproliferative glomerulonephritis should be considered. No specific treatment of PSGN exists; however, the patient should be monitored for hypertension, which should be treated if present. A diuretic is preferred because the mechanism of hypertension is sodium and water retention. The patient in this case would most likely be treated with Lasix for her mild hypertension. Antibiotic therapy is warranted only if it is necessary to treat the streptococcal infection. Steroids are not usually indicated in the treatment of PSGN. In rare cases, a rapidly progressive form of PSGN may occur and can cause renal failure. In 98% of cases, however, a full recovery is expected. The proteinuria may persist for weeks and the hematuria for up to 2 years and this should be explained to the family.

9. A 12-year-old girl presents to you for evaluation of enuresis. She complains of daytime and nighttime accidents, stating that she often cannot sense when she has to urinate. She has never been fully potty trained per the parents. She states that she does have bowel continence. She denies any pain in the back or lower extremity. You ascertain that she had quite a few febrile episodes without apparent cause, as a young child. There is no contributory family history. You find no abnormalities in her physical examination. It is appropriate to obtain all of the following studies *except:*

a. Renal ultrasonography
b. Voiding cystourethrogram
c. Urinalysis
d. Magnetic resonance imaging (MRI) spine

Answer
The answer is d. Enuresis is a common problem in children; approximately 15% of 5-year-old children present with bed-wetting. The incidence decreases with age and resolves spontaneously at a rate of approximately 15% per year. When evaluating these children, key issues to ascertain in the history include the presence of daytime symptoms, family history of enuresis, fluid intake summary, voiding diary (specifically obtaining information to ascertain bladder capacity), stooling diary (to determine if there is associated constipation or encopresis), medical history, and social history (especially in secondary enuresis). Physical examination (to evaluate for lumbosacral abnormalities such as tuft of hair over the sacrum, sacral dimple, etc.) and abdominal/rectal examination should be performed, and growth measurements (to ascertain for chronic kidney disease) should be taken. Evaluation should include a urinalysis to determine the urinary concentrating ability in order to exclude diabetes insipidus, diabetes mellitus, or urinary tract infection. Urologic imaging, including a renal ultrasonography and voiding cystourethrogram, should be performed in children who have significant daytime complaints, history of prior urinary tract infections, or signs of structural urologic abnormalities (such as neurogenic bladder, tethered cord, and vesicoureteral reflux). MRI of the spine should be reserved for children who have abnormalities of the lumbosacral spine on physical examination, symptoms of encopresis, neurologic abnormalities of the lower extremities, or evidence of neurogenic or neuropathic bladder on a voiding cystourethrogram.

10. A 14-year-old boy presents to the emergency room in northern Minnesota in December with a feeling of tingling in his fingers and toes as well as cramping in his legs. He had been playing football outdoors for approximately 6 hours that afternoon. On physical examination, you see redness in the fingertips and toes; however, neurologic examination only reveals a decrease in sensation to his fingertips with motor examination intact. The expected electrolyte abnormality causing his symptoms is *most* likely:

a. Hypernatremia
b. Hypokalemia
c. Hypermagnesemia
d. Hyperphosphatemia

Answer
The answer is b. Hypothermia causes an intracellular shifting of potassium, which causes hypokalemia. If a patient is near death, hyperkalemia resulting from tissue necrosis ensues. When managing a patient with hypothermia, it is imperative to initiate resuscitation immediately including evaluation for cardiac electroconductive changes. Despite prolonged resuscitation, complete recovery is possible because of the neuroprotective effects of hypothermia. Management should include passive external rewarming (removal of wet/cold clothing) and active external rewarming (use of heating blankets, forced warm air, warm bath). Internal rewarming should be reserved for severe cases. Cardiac arrhythmias can be treated with defibrillation but may be refractory until rewarming has occurred. Electrolyte abnormalities should be corrected intravenously.

11. A 15-month-old African-American female infant presents to you for failure to thrive. On physical examination, you note bowing of her legs and as part of the evaluation, obtain x-rays that show fraying and cupping of the metaphyseal regions of both femurs, both tibias, and both fibulas. There is no acute fracture. The mother states that the infant is still breast-fed and drinks only about 360 mL of milk/day. She does not eat other dairy foods. The mother also states that the patient is not exposed much to sunlight. She is otherwise developmentally normal per the mother. Which of the following electrolyte profiles is this child *most* likely to have?

a. Ca = 10.1 mg/dL, PO_4 = 2.3 mg/dL, parathyroid hormone (PTH) = 85 IU/mL, Na = 140 mEq/L, K = 4.5 mEq/L, Cl = 99 mEq/L, HCO_3 = 27 mEq/L
b. Ca = 8.2 mg/dL, PO_4 = 4.5 mg/dL, PTH = 189 IU/mL, Na = 140 mEq/L, K = 4.5 mEq/L, Cl = 99 mEq/L, HCO_3 = 21 mEq/L
c. Ca = 13.1 mg/dL, PO_4 = 4.0 mg/dL, PTH = 185 IU/mL, Na = 140 mEq/L, K = 4.5 mEq/L, Cl = 99 mEq/L, HCO_3 = 27 mEq/L
d. Ca = 8.1 mg/dL, PO_4 = 7.0 mg/dL, PTH = 189 IU/mL, Na = 140 mEq/L, K = 4.5 mEq/L, Cl = 99 mEq/L, HCO_3 = 20 mEq/L

Answer
The answer is b. This infant likely has *vitamin D–deficient rickets* resulting from nutritional causes. The electrolyte abnormalities seen in vitamin D–deficient rickets include:

- A low normal to normal serum calcium
- Low normal to normal phosphate
- Elevated alkaline phosphatase
- Elevated parathyroid hormone (PTH)
- Decreased 25 (OH) vitamin D levels
- Low normal to slightly decreased $1,25(OH)_2$ vitamin D levels

An increased anion gap metabolic acidosis may be present because of malnutrition. The choice a represents X-linked hypophosphatemic rickets, which occurs in male, rather than female patients. The specific electrolyte abnormalities include a depressed serum phosphate, elevated alkaline phosphatase, and normal or decreased 1,25(OH)2 vitamin D levels. The serum calcium, PTH, 25 (OH) vitamin D, and electrolytes are normal. Choice *c* represents hyperparathyroidism, as exhibited by elevated serum calcium, normal phosphorus, elevated serum PTH, and normal electrolyte levels. Choice *d* represents renal osteodystrophy, otherwise known as renal rickets, as hallmarked by elevated serum phosphorus and PTH levels, as well as depressed serum calcium levels and possible presence of acidosis.

12. A 7-year-old girl who was adopted from China presents to you for evaluation of episodic gross hematuria and persistent microscopic hematuria. She states that the hematuria is painless and occurs approximately once a month, lasting approximately 2 days each time. You discover significant proteinuria on your evaluation and you perform a renal biopsy, which confirms a diagnosis of membranous nephropathy (MN). A laboratory evaluation should be undertaken to evaluate for which of the following?
a. Hepatitis B
b. Wilson disease
c. Human immunodeficiency virus
d. Shigellosis

Answer
The answer is **a.** MN may be idiopathic, but is often secondary to a variety of causes. Hepatitis B can be associated with MN and typically occurs in children from endemic areas who have not been vaccinated against the virus. Typically, these children are asymptomatic without active disease, but have positive hepatitis B surface antigen, hepatitis Be antigen.

MN is present in approximately 10% to 20% of patients with systemic lupus erythematosus. Children may present without any systemic findings and with only renal disease. Screening ANA and appropriate evaluation should be performed in all children with MN. Malignancies, specifically lung and colon cancer, can cause the renal findings of MN but these occur in adults, and generally not in children. Medications such as penicillamine or gold, as used in patients with rheumatoid arthritis, and nonsteroidal anti-inflammatory drugs, can cause MN. Wilson disease and Shigellosis do not typically cause renal manifestations. Human immunodeficiency virus can cause various forms of nephropathy but is classically associated with a collapsing form of focal segmental glomerulosclerosis.

13. You are asked to see a patient in the intensive care unit. A 15-year-old girl presented unconscious after a suspected suicide attempt by ingestion. Her serum chemistries are as follows:

Na = 143 mEq/L   Blood urea nitrogen (BUN) = 35 mg/dL

K = 5.4 mEq/L   Creatinine = 1.2 mg/dL

Cl = 102 mEq/L   Glucose = 126 mg/dL
HCO$_3$ = 12 mEq/L

What is the *most* likely agent she ingested?
a. Ethylene glycol
b. Tylenol
c. Iron
d. Acetazolamide

Answer
The answer is **a.** This patient has metabolic acidosis with an elevated anion gap (Na − [Cl + HCO$_3$]) of 19. The usual differential diagnosis includes salicylate, methanol, ethanol, or ethylene glycol ingestion; lactic acidosis that may be secondary to malignancy, systemic hypoperfusion or metformin therapy for type II diabetes mellitus; diabetic ketoacidosis; or renal failure causing uremia. A key feature to ascertain when addressing an acid–base abnormality is whether there is an elevated anion gap. If nonanion gap acidosis is present, diarrhea or renal tubular acidosis should be considered in the differential diagnosis.

14. A 3-year-old white girl with a known history of steroid-responsive nephrotic syndrome presents to the emergency room with shortness of breath and fever. She had relapsed recently and is currently receiving 2 mg/kg per day of oral steroids. Physical examination reveals temperature of 3 8.1°C (100.58°F), HR 150/minute, RR 28/minute, and BP 118/74 mm Hg; periorbital edema is present; chest auscultation reveals decreased breath sounds in the right base; abdominal examination reveals ascites with marked abdominal tenderness and evidence of rebound tenderness.

The most important next step in your evaluation is:
a. Ventilation/perfusion lung scan
b. Paracentesis
c. Blood culture
d. Renal ultrasonography

Answer
The answer is **b.** Spontaneous bacterial peritonitis is the most common life-threatening complication of nephrosis. A paracentesis should be performed and the fluid sent for cell count, Gram stain, and culture. Empiric antibiotic therapy can be initiated and geared toward the most common bacterial causes, specifically Pneumococcus and *Escherichia coli*. A complete blood count and blood cultures should also be obtained prior to the initiation of antibiotics.

Another complication of nephrosis is thrombosis. Because of urinary losses of antithrombin, increased platelet activation, and the presence of high-molecular-weight fibrinogen, patients with nephrotic syndrome are at risk for thromboembolic phenomenon, such as pulmonary embolus, deep venous thrombosis, or renal vein thrombosis. As such, in an acute setting, a ventilation/perfusion lung scan, venography, or MRI may be warranted. Renal ultrasonography with Doppler may yield false-positive and false-negative results, and hence, is not the test that would be utilized to assess for possible thrombosis.

Other long-term complications of nephrotic syndrome may include an increased susceptibility to infections secondary to immunosuppressant agents and hypercholesterolemia. Patients may be refractory to treatment and develop frequent episodes of nephrosis, which may impair growth and cause kwashiorkor. Side effects of long-term steroid use may occur as well.

15. A 13-year-old white girl presents for evaluation of leg cramps, which have become progressively worse over the past few weeks. The patient also has noted tingling in her fingers. She states that recently, she has been waking up at night to urinate and has been craving for salty foods. You obtain laboratory evaluation results, which show serum potassium of 2.3 mmol/L, bicarbonate of 32 mmol/L, and serum magnesium of 1.0 mg/dL. The long-term treatment of this disorder involves all of the following *except*:
a. Oral potassium
b. Oral magnesium
c. Thiazide diuretics
d. Potassium-sparing diuretics

Answer

The answer is c. This patient has Gitelman syndrome, which is an autosomal-recessive disorder that usually presents in late childhood and adolescence. Patients usually present with cramping of the arms and legs, which is secondary to hypokalemia and hypomagnesemia. Up to 10% of patients may present with tetany, usually related to an acute illness (diarrhea, vomiting), which worsens the hypomagnesemia. Some patients may present with severe fatigue, BP readings that are lower than average, and polyuria/nocturia as a result of some salt wasting.

The genetic defect in Gitelman syndrome is a mutation in the gene coding for the thiazide-sensitive Na-Cl cotransporter in the distal tubule. A defect in this transporter causes magnesium wasting and a marked decrease in calcium excretion, which is similar to that induced by thiazide therapy and the opposite of the hypercalciuria seen in the classic Bartter syndrome.

Treatment involves correction of the electrolyte abnormalities, specifically oral magnesium and potassium supplements. Treatment is lifelong. Treatment with a thiazide diuretic may be beneficial in Bartter syndrome, in which urinary calcium wasting occurs, but not in Gitelman syndrome. Additionally, a nonsteroidal anti-inflammatory drug and/or a potassium-sparing diuretic (such as spironolactone or amiloride) may raise the plasma potassium concentration toward normal level, largely reverse the metabolic alkalosis, and partially correct the hypomagnesemia.

Classic Bartter syndrome generally presents in the toddler years and may be associated with growth and mental retardation. Children present with hypokalemia, metabolic alkalosis, polyuria, polydipsia, and decreased urinary concentrating ability. Urinary calcium excretion is increased and the plasma magnesium level is normal or mildly reduced. This is caused by a primary defect in sodium chloride reabsorption in the medullary thick ascending limb of the loop of Henle. The treatment of Bartter syndrome involves electrolyte correction. However, because these patients have hypercalciuria, some benefit from a thiazide diuretic may be observed.

16. An 8-year-old boy presents to your office with complaints of burning in his hands and feet, especially following his summer baseball games. The palms and soles burn intensely and the mother also notes that he does not sweat. One of the mother's brothers complained of similar findings as a youngster and is on dialysis at the age of 45 years, and a second brother is on a cardiac transplantation list with severe cardiomyopathy. Which skin lesions might you see in this child?
a. *Café au lait* spots over the chest and abdomen
b. Ash leaf spots
c. Angiokeratomas in the groin region
d. Spider angiomas in the chest and abdominal area

Answer

The answer is c. This history is highly suggestive of *Fabry disease* and the characteristic skin lesions are *angiokeratomas* in the groin and umbilical region. This is an *X-linked recessive* disorder and is caused by the absence of the enzyme α-galactosidase A. The patient usually presents by the age of 10 years with symptoms of burning of the palms and feet and skin lesions. As time progresses, the patients develop either renal or cardiac disease as a result of the accumulation of globotriaosylceramide, which is the substrate for galactosidase A. The diagnosis can be confirmed by measuring galactosidase A in leukocytes. Enzyme therapy is now available, which may prevent cardiac and renal complications.

SUGGESTED READINGS

1. Avner ED, Harmon WE, Niaudet P. *Pediatric nephrology*, 5th ed. Philadelphia: Lippincott Williams & Wilkins, 2003.
2. Brenner & Rector's. *The kidney*, 7th ed. Philadelphia: Elsevier, 2004.
3. Conley S. Fluid and electrolyte therapy: hypernatremia. *Pediatr Clin North Am* 1990;37(2):365–370.
4. Hogg RJ. Evaluation and management of proteinuria and nephrotic syndrome in children: recommendations from a pediatric nephrology panel established at the National Kidney Foundation conference on Proteinuria, Albuminuria, Risk, Assessment, Detection, and Elimination (PARADE). *Pediatrics* 2000;105(6):1242–1249.
5. Perry PL, Belsha CW. Fluid and electrolyte therapy: hypernatremia. *Pediatr Clin North Am* 1990;37(2):351–361.
6. Warshaw B. Nephrotic syndrome in children. *Pediatric Ann* 1994; 23(9):49.

Chapter 16

Adrenal Disorders

Anzar Haider

Adrenal disorders represent a classical bio-feedback system and underscore the importance of physiology and biochemistry in understanding the disease process.

ANATOMY

The adrenal gland is a pyramidal-shaped organ that lies above the upper pole of the kidneys. It functionally consists of two endocrine tissues; the outer one derived from mesodermal tissue, develops into the *adrenal cortex*; and the inner one derived from ectodermal neural crests forms the *medulla*.

The fetal adrenal cortex forms by the fifth week of gestation, consisting of two distinct zones, an outer zone "adult/definite zone" that produces glucocorticoids and mineralocorticoids, and a much larger "fetal zone" that mainly produces androgens (dehydroepiandrosterone [DHEA]) for the synthesis of estrogen by the placenta. The fetal zone regresses after birth and the adult/definite zone then proliferates and androgen-specific reticularis zone develops by 5 to 6 years of age.

PHYSIOLOGY AND REGULATION OF THE ADRENAL CORTEX

The adrenal cortex in older children and adults is divided into three zones:

- Zona glomerulosa: Outer zone that principally produces aldosterone
- Zona fasciculata: Middle zone that synthesizes glucocorticoids
- Zona reticularis: Inner zone that principally secretes androgens (DHEA and androstenedione)

All adrenal hormones are synthesized from cholesterol by a series of P450 (CYP) and hydroxysteroid dehydrogenase (HSD) enzymes. Aldosterone is regulated by the renin-angiotensin system and is influenced by sodium levels and blood pressure. Cortisol secretion is under the control of adrenocorticotrophic hormone (ACTH), which in turn is stimulated by corticotropin releasing hormone (CRH) from the hypothalamus. No direct stimulatory signal accounts for the release of adrenal androgen secretion; however, ACTH does have a permissive role in the secretion of adrenal androgens.

DISORDERS OF ADRENAL CORTEX

Adrenal cortical secretions consist of glucocorticoid, mineralocorticoid, and androgen and can be broadly classified into hypofunctional and hyperfunctional states.

Adrenal insufficiency (hypofunction) is termed primary when the defect is in the adrenal gland itself, and secondary if the defect is in the pituitary region.

Primary Adrenal Insufficiency (Low Cortisol, High Adrenocorticotrophic Hormone)

Patients with primary adrenal insufficiency may present in adrenal crises with cardiovascular collapse and can be fatal. Clinical features are the result of combined defects in glucocorticoid and mineralocorticoid secretion. There are congenital and acquired causes.

Congenital Primary Adrenal Insufficiency

Causes of primary adrenal insufficiency include:

- Congenital adrenal hypoplasia
- Congenital adrenal hyperplasia (CAH)
- Familial glucocorticoid deficiency (ACTH resistance)
- Metabolic disease: Adrenoleukodystrophy, Wolman disease, Smith Lemli Opitz

Infants with *congenital adrenal hypoplasia* present in the newborn period, typically 2 weeks after birth, with hypoglycemia, jaundice, failure to thrive, and vomiting. These patients have severe glucocorticoid, mineralocorticoid, and androgen deficiency. Thus, they may present with dehydration, hypotension, hyponatremia, and hyperkalemia.

Males are generally affected, as this is caused by an X-linked mutation in the DAX-1 gene on chromosome Xp21. This gene is important in the development of the adrenal glands and gonads. The gene is contiguous to the glycerol kinase and Duchenne muscular dystrophy gene. Recently, an autosomal gene (SF-1) also has been identified; heterozygous mutation causes adrenal and gonadal hypoplasia.

Congenital adrenal hyperplasia is a group of inherited autosomal recessive disorders of one of the enzyme in the cortisol pathway that results in hyperplasia of the adrenal gland with low cortisol and an elevated ACTH level. Adrenal steroidogenesis pathway is depicted in (Fig. 16.1). Enzyme defects are discussed later in detail.

Familial glucocorticoid deficiency is transmitted in autosomal recessive manner. Patients have ACTH resistance and may have mutations in the MC2 receptor.

Adrenoleukodystrophy (ALD) is an X-linked disorder characterized by progressive CNS demyelination and adrenal failure. Signs of adrenal failure may be the initial and only manifestation of this disorder, although neurologic symptoms may precede the adrenal deficiency. It is caused by a gene mutation on chromosome Xq28. The diagnosis is established by finding an elevated level of very long chain fatty acids (VLCFA) in the plasma. This condition should be ruled out in all males presenting with adrenal insufficiency.

Triple A syndrome (Allgrove syndrome) consists of ACTH resistance, achalasia, and alacrima. Many patients may have neurologic symptoms as well. This syndrome is caused by mutation in the AAAS gene whose product ALADIN is expressed in the central nervous (CNS) and gastrointestinal systems.

Acquired Primary Adrenal Insufficiency

Causes of acquired primary adrenal insufficiency include:

- Autoimmune adrenalitis (isolated)
- Autoimmune polyglandular syndrome (APS) Type 1 and Type 2
- Adrenal infections (TB, HIV, fungal, sepsis)
- Adrenal hemorrhage, infarction, and infiltration
- Medications (mitotane, ketoconazole, megestrol, medroxyprogesterone)

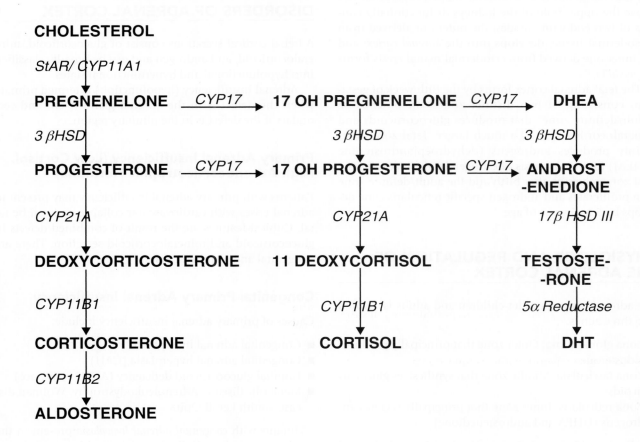

3 βHSD, 3β-OH steroid dehydrogenase; DHEA, dehydroepiandrosterone; DHT, Dihydrotestosterone.

Figure 16.1 The adrenal steroidogenesis pathway.

Autoimmune adrenalitis is the most common cause of acquired adrenal insufficiency. It may occur as an isolated problem or as a part of the autoimmune polyglandular syndrome (APS). There are two types associated with adrenal insufficiency:

Type I APS typically presents in younger patients (first decade of life) and is also called APECED (autoimmune polyendocrinopathy with cutaneous ectodermal dysplasia). This is caused by a mutation in the AIRE gene on chromosome 21. It is characterized mainly by:

- Hypoparathyroidism
- Adrenal insufficiency
- Mucocutaneous candidiasis
- Other minor manifestations: primary hypogonadism, Hashimoto thyroiditis, vitiligo, alopecia

Type II APS is characterized by:

- Hypothyroidism
- Adrenal insufficiency
- Type I diabetes mellitus

Other endocrine organs also may be affected. It occurs in late adolescence and appears to have an autosomal dominant pattern of transmission. Adrenal failure is typically the first manifestation.

Secondary Adrenal Insufficiency (Low Cortisol, Low Adrenocorticotrophic Hormone)

Signs and symptoms of secondary adrenal insufficiency are non-specific and milder than in primary adrenal insufficiency. These can also be classified into congenital and acquired.

Congenital causes include:

- Hypopituitarism
- Septo-optic dysplasia
- Cerebral midline defects
- Isolated ACTH defect

Acquired causes include:

- Craniopharyngioma
- Cranial irradiation
- Infiltrative pituitary and hypothalamic lesions (Langerhans cell histiocytosis, sarcoidosis)
- Hypophysitis
- Surgery to the hypothalamic-pituitary area
- Steroid therapy

Mineralocorticoid function in these disorders is intact; thus, these patients do not present with salt wasting and cardiovascular collapse. ACTH deficiency typically presents in the context of multitrophic hypothalamic pituitary disease. Neonates may present with hypoglycemia, poor feeding, and jaundice. Older children may have nonspecific symptoms of inappropriate fatigue, anorexia, weakness, ill-defined abdominal pain, nausea, and prolonged

recovery from illness. Symptoms of orthostatic hypotension, salt craving, and generalized skin pigmentation—characteristics of primary adrenal insufficiency—are *not* found in secondary adrenal insufficiency.

Laboratory Investigations of Adrenal Insufficiency

Laboratory findings may include a low morning cortisol concentration, associated with an elevated ACTH concentration in primary, but a normal or low ACTH in secondary adrenal insufficiency. Mineralocorticoid insufficiency occurs in *primary* adrenal insufficiency and can be diagnosed by an increased plasma renin activity, low aldosterone, sodium, and bicarbonate levels, and high potassium level. Since mineralocorticoid activity is normal in secondary adrenal insufficiency, hyperkalemia is not present, but hyponatremia occurs because of decreased water excretion from a lack of glucocorticoid activity.

Treatment of Adrenal Insufficiency

Hydrocortisone 10 to 15mg/m^2/day should be given two to three times a day to replace glucocorticoid deficiency. Fludrocortisone should be added in mineralocorticoid deficiency (typically found in primary adrenal insufficiency states).

Glucocorticoid Excess (Hypercortisolism)

Cushing syndrome is a disorder of excess glucocorticoid secretion and the effect of prolonged exposure to cortisol. Cushing syndrome is rare in children. The most common cause in children is exogenous administration of pharmacological dose of glucocorticoid.

Endogenous Cushing syndrome includes *Cushing disease* if the source is increased production from the pituitary caused by an ACTH-secreting pituitary microadenoma. This accounts for 75% of all cases of Cushing syndrome in children over 7 years of age. In children under 7 years of age, adrenal sources of Cushing syndrome are common (adrenal adenoma, carcinoma, or bilateral hyperplasia). Most adrenal tumors in children presenting with Cushing syndrome are malignant.

Clinical features include weight gain, growth deceleration, fatigue, muscle weakness, and emotional lability. The patient may have increased facial plethora, easy bruising, violaceous striae, hirsutism, and hypertension. Growth failure in Cushing syndrome is the most important distinguishing feature from exogenous obesity and can obviate the need for an expensive workup for obesity.

Elevated values of midnight salivary cortisol, 24-hour urinary free cortisol, and cortisol level drawn in the early morning following overnight dexamethasone administration (overnight dexamethasone test) can be used to screen for hypercortisolemia. The low-dose, high-dose dexamethasone suppression test can be employed to distinguish pituitary versus adrenal source. Cortisol values are not suppressed in disorders of adrenal origin.

Iatrogenic Cushing syndrome is treated by gradual withdrawal of the exogenous glucocorticoid and employing minimal effective dose or alternate day dosing.

Mineralocorticoid Deficiency

Mineralocorticoid deficiency causes salt wasting with vomiting, dehydration, hyponatremia, hyperkalemia, and acidosis. Etiologies of mineralocorticoid deficiency include congenital adrenal hypoplasia, primary adrenal insufficiency, congenital adrenal hyperplasia (StAR protein deficiency, 3βHSD, CYP21), CYP11B2 (aldosterone synthase deficiency) (see Fig. 16.1), and aldosterone resistance (pseudohypoaldosteronism). Treatment of the latter condition includes salt replacement and resin exchange.

Mineralocorticoid Excess

Mineralocorticoid excess causes hypertension. CYP11B1 and CYP17 enzyme deficient patients also have been associated with hypokalemia. Virilization in girls may also be present at birth in CYP11B1 defect. Hypertension occurs because of elevated 11-deoxycorticosterone (DOC) levels. *CYP17* defect causes cortisol and androgen deficiency. In this disorder, there is a blockage in conversion from mineralocorticoid to glucocorticoid and androgen pathway. Patients with 46XY may have incompletely virilized, phenotypically female or ambiguous genitalia. Affected females have normal external genitalia but fail to progress into normal sexual development in adolescence.

An *11βHSD* defect causes apparent mineralocorticoid excess (AME) because of excess accumulation of cortisol from failure to metabolize to inactive cortisone.

Liddle syndrome results from an activating mutation of epithelial sodium channel. It is transmitted in an autosomal dominant mode and is characterized by low renin, low aldosterone, and hypertension.

Adrenal Androgen (Sex Steroid) Excess

Adrenal causes of androgen excess include premature adrenarche, adrenal tumors, and congenital adrenal hyperplasia (CYP21, CYP11B1, 3βHSD in females).

Premature adrenarche may results from an early activation of adrenal androgen and typically presents between the ages of 5 and 8 years. It is a benign condition and is characterized by pubic hair and body odor development. Patients subsequently develop normal puberty.

An *adrenocortical tumor* produces excess androgen with features of virilization (clitoral enlargement, hirsutism) in females, early adrenarche, deepening of the voice, and accelerated growth. In males, the testes may be small, yet they have secondary features of puberty. Adrenal androgens (androstenedione and DHEAS) may be elevated. Luteinizing

hormone (LH) and follicle stimulating hormone (FSH) may be low. Computed tomography and/or magnetic resonance imaging may identify the tumor. Treatment involves surgical resection of the tumor.

Congenital Adrenal Hyperplasia

The clinical features of congenital adrenal hyperplasia (CAH) vary with the extent and locations of the enzyme defect and are outlined in Table 16.1.

CAH with enzymatic deficiency in CYP21, CYP11, 3βHSD causes increased androgen levels resulting in ambiguous genitalia at birth and postnatal virilization in females.

21-Hydroxylase Deficiency (CYP21)

21-Hydroxylase deficiency (CYP21) is the most common form of CAH, accounting for 95% of cases; the overall incidence is 1 per 15,000 births. This disorder results from a mutation in CYP21A gene present on chromosome 6. The severity of the defects in the enzyme determines the phenotype of this disorder. Three main forms occur clinically:

- Classic salt wasting form (<1% enzyme activity)
- Simple virilizing form (1%–2% enzyme activity)
- Non-classical (Late onset) (20%–60% enzyme activity)

Classical Salt Wasting

The enzymatic defect causes cortisol deficiency, which by classic biofeedback mechanism, increases ACTH secretion, resulting in increased adrenal androgens (androstenedione and DHEA), which peripherally are converted to testosterone. This causes virilization of the external genitalia in the female, who may have an enlarged clitoris with fusion of labioscrotal folds forming a urogenital sinus. The internal genitalia are normal with normal development of ovaries and Müllerian structures. The enzyme defect also causes aldosterone deficiency, resulting in salt wasting, which manifests as vomiting, lethargy, and weight loss. Male infants have normal-appearing genitalia and present at 2 to 3 weeks of age with vomiting and weight loss as clinical features of salt wasting.

Classical Simple Virilizing

The simple virilizing form of 21-hydroxylase deficiency presents with ambiguity of genitalia in females but normal genitalia in males. There is no salt loss, since the aldosterone pathway is not severely affected. Later in infancy or childhood, males and females in whom virilization has been missed may present with premature development of pubic and axillary hair, acne, enlarged phallus, accelerated growth, and advanced bone age.

Nonclassical CAH

Patients with this form of 21-hydroxylase deficiency present anytime postnatally with features of androgen excess.

TABLE 16.1

CHARACTERISTICS OF CLINICAL FORMS OF CONGENITAL ADRENAL HYPERPLASIA

Disease	21 Hydroxylase			11β Hydroxylase	3βHSD	17α Hydroxylase	Lipoid Hyperplasia
	Salt Wasting	Simple Virilizing	Late Onset				
Gene mutation	CYP21A	CYP21A	CYP21A	CYP11B1	HSD3B2	CYP17	CYP11A1
Genital ambiguity	Yes in XX	Yes in XX		Yes in XX	Yes in XX	Yes in XY	Yes in XY
	No in XY	No in XY		No in XY	Yes in XY		
HCO3	↓			*↑	↓	↑	↓
Na$^+$ level	↓			*↑	↓	↑	↓
K$^+$ level	↑			*↓	↑	↓	↑
Androgen	↑	↑	↑	↑	↑ in XX ↓ in XY	↓	↓
Blood pressure	↓			*↑	↓	↑	↓
Diagnostic analyte	17-OHP	17-OHP	17-OHP	DOC, 11-deoxycortiol	DHEA 7-Preg	DOC Corticosterone	All low
Therapy	Gluco and mineralo	Gluco and mineralo	Gluco	Gluco	Gluco and mineralo	Glucocorticoid	Gluco and mineralo

*, Postneonatal period; ↓, decreased; ↑, increased; 17-OHP,17-hydroxyprogesterone; 17 preg, 17-hydroxypregnenolone; DHEA, dehydroepiandrosterone; DOC, deoxycorticosterone; gluco, glucocorticoid; mineralo, mineralocorticoid.

Females affected are born with normal genitalia, but develop features of excess androgen with or without polycystic ovarian syndrome (PCOS). Males may have premature pubarche. Patients have smaller testes for the size of their phallus.

Diagnosis of 21-Hydroxylase Deficiency

Measurement of 17-hydroxyprogesterone (random or ACTH-stimulated) serves as the ideal screening tool in the diagnosis of congenital adrenal hyperplasia. 17-Hydroxyprogesterone levels 10,000 ng/dL are typical of the classic form, whereas elevations closer to 1000 ng/dL are seen in the nonclassic type.

Many states in the United States have adopted screening tests to identify affected patients before they become ill. Early screening for congenital adrenal hyperplasia detects the 70% of boys and 25% of girls who are missed on clinical examination. Early diagnosis and treatment prevents adrenal crisis and infant death, and allows earlier gender assignment.

11-Hydroxylase Deficiency (CYP 11 B1)

Deficiency of CYP 11B1 accounts for approximately 5 % of cases of CAH. In this disorder, enzymatic blockage causes overproduction of 11-deoxycortisol and deoxycorticosterone (DOC). The 11-deoxycortisol is diverted to androgen which causes virilization of the female fetus. The elevated DOC induces sodium retention with increase plasma volume resulting in renin suppressed hypertension and hypokalemia, which may be evident after the neonatal period.

3 βHSD2 Deficiency

Deficiency of 3βHSD accounts for 3% of cases of CAH. Decreased activity of this enzyme causes reduced conversion of pregnenolone to progesterone, 17- hydroxypregnenolone to 17-hydroxyprogesterone and DHEA to androstenedione, resulting in decreased synthesis of aldosterone, cortisol, and androstenedione, respectively. The DHEA is a weak androgen, but an excess accumulated level is enough to cause virilization in females. Males have incomplete masculinization with varying degree of genitalia ambiguity.

Treatment and Monitoring

The principle of therapy is to replace the deficient hormone and reduce the excess hormone. Glucocorticoid administration replaces cortisol, reduces ACTH secretion, and suppresses adrenal androgens, resulting in prevention of further virilization. Oral hydrocortisone at a dose of 10 to 15 mg/m^2 provides an optimum maintenance dose in growing children.

During periods of stress (fever >38°C, illness), the dose should be doubled or tripled and may even be given four to five times during major stress (e.g., surgery). If the patient is not able to tolerate orally, then 50 mg/m^2 intramuscular hydrocortisone injections should be considered.

The efficacy of treatment is best monitored by measuring 17-hydroxyprogesterone and androstenedione in patients with 21-hydroxylase deficiency. Patients should also be monitored for signs of overdose such as rapid weight gain, hyperpigmentation, and growth deceleration.

Infants with the salt-wasting form require supplement with a mineralocorticoid (0.1–0.2 mg Florinef) and 1 to 2 g

NaCl in addition to glucocorticoids. Older children may not require salt supplement. Plasma renin activity may be monitored to assess the efficacy of treatment.

Abnormal external genitalia in females with the classic form of the disease may require genitoplasty.

Hypertension in patients with 11-hydroxylase or 17-hydroxylase may be treated with a calcium channel blocker.

Gonadal hormone therapy may be needed for sex steroid replacement therapy in patients with 3βHSD or StAR protein defect.

Adrenal Androgen Deficiency

Isolated adrenal androgen deficiency may not be significant if gonadal androgen production is intact. Androgen defect in both gonadal and adrenal can present with ambiguous genitalia or feminization of external genitalia. Examples include StAR protein, 3 βHSD, and 17-hydroxylase deficiency.

DISORDERS OF ADRENAL MEDULLA

Pheochromocytoma is a catecholamine-producing tumor of the chromaffin cells derived from neuroectodermal tissue in the adrenal medulla or the extra-adrenal tissue. This tumor follows the "rule of tens":

- Ten percent are extra-adrenal.
- Ten percent are malignant.
- Ten percent occur in children.
- Ten percent are bilateral.
- Ten percent are familial. (Recent data suggest that 25% may be familial.)

Clinical manifestations of pheochromocytoma include the classic triad of palpitations, diaphoresis, and headache. Ninety percent of patients have labile or sustained hypertension. Other features may include episodic anxiety or panic attacks, vomiting, pallor, hyperglycemia, and hypercalcemia.

The diagnosis is established by demonstrating elevated fractionated urinary catecholamines, metanephrine, normetanephrine, and elevated plasma metanephrine and normetanephrine levels. Magnetic resonance imaging is used to localize the tumor.

Familial forms of pheochromocytoma occur as part of the multiple endocrine neoplasia syndromes (MEN 2A and MEN 2B), Von Hippel-Lindau syndrome, and neurofibromatosis, all of which are inherited in an autosomal-dominant fashion.

MEN syndrome type 1 is *not* associated with pheochromocytoma and is characterized by:

- Hyperparathyroidism
- Pancreatic tumors (insulinoma, glucagonoma)
- Pituitary tumors

MEN syndrome type 2A is characterized by:

- Medullary thyroid carcinoma
- Hyperparathyroidism
- Pheochromocytoma

MEN syndrome type 2B includes:

- Medullary thyroid carcinoma
- Pheochromocytoma
- Mucosal neuromas

Von Hippel-Lindau syndrome is characterized by:

- Visual defects
- Ocular defects (retinal angioma)
- Nephron (renal) carcinoma
- Hemangioblastoma of the cerebellum
- Increased intracranial pressure
- Pheochromocytoma
- Pancreatic cysts
- Ectopic erythropoietin production
- Liver cysts

REVIEW EXERCISES

QUESTIONS

1. The principal hormones of the adrenal cortex include all of the following *except:*
a) Renin
b) Aldosterone
c) DHEA
d) Androstenedione
e) Cortisol

Answer
The answer is a. Renin is produced by the kidney and the only hormone listed not produced by the adrenal gland.

2. 21-Hydroxylase deficiency is associated with all of the following *except:*
a) Genital ambiguity
b) Growth failure
c) Infertility
d) Irregular menses
e) Acne

Answer
The answer is b. Growth failure is not a clinical feature of congenital adrenal hyperplasia. Growth acceleration can be a feature of the simple virilizing form of this disorder. All the other features occur in CAH.

3. The clinical features of Cushing syndrome include all of the following *except:*
a) Hypertension
b) Obesity and striae

c) Alopecia
d) Growth failure
e) Precocious body hair distribution

Answer
The answer is c. Alopecia is not a feature of Cushing syndrome.

4. Pheochromocytoma is associated with all of the following syndromes *except*:
a) Neurofibromatosis
b) Von Hippel-Lindau syndrome
c) MEN 1
d) MEN 2A
e) MEN 2B

Answer
The answer is c. Pheochromocytoma is associated with MEN 2A and 2B, as well as neurofibromatosis and Von Hippel-Lindau syndrome. MEN 1 consists of hyperparathyroidism, pancreatic tumors, and pituitary tumors.

SUGGESTED READINGS

1. Bethin KE, Muglia LJ. Adrenal insufficiency. In: Radovick S, MacGillivray MH, eds. *Pediatric endocrinology: a practical clinical guide.* Totowa, NJ: Humana Press, 2003:203–226.
2. Consensus statement on management of 21-hydroxylase deficiency from the Lawson Wilkins Pediatric Endocrine Society and the European Society for Pediatric Endocrinology. *J Clin Endocrinol Metab* 2002;97:4048–4053.
3. Speiser P. Congenital adrenal hyperplasia. *N Engl J Med* 2003;349:776–778.

Chapter 17

Thyroid Disease

Douglas G. Rogers

EMBRYOGENESIS

During embryogenesis, epithelial cells on the pharyngeal floor thicken to form a diverticulum. At about the fourth gestational week, the diverticulum elongates, and the primordial thyroid cells migrate caudally until they fuse with the ventral aspect of the fourth pharyngeal pouch. Two lobes connected by an isthmus are typically located anterior to the third tracheal cartilage. The thyroglossal duct that results from the migration normally involutes. Retention and growth of thyroid tissue at the lower end of the duct occasionally result in a pyramidal lobe. Thyroglobulin is produced by the eighth gestational week; trapping of iodine occurs by week 10, followed by iodination of tyrosine. Colloid formation and pituitary secretion of thyroid-stimulating hormone (TSH) occur by week 12.

Fetal thyroid development is completely independent of the mother's pituitary–thyroid axis because negligible amounts of maternal TSH or thyroxine (T_4) cross the placenta.

NORMAL THYROID PHYSIOLOGY

The secretion of T_4 is controlled by TSH, which is secreted by the pituitary gland. TSH secretion, in turn, is controlled by thyrotropin-releasing hormone (TRH), which is produced in the hypothalamus. The secretion of both TSH and TRH is modulated by serum levels of T_4 in a negative feedback loop. Circulating T_4 is predominantly bound by thyroxine-binding globulin and thyroxine-binding prealbumin. T_4 is deiodinated in peripheral tissues to the more bioactive hormone triiodothyronine (T_3). T_3 affects almost every tissue in the body. T_3 binds to its receptors in the cell nucleus, and subsequent alteration of gene transcription by this complex leads to increases in the consumption of oxygen, formation of adenosine triphosphate, and cellular concentration of cyclic adenosine monophosphate.

Within 30 minutes after delivery, TSH levels in the normal neonate rapidly rise to about 80 μU per mL (80 mU/L) and then slowly decline during the next 3 days. In response, T_4 and T_3 levels rise dramatically by 24 hours of age, then slowly decline during the next few weeks.

CONGENITAL HYPOTHYROIDISM

The mental development of children with congenital hypothyroidism is related to the adequacy of treatment. Beginning treatment before 3 months of age improves the mental development of these children. Because of the paucity of early signs and symptoms in infants with congenital hypothyroidism (Table 17.1), early diagnosis and treatment were often delayed before the introduction of population screening.

Population screening for congenital hypothyroidism, by means of a T_4 radioimmunoassay of blood spots on filter paper, was begun in 1974 and combined with screening for phenylketonuria. Refinements in the initial screening program developed rapidly, and most industrialized nations now have such screening programs. In North America, the total T_4 level is measured in all newborns. Generally, if the T_4 level of a neonate falls within the lowest 10th percentile, both the T_4 and TSH levels are reassayed.

Newborn screening programs detect about one infant with congenital hypothyroidism for every 4000 live births. Up to five false-positive results may be obtained for every one confirmed case of congenital hypothyroidism. However, newborn screening programs are statistically unable to detect congenital hypothyroidism in about three

TABLE 17.1

SIGNS AND SYMPTOMS OF CONGENITAL HYPOTHYROIDISM AT AGE 5 WEEKS

Prolonged jaundice
Umbilical hernia
Constipation
Macroglossia
Feeding problems
Distended abdomen
Hypotonia
Hoarse cry
Large posterior fontanelle
Dry skin
Hypothermia
Goiter

In decreasing order of frequency.

infants for every 100,000 live births (about 12% of all infants with congenital hypothyroidism).

Of infants with congenital hypothyroidism:

- Seventy-five percent have sporadic thyroid dysgenesis.
- Ten percent have thyroid enzyme defects.
- Ten percent have transient hypothyroidism.
- Five percent have hypothalamic-pituitary hypothyroidism.

Thyroid enzyme defects are inherited in an autosomal-recessive pattern.

Any infant in whom congenital hypothyroidism has been identified by a state screening program should immediately be examined by a physician for signs of congenital hypothyroidism (see Table 17.1). The infant's serum free T_4 and TSH levels should be measured for confirmation. Infants with a deficiency of thyroxine-binding globulin are identified by state screening programs, but on confirmation testing, their free T_4 levels are found to be normal. The screening test results of infants whose mothers are receiving antithyroid medication also may be abnormal.

Therapy with levothyroxine should begin without delay after confirmatory blood tests have been obtained but before results become available. If the confirmatory tests show normal thyroid function, therapy is discontinued. The starting daily dose of levothyroxine is approximately 10 μg/kg.

Once treatment has been initiated, the T_4 and TSH levels should be followed monthly during the first year of life, every other month during the second year, and biannually thereafter. Dose increases of 0.0125 mg (one half of a 0.025-mg tablet) should be initiated when indicated, and measurements of T_4 and TSH should be repeated 1 month after the increase. The tablets are easily crushed and can be added to breast milk, formula, or water, or stirred into cereal. However, levothyroxine should not be mixed with soy-based formulas. Because the half-life of T_4 is about 6 days, a period of 4 weeks is required for serum T_4 values to reach a steady state. Normalization of elevated TSH levels may take even longer.

Even with adequate diagnosis and therapy, the intelligence quotient (IQ) of some children with congenital hypothyroidism is lower than predicted. Factors contributing to a decreased IQ include:

- Markedly low level of T_4 at birth
- Markedly delayed bone age at birth
- Delayed treatment
- Serum T_4 level <8 μg/dL (103 nmol/L) during the first year of therapy

Occasionally, an infant appears to have congenital hypothyroidism on screening but has a normal T_4 value and a TSH value above 10 μU/mL (10 mU/L) on confirmatory testing. Some pediatric endocrinologists choose not to treat, but follow such infants carefully and treat them if the TSH levels increase with time. Alternatively, a cautious approach is to treat these infants with levothyroxine until they are more than 2 years old. At this time, therapy can be stopped for 3 months and measurement of the T_4 and TSH levels repeated.

ACQUIRED HYPOTHYROIDISM

Causes of acquired hypothyroidism in children include:

- Autoimmune thyroiditis
- Drugs (e.g., lithium, amiodarone)
- Endemic goiter secondary to nutritional iodide deficiency
- Irradiation of the thyroid gland
- Surgical excision of the thyroid gland

A common cause of acquired hypothyroidism in children is *autoimmune thyroiditis*, which occurs in genetically predisposed persons. Clinical disease is triggered or aggravated by unidentified factors. The thyroid gland becomes enlarged but is usually not painful. Histologic changes include lymphocytic infiltration, formation of lymphoid follicles, and follicular cell hyperplasia. Antibodies to thyroid peroxidase (so-called microsomal antibodies) are characteristic of Hashimoto (chronic lymphocytic) thyroiditis. However, the antibodies are not responsible for the actual destruction of thyroid cells, which is probably caused by cytotoxic lymphocytes. Symptoms and signs of acquired hypothyroidism in children are listed in **Table 17.2**. The growth chart of an actual child with acquired hypothyroidism is shown in **Figure 17.1**.

Once a child is suspected of having hypothyroidism, the serum T_4 and TSH levels should be measured. *If the T_4 level is low and the TSH level is high, the diagnosis of hypothyroidism is confirmed, and levothyroxine therapy should be started.* Measuring the thyroid antibodies is unnecessary because the result of this test does not alter the treatment regimen.

In children with a goiter and normal T_4 and TSH levels, positive titers of microsomal thyroid antibodies confirm the diagnosis of Hashimoto thyroiditis and explain the thyromegaly. If a child or adolescent with Hashimoto thyroiditis has a noticeable goiter, treatment with levothyroxine may reduce it to some degree but usually does not eliminate it.

Levothyroxine treatment should be started at a dose of 0.05 mg daily, which is generally smaller than the dose required to attain euthyroidism. Initial treatment with larger doses of levothyroxine may cause headaches and abrupt personality changes. The T_4 and TSH levels should be determined no sooner than 1 month after a change in dose. TSH levels in the normal range are desirable; a TSH level below normal indicates excessive treatment.

Parents and teachers should be warned that the previously quiet, docile, hypothyroid child will soon become more active and even rambunctious. The dramatic change in personality that can occur after the initiation of therapy may be more than teachers, and even some parents, can readily accommodate.

EUTHYROID SICK SYNDROME

T_4 is converted in peripheral tissues to bioactive T_3 by the 5'-deiodinase enzyme. This enzyme is also responsible for clearing the small amounts of inactive reverse T_3 that are a byproduct of T_4 metabolism. During *acute or chronic severe illness, surgery, trauma, or malnutrition*, the activity of the deiodinase enzyme is decreased, so that the amount of T_3 produced is decreased and reverse T_3 accumulates. TSH secretion is also decreased and does not respond to falling levels of T_4. *Low levels of T_4 and T_3, in addition to normal to low levels of TSH, are common in stressed children.* Sick euthyroid patients do not require thyroid hormone replacement.

HYPERTHYROIDISM

Hyperthyroidism can be caused by:

- Increased production of thyroid hormone
- Increased release of thyroid hormone

The conditions associated with increased production or merely increased release of thyroid hormone are listed in **Table 17.3**.

A scan demonstrating the uptake of radioactive iodine can clearly differentiate between the two types of hyperthyroidism. *In cases of excess thyroid hormone production, uptake is increased. In cases of increased release, uptake is decreased.*

In Graves disease, an autoimmune disorder, antibodies develop that stimulate TSH receptors and therefore the production of T_4.

Hyperthyroid children may note tiredness or easy fatigability. Hyperthyroidism in children can easily be mistaken for an anxiety disorder, anorexia nervosa, or another psychiatric illness. Common symptoms and signs of Graves disease in adolescents are presented in **Table 17.4**.

TABLE 17.2	
SYMPTOMS AND SIGNS OF ACQUIRED HYPOTHYROIDISM IN CHILDREN	
Symptoms	**Signs**
Weakness	Goiter
Lethargy	Growth retardation
Decreased appetite	Delayed dentition
Cold intolerance	Delayed or precocious puberty
Constipation	Galactorrhea
Dry skin	Carotenemia
Mild obesity	Pale, dry skin
	Myopathy and muscular hypertrophy

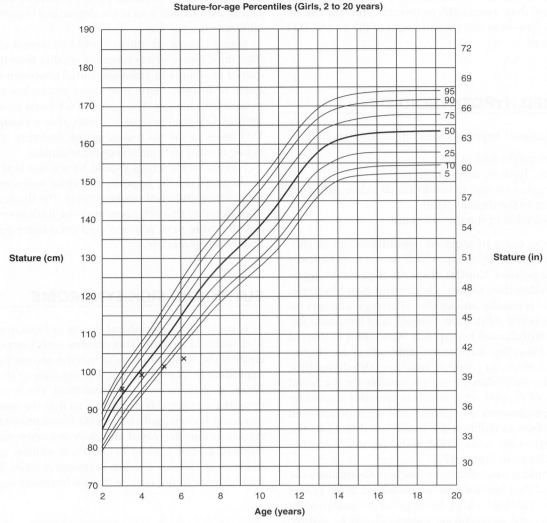

Figure 17.1 Growth curve of a child with acquired hypothyroidism. Note the insidious decline in growth velocity.

TABLE 17.3
CAUSES OF HYPERTHYROIDISM

Excess production of T_4
  Graves disease
  Toxic adenoma
  McCune-Albright syndrome
  TSH-producing pituitary tumor
  Pituitary resistance to thyroid hormone
Excess release of T_4
  Subacute thyroiditis
  Hashimoto toxic thyroiditis
  Iodine-induced hyperthyroidism

T_4, thyroxine; TSH, thyroid-stimulating hormone.

TABLE 17.4
SIGNS AND SYMPTOMS OF GRAVES DISEASE IN ADOLESCENTS

Goiter
Tachycardia
Nervousness
Increased pulse pressure
Proptosis
Increased appetite
Tremor
Weight loss
Heat intolerance

In decreasing order of frequency.

Graves disease often can be diagnosed clinically in the presence of goiter, exophthalmos, weight loss, and tachycardia. The diagnosis can be documented by an elevated level of free T_4 and a low level of TSH. TSH assays are now capable of differentiating low levels from normal levels. In less obvious cases, the uptake of radioactive iodine is helpful in determining the presence and cause of hyperthyroidism (uptake increased in cases of Graves disease).

Graves disease can be treated with antithyroid medications, radioactive iodine ablation, or surgical excision of the thyroid. The administration of β-blockers (e.g., 10–20 mg of propranolol every 8 hours) relieves many of the symptoms of hyperthyroidism and may make patients more comfortable.

Propylthiouracil and *methimazole* interfere with several steps in the synthesis of thyroid hormone. Propylthiouracil also blocks the peripheral conversion of T_4 to T_3. The dosage of propylthiouracil is 5 to 10 mg/kg per day, given every 8 hours. The dosage of methimazole is 0.5 mg/kg per day, given once daily.

Both propylthiouracil and methimazole are associated with side effects, including:

- Rash
- Arthritis
- Leukopenia
- Hepatic toxicity

Because of these side effects, about 5% of patients stop taking their medication. Patients must be warned about side effects and instructed to return to their physician for a complete blood cell count if a sore throat or fever develops. If jaundice develops, patients must discontinue the medication immediately and contact their physician.

A remission, evidenced by the resolution of goiter, occurs in 45% of patients taking these drugs, who then no longer require antithyroid medication. If remission does not occur within 3 years after the initiation of treatment, radioactive iodine ablation or subtotal thyroidectomy should be performed.

Ablation with radioactive iodine does not increase the risk for thyroid neoplasia, nor does it appear to cause any teratogenic effects in the progeny of those to whom it is administered. Thyroid antibody titers increase after radioactive iodine ablation, and the increase may be responsible for the temporary worsening of eye symptoms in patients with Graves disease that sometimes occurs after radioactive iodine ablation. Besides leaving a scar, thyroidectomy may damage the recurrent laryngeal nerve or cause hypoparathyroidism.

NEONATAL GRAVES DISEASE

Pregnant women with Graves disease or a history of Graves disease may transfer thyroid-stimulating immunoglobulin G to the fetus. Affected infants may exhibit any of the signs

TABLE 17.5

SIGNS AND SYMPTOMS OF NEONATAL GRAVES DISEASE

Premature birth
Low birth weight
Goiter
Restlessness and irritability
Fever, flushing
Tachycardia, cardiomegaly, heart failure
Lid retraction, proptosis, periorbital edema
Poor weight gain or weight loss
Increased gastrointestinal motility, frequent stooling

listed in **Table 17.5**. An elevated level of free T_4, a low level of TSH, and positive thyroid-stimulating immunoglobulins confirm the diagnosis. Treatment with 5 to 10 mg of propylthiouracil per kilogram per day or 0.5 mg of methimazole per kilogram per day should be initiated in these children.

Prednisone may be required to stabilize severely ill neonates while they are thyrotoxic. As the T_4 levels become suppressed, levothyroxine should be given to maintain normal levels of T_4 and TSH. After 6 months, the antithyroid medication and levothyroxine can be discontinued.

SUBACUTE THYROIDITIS

Painful enlargement of the thyroid gland in association with signs and symptoms of hyperthyroidism may occur as a postviral syndrome. The T_4 level is elevated, and the TSH level is suppressed. Scanning with radioactive iodine reveals little uptake. Although no thyroid hormone is produced, an increased dysfunctional release of vast stores of thyroid hormone from the inflamed gland takes place. Antithyroid medications such as propylthiouracil have no effect on subacute thyroiditis. Treatment is limited to the administration of β-blockers, aspirin, and in extreme cases glucocorticoids.

THYROID NODULES

Thyroid nodules are uncommon in children, whereas the prevalence is 5% in adults more than 50 years of age. The risk that a solitary thyroid nodule is malignant in a child or an adolescent is approximately 33%.

In children and adolescents with a thyroid nodule, a history of endocrine tumors indicative of multiple endocrine neoplasia type 2 (see Chapter 16) in family members should be sought, in addition to a history of previous radiation therapy to the head or neck.

Solid thyroid nodules in children should be surgically excised. Before excision, a thyroid scan can be performed with ^{123}I. "Hot" nodules are usually not malignant, but some

TABLE 17.6

EXPECTED BLOOD TEST RESULTS IN PEDIATRIC THYROID DISORDERS

Condition	Free T_4	TSH	Antibodies
Congenital hypothyroidism			
Athyrotic	Low	High	Absent
Nonathyrotic	Normal/low	High	Absent
Acquired hypothyroidism	Low	High	Microsomal hypothyroidism
Euthyroid sick syndrome	Low	Normal/low	Absent
Graves disease	High	Low	TSI
Neonatal Graves disease	High	Low	TSI in infant and mother
Subacute thyroiditis	High	Low	Absent

T_4, thyroxine; TSH, thyroid-stimulating hormone; TSI, thyroid-stimulating immunoglobulin.

exceptions have occurred. Simple cysts are usually not malignant, but exceptions are also possible in these cases.

Ultrasonographic examination of the thyroid is warranted for "cold" nodules. A cold nodule that is found to be solid, complex cystic, or mixed on ultrasonography should be regarded as malignant until shown to be otherwise. Fine needle biopsy of solitary thyroid nodules in adults has proved helpful; however, its efficacy has not yet been proved in children.

SUMMARY

The results of blood tests in various thyroid disorders are summarized in Table 17.6.

REVIEW EXERCISES

QUESTIONS

1. The incidence of congenital hypothyroidism in otherwise normal newborns is closest to:
a. 1 in 10,000
b. 1 in 100,000
c. 1 in 4000
d. 1 in 400

Answer
The answer is c.

2. Which of the following conditions is *least* likely to be associated with a goiter?
a. Hashimoto lymphocytic thyroiditis
b. Graves disease
c. Subacute thyroiditis
d. Congenital hypothyroidism

Answer
The answer is d. Only 2% of children with congenital hypothyroidism have a goiter. These children probably have an enzyme defect that interferes with thyroid hormone synthesis. Most children with congenital hypothyroidism have thyroid aplasia or hypoplasia.

3. Which of the following tests best differentiate subacute thyroiditis from Graves disease?
a. Free T_4
b. TSH
c. Radioactive iodide uptake scan
d. Erythrocyte sedimentation rate

Answer
The answer is c. Both Graves disease and subacute thyroiditis are associated with suppressed TSH levels and elevated free T_4 levels. The erythrocyte sedimentation rate is usually elevated in subacute thyroiditis, but an elevated erythrocyte sedimentation rate is a nonspecific finding. The uptake of radioactive iodide is always increased in active Graves disease, whereas uptake is always low in subacute thyroiditis.

4. The risk that a solitary solid thyroid nodule in a child is malignant is approximately:
a. 1%
b. 3%
c. 33%
d. 60%

Answer
The answer is c.

5. A low total T_4 level and normal TSH level in an otherwise normal child is most likely caused by:
a. Thyroid-binding globulin deficiency
b. Subclinical hypothyroidism
c. Pituitary resistance to T_4
d. Subacute thyroiditis

Answer
The answer is a. Subclinical hypothyroidism is associated with a normal T_4 level and a slightly elevated TSH level. Pituitary resistance to T_4 is associated with elevated T_4 and normal TSH levels. Subacute thyroiditis is associated with an elevated T_4 level and a suppressed TSH level.

SUGGESTED READINGS

1. American Academy of Pediatrics: Section of Endocrinology, Committee on Genetics, and American Thyroid Association Committee on Public Health. Newborn screening for congenital hypothyroidism: recommended guidelines. *Pediatrics* 1993;91: 1203–1209.
2. Clayton GW. Thyrotoxicosis in children. In: Kaplan SA, ed. *Clinical pediatric and adolescent endocrinology.* Philadelphia: Saunders, 1982: 110–117.
3. Dallas JS, Foley TP. Hypothyroidism. In: Lifshitz F, ed. *Pediatric endocrinology: a clinical guide,* 2nd ed. New York: Marcel Dekker, 1990:469–481.
4. Dallas JS, Foley TP. Hyperthyroidism. In: Lifshitz F, ed. *Pediatric endocrinology: a clinical guide,* 2nd ed. New York: Marcel Dekker, 1990: 484–486.
5. Fisher DA. Screening for congenital hypothyroidism. *Trends Endocrinol Metab* 1991;2:129–133.
6. Hung W. Nodular thyroid disease and thyroid carcinoma. *Pediatr Ann* 1992;21:50–57.
7. Rogers DG. Thyroid disease in children. *Am Fam Physician* 1994;50: 344–350.
8. Singer PA, Cooper DS, Levy EG, et al. Treatment guidelines for patients with hyperthyroidism and hypothyroidism. *JAMA* 1995; 273:808–812.

Chapter 18

Calcium and Phosphorus Metabolism

Robert J. Cunningham III

This chapter discusses the complex systems that control the homeostasis of calcium and phosphorus. The aim is to provide an understanding of the relationships between vitamin D, parathyroid hormone (PTH), calcium, and phosphorus. Diseases that disturb the balance of this system are also discussed.

Calcium ions are critical for normal neuromuscular function and must be maintained at very precise concentrations to allow normal function. The two systems that control calcium metabolism are schematically outlined in **Figure 18.1.** The system responsible for the long-term control of calcium metabolism is the vitamin D pathway. Vitamin D_3 (cholecalciferol) is formed in the skin on exposure to ultraviolet light. It is then transported to the liver, where it undergoes chemical conversion to 25-D_3 (25-hydroxy-cholecalciferol). 25-D_3 in turn circulates to the renal

cortex, where it is converted by the addition of a second hydroxyl group to 1,25-D_3 (1,25-dihydroxycholecalciferol). This compound is transported to the cells of the small intestine, stimulates protein synthesis, and ultimately leads to an increase in calcium absorption from the gastrointestinal tract. The entire process requires time, approximately 24 hours, because proteins must be synthesized in the intestinal cells in response to the stimulus provided by 1,25-D_3.

PTH provides a rapid response system that allows a nearly instantaneous increase in ionized calcium (Fig. 18.1, upper right panel). When the serum level of ionized calcium decreases, the parathyroid gland is stimulated to produce and release PTH. The released PTH mobilizes calcium directly from bone, so that the serum level of calcium increases immediately. PTH also induces an increase

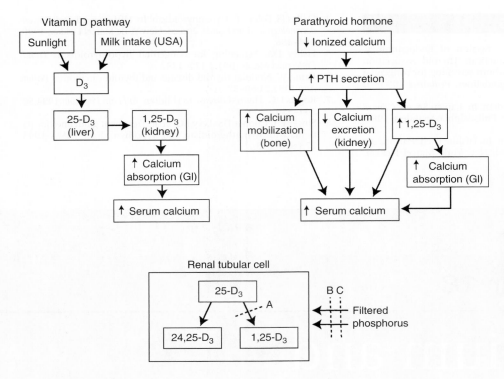

Figure 18.1 The two systems that control calcium and phosphorus metabolism are the vitamin D pathway (*upper left panel*) and the parathyroid hormone (PTH) (*upper right panel*). The renal tubular cell is the site of 1 α-hydroxylation of 25-D$_3$ and also the site of phosphorus reabsorption. **Line A** represents the defect that occurs in vitamin D-dependency rickets. **Line B** represents the block in the transport of filtered phosphate into the renal tubular cell that occurs in vitamin D-resistance rickets. **Line C** represents the decrease in phosphate reabsorption that is caused by PTH. GI, gastrointestinal.

in 1α-hydroxylase activity by stimulating the transcription of RNA. This increases the production of 1,25-D$_3$ and hence increases the absorption of calcium which feeds back to *turn off* the secretion of PTH.

Another effect of PTH is to cause a decrease in renal phosphate reabsorption so that there is some phosphate wasting in patients who have long-term elevated PTH levels.

VITAMIN D–DEFICIENCY RICKETS

A number of factors predispose to the development of vitamin D deficiency:

- Lack of exposure to sunlight
- Lack of intake of commercial milk products
- Anticonvulsant therapy (particularly with phenobarbital or phenytoin)
- Intestinal malabsorption syndromes, particularly those that cause fat malabsorption (e.g., cystic fibrosis)

Exposure to sunlight results in the formation of vitamin D$_3$ in the skin cells; therefore, children with significant exposure to sunlight have adequate levels of vitamin D$_3$ and rarely have vitamin D–deficiency rickets. Therefore, deficiency rickets is seen more often in the northern climates; in patients who, for cultural or religious reasons, have most of their skin surface covered with clothing; and in individuals with darker skin. In Siberia, school children are stripped to their underwear and made to stand in front of an ultraviolet light for 30 minutes three times a week during the winter. In this way, they receive adequate exposure to ultraviolet light

to prevent vitamin D deficiency. By law, commercial milk products sold in the United States are fortified with vitamin D, and children who consume commercial milk products are unlikely to have vitamin D deficiency. Patients who consume skim milk are at greater risk of developing vitamin D deficiency, not because the milk is unfortified, but because the lower fat content of skim milk causes a lower absorption than milk with a higher fat content. Breast-fed infants are also at higher risk, particularly if the mother has a low intake of vitamin D, is dark skinned, or has limited exposure to sunlight. Anticonvulsant therapy does not influence the synthesis of vitamin D, but rather stimulates the P-450 system in the liver and accelerates the catabolism of 1, 25-D$_3$; this accelerated breakdown may result in deficiency rickets. Vitamin D is fat-soluble; therefore, vitamin D deficiency may develop in patients who depend on an oral intake of vitamin D and have a fat malabsorption syndrome.

Rickets develops in stages. The stage I is that, as a consequence of vitamin D$_3$ deficiency, there is insufficient absorption of calcium from the diet, and with time, the serum calcium levels fall. The fall leads to the synthesis and release of PTH and the mobilization of calcium from bone. In stage II, phosphorus reabsorption is decreased, and the renal tubular concentration of phosphate decreases. However, no 25-D$_3$ is presented to the renal tubular cells, so that no conversion of 25-D$_3$ to 1,25-D$_3$ and no increase in calcium absorption takes place. Therefore, calcium levels are maintained only by the continued release of PTH, and the mobilization of calcium from bone continues. As the disease progresses to stage III, the serum calcium levels fall, and the calcification of bony matrix becomes inadequate. The product of calcium and phosphorus (calcium × phosphorus) must be higher than 35 to 40 mg/dL for normal mineralization of bone to proceed. The calcium and phosphorus precipitate into a cartilaginous matrix; if the concentration of either is inadequate, precipitation may not occur.

The clinical signs and symptoms of vitamin D deficiency include:

- Tetany
- Growth retardation
- Frontal bossing
- Rachitic rosary
- Widening of the wrists or knee joints
- Subluxation of the wrists, knees, or ankles at the epiphyseal plates
- Seizures

Seizures result from hypocalcemia and are a common presenting symptom in infants and often occur in the springtime. Vitamin D deficiency develops during the winter with a lack of sunlight exposure and then in the springtime, vitamin D is synthesized as the infant is exposed to sunlight. This triggers an avid deposition of calcium into bone and this may happen so rapidly that the ionized calcium in the serum falls with resulting hypocalcemic seizures. Tetany may also result from hypocalcemia but is less often a presenting symptom. Growth retardation results from poor bone mineralization and the failure of unmineralized bone to grow. The frontal bossing, rachitic rosary, and widening of the wrist or knee joints all have the same underlying cause. The cartilaginous matrix proliferates, and this tissue *mounds up on itself*, causing the formation of lumps at the costochondral junctions (the rosary), the frontal bossing, and the widening of the wrists and knees. The cartilaginous matrix is not calcified and therefore has little compressive strength. It is susceptible to trauma, and bending or subluxation may occur during minor trauma, which is why rachitic patients may have *bent* joints.

The radiologic findings correspond to the clinical findings and include widening of the epiphyses and *fraying* at the epiphyseal junctions (Fig. 18.2). The bony metaphyses may also be widened, the long bones may have a *ball* of matrix at the growing ends, and fractures may be visualized. Bone mineralization does not proceed normally and PTH breaks down bone that has already formed. Both processes predispose to fractures.

Laboratory findings in vitamin D–deficiency rickets include:

- Low serum level of calcium
- Low serum level of phosphorus
- High level of alkaline phosphatase
- High serum level of PTH
- Low serum level of 25-D$_3$

The treatment of vitamin D–deficiency rickets is the administration of vitamin D$_3$, which provides a substrate for

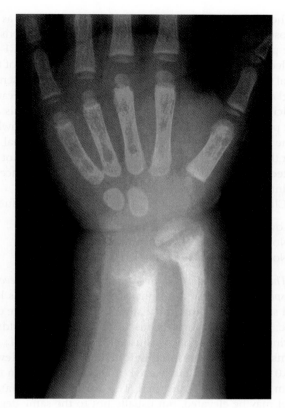

Figure 18.2 Radiograph of the wrist of a child with vitamin D–deficiency rickets. Note the widening and fraying at the epiphyses of the ulna and radius.

the formation of 1,25-D$_3$ and allows an equilibration of the calcium, phosphorus, 1,25-D$_3$, and PTH levels.

TYPE I RICKETS (VITAMIN D–DEPENDENT RICKETS)

Vitamin D–dependent rickets is the result of a deficiency of the enzyme that converts 25-D$_3$ to 1,25-D$_3$ (Fig. 18.1, line A). This is a rare inherited disorder. The deficiency results in inadequate absorption of calcium from the gastrointestinal tract and a symptom complex virtually identical to that of deficiency rickets. The radiologic and laboratory findings are identical to those seen in vitamin D–deficiency rickets. The exception is that the condition of patients with vitamin D–dependent rickets is not improved by the administration of vitamin D$_3$, and they require treatment once daily with 1,25-D$_3$.

TYPE II RICKETS (HYPOPHOSPHATEMIC RICKETS OR VITAMIN D–RESISTANT RICKETS)

Vitamin D–resistant rickets is not a disease of vitamin D metabolism but rather represents a phosphate *leak* at the level of the proximal tubule (see Fig. 18.1). It is inherited as an autosomal-dominant or sex-linked dominant characteristic. The primary defect is an inability to degrade the FGF-23 molecule that causes a *leak* of phosphate at the level of the renal tubule. This, in turn, results in a persistently low serum level of phosphate. Bone mineralization is defective because (calcium × phosphorus) is <35 mg/dL and minerals are not precipitated into the cartilaginous matrix of growing bone normally. Calcium metabolism is usually normal, so that the serum calcium levels are normal and PTH is not secreted. Thus, no active bone reabsorption takes place to maintain the normal serum levels of calcium.

Clinical features of vitamin D–resistant rickets include:

- Low serum level of phosphorus
- Normal serum level of calcium
- Normal or elevated level of PTH

The pathognomonic laboratory finding is a low serum level of phosphate. The serum phosphate level in newborns is low and should be measured if a sibling or parent has the disease. The serum phosphorus level in healthy children during the first year of life is usually 5.5 to 7.0 mg/dL; patients with hypophosphatemic rickets may have levels <3.0 mg/dL; this is rarely seen otherwise. The serum calcium level is usually normal. The alkaline phosphatase level may be elevated, but usually not to the same degree that it is in deficiency or dependent rickets because the serum calcium level is never low; therefore, PTH is not secreted and active bone reabsorption is decreased.

The radiologic findings in hypophosphatemic (vitamin D–resistant) rickets include:

- Widening of the epiphyseal plates
- Fraying of the epiphyseal plates
- Osteopenia

These clinical and radiologic findings are characteristically much more prominent in the lower extremities.

Unlike vitamin D–deficiency or –dependent rickets, resistant rickets is not usually characterized by changes associated with the action of PTH.

Resistant rickets is treated with phosphate supplements. Neutral phosphate solutions are administered on a thrice-daily schedule, but a limiting factor is that they cause diarrhea, and it is difficult to drive the serum phosphorus level >3.0 mg/dL. These patients also require 1,25-D$_3$, but it is imperative that the urinary calcium excretion be monitored for children. Some patients will develop significant hypercalcuria on 1,25-D$_3$ therapy. This may lead to nephrocalcinosis, scarring, and loss of renal function over time so it is essential to periodically monitor urinary calcium excretion.

RENAL INSUFFICIENCY RICKETS

In renal insufficiency, both the vitamin D and PTH systems are awry! The serum level of phosphate is elevated because the capacity for excretion is reduced as renal function deteriorates. There is a decrease in the synthesis of 1,25-D$_3$; therefore, calcium absorption from the gastrointestinal tract is severely reduced.

Presenting clinical signs are growth failure and bowing of legs. Pathologic fractures may also be a presenting symptom, and hypocalcemic tetany is occasionally seen.

The laboratory findings of renal insufficiency rickets are as follows:

- High serum level of phosphorus
- Low serum level of calcium
- High serum level of PTH
- Elevated levels of serum creatinine and blood urea nitrogen

The characteristic laboratory finding is an elevated serum level of phosphorus. Renal insufficiency rickets is the *only* form of rickets in which the serum level of phosphate is high. The serum calcium level is low, the alkaline phosphatase level is elevated, and the serum creatinine and blood urea nitrogen levels are also elevated. The radiographic findings are similar to those described for deficiency rickets, but the changes are often more severe because PTH, vitamin D, and the kidneys are all involved, and none of these are functioning normally.

The treatment of renal insufficiency rickets involves three steps:

1. Reduction of the serum phosphorus level. This is accomplished by giving phosphate binders and utilizing the gastrointestinal tract to eliminate phosphorus because the kidney is no longer capable of doing so. Binders frequently used are calcium carbonate (Tums), calcium acetate, and aluminum hydroxide in severe cases of hyperphosphatemia.
2. Administration of calcium supplements.
3. Provision of 1,25-D$_3$.

The reason why it is necessary to lower the phosphorus level before calcium supplements are given is that if (calcium × phosphorus) is >75 mg/dL, then the precipitation of calcium phosphate may occur in tissues other than bone—for example, in the skin or conjunctival surfaces.

HYPOPARATHYROIDISM

Hypoparathyroidism is usually diagnosed shortly after birth but is usually transient. The placenta serves as a calcium pump, and consequently the fetus lives in a calcium-rich environment. After birth, as the calcium level falls, no PTH is synthesized, and the infant's response to hypocalcemia is delayed. Once the parathyroid glands are activated and the hormone is synthesized for the first time, the problem resolves.

Presenting symptoms of hypoparathyroidism include:

- Seizures
- Stridor secondary to laryngeal spasm
- Heart failure
- Neuromuscular irritability

All these symptoms are caused by hypocalcemia secondary to inadequate secretion of PTH.

Laboratory findings in hypoparathyroidism include:

- Low serum level of calcium
- High serum level of phosphorus
- Low level of PTH (or levels are normal in the face of low serum calcium)

Hypoparathyroidism is treated with calcium supplements and additionally with 1,25-D$_3$ if calcium supplements alone fail to normalize the serum calcium level. Intravenous calcium is recommended if the QT interval is prolonged, but most patients can be treated with oral calcium gluconate.

Apart from the newborn period, hypoparathyroidism is rarely seen.

PSEUDOHYPOPARATHYROIDISM

A syndrome of pseudohypoparathyroidism is often not recognized until children are 5 to 10 years of age. It is caused by a genetic resistance to the action of PTH. Messenger molecules, specifically cyclic adenosine monophosphate (cAMP), are not produced normally, so that even if PTH is secreted, it is unrecognized at the cellular level. Two types of pseudohypoparathyroidism have been described.

Children with type I pseudohypoparathyroidism, the more commonly recognized variety of this disorder, demonstrate the following characteristics:

- Cherubic appearance resulting from a round facies
- Brachydactyly or spade-like hands
- Short stature
- Developmental delay (occasional)

The characteristic laboratory findings are as follows:

- Low serum level of calcium
- High serum level of phosphorus
- Very elevated serum level of PTH

Children with type II hypoparathyroidism do not have the clinical features as shown earlier, but do present with hypocalcemia. It appears that cAMP is generated normally in these patients, but there is a specific intracellular resistance that blunts the renal cellular response to PTH.

No radiographic findings are characteristic. The treatment involves calcium supplementation and occasionally the administration of 1,25-D$_3$ to maintain normal serum levels of calcium.

HYPERPARATHYROIDISM

Hyperparathyroidism is very rare in childhood; the most common cause is renal failure, in which increased parathyroid activity is part of the *renal rickets* picture. Malignancy is a cause of hyperparathyroidism in adults and must be considered if hyperparathyroidism develops in a child. The characteristic findings of hyperparathyroidism are as follows:

- High serum level of calcium
- Low serum level of phosphorus
- Elevated serum level of PTH

Hyperparathyroidism causes few clinical symptoms, and it is often discovered during a *routine* laboratory evaluation. The most important aspect of evaluating a pediatric patient with hypercalcemia is to distinguish hyperparathyroidism from other, more common causes of hypercalcemia in children. These include:

- Sarcoidosis
- Immobilization hypercalcemia
- Vitamin D intoxication
- Nonmetastatic cancers
- Williams syndrome in neonates with hypercalcemia

Subtotal parathyroidectomy is the treatment of choice for hyperparathyroidism. In cases of hypercalcemia with another cause, treatment of the underlying disorder is the key to restoring normal calcium metabolism.

FAMILIAL HYPOCALCIURIC HYPERCALCEMIA

This is a disorder that is inherited in an autosomal-dominant manner and results from a disorder in the calcium-sensing receptor such that higher than normal levels of serum calcium are required to suppress PTH secretion. The characteristics of this disorder are as follows:

- High serum level of calcium
- Low serum level of phosphorus
- Low urinary calcium excretion

The key to diagnosis is the discovery of hypercalcemia in a parent. The patients are usually asymptomatic and treatment is generally not required.

REVIEW EXERCISES

QUESTIONS

1. Which of the following medications is associated with rickets?
a) Propranolol
b) Phenobarbital

c) Fluoxetine (Prozac)

d) Paroxetine (Paxil)

Answer

The answer is b. Anticonvulsants accelerate the breakdown of 1,25-D_3. The other anticonvulsant that has been associated with rickets is phenytoin.

2. You are caring for a 16-month-old girl whose mother has vitamin D-resistant rickets. The parents want to know if the child has the same disease as her mother. Which of the following tests would be *most* helpful in answering this question?

a) Hand and wrist radiography for bone age

b) Determination of the PTH level

c) Determination of the serum phosphorus level

d) Determination of the alkaline phosphatase level

Answer

The answer is c. Determination of the serum level of phosphorus is the best test to perform. The phosphorus level will be abnormally low in newborns.

3–6. Match the chemical profiles with the *most* likely cause of *rickets*.

a) Vitamin D–deficiency rickets

b) Vitamin D–resistant rickets

c) Renal insufficiency rickets

d) Hyperparathyroidism

3. Ca = 10.1 mg/dL, PO_4 = 3.0 mg/dL,
PTH = 85 IU/mL, Na = 140 mEq/L, K = 4.5 mEq/L,
Cl = 99 mEq/L, HCO_3 = 27 mEq/L.

4. Ca = 8.2 mg/dL, PO_4 = 4.5 mg/dL,
PTH =189 IU/mL, Na = 140 mEq/L, K = 4.5 mEq/L,
Cl = 99 mEq/L, HCO_3 =21 mEq/L.

5. Ca = 13.1 mg/dL, PO_4 = 4.0 mg/dL,
PTH =185 IU/mL, Na = 140 mEq/L, K = 4.5 mEq/L,
Cl = 99 mEq/L, HCO_3 = 27 mEq/L.

6. Ca = 8.1 mg/dL, PO_4 = 7.0 mg/dL,
PTH =189 IU/mL, Na = 140 mEq/L, K = 4.5 mEq/L,
Cl = 99 mEq/L, HCO_3 = 20 mEq/L.

Answers

3. The answer is b.

4. The answer is a.

5. The answer is d.

6. The answer is c.

The key to questions 3 through 6 is the phosphorus level, which helps distinguish the variants of rickets. All profiles tend to be associated with a low serum level of calcium, so this is not helpful. Rather, look for a high serum level of phosphorus. This is associated with renal insufficiency, the only variant in which the serum phosphorus level is elevated. Next, look for the lowest serum level of phosphorus (usually <3.0 mg/dL). The lowest level of phosphorus generally indicates vitamin D–resistant rickets (hypophosphatemic rickets). Then, the others can be distinguished. Hyperparathyroidism is the only diagnosis in which the calcium level is elevated. Deficiency rickets is associated with a low calcium level and a phosphorus level that is slightly depressed, but not as much as in vitamin D–resistant rickets.

SUGGESTED READINGS

1. Bishop N. Rickets today—children still need milk and sunshine. *N Engl J Med* 1999;341:602–603.
2. Chesney RW. Vitamin D deficiency and rickets. *Rev EndocrMetab Disord* 2001;2:145–151.
3. Joiner T, Foster C, Shope T. The many faces of vitamin D deficiency rickets. *Pediatr Rev* 2000;21:296–304.
4. Narchi H, El Jamil M, Kulaylat N. Symptomatic rickets in adolescence. *Arch Dis Child* 2001;84:501–503.
5. Portale AA, Miller WL. Hereditary rickets revealed. *Kidney Int* 1998;54:1762–1764.
6. Yoshida T, Monkawa T, Tenenhouse HS, et al. Two novel 1-α-hydroxylase mutations in French-Canadians with vitamin D dependency rickets type 1. *Kidney Int* 1998;54:1437–1443.

Chapter 19

Short Stature and Growth Hormone Therapy

Douglas G. Rogers

Short stature is a common complaint. Of every 20 children, the height of one will be below the fifth percentile channel on a standard growth curve. Differentiating between normal variations of growth and pathologic conditions that cause short stature can be difficult. The purpose of this chapter is to review the diagnostic evaluation that can differentiate between normal variations and pathologic conditions.

GENERAL CONSIDERATIONS

Analysis of the growth curve is critical in the evaluation of a child with short stature. Important information obtained from the growth curve includes:

- Absolute height
- Growth rate
- Ratio of weight to height

  Other tools helpful in the evaluation include:

- Relative proportions of the lower and upper body segments
- Bone age

Although the height of many children is below the fifth percentile channel on a growth curve, in only a few of them is the *growth rate* also below normal. *Measuring a child's height over a 6-month period of time to determine the growth rate, is the first and most important step in evaluating a child with short stature.* Because linear growth normally occurs at a relatively constant rate of between 5 and 7 cm annually after the first 3 years of life, an annualized growth rate of <5 cm is considered abnormal. A normal growth rate, regardless of a child's height (even if it is below the fifth percentile), is unlikely to be associated with an underlying pathologic condition.

The *weight-to-height ratio* can help distinguish between endocrine causes (i.e., growth hormone deficiency) of short stature and other chronic conditions that may interfere with growth (i.e., renal or gastrointestinal disease). In general, weight gain is relatively preserved in children with endocrine conditions, whereas it is impaired in those with chronic conditions not of endocrine origin.

An assessment of the *relative proportions of the upper and lower body segments* can help differentiate conditions that involve both the upper and lower body segments from those that involve one more than the other. Conditions that affect the trunk and lower extremities equally include:

- Growth hormone deficiency
- Hypothyroidism
- Inadequate caloric intake
- Gastrointestinal disorders
- Chronic renal disorders

Conditions that affect the trunk more than the lower extremities (decreased upper body–to–lower body ratio) include the spondylodysplasias. In contrast, the skeletal dysplasias, such as achondroplasia, are associated with an increased upper body–to–lower body ratio.

The *bone age* is utilized to assess skeletal maturity. Most conditions associated with a poor growth rate result in delayed skeletal maturation and thus a delayed bone age. A notable exception to this is Cushing's syndrome which may cause growth failure while the bones continue to mature. A delayed bone age does not indicate a specific diagnosis.

CLINICAL ENTITIES ASSOCIATED WITH NORMAL VARIATIONS IN GROWTH

Children who are short but have a *normal growth rate* generally exhibit either of two normal growth patterns:

■ Familial short stature (Fig. 19.1)
■ Constitutional delay/delayed onset of puberty (Fig. 19.2)

Children with *familial short stature* characteristically have:

■ Short parents and a short final adult height
■ *Normal* bone age consistent with chronologic age
■ Normal onset of puberty

Children with *constitutional delay of growth* characteristically have a:

■ Delayed bone age
■ Delayed onset of puberty
■ Parent(s) in whom puberty may have been delayed
■ Normal final adult height

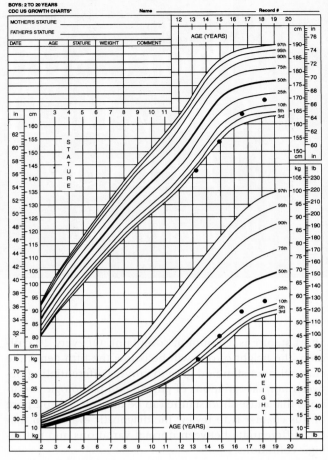

Figure 19.2 Typical growth curve of a child with constitutional delay of growth.

PATHOLOGIC CLINICAL ENTITIES CAUSING SHORT STATURE

Once it has been established that a child's growth rate is subnormal (<5 cm per year), chronic conditions or illnesses that can cause growth failure must be eliminated from the differential diagnosis. Many chronic conditions are associated with growth failure (e.g., congenital heart disease, cystic fibrosis, sickle cell anemia, achondroplasia). Most of them can easily be eliminated from the differential diagnosis by means of a careful history and physical examination. However, the manifestations of some chronic conditions or illnesses can be so subtle that they may not be revealed by a thorough history and physical examination. These include:

■ Turner syndrome (Fig. 19.3)
■ Growth hormone deficiency (Fig. 19.4)
■ Cushing syndrome (Fig. 19.5)
■ Crohn disease (Fig. 19.6)
■ Celiac disease
■ Hypothyroidism
■ Chronic renal disease

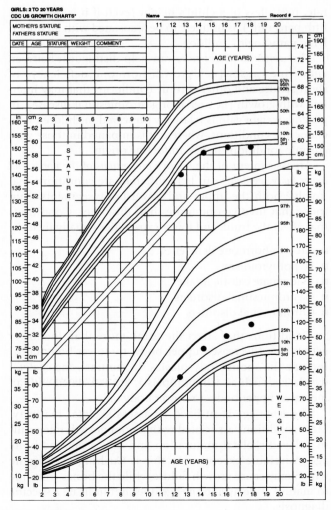

Figure 19.1 Typical growth curve of a child with familial short stature.

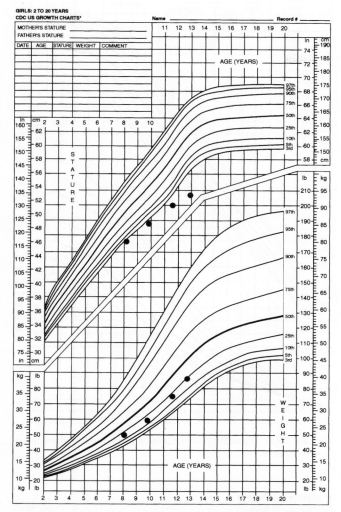

Figure 19.3 Typical growth curve of a child with Turner syndrome.

- Renal tubular acidosis
- Hypochondroplasia

Even in patients with subtle manifestations of these conditions, it is frequently possible to ascertain additional historical factors that may pinpoint the diagnosis (Table 19.1). In some cases, growth failure may be the only obvious manifestation; for example, inflammatory bowel disease may result in growth impairment before the gastrointestinal features develop.

Specific physical examination findings may suggest the presence of some of these entities (Table 19.2). It is important to remember that although most girls with Turner syndrome have some dysmorphic features that are clues to the diagnosis, growth failure may be the only manifestation. Once growth failure has been documented in a child and no obvious cause can be determined by the history or physical examination, initial laboratory tests should be performed to rule out subtle chronic conditions as the cause of growth failure (Table 19.3). For a child with growth failure and open growth plates (based on bone

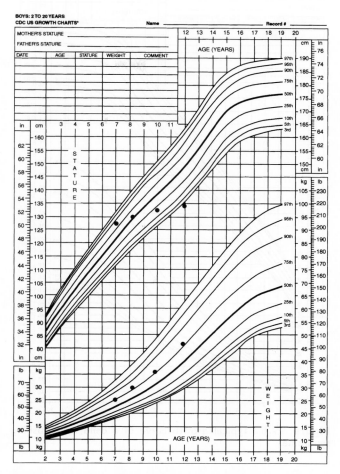

Figure 19.4 Typical growth curve of a child with growth hormone deficiency.

age) but no indication of a chronic condition that might be causing growth failure, the next step would be to evaluate the child's ability to secrete growth hormone.

GROWTH HORMONE DEFICIENCY

Growth hormone deficiency can be congenital or acquired. Congenital deficiency may result from perinatal asphyxia or prenatal embryologic malformations. Associated central nervous system abnormalities, midline abnormalities, and micropenis in males are sometimes present when growth hormone deficiency is secondary to embryologic malformations. Infants with congenital growth hormone deficiency often have neonatal hypoglycemia. They exhibit decelerated growth with normal weight gain after the first year of life. Causes of acquired growth hormone deficiency include:

- Tumors (craniopharyngioma)
- Infection
- Trauma
- Irradiation
- Surgical damage

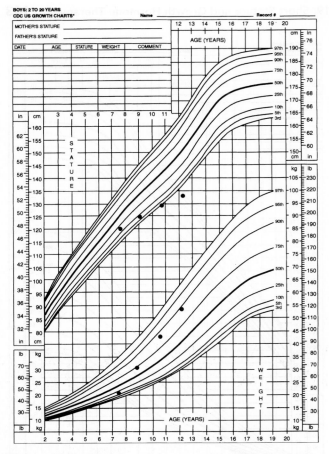

Figure 19.5 Typical growth curve of a child with Cushing syndrome.

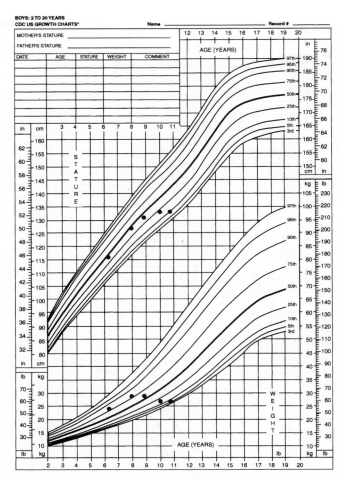

Figure 19.6 Typical growth curve of a child with inflammatory bowel disease.

TABLE 19.1

IMPORTANT HISTORICAL FEATURES AND ASSOCIATED CLINICAL ENTITIES IN THE EVALUATION OF PATHOLOGIC SHORT STATURE

Historical Feature	Associated Clinical Entity
Height consistently short versus recent onset of growth failure	Can help distinguish nonpathologic short stature from abnormal growth rate
Nocturia	Diabetes insipidus
Headache on awakening	Increased intracranial pressure/ brain tumor resulting in acquired growth hormone deficiency
Gastrointestinal symptoms: diarrhea, abdominal pain	Inflammatory bowel disease
History of previous urinary tract infections	Chronic renal disease
Remote history of central nervous system infection or tumor	Pituitary disorder resulting in growth hormone deficiency
Remote history of radiation to head or neck	Thyroid or pituitary disease resulting in hypothyroidism or growth hormone deficiency

TABLE 19.2

SPECIFIC PHYSICAL EXAMINATION FINDINGS AND ASSOCIATED CLINICAL ENTITIES IN THE EVALUATION OF PATHOLOGIC SHORT STATURE

Physical Finding	Associated Clinical Entity
Disproportionate shortening of limbs in comparison with trunk	Skeletal dysplasia (achondroplasia or hypochondroplasia)
Disproportionate shortening of trunk in comparison with limbs	Spondylodysplasia
Midline facial deformities (cleft lip, cleft palate)	May be associated with pituitary dysfunction and growth hormone deficiency
Abnormalities in peripheral vision	Tumor involving the optic chiasm interfering with hypothalamic and pituitary function
Markedly delayed pubertal status in a girl	Turner syndrome
Webbed neck, upcurving finger nails	Turner syndrome
Dysmorphic features	Various syndromes (Prader-Willi, trisomy 21, Russell-Silver, 18 p-)

TABLE 19.3

INITIAL LABORATORY TESTS IN THE EVALUATION OF PATHOLOGIC SHORT STATURE

Laboratory Test	Clinical Entity
Karyotype (girls only)	Turner syndrome
Complete blood cell count	Crohn disease
Erythrocyte sedimentation rate	
Transglutaminase antibodies	Celiac disease
Endomysial antibodies	
T_4, TSH	Hypothyroidism
Urinalysis	Chronic renal disease
Complete metabolic panel	Renal tubular acidosis, rickets

T_4, thyroxine; TSH, thyroid-stimulating hormone.

Growth hormone levels obtained at random are not clinically useful. Exercise can be used to stimulate a screening growth hormone level. Growth hormone stimulates the secretion of insulin-like growth factor 1 (IGF-1) and IGF-binding protein 3 (IGFBP-3). Serum levels of these two proteins can be used to screen for growth hormone deficiency, but the tests are not specific.

Failure to release growth hormone in response to two stimuli known to cause the release of growth hormone indicates that a patient has classic growth hormone deficiency. Substances commonly used to stimulate the release of growth hormone include clonidine, glucagon, arginine, growth hormone–releasing hormone, and insulin. A child who cannot produce growth hormone to a level >7 ng/mL after receiving two of these substances is considered to have classic growth hormone deficiency.

Children with classic growth hormone deficiency should undergo magnetic resonance imaging of the pituitary before growth hormone therapy is initiated. Frequently, the pituitary gland is small, ectopic, or even absent. The presence of a brain tumor (i.e., craniopharyngioma) must be excluded before growth hormone therapy is begun.

Overnight serum sampling every 20 minutes for growth hormone levels has been proposed to identify children with neurosecretory growth hormone deficiency. These children have growth failure but normal results on growth hormone stimulation testing. Many of them respond very well to growth hormone therapy, as do children with classic growth hormone deficiency.

GROWTH HORMONE THERAPY

Growth hormone treatment should be reserved for those children who require it and in whom success is anticipated. Growth hormone therapy has been approved by the U.S.

Food and Drug Administration for children with any of the following causes of growth failure:

- Classic growth hormone deficiency
- Neurosecretory growth hormone deficiency
- Turner syndrome
- Chronic renal failure
- Noonan syndrome
- Prader-Willi syndrome
- Intrauterine growth retardation
- Wasting syndrome secondary to human immunodeficiency virus infection
- Idiopathic short stature when the child is shorter than 2.25 standard deviations below the mean height for age

A subcutaneous injection of growth hormone is administered each night at an initial dose of 0.04 mg/kg (0.05 mg/kg for children with Turner syndrome, chronic renal failure, or intrauterine growth retardation). Doses up to 0.1 mg/kg have recently been approved for adolescents with growth hormone deficiency.

Side Effects of Treatment with Growth Hormone

Known side effects include:

- Pseudotumor cerebri
- Edema
- Glucose intolerance
- Slipped femoral capital epiphysis
- Rapid growth of nevi
- Worsening of scoliosis

Probable side effects include arthritis, transplant (kidney) rejection, leukemia in children who have previously received radiation therapy, acute pancreatitis, increased risk for future development of type 2 diabetes, and colon cancer.

REVIEW EXERCISES

QUESTIONS

1. The most common cause of short stature in children is:
a. Growth hormone deficiency
b. Turner syndrome
c. Russell-Silver syndrome
d. Familial short stature

Answer
The answer is d.

2. Short stature and growth failure may be the presenting complaint for which of the following conditions:
a. Juvenile rheumatoid arthritis
b. Insulin-dependent diabetes mellitus

c. Crohn disease
d. Leukemia

Answer

The answer is c. Other conditions that may initially present with growth failure include kidney disease (especially renal tubular acidosis) and celiac disease. Although growth failure may occur in juvenile rheumatoid arthritis, diabetes mellitus type I, and leukemia, it is not the initial presenting problem in these conditions.

3. Short stature and growth failure may be the presenting complaint for which of the following brain tumors:
a. Hypothalamic hamartoma
b. Craniopharyngioma
c. Pinealoma
d. Posterior fossa meduloblastoma

Answer

The answer is b. Growth failure may be the first sign of a craniopharyngioma. Although growth failure may occur with the other types of brain tumors, it is usually not the presenting sign in these cases.

4. Growth hormone is currently approved by the U.S. Food and Drug Administration to treat short stature and growth failure caused by:
a. Familial short stature and growth hormone deficiency
b. Delayed puberty and growth hormone deficiency
c. Chronic renal failure, Turner syndrome, and growth hormone deficiency
d. Down syndrome and growth hormone deficiency

Answer

The answer is c. Growth hormone therapy is approved for growth failure in growth hormone deficiency, chronic renal failure, Turner syndrome, Prader-Willi syndrome, wasting syndrome secondary to human immunodeficiency virus infection, and intrauterine growth retardation.

5. Which of the following potential side effects has *not* been attributed to growth hormone treatment?
a. Hepatitis
b. Pseudotumor cerebri
c. Growth of nevi
d. Slipped femoral capital epiphysis

Answer

The answer is a. Other side effects of growth hormone therapy include worsening of scoliosis, glucose intolerance, arthralgia, and edema.

SUGGESTED READINGS

1. American Academy of Pediatrics: Committee on Drugs and Committee on Bioethics. Considerations related to the use of recombinant human growth hormone in children. *Pediatrics* 1997;99:122–129.
2. Lawson Wilkins Pediatric Endocrine Society: Drug and Therapeutics Committee. Guidelines for the use of growth hormone in children with short stature. *J Pediatr* 1995;127:857–867.
3. Lindgren AC, Hagenäs L, Müller J, et al. Growth hormone treatment of children with Prader-Willi syndrome affects linear growth and body composition favourably. *Acta Paediatr* 1998;87:28–31.
4. Rosenfeld RG, Tesch LG, Rodriguez-Rigau L, et al. Recommendations for the diagnosis, treatment, and management of individuals with Turner syndrome. *Endocrinologist* 1994;4:351–358.

Chapter 20

BOARD SIMULATION:
Endocrinology

Elumalai Appachi

QUESTIONS

1. The parents of a 10-year-old girl (Fig. 20.1) are concerned about her height. She is shorter than her classmates, and the parents request growth hormone therapy. Which of the following statements is *true* regarding the diagnosis and management of her condition?
a) A skeletal survey is required to rule out hypochondroplasia.
b) Growth hormone therapy is indicated because she may have growth hormone deficiency.
c) The parents should be reassured that her growth will catch up during the adolescent growth spurt.
d) Chromosomal analysis will reveal the diagnosis.
e) None of the above.

Answer

The answer is d. Most patients with Turner syndrome have a 45,X chromosome complement, although 15% display mosaicism (45,X/46,XX). This condition occurs in 1 of 1500 to 2500 liveborn female infants. Most pregnancies with a Turner syndrome karyotype abort spontaneously. The major clinical manifestations, commonly present at birth, include lymphedema of the dorsa of the hands and feet (see Fig. 20.1) and loose skin folds at the nape of the neck. In childhood, short stature, webbing of the neck, a broad chest, cubitus valgus, and extremely convex fingernails are the predominant features. Sexual maturation fails to occur at the expected age. Associated cardiac anomalies include bicuspid aortic valve, coarctation of aorta, aortic stenosis, and mitral valve prolapse. Renal anomalies include pelvic kidney, horseshoe kidney, absence of one kidney, and double collecting systems. Any short female child should be investigated for Turner syndrome. Although growth hormone deficiency has not been established in this syndrome, treatment with growth hormone helps to increase the child's height. Hypochondroplasia resembles achondroplasia but is a milder disorder. Children with hypochondroplasia display a characteristic phenotype, and radiography is diagnostic.

2. A 2-week-old boy is seen in the emergency department because he has been vomiting for the past 24 hours. On examination, the infant is lethargic and his skin is mottled. He is given two boluses of normal saline solution with no improvement. The infant's laboratory data include the following values:
a) Na = 121 mmol/L
b) K = 6.1 mmol/L
c) Blood urea nitrogen = 40 mg/dL
d) HCO_3 = 12 mmol/L
e) Blood glucose = 40 mg/dL

Appropriate management would include all of the following *except:*
a) Administering intravenous hydrocortisone
b) Administering 2 to 4 mL/kg of 10% dextrose intravenously
c) Administering dopamine infusion
d) Measuring serum 17-hydroxyprogesterone
e) Administering broad-spectrum antibiotics

Answer

The answer is c. Congenital adrenal hyperplasia is an autosomal-recessive disorder. Ninety percent of affected patients have 21-hydroxylase deficiency. Patients with the salt-wasting variety of congenital adrenal hyperplasia present with failure to thrive, dehydration, vomiting, and anorexia. In female infants, virilization of the external genitalia leads to an early diagnosis; the condition is often diagnosed later in male infants with the salt-wasting variety (2–3 weeks of life) because the external genitalia may appear normal. Hydrocortisone (10–20 mg/m² every 24 hours) is recommended as a replacement therapy and to prevent virilization. Sodium supplementation and the administration of mineralocorticoid are

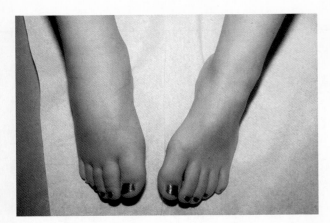

Figure 20.1   The girl in question 1. See explanation for question 1 for details.

necessary to maintain a normal electrolyte balance. The infant in question requires another normal saline bolus and the administration of hydrocortisone; dopamine is not indicated.

3. An 8-year-old girl with insulin-dependent diabetes presents with a 3-day history of abdominal pain and vomiting. She was treated in the emergency department 1 week ago for hypoglycemia. Examination reveals rapid breathing, dry mucous membranes, and poor peripheral perfusion. Appropriate management would include all of the following *except:*
a) Initiating fluid resuscitation judiciously, with close monitoring of the neurologic status
b) Monitoring serum potassium frequently
c) Remembering that sodium bicarbonate therapy is not routinely indicated and may cause intracellular acidosis
d) Administering 0.1 U/kg of regular insulin subcutaneously
e) Advising her to rotate the sites of insulin injection at the time of discharge

Answer
The answer is d. The administration of fluid and electrolytes to replete the intravascular volume and correct electrolyte abnormalities is the most important step in the management of diabetic ketoacidosis. Insulin therapy helps arrest the metabolic derangement and reverses the catabolic state. *Intravenous, rather than subcutaneous,* infusion of insulin is the standard of care for diabetic ketoacidosis. Because diabetic ketoacidosis causes hyperosmolar dehydration, the administration of 0.9% saline solution is hypotonic, relative to the patient's osmolality. A gentle and gradual decrease in osmolality is required to prevent the development of cerebral edema, one of the major complications of diabetic ketoacidosis therapy. The administration of a total fluid volume of 4 L/m^2 per day is associated with a decreased incidence of cerebral edema. Because the total body potassium is depleted in diabetic

ketoacidosis, potassium replacement must be started early in the therapy to avoid life-threatening hypokalemia. Bicarbonate therapy is not routinely recommended during the management of diabetic ketoacidosis because it causes alkalosis, which in turn shifts the oxygen dissociation curve to the left and reduces oxygen delivery to tissues. It also causes intracellular acidosis with the production of carbon dioxide, which diffuses across the blood–brain barrier and exacerbates the cerebral acidosis. The patient in question should rotate the insulin injection sites because her erratic insulin absorption is contributing to the episodes of hypoglycemia and hyperglycemia.

4. The parents of a 2-year-old girl who was brought into your clinic express concern about the development of pubic hair in the child. Appropriate management should include:
a) Measurement of her bone age
b) Reassurance of the parents that the condition is probably benign but should be followed up closely
c) Measurement of serum androgens and 17-hydroxyprogesterone
d) All of the above
e) None of the above

Answer
The answer is d. Precocious puberty is defined as the development of secondary sexual characteristics before the age of 8 years in girls and 9 years in boys. Premature adrenarche is the appearance of pubic hair before the age of sexual maturation. It is much more common in girls than in boys and is an early maturational event of adrenal androgen production. Premature adrenarche is a benign condition and does not require therapy. However, if the child shows evidence of a systemic androgen effect (e.g., acceleration of growth, clitoromegaly, advanced bone age, cystic acne), further investigations are warranted. The measurement of androgen and 17-hydroxyprogesterone is necessary to rule out nonclassic forms of congenital adrenal hyperplasia.

5. A 21-month-old toddler is brought to you for a routine physical examination. You note that she has recently gained an excessive amount of weight. Examination shows a markedly obese child with a blood pressure of 130/90 mm Hg. Urinalysis shows glycosuria. Which of the following is the *best* course of action?
a) Taking a detailed dietary history and advising the family about caloric restriction
b) Ordering an abdominal ultrasound as it is diagnostic
c) Measuring serum Cortisol in the morning and evening to evaluate diurnal rhythm
d) Administering insulin 0.1 U/kg subcutaneously
e) Measuring urinary excretion of free Cortisol

Answer
The answer is e. The features of Cushing syndrome, which result from adrenal cortical hyperfunction, are

obesity, hypertension, and glucose intolerance. The most common cause of Cushing syndrome in infants is a malignant, functioning adrenocortical tumor. Most of the tumors occur in children younger than 3 years. Other causes of Cushing syndrome in childhood include primary pigmented nodular adrenocortical disease and nodular hyperplasia, both of which are independent of adrenocorticotropic hormone (ACTH) secretion. ACTH-dependent Cushing syndrome is caused by microadenomas of the pituitary and the ectopic production of ACTH in islet cell carcinoma of the pancreas, neuroblastoma, and occasionally Wilms tumor. The clinical manifestations of Cushing syndrome include obesity, masculinization, hypertrichosis, acne, and impaired growth. The diurnal variation of cortisol production is lost in Cushing syndrome, but diurnal variation is lacking in children younger than 3 years. The urinary excretion of cortisol is almost always increased. Ultrasonography may not be able to identify the tumors, and CT scan is required to make the diagnosis. Other findings include polycythemia, lymphopenia and eosinopenia, altered glucose tolerance, advanced bone age, pathologic fracture, and absence of the thymic shadow on chest x-ray films.

6. A 16-year-old adolescent (Fig. 20.2) is losing weight despite having a good appetite. She is a long-distance runner at school and seems to tire easily. She exhibits emotional lability, and her grades at school have suffered lately. The *most* appropriate plan of action is to:
a) Order thyroid function tests.
b) Refer her for a psychiatric evaluation.
c) Commence a workup for inflammatory bowel disease.

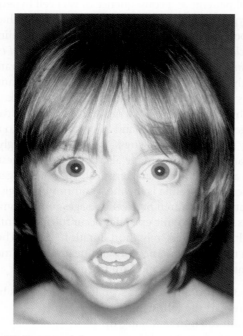

Figure 20.2 The adolescent in question 6. See explanation for question 6 for details.

d) Hospitalize her for intensive nutritional therapy under supervision.
e) None of the above

Answer
The answer is a. The peak incidence of thyrotoxicosis (Graves disease) occurs during adolescence. The symptoms develop slowly, and the earliest sign can be a poor school performance. Emotional lability, hyperactivity, and tremors are also early features. Increased appetite with poor weight gain is a prominent feature. Goiter is found in almost all patients; exophthalmos (see Fig. 20.2) may be mild. Proximal muscle weakness, palpitations, and breathing difficulties may occur. The serum levels of thyroxine (T_4), tri-iodothyronine (T_3), free T_4, and free T_3 are all elevated. The level of thyroid-stimulating hormone is suppressed and may be undetected. The diagnosis of hyperthyroidism should be considered in any young adolescent girl with poor school performance, emotional lability, and weight loss.

7. A 2-month-old boy is brought to your clinic for routine immunizations. The infant exhibits signs of hypothyroidism. The following statements are true regarding congenital hypothyroidism *except:*
a) He may have had prolonged physiologic jaundice in the neonatal period.
b) Goiter is almost always present in congenital hypothyroidism.
c) Plain radiography may show the absence of distal femoral epiphysis.
d) The incidence of congenital hypothyroidism is lower in the African American population.
e) Deficiency of thyroid-stimulating hormone is a rare cause of this condition.

Answer
The answer is b. The incidence of congenital hypothyroidism is 1/4000 infants worldwide but lower in African Americans. Thyroid dysgenesis accounts for almost all cases of congenital hypothyroidism, and the presence of goiter is rare. Other causes of congenital hypothyroidism include thyrotropin receptor-blocking antibody, defective synthesis of thyroxine, defects in iodine transport, and thyroid peroxidase defects of organification and coupling. Thyrotropin deficiency is rare and associated with other pituitary abnormalities. Although clinicians depend on neonatal screening, awareness of the early symptoms of hypothyroidism is necessary to make a timely diagnosis. Affected infants exhibit feeding difficulties, sluggishness, sleepiness, and prolonged physiologic jaundice. Constipation, edema of the extremities and genitalia, and refractory anemia are other features.

8. A 5-year-old boy (Fig. 20.3) with a known metabolic disorder is seen in your clinic with recurrent otitis media.

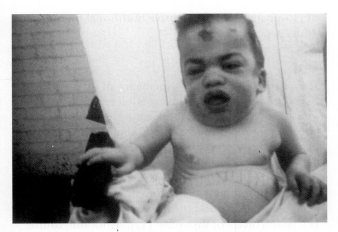

Figure 20.3 The boy in question 8. See explanation for question 8 for details.

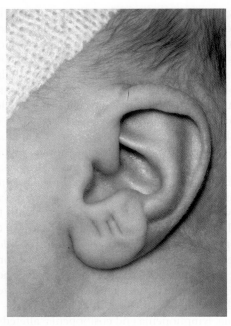

Figure 20.4 The neonate in question 9. See explanation for question 9 for details.

The following statements are true regarding his condition *except:*

a) Progressive neurologic deterioration is common.
b) It is inherited in an autosomal-recessive pattern.
c) He has extensive bone and joint disease.
d) Congestive heart failure develops secondary to valvular heart disease.
e) Abnormal physical features are present at birth.

Answer

The answer is e. Hurler syndrome is a type I mucopolysaccharidosis with an autosomal-recessive inheritance. This is a severe form of mucopolysaccharidosis. The infant with Hurler syndrome appears normal at birth; the abnormal features develop during infancy. These include hepatosplenomegaly, coarse facial features, multiple skeletal deformities, and corneal clouding. A large tongue causes airway difficulties. Severe neurologic degeneration with developmental delay is common. Recurrent ear and respiratory infections develop in many patients. Cardiac abnormalities, including acute cardiomyopathy and valvular heart disease, can be life-threatening. Bone marrow transplantation increases long-term survival and relieves symptoms but does not reverse the skeletal abnormalities. Enzyme replacement therapy with recombinant αL-iduronidase is available in specialized centers that care for children with Hurler syndrome.

9. A 1-week-old neonate (Fig. 20.4) is recovering from an omphalocele repair. He was a full-term infant born by cesarean delivery with a birth weight of 5 kg. A generalized seizure develops, and his rapid blood glucose measurement is 24 mg/dL. Which of the following is *true* regarding this infant's condition?

a) He is at increased risk for the development of Wilms tumor.
b) He has transient hypoglycemia of the newborn.
c) He has ketotic hypoglycemia.

d) He has panhypopituitarism.
e) None of the above.

Answer

The answer is a. Beckwith-Wiedemann syndrome is characterized by macrosomia, omphalocele, macroglossia, and visceromegaly. Infants have characteristic transverse ear lobe creases (see Fig. 20.4). Hypoglycemia develops in 50% of patients as a consequence of islet cell hyperplasia and hyperinsulinism. The absence of ketones in the face of hypoglycemia is a diagnostic clue to hyperinsulinism. *These children are predisposed to a subset of childhood tumors, including Wilms tumor and adrenocortical tumors.* Transient hypoglycemia is more common in premature infants and infants who are small for their gestational age. It is thought to result from inadequate storage of the liver glycogen, muscle protein, and body fat required to meet energy needs at times of stress. Infants with hypoglycemia and panhypopituitarism are also small for their gestational age, and boys characteristically have microgenitalia. Ketotic hypoglycemia is the most common hypoglycemia presenting in children between the ages of 18 months and 5 years. Hypoglycemic episodes occur following intercurrent illness and relatively short duration fasting. The condition resolves spontaneously and treatment is aimed at preventing hypoglycemia with frequent feeds.

10. A 3-year-old toddler is seen for bowlegs. His blood work reveals the following:

a) Serum calcium = 8.5 mg/dL
b) Phosphate = 3 mg/dL
c) Alkaline phosphatase = 850 U/dL

All of the following statements are true regarding the etiology of the toddler's diagnosis *except:*

a) Anticonvulsant therapy is a recognized cause
b) Cystic fibrosis is a recognized cause
c) Inadequate exposure to the sun may cause this condition.
d) This condition is rare in low-birth-weight infants and in adolescents.
e) Chronic renal failure is a recognized cause

Answer

The answer is d. Predominant causes of rickets include nutritional deficiency, inadequate exposure to sunlight, or both in some cases. Rickets may develop in breast-fed infants of mothers who are not exposed to sunlight. Darkly pigmented children are more susceptible to rickets. Causes of secondary rickets include chronic renal failure, malabsorptive diseases such as celiac disease and cystic fibrosis, and anticonvulsant therapy, especially with phenytoin and phenobarbital. Rickets with vitamin D deficiency develops during the phases of rapid growth, as in low-birth-weight infants and adolescents. The clinical manifestations of rickets include craniotabes, delayed eruption of the teeth, enlarged and prominent costochondral junctions, bowlegs or knock-knees, and poor muscle tone. Typical laboratory values include *low serum calcium, low serum phosphate, increased alkaline phosphatase,* and increased excretion of cyclic adenosine monophosphate in the urine.

11. A 6-year-old boy (**Fig. 20.5**) is brought to you because of parental concern about nocturnal enuresis. He has developmental delay and has been gaining weight progressively. On further questioning, the parents reveal that he was small for his gestational age at birth and had feeding problems during the first few months of life. All of the following statements are true regarding the boy's condition *except:*

a) He may continue to gain weight and remain obese.
b) He is at increased risk for right-sided heart failure.
c) He may have mild-to-moderate mental retardation.
d) New onset diabetes mellitus may be the cause of the nocturnal enuresis.
e) He may develop precocious puberty.

Answer

The answer is e. Children with Prader-Willi syndrome (**Fig. 20.5**) become obese after a period of failure to thrive in infancy. Gross obesity results in sleep apnea, chronic hypoxemia, and right-sided heart failure secondary to the development of pulmonary hypertension. Mild to moderate psychomotor retardation is very common, as are multiple endocrine abnormalities. Insulin-dependent diabetes mellitus may present as nocturnal enuresis. Hypogonadotropic hypogonadism presents as delayed puberty. The condition is sporadic, but a paternally derived deletion of the long arm of chromosome 15 is found in >50% of children with Prader-Willi syndrome.

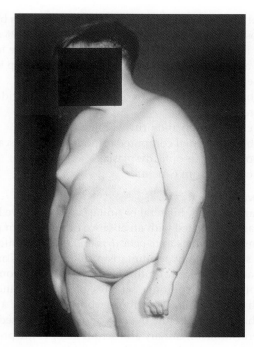

Figure 20.5 The boy in question 11. See explanation for question 11 for details.

12. A 12-year-old boy presents with a 2-week history of swelling in his left eye. On examination, he has thoracic scoliosis, *café au lait* spots, and moderate hypertension. All of the following statements are true regarding his condition *except:*

a) He may have mild learning disability.
b) Cutaneous nodules characteristically develop during adolescence.
c) He may have an optic glioma on the left side with minimal visual disturbance.
d) He should undergo a workup for pheochromocytoma.
e) All his daughters will be carriers of his condition.

Answer

The answer is e. Neurofibromatosis is an autosomal-dominant condition; therefore, the offsprings of affected individuals have a 50% chance of being affected. The incidence is 1 in 4000. The diagnosis is based on the presence of six or more *café au lait* spots, axillary or inguinal freckling, two or more Lisch nodules of the iris (see Fig. 35.3), and cutaneous neurofibromas. Cutaneous neurofibromas typically develop during adolescence. Optic gliomas are present in 15% of patients, who are usually asymptomatic with nearly normal vision. Plexiform neuroma of the eyelid is strongly associated with ipsilateral optic glioma. Hypertension may be caused by renal vascular stenosis or pheochromocytoma. The other features of neurofibromatosis include scoliosis, learning difficulties, precocious puberty, and malignant neoplasms.

13. You are called to the neonatal nursery to see a jittery newborn. The examination reveals a healthy-looking infant except for microphallus and jitteriness. His blood glucose is 15 mg/dL. An intravenous bolus of 10% dextrose in water is given and an infusion of dextrose in water is administered. The next *most* appropriate step is to:

a) Measure urine 17-ketosteroids.
b) Obtain urinalysis for an organic and amino acid screening.
c) Measure serum and urine ketones.
d) Obtain a cranial computed tomography (CT) scan to look for septo-optic dysplasia.
e) Measure serum C-peptide.

Answer

The answer is d. Bilateral or unilateral optic nerve hypoplasia associated with an absence of the septum pellucidum is known as *septo-optic dysplasia*. Affected infants have signs of panhypopituitarism, and their discs are pale and hypoplastic on funduscopy. Affected neonates exhibit apnea, hypotonia, seizures, prolonged jaundice, and hypoglycemia. Typically, newborn boys have a microphallus. Because the hypoglycemia is not caused by hyperinsulinism, urinary and serum ketones are present. The urinary excretion of 17-ketosteroids is increased in congenital adrenal hyperplasia and adrenocortical tumors. The measurement of organic and amino acids has a role in the workup of hypoglycemia but is not warranted in this instance.

14. A 4-year-old child is brought to the emergency department with tetany. The serum calcium level is 6.0 mg/dL, phosphate 9.6 mg/dL, and alkaline phosphatase 586 U/dL. All of the following statements are true regarding pseudohypoparathyroidism *except:*

a) Cranial CT scan may show calcification of the basal ganglia.
b) He is at risk for gonadal dysfunction during adult life.
c) The parathyroid hormone (PTH) levels will be low.
d) He is at risk for moderate learning disability.
e) A slit-lamp examination may reveal cataracts.

Answer

The answer is c. The patient in question exhibits signs and symptoms of hypoparathyroidism. The parathyroid glands are normal and can synthesize and secrete PTH in pseudohypoparathyroidism. A genetic defect in the hormone receptor adenylate cyclase system results in unresponsiveness to the hormone, whether PTH is administered endogenously or exogenously. Tetany is the most common presenting sign. Affected children have brachydactyly with short metacarpals, moderate mental retardation, calcium deposits in the subcutaneous tissues and basal ganglia, and lenticular cataracts. Other endocrine abnormalities include hypothyroidism and gonadal dysfunction. The diagnosis is based on a demonstration of reduced excretion of urinary phosphate and cAMP after an intravenous infusion of PTH. A definitive diagnosis is based on genetic studies.

15. A 1-month-old infant is brought in with constipation and poor weight gain. Examination reveals facial wasting with an inverted V-shaped upper lip and generalized hypotonia. The following statements are true regarding this infant's condition *except:*

a) Electrocardiography may show cardiac conduction abnormalities.
b) The serum creatine kinase levels will be markedly elevated.
c) He is at risk for the development of diabetes mellitus later.
d) Slit lamp examination of his eyes may show cataracts.
e) He inherited this condition from his mother.

Answer

The answer is b. Myotonic dystrophy is the second most common form of muscular dystrophy in the United States, Europe, and Australia. It is inherited as an autosomal-dominant trait. Multiple organ systems are involved, given the defects in striated, smooth, and cardiac muscles. The facial appearance is characteristic, with an inverted V-shaped upper lip, thin cheeks, and a thinned-out temporalis muscle. Progressive weakness develops in the distal muscles; in contrast, the weakness is primarily in the proximal muscles in other muscular dystrophies. Myotonia (delayed relaxation of a muscle after contraction) is a classic feature of this condition and develops after 3 years of age. Smooth-muscle involvement in the gastrointestinal system results in slow gastric emptying and constipation. In women with this condition, uterine contractions during labor may be ineffectual. Cardiac involvement is in the form of heart block and occasional arrhythmias. Endocrine abnormalities include hypothyroidism, diabetes mellitus, and adrenocortical insufficiency. Testicular atrophy and testosterone deficiency cause infertility in men. Cataracts and mild to moderate mental retardation are additional features. The creatine kinase levels are usually normal or mildly elevated. Muscle biopsy and electromyography showing myotonia provide important diagnostic information. The genetic defect involves chromosome 19 and the mother is the transmitting parent in 94% of cases, a finding that is not explained by male infertility alone.

SUGGESTED READINGS

1. Argao EA, Heubi JE. Fat-soluble vitamin deficiency in infants and children. *Curr Opin Pediatr* 1993;5:562.
2. Cnossen MH, de Goede-Bolder A, van den Broek KM, et al. A prospective 10-year follow-up study of patients with neurofibromatosis type 1. *Arch Dis Child* 1998;78:408.
3. Elliott M, Maher ER. Beckwith-Wiedemann syndrome. *J Med Genet* 1994;31:560.
4. Finberg L. Fluid management of diabetic ketoacidosis. *Pediatr Rev* 1996;17:46.
5. Fisher DA. Management of congenital hypothyroidism. *J Clin Endocrinol Metab* 1991;72:523.

6. Forest MG. Prenatal diagnosis, treatment, and outcome in infants with congenital adrenal hyperplasia. *Curr Opin Endocrinol Diabetes* 1997;4:209.

7. Magiakou MA, Mastorakos G, Oldfield EH, et al. Cushing's syndrome in children and adolescents. *N Engl J Med* 1994;331:629.

8. Margalith D, Tze WJ, Jan JE. Congenital optic nerve hypoplasia with hypothalamic-pituitary dysplasia. *Am J Dis Child* 1985;139:361.

9. Moxley RT III. Myotonic disorders in childhood: diagnosis and treatment. *J Child Neurol* 1997;12:116.

10. Muller J. Hypogonadism and endocrine metabolic disorders in Prader Willi syndrome. *Acta Paediatr Suppl* 1997;423:58.

11. Nakamoto JM, Sandstrom AT, Van Dop C, et al. Pseudohypoparathyroidism type Ia from maternal but not paternal transmission of a Gs gene mutation. *Am J Med Genet* 1997;77:261.

12. Peters C, Shapiro EG, Krivit W. Hurler syndrome: past, present, and future. *J Pediatr* 1998;133:79.

13. Plotnick L, Attie KM, Blethen SL, et al. Growth hormone treatment of girls with Turner syndrome: the National Cooperative Growth Study experience. *Pediatrics* 1998;102:479.

14. Sills IN. Hyperthyroidism. *Pediatr Rev* 1994;15:417.

15. Styne DM. New aspects in the diagnosis and treatment of pubertal disorders. *Pediatr Clin North Am* 1993;44:505.

Chapter 21

Respiratory Diseases of the Newborn

Craig H. Raskind

OVERVIEW

Respiratory diseases in the neonate often present as respiratory distress. Respiratory distress is a clinical mosaic composed of a combination of signs and symptoms that include elements of tachypnea, intercostal, subcostal and suprasternal retractions, nasal flaring, grunting, and cyanosis. It is one of most common reasons for admissions to the neonatal intensive care unit (NICU). The most common causes for NICU admission include transient tachypnea of the newborn (TTN) and infection (i.e., sepsis, pneumonia). Respiratory distress as a diagnostic sign has an expansive differential that includes multiple disease etiologies. These etiologies can be broadly divided into two classifications: *nonrespiratory disorders* and *respiratory diseases*.

Etiologies of *nonrespiratory disorders* causing respiratory distress are extensive and include:

- Cardiovascular
  - Congenital heart disease
- Congestive heart failure with secondary pulmonary edema
- Hematologic
  - Severe anemia
  - Polycythemia/hyperviscosity syndrome
- Metabolic
  - Metabolic acidosis
  - Hypoglycemia
  - Hypothermia
- Neuromuscular
  - Central nervous system
    - Cerebral edema
    - Intracranial hemorrhage
    - Meningitis
    - Spinal muscular atrophy
    - Drug exposure
  - Peripheral nervous system
    - Myasthenia gravis
  - Muscular
    - Muscular dystrophy

Although it is essential and critical to consider cardiac disease at the outset of a neonatal evaluation, it is an uncommon cause of symptomatology immediately following birth.

Respiratory diseases causing respiratory distress during the neonatal period may be divided into four general categories:

1. Parenchymal conditions
2. Developmental abnormalities
3. Mechanical abnormalities
4. Airway abnormalities

Parenchymal conditions include transient tachypnea of the newborn (TTN), respiratory distress syndrome (RDS), bacterial pneumonia, meconium aspiration syndrome (MAS), and persistent pulmonary hypertension of the newborn (PPHN). Developmental abnormalities include congenital diaphragmatic hernia (CDH), congenital cystic adenomatoid malformation (CCAM), pulmonary sequestration, tracheoesophageal fistula (TEF), pulmonary hypoplasia, and infantile lobar emphysema. Mechanical abnormalities include all forms of pulmonary air-leak syndromes. Airway abnormalities may include any intrinsic or extrinsic causes leading to airway obstruction. Further elaboration and discussion on many of these conditions follow the questions listed in the following.

REVIEW EXERCISES

QUESTIONS

1. Embryologically the lung is derived from:
a) Lateral folds of embryonic mesoderm
b) Medial pharyngeal groove of the foregut endoderm
c) Epithelial cells of the neural crest
d) Subdivision of primordial mesenchyme
e) None of the above

Answer

The answer is b. Lung development begins during the third week of gestation. It is during the embryonic period of fetal development that the lung bud differentiates from a ventral outpouching from the floor of the primitive foregut endoderm (Fig. 21.1).

Lung organogenesis can be divided into five distinct periods:

■ Embryonic (weeks 3–6)
■ Pseudoglandular (weeks 6–16)
■ Canalicular (weeks 16–26)
■ Saccular (weeks 26–36)
■ Alveolar (weeks 36–maturity)

During the embryonic and pseudoglandular periods the major conducting airways are established and elaborated upon through branching morphogenesis. The canalicular and saccular periods include vascularization of

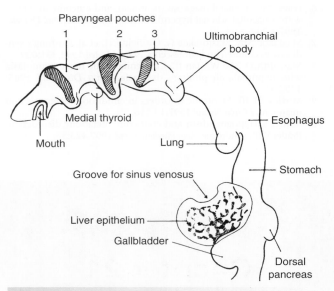

Figure 21.1 Medial pharyngeal groove of foregut endoderm (caudal end). (From Skandalakis JE, Gray SW. *Embryology for surgeons*, 2nd ed. Baltimore: Williams & Wilkins, 1994, with permission.)

terminal respiratory units to form the adult respiratory unit and cytodifferentiation of bronchiolar and alveolar cells leading to the appearance of Type I and Type II surfactant-producing pneumocytes. Finally, it is during the alveolar period that a marked reduction of interstitial tissue and maturation of alveolar organization (alveolarization) occur. Subsequent alveolar development and lung growth, including further subdivision and proliferation of alveoli, continue well beyond infancy until approximately 2 to 6 years of age. As each stage of lung development is important for subsequent growth and maturation, defects in morphogenesis may be traced to aberrant or arrested development during these periods. For example, tracheoesophageal fistula and tracheal stenosis arise during the embryonic period. Congenital diaphragmatic hernia (CDH), congenital cystic adenomatoid malformation (CCAM), and bronchogenic cysts arise during the pseudoglandular period.

2. A term male newborn is delivered by repeat caesarean section (C/S). Rupture of membranes occurs at delivery. APGARs are 9 at 1 minute and 9 at 5 minutes. At 15 minutes of life the infant is noted to have tachypnea and mild intercostal retractions. He is acyanotic with peripheral oxygen saturation at 88% to 90% on room air. There is no cardiac murmur. Chest radiograph shows expansion of the lungs to 8 to 10 anterior ribs, perihilar streaking, and a fluid density in the right horizontal fissure. Of the following, the *best* therapy for this infant is:
a) Intravenous furosemide
b) Intravenous ampicillin and gentamicin
c) Tracheal intubation and surfactant

d) Intravenous prostaglandin E1
e) Supplemental oxygen by nasal cannula

Answer

The answer is e. This infant most likely had transient tachypnea of the newborn (TTN), which is the most common cause of respiratory distress in newborns. It affects both term and preterm neonates. It results from the delayed clearance of fetal lung fluid after birth. This delayed clearance results from a combination of factors, including inhibition of apical Na^+ channels activation through which lung fluid is reabsorbed, lack of inhibition of chloride-mediated lung fluid secretion, and absent or decreased mechanical forces associated with labor that are either absent with cesarean delivery or decreased with precipitous vaginal delivery. Symptoms may include a combination of grunting, nasal flaring, intercostal, subcostal, or suprasternal retractions, and tachypnea, with or without cyanosis. Resolution typically occurs by 48 to 72 hours after birth. This condition is usually benign and self-limiting, although not universally. Risk factors for TTN include:

- Cesarean delivery without a trial of labor
- Late-preterm delivery
- Maternal diabetes
- Precipitous delivery
- Fetal distress
- Maternal sedation
- Perinatal depression

Roentgenographic evaluation (Fig. 21.2) generally demonstrates good lung volumes, increased interstitial

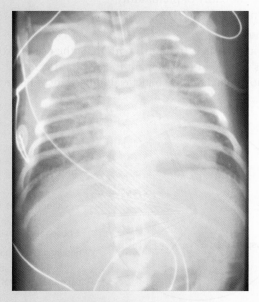

Figure 21.2 Chest radiograph showing perihilar streaking and increased interstitial markings, typical for transient tachypnea of the newborn.

markings, perihilar streaking without air bronchograms, fluid in fissure(s), and only occasionally pleural effusion. Arterial blood gas testing may indicate mild hypoxemia with or without hypercarbia. The differential diagnosis includes RDS, pneumonia, air leak syndromes, and congenital lung malformations. Treatment is supportive and may include oxygen supplementation, continuous positive airway pressure (CPAP), intravenous fluid administration, and close monitoring.

3. A 1600 g infant is born at 32 weeks gestation. The pregnancy was complicated by preterm labor and precipitous delivery. The mother received no antenatal steroids and her membranes ruptured just prior to delivery. At 1 to 2 hours of age, the infant develops tachypnea, grunting, nasal flaring, and subcostal retractions. Of the following, the *most* likely radiographic finding in this infant would be:

a) Fine reticulogranular pattern
b) Diffuse coarse infiltrates
c) Pleural effusion
d) Raised thymic silhouette (sail sign)
e) Fluid in the fissures

Answer

The answer is a. Respiratory distress syndrome (RDS) is the most common cause of *severe* respiratory distress in the newborn. It is a disease of both biological and biochemical immaturity, characterized by pulmonary surfactant deficiency. This deficiency leads to alveolar collapse at low lung volumes. The resultant atelectasis leads to ventilation-perfusion mismatching within the lung and pulmonary edema. These changes in turn lead to decreased lung compliance and altered gas exchange patterns, including hypoxemia, hypercarbia, and acidosis. The incidence of RDS is inversely proportional to gestational age, affecting nearly 100% of neonates delivered between 23 and 25 weeks of gestation, approximately 60% among neonates delivered by 29 weeks of gestation, 20% to 30% among those delivered at 29 to 34 weeks gestation, nearly 5% among those delivered at 34 to 37 weeks, and <1% among those delivered at >37 weeks. Onset of symptoms may be evident immediately after birth, or may develop or worsen within minutes to hours after birth and present with symptoms of respiratory distress. Symptoms may include tachypnea, grunting, nasal flaring, suprasternal, subcostal and intercostal retractions, and cyanosis. Roentgenographic evaluation (Fig. 21.3) demonstrates a characteristic fine reticulogranular pattern ("ground-glass" appearance) with air-bronchograms indicative of diffuse atelectasis. Peak severity occurs at 72 to 96 hours after birth. Recovery usually coincides with brisk urinary diuresis. Preventive strategies include maternal treatment with tocolytic agents to arrest premature labor and maternal antenatal corticosteroid therapy to accelerate fetal lung

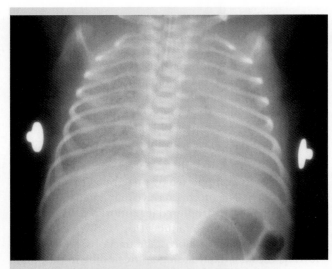

Figure 21.3 Radiograph showing a fine reticulogranular pattern, characteristic of respiratory distress syndrome.

maturity. Efficacy of the latter is best when administered 24 to 48 hours prior to delivery. When delivery occurs 7 to 14 days after maternal dosing, efficacy is limited, if at all efficacious. Complications associated with RDS include the development of air-leak syndromes (20%–50%) and increased incidence of chronic lung disease. Medical management of RDS may necessitate where indicated use of oxygen therapy, mechanical respiratory support, intravenous fluid and electrolyte therapy, and intratracheal surfactant replacement therapy. The use of exogenous surfactant replacement therapy is associated with decreased mortality, frequency of associated air-leak syndromes, and duration of mechanical ventilation. It has been demonstrated to reverse atelectasis and improve pulmonary functional residual capacity with a resultant improvement in gas exchange patterns, including oxygenation. Surfactant is commonly administered prophylactically to patients less than 29 weeks gestation at high risk for RDS and as rescue treatment in established moderate to severe RDS disease. The differential diagnosis includes TTN, pneumonia, and pleural effusion.

4. A pregnant woman is counseled to have a repeat cesarean section as her pregnancy approaches term. To avoid delivering a newborn who has immature lungs and consequent respiratory distress syndrome, she undergoes antenatal assessment of her amniotic fluid. Of the following, the amniotic fluid test *most* likely to predict fetal lung maturity is:
a) Phosphatidylglycerol
b) Alpha-fetoprotein
c) Surfactant protein A
d) Thyroxine
e) Sphingomyelin

Answer
The answer is a. Produced by type II pneumocytes, pulmonary surfactant is a complex mixture of both phospholipids and associated proteins. Its presence reduces alveolar surface tension, thereby helping maintain alveolar stability at low lung volumes (i.e., prevention of alveolar collapse at the end of expiration). This in turn prevents atelectasis while promoting efficient ventilation and oxygenation. Of its many components (Fig. 21.4), phosphatidylglycerol (PG) is a late-appearing surfactant component; when present in the amniotic fluid, the risk of developing RDS is <0.5%. Another biochemical marker useful in predicting lung maturation and adequacy of lung function at birth is the lecithin:sphingomyelin ratio (L:S ratio). Both lecithin (also known as phosphatidylcholine) and sphingomyelin are phospholipids found in the amniotic fluid. Although sphingomyelin remains at constant levels throughout gestation, lecithin, an active component of surfactant, is found in increasing amounts throughout gestation. The L:S ratio increases from approximately (1:1) at 31 to 32 weeks gestation to (2:1) by 35 weeks gestation. A ratio of greater than (2:1) indicates fetal lung maturity among nearly all nondiabetic pregnancies. For infants born to diabetic mothers (IDMs), an L:S ratio of 2.5:1 or greater is preferred for declaring fetal lung maturity.

5. The treatment of respiratory distress syndrome (RDS) with exogenous administration of surfactant is *most* likely to increase the incidence of:
a) Intraventricular hemorrhage
b) Bronchopulmonary dysplasia
c) Pulmonary hemorrhage
d) Retinopathy of prematurity
e) Pneumothorax

Answer
The answer is c. In infants with RDS, the use of exogenous surfactant replacement therapy has been well demonstrated to have beneficial impact, including reversal

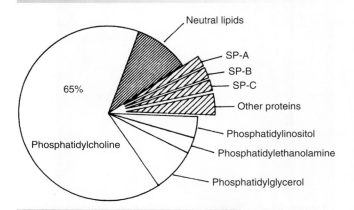

Figure 21.4 Biochemical components of pulmonary surfactant, including lipids and associated proteins.

of atelectasis, increase in functional residual capacity, and improvement in oxygenation. However, its use is not without potential complications. Most adverse effects that occur during intratracheal administration are transient, and include bradycardia, airway obstruction, and oxygen desaturation. Additionally, the clinician must anticipate the resultant hyperoxia, hypocarbia, and risk for development of pulmonary air leaks when reduction of mechanical ventilatory support is not commensurate with favorable pulmonary compliance changes. Likewise, risk for pulmonary hemorrhage may be associated with and without the persistence of a patent ductus arteriosus potentiated by these pulmonary compliance improvements.

6. Before delivery of an infant at 41 weeks gestation, the obstetrician remarks that the amniotic fluid contains thick particulate meconium. As the infant is placed upon the warmer after the delivery, he appears limp and pale with depressed respirations.

Of the following, the *most* important initial step in resuscitation of the infant is to:
a) Determine the infant's APGAR score.
b) Initiate tracheal intubation with suctioning.
c) Provide positive pressure ventilation.
d) Suction the hypopharynx.
e) Aspirate the gastric contents.

Answer

The answer is b. Meconium-stained amniotic fluid (MSAF) is present in 10% to 15% of all births. Although passage of meconium is rare before 37 weeks gestation, its presence in the amniotic fluid is often a warning sign of fetal distress. Meconium aspiration syndrome (MAS), in which fetal aspiration of meconium results in severe respiratory distress and disease occurs in 5% to 15% of neonates born through MSAF (an overall incidence of 2% among all live births), with a mortality rate of 5% to 20%. Meconium, the first intestinal discharge of a neonate, is a sterile mixture of lanugo, vernix, cellular debris, bile acids and pigments, gastric and pancreatic secretions, mucus, and blood. It appears in the fetal ileum at 10 to 16 weeks gestation. In utero meconium passage is associated with antepartum or intrapartum fetal hypoxia, acidosis, or both, leading to increased intestinal peristalsis and rectal sphincter relaxation, resulting in its passage. Associated gasping respiratory efforts of the fetus and laryngeal incompetence lead to aspiration of the MASF into the large and small airways of the lungs. Once aspirated, this meconium can result in obstruction of the airways. This airway obstruction may be either partial or complete. Where partial, this viscous particulate matter leads to air trapping and hyperinflation through a ball-valve effect, increasing the potential for the development of air leaks. If the airway obstruction is complete, the meconium leads to alveolar collapse, atelectasis, and ventilation-perfusion mismatching. Additionally, a chemical pneumonitis develops

with noted leukocyte infiltration, protein leak, bronchiolar edema, and alveolar necrosis. Surfactant inactivation secondary to this protein leak leads to decreased pulmonary compliance with resultant oxygen requirement, hypercarbia, and acidosis. These combined changes may result in pulmonary air leaks in 10% to 30% of affected patients and increased risk for development of hypoxic pulmonary vasoconstriction and pulmonary hypertension (PPHN). Risk factors associated with MAS include:

- Postdate gestation
- Fetal distress
- In utero hypoxia

Medical management of MAS is supportive and may require various ventilation modalities, including HFOV, high concentrations of oxygen, use of inhaled nitric oxide (iNO) as a direct pulmonary vasodilator, intratracheal surfactant administration, and antibiotic treatment. Prevention of MAS may include maternal intrapartum amnioinfusion (which is controversial). *According to Neonatal Resuscitation Program (NRP) 2006 guidelines, when faced with an infant born with meconium-stained amniotic fluid, indication for direct tracheal suctioning is limited to the "nonvigorous" neonate.* A nonvigorous neonate is defined by the presence of depressed respirations, poor muscle tone, and/or a heart rate <100 beats per minute. *Additionally, these guidelines identify initiation of tracheal intubation with suctioning as the initial step in resuscitation of the nonvigorous infant born with meconium-stained amniotic fluid.* Differential diagnoses for MAS include TTN, RDS, and congenital pneumonia.

7. A newborn whose estimated gestational age is 42$^+$ weeks is stained with meconium. Tracheal intubation reveals meconium below the vocal cords. The infant has respiratory distress. A chest radiograph (CXR) is obtained. Of the following, the *most* likely radiographic finding is:
a) Decreased lung volumes
b) Coarse, patchy infiltrates
c) Pleural effusion
d) Reticulogranular pattern
e) Mediastinal shift

Answer

The answer is b. Roentgenographic evaluation of meconium aspiration syndrome demonstrates characteristic patchy pulmonary infiltrates surrounded by areas of hyperinflation (Fig. 21.5); when surfactant inactivation is prominent, initial presentation may include streaky, linear densities or decreased lung volumes with homogenous densities.

8. A 3-hour-old infant delivered at term has respiratory distress. The clinical history is significant for meconium-stained amniotic fluid. CXR shows bilateral diffuse coarse infiltrates. The infant is receiving mechanical

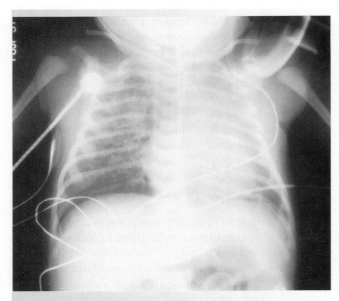

Figure 21.5 Radiograph of an infant with meconium aspiration syndrome. Note the bilateral coarse, patchy infiltrates and areas of hyperinflation.

ventilation with FiO_2 1.0 and a high mean airway pressure. Arterial blood gas (ABG) reveals PaO_2 of 35 mm Hg. Of the following, the manifestation *most* helpful for the diagnosis of persistent pulmonary hypertension of the newborn (PPHN) is:

a) Elevated $PaCO_2$
b) Differential oxygen saturations between right arm and leg
c) Precordial hyperactivity
d) Response to inhaled nitric oxide
e) Tricuspid regurgitation

Answer

The answer is d. Persistent pulmonary hypertension of the newborn (PPHN) is a clinical syndrome with an abnormal persistence of elevated pulmonary vascular resistance (PVR). This persistence of PVR may be as a result of either maladaption or maldevelopment of the pulmonary vascular bed. The incidence of PPHN is approximately 1 in 1000 live births. Its pathophysiology includes failure of the normal decline in PVR expected after birth, leading to a persistence of elevated pulmonary vascular resistance. The elevated PVR is often evidenced on echocardiography by right to left shunting at the atrial level and/or at the ductus arteriosus. The resultant decrease in pulmonary blood flow leads to hypoxemia and development of acidosis. When maladaption of the pulmonary vasculature occurs, the neonate appears to have normal pulmonary vascular anatomy, with a continued persistence of the PVR. Related conditions leading to pulmonary vascular maladaption include:

- Bacterial sepsis
- Perinatal hypoxia/asphyxia
- Pneumonia
- MAS
- Hypothermia
- Postdate gestation

When PPHN results from pulmonary maldevelopment, the pulmonary vascular architecture appears abnormal with excessive muscularization of pulmonary arterioles. Disorders associated with pulmonary maldevelopment include:

- Pulmonary hypoplasia (i.e., congenital diaphragmatic hernia [CDH])
- Intrauterine hypoxia
- Alveolar-capillary dysplasia
- Premature ductus arteriosus closure of the fetus

Clinical presentation typically occurs among term or postdates neonates, usually within the first 24 hours of life. Symptoms include respiratory distress and severe cyanosis. The diagnosis of PPHN is verified by the presence of severe hypoxemia (low PaO_2) on arterial blood sampling. On roentgenographic evaluation, parenchymal lung disease may be identified and oligemic appearing lungs secondary to decreased pulmonary blood flow may be apparent. With the absence of significant shunting at the PFO, the clinician may appreciate pre- and postductal splitting with $\Delta SPaO_2$ >10%. Echocardiography will often demonstrate elevated right-sided cardiac pressures equivalent to systemic levels, tricuspid regurgitation with right to left shunting at the patent ductus arteriosus and leftward-deviation of the interventricular septum.

Medical management of PPHN includes treatment of the underlying suspected cause(s), use of broad-spectrum antibiotics where sepsis is suspected and MAS is present, use of sedation to maximize oxygen saturation and oxygen delivery, and cardiac output support through volume expansion and inotropes. Augmentation of systemic vascular resistance may preferentially drive pulmonary blood flow and circulation through the pulmonary circuit and diminish right to left shunting. Promotion of pulmonary vasodilation may be enhanced through the use of high tension FiO_2 and inhaled nitric oxide (iNO). *When initiation of iNO therapy is indicated, often a rapid and dramatic improvement in arterial oxygenation is appreciated, a characteristic response in many patients with PPHN.* Historical use of either respiratory or metabolic alkalosis to promote pulmonary vasodilatation has fallen into disfavor among clinicians. In the most severe cases, therapeutic rescue with extracorporeal membrane oxygenation, in spite of significant associated morbidities, may prove both lung sparing and life saving in highly selective cases.

9. Newborns who do not demonstrate a difference in the preductal and postductal values for SpO_2 and PaO_2 cannot have PPHN.

a) True
b) False

Answer

The answer is b. Persistent pulmonary hypertension of the newborn (PPHN) is a clinical syndrome with an abnormal persistence of elevated pulmonary vascular resistance (PVR). This persistence of PVR may be as a result of either maladaption or maldevelopment of the pulmonary vascular bed. The incidence of PPHN is approximately 1 in 1000 live births. Its pathophysiology includes failure of the normal decline in PVR expected after birth, leading to a persistence of elevated pulmonary vascular resistance. The elevated PVR is often evidenced on echocardiography by right-to-left shunting at the atrial level and/or at the ductus arteriosus. The resultant decrease in pulmonary blood flow leads to hypoxemia and development of acidosis. When maladaption of the pulmonary vasculature occurs, the neonate appears to have normal pulmonary vascular anatomy, with a continued persistence of the PVR. Related conditions leading to pulmonary vascular maladaption includes:

- Bacterial sepsis
- Perinatal hypoxia/asphyxia
- Pneumonia
- MAS
- Hypothermia
- Postdate gestation

When PPHN results from pulmonary maldevelopment, the pulmonary vascular architecture appears abnormal with excessive muscularization of pulmonary arterioles. Disorders associated with pulmonary maldevelopment include:

- Pulmonary hypoplasia (i.e., congenital diaphragmatic hernia [CDH])
- Intrauterine hypoxia
- Alveolar-capillary dysplasia
- Premature ductus arteriosus closure of the fetus

Clinical presentation typically occurs among term or post-date neonates, usually within the first 24 hours of life. Symptoms include respiratory distress and severe cyanosis. The diagnosis of PPHN is verified by the presence of severe hypoxemia (low PaO_2) on arterial blood sampling. On roentgenographic evaluation, parenchymal lung disease may be identified and oligemic appearing lungs secondary to decreased pulmonary blood flow may be apparent. With the absence of significant shunting at the PFO, the clinician may appreciate pre- and postductal splitting with $\Delta SPaO_2$ >10%. Echocardiography often demonstrates elevated right-sided cardiac pressures equivalent to systemic levels, tricuspid regurgitation with right-to-left shunting at the patent ductus-arteriosus, and leftward deviation of the interventricular septum.

Medical management of PPHN includes treatment of the underlying suspected cause(s), use of broad-spectrum antibiotics in which sepsis is suspected and MAS is present, use of sedation to maximize oxygen saturation and oxygen delivery, and cardiac output support through volume expansion and inotropes. Augmentation of systemic vascular resistance may preferentially drive pulmonary blood flow and circulation through the pulmonary circuit and diminish right to left shunting. Promotion of pulmonary vasodilation may be enhanced through the use of high tension FiO_2 and inhaled nitric oxide (iNO). *When initiation of iNO therapy is indicated, often a rapid and dramatic improvement in arterial oxygenation is appreciated, a characteristic response in many patients with PPHN.* Historical use of either respiratory or metabolic alkalosis to promote pulmonary vasodilatation has fallen in disfavor among clinicians. In the most severe cases, therapeutic rescue with extracorporeal membrane oxygenation, in spite of significant associated morbidities, may prove both lung sparing and life saving in highly selective cases.

10. A neonate born at 38 weeks gestation has tachypnea, expiratory grunting, nasal flaring, subcostal retractions, and cyanosis shortly after birth. The mother had rupture of membranes 36 hours prior to vaginal delivery and has developed uterine tenderness and fever. Of the following, the *most* likely chest radiographic finding in this infant is:
a) Mediastinal displacement
b) Diffuse reticulogranular pattern
c) Lung overinflation with coarse densities
d) Prominent perihilar streaking
e) Fine curvilinear lucencies

Answer

The answer is c. Neonatal pneumonia is suspected in as many as 20% to 60% of stillbirths and liveborn neonatal deaths by autopsy. Causative agents can be acquired in utero, perinatally or postnatally. Transmission of organisms may occur through transplacental passage, aspiration of contaminated amniotic fluid, hematogenous spread, or inhalation. Identified risk factors for neonatal pneumonia include prolonged rupture of membranes, maternal fever, chorioamnionitis, maternal Group B Streptococcus (GBS) *(Streptococcus agalactiae)* colonization, preterm labor, prematurity, and fetal asphyxia.

The causative agent is often related to time of acquisition. In the case of intrauterine acquisition, whether from maternal colonization or infection, a variety of infectious agents may be conferred to the neonate. Associated viral agents include rubella, cytomegalovirus (CMV), varicella zoster virus (VZV), and the human immunodeficiency virus (HIV). Other organisms include the spirochete bacterium *Treponema pallidum*, the parasitic protozoan *Toxoplasma gondii*, and *Listeria monocytogenes*. Perinatal acquisition include *E. coli*, GBS, *Neisseria gonorrhea*, *Chlamydia trachomatis*, and Herpes simplex virus 1 and 2 (HSV). Postnatal acquisition involves the respiratory viruses of adenovirus and human respiratory syncytial virus (RSV), *Staphylococcus aureus*, and gram-negative enteric bacteria such as *Pseudomonas aeruginosa* and *Serratia marcescens*.

Clinical presentation of neonatal pneumonia often includes symptoms of respiratory distress, including increased work of breathing, tachypnea, thoracic retractions, and nasal flaring. Some patients may present with overt episodes of apnea and cyanosis, whereas others present insidiously with temperature instability and occasional oxygen desaturation. Poor feeding and lethargy are additional associated findings. With early-onset disease (<7 days of age), in utero and perinatal acquisition are suspect and include GBS, *E. coli*, *Klebsiella* sp., or *Listeria*. Late-onset disease (≥7 days of age) includes gram-negative enteric bacterial and fungal agents, *Chlamydia trachomatis*, and HSV. Late onset disease often presents as systemic disease. Although the diagnosis of congenital pneumonia can be established through roentgenographic evaluation, abnormal findings on AP films may be delayed for 24 to 72 hours post onset of symptoms. Findings on CXR often include either lung overinflation with coarse densities or may be indistinguishable from RDS, especially in the case of GBS pneumonia (Fig. 21.6). Not surprisingly, the differential diagnoses should include RDS and TTN.

11. The most appropriate initial combination of antibiotics to treat neonatal pneumonia is:
a) Vancomycin and gentamicin
b) Cefotaxime and metronidazole
c) Ampicillin and gentamicin
d) Erythromycin and dicloxacillin
e) Cefaclor monotherapy

Answer
The answer is c. Management of neonatal pneumonia includes the need for varying degrees of respiratory support when indicated, and close cardiorespiratory and SpO₂ monitoring. The laboratory evaluation optimally includes culture and gram-stain testing of blood and tracheal secretions specimens (when feasible). Associated laboratory anomalies include neutropenia or leukocytosis,

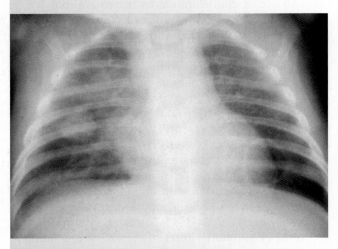

Figure 21.6 Radiograph of an infant with congenital pneumonia. Note the lung overinflation and bilateral coarse densities.

bandemia, thrombocytopenia, and a high C-reactive protein level. Where bacterial infection is suspected, prompt initiation of broad-spectrum antibiotic coverage with ampicillin and either an aminoglycoside or third-generation cephalosporin is reasonable while pending laboratory results. When suspicion for viral or fungal agents is high and associated morbidities even greater, additional consideration for initiation of treatment with antiviral and/or antifungal agents are appropriate.

12. After successful intubation and manual ventilation of a 26-week gestation infant at delivery, the patient is pink and vital signs are stable. His color abruptly turns blue. Breath sounds are diminished on the right, normal on the left, and heart rate rapidly falls. The colorimetric carbon dioxide detector continues to display cyclical color changes. Of the following, which intervention is *most* likely to resolve these findings?
a) Intravenous bolus of normal saline
b) Endotracheal administration of epinephrine
c) Needle thoracotomy
d) Reintubation
e) Surfactant therapy

Answer
The answer is c. Pulmonary air-leak syndromes occur in as many as 2% of term infants. The most common forms include pneumothorax and pneumomediastinum. Other pulmonary air-leak syndromes include pulmonary interstitial emphysema (PIE), pneumopericardium, pneumoperitoneum, and subcutaneous emphysema. The pathophysiology of these conditions involve uneven alveolar ventilation, air trapping, and/or high transpulmonary pressure swings that in turn lead to alveolar overdistension and rupture. Escaping alveolar air subsequently tracks along the root of the lung via perivascular connective tissue sheaths. Accumulated air may be resorbed or may rupture into either pleural spaces (pneumothorax) or mediastinal spaces (pneumomediastinum). Pulmonary air-leak syndromes may additionally result from direct mechanical trauma to the airway, such as from an aberrantly directed suction catheter.

In the case of a pneumothorax, air dissects and leaks into the pleural space within the thorax between visceral and parietal pleural reflections. This occurs spontaneously in 1% to 2% of healthy term births secondary to high transpulmonary pressure swings associated with the first breaths. Often these infants are asymptomatic.

Pulmonary interstitial emphysema (PIE) occurs when air dissects, accumulates, and remains trapped in the lung parenchyma, within pulmonary interstitium, lymphatics, perivascular, or subpleural spaces. PIE is more common among premature infants, usually in those younger than 32 weeks gestation and weighing <1200 g. This condition often occurs within the first 72 hours of life, although it may be observed as a complication of prolonged positive pressure ventilation in the older premature infant. PIE may precede the development of a pneumothorax with rupture of subpleural lymphatic blebs into the pleural space; its presence is associated with an increased mortality rate.

Risk factors associated with the development of pulmonary air-leak syndromes include conditions with:

- Poor lung compliance (i.e., TTN, RDS, MAS, pneumonia, pulmonary hypoplasia, and CDH)
- Asynchronous ventilation
- Use of high ventilatory pressures
- Rapidly improving lung compliance (i.e., postsurfactant administration)

The clinical presentation of a pneumothorax is often dependent upon the effects of trapped air on the degree of lung collapse and cardiovascular compromise. Patients may present with varying degrees of respiratory distress, tachypnea, increased work of breathing, muffled heart sounds, cyanosis, and increased diastolic blood pressures. Often the affected side of the thorax has decreased breath sounds, and anterior-posterior thoracic diameter is increased. When tension pneumothorax is evident, mediastinal shift is often appreciated both on physical exam (i.e., shifted PMI) and CXR (Fig. 21.7). Severe sequela includes acute development of bradycardia with resultant drop in cardiac output, impaired venous return, hypotension, cardiovascular collapse and ensuing systemic hypoxemia and acidosis. Diagnostic evaluation includes physical exam, CXR, and transillumination of the thorax. Depending upon severity and acuity of presentation, treatment may be limited to observation and include the use of "nitrogen washout" (FiO_2 1.00 for 8–12 hours),

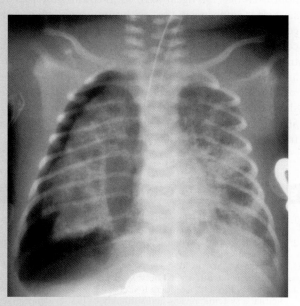

Figure 21.7 Right-sided pneumothorax with extra-pulmonary air and mediastinal shift.

emergent needle-thoracotomy, chest tube insertion, and ventilatory supportive measures.

For PIE, initial presentation may be limited to characteristic radiographic features of small cystic or linear lung parenchymal lucencies, often preceding increasing ventilatory requirements. Management is directed at treatment of the underlying lung disease and reducing the factors associated with barotrauma (high peak inspiratory pressures, positive end-expiratory pressure, and longer inspiratory times).

13. Shortly after birth, a term infant presents with tachypnea, worsening retractions, and persistent cyanosis. The abdomen appears scaphoid. Bag and mask ventilation is initiated. Auscultation reveals decreased breath sounds on the left and heart tones that are louder on the right. The *most* likely explanation for these findings is:
a) Dextrocardia with situs solitus
b) Congenital cystic adenomatoid malformation
c) Esophageal atresia with tracheoesophageal fistula
d) Pneumothorax
e) Diaphragmatic hernia

Answer

The answer is e. Congenital diaphragmatic hernia (CDH) (Fig. 21.8) results from a developmental diaphragmatic defect (persistence of the pleuroperitoneal canal in the posterolateral portion of the diaphragm) that occurs prior to the eighth week of embryonic life. The incidence of CDH is approximately 1 in 2000 to 5000 births. Considered both heterogenous and complex, this birth defect allows for the abdominal viscera to enter the thoracic cavity during fetal development. Ninety-five percent of these defects occur through the posterolateral foramen of Bochdalek. Two-thirds of patients are male, 80% of defects are left-sided, with a recurrence risk in future pregnancies of 2%. Mortality rates are highly variable and range from 25% to 75%. Increased mortality rates are associated with major malformations, liver herniation, greater degree of pulmonary hypoplasia, and presence of PPHN. As many as one third of CDH patients have associated cardiac, renal, GI, limb, and chromosomal abnormalities.

The classic pathophysiologic model of CDH centers around the thoracic displacement of herniated abdominal viscera, leading to lung compression. Resultant development of pulmonary hypoplasia and abnormal lung vasculature in turn relate to subsequent hypoxemia, respiratory failure, and surfactant deficiency. Clinical presentation includes notable respiratory distress that often follows shortly after birth. On physical exam, the abdomen appears scaphoid, a finding characteristic in patients with CDH. Air entry is typically reduced on the affected side of the thorax with heart sounds displaced to the contralateral side; as most defects are left-sided, air entry would be decreased on the left with heart sounds louder on the right.

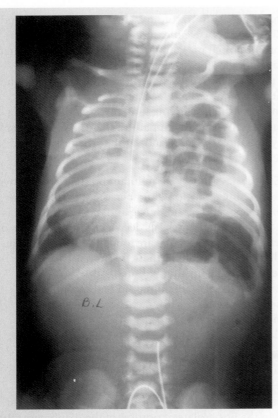

Figure 21.8 An infant with a left-sided congenital diaphragmatic hernia. Note the presence of multiple bowel loops and stomach in the left hemithorax, deviation of the trachea and cardiac silhouette across the midline, and the lack of bowel gas in the abdomen.

14. The *most* appropriate initial treatment for the infant in question 13 is:
a) Increased bag-mask ventilation
b) Extracorporeal membrane oxygenation (ECMO)
c) Intubation and gastric decompression
d) Sodium bicarbonate infusion
e) Immediate surgical repair

Answer

The answer is c. Management and treatment of CDH includes *immediate intubation after birth and initiation of gastric decompression* to prevent intestinal distension, avoiding any exacerbation of worsening cardiovascular compromise. Management approaches are varied and have historically included the use of HFOV, surfactant administration, and iNO therapies. The institution of well-defined treatment guidelines including lung-sparing mechanical ventilation practice strategies, tolerance of postductal acidosis and hypoxemia, predetermined selective criterion for use of ECMO, and elective surgical repair on medically stabilized patients have been employed with improved success and with increased survival rates. Difficulties remain in predicting outcomes for patients diagnosed with CDH. Estimates of fetal lung size to predict outcomes have been used with mixed success, and include use of lung area to head circumference ratio and most recently prenatal lung volumetric MRI studies. Progress continues to be made toward stratifying risk factors as the development of therapies to further improve outcome move forward.

15. All listed conditions are associated with intrinsic airway abnormalities that may lead to airway obstruction *except:*
a) Vascular ring
b) Choanal atresia
c) Beckwith-Wiedemann syndrome
d) Laryngomalacia
e) Pierre-Robin sequence

Answer

The answer is a. A number of conditions may affect the neonatal airway and lead to varying degrees of airway obstruction evident after birth. These congenital airway abnormalities may be divided into either intrinsic or extrinsic components. Abnormalities intrinsic to the airway may affect the nose and nasopharynx, mouth and jaw, tongue, or larynx. Those affecting the nose and nasopharynx include choanal atresia and edema secondary to suctioning. Affecting the mouth and jaw include the Pierre-Robin sequence and mandibular hypoplasia. When the tongue is affected with macroglossia, etiologies include Trisomy 21 and Beckwith-Wiedemann syndrome and when affected by mass-effect includes a thyroglossal duct cyst. Laryngeal involvement includes laryngomalacia, the most common cause of neonatal airway obstruction when inspiratory stridor is a prominent feature; other conditions include epiglottis abnormalities, laryngeal web, vocal cord paralysis/paresis, and laryngospasm (i.e., with symptomatic hypocalcemia). When intrinsic to the trachea and bronchi, conditions include tracheomalacia or bronchomalacia, tracheal, bronchial or subglottic stenosis, tracheal cyst, and congenital lobar emphysema. Conditions with *extrinsic* effects upon the airway include airway compression secondary to thyroid enlargement, vascular ring or aberrant blood vessel(s), hemangioma, cystic hygroma, tracheoesophageal fistula, and mediastinal mass.

SUGGESTED READINGS

1. Burg FD, Ingelfinger, Polin RA, et al. *Gellis and Kagan's current pediatric therapy,* 18th ed. Philadelphia: Saunders, 2006.
2. Chernick V, Boat T, Wilmott R, et al. *Kendig's disorders of the respiratory tract in children,* 7th ed. Philadelphia: Saunders, 2006.
3. Faranoff AA, Martin RJ. *Neonatal-perinatal medicine: diseases of the fetus and infant,* 8th ed. St. Louis: Mosby, 2005.
4. Logan JW, Rice HE, Goldberg RN, et al. Congenital diaphragmatic hernia: a systemic review and summary of best-evidence practice strategies. *J Perinatol* 2007;27:535–549.
5. Spitzer AR. *Intensive care of the fetus and neonate,* 2nd ed. Philadelphia: Elsevier, 2005.

Chapter 22

Neonatal Sepsis and Congenital Infections

Camille Sabella

Approximately 10% of liveborn infants contract an infection in the neonatal period.

In comparison with older children and adults, neonates have less effective neutrophil function and natural killer-cell activity, lower antibody levels, and abnormal T-cell function and cytokine regulation. The relatively immunodeficient state of neonates, together with the increased survival of infants born ever more prematurely, contributes to a high risk for infection.

This chapter discusses three broad categories of neonatal infection:

- Bacterial sepsis
- Viral infections that mimic bacterial sepsis
- Congenital (acquired in utero) infection

NEONATAL BACTERIAL SEPSIS

The overall incidence of neonatal bacterial sepsis is between 1 and 5/1000 live births. Classically, neonatal sepsis has been divided into early-onset and late-onset forms. Infants with *early-onset* sepsis manifest the symptoms within the first 5 days of life, usually have a mother with a history of obstetric complications, and invariably acquire the infection by the vertical transmission of organisms that normally colonize the maternal genital or gastrointestinal tract.

Infants with *late-onset* sepsis manifest the symptoms after day 5 of life. These neonates can be further divided into two distinct groups:

- Healthy term neonates without risk factors for sepsis who present between day 5 of life and 3 months of age, usually with bacteremia and meningitis
- High-risk hospitalized neonates in whom healthcare associated infections develop

The risk factors for bacterial sepsis associated with pregnancy and delivery include:

- Prematurity and a low birth weight
- Prolonged interval after rupture of the membranes (>18 hours)
- Maternal peripartum fever
- Depressed respiratory function at birth

Certain risk factors are associated with an intensive care environment, including the following:

- Mechanical ventilation
- Surgical/invasive procedures
- Indwelling catheters
- Total parenteral nutrition
- Widespread use of broad-spectrum antimicrobial agents
- H2 blockers

Premature, low-birth-weight infants are at the highest risk for infection; the incidence of early-onset sepsis is 4- to 25-fold higher in these infants than in full-term infants with a normal birth weight. The incidence of late-onset sepsis is also higher in premature infants because they are at risk for hospital-acquired infection.

Bacteriology of Neonatal Sepsis

The most common causes of early-onset neonatal sepsis in the United States are as follows:

- Group B streptococci
- *Escherichia coli*
- *Listeria monocytogenes*

Although traditionally group B streptococci accounted for most cases of early-onset sepsis, there has been a recent decline in the incidence of early-onset neonatal group B streptococcal infection. This decline is a result of the successful implementation of routine maternal screening for, and maternal intrapartum antimicrobial prophylaxis against, this organism. Therefore, *E. coli* is now likely the most common cause of early-onset sepsis in this country. Other, less common pathogens include viridans streptococci and nontypeable *Haemophilus influenzae*.

Group B streptococci and *L. monocytogenes* remain important causes of late-onset neonatal sepsis in previously healthy infants. In high-risk neonates who are hospitalized, the most important causes of late-onset sepsis, in decreasing order of relative frequency, are as follows:

■ Coagulase-negative staphylococci
■ Gram-negative bacilli (*E. coli, Klebsiella* spp., *Enterobacter* spp.)
■ Candida species
■ *Staphylococcus aureus*
■ Enterococci

Coagulase-negative staphylococci are the most common cause of late-onset neonatal sepsis in hospitalized high-risk neonates, accounting for almost 50% of hospital-acquired infections in neonatal intensive care settings.

Clinical Manifestations

The clinical features of neonatal sepsis are subtle and nonspecific. Respiratory distress, lethargy, an unstable temperature, apnea, jaundice, feeding intolerance, and tachycardia are common. Regardless of the specific pathogen causing the sepsis, the clinical manifestations are similar and also do not differ from those of noninfectious illnesses in neonates. Finally, it is important to remember that the characteristics of neonatal meningitis are indistinguishable from those of sepsis. The specific epidemiologic and clinical features of disease caused by the most common pathogens are discussed in the subsequent text.

Group B Streptococci

Group B streptococci are important causes of both early- and late-onset sepsis, with an incidence of 0.3/1000 live births for each. These organisms are frequent inhabitants of the maternal genital and gastrointestinal tracts; 15% to 40% of all pregnant women are colonized with group B streptococci. This colonization may be constant or intermittent, and the presence of colonization in a pregnant woman in one pregnancy does not predict colonization in another pregnancy. Although 50% to 70% of mothers in whom organisms are colonized transmit the organisms to their infants if intrapartum antimicrobial prophylaxis is not given, early-onset group B streptococcal sepsis develops in only 1% to 2% of the colonized infants. The risk increases dramatically in infants with any high-risk gestational factors, which include:

■ Prematurity (Increased sevenfold for babies with birth weight <2500 g and gestation <37 weeks)
■ Prolonged rupture of membranes (>18 h)
■ Chorioamnionitis/maternal fever
■ Group B streptococcal bacteriuria

■ Previous Group B Streptococcal–infected infant
■ Deficiency of transplacentally acquired serotype specific Group B Streptococcal capsular polysaccharide serum antibody

The most common manifestations of early-onset group B streptococcal sepsis are pneumonia and apnea, and they usually occur within the first 24 hours of life. Septic shock occurs in 25% of affected infants, and meningitis in 5% to 10%. The radiographic appearance of group B streptococcal pneumonia is indistinguishable from that of respiratory distress syndrome or other infections. The case fatality rate for early-onset group B streptococcal sepsis is 10% to 15%.

Late-onset group B streptococcal sepsis usually affects term infants between 1 and 12 weeks of age who have had an unremarkable early neonatal history. Bacteremia and purulent meningitis are the most common features, although focal infections such as osteomyelitis and adenitis can also occur. The case fatality rate is 2% to 6%; however, long-term neurologic sequelae develop in 25% to 50% of the survivors of group B streptococcal meningitis.

Escherichia coli

The incidence of neonatal sepsis caused by *E. coli* is approximately 1/1000 live births. Most of these infants present within the first few days of life. The K1 capsular antigen of the organism is associated with neonatal infection, and the antigen is detected in 80% of the cases of meningitis.

Vertical transmission appears to be the major route by which infants acquire the organism. *Infants with galactosemia are particularly susceptible to* E. coli *infection.*

The clinical features of sepsis and meningitis caused by *E. coli* are similar to those of infections caused by group B streptococci and other pathogens. It should be pointed out that gram-negative neonatal meningitis is associated with a higher incidence of brain abscess. Therefore, the cerebrospinal fluid (CSF) of an infant (that has not been sterilized with appropriate antibiotics) with gram-negative meningitis should prompt a search for a brain abscess. *A gram-negative organism that causes neonatal meningitis,* Citrobacter koseri *(formerly diversus), is strongly associated with the development of brain abscess.* The case fatality rate for sepsis and meningitis caused by *E. coli* is 15% to 25%, but significant neurologic sequelae develop in 30% to 50% of survivors.

Listeria monocytogenes

L. monocytogenes is a gram-positive bacillus that is rarely associated with sporadic neonatal sepsis, but it has been associated with several food-borne outbreaks of perinatal disease that have resulted in substantial morbidity and mortality.

As in group B streptococcal infection, early- and late-onset neonatal diseases have been described. The incidence of prematurity and gestational complications is relatively high in infants with early-onset disease. Most, but not all, mothers of these infants have experienced an influenza-like illness, representing maternal listeriosis, during the third trimester of pregnancy. Late-onset infection affects full-term neonates of uncomplicated pregnancies.

Pneumonia, septicemia, and meningitis are the most common features of early-onset disease. An erythematous rash, characterized by widespread granulomatous lesions of the skin and other organs, may accompany severe disease, and is termed *granulomatosis infantisepticum. The blood monocyte count is elevated in approximately 50% of infected infants.*

Infants with late-onset infection typically present with bacteremia and meningitis. They may present anytime between the first and eighth weeks of life. CSF characteristics of infants with meningitis include a polymorphonuclear *(not mononuclear)* leukocytosis with an elevated protein level; 60% of infants have a normal CSF glucose level.

The mortality rate for early-onset listeriosis is approximately 25%, whereas that for late-onset disease is approximately 5%.

Diagnosis

The isolation of an organism from the blood or CSF provides definitive evidence of bacterial sepsis. The utility of rapid diagnostic tests such as latex particle agglutination to detect group B streptococcal and *E. coli* infections is limited by poor sensitivity and specificity. Because 25% to 30% of neonates with bacterial sepsis also have meningitis, a lumbar puncture should be performed whenever sepsis is documented. Even in the absence of a blood culture that is positive for bacteria, examination of the CSF should be strongly considered whenever sepsis is suspected because the blood cultures of 10% to 15% of neonates with meningitis are negative for the bacteria. The hematologic findings associated with neonatal sepsis include an elevated ratio of immature neutrophils to total neutrophils (>0.2), neutropenia, an elevated total neutrophil count, and thrombocytopenia.

Therapy

Antimicrobial therapy for early-onset neonatal sepsis must include coverage for group B streptococci, *E. coli*, and *L. monocytogenes*. Administration of ampicillin/gentamicin provides such coverage. Although gentamicin has no activity against group B streptococci and *L. monocytogenes*, when it is administered with penicillin, the combination is synergistic.

Antimicrobial coverage for late-onset infection acquired in the neonatal intensive care nursery setting usually includes a combination of oxacillin or vancomycin to provide coverage against gram-positive organisms, including coagulase-negative staphylococci, and an aminoglycoside or third-

generation cephalosporin to provide broad gram-negative coverage. Once the organism has been recovered and sensitivity results are available, the regimen can be re-evaluated.

Initial antimicrobial therapy for an infant with late-onset sepsis or meningitis that has not been acquired nosocomially usually includes a combination of ampicillin and an aminoglycoside or third-generation cephalosporin, such as cefotaxime. *Ampicillin is required in this situation to cover the possibility of* L. monocytogenes *infection, against which cephalosporins have no activity.*

Prevention

Most preventive efforts are focused on group B streptococci infection. Currently, group B streptococcal screening with vaginal and rectal cultures is recommended for all pregnant women at 35 to 37 weeks' gestation, with the exception of mothers who have had group B streptococcal bacteriuria during the current pregnancy or those having had a previous infant with group B streptococcal disease. Mothers who are shown to be carriers of group B streptococci during the current pregnancy should receive intrapartum prophylaxis, unless a planned cesarean delivery is performed in the absence of labor or membrane rupture. Maternal intrapartum antimicrobial prophylaxis is also indicated for mothers with:

- Group B streptococcal bacteriuria during current pregnancy
- Previous infant with group B streptococcal disease

If the group B streptococcal status of the mother is unknown at the time of delivery, maternal intrapartum prophylaxis is indicated if any of the following are present:

- Delivery at less than 37 weeks gestation
- Membranes ruptured for 18 hours or longer
- Intrapartum fever (temperature ≥38°C [100.4°F])

VIRAL SEPSIS

Important viral agents acquired at birth (natal infection) or after birth but during the neonatal period (postnatal infection) that may mimic bacterial neonatal sepsis include:

- Herpes simplex virus (HSV)
- Enteroviruses
- Cytomegalovirus (CMV)

Herpes Simplex Virus

Neonatal HSV infection is the most feared consequence of gestational genital HSV infection. Because HSV infection closely mimics bacterial sepsis, a delayed diagnosis is common, and despite the availability of antiviral therapy, the associated mortality and morbidity remain high.

Most neonates acquire the virus from an infected maternal genital tract at the time of delivery. HSV 2 accounts for most cases of neonatal HSV infection; approximately 30% of the cases are caused by HSV 1. Viral transmission can follow either primary or recurrent maternal infection. The transmission rate during primary maternal infection is estimated to be 35% to 50%, but 3% to 5% during recurrent maternal infection. The higher rates are likely the consequence of a high viral titer, involvement of the cervix, and the lack of transplacental antibody in the primary maternal infection. *Most neonates with HSV infection are born to asymptomatic mothers with no past history of genital HSV infection.* This finding is explained by the high prevalence of "silent" maternal genital HSV infection.

There are three clinical forms of neonatal HSV infection (Table 22.1):

■ Disseminated disease
■ Central nervous system (CNS) disease
■ Localized disease involving the skin, eyes, and/or oral mucosa (SEM)

Infants with *disseminated disease* usually present during the first 2 weeks of life with nonspecific symptoms. Irritability, apnea, poor feeding, unstable temperature, jaundice, hepatosplenomegaly, disseminated intravascular coagulation, hepatic failure, seizures, and shock are common features. A vesicular rash occurs in about 60% of the cases but is often absent at the time of presentation. Seizures occur in 22% of patients with disseminated disease. Even with appropriate antiviral therapy, the mortality rate associated with this form of HSV infection is 30%.

Neonates with disease localized to the *CNS* most commonly present between the second and third weeks of life, usually with lethargy, fever, and seizures. CSF pleocytosis with an elevated CSF protein is the rule. Approximately 65% of these infants have skin vesicles at any time during the course of the disease. It is important to remember that neonatal HSV causes *diffuse* encephalitis, without localization to the temporal lobes, unlike HSV encephalitis beyond the neonatal period. The mortality rate for this form

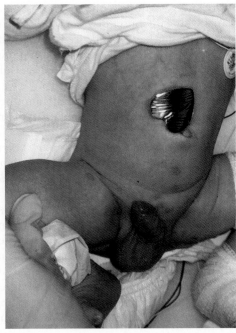

Figure 22.1 A neonate with multiple vesicular lesions on the abdomen and perineum. Results of direct fluorescent antibody testing and viral culture of the vesicular fluid were positive for herpes simplex virus type 1. (See color insert.)

of disease is 5%, but at least two thirds of the survivors have long-term neurologic sequelae.

Neonates with HSV disease *localized to the SEM* usually present between 1 and 2 weeks after birth with vesicular lesions, forming singly or in clusters, on an erythematous base (Fig. 22.1). Ocular involvement, in the form of keratitis, conjunctivitis, or chorioretinitis, occurs in 10% to 15% of these infants. Patients with SEM disease have the best prognosis; infants treated early in the course with antiviral agents uniformly survive. However, cutaneous lesions may recur in 10% to 15% of treated infants during the first year of life, and they are at risk for long-term neurologic sequelae. If SEM disease is not treated, it progresses to the disseminated and CNS form.

TABLE 22.1

CLINICAL FEATURES OF THE THREE MAJOR FORMS OF NEONATAL HERPES SIMPLEX VIRUS INFECTION

	Disseminated	Central Nervous System Disease	Localized Skin, Eye, Oral Mucosal Disease
Relative frequency	25%	30%	45%
Average age at presentation (days)	7–12	16–19	7–12
Major clinical features	Apnea, irritability, coagulopathy, shock, hepatic failure, seizures/encephalitis	Fever, seizures, lethargy, diffuse encephalitis	Vesicular lesions of skin and oral mucosa, ocular involvement
Frequency of vesicular lesions	58%	63%	83%
Mortality rate with antiviral therapy	30%	5%	0%

The diagnosis of neonatal HSV infection is difficult, especially in the absence of vesicular lesions. Therefore, a high index of clinical suspicion is warranted in any neonate in whom sepsis is suspected, especially in the setting of negative bacterial cultures. Viral culture is the most reliable method of making the diagnosis. The virus can be isolated from cutaneous lesions or from the nasopharynx, CSF, conjunctivae, or maternal genital tract. When vesicular lesions are present, a direct fluorescent antibody test can provide a rapid diagnosis. Polymerase chain reaction testing for HSV DNA in the CSF is sensitive and is the diagnostic method of choice for establishing CNS disease.

Parenteral *acyclovir* is the antiviral agent of choice in the treatment of neonatal HSV infection. The currently recommended dosage of acyclovir is 60 mg/kg per day given in three divided doses. The duration of the therapy is 14 days for SEM disease and 21 days for disseminated or CNS disease. Neonates treated with this dosage of acyclovir should be monitored closely for the development of *neutropenia*. It must be stressed that despite appropriate and timely antiviral therapy, the mortality and morbidity rates associated with these infections remain high.

Enteroviruses

Nonpolio enteroviruses are a common cause of benign febrile infections in older infants and children but have the potential to cause more severe infections in neonates. These viruses are transmitted by the fecal–oral and oral–oral routes, and newborns most commonly acquire them during the birth process. In temperate climates, enteroviral diseases are most common in the summer and fall. Echoviruses 9, 11, 30, and Coxsackie virus B are the most common causes of enteroviral neonatal disease.

Most neonatal enteroviral infections are mild and cause nonspecific symptoms. However, 20% of infections are severe and life threatening, and these occur in neonates who acquire the infection without the maternal antibody. Fever, feeding intolerance, abdominal distension, and irritability are the common presenting features. Diarrhea, vomiting, shock, disseminated intravascular coagulation, hepatomegaly, jaundice, and apnea may follow. A rash is present in 40% of the infants; macular and maculopapular rashes are most common, but petechial and vesicular exanthems have also been described. Hepatitis, hepatic necrosis, myocarditis (especially with coxsackievirus B), and meningoencephalitis may be evident.

Distinguishing the enteroviral illness from HSV infections and bacterial sepsis is difficult. The following features are more *suggestive* of an enteroviral infection:

- Recent maternal history of a febrile illness and abdominal pain
- Lack of obstetric complications
- Illness in the summer or fall
- Presence of myocarditis or hepatitis

Isolation of the virus from the nasopharynx, throat, stool, rectal swab, blood, urine, or CSF confirms the diagnosis. Polymerase chain reaction assays for the presence of enterovirus RNA on CSF is more sensitive than the viral culture in infants with meningoencephalitis. The management of these infants relies on meticulous intensive care. A neonate with myocarditis, encephalitis, or hepatic involvement has a poor prognosis.

Cytomegalovirus

CMV infections that are acquired perinatally or postnatally (breast-feeding, blood transfusions) occasionally result in a sepsis-like syndrome. Most term healthy infants who acquire this virus at or shortly after birth are asymptomatic. However, in full-term infants who are ill and in premature infants, a syndrome may develop that is manifested by a gray pallor, septic appearance, hepatosplenomegaly, neutropenia, lymphocytosis, and hemolytic anemia. Low-birth-weight infants born to CMV-negative mothers who receive blood transfusions from one or more seropositive donors are at highest risk for this syndrome. Infection can be prevented by using only CMV-seronegative donor blood; acquisition of the virus is thereby eliminated.

CONGENITAL (INTRAUTERINE) INFECTIONS

Intrauterine infections can result in resorption of the embryo, abortion, stillbirth, premature delivery, fetal malformation and growth retardation, asymptomatic infection, and chronic postnatal infection. These infections may be apparent at or shortly after birth, or they may present months to years later. The clinical manifestations of the intrauterine infections are listed in Table 22.2. It is important to remember that different agents may cause similar clinical features. However, infections with certain microorganisms are *more likely* to result in specific congenital anomalies (Table 22.3).

Cytomegalovirus Infection

CMV infection is the *most common* congenital infection, affecting approximately 1% of all newborns in the United States. It can be acquired by the fetus during either a primary or recurrent maternal CMV infection. The risk of infection to the fetus during a primary CMV infection of a nonimmune mother is approximately 40%; the risk is 1% for the fetus of a seroimmune mother. The risk for symptomatic infection is greater after a primary CMV infection than after a recurrent maternal CMV infection.

Most infants (90%) with congenital CMV infection are *asymptomatic* at birth. Nevertheless, up to 20% of these infants are at risk for long-term neurologic developmental

TABLE 22.2

CLINICAL MANIFESTATIONS OF CONGENITAL INFECTION

Jaundice
Hepatosplenomegaly
Hematologic manifestations
   Thrombocytopenia
   Anemia
Exanthems
   Petechiae
   Purpura
Central nervous system manifestations
   Microcephaly
   Hydrocephalus
   Intracranial calcifications
   Meningoencephalitis
   Sensorineural hearing loss
Eye manifestations
   Chorioretinitis
   Cataracts
   Microphthalmia
Bone lesions
Adenopathy
Pneumonitis
Cardiac anomalies

abnormalities, such as sensorineural hearing loss, mental retardation, motor defects, and chorioretinitis.

The most common manifestations of symptomatic CMV infection in infants are listed in Table 22.4. Approximately half of the 10% of infants who are sympto-

TABLE 22.3

SPECIFIC CONGENITAL MANIFESTATIONS WITH MOST LIKELY RESPONSIBLE INFECTION(S)

Congenital Manifestation	Most Likely Infectious Agent
Adenopathy	Treponema *pallidum*
	Rubella virus and Toxoplasma *gondii* (less likely)
Maculopapular exanthem	*T. pallidum*
	Enterovirus (perinatally acquired)
Bone lesions	Rubella virus
	T. pallidum
Congenital heart defects	Rubella virus
Intracranial calcifications	*T. gondii* (parenchymal calcifications)
	Cytomegalovirus (periventricular calcifications)
Focal chorioretinitis	*T. gondii*
	Cytomegalovirus
Salt and pepper retinitis	Rubella virus
	T. pallidum
Cataracts	Rubella virus
	T. gondii (less likely)

TABLE 22.4

COMMON MANIFESTATIONS OF SYMPTOMATIC CONGENITAL CYTOMEGALOVIRUS INFECTION

Petechiae
Jaundice
Hepatosplenomegaly
Microcephaly
Small-for-gestational-age
Prematurity
Inguinal hernia
Chorioretinitis

In decreasing order of frequency.

matic present with typical generalized *cytomegalic inclusion disease*, characterized by intrauterine growth retardation, hepatosplenomegaly, jaundice, thrombocytopenia, petechiae, microcephaly, and chorioretinitis. The presentations of the other half of the symptomatic infants are milder or atypical.

Although chorioretinitis occurs less frequently in congenital CMV infection than in congenital toxoplasmosis, the retinal lesions of the two conditions cannot be distinguished at birth by location or appearance. However, unlike the chorioretinitis associated with congenital *Toxoplasma* infection, which is associated with congenital CMV, infection rarely progresses or becomes reactivated postnatally. *In the classic description of cerebral calcifications in congenital CMV infection, the lesions have a periventricular distribution, whereas the distribution is more parenchymal in congenital toxoplasmosis* (Fig. 22.2).

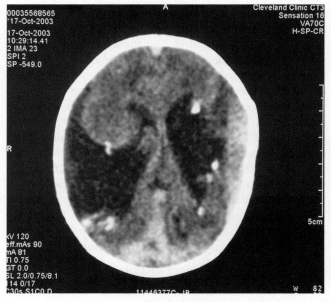

Figure 22.2 A neonate born with large porencephalic cyst and periventricular calcifications. Urine culture at birth grew cytomegalovirus.

Common laboratory abnormalities in neonates with symptomatic CMV include:

- Elevated levels of transaminases
- Thrombocytopenia
- Conjugated hyperbilirubinemia
- Hemolysis
- Increased CSF protein levels

Congenital CMV infection is diagnosed by isolating the virus from the urine. The virus is readily excreted in the urine of congenitally infected neonates, and its isolation in the first 2 to 3 weeks of life provides definitive evidence of congenital infection. CMV-specific immunoglobulin G (IgG) is an indicator of maternal infection but it does not distinguish the congenital infection from a previous one. The sensitivity and specificity of the tests for CMV-specific IgM are poor, and the tests are not reliable in confirming or ruling out a diagnosis of congenital CMV infection.

The mortality rate associated with symptomatic CMV infection is 10% to 15%, but the mortality rate of infants born with cytomegalic inclusion disease approaches 30%. Most surviving infants with symptomatic CMV disease have long-term permanent sequelae, including visual defects, hearing loss, motor and intellectual retardation, and seizure disorders. Although all infants born with asymptomatic CMV infection survive, it is important to remember that hearing loss and intellectual problems eventually develop in up to 10% of these children.

Rubella

Almost all cases of congenital rubella are the consequence of a maternal *primary* rubella. Congenital rubella remains a significant problem in populations that are not adequately immunized against rubella. The overall risk for fetal infection during the primary maternal infection is approximately 20%; however, the risk is at least 70% when the maternal infection occurs in the first trimester.

Sixty percent of infants born with congenital rubella are asymptomatic at birth. However, because this virus causes a silent and progressive infection, neurologic and other permanent sequelae often become evident with time. The clinical manifestations of congenital rubella can be classified as transient, permanent, and developmental (late in onset):

- *Transient manifestations* usually clear spontaneously within days to weeks. They include hepatosplenomegaly, hepatitis, jaundice, thrombocytopenia, "blueberry muffin" lesions (sites of dermal erythropoiesis), hemolytic anemia, adenopathy, rash, meningoencephalitis, and bony radiolucencies. These infants are usually affected by severe intrauterine growth retardation.
- *Permanent manifestations* include abnormalities of the heart, eyes, and CNS and deafness. Congenital heart disease occurs in more than 50% of infants infected during

the first trimester. *The most common lesions are patent ductus arteriosus, pulmonary artery stenosis, and pulmonary valvular stenosis.* Retinopathy and cataracts are the most common ocular abnormalities. The retinopathy is in a "salt and pepper" distribution (unlike that associated with CMV and *Toxoplasma* congenital infections), and cataracts (bilateral in half of the cases) are present in approximately one third of the cases. Microcephaly, mental and motor retardation, and encephalitis are possible CNS manifestations. Deafness is probably the most common manifestation of congenital rubella syndrome, occurring in approximately 80% of those infected.

- *Developmental* and late-onset manifestations may not be identified for years after birth, and include insulin-dependent diabetes mellitus, thyroid dysfunction, and late-onset ocular and auditory defects. In addition, some of the "permanent" manifestations, especially intellectual and behavioral manifestations, may become apparent with time and also progress.

Rubella virus can be cultured from the urine, CSF, or nasopharynx when the diagnosis is suspected. The virus is shed from these sites for 1 year or longer. Rubella-specific IgG and IgM antibody titers in neonatal serum are also helpful in establishing the diagnosis.

Toxoplasmosis

Toxoplasma gondii is a coccidian protozoan that can be transmitted to a fetus when the mother becomes infected during gestation. The incidence of a congenital infection varies by geographic location; in the United States, it is 1 in 1000 to 8000 live births. The organism is acquired by the ingestion of food containing cysts or by the exposure to oocytes excreted by cats. Undercooked pork, beef, and lamb serve as important sources of infection. Oocytes are ingested with the material contaminated by feces of severely infected cats.

Congenital infection occurs when a pregnant mother is severely infected with the organism (primary infection). The risk for transmission to the fetus depends on the timing of the maternal infection. If the mother is not treated, the risk is approximately 15% when the infection occurs in the first trimester, but approaches 60% if the infection is acquired during the third trimester. However, the manifestations are severe in most cases when the fetus becomes infected in the first trimester, whereas they are mild or inapparent when the fetus becomes infected during the third trimester.

Infants with congenital toxoplasmosis may present with severe neonatal disease, or signs of reactivated infection may develop at any time during infancy or later. The classic triad of congenital *Toxoplasma* infection includes:

- Chorioretinitis
- Hydrocephalus
- Cerebral calcifications

The cerebral calcifications associated with congenital toxoplasmosis develop throughout the brain, whereas a periventricular pattern is seen in congenital CMV infection. Other manifestations in the early neonatal period include a small-for-gestational-age, prematurity, retinal scarring, hepatomegaly, thrombocytopenia, and jaundice. *Although the majority of infants with Toxoplasma infections are asymptomatic at birth, 80% of these infant will develop neurologic or ocular manifestations later in life.* The chorioretinitis is a *focal* necrotizing retinitis that can be recurrent and progressive, and may develop later in life without any other manifestations of *Toxoplasma* infection.

Prenatal diagnosis of *Toxoplasma* infection is possible through the isolation of *Toxoplasma* DNA in amniotic fluid or fetal blood, by the isolation of the parasite by mouse inoculation or tissue culture, or by finding increased size of lateral ventricles via serial fetal ultrasonography.

Postnatal diagnosis of a congenital *Toxoplasma* infection most frequently relies on serologic assays on the infant and mother. Persistent or rising IgG antibody titers in an infant, or positive results of specific IgM or IgA assays help establish the diagnosis. Other helpful modalities in the diagnosis of congenital *toxoplasma* include nucleic acid assays on the amniotic fluid, blood and CSF of the infant, histopathology of the placenta or infected organ/tissue, or by mouse inoculation assays of the infant's blood, placenta, or umbilical cord.

Infants suspected of having congenital toxoplasma infection should have a careful clinical evaluation, computed tomography of the brain, a retinal examination by an ophthalmologist, as well as specific serologic testing of the serum and CSF.

All infected infants, whether they manifest signs of infection, should be treated with a combination of *pyrimethamine and sulfadiazine.* Therapy is continued for 1 year. The early institution of a specific therapy decreases the severity of the disease and the frequency of sequelae. The prognosis is variable depending on the degree of involvement, promptness of therapy, and presence of comorbid factors.

Spiramycin therapy is used during pregnancy to decrease transmission from mother to fetus. Pyrimethamine and sulfadiazine are utilized in pregnant mothers if fetal infection is confirmed after 17 weeks gestation.

Congenital Syphilis

Treponema pallidum, the causative agent of syphilis, belongs to the family Spirochaetaceae. Untreated syphilis in pregnant women can result in congenital syphilis. The incidence of congenital syphilis increased dramatically in the late 1980s and early 1990s, along with the rate of infection among young women of childbearing age. This resurgence was likely the consequence of an increase in illegal drug use and the exchange of sex for drugs, and also of the concomitant epidemic of the human immunodeficiency virus

infection. However, the rates of congenital syphilis have declined steadily since 1990, to the lowest recorded levels by 1998.

Congenital infection usually represents transplacental infection of the fetus, although the infection may be acquired at the time of delivery. The infection is more readily transmitted from the pregnant mother to the fetus if the mother is in the early stages of untreated infection. Therefore, mothers with primary or secondary syphilis are significantly more likely to transmit the infection (60%–90%) than mothers with early latent (40%) or late latent (<10%) syphilis.

Congenital infection results in perinatal death in 30% to 40% of infected fetuses; most of these infants are stillborn. Most liveborn infants are asymptomatic at birth. Without specific therapy, symptoms develop in many of them within the neonatal period and beyond. Because congenital syphilis is a consequence of hematogenous dissemination of the organism, the clinical features are similar to those of secondary syphilis. The manifestations of congenital syphilis can be divided into "early" and "late" features.

Early features (Table 22.5) appear during the first 2 years of life, often within the first 3 months. These include mucocutaneous manifestations such as snuffles (syphilitic rhinitis) and a desquamating maculopapular rash, especially on the palms, soles, mouth, and anus. Vesiculobullous lesions *(pemphigus syphiliticus)*, which may rupture and leave a macerated appearance, may be present and are unique to congenital syphilis. Abnormalities of the long bones, including periostitis and osteochondritis (Fig. 22.3), are among the most common features of congenital syphilis, present in 90% of symptomatic and 20% of asymptomatic infants. The neurologic involvement may be subclinical, and examination of the CSF may show a pleocytosis, elevated protein level, or reaginic antibody.

TABLE 22.5

***EARLY* MANIFESTATIONS OF CONGENITAL SYPHILIS**

Mucocutaneous manifestations
    Syphilitic rhinitis (snuffles)
    Maculopapular desquamating rash
    Vesicular or bullous rash (Pemphigus *syphiliticus*)
Bony abnormalities
    Periostitis
    Osteochondritis
    Osteomyelitis
Hepatosplenomegaly
Lymphadenopathy
Thrombocytopenia
Coombs-negative hemolytic anemia
Jaundice
Meningoencephalitis
Pneumonitis
Glomerulonephritis

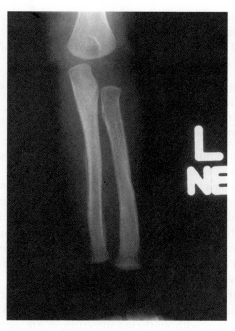

Figure 22.3 Radiograph of the arm in an infant with congenital syphilis. Transverse lucent bands are evident in the metaphyses of the distal radius and ulna. Periosteal new bone can be visualized in the ulnar diaphysis and metaphysis.

Hepatosplenomegaly, lymphadenopathy, and less commonly pneumonia (Fig. 22.4) are some other early manifestations of congenital syphilis.

Late manifestations (Table 22.6) of congenital syphilis appear after 2 years of age and represent latent infection. Interstitial keratitis, deafness, dental anomalies, neurosyphilis, and skeletal abnormalities are the major features. The triad of incisor defects, interstitial keratitis, and deafness is referred to as the Hutchinson triad.

Because of the silent nature and severe long-term sequelae of untreated congenital syphilis, all pregnant mothers undergo serologic testing in early pregnancy and at delivery.

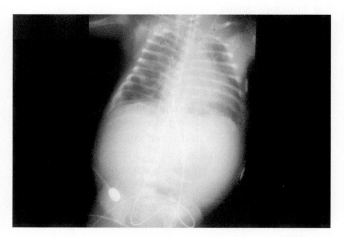

Figure 22.4 Chest and abdominal radiograph of an infant with congenital syphilis showing bilateral pulmonary infiltrates and hepatosplenomegaly.

TABLE 22.6
LATE MANIFESTATIONS OF CONGENITAL SYPHILIS

Skeletal abnormalities
   Frontal bossing
   Anterior bowing of midsection of tibia
Neurosyphilis
Deafness
Ocular abnormalities
   Interstitial keratitis
   Retinitis
   Optic atrophy
Dental anomalies
   Peg-shaped upper central incisors (Hutchinson teeth)
   Abnormal enamel
   Mulberry molars

Mothers at high risk for infection should also be tested at the beginning of the third trimester. It is imperative that no newborn leave the hospital without verification of the maternal serologic status.

Nontreponemal serologic tests include the venereal disease research laboratory (VDRL) slide test and the rapid plasma reagin (RPR) card test. These detect the presence of nonspecific lipoidal antigens, and they provide sensitive tools for the detection of treponemal antibodies and quantitative markers of disease activity. The results of nontreponemal tests must be confirmed by more specific treponemal antibody tests, such as the fluorescent treponemal antibody absorption (FTA-ABS) test.

Congenital syphilis is difficult to diagnose. Many infected infants are asymptomatic, and positive results of the serologic tests in an infant do not distinguish between the maternal and congenital infections because the antibodies are transferred passively. A positive result of the nontreponemal antibody test in an infant that does not disappear by 6 months of age, a rising antibody titer after birth, or a titer in an infant that is fourfold higher than the mother's titer are all highly suggestive of congenital infection. In addition, a mother who is infected late in pregnancy may transmit the infection to the newborn without herself having positive serologies.

Any infant born to a mother with a positive nontreponemal test result that is confirmed by treponemal testing, and any infant with clinical evidence of congenital syphilis, must be evaluated fully for the infection. An evaluation for congenital syphilis should include:

- Physical examination
- Quantitative nontreponemal and treponemal testing of the infant's serum (umbilical cord blood not reliable)
- Determination of antitreponemal IgM antibody if available
- CSF VDRL test, cell count, and protein levels
- Radiography of the long bones
- Complete blood cell count and platelet count

■ Chest radiography and liver function tests if clinically indicated

Infants should be treated for congenital syphilis if they have a proven or probable disease. In general, any infant who warrants evaluation for congenital syphilis should be treated if the test results do not rule out infection, the infant cannot be fully evaluated, or follow-up cannot be ensured. Infants born to mothers who are infected but have not been treated, have been treated inadequately, have been treated within 1 month of delivery, or have not demonstrated a fourfold decrease in the titer of nontreponemal antibody also require treatment. CSF features of neurosyphilis include an increased protein concentration, pleocytosis, and a positive result for CSF VDRL test. However, a negative result CSF VDRL test does not rule out congenital neurosyphilis.

For neonates with proven or presumptive congenital syphilis, aqueous crystalline penicillin G for 10 to 14 days is the preferred therapy. Alternatively, procaine penicillin G can be used, although adequate CSF concentrations may not be achieved with this regimen. The treatment given for infants who are asymptomatic, who appear normal on evaluation, and whose follow-up can be ensured but whose mothers have not been treated, or have been treated inadequately, or have been treated within 1 month of delivery, or have not demonstrated a fourfold decrease in antibody titer is controversial. Many experts recommend treating these infants with aqueous penicillin G for 10 to 14 days, whereas others recommend treating them with a single dose of benzathine penicillin.

Infants treated for congenital syphilis should undergo careful evaluation at 1, 2, 3, 6, and 12 months of age. Nontreponemal antibody titers should decline by 3 months of age and disappear by 6 months of age with appropriate therapy. Infants with CSF abnormalities secondary to congenital syphilis should undergo repeated CSF examinations at 6-month intervals to document clearance. Re-treatment is indicated if the results of the VDRL tests of CSF remain positive at 6 months or if the cell counts remain abnormal at 2 years or if they do not decrease at each examination.

Parvovirus Infection

Human parvovirus (HPV) is the agent that causes erythema infectiosum. This virus can also cause fetal infection when a susceptible pregnant mother becomes infected.

Most children become infected with HPV early in life, and at least 50% of women in the United States are seropositive for HPV before pregnancy. The virus is transmitted by the respiratory route, and the likelihood of transmission after close exposure is estimated to be 50%. When the fetus becomes infected, the risk for fetal loss is estimated to be 2% to 6%. Because many pregnant women are seropositive before pregnancy, and because the rate of transmission to susceptible contacts with close exposure is approximately 50%, the estimated overall risk for fetal loss associated with this infection is 1% to 2%. Fetal infection with HPV can result in:

■ An asymptomatic newborn without untoward effect
■ Spontaneous abortion
■ Stillborn child with hydrops fetalis
■ Liveborn child with hydrops fetalis

HPV infection has *not* been proved to cause congenital anomalies.

Most women with pregnancies complicated by HPV infection deliver normal, asymptomatic newborns. Nonimmune hydrops fetalis is one possible consequence of congenital infection. This is manifested as generalized edema, caused by the extravasation of fluid from the intravascular compartment as a direct consequence of severe cardiovascular failure induced by severe fetal anemia.

Pregnant mothers who are exposed to children at home or work should be counseled about the risks of HPV infection. Children with erythema infectiosum are *not* contagious at the time the classic rash appears. Given the high prevalence of HPV infection in the community, the high rate of silent infection, and the low risk for adverse effects on the fetus, the exclusion of pregnant women from the workplace because of outbreaks of erythema infectiosum is *not* recommended. Pregnant mothers who have been in contact with children incubating erythema infectiosum should be advised of the low risk of infection and may be offered serologic testing. Fetal ultrasonography may be helpful in these situations.

REVIEW EXERCISES

QUESTIONS

1. Of the following, the organism *least* likely to cause early-onset neonatal sepsis is:
a) *L. monocytogenes*
b) Group B streptococci
c) *Streptococcus pneumoniae*
d) *E. coli*

Answer
The answer is c. The most common causes of sepsis and meningitis *beyond* the neonatal period—namely, *S. pneumoniae* and *Neisseria meningitidis*—are rare causes of sepsis and meningitis in the neonatal period. Group B streptococci and *E. coli* account for most cases of early-onset sepsis. *L. monocytogenes* is a less frequent but nevertheless important cause of early-onset sepsis.

2. All of the following are important causes of late-onset neonatal sepsis *except:*
a) *Streptococcus pyogenes*
b) Coagulase-negative staphylococci

c) *S. aureus*
d) Gram-negative bacilli
e) *Candida albicans*

Answer

The answer is a. Neonates with late-onset infection manifest symptoms after the first 5 days of life. Two distinct groups of neonates are at risk for late-onset sepsis. The first group includes term neonates who have no gestational complications and in whom symptoms develop after their discharge from the hospital. Infections with group B streptococci, *L. monocytogenes*, and rarely *Salmonella* species most commonly develop in these infants. The second group of neonates includes high-risk newborns hospitalized for a prolonged period, usually because of prematurity. These infants are at risk for nosocomial infection with such organisms as coagulase-negative staphylococci (most common), gram-negative bacilli, *S. aureus*, and *C. albicans*. *An extremely rare cause of neonatal sepsis is* S. pyogenes, also known as *group A streptococci*.

3. Which of the following is a *true* statement concerning early-onset group B Streptococcus (GBS) neonatal sepsis?
a) Pneumonia and apnea are the most common clinical findings.
b) Meningitis is present in 80% of the cases.
c) The case fatality rate is lower than with late-onset GBS infection.
d) Septic shock occurs in 75% of the cases.
e) The mean age of onset is 72 hours of life.

Answer

The answer is a. Infants with early-onset GBS sepsis most commonly present with respiratory distress and apnea within the first 24 hours of life (mean age of onset 8 hours). Pneumonia is the most common clinical entity associated with early-onset infection. Septic shock and meningitis are present in 25% and 5% to 10% of patients with early-onset GBS infection, respectively. The mortality rate with early-onset infection is 10% to 15%. In contrast, late-onset GBS infection has a mean age of onset of 27 days, clinically manifests with fever, bacteremia, and meningitis, and has focal sites of infection such as bones and joints. The mortality rate with late-onset infection is 2% to 6%.

4. Which of the following is a *true* statement concerning congenital CMV infection?
a) Chorioretinitis is the most common clinical manifestation.
b) Fetal infection occurs only after primary maternal infection.
c) Infected neonates shed virus in the urine.
d) Long-term sequelae do not occur in infected neonates who are asymptomatic.

e) Fifty percent of infected neonates exhibit signs and symptoms of infection.

Answer

The answer is c. CMV infection is the most common congenital infection, occurring in 1% of all newborn infants. Infection can follow primary or recurrent maternal infection. Of the infected infants, 90% are asymptomatic at birth; however, long-term neurologic developmental abnormalities, mainly in the form of sensorineural hearing loss, mental retardation, and motor defects, affect 5% to 20% of these asymptomatic infants. Chorioretinitis occurs in approximately 10% of symptomatic infants. Neonates with congenital CMV infection excrete large amounts of virus in the urine, which serves to support the diagnosis in suspected cases.

5. A newborn infant has microcephaly, is small-for-gestational age, and has a widespread petechial rash, bilateral cataracts, and pulmonic stenosis. The *most* likely cause of these findings is:
a) Rubella
b) CMV infection
c) Toxoplasmosis
d) *T. pallidum* infection
e) Enterovirus infection

Answer

The answer is a. The presence of defects and manifestations at birth supports congenital infection. Enteroviral infection can develop in the immediate neonatal period after perinatal transmission but does not cause congenital defects. The findings of microcephaly, a small-for-gestational-age, and a widespread petechial rash can be consistent with the other infections listed. Cataracts and congenital heart disease are *most* consistent with congenital rubella. Congenital heart disease is common in infants infected during the first trimester; patent ductus arteriosus and pulmonary artery and valvular stenosis are the cardiac lesions most frequently associated with rubella.

6. A 1-year-old infant has chorioretinitis, which has progressed throughout the first year of life, and cerebral calcifications. The *most* likely congenital infection in this child is:
a) Rubella
b) CMV infection
c) Syphilis
d) Toxoplasmosis

Answer

The answer is d. The classic triad of congenital *Toxoplasma* infection includes chorioretinitis, hydrocephalus, and cerebral calcifications. The chorioretinitis associated with the *Toxoplasma* infection is a focal necrotizing retinitis that can be recurrent and progressive. Manifestations of chorioretinitis in infected individuals may not become apparent until late in life.

7. Which of the following is true regarding congenital *Toxoplasma* infection?
a) The incidence is constant despite geographic location.
b) Prenatal diagnosis is not possible.
c) Treatment of infected pregnant women is not recommended.
d) Neurological and visual problems become apparent in the majority of infected asymptomatic infants.

Answer
The answer is d. Although most infants with congenital toxoplasma infection are asymptomatic, 80% develop neurologic and ocular manifestations later in life. This includes chorioretinitis, which may be persistent or intermittent and may be present without other manifestations. The incidence of congenital toxoplasmosis varies by geographic region, likely related to increased risk factors in certain areas of the world. Prenatal diagnosis is possible through the isolation of *Toxoplasma* DNA in amniotic fluid or fetal blood, the isolation of the parasite by mouse inoculation or tissue culture, or finding increased size of lateral ventricles via serial fetal ultrasonography.
Treatment of infected mothers with spiramycin decreases the risk of transmission to the fetus. Treatment of mothers when transmission has been established improves the outcome of congenital toxoplasmosis.

8. A copious nasal discharge, lymphadenopathy, and evidence of periostitis of the tibia develop in a 1-week-old infant. The laboratory test that will *most* likely reveal the diagnosis is:
a) Urine culture for CMV
b) Serum RPR
c) *Toxoplasma* IgM assay
d) Polymerase chain reaction testing for human immunodeficiency virus
e) Direct fluorescent antibody testing for respiratory syncytial virus

Answer
The answer is b. This infant has snuffles, seen in approximately 25% of infants with congenital syphilis, and bony lesions, which are also frequently encountered manifestations of congenital syphilis. Lymphadenopathy is more often associated with congenital syphilis than with other congenital infections. Nontreponemal antibody testing with RPR or VDRL will likely confirm the diagnosis, although the results of serologic tests can be negative in the mother and infant with recent infection.

SUGGESTED READINGS

1. American Academy of Pediatrics. Parvovirus B19. In: Pickering LK, Baker CJ, Long SS, McMillan JA, eds. *Red Book 2006 Report of the Committee on Infectious Diseases*, 27th ed. Elk Grove Village, IL: American Academy of Pediatrics, 2006:484–487.
2. American Academy of Pediatrics. Syphilis. In: Pickering LK, Baker CJ, Long SS, McMillan JA, eds. *Red Book 2006 Report of the Committee on Infectious Diseases*, 27th ed. Elk Grove Village, IL: American Academy of Pediatrics, 2006:631–644.
3. Arav-Broger R, Pass RF. Diagnosis and management of cytomegalovirus infection in the newborn. *Pediatr Ann* 2002;31: 719–725.
4. Bizzarro MJ, Raskind C, Baltimore RS, Gallagher PG. Seventy-five years of neonatal sepsis at Yale: 1928–2003. *Pediatrics* 2005;116: 595–602.
5. Darville T. Syphilis. *Pediatr Rev* 1999;20:160–165.
6. Edwards MS, Baker CJ. *Streptococcus agalactiae* (group B streptococcus). In: Long SS, Pickering LK, Prober CG, eds. *Principles and practice of pediatric infectious diseases*. Philadelphia: Churchill Livingstone, 2003:725–730.
7. Kimberlin DW, Lin CY, Jacobs RF, et al. Natural history of neonatal herpes simplex virus infection in the acyclovir era. *Pediatrics* 2001;108:223–229.
8. Kimberlin DW, Lin CY, Jacobs RF, et al. Safety and efficacy of high-dose intravenous acyclovir in the management of neonatal herpes simplex virus infection. *Pediatrics* 2001; 108:230–238.
9. Posfay-Barbe KM, Wald ER. Listeriosis. *Pediatr Rev* 2004;25: 151–157.
10. Prober CG, Arvin AM. Perinatal viral infections. *Eur J Clin Microbiol* 1987;6:245–261.
11. Remington JS, McLeod R, Thulliez P, et al. Toxoplasmosis. In: Remington JS, Klein JO, eds. *Infectious diseases of the fetus and newborn infant*, 5th ed. Philadelphia: Saunders, 2001:205–346.
12. Stoll BJ, Hansen N, Fanaroff AA, et al. Changes in pathogens causing early-onset sepsis in very-low birth-weight infants. *N Engl J Med* 2002;347:240–247.
13. Stoll BJ, Hansen N, Fanaroff AA, et al. Late-onset sepsis in very-low-birth weight neonates: the experience of the NICHD neonatal research network. *Pediatrics* 2002;110:285–291.
14. Valeur-Jensen AK, Westergaard T, Jensen IP, et al. Risk factors for parvovirus B19 infection in pregnancy. *JAMA* 1999;281:1099–1105.
15. Whitley R, Arvin A, Prober C, et al. Predictors of morbidity and mortality in neonates with herpes simplex virus infection. *N Engl J Med* 1991;324:450–454.

Chapter 23

BOARD SIMULATION:
Neonatology

Elumalai Appachi

QUESTIONS

1. A 4-week-old male infant presents with fever and irritability for 3 days. On examination he lies motionless and has an erythematous rash, bullae, and peeling of the skin. He has circumoral erythema and has crusting and fissuring around the mouth, eyes, and nose (**Fig. 23.1**). Which of the following is *true* regarding the diagnosis and management of this illness?
a) It is almost always acquired in utero.
b) It is usually associated with pharyngitis, conjunctivitis, or impetigo.
c) Fluid restriction is required to prevent bullae formation.
d) The skin lesions heal and leave a pigmented whorl-like pattern.
e) Ampicillin is the drug of choice.

Answer

The answer is b. Staphylococcal scalded skin syndrome is a toxin-mediated complication of *Staphylococcus aureus* infection, characterized by bullous impetigo, generalized scarlatiniform erythematous rash, and systemic manifestations. The skin is extremely tender and the affected infant barely moves as movement aggravates the pain. Conjunctivitis, pharyngitis, and pneumonia are common associated features. The disease is more common in infants and young children, and the foci of infection include the nasopharynx, umbilicus, urinary tract, superficial abrasion, and rarely, the blood. The intact bullae contain sterile fluid (since toxin-mediated) but cultures should be obtained from the blood and all suspected sites of localized infection. Separation of the epidermis at the site of pressure on the skin (Nikolsky sign) is common and at times large areas of the epidermis peel away easily. Systemic therapy with semisynthetic penicillinase-resistant penicillin is the drug of choice. Recovery is rapid and healing occurs without scarring.

2. This full-term infant was born to a 24-year-old primigravida. During routine postnatal examination you notice this abnormality (**Fig. 23.2**). All of the following are true regarding this condition *except:*
a) Chromosomal analysis should be performed on the infant and parents.
b) The infant may develop moderate to severe learning disability.
c) The risk of having this condition in future pregnancies is 50%.
d) An echocardiogram should be performed on this infant.
e) Thyroid hormone abnormality is commonly found in this condition and therefore thyroid function needs to be evaluated.

Answer

The answer is c. The picture shows Brushfield spots, or speckled irises, which are one of the presenting features of Down syndrome (trisomy 21). Other common features include hypotonia, mental and growth retardation, cardiac malformations, midgut anomalies, and thyroid abnormalities. The incidence of Down syndrome or trisomy 21 is 1/600 to 800 live births. Approximately 4% to 5% of children with Down syndrome have a translocation involving the chromosome 21. One of the parents is a translocation carrier in about half of the cases. Hence it is important to get chromosomal analysis done in the child and parents. The risk for future pregnancies is much lower than 50%.

3. The parents of this neonate are concerned about the birthmark (**Fig. 23.3**). All of the following are true statements about this neonate and her condition *except:*
a) The birthmark will disappear slowly as she grows older.
b) Imaging of her brain is part of the initial workup.
c) She is at risk of developing a seizure disorder.

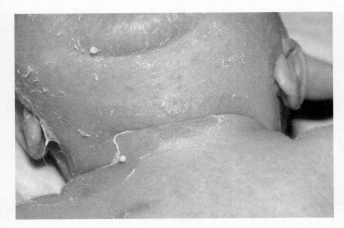

Figure 23.1 The infant in question 1. See explanation of question 1 for details. (See color insert.)

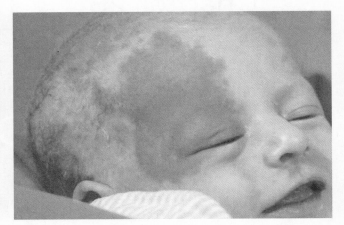

Figure 23.3 The "birthmark" of the neonate in question 3. See explanation of question 3 for details. (See color insert.)

d) She may develop moderate to severe learning disability.

e) Future pregnancies are not at increased risk.

Answer

The answer is a. Sturge-Weber syndrome is a sporadic condition characterized by facial port-wine stain, seizures, hemiparesis, and moderate-to-severe mental retardation. The port-wine stain has to be differentiated from the salmon patch, a benign condition. Port-wine stains do not regress. The facial nevus is usually unilateral and tends to involve the upper face, but occasionally may involve the whole upper half of the body. Ocular manifestations include buphthalmos and glaucoma of the eye on the side of the port-wine stain. Tonic-clonic seizures, which may be intractable, develop during infancy. Mental retardation develops in more than 50% of the cases. X-ray of the skull shows a characteristic calcification "railroad pattern" and a computed tomography (CT) scan of the brain shows ipsilateral atrophy of the brain. Functional hemispherectomy or lobectomy has shown to control the seizures and delay the development of mental

retardation. The most effective therapy for the port-wine stain is flash-lamp-pumped pulsed dye laser.

4. Examination of a neonate reveals this physical feature (Fig. 23.4). The following are true regarding his condition *except*:

a) An echocardiogram should be performed to evaluate for any associated cardiac anomalies.

b) He may develop pancytopenia.

c) Chromosomal studies should be performed

d) Future pregnancies are not at risk

e) He may have an increased predisposition to malignancies.

Answer

The answer is d. Fanconi anemia is an autosomal-recessive condition characterized by physical abnormalities including short stature, café au lait spots, and abnormalities in hands and arms. The upper limb abnormalities include absent thumb and absent radius. Pancytopenia develops because the marrow is usually aplastic. A small percentage of patients may have associated internal organ

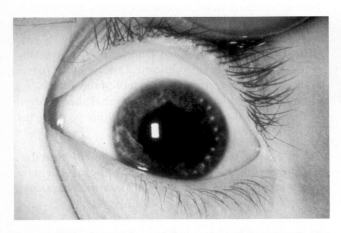

Figure 23.2 The infant in question 2. See explanation of question 2 for details. (See color insert.)

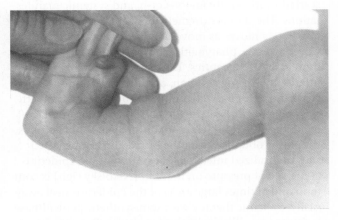

Figure 23.4 The physical feature of the neonate in question 4. See explanation of question 4 for details.

abnormalities including heart defects. Children with this disorder are at increased risk for developing leukemia and other malignancies. Chromosomal breakage studies are required because chromosomal breaks occur; parents need genetic counseling for future pregnancies.

5. A 5-day-old neonate is brought to the emergency department with a history of poor feeding, fever, irritability, and a brief seizure. A rash is noted on his trunk (Fig. 23.5). He is a full-term neonate born by normal vaginal delivery. He has been bottle-fed and was doing well until today. All of the following are true regarding his diagnosis and management *except:*
a) A sepsis workup, including blood, urine, and cerebrospinal fluid cultures should be performed.
b) Treatment with broad-spectrum intravenous antibiotics should be administered.
c) Acyclovir therapy should be initiated only after the results of a herpes simplex polymerase chain reaction test on the cerebrospinal fluid has returned.
d) Imaging studies of the brain and an electroencephalogram should be obtained.
e) He may have acquired this illness during the delivery.

Answer
The answer is c. Perinatal herpes infection occurs predominantly during delivery and in most cases is caused by herpes simplex virus type 2. Symptoms manifest in the first month of life with localized skin, eye, and mouth infection, disseminated disease, or encephalitis. Vesicular skin lesions are present in most cases, but may be absent in neonates presenting with disseminated infection or encephalitis. The lesions may be present at the site of fetal monitoring. Symptoms of central nervous system involvement include lethargy, poor feeding, and seizures. Systemic herpes infection should be suspected in any sick neonate having sepsis with negative bacterial cultures or who is nonresponsive to antibiotics. The typical clinical picture and isolation of the virus make the diagnosis. The use of polymerase chain reaction analysis of the cerebrospinal fluid for the isolation of the virus may be important in the absence of skin lesions. Treatment with intravenous acyclovir should be started immediately upon clinical suspicion of the diagnosis.

6. Routine postnatal examination of a neonate revealed the physical finding shown in **Figure 23.6**. Which of the following is a *true* statement regarding this condition?
a) It is less common in male infants.
b) He requires investigation for renal abnormalities.
c) Rectal biopsy is required to confirm the diagnosis.
d) Most infants with this condition have an associated cardiac anomaly.
e) An urgent upper gastrointestinal contrast study is required.

Answer
The answer is b. Prune belly syndrome occurs predominantly in male infants (95%). The syndrome comprises characteristic deficiency of the abdominal wall musculature, undescended testes, and urinary tract abnormalities. Oligohydramnios and pulmonary hypoplasia are common. Cardiac anomalies occur in 10% of infants, whereas musculoskeletal abnormalities occur in over 50%. Urinary tract infections are frequent and all patients with this condition require antibiotic prophylaxis. The renal abnormalities include dysplastic kidneys, vesicoureteric reflux with dilated ureters, and abnormal urethra. The prognosis depends on the severity of pulmonary hypoplasia and the dysplasia of the kidneys.

7. The parents of a healthy, full-term 2-day-old neonate are concerned about a rash (shown in Fig. 23.7) that has developed over the last 24 hours. Which of the following is *true* regarding this infant?

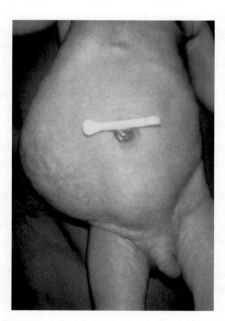

Figure 23.6 The physical finding of the neonate in question 6. See explanation of question 6 for details.

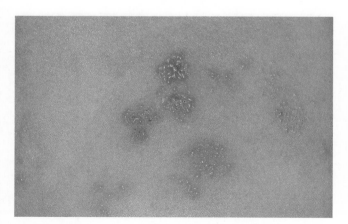

Figure 23.5 The rash on the neonate in question 5. See explanation of question 5 for details. (See color insert.)

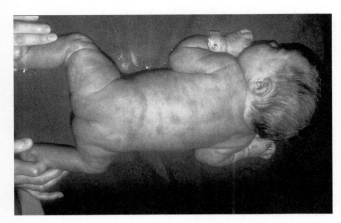

Figure 23.7 The rash on the neonate in question 7. See explanation of question 7 for details. (See color insert.)

a) Parenteral acyclovir therapy should be commenced immediately.
b) He is at risk of developing a seizure disorder later in life.
c) The culture of the fluid from the pustule may grow *Staphylococcus* species.
d) Microscopic examination of the fluid from his rash may reveal many polymorphonuclear cells.
e) The parents should be assured that this is a benign condition and does not require any treatment.

Answer

The answer is e. Erythema toxicum (see Fig. 1.1) is a benign skin eruption occurring commonly in full-term neonates. The characteristic lesion has a 1- to 2-mm papule or a pustule with a surrounding erythema. The eruption is generalized but spares the palms and soles. The eruption commonly occurs on the second day of life and new crops commonly occur for a few days more. It is a self-limited condition that resolves spontaneously. The fluid in the pustule contains many eosinophils with negative bacterial culture. The cause is unknown. This condition has to be differentiated from herpes simplex, bacterial, and candidal infection, as well as transient neonatal pustular melanosis.

8. The parents of this neonate are concerned about the feature shown in **Figure 23.8**. The *best* management plan for this neonate is to:
a) Obtain chromosomal analysis for karyotyping.
b) Start hydrocortisone therapy.
c) Obtain an abdominal ultrasonography to rule out renal abnormalities.
d) Start local testosterone therapy.
e) Reassure the parents that future pregnancies are not at risk.

Answer

The answer is a. The presence of ambiguous genitalia in a neonate poses great difficulty in counseling parents.

Chromosomal analysis usually should be done first to ascertain the gender of the given child. Abdominal ultrasonography may be helpful to identify the uterus. The infant in the vignette needs further workup for congenital adrenal hyperplasia or hermaphrodism and further therapy is based on the final endocrinological diagnosis. The risk for future pregnancy is dependant on the diagnosis and one cannot reassure the parents that there will be no future risk.

9. A 2-day-old breast-fed neonate presents with bilious vomiting, lethargy and without abdominal distension. Appropriate management of this neonate should include each of the following *except:*
a) Stop the feeds.
b) Place a nasogastric tube.
c) Administer a fluid bolus to improve intravascular volume.
d) Consult a pediatric surgeon immediately.
e) Obtain an abdominal ultrasound to rule out infantile hypertrophic pyloric stenosis.

Answer

The answer is e. Duodenal obstruction presents with bilious vomiting without abdominal distension usually in the first day of life. Duodenal atresia may also be associated with Down syndrome, malrotation, congenital heart disease, and esophageal atresia. The radiologic finding is called the double-bubble appearance (see Fig. 63.3), which is caused by the proximal duodenum, and gas-filled stomach. Prenatal diagnosis of duodenal atresia is possible with fetal ultrasonography. The initial treatment is nasogastric decompression of the stomach and intravenous fluid replacement. Surgical repair follows the period of stabilization. Hypertrophic pyloric stenosis does not present at this age and usually presents with nonbilious vomiting, failure to thrive, and a hungry infant.

10. A 3-day-old neonate presents with abdominal distension, delayed passage of meconium, and vomiting. The

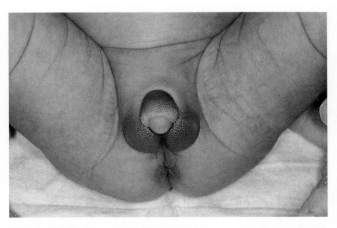

Figure 23.8 The physical feature of the neonate in question 8. See explanation of question 8 for details.

infant's mother has gestational diabetes. Which of the following is a *true* statement regarding meconium ileus?
a) Physical examination may show features of trisomy 21.
b) A negative sweat chloride test does not rule out cystic fibrosis (CF) in the neonatal period.
c) Meconium peritonitis is a rare complication of the meconium ileus.
d) The overall prognosis is excellent.
e) Surgery is the treatment of choice in all the cases.

Answer
The answer is b. Meconium ileus is commonly associated with the diagnosis of CF. Clinically, the infant presents with intestinal obstruction. Meconium is sticky in the absence of pancreatic enzymes and clings to the intestinal wall. The sweat chloride test may be negative in the neonatal period and does not rule out the diagnosis of CF; genetic testing is necessary to confirm the diagnosis of CF. Meconium ileus is not specifically associated with Down syndrome. Treatment with Gastrografin enema is usually successful; surgical intervention is opted for if Gastrografin enema therapy fails or there is evidence of peritonitis. Meconium peritonitis is a common complication of meconium ileus. The overall prognosis depends on the severity of the CF.

11. A 4-hour-old term neonate is found to be tachypneic, pale, and has poor peripheral perfusion. The baby was born by normal vaginal delivery without apparent prenatal problems. The complete blood count shows hemoglobin 8 g/dL, hematocrit 25%, and platelets 240/mm^3. The mother's blood group is O Rh-positive. The first *best* plan of action is to:
a) Urgently transfuse the infant with 10 to 15 mL/kg of O Rh-negative blood.
b) Administer erythropoietin therapy to the infant immediately.
c) Place the infant on 100% oxygen and observe the baby in the nursery.
d) Administer Rh immunoglobulin (RhoGAM) to the mother.
e) Arrange for an exchange transfusion for the infant.

Answer
The answer is a. Transplacental hemorrhage is probably a common condition that goes unnoticed until it is severe. Acute blood loss presents as pallor, associated with circulatory shock, respiratory distress, and poor perfusion. It can be proved by the Kleihauer-Betke test, which demonstrates the presence of fetal hemoglobin and fetal red cells in the maternal blood. The infant in the vignette should first be acutely transfused with blood.

12. A 1-month-old infant is seen in the outpatient clinic for a routine visit. The mother gives a history of poor feeding and unsatisfactory weight gain. She states that the infant's 5-year-old sibling had a similar history at this age. On further questioning, the mother reveals that

the sibling has delayed development. On examination, the infant has facial dysmorphic features that include maxillary hypoplasia and an absent philtrum. Which of the following is *true* regarding the infant's condition?
a) It is rarely associated with congenital heart disease.
b) The infant is at minimal risk for developmental delay.
c) Future pregnancies are not at risk.
d) Major/minor components of this condition are expressed in 1 to 2/1000 live births.
e) None of the above.

Answer
The answer is d. Alcohol has been implicated in causing fetal anomalies if consumed during pregnancy. A specific clinical pattern has been described, including a characteristic facial appearance, called fetal alcohol syndrome. Major and minor components of the condition are expressed in 1 or 2/1000 live births. Features of the syndrome include intrauterine growth retardation, facial abnormalities (e.g., short palpebral fissures, maxillary hypoplasia, thin upper lip), congenital cardiac defects (e.g., septal defects), and delayed development and mental retardation. Fetal alcohol syndrome is a common cause of mental retardation. The offspring of future pregnancies are at risk if alcohol consumption is continued during the next pregnancy. The management of these infants is supportive, and the prognosis is poor in a full-blown syndrome.

13. A 7-day-old neonate presents with jaundice and rash. The infant was small for his gestational-age at birth and has not gained any weight. On examination, he is irritable and exhibits hypertonia, and the red reflex is absent. All of the following are true regarding congenital rubella syndrome, *except*:
a) An echocardiogram should be obtained.
b) A hearing assessment is indicated.
c) The diagnosis can be confirmed by isolating the virus from the urine.
d) It can be difficult to differentiate rubella syndrome from congenital cytomegalovirus infection.
e) The prognosis is good with medical treatment.

Answer
The answer is e. Rubella virus acquired during the first trimester of pregnancy causes congenital rubella syndrome in the fetus. Congenital defects occur in approximately 90% of infants if the maternal infection is acquired before week 11 of pregnancy. The incidence of congenital rubella syndrome is on the decline, and the syndrome has been targeted for elimination by the rigorous implementation of vaccination. The manifestations include intrauterine growth retardation, cataracts, microphthalmia, congenital heart defects (e.g., patent ductus arteriosus, pulmonary artery stenosis), sensorineural deafness, meningoencephalitis, anemia, and thrombocytopenia. The development of severe motor and mental

retardation is common. The diagnosis is established by demonstrating rubella-specific immunoglobulin M or culturing the rubella virus from the nasopharynx or urine of an affected infant with classic clinical features. The prognosis for infants with congenital rubella syndrome is very poor given the likelihood of neurologic deterioration.

SUGGESTED READINGS

1. Alter BP, Young NS. The bone marrow failure syndromes. In: Nathan DG, Orkin SH, eds. *Hematology of infancy and childhood,* 5th ed. Philadelphia: Saunders, 1998:237–335.
2. De Almeida V, Bowman JM. Massive fetomaternal hemorrhage: Manitoba experience. *Obstet Gynecol* 1994;83:323.
3. Diamond M, Sigmundson HK. Sex reassignment at birth. *Arch Pediatr Adolesc Med* 1997;151:298.
4. Fuchs JR, Langer JC. Long term outcome after neonatal meconium obstruction. *Pediatrics* 1998;101:E7.
5. Jacobs AH, Walton RG. The incidence of birthmarks in the neonate. *Pediatrics* 1976;58:281.
6. Kays DW. Surgical conditions of the neonatal intestinal tract. *Clin Perinatol* 1996;23:353.
7. Kuhnle U, Bullinger M. Outcome of congenital adrenal hyperplasia. *Pediatr Surg Int* 1997;12:511.
8. Manivel JC, Pettmato G, Reinberg Y, et al. Prune belly syndrome: clinicopathological study of 28 cases. *Pediatr Pathol* 1989;9:691.
9. Melish ME, Glasgow LA. Staphylococcal scalded skin syndrome: the expanded clinical syndrome. *J Pediatr* 1971;78:958.
10. Rimoin DL, Connor JM, Pyeritz RE. *Emery and Rimoin's principles and practice of medical genetics,* 3rd ed. New York: Churchill Livingstone, 1997.
11. Shalaby-Rana E, Lowe LH, Blask AN, et al. Imaging in pediatric urology. *Pediatr Clin North Am* 1997;44:1065.
12. Van der Horst CMAM, Koster PHL, De Borgie CAJM, et al. Effect of the timing of treatment of port-wine stains with the flash-lamp-pumped pulsed dye laser. *N Engl J Med* 1998;338:1028.

Chapter 24

Recognition of Cardiovascular Disorders

Daniel J. Murphy Jr.

HEART MURMURS

Auscultation is a critical component of the physical examination of the infant or child. A proper examination is conducted in a quiet environment so that the examiner's attention is focused entirely on the auscultatory findings. In general, a "pediatric" stethoscope is not necessary, and in some cases "neonatal" stethoscopes with long tubing and a small head may be inferior to an "adult" stethoscope, which transmits sounds more reliably. It is important to examine all areas of the body and listen over the precordium in addition to the right side of the chest and both sides of the back. Finally, the examiner should note any changes in the heart sounds caused by respiration or a change in the patient's position. Children should be examined in the supine and standing positions so that the effect of a change in position on murmurs can be appreciated.

In addition to noting the characteristics of any murmurs, the examiner should assess the patient's overall clinical condition, measure the heart rate and blood pressure, and palpate the pulses in all the four extremities. The strength of the precordial impulse and the presence or absence of a thrill should also be noted. Finally, the first and second heart sounds (S_1 and S_2) should be characterized. Split heart sounds and the effect of respiration on the S_2 should be noted. A split S_1 is normal. The S_2 normally splits variably with respiration. *A fixed split of the S_2 is characteristic of atrial septal defect.* Any additional sounds—for example, clicks—should also be noted.

Most murmurs in infants and children are innocent murmurs that are not caused by any structural abnormality or pathologic flow (Table 24.1). The most common murmur in the newborn is a *pulmonary branch stenosis* murmur resulting from the relatively small size of the branch pulmonary arteries at birth. This is a systolic ejection murmur heard over the precordium and also in the right side of the chest and both sides of the back. The presence of a systolic ejection murmur in the right and left axillae is characteristic of a pulmonary branch stenosis murmur. This type of murmur is generally inaudible after the age of 4 months.

The *Still murmur* is a vibratory, musical, or buzzing noise heard during ejection, generally along the left sternal border. It can be heard at any age and is more prominent during an increase in cardiac output (e.g., fever, exercise). The Still murmur is loudest when the patient is in a supine position and becomes attenuated or inaudible when the patient stands. *Any ejection murmur that increases in intensity when the patient is standing is likely pathologic and should prompt further investigation.*

A venous hum is commonly heard in younger children in the upright position. This murmur is a continuous blowing sound created by the flow of blood in the large veins from the neck into the thorax. The murmur of a venous hum can be abolished by compressing the jugular veins on the ipsilateral side or by turning the patient's head. This murmur could be confused with a patent ductus arteriosus.

Physiologic changes, especially in the perinatal period, affect the clinical examination findings, especially the features of murmurs. At birth, because the pulmonary artery resistance is elevated, the right ventricular and left ventricular pressures are nearly equal. Therefore, little blood flows from the left ventricle to the right ventricle in an infant with a ventricular septal defect immediately after birth, so that the holosystolic murmur of ventricular septal defect is rare during the first several days of life. As the pulmonary vascular resistance decreases during the first week, the volume and velocity of the flow through the ventricular septal defect increase to produce the typical holosystolic, harsh murmur associated with ventricular septal defect. On the other hand, stenotic lesions (e.g., aortic stenosis, pulmonary stenosis) are associated with high-velocity, disturbed flow during the systolic ejection period and cause systolic ejection murmurs immediately after birth.

In the newborn, in whom the pulmonary resistance and right ventricular pressure are elevated, moderate tricuspid regurgitation is common. In this setting, the jet of tricuspid regurgitation produces at the lower left sternal border a holosystolic murmur that is indistinguishable from the typical murmur of a ventricular septal defect. As the pulmonary resistance decreases, the murmur of the tricuspid regurgitation becomes less intense, lower in pitch, and eventually inaudible, usually during the first day or two after birth.

TABLE 24.1

INNOCENT MURMURS IN INFANTS AND CHILDREN

	Neonatal	Still	Venous Hum	Pulmonary Flow
Pitch	Medium to high	Low	High	Medium
Intensity	1–2/6	1–3/6	1–3/6	1–3/6
Time in cycle	Midsystolic	Midsystolic	Continuous	Midsystolic
Quality	Soft ejection	Vibratory, musical, buzzing	Soft blowing	Soft blowing
Location	1st and 2nd ICS, RSB, LSB, back	LLSB	Right and Left infraclavicular areas	2nd LICS
Increased by	Increased cardiac output	Supine, fever, exercise	Sitting, standing	Supine, expiration, ↑CO
Decreased by	Decreased cardiac output	Standing, valsalva	Supine, head turn, jugular compression	Upright, inspiration, ↓CO
Age appears	Birth–1 week	1–10 years	2–5 years	7–10 years
Age disappears	3–4 months	Puberty	7–10 years	Persists in adults
Produced by	Relatively small pulmonary arteries	Vibration in LVOT	Flow in jugular veins	Flow in RVOT
Confused with	Pulmonary branch stenosis	Hypertrophic cardiomyopathy	PDA	ASD or mild PS

ASD, atrial septal defect; CO, cardiac output; ICS, intercostal space; LICS, left intercostal space; LLSB, lower left sternal border; LSB, left sternal border; LVOT, left ventricular outflow tract; PDA, patent ductus arteriosus; PS, pulmonary stenosis; RSB, right sternal border; RVOT, right ventricular outflow tract.

In the normal newborn, systolic ejection murmurs can be caused by:

- Patent ductus arteriosus
- Peripheral pulmonary stenosis
- Flow through the right ventricular outflow tract (pulmonary flow murmur)
- Vibration in the left ventricular outflow tract (Still murmur)

In comparison with innocent murmurs, pathologic murmurs tend to be louder, usually grade 3 or higher, and harsher. Holosystolic murmurs are always pathologic, as are murmurs associated with systolic clicks or an abnormal S_2. Further evaluation is recommended for all children with a:

- Diastolic murmur
- Holosystolic or pansystolic murmur
- Late systolic murmur
- Very loud murmur
- Continuous murmur, except for a venous hum

Most studies have shown that a pediatric cardiology consultation is more cost-effective than echocardiography performed without consultation as an initial step in the evaluation of a heart murmur.

SYNDROMES AND CONGENITAL HEART DISEASE

Congenital heart defects are a prominent feature of many chromosomal and genetic disorders (Table 24.2). The most commonly encountered syndromes are Down, Turner, Noonan, Williams, and DiGeorge. *Each has a 33% to 90% incidence of associated congenital cardiac defects, and the spectrum of heart defects is unique for each syndrome.* Fetal or postnatal screening with echocardiography is reasonable for these syndromes and others associated with multiple congenital anomalies.

FAMILIAL CARDIOVASCULAR DISEASE

There are a number of familial cardiovascular disorders that pose a significant risk to children and adolescents. A careful family history is essential and a family history positive for the following should prompt the practitioner to pursue further cardiac evaluation:

- Dilated cardiomyopathy
- Hypertrophic cardiomyopathy
- Marfan syndrome
- Muscular dystrophy
- Long QT syndrome (congenital deafness, familial seizures, or syncope)
- Sudden or premature death

TABLE 24.2

SYNDROMES AND CONGENITAL HEART DISEASE

Syndrome	Congenital Heart Disease
Down (40%–50%)	AV canal defect, VSD, TOF
Turner (35%)	Coarctation, bicuspid aortic valve, AS
Noonan (80–90%)	Pulmonary stenosis, ASD, HCM
Williams (60%)	Supravalvar aortic stenosis, coarctation
DiGeorge (35%)	Conotruncal malformations (interrupted aortic arch, truncus arteriosus, TOF)
Alagille (95%)	Pulmonary artery stenosis, TOF, PS
Asplenia	Complex cyanotic CHD
CHARGE	VSD, ASD
Cri-du-chat (5p-)	Various congenital cardiac defects
De Lange	TOF, VSD
Diabetes (maternal)	Hypertrophic cardiomyopathy, VSD, TGA
Ellis van Creveld	Common atrium (ASD)
Fanconi	PDA, VSD
Fetal alcohol	VSD, ASD, TOF
Fetal hydantoin	ASD, VSD, coarctation
Goldenhar	TOF
Holt-Oram	ASD, VSD
Laurence-Moon-Biedl	TOF, VSD
Marfan	Aortic root aneurysm, mitral prolapse
Multiple lentigines (leopard)	Pulmonary stenosis
Polysplenia	Complex CHD
Rubella	PDA, peripheral pulmonary stenosis
Rubinstein-Taybi	PDA
Smith-Lemli-Opitz	VSD, PDA
Thrombocytopenia-absent radius	ASD, TOF
Tuberous sclerosis	Cardiac rhabdomyomas

AS, aortic stenosis; ASD, atrial septal defect; AV, atrioventricular; CHARGE, coloboma of the eye, heart defects, atresia of the choanae, renal anomalies and retardation of growth and/or development, genital anomalies in moles and ear abnormalities or deafness; CHD, congenital heart disease; HCM, hypertrophic cardiomyopathy; PDA, patent ductus arteriosus; PS, pulmonary stenosis; TGA, transposition of the great arteries; TOF, tetralogy of Fallot; VSD, ventricular septal defect.

PREPARTICIPATION SCREENING AND DIAGNOSIS OF CARDIOVASCULAR DISEASE IN ATHLETES

The objective of preparticipation screening of the young athlete is the identification of "silent" cardiovascular abnormalities that can progress or cause sudden cardiac death. Such abnormalities may be suspected based upon a family history of heart disease or sudden unexpected death, cardiac symptoms or abnormal physical findings.

The personal history should include all of the following:

- History of heart disease, including Kawasaki disease
- Heart murmur
- Systemic hypertension
- Fatigue
- Syncope/near-syncope
- Excessive/unexplained exertional dyspnea
- Exertional chest pain
- Medication history
- Illicit drug use (including performance enhancing drugs)

Physical examination should include identification of the following:

- Heart murmur (supine/standing)
- Femoral arterial pulses
- Stigmata of Marfan syndrome
- Brachial blood pressure measurement (sitting)

Suspicion of the presence of a cardiac abnormality should prompt referral to a cardiovascular specialist and appropriate diagnostic evaluation before the athlete is allowed to participate in training and competitive sports.

CHEST PAIN

Chest pain is common in children and rarely associated with cardiac abnormalities. In most published series, musculoskeletal or idiopathic chest pain accounts for symptoms in more than half the children who present with chest pain. Additional causes of chest pain include lower respiratory infection (pneumonia), other pulmonary abnormalities (asthma, chronic cough), gastrointestinal disorders (especially gastroesophageal reflux), and trauma. Chest pain at rest is rarely associated with a cardiac cause. Chest pain with exercise may be of cardiac origin and should be evaluated further.

The history and physical examination are most useful in determining the underlying cause of chest pain. Laboratory tests are rarely helpful, although chest roentgenography can be of value in evaluating pulmonary causes of chest pain. Electrocardiographic abnormalities may be present in up to 10% of children with chest pain, but the electrocardiographic findings are usually nonspecific and unrelated to the symptoms or cause of the chest pain.

Children with chest pain should be referred for further evaluation if they are in significant distress, have a history of significant trauma, or the pain is associated with syncope, dizziness, palpitations, or exertion. In addition, *a history of structural heart disease or previous Kawasaki disease should prompt a further investigation of the chest pain.*

NEONATAL CYANOSIS

Almost all newborns have cyanosis of the hands and feet. Acrocyanosis, or peripheral cyanosis, is associated with

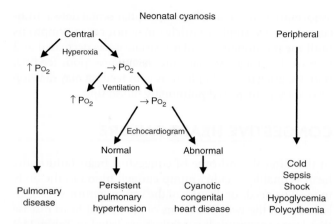

Figure 24.1 Treatment flow diagram for evaluating the cyanotic newborn.

pale or cool extremities and pink mucous membranes. The partial oxygen pressure (P_{O_2}) is usually >60 mm Hg, and the oxygen saturation is generally >93%. Causes of peripheral cyanosis include cold, stress, sepsis, shock, polycythemia, and hypoglycemia.

Central cyanosis is present when the P_{O_2} is <60 mm Hg or the oxygen saturation is <94%. Some form of hypoventilation or pulmonary disease is found in most infants with central cyanosis, including respiratory distress syndrome, pneumonia, aspiration, and pneumothorax. Clinical examination and chest roentgenography are valuable in the initial evaluation of the cyanotic infant. In addition, treatment with 100% inspired oxygen (the hyperoxia test) can be useful in distinguishing the pulmonary causes from cardiac causes of hypoxemia. If the P_{O_2} rises above 50 mm Hg, pulmonary disease is the most likely cause of cyanosis. If the administration of oxygen does not significantly increase the arterial P_{O_2}, the infant should be ventilated. A rise in the P_{O_2} in response to oxygen and ventilation may indicate that the initial abnormality was hypoventilation, pulmonary disease, or persistent pulmonary hypertension. If the administration of oxygen and ventilation do not increase the arterial P_{O_2}, cyanotic congenital heart disease is most likely, and echocardiography should be performed (Fig. 24.1).

MODES OF PRESENTATION

Cyanosis and shock are the most common modes of presentation at birth in infants with congenital heart disease. Heart murmur is a less important feature of congenital heart disease in the newborn, and the absence of a murmur should not delay appropriate evaluation.

Between birth and 3 days of age, infants with transposition of the great arteries, obstructive lesions of the left side of the heart (such as critical aortic stenosis or hypoplastic left heart syndrome), and obstructive lesions of the right side of the heart become symptomatic. The pulmonary resistance is elevated at birth, and shunting lesions (e.g., atrioventricular canal defect, ventricular septal defect, truncus arteriosus, single ventricle) may not cause symptoms until the pulmonary vascular resistance has decreased at 2 to 6 weeks of age. At that time, tachypnea, poor feeding, poor weight gain, or diaphoresis with feeding may develop secondary to increased pulmonary blood flow.

CONGESTIVE HEART FAILURE

In the clinical syndrome of congestive heart failure, the heart is unable to either pump enough blood to the body to meet its needs or dispose of the venous return, or a combination of the two. The forms of congenital heart disease that cause congestive heart failure are listed in Table 24.3 according to the age at which symptoms generally appear. In addition to congenital heart defects, acquired heart diseases, such as myocarditis, metabolic abnormalities, dilated cardiomyopathy, and chronic tachycardia, can cause signs of heart failure. Miscellaneous metabolic abnormalities, such as severe anemia and acute hypertension, can also cause signs of congestive heart failure.

In infants, poor feeding and poor weight gain are associated with congestive heart failure. In addition, because the pulmonary arterial or venous flow of most such infants is increased, tachypnea and dyspnea also develop with exertion. Wheezing is common in infants and children with heart failure; rales are rare. Fluid overload produces hepatomegaly and facial puffiness, especially around the eyelids. *Peripheral edema is rarely encountered in infants or children with congestive heart failure.*

The management of congestive heart failure includes administering oxygen if pulmonary edema has caused hypoxemia. Diuretics are a mainstay of therapy in congestive heart failure with fluid retention. The standard regimen is furosemide 0.5 to 2.0 mg/kg given two or three times a day. Furosemide toxicity includes hypokalemia, hypochloremic alkalosis, hyperostosis, and nephrocalcinosis in premature infants. The rapid intravenous administration of furosemide can cause ototoxicity. Spironolactone is also used in conjunction with diuretics for its potassium sparing and neurohormonal effects.

Digoxin is occasionally given to patients with congestive heart failure, but is used in conjunction with diuretics and angiotensin-converting enzyme (ACE) inhibitors. The loading dose of digoxin is 20 to 40 µg/kg given over 12 to 24 hours. A maintenance dose of 8 to 10 µg/kg per day in one or two doses (5 µg/kg per day for premature infants) is standard. Signs of digoxin toxicity include:

- Atrioventricular block
- Sinus bradycardia
- Supraventricular arrhythmias
- Nausea
- Vomiting
- Drowsiness

Digitalis toxicity is increased by:

- Renal disease
- Hypokalemia
- Hypocalcemia
- Myocarditis
- Hypoxia
- Alkalosis

A number of drugs *increase* the digoxin levels, including the following:

- Quinidine
- Amiodarone
- Verapamil
- Carvedilol
- Erythromycin

Drugs that reduce afterload and attenuate the neurohormonal effects of heart failure include ACE inhibitors and angiotensin receptor blockers (ARBs). They are most effective in cases of reduced cardiac function and are contraindicated in cases of fixed or dynamic left ventricular outflow tract obstruction (e.g., aortic stenosis, hypertrophic cardiomyopathy). ACE inhibitors include captopril (0.5–6.0 mg/kg per day orally every 6–12 hours) and enalapril (0.1 mg/kg twice daily). They should be started at low doses and gradually increased as they are tolerated. ACE inhibitor toxicity includes hyperkalemia, proteinuria, neutropenia, hypotension, lethargy, dizziness, and syncope. Aspirin may attenuate the effect of ACE inhibitors.

TABLE 24.3

DEVELOPMENT OF CONGESTIVE HEART FAILURE IN ASSOCIATION WITH CONGENITAL HEART DISEASE

Age	Forms of Congenital Heart Disease
At birth	Hypoplastic left heart syndrome Volume overload (large systemic arteriovenous fistula, severe valvular regurgitation)
1–7 days	Transposition of the great arteries PDA in premature infants Hypoplastic left heart syndrome Total anomalous pulmonary venous connection (obstructed) Systemic arteriovenous fistula Critical aortic stenosis
1–4 weeks	Coarctation of the aorta Critical aortic stenosis Large left-to-right shunt lesions (VSD, PDA) in premature infants All other lesions listed above
4–6 weeks	Large left-to-right shunt lesions (VSD, AV canal, single ventricle) Anomalous left coronary artery from the pulmonary artery

AV, atrioventricular; PDA, patent ductus arteriosus; VSD, ventricular septal defect.

β-Blockers are now standard therapy for adults with heart failure, but there is no evidence of the efficacy of these medications in children. Carvedilol administration in children has been associated with a high incidence of adverse effects, including dizziness, hypotension, and headache. If used, β-blockers must be initiated at low doses and carefully titrated upward.

CARDIOGENIC SHOCK

Cardiogenic shock occurs when the cardiac output is inadequate to supply end-organ needs. Clinical manifestations include pallor, tachycardia, tachypnea, hypotension with a narrow pulse pressure, oliguria, metabolic acidosis, and altered mental status.

In newborns, the various causes of cardiogenic shock include sepsis, myocarditis, tachyarrhythmias, and cardiac structural abnormalities. Congenital heart defects that cause cardiogenic shock include obstructive lesions of the left side of the heart (hypoplastic left heart syndrome, aortic stenosis, coarctation, total anomalous pulmonary venous connection). In infants and older children, cardiogenic shock is more commonly the consequence of sepsis, myocarditis, or myocardial infarction.

The management of cardiogenic shock includes intubation and mechanical ventilation and the administration of positive inotropic agents, such as dopamine (5–15 μg/kg per minute) or dobutamine (2.5–20 μg/kg per minute). Diuretics can be useful in cases of pulmonary edema or fluid overload. Afterload-reducing agents such as nitroprusside (0.5–5.0 μg/kg per minute) can be used to decrease the cardiac expenditure of energy. Myocardial phosphodiesterase inhibitors, such as milrinone (50 μg/kg load, then 0.375–0.75 μg/kg per minute), are used for additional inotropic support and afterload reduction.

COMPLICATIONS OF CYANOTIC CONGENITAL HEART DISEASE

When cyanotic congenital heart disease is not corrected, a persistent right-to-left shunt predisposes the patient to a variety of long-term complications. Chronic arterial hypoxemia causes erythrocytosis. Symptoms of erythrocytosis are rare until the hematocrit rises above 65% unless a relative anemia secondary to iron deficiency is present. In any hypoxemic patient, the red cell indices should be measured and iron administered if the mean cell volume and mean cell hemoglobin concentration are subnormal. Longstanding cyanosis causes clubbing of the digits. Chronic renal insufficiency also develops in a substantial percentage of long-term cyanotic patients. *A right-to-left intracardiac shunt predisposes these patients to stroke and brain abscess.* Finally, disorders of bleeding can develop secondary to platelet dysfunction.

Hypercyanotic spells, a unique but potentially fatal complication, occur in infants and children with uncorrected tetralogy of Fallot. The peak age for hypercyanotic spells is 2 to 4 months. These can develop in the early morning after feeding, exercise, crying, or defecation. The increase in cyanosis is accompanied by an increased rate and depth of respiration and irritability. Consciousness may be lost. Treatment of a hypercyanotic spell includes placing the child in a knee-chest position, administering oxygen and sedation, infusing intravenous fluids, and administering intravenous phenylephrine to raise the blood pressure. Hypercyanotic spells can be prevented by avoiding dehydration, treating iron deficiency, or prophylactically administering β-blockers (propranolol 2–4 mg/kg per day). In addition to normal daily activities, pain symptoms, the induction of anesthesia, and dehydration can cause hypercyanotic spells in the medical setting. Care must be taken before surgical procedures are undertaken in infants and children with uncorrected tetralogy of Fallot.

COR PULMONALE

In cor pulmonale, right ventricular hypertrophy and dilation develop secondary to pulmonary hypertension. Frequent causes of pulmonary hypertension in children include:

- Large left-to-right shunt
- Alveolar hypoxia, such as that associated with pulmonary parenchymal disease
- Airway obstruction
- High altitude
- Pulmonary venous hypertension
- Primary pulmonary hypertension

The clinical manifestations of cor pulmonale include dyspnea, fatigue, and syncope. The physical examination reveals a single loud S_2, hepatomegaly, and jugular venous distension. Electrocardiography reveals deviation of the right axis and right ventricular hypertrophy.

The management of cor pulmonale includes treating the underlying cause of pulmonary hypertension. Possible treatments include relief of airway obstruction, administration of oxygen for chronic hypoxia, administration of diuretics for pulmonary edema, and ventilation. Surgery should be performed to correct any operable structural cardiac abnormalities. If the pulmonary hypertension can be reversed, the cor pulmonale resolves.

REVIEW EXERCISES

QUESTIONS

1. All of the following may cause chest pain in children *except:*
a) Asthma
b) Costochondritis

c) Pericarditis
d) Upper respiratory infection
e) Gastroesophageal reflux

Answer
The answer is d. *Lower* respiratory infection (pneumonia), other pulmonary abnormalities (asthma, chronic cough), and the other entities listed commonly cause chest pain. Cardiac causes of chest pain are rare in children.

2. All of the following cardiac conditions can present with heart failure in the first 6 weeks of life *except:*
a) Complete atrioventricular canal defect
b) Coarctation of the aorta
c) Pulmonary stenosis
d) Ventricular septal defect
e) Hypoplastic left heart syndrome

Answer
The answer is c. Infants with obstructive lesions of the left side of the heart (aortic stenosis, coarctation of the aorta, hypoplastic left heart syndrome) commonly present with symptoms of congestive heart failure or cardiogenic shock. Large shunt lesions cause pulmonary overcirculation and symptoms of heart failure. Pulmonary stenosis can cause cyanosis if a right-to-left shunt is present, but even if severe it rarely causes symptoms of congestive heart failure.

3. The following statements are true of furosemide therapy *except:*
a) It should be given rapidly intravenously.
b) The usual dose is 0.5 to 2.0 mg/kg.
c) It can cause hypokalemia.
d) It can cause hyperostosis and nephrocalcinosis in newborns.
e) It can cause hypochloremic alkalosis.

Answer
The answer is a. Furosemide should be given slowly intravenously because of the risk for ototoxicity that is associated with rapid intravenous administration. The other statements are all true.

4. An ACE inhibitor would be indicated for which of the following?
a) Pulmonary stenosis
b) Dilated cardiomyopathy
c) Atrial septal defect
d) Hypertrophic cardiomyopathy
e) Aortic stenosis

Answer
The answer is b. ACE inhibitors are useful in cases of reduced cardiac function. In hypertrophic cardiomyopathy, the systolic ventricular function is generally normal,

and the afterload reduction is contraindicated because it can provoke the left ventricular outflow tract obstruction. Afterload reduction is also contraindicated in cases of fixed outflow tract obstruction (e.g., aortic stenosis). Atrial septal defect causes right ventricular volume overload, and pulmonary stenosis causes right ventricular pressure overload. An ACE inhibitor would not be useful in either situation.

5. A 3-month-old girl with known congenital heart disease has been having brief intermittent episodes of cyanosis. Today, a few minutes after feeding, tachypnea, cyanosis, and persistent irritability developed. The *most* likely diagnosis is:
a) Breath-holding
b) Colic
c) Congestive heart failure
d) Hypercyanotic spell
e) Seizure

Answer
The answer is d. This is a fairly typical presentation in an infant with tetralogy of Fallot. She likely had mild "spells" previously. Without treatment, severe spells can cause seizures and death. Although β-blockers can be used to prevent hypercyanotic spells, the occurrence of spells is generally an indication for surgical intervention to increase the pulmonary blood flow.

6. Hypercyanotic spells can be provoked by any of the following *except:*
a) Pain
b) Induction of anesthesia
c) Dehydration
d) Iron deficiency
e) Squatting

Answer
The answer is e. Squatting has been noted to prevent or abort hypercyanotic spells in older children. All the other factors can precipitate spells through tachycardia, hypovolemia, or tissue hypoxia.

7. The treatment of hypercyanotic spells includes which of the following?
a) Isoproterenol
b) Adenosine
c) Digoxin
d) Oxygen
e) Furosemide

Answer
The answer is d. Oxygen is administered to reduce the hypoxemia. The intracardiac volume is increased by placing the infant in the knee-chest position or by administering intravenous fluid.

SUGGESTED READINGS

1. Artman M, Parrish MD, Graham TP. Congestive heart failure in childhood and adolescence: recognition and management. *Am Heart J* 1983;105:471–480.
2. Danford DA, Nasir A, Gumbiner C. Cost assessment of the evaluation of heart murmurs in children. *Pediatrics* 1993;91:365–368.
3. Danford DA. Sorting through the haystack-decision analysis and the search for heart disease among children with murmur. *J Pediatr* 2002;141:465–467.
4. Diwakaran A. Index of suspicion. Case 1. Cyanotic congenital heart disease. *Pediatr Rev* 1999;20:246–247.
5. McCrindle BW, Shaffer KM, Kan JS, et al. Cardinal clinical signs in the differentiation of heart murmurs in children. *Arch Pediatr Adolesc Med* 1996;150:169–174.
6. Owens TR. Chest pain in the adolescent. *Adolesc Med* 2001;12:95–104.
7. Pelech AN. Evaluation of the pediatric patient with a cardiac murmur. *Pediatr Clin North Am* 1999;46:167–188.
8. Reich JD, Miller S, Brogdon B, et al. The use of pulse oximetry to detect congenital heart disease. *J Pediatr* 2003;142:268–272.
9. Selbst SM. Pediatric chest pain: a prospective study. *Pediatrics* 1988;82:319–323.
10. Selbst SM. Pediatric chest pain: a prospective study. *Clin Pediatr* 1990;29:615–618.
11. Selbst SM. Consultation with the specialist: chest pain in children. *Pediatr Rev* 1997;18:169–173.
12. Shaddy RE. Optimizing treatment for chronic congestive heart failure in children. *Crit Care Med* 2001;29:S237–S240.
13. Singh A, Silberbach M. Cardiovascular preparticipation sports screening. *Pediatr Rev* 2006;27:418–423.
14. Swenson JM, Fischer DR, Miller SA, et al. Are chest radiographs and electrocardiograms still valuable in evaluating new pediatric patients with heart murmurs or chest pain? *Pediatrics* 1997;99:1–3.
15. Yi MS, Kimball TR, Tsevat J, et al. Evaluation of heart murmurs in children: cost-effectiveness and practical implications. *J Pediatr* 2002;141:504–511.

Chapter 25

Congenital Heart Disease

Athar M. Qureshi

In this chapter, some basic congenital heart lesions that are not only important from the perspective of the general pediatric board certification examinations, but also as a basis for understanding congenital heart disease in general pediatric practice, are discussed.

It is extremely important to understand the anatomy and physiology of each congenital lesion. By doing so, establishing the predominant physiologic effects and clinical presentation becomes easy. To achieve this goal, it is important to remember a few significant points:

- Blood flows down the path of least resistance.
- In general, pulmonary vascular resistance is lower that systemic vascular resistance. (*Exceptions* to this rule are fetal and newborn circulations, Eisenmenger syndrome, and pulmonary hypertension from various causes.)
- For cyanosis to occur from cardiac causes, there must be a right-to-left shunt occurring in the heart or between blood vessels.
- Delivery of deoxygenated blood, although not ideal, is better than little or no blood supply and can prevent shock-like states.

NONCYANOTIC HEART LESIONS

Ventricular Septal Defects

Ventricular septal defects (VSDs) can occur anywhere in the ventricular septum. *VSDs are the most common form of congenital heart disease (excluding bicuspid aortic valves)*. The physiologic effect of a VSD is determined by the size of the defect and the relative resistances of the systemic and pulmonary circulations. Small and moderate-sized VSDs often close spontaneously or get smaller over time. Even if a VSD remains small, it does not lead to congestive heart failure. Occasionally, small defects may be a nidus for infective endocarditis.

Large defects cause significant congestive heart failure, or "pulmonary overcirculation." Generally the pulmonary vascular resistance drops in the first few weeks and months of life. As the pulmonary vascular resistance drops, more blood is shunted from left to right, resulting in pulmonary overcirculation and enlargement of the left side of the heart. *Symptoms of congestive heart failure in infants are tachypnea, poor feeding, sweating with feeds, failure to thrive, and lethargy*. The growth chart of such infants is an invaluable tool in assessing the overall physiologic effect of the VSD. On physical exam, these infants may appear small, and have hepatomegaly. It is uncommon to hear rales or crackles in small babies with VSDs and congestive heart failure.

Cardiac examination can reveal a hyperdynamic precordium. Initially a systolic ejection murmur is heard and as the pulmonary vascular resistance drops, a *holosystolic murmur* may be heard. In very large defects, the murmur may remain systolic ejection in quality or not carry throughout systole, as there is little pressure difference between the two circulations. A diastolic rumble at the apex reflecting the large volume of shunted blood crossing the mitral valve as it is returned from the lungs may be heard in advanced congestive heart failure.

The CXR shows cardiomegaly and increased pulmonary vascular markings dilation of the pulmonary arteries. The electrocardiogram reflects left ventricular and atrial enlargement and sometimes left and right ventricular hypertrophy. Definitive diagnosis is made by transthoracic echocardiography.

The treatment of significant VSDs involves medical management initially before eventual surgical repair. Maximizing growth and feeding is an important initial step. Remember, feeding for any infant requires a lot of energy "relative" to an infant's body size. Patients with significant congenital heart disease require more calories to grow. This, in combination with the fact that they may tire or take breaks with feeds because of the additional amount of work needed to feed results in failure to thrive. In addition, some babies with congenital heart disease have genetic defects and gastroesophageal reflux, which can result in feeding difficulties. Thus maximizing caloric intake (preferably by increasing caloric density and not overall fluid intake) is essential. In addition, some babies with congenital heart disease may require nasogastric feeding before or after surgery. Nasogastric feeds take away the extra effort and energy required during feeding in these infants.

Medical treatment includes:

- Diuretics: Help treat the pulmonary overcirculation and fluid overload
- Digoxin: Helps with ventricular contractility
- Angiotensin converting enzyme (ACE) inhibitors: Alter the balance of resistances between the two circulations

By decreasing the systemic vascular resistance with ACE inhibitors, less blood is shunted to the pulmonary circulation, thus decreasing the extra blood flow to the lungs and heart.

Today, surgery in these infants is performed between 3 and 6 months of age routinely to prevent long standing pulmonary hypertension. Surgery beyond 2 years of age may increase the risk of pulmonary hypertension even after repair.

Atrial Septal Defects

Like VSDs, atrial septal defects can occur anywhere in the atrial septum. The most common ASD is called a secundum ASD. The left-to-right shunt is mainly dependent on the differences between the compliance of the two ventricular ventricles. Because the compliance difference between the two ventricles is not of a high magnitude, these children are asymptomatic and not at risk for early pulmonary hypertension, despite the increased pulmonary blood flow. Also, unlike patients with VSDs and PDAs, the right side of the heart is enlarged. *It is important to remember that the vast majority of patients with ASDs are asymptomatic in childhood. Only rarely do children with ASDs encounter problems early on in life, such as congestive heart failure or frequent lower respiratory tract infections*.

Examination reveals a systolic ejection murmur in the pulmonary area, indicative of excessive flow across the pulmonary valve. A diastolic rumble may be heard at the right and left lower sternal border because of extra flow across the tricuspid valve. *The hallmark of atrial septal defects is a fixed splitting of the second heart sound*. Normally the right ventricle empties slightly later than the left ventricle, thus accounting for the pulmonary component (P2) of the second heart sound (S2) to come after the aortic component (A2). This split is increased in inspiration because of the increase in venous return to the right ventricle. In patients with ASDs, the right ventricle is always volume loaded, both in expiration and inspiration, thus leading to a fixed, split second heart sound that does not vary with respiration. The CXR shows cardiomegaly with increased pulmonary flow. The EKG shows an RSR' pattern in VI, indicating right ventricular volume load. Transthoracic echocardiography allows accurate delineation of the anatomy.

Medical therapy is almost never needed in childhood. The majority of secundum ASDs are closed in the catheterization laboratory electively between the ages of 3 and 5 years. A small minority of secundum ASDs (because of large size and/or proximity to other structures) in addition to other forms of ASDs are closed surgically. Left untreated, significant ASDs can lead to pulmonary hypertension much later on in life.

Atrioventricular Canal Defects

Atrioventricular canal defects (AV canal defects) are a heterogeneous group of defects that result from defects in the endocardial cushion development. There are numerous subtypes and classifications, the most common form being the complete AV canal defect. In this lesion, there is a primum ASD and inlet VSD, resulting in defects in the atrial and ventricular septums that are in continuity. *It is important to remember that about 40% to 50% of patients with Down syndrome have congenital heart disease. Of those patients, 40% to 50% have AV canal defects.*

Infants with complete AV canal defects have clinical presentations similar to that of infants with large VSDs. Likewise, the CXR is similar to that of infants with large VSDs. The electrocardiogram shows features of VSDs and ASDs. The classic eletcrocardiographic feature is left axis deviation and a frontal plane axis that is superiorly oriented. Diagnosis is made by echocardiography.

Medical therapy is similar to that for infants with large VSDs. Surgical repair is usually performed between 3 and 6 months of life. In addition to feeding difficulties encountered with this lesion, infants with Down syndrome may have more feeding difficulties.

Patent Ductus Arteriosus

Children with a patent ductus arteriosus (PDA) may present any time in life. Closure of PDAs in term newborns normally occurs soon after birth. PDAs are frequently encountered lesion in premature babies. In premature babies, initially there may be predominantly right-to-left shunting of blood. In these babies, the PDA acts as a "pop-off" for the high resistance pulmonary circulation. PDAs in these circumstances should not be closed, as closure could result in a further increase in pulmonary hypertension, and an extra strain on the right ventricle. As the pulmonary vascular resistance falls, there is a predominant left-to-right shunt. The left side of the heart enlarges. Neonates become more tachypneic or if ventilated, their ventilatory support parameters increase, and hepatomegaly develops. There is a wide pulse pressure and the pulses are bounding because of the "runoff" in diastole in the aorta.

The cardiac exam reveals a hyperactive precordium. *A continuous machinery-like murmur* (systolic and diastolic component) is heard in the left infraclavicular region and throughout the precordium. The CXR shows cardiomegaly and the EKG is consistent with left ventricular and atrial volume overload. Echocardiography is diagnostic and provides accurate assessment of the degree of shunting in systole and diastole, and the relative resistances of the pulmonary and systemic circulations.

In premature babies, closure can be achieved with non-steroidal anti-inflammatory medications (NSAIDs) such as indomethacin and ibuprofen. NSAIDs are contraindicated in neonates with severe thrombocytopenia and impaired renal function. Fluid restriction is also advantageous. If these measures fail, surgical ligation is indicated for clinically significant PDAs in the newborn period.

Infants and older children with PDAs are often asymptomatic and a PDA is only diagnosed upon hearing a murmur on routine physical exam. If the PDA is large, they may present with congestive heart failure and failure to thrive. The vast majority of these PDAs are closed in the catheterization laboratory with coils or devices.

CYANOTIC HEART LESIONS

Tetralogy of Fallot

Tetralogy of Fallot is the most common cause of cyanotic congenital heart disease. It is a conotruncal abnormality, and *it is associated with DiGeorge syndrome.* The four components of the defect are:

1. A VSD
2. An overriding aorta
3. Pulmonary stenosis (or right ventricular outflow tract obstruction at other levels)
4. Right ventricular hypertrophy

The clinical presentation is variable. Patients with minimal right ventricular outflow tract obstruction may only be detected upon auscultation of a murmur. Infants with severe right ventricular outflow tract obstruction are cyanotic.

Infants may be cyanotic or pink on exam, depending on the degree of obstruction to pulmonary blood flow. The cardiac examination reveals an increased right ventricular impulse. There is a harsh, high frequency systolic ejection murmur (from the right ventricular outflow tract obstruction) heard at the left middle and upper sternal border, which radiates to the lung fields and back. The CXR shows a "boot-shaped" heart (the hypertrophic right ventricle causes the apex to be "lifted up") and decreased pulmonary vascular markings resulting from decreased pulmonary flow (Fig. 25.1). The electrocardiogram is consistent with right ventricular hypertrophy. Transthoracic echocardiography defines the precise anatomy of the components of the defect and other associated lesions.

Hypercyanotic episodes, or "Tet spells," are also discussed in Chapter 24. These are bouts in which infants are

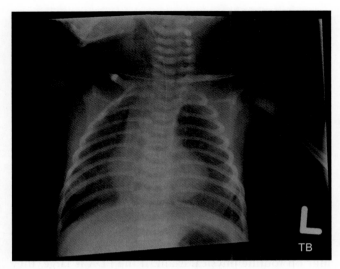

Figure 25.1 CXR (AP view) in a patient with tetralogy of Fallot. Note the dark lung fields (decreased pulmonary blood flow) and upturned cardiac apex, representing a "boot-shaped heart."

inconsolable and extremely cyanotic. The exact etiology of these spells is unknown, although various theories have been proposed. Treatment includes consoling the patient (handing the baby over to a parent), and assuming a knee-chest position. The knee-chest position increases the systemic vascular resistance, thereby forcing more blood to flow to the lungs and less deoxygenated blood to flow to the systemic circulation. Oxygen, fluid resuscitation, administration of morphine, phenylephrine (increases systemic vascular resistance and forces more blood to the lungs), and beta-blockers (decreasing heart rate and thus potentially decreasing the obstruction to pulmonary blood flow) are options for medical therapy *It is important to remember that the murmur during a "tet spell" is actually softer and not louder. This is because less blood flows across the right ventricular outflow tract (cause of the murmur) in a "tet spell."*

Treatment is eventual surgery within the first year of life. For severe hypercyanotic episodes, a palliative systemic to pulmonary artery shunt (i.e., Blalock-Taussig [BT] shunt) improves oxygenation before an eventual complete repair of the lesion can be performed.

Transposition of the Great Arteries

Transposition of the great arteries (TGA) is the most common form of cyanotic congenital heart disease diagnosed in the newborn period. This is because many patients with tetralogy of Fallot are not severely cyanotic and are diagnosed later in life. Babies with TGA, however, are profoundly cyanotic. The pulmonary and systemic circulations are in parallel and not in a circuit. Thus, long-term survival is not possible unless there is a communication between the two circulations, which may occur at the atrial or ventricular levels or via a patent ductus arteriosus. It is more common in males and

in infants of diabetic mothers. The cardiac exam may only reveal a systolic ejection murmur. The CXR shows normal or increased pulmonary vascular markings (no obstruction to pulmonary flow) and a classic "egg on a string" shaped heart (Fig. 25.2). This is because of a narrow mediastinum from the direct anterior-posterior relationship of the great arteries. Transthoracic echocardiography is diagnostic.

Prostaglandin is essential early on in the infant to maintain patency of the arterial duct and promote mixing. If the atrial communication is not sufficiently large, a balloon atrial septostomy is performed to enlarge the atrial communication. An arterial switch operation (translocating the great vessels above the semilunar valves to the respective ventricles with coronary artery translocation) is performed in the first couple of weeks of life.

Total Anomalous Pulmonary Venous Return

Total anomalous pulmonary venous return (TAPVR) refers to a condition in which the pulmonary veins drain anomalously to the systemic venous system instead of to the left atrium. TAPVR may be:

- Supracardiac (drainage to the innominate vein or superior vena cava [SVC])
- Cardiac (drainage to the coronary sinus), or
- Infracardiac (drainage to the inferior vena cava)

A prominent right ventricular impulse is felt because of the enlarged right ventricle. All of these infants have an ASD, which can be reflected on examination. A gallop rhythm may be heard as well. The CXR shows cardiomegaly and increased pulmonary blood flow. In supracardiac TAPVR a "snowman" appearance on CXR is seen. There are two shadows seen, a wide superior shadow from the pulmonary venous confluence and enlarged innominate vein and superior vena cava, and an inferior shadow representing the heart.

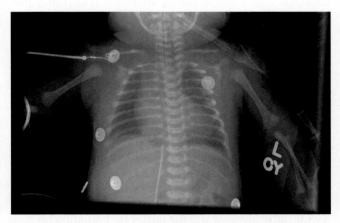

Figure 25.2 CXR (AP view) in an infant with transposition of the great arteries. The somewhat narrow mediastinum gives the appearance of an "egg on a string."

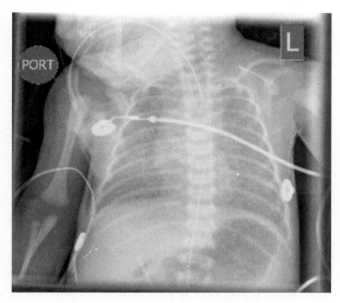

Figure 25.3 CXR of a neonate with *obstructed* total anomalous pulmonary venous return (TAPVR). Note the reticular pattern seen in both lung fields from pulmonary edema because of severe obstruction of the pulmonary venous drainage. The lung field findings mimic that seen with interstitial pneumonia and respiratory distress syndrome. In *obstructed* TAPVR, the heart size is small, because of little pulmonary venous drainage getting back to the heart.

Supracardiac and infracardiac types of TAPVR may become obstructed. In obstructed TAPVR, the heart size is normal on CXR (not getting enough blood return from the lungs) and there are prominent pulmonary vascular markings because of pulmonary venous obstruction (Fig. 25.3). A reticular pattern is seen in the lungs because of pulmonary venous congestion. The clinical picture and CXR can be confused with an infant with respiratory distress syndrome or interstitial pneumonia. Because of poor output, this can lead to shock quickly. Emergent surgical repair is indicated if an infant has obstructed TAPVR, otherwise elective surgery is performed.

Obstructive Left-Sided Lesions

Obstruction of the left-sided structures may occur at any level or at multiple levels. *Infants with critical aortic stenosis or critical coarctation of the aorta present in shock.* This is true also for babies with the extreme form of left-sided obstruction, *hypoplastic left heart syndrome.* Physical exam reveals pallor, cool extremities, absent or weak pulses, and signs of decreased perfusion to vital organs, i.e., poor urine output. In addition, they are acidotic. *Maintaining patency of the arterial duct with prostaglandin is life-saving in these infants.* Though this means deoxygenated blood will be supplying a portion of the systemic circulation, this is well tolerated by infants and is sufficient to maintain cardiac output and perfusion to vital organs.

Coarctation of the aorta may present early or later on in life. If not critical, these patients do not present in shock. Weak or absent lower extremity pulses with upper extremity hypertension is characteristic. *There is a significant blood pressure discrepancy in the upper extremity blood pressure compared to the lower extremity blood pressure.* A radio femoral delay in pulses may be present. The CXR may show a 3 sign (from the narrowed segment of aorta). Later in life, collateral vessels develop to supply the lower body beyond the narrowed aortic segment and can cause erosion of some ribs, leading to "rib notching" on the CXR. Treatment is surgical and in some cases in the angioplasty or stent placement in the catheterization laboratory.

Coronary Anomalies

There are numerous coronary anomalies that are beyond the scope of this text. However, two anomalies merit brief discussion. The normal coronary artery branching pattern is depicted in Figure 25.4.

The first anomaly is *anomalous left coronary artery form the pulmonary artery (ALCAPA).* In this lesion, the left coronary artery arises from the pulmonary artery instead of the aorta (Fig. 25.5). Initially, babies may be relatively asymptomatic. Although the left coronary artery is receiving deoxygenated blood, it is initially perfused at a relatively higher pressure in a newborn because of the elevated pulmonary vascular resistance. As the pulmonary vascular resistance drops, the effect of deoxygenated

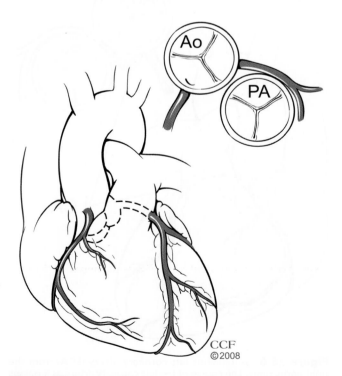

Figure 25.4 Normal coronary artery branching pattern. (See color insert.)

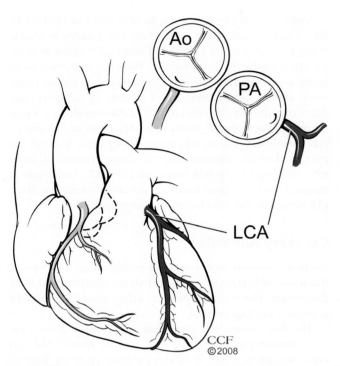

Figure 25.5 Anomalous left coronary artery from the pulmonary artery (ALCAPA). The left coronary artery (LCA) is perfused with deoxygenated blood (blue color), leading to ischemic changes. (See color insert.)

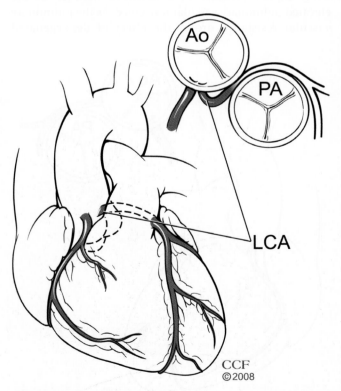

Figure 25.6 Anomalous left coronary artery (LCA) from the right aortic sinus. The course of the left coronary artery as it passes between the aorta and pulmonary artery is seen. This can lead to compression of the LCA, *exertional symptoms*, and sometimes sudden death. (See color insert.)

blood to the myocardium is compounded with the lower perfusion pressure in the coronary artery. These infants are extremely "irritable," especially when they feed, in essence from angina during this period of exertion. Cardiomegaly is seen on CXR and the electrocardiogram shows ischemia. Surgical correction is warranted soon after diagnosis.

The second important coronary anomaly to remember is an anomalous coronary artery originating from an *inappropriate aortic sinus*. The most common of these defects is the left coronary artery from the right sinus of valsalva (Fig. 25.6). Although the left coronary artery comes off the aorta, its anatomy and course is abnormal. It may also become compressed between the two great vessels during activity, resulting in chest pain or syncope with activity. *It is important to remember that chest pain and syncope during exertion are red flags that warrant cardiac evaluation.* The definitive diagnosis is made by angiography, although nowadays noninvasive testing such as a computed tomography scan or magnetic resonance imaging can pinpoint the diagnosis as well. Treatment is surgical.

REVIEW EXERCISES

QUESTIONS

1. A 1-month-old previously well male infant presents with poor feeding. His parents state that 5 minutes after starting to feed he becomes sweaty and fatigued.

Physical examination reveals a HR = 165 bpm, RR = 90 bpm, BP = 80/63, O2 sat = 97%. The infant is pink and tachypneic and has hepatomegaly. There is a harsh holosystolic murmur at the left sternum. There are normal pulses in all four extremities. Of the following, the *most likely* diagnosis is:
a) Atrial septal defect
b) Tetralogy of Fallot
c) Ventricular septal defect
d) Hypoplastic left heart syndrome

Answer
The answer is c. This infant has signs and symptoms of congestive heart failure or pulmonary overcirculation caused by a VSD. It is exceedingly rare for an ASD to lead to congestive heart failure. Patients with tetralogy of Fallot present with cyanosis and the murmur heard is a systolic ejection murmur from pulmonary stenosis or right ventricular outflow tract obstruction. Infants with hypoplastic left heart syndrome present in shock.

2. Appropriate medical therapy for the infant in question #1 might include all of the following *except:*
a) Digoxin
b) Oxygen

c) Furosemide
d) Angiotensin converting enzyme (ACE) inhibitor

Answer

The answer is b. Diuretics such as Lasix help treat infants whose lungs and liver become congested because of heart failure. Digoxin helps with cardiac contractility and ACE inhibitors decrease the systemic vascular resistance, thus promoting more blood flow to the systemic circulation and less blood flow to the lungs. Oxygen is a pulmonary vasodilator and would increase pulmonary blood flow, thus making the congestive heart failure worse. Moreover, oxygen is also a systemic vasoconstrictor, forcing more blood to go to the pulmonary circulation than systemic circulation.

3. A 5-year-old child undergoes a cardiac catheterization and the hemodynamic data reveals saturations as follows: SVC 70%, RA of 85%, RV 86%, MPA 85%, LPA 85%, RPA 85%, aorta 98%. These data are *most likely* consistent with a diagnosis of:
a) Ventricular septal defect
b) Patent ductus arteriosus
c) Atrial septal defect
d) No structural heart disease

Answer

The answer is c. It is important to understand basic cardiac catheterization and hemodynamic data. Generally, the saturation in normal individuals in the right side of the heart is in the 70% range. Of course, normal individuals are fully saturated in the left sided of the heart, with saturations close to or equal to 100%. When encountered with a problem like this, a quick drawing of the heart makes interpreting the data easy. In this case, the right atrial saturation is higher than it should be. (It should be the same as the SVC saturation, i.e., 70%.) Therefore, an ASD must have accounted for that because of the left-to-right shunt. When trying to identify a lesion in a question like this, identify the first chamber or vessel in which the saturation increased. Had the first saturation increase (or "step-up" in saturation) been in the right ventricle, this would have been a VSD. Similarly, if the "step-up" in saturation occurred in the pulmonary artery, this patient would have had a PDA.

4. A 5-day-old infant presents with severe tachypnea, and mild cyanosis. On examination, he has poor perfusion, hepatomegaly and a 2/6 systolic ejection murmur at the left upper sternal border. He becomes acidotic over the next few hours. His CXR shows a reticular pattern with a small heart size. The most likely diagnosis is:
a) Obstructed total anomalous pulmonary venous return
b) Transposition of the great vessels
c) Interstitial pneumonia
d) VSD

Answer

The answer is a. This infant has signs of obstructed total anomalous pulmonary venous return. Because of the obstructed pulmonary venous return, the baby presents with tachypnea and rapidly develops pulmonary edema and then shock. The heart size is small because of little pulmonary venous return. The cardiac signs initially may be very subtle, and it is often difficult to initially distinguish this from interstitial pneumonia or RDS on the CXR. Transposition of the great arteries presents with profound cyanosis. Infants with VSDs present with signs of congestive heart failure, not shock.

5. The finding *most* suggestive of neonatal coarctation of the aorta is:
a) BP higher in the arms than legs
b) O_2 saturation lower in the arms than the legs
c) Bounding femoral pulses
d) Wide pulse pressure

Answer

The answer is a. Patients with coarctation of the aorta have increased upper extremity blood pressure and decreased or absent lower extremity pulses. *If the coarctation is critical,* infants present in shock and the PDA supplies the aorta distal to the coarctation, leading to lower saturation in the lower extremities, not in the upper extremities. Wide pulse pressure and bounding pulses are seen in patients with PDAs.

6. You are reviewing the catheterization data on a patient who just came up to the pediatric ward. The data show the following pressures: RA mean 6 mm Hg; RV 25/06 mm Hg; PA 22/10,16 mm Hg; LV 130/5,14 mm Hg; ascending aorta 80/50,65 mm Hg; descending aorta 80/50,65 mm Hg. These data are *most likely* consistent with a diagnosis of:
a) Pulmonary stenosis
b) Coarctation of the aorta
c) Aortic stenosis
d) No structural heart disease

Answer

The answer is c. Similar to Question 3, figure out where the change occurred, and the diagnosis becomes very easy. In this patient the systolic pressure from the LV to aorta decreased. (The systolic pressures in the LV and aorta should be the same.) Thus narrowing of the aortic valve, aortic stenosis must have accounted for this finding. Similarly, the systolic pressure in the right ventricle and pulmonary arteries should be the same.

7. You are seeing a 3-month-child who has had poor growth and feeding. His parents report that he has recurrent episodes of sweating with feeds, tachypnea, and irritability mostly when he feeds. In addition, he is noted to be extremely pale with these episodes. Despite "rocking and consoling him," he remains irritable during and immediately after feeds. The infant is pink and tachypneic. The liver is enlarged. There is a high pitched holosystolic murmur at the apex. His CXR reveals cardiomegaly. His EKG shows q waves in leads 1, aVL, V5, and V6, along with ST elevation in V5 and V6. Of the following, the *most likely* diagnosis is:

a) Colic
b) Atrial septal defect
c) Ventricular septal defect
d) Anomalous left coronary artery from the PA

Answer

The answer is d. This infant is experiencing angina when he feeds. Although irritability in infants is common, clues in this question are irritability, sweating with feeds, and tachypnea. The cardiac exam is abnormal because the holosystolic murmur is from mitral valve regurgitation resulting from ischemia of the mitral valve–supporting apparatus. The EKG shows an ischemic pattern. This infant has an anomalous left coronary artery from the pulmonary artery (ALCAPA). Although rare, this presentation is important to remember.

SUGGESTED READINGS

1. Allen HD, Driscoll DJ, Shaddy RE, Feltes TF, eds. *Moss and Adams' heart disease in infants, children, and adolescents: including the fetus and young adult,* 7th ed. Baltimore: Lippincott Williams & Wilkins, 2007.
2. Keane JF, Lock JE, Fyler DC, Nadas AS, eds. *Nadas' pediatric cardiology,* 2nd ed. Philadelphia: Saunders, 2006.
3. Kliegman R, Nelson WE, Behrman RE, et al., eds. *Nelson textbook of pediatrics,* 18th ed. Philadelphia: Saunders, 2007.
4. Silberbach M, Hannon D. Presentation of congenital heart disease in the neonate and young infant. *Pediatr Rev* 2007;28:123–131.

Chapter 26

Acquired Heart Disease

Daniel J. Murphy Jr.

INFECTIVE ENDOCARDITIS

Infective endocarditis remains a serious illness in children. Causative bacteria include:

- Viridans streptococci (40%)
- *Staphylococcus aureus* (30%)
- *Staphylococcus epidermidis* (5%)
- Fungal pathogens (1%–10%)

Less often, endocarditis can be caused by enterococci, pneumococci, *Pseudomonas* spp., and a variety of other less common organisms, including those of the HACEK group (*Haemophilus parainfluenzae, Haemophilus aphrophilus, Actinobacillus actinomycetemcomitans, Cardiobacterium hominis, Eikenella* species, and *Kingella* spp.). In addition to bacteria, a variety of fungi can cause infective endocarditis (*Candida* spp. and *Aspergillus*), especially in patients treated with broad-spectrum antibiotics and steroids, premature infants, and patients with indwelling catheters.

Pertinent historical features in the patient with infective endocarditis include an underlying heart defect, a recent dental procedure or disease, and a previous episode of endocarditis. The illness is generally indolent, with an insidious onset that develops over weeks to months. Anorexia, lethargy, fever, weight loss, and night sweats are prominent historical features. Common clinical manifestations include:

- Heart murmur suggesting valvular regurgitation
- Splenomegaly
- Skin manifestations, such as petechiae and splinter hemorrhages

Classic findings, such as Janeway lesions (painless lesions on the palms and soles), Osler nodes (painful lesions on the pads of the fingers and toes), and Roth spots (retinal hemorrhages), are seen less often. *The key to the diagnosis of endocarditis is a blood culture positive for the causative organism.* At least three blood cultures should be obtained and need not be timed to fever spikes. The first blood culture is positive in >90% of the patients with subacute endocarditis. Supporting laboratory findings include anemia, leukocytosis with a left shift, elevated acute phase reactants, and microscopic hematuria.

For a select group of patients the American Heart Association recommends prophylactic antibiotics to prevent the development of bacterial endocarditis. Endocarditis prophylaxis is indicated for patients undergoing dental procedures that involve manipulation of gingival tissue or the periapical region of teeth or perforation of the oral mucosa, tonsillectomy or adenoidectomy, a surgical procedure, or biopsy involving the respiratory mucosa. In a significant change from prior guidelines, patients undergoing genitourinary and gastrointestinal procedures no longer require endocarditis prophylaxis.

According to the current guidelines, patients with the following conditions should receive prophylactic antibiotics:

- Prosthetic cardiac valve
- Previous infective endocarditis
- Unrepaired cyanotic CHD, including shunts and conduits
- Completely repaired CHD with prosthetic material or device within 6 months
- Repaired CHD with residual defects at the site or adjacent to the site of prosthetic patch or device.
- Cardiac transplant recipients with valvulopathy

Except for the conditions listed in the preceding, antibiotic prophylaxis is no longer recommended for any other form of CHD. A heart murmur alone is not an indication for antibiotic prophylaxis. Specifically, patients with innocent heart murmurs do not require pretreatment.

According to the current recommendations, standard general prophylaxis for dental, oral, respiratory tract, or esophageal procedures includes amoxicillin (50 mg/kg orally 1 hour before the procedure; maximum dose, 2.0 g), clindamycin (20 mg/kg orally 1 hour before the procedure; maximum dose, 600 mg), or cephalexin (50 mg/kg orally 1 hour before the procedure; maximum dose, 2.0 g). For patients unable to take oral medications, intramuscular or intravenous ampicillin, intravenous clindamycin, or intravenous or intramuscular cefazolin or ceftriaxone are acceptable.

ACUTE RHEUMATIC FEVER

Acute rheumatic fever is an immunologic disease, the delayed sequela of group A streptococcal infection of the pharynx. *Streptococcal skin infections or infections at other sites do not cause the subsequent development of acute rheumatic fever.* The causative *Streptococcus* organism belongs to the mucoid group A type 18 (M-18). Acute rheumatic fever generally develops 1 to 5 weeks following streptococcal pharyngitis; however, a history of clinical infection may not be obtained. The latent period between the streptococcal infection and the development of isolated chorea may be as long as 2 to 6 months.

The diagnosis of acute rheumatic fever is made according to the revised Jones criteria (Table 26.1). The diagnosis requires evidence of a recent streptococcal infection (elevated antistreptolysin O [ASO] titer or a throat culture positive for group A streptococcus) in addition to the presence of either two major criteria or one major criterion and two minor criteria. *Remember that arthralgia cannot be used as a minor criterion when polyarthritis is a major finding, and a prolonged PR interval cannot be used when carditis is a major finding.*

The treatment of acute rheumatic fever includes the administration of 0.6 to 1.2 million units of benzathine penicillin G intramuscularly. Anti-inflammatory medications can be given but should be withheld until a definitive diagnosis is established. Bed rest is generally advised during the inflammatory process. For severe carditis or resistant symptoms, steroids can be administered. The prevention of subsequent acute rheumatic fever is highly desirable, and a regimen of 1.2 million units of benzathine penicillin G given intramuscularly every 21 to 28 days is recommended. Less effective alternatives include 250 mg of oral penicillin twice a day or 250 mg of oral erythromycin twice

TABLE 26.1

REVISED JONES CRITERIA FOR THE DIAGNOSIS OF ACUTE RHEUMATIC FEVER

Major	Minor
Carditis (40%–50%)	Previous acute rheumatic fever
Polyarthritis (60%–85%)	Arthralgia
Chorea (15%)	Fever
Subcutaneous nodules (2%–10%)	Prolonged PR interval
Erythema marginatum (10%)	Elevated acute phase reactants

Either two major or one major and two minor criteria plus evidence of a recent streptococcal infection.

a day. Prophylactic antibiotics are generally continued through childhood. Lifetime prophylaxis is recommended for patients with valvular involvement or in high-risk occupations, such as teaching.

KAWASAKI DISEASE

Kawasaki disease is an immunologically mediated disease of unknown cause. It most commonly affects children between the ages of 6 months and 2 years and presents as total body inflammation.

Because the etiologic agent in Kawasaki disease has not been identified, the diagnosis is based on specific criteria (Table 26.2). *For a diagnosis of Kawasaki disease, the presence of fever for 5 days or more must be documented, in addition to at least four of the other five features.* Skin changes include papular and maculopapular rashes and erythema multiforme. Conjunctivitis is usually bilateral. Oral pharyngeal changes generally include erythematous involvement of the anterior oral pharynx, cracking of the lips, and reddening of the tongue (strawberry tongue). In addition to the diagnostic criteria, frequently associated clinical findings include severe irritability, abdominal pain, and diarrhea. Other associated findings include:

- Urethritis with sterile pyuria (70%)
- Aseptic meningitis (50%)
- Hepatitis (30%)
- Arthralgia and arthritis (10%–20%)
- Hydrops of the gallbladder (15%)
- Myocarditis with congestive heart failure (5%)
- Uveitis

Typical laboratory findings include leukocytosis, anemia, elevation of acute phase reactants (e.g., erythrocyte sedimentation rate and C-reactive protein), and thrombocytosis. Mild to moderate elevations in serum transaminases occur in 40% of patients, sterile pyuria in 33%, and cerebrospinal fluid (CSF) pleocytosis in 50% of those who undergo lumbar puncture.

The most serious clinical complication of Kawasaki disease is the development of coronary artery aneurysms, seen in approximately 20% of untreated children. Coronary artery aneurysms are diagnosed by echocardiography. Congestive heart failure or arrhythmias can also develop in children with Kawasaki disease. An echocardiogram is required when the diagnosis of Kawasaki disease is considered.

Patients with Kawasaki disease are treated with intravenous immune globulin 2 g/kg as a continuous infusion. In addition, aspirin 80 to 100 mg/kg per day in four divided doses should be administered as soon as Kawasaki disease is suspected. Once the patient is afebrile or when signs of acute inflammation resolve, the aspirin dose is reduced to 3 to 5 mg/kg per day and continued for 6 to 8 weeks. If coronary artery aneurysms develop, aspirin is continued indefinitely. Corticosteroids are *not* currently recommended for the treatment of Kawasaki disease. However, in cases of resistant or recurrent disease, steroids can be administered.

PERICARDITIS

Pericarditis is an acute inflammation of the pericardium. It is usually idiopathic or secondary to viral infection. Other causes include acute rheumatic fever, bacterial infection (purulent pericarditis), tuberculosis, collagen-vascular disease, and uremia. Pericarditis can also follow cardiac surgery or treatment of malignancy.

The patient may have a history of a preceding upper respiratory illness or a predisposing feature. The hallmarks of the illness include fever and chest pain. The pain is generally precordial, with radiation to the shoulder or neck. It tends to be constant but may be worse when the patient is in the supine position and exacerbated by swallowing or breathing. Clinical examination may reveal a pericardial friction rub. The signs of cardiac tamponade including tachycardia, pulsus paradoxus, jugular venous distension, and hepatomegaly. Distant heart tones may develop if a large pericardial effusion is present. In most cases, pericarditis produces only a small effusion. The electrocardiogram (Fig. 26.1) characteristically shows global ST elevation with flattened or inverted T waves. In addition, a depressed PR segment may be present. Echocardiography may demonstrate a pericardial effusion, but the absence of pericardial effusion indicated on the echocardiogram does not exclude the diagnosis of pericarditis, and echocardiography is not routinely required.

The management of pericarditis is generally symptomatic. Nonsteroidal anti-inflammatory medications are given for pain and fever. Cases complicated by a large pericardial fluid collection or cardiac tamponade require pericardiocentesis. The presence of purulent or tuberculous pericarditis is an indication for urgent surgical drainage and intravenous antibiotics. Corticosteroids are generally not necessary for the treatment of uncomplicated pericarditis but are useful in cases of severe rheumatic carditis or resistant postpericardiotomy syndrome.

TABLE 26.2

DIAGNOSTIC CRITERIA FOR KAWASAKI DISEASE

Fever for 5 days or longer
Skin changes (rash)
Extremity changes (erythema, induration, desquamation)
Bilateral nonpurulent conjunctivitis
Oropharyngeal changes (cracked red lips, "strawberry" tongue)
Lymphadenopathy (>1.5 cm)

Patient must have fever and at least four of the remaining five features given above.

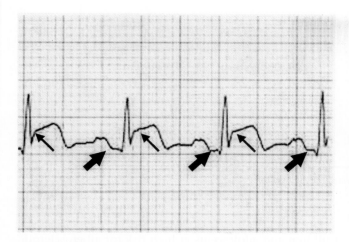

Figure 26.1 Electrocardiogram in pericarditis. Typical features include global elevation of the ST segment (*thin arrows*) and depression of the PR segment (*thick arrows*).

MYOCARDITIS

Myocarditis is an inflammation of the myocardium that is usually caused by a viral infection; coxsackievirus B (various serotypes), rhinovirus, adenovirus, influenza virus, Epstein-Barr virus, and varicella zoster virus are most frequently implicated. Other infectious agents that can cause inflammation or infection of the myocardium include rickettsiae, bacteria, fungi, and parasites. Noninfectious causes include acute rheumatic fever, inflammatory and rheumatic diseases, and various toxins.

The clinical manifestations of myocarditis depend on the severity of the infection. A history of a preceding upper respiratory or other viral prodrome may be obtained. Signs of congestive heart failure may be evident, specifically a third heart sound (S_3) gallop. Nonspecific electrocardiographic features include low QRS voltage, ST-T–wave changes, conduction disturbances, and pseudoinfarction.

The treatment of myocarditis is supportive and symptomatic. Restricted activity or bed rest is generally recommended until all signs of inflammation have resolved. Diuretics (furosemide 1 mg/kg) may be given. In more severe cases, oxygen may be administered or intravenous inotropic agents infused (e.g., dopamine, dobutamine). Treatment with immunosuppressive agents, corticosteroids, or intravenous immune globulin has not been reproducibly demonstrated to be efficacious and remains controversial.

DILATED CARDIOMYOPATHY

The term *dilated cardiomyopathy* is used to describe a weakened myocardium with reduced systolic function. The pathologic examination generally demonstrates myocardial fibrosis and necrosis secondary to infectious, toxic, or metabolic agents. Viruses have been implicated in the

development of dilated cardiomyopathy. *The antineoplastic agent Adriamycin has been associated with the late development of dilated cardiomyopathy.* Patients who receive a total dose of more than 500 mg/m^2, especially with adjunctive radiation therapy, are at increased risk for the development of late dilated cardiomyopathy. Finally, a number of genetically determined familial forms of dilated cardiomyopathy are known to exist and may account for up to 30% of the patients.

A history of prior viral illness may be obtained in some patients who present with cardiomyopathy. Generally, the earliest signs are congestive heart failure, weakness, and fatigue. The electrocardiogram demonstrates left ventricular hypertrophy and *ST-T-wave changes.* The chest roentgenogram demonstrates cardiomegaly with increased pulmonary venous markings. The most useful diagnostic test is echocardiography, which generally demonstrates a dilated left ventricle with diminished systolic ventricular function.

The treatment of dilated cardiomyopathy includes the administration of diuretics, digoxin, and angiotensin-converting enzyme inhibitors. β-Blockers have not been routinely used in children, and there is no published evidence of their efficacy. Anticoagulation may be necessary to prevent the development of intracardiac thrombus. Cardiac transplantation is an option when more conservative medical management strategies fail.

HYPERTROPHIC CARDIOMYOPATHY

Hypertrophic cardiomyopathy is a genetically transmitted abnormality of the myocardial proteins that results in hypertrophy of the ventricular myocardium, especially the intraventricular septum. The disease is transmitted as an autosomal-dominant trait. Although the systolic function is preserved, diastolic function is usually impaired. In addition, septal hypertrophy can cause left ventricular outflow obstruction in a significant percentage of affected persons.

Septal and left ventricular hypertrophy can develop in the newborn infants of mothers with diabetes. Although these infants may be symptomatic, the hypertrophy usually resolves within several weeks. Hypertrophic cardiomyopathy is occasionally seen in infants and young children, especially in association with Noonan syndrome; however, most familial cases of hypertrophic cardiomyopathy remain undetected until adolescence or young adulthood. The family history is positive in 30% of patients. Symptoms include exercise intolerance, arrhythmias, syncope, and sudden death. The clinical findings of hypertrophic cardiomyopathy are subtle and 25% have no auscultatory abnormalities. Most suggestive is a systolic ejection murmur produced by left ventricular outflow tract obstruction. The murmur is increased by maneuvers and agents that increase contractility or decrease preload or afterload (e.g., exercise, standing,

TABLE 26.3

HYPERLIPIDEMIA IN CHILDREN

	Total Cholesterol	LDL Cholesterol	Treatment
Desirable	<170 mg/dL	<110 mg/dL	None
Borderline	110–130 mg/dL	110–130 mg/dL	Diet therapy
High	>200 mg/dL	>130 mg/dL	Diet therapy
		>190 mg/dL	Drug therapy
Other concerns	Triglycerides >150 mg/dL		
	HDL-C <35 mg/dL		

HDL-C, high-density lipoprotein cholesterol; LDL, low-density lipoprotein.

the straining phase of the Valsalva maneuver, digitalis, amyl nitrate, and nitroglycerin). The murmur is decreased by squatting, handgrip, β-blockade, and general anesthesia. A holosystolic murmur at the apex suggests the presence of mitral regurgitation. Third and fourth heart sounds are often audible. The electrocardiographic pattern is abnormal in most cases, demonstrating left ventricular hypertrophy, *ST-T-wave changes*, pre-excitation, and arrhythmias. The echocardiogram is diagnostic and generally shows asymmetric hypertrophy of the left ventricular myocardium.

Children and adolescents with hypertrophic cardiomyopathy are restricted from participating in highly competitive sports. If significant left ventricular outflow tract obstruction is present, surgical myectomy is recommended. Medical treatment of patients with congestive heart failure occasionally includes the administration of β-blockers or calcium channel blockers, although the response to medical therapy is limited. Antibiotic prophylaxis is recommended for all patients with hypertrophic cardiomyopathy. In cases of syncope or significant arrhythmia, antitachycardia/defibrillator systems are implanted.

PREVENTIVE CARDIOLOGY

Atherosclerotic cardiovascular disease is the leading cause of death and disability in the United States, and atherosclerotic lesions are present at autopsy in children and young adults. Therefore, primary prevention of atherosclerotic cardiovascular disease should begin in childhood. Appropriate health promotion goals include:

- An overall healthy eating pattern
- Appropriate body weight
- Desirable lipid profile
- Desirable blood pressure
- No new initiation of cigarette smoking
- No exposure to environmental tobacco smoke
- Complete cessation for those who smoke
- Physical activity every day
- Reduce sedentary time (e.g., television watching, video games)

Children and adolescents at high risk for atherosclerotic disease should be identified through:

- Family history of obesity, hypertension, dyslipidemia, and premature cardiovascular disease
- Height, weight, and blood pressure recordings
- Diet and physical activity assessment
- Cigarette smoking assessment starting at 9 to 10 years of age
- Targeted screening of fasting lipids in children older than 2 years

Table 26.3 lists desirable lipid levels and recommended treatment of children and adolescents with hyperlipidemia. Treatment of all children with hypercholesterolemia begins with diet intervention. Pharmacologic intervention should be considered for patients 8 years and older with an LDL concentration of ≥190 mg/dL (or ≥160 mg/dL with a family history of early heart disease or ≥2 additional risk factors or ≥ 130 mg/dL with diabetes mellitus. There are no studies of long-term safety or efficacy of lipid lowering drugs in the pediatric population, but lovastatin and atorvastatin are approved for use in children older than 10 years. Potentially serious adverse effects include hepatitis, myositis, and rhabdomyolysis.

REVIEW EXERCISES

QUESTIONS

Case 1

A 4-year-old girl is seen 10 days following an upper respiratory infection. Her knees and ankles are swollen and painful, and her temperature is 40°C (104°F). The cardiac examination is significant for a grade 6/6 systolic murmur at the apex.

1. These findings are consistent with which of the following?
a) Acute rheumatic fever
b) Septic arthritis
c) Juvenile rheumatoid arthritis

d) Pericarditis
e) Kawasaki disease

Answer
The answer is a. This patient fulfills the Jones criteria, having two major (carditis, arthritis) and one minor (fever) features. The apical murmur is most likely caused by mitral regurgitation. Evidence of a recent group A streptococcal infection (ASO titer) should be sought.

2. The *most* appropriate treatment of this patient would be:
a) Intravenous steroids
b) Oral aspirin and prednisone
c) Oral aspirin and intramuscular penicillin
d) Intravenous digoxin
e) Intravenous furosemide

Answer
The answer is c. Salicylates are given for symptomatic relief, usually as aspirin 80 to 120 mg/kg per day given every 4 hours. Steroids are reserved for patients with severe carditis or for symptoms that are unresponsive to aspirin. Neither steroids nor aspirin alter the long-term outcome of patients with carditis. Penicillin is given initially as primary prophylaxis. Anticongestive treatment is not indicated.

Case 2
A 2-year-old boy presents with fever of 5 days duration, swollen hands and feet, strawberry tongue, maculopapular rash, and conjunctivitis.

3. The *most* likely diagnosis is:
a) Lyme disease
b) Kawasaki disease
c) Stevens-Johnson syndrome
d) Mononucleosis
e) Acute rheumatic fever

Answer
The answer is b. This patient exhibits the diagnostic features of Kawasaki disease, lacking only lymphadenopathy, which is the least likely of the diagnostic criteria to be present. The clinical findings can be similar to those in Stevens-Johnson syndrome and scalded skin syndrome. Other clinical and laboratory features will likely strengthen the diagnostic impression.

4. Treatment should include:
a) Hospitalization
b) Aspirin
c) Intravenous immune globulin
d) All of the above
e) None of the above

Answer
The answer is d. As soon as the diagnosis of Kawasaki disease is considered, echocardiography should be per-

formed, with specific attention directed to the coronary arteries. Once the diagnosis has been established, the child should be hospitalized and treated with aspirin and intravenous immune globulin.

Case 3
A 12-year-old boy presents with a 24-hour history of sharp, pleuritic chest pain that is worse in the supine position. His temperature is 38.5°C (101.3°F), and a pericardial friction rub is heard.

5. The *most* likely diagnosis is:
a) Musculoskeletal chest pain
b) Pericarditis
c) Bacterial endocarditis
d) *Mycoplasma* pneumonia
e) Pulmonary embolus

Answer
The answer is b. The description of the pain and the presence of fever and a friction rub are all consistent with pericarditis. Musculoskeletal chest pain is usually short-lived and not associated with abnormal physical findings. Pneumonia can cause chest pain and fever with a pleural friction rub. However, positional pain is uncommon in pneumonia.

6. The *most* useful diagnostic test is:
a) Chest roentgenography
b) Sedimentation rate
c) Electrocardiography
d) Arterial blood gas determination
e) Complete blood cell count

Answer
The answer is c. The electrocardiographic features may be abnormal. In the case described, echocardiogram is not required. If the physical examination findings raised questions regarding pneumonia, chest roentgenography would be useful.

7. Treatment should include:
a) Nonsteroidal anti-inflammatory medication
b) Corticosteroids
c) Pericardiocentesis
d) Hospitalization
e) All of the above

Answer
The answer is a. Most patients with idiopathic or viral pericarditis respond to anti-inflammatory medication. Steroids are rarely indicated and can cause recurrent, steroid-dependent pericarditis. Some forms of pericarditis (e.g., after cardiotomy, malignancy) may be associated with a significant pericardial effusion. If signs of cardiac tamponade are present (tachycardia, pulsus paradoxus), pericardiocentesis is indicated.

SUGGESTED READINGS

1. Batra AS, Lewis AB. Acute myocarditis. *Curr Opin Pediatr* 2001;13: 234–239.
2. Belay B, Belamarich P, Racine AD. Pediatric precursors of adult atherosclerosis. *Pediatr Rev* 2004;25:4–15.
3. Belay B, Belamarich PF, Tom-Revzon C. The use of statins in pediatrics: knowledge base, limitations, and future directions. *Pediatrics* 2007;119:370–380.
4. Brook MM. Pediatric bacterial endocarditis: treatment and prophylaxis. *Pediatr Clin North Am* 1999;46:275–287.
5. Burch M. Heart failure in the young. *Heart* 2002;88:198–202.
6. Capitano B, Quintillani R, Nightingale CH, et al. Antibacterials for the prophylaxis and treatment of bacterial endocarditis in children. *Pediatr Drugs* 2001;3:703–718.
7. Dajani AS, Taubert KA, Gerber MA, et al. Diagnosis and treatment of Kawasaki disease in children. *Circulation* 1993;87:1776–1780.
8. Daniels SR, Greer FR. Lipid screening and cardiovascular health in childhood. *Pediatrics* 2008;122:198–208.
9. Ferrieri P, Gewitz MH, Gerber MA, et al. Unique features of infective endocarditis in childhood. *Pediatr* 2002;109:931–943.
10. Hoyer A, Silberbach M. Infective endocarditis. *Pediatr Rev* 2005; 26:394–399.
11. Kavey RE, Allada V, Daniels SR, et al. Cardiovascular risk reduction in high-risk pediatric patients. *Circulation* 2006;114:2710–2738.
12. Laupland KB, Dele Davies H. Epidemiology, etiology and management of Kawasaki disease: state-of-the-art. *Pediatr Cardiol* 1999;20: 177–183.
13. Melish ME. Kawasaki syndrome. *Pediatr Rev* 1996;17:153–162.
14. Morrow WR. Cardiomyopathy and heart transplantation in children. *Curr Opin Cardiol* 2000;15:216–223.
15. Newberger JW, Takahashi M, Gerber MA, et al. Diagnosis, treatment and long-term management of Kawasaki disease: a statement for health professionals from the committee on rheumatic fever, endocarditis, and Kawasaki disease, council on cardiovascular disease in the young, American Heart Association. *Pediatr* 2004; 114:1708–1733.
16. Rowley AH, Shulman ST. Kawasaki syndrome. *Pediatr Clin North Am* 1999;46:313–329.
17. Takahashi M. Kawasaki disease. *Curr Opin Pediatr* 1997;9:523–529.
18. Tissieres P, Gervaix A, Beghetti M, Jaeggi ET. Value and limitations of the von Reyn, Duke and Modified Duke Criteria for the diagnosis of infective endocarditis in children. *Pediatrics* 2003;112: e467–e471.
19. Towbin JA. Myocarditis and pericarditis in adolescents. *Adolesc Med* 2001;12:47–67.
20. Wald ER. Acute rheumatic fever. *Curr Probl Pediatr* 1993;23: 264–270.
21. Wigle ED, Rakowski H, Kimball BP, et al. Hypertrophic cardiomyopathy: clinical spectrum and treatment. *Circulation* 1995;92: 1680–1692.
22. Wilson W, Taubert KA, Gewitz M, et al. Prevention of infective endocarditis: guidelines from the American Heart Association. *Circulation* 2007;116:1736–1754.

Chapter 27

Disorders of Cardiac Rate and Rhythm

Richard Sterba

An evaluation of abnormalities in the cardiac rate or rhythm may be initiated during a patient interview, auscultation of the heart, or palpation of the peripheral pulses. We rely on electrocardiogram (EKG) to make the definitive diagnosis of clinically suspected abnormalities. Electrocardiography, although simple and inexpensive to perform, provides a great deal of information about the components and function of the electrical system of the heart. Information regarding atrial conduction properties or atrial hypertrophy can be identified by studying the P-wave morphology. Cardiac conduction from the sinus node through the atrium, atrioventricular (AV) node, and His-Purkinje system occurs during the PR interval. Therefore, abnormalities in the conduction from the atrium to the ventricle can be identified by abnormalities in the duration of the PR interval. Change in the shape or size of the P wave is present if atrial hypertrophy exists. The QRS complex represents ventricular depolarization, and therefore contains information regarding intraventricular conduction and ventricular hypertrophy. Both right and left ventricular hypertrophies have well-described changes in their QRS waveform and voltage. The QT interval records ventricular repolarization.

VARIABILITY IN SINUS RHYTHM

The heart rate generated by the sinus node varies with age. Newborns typically have a faster heart rate, in the range of 100 to 180 beats/minute. By the age of 5 years, the heart rate generally decreases to approximately 60 to 120 beats/minute in a quiet and restful situation. Through adolescence and early adulthood, the sinus rate falls to the normal adult range, and typically varies between 50 and 100 beats/minute. The sinus node and heart rate follow signals from the body to generate an appropriate cardiac output. In stressful situations, the heart rate should increase. During sleep or rest it will decrease. To diagnose the abnormalities of the heart rate correctly, one must be aware of the outside influences and disease states that can affect the heart rate.

Sinus arrhythmia is the normal variation that occurs in the heart rate while a patient is breathing. Some parents who check their child's heart rate while the child is asleep will notice this subtle variation in pulse rate and be concerned that extra heartbeats are present. Although called sinus *arrhythmia*, it is a normal phenomenon, and should not be interpreted as an abnormality in sinus node function.

Sinus bradycardia is the most common type of bradycardia seen in pediatrics. Sinus bradycardia can be seen in well-trained athletes. Sinus bradycardia is not uncommonly seen in patients with hypothyroidism, or those with eating disorders, such as anorexia. True sinus node dysfunction resulting in significant sinus bradycardia and its symptoms is unusual in pediatric patients. This is discussed further in the subsequent section on Bradycardia.

Normal heart rates above the expected normal ranges are labeled sinus tachycardia. Sinus tachycardia can be seen at rates over 200 beats/minute in expected situations. This extreme sinus tachycardia can be seen in patients who are very febrile, or during peak exercise. Patients with critical diseases who are receiving inotropic agents can also have an elevated sinus rate. There is generally a subtle variation in the R-R interval during sinus tachycardia, and this phenomenon is not commonly seen in patients with true supraventricular tachycardia (SVT).

TACHYCARDIAS

Tachycardias, typically paroxysmal tachycardias, are the most common significant arrhythmias seen in pediatric patients. In general, heart rates faster than 220 beats/minute should be considered abnormal. Sinus, supraventricular, and ventricular tachycardias cannot always be differentiated on the basis of their clinical presentation alone. Therefore, a 12-lead EKG is an important tool in defining the specific type of tachycardia in an individual patient.

A rapid, regular, narrow QRS rhythm is called *supraventricular tachycardia*, and is the most common abnormal tachycardia seen in pediatrics (Fig. 27.1). SVT accounts for at least 90% of the cases of abnormal tachycardia. SVT is typically paroxysmal. This statement means that the tachycardia has a sudden onset and offset, and is not consistently present. Pediatric patients older than 5 years can often describe the sudden onset of tachycardia quite well. The electrophysiologic mechanisms responsible for SVT include AV re-entrant tachycardia (tachycardia secondary to an accessory AV connection) and AV nodal re-entry tachycardia. These two mechanisms account for approximately 90% of the cases of SVT seen in a pediatric electrophysiologic practice. Less commonly, ectopic atrial tachycardia, atrial flutter, or junctional tachycardia is seen. Patients with paroxysmal SVT may describe the sensation as a fast heart rate that starts suddenly and stops suddenly. In most cases, arrhythmia is not life threatening, and can be characterized as a nuisance. Should an episode of SVT last for a significant time, generally hours, hemodynamic

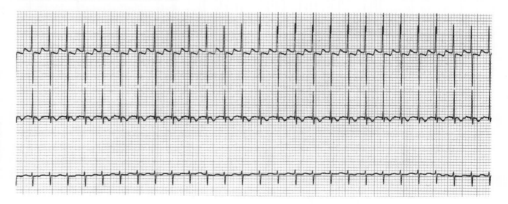

Figure 27.1 This electrocardiogram (EKG) demonstrates the typical supraventricular tachycardia (SVT) seen in pediatrics. The rhythm is regular. The QRS complex is narrow (or normal). A "P" wave is not seen clearly on this EKG.

compromise can develop, and the patient may present critically ill. Some newborns who present with SVT and patients who have SVT in association with significant structural heart disease can present in a more compromised condition. Infants and newborns present with critical illness because the parents are not aware of the SVT and notice signs such as poor feeding and poor color that generally occur later in the episode of supraventricular tachycardia. The rate of SVT in newborns ranges from 240 to 300 beats/minute. The heart rate during SVT in children and adolescents ranges from 180 to 250 beats/minute. Because most patients with SVT have a structurally normal heart, they usually do not present with cardiac collapse or syncope, but rather with the sensation of a rapid heartbeat that is frequently associated with chest tightness. Tachycardia may be brought to the attention of a primary care physician only after a prolonged episode or frequent episodes. Patients with symptoms suggestive of SVT would benefit from a cardiac consultation.

The acute treatment of SVT depends on the patient's presentation. Critically ill patients should be treated appropriately, with placement of an intravenous line and infusion of adenosine. If intravenous access is not available, the patient can be returned to sinus rhythm with synchronized cardioversion. In more stable patients, the use of vagal maneuvers, such as the Valsalva maneuver, or diving reflex can terminate episodes of SVT. To induce a vagal stimulus, one can also place a washcloth in a basin of ice-cold water and then firmly press the chilled washcloth over the patient's face. Vagal maneuvers terminate SVT by slowing the conduction through the AV node, which is a critical part of the re-entrant circuit. The preferred medical treatment of an acute episode of SVT is intravenous adenosine. The recommended dose is 0.1 mg/kg bolus preferably through a centrally placed intravenous line. This medication terminates SVT by blocking the conduction through the AV node. Again, the AV node is a critical portion of the re-entry tachycardia loop. Tachycardia will terminate abruptly, and it is not uncommon to see a significant pause in the heart rate, and then perhaps in the sinus tachycardia. If tachycardia recurs after an infusion of adenosine, other antiarrhythmic medications (e.g., digoxin, β-blockers, intravenous procainamide, or other antiarrhythmics) can be added to the antiarrhythmic regimen to help maintain sinus rhythm. Transesophageal atrial pacing can also be performed to terminate SVT. This method is an excellent alternative for patients who have a tachycardia such as atrial flutter or intra-atrial re-entry tachycardia.

The long-term treatment of SVT depends on its mechanisms. Three options can generally be offered to the family and patients who have SVT. Patients with hemodynamically uncompromising, infrequent, and short episodes of tachycardia can be managed with observation alone. They are instructed in the use of vagal maneuvers should episodes of tachycardia occur. The second option is antiarrhythmic medications. Medications commonly used in pediatrics include β-blockers, digoxin, calcium channel blockers, flecainide, and sotalol. The typical re-entrant SVTs seen out-

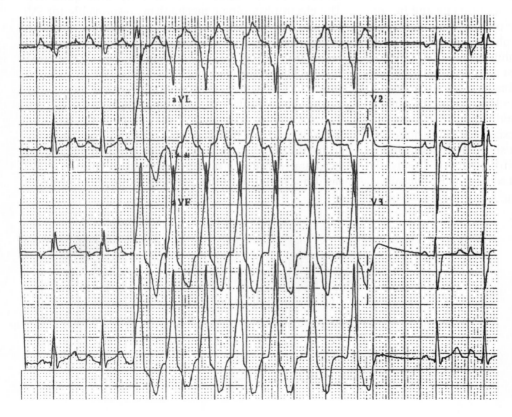

Figure 27.2 This rhythm strip demonstrates ventricular tachycardia. There is a sudden onset of a wide QRS tachycardia. No P wave is visible during the tachycardia. The tachycardia ends with a widening of the last two R-R intervals. This is typically seen in the type of ventricular tachycardia called repetitive monomorphic ventricular tachycardia.

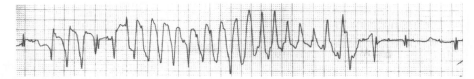

Figure 27.3 This rhythm strip demonstrates unusual but classic ventricular arrhythmias seen in patients with the long QT syndrome during a syncopal episode. The QRS complex is bizarre and constantly changing in its pattern. The term *torsades de pointes* means a twisting of the points and is the original description of this unusual ventricular tachycardia.

side the newborn age will not disappear as the child grows older. For that reason, many families prefer a more invasive approach with the use of an electrophysiologic procedure and ablation of the offending cardiac tissue. During this type of procedure, a catheter is positioned in the heart near the accessory or abnormal electrical tissue that is the underlying substrate for the arrhythmia. Myocardial destruction by tissue modification or destruction with heating (radiofrequency [RF] ablation) or cryoblation can destroy the abnormal electrical tissue and render the tachycardia noninducible. Many patients are cured after this type of procedure. The risk is considered low, and major complications develop in <2% of the procedures. SVT in pediatric patients should be considered a nuisance that is typically not life threatening, and can be controlled well either with medication or with ablation procedures.

Other SVTs include atrial flutter, atrial fibrillation, ectopic atrial tachycardia, and junctional tachycardias. Adenosine is not effective in terminating these arrhythmias, because the AV node is not a critical part of the tachycardia circuit. In an acute situation, these types of SVTs can be terminated with intravenous medications such as procainamide or amiodarone. They respond nicely to cardioversion or atrial overdrive pacing. Many of these arrhythmia circuits can also be destroyed during an ablation procedure.

Ventricular tachycardia (Fig. 27.2) is a rapid, regular, wide QRS tachycardia that occurs infrequently in pediatric patients. Approximately 5% of patients who present with paroxysmal tachycardia have ventricular tachycardia as the underlying mechanism. Although SVT can be considered a nuisance in children, ventricular tachycardia should never be considered a nuisance, and should be considered a potentially life-threatening event. These patients require careful evaluation in an appropriate center where definitive studies can be performed to rule out structural heart defects, cardiomyopathic states, or a possible tumor in the heart. Patients presenting with ventricular tachycardia may respond to intravenous lidocaine, procainamide, or amiodarone. In critically ill patients, synchronized cardioversion should be performed. The long-term treatment of patients

with ventricular tachycardia may include medications, RF ablation, or perhaps implantation of a defibrillator.

Ventricular fibrillation can certainly occur in pediatric patients. It is typically seen in patients with electrocardiographic abnormalities such as a long QT interval (Fig. 27.3) or a Brugada syndrome. Cardiomyopathies or structural heart abnormalities that cause significant ventricular dysfunction are also associated with ventricular fibrillation or ventricular tachycardia that degenerates into ventricular fibrillation. Patients with ventricular fibrillation require cardiopulmonary resuscitation (CPR), immediate defibrillation, and transfer to an appropriate center for further evaluation.

BRADYCARDIAS

The most common cause of abnormal bradycardia (Fig. 27.4) in infants and children is a complete heart block (or complete AV block). The EKG shows a complete disassociation between the P wave and QRS complex. Typically, the heart rate is regular. The QRS morphology may be normal or widened. Complete AV block can be congenital, and can occur in patients who have no structural heart abnormalities. *Congenital complete AV block is strongly associated with maternal systemic lupus erythematosus.* The mother of an infant who presents with a complete heart block should be evaluated for this condition. The most common structural heart disease associated with congenital complete AV block is corrected transposition of the great vessels (L-TGA or ventricular arterial discordance). The treatment of a complete heart block depends on the heart rate and the symptoms. Patients with the slowest heart rate and those with wide QRS escape rhythms fall into a higher risk group, and may need implantation of a pacemaker at earlier ages. Many patients with complete AV block are asymptomatic and can be followed up clinically. Scenarios in this situation that would lead to the recommendation for a pacemaker implantation include significant bradycardias, syncope, exercise intolerance, or ventricular arrhythmias.

Figure 27.4 A rhythm strip demonstrating complete (or third-degree) heart block. The P-P interval is equal. The QRS-QRS interval is equal. No consistent association is seen between the P wave and QRS complex.

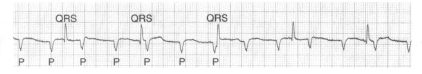

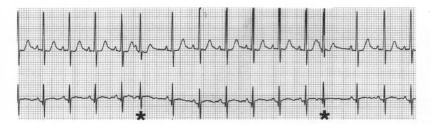

Figure 27.5 This rhythm strip demonstrates two premature atrial contractions (PACs, *). Note the early-occurring P wave. The P wave associated with the second PAC distorts the T wave of the preceding beat.

Patients who have structural heart disease usually do not tolerate a complete heart block well, and need a pacemaker implanted early in their life. Patients who present with heart block and demand acute treatment could be treated with an infusion of Isoproterenol to increase the heart rate. Transcutaneous pacing or insertion of a temporary pacing catheter can be performed.

IRREGULAR RHYTHMS

Many different types of irregular rhythms are seen in pediatric patients. Both premature atrial and ventricular contractions are common. It has been estimated that between 10% and 25% of adolescent patients have premature beats. Premature contractions are not typically associated with structural heart abnormalities.

Premature atrial contractions (PACs) (Fig. 27.5) can be diagnosed by the early occurrence of a P wave that may have a different form of morphology from a sinus P wave. Some PACs are blocked and not conducted to the ventricle. These patients may be thought to have bradycardia or pauses if the blocked P waves are not seen on the EKG. Some premature beats conduct to the ventricle with an aberrant or widened QRS complex. These PACs with widened QRS complexes can be misinterpreted as premature ventricular contractions (PVCs).

Premature ventricular contractions (Fig. 27.6) are early wide QRS complexes that are not preceded by P waves. Bigeminy—in which a sinus beat is followed by a premature ventricular beat and then the pattern is repeated—is frequently seen. Unifocal PVCs (every PVC looks similar) are the most common type of PVC encountered. Because PVCs can originate from any part of the ventricles, the morphology changes from patient to patient.

The evaluation of PVCs should include echocardiography and Holter monitoring. A stress test may be helpful in the evaluation of PVCs. PVCs that are unifocal disappear with exercise, are associated with a structurally and func-

tionally normal heart, are typically considered benign, and do not require therapy. Many patients with frequent unifocal PVCs must have frequent follow-ups to make sure there is no deterioration in cardiac function. Multifocal PVCs that are associated with structural or postoperative heart abnormalities or paired PVCs (called couplets) are considered more worrisome, and a more detailed workup is required. Therapy for symptomatic or troublesome premature contractions could include antiarrhythmic medications. Certainly all patients with PACs or PVCs should be advised to avoid cardiac stimulants such as caffeinated beverages.

Abnormal conduction from the atrium to the ventricle can also cause an irregular rhythm. This is most commonly seen in a type of second-degree heart block called *Wenckebach AV block*. In this condition, QRS complexes are regularly omitted after sinus P waves. An atypical pattern could be three P waves for every two QRS complexes, or four P waves for every three QRS complexes. The typical electrocardiographic pattern is one of equal intervals between P waves and a progressive prolongation of the PR interval before a P wave is not conducted to the ventricle. Second-degree heart block can be seen in healthy teenagers, especially athletes, when they are resting or sleeping. Although typically not a long-term medical problem, the occasional case has been reported in which a second-degree heart block progressed to a third-degree heart block.

SYNCOPE

Syncope is defined as an abrupt, short loss of consciousness in postural tone that is followed by rapid and spontaneous recovery. *The most common form of syncope seen in the pediatric population is vasovagal, neurocardiogenic, or neurally mediated syncope commonly described as a faint.* Careful history, especially from an eyewitness, can be diagnostic. Typically the patient is in an upright position and may experience dizziness, tunnel vision, diaphoresis, and nausea. Some patients complain of palpitations. The patient

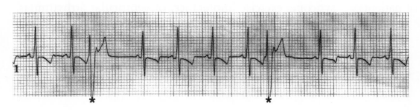

Figure 27.6 Premature ventricular contractions (*). An early wide QRS not preceded by a P wave is demonstrated.

collapses, and is usually described as pale. Once the patient is in the supine position, recovery is rapid. Syncopal episodes can be precipitated by prolonged standing (especially in a fasting state), venipuncture, or hair grooming. Occasionally reflex syncope follows micturition, swallowing, coughing, or defecation. Physiologically, both centrally mediated hypotension and bradycardia occur, leading to cerebral hypoperfusion.

Patients with a history of syncope need to have a careful history recorded. The physician caring for the patient needs to know the history of the event. The physician must try to obtain a history of the event from an observer and acquire a thorough family history to rule out the possibility of an inherited disorder that could be associated with syncope or sudden cardiac death. A normal cardiovascular system should be assured and electrocardiography should be considered a very important test. Many times with a classic history, a normal physical examination and a normal EKG, further testing may not be needed. Head-up tilt table testing can elicit an episode of vasodepressor syncope in many patients who present with neurally mediated syncope. The test can have both false-positive and -negative results. It is a very helpful test to consider in patients who have an atypical presentation of syncope.

Patients in whom syncope occurs without warning or is associated with tachycardia or exercise require a detailed evaluation to rule out cardiac causes. Tachycardias, especially atrial fibrillation associated with Wolff-Parkinson-White (WPW) syndrome (**Fig. 27.7**) or ventricular tachycardia can cause syncope. As described, SVT alone usually does not cause syncope. Bradycardia associated with sinus node dysfunction or third-degree heart block, and tachycardias associated with a long QT syndrome, Brugada syndrome, or arrhythmogenic right ventricular dysplasia are associated with syncope and sudden cardiac death. An EKG and perhaps extended ambulatory electrocardiographic monitoring can be helpful in defining these abnormalities. One cannot state too firmly that the EKG is a most important, cost-effective, and invaluable tool in identifying an arrhythmogenic substrate in patients with syncope.

The treatment of neurocardiogenic syncope should be kept simple. The physiology of the event should be explained to the patient and the parents. The family should be reassured. Patients who experience prodromal symptoms should be instructed to assume a supine position to prevent a severe syncopal episode and possible injury. Intake of both fluids and sodium should be increased. Medications such as mineralocorticoids (Florinef), midodrine, β-

blockers, serotonin reuptake inhibitors, and disopyramide have all been reported to be beneficial in treating patients with recurrent syncope. Unfortunately, none of these reports is based on controlled studies. In many patients, syncope ceases to be a problem without therapy.

Structural heart defects such as aortic stenosis, hypertrophic cardiomyopathy, and pulmonary hypertension that limit the cardiac output can be associated with syncope. These abnormalities should be suspected on the basis of the abnormal findings of a physical examination. An echocardiogram can confirm the clinically suspected abnormalities. There are other noncardiac causes of syncope, such as hypoglycemia (almost exclusively in diabetics) and migraine syndromes. Syncope can be psychogenic. Atonic seizures can be difficult to distinguish from neurocardiogenic syncope.

LONG QT SYNDROME

Long QT syndrome is an autosomal-dominant disorder that is associated with *syncope and sudden cardiac death*. Patients typically present with episodes of syncope. Exertional syncope or emotional syncope is seen commonly in patients who have a prolonged QT interval. *A family history of syncope, sudden cardiac death, drowning, and deafness are somewhat unique to this syndrome.* An electrocardiographic abnormality of prolonged QT interval is caused by abnormal fluxes of either sodium or potassium ions across cell membranes during myocardial repolarization. This channelopathy leads to the prolongation of the QT interval and the T wave abnormalities in patients with these abnormalities (**Fig. 27.8**). On an EKG, corrected QT intervals of <410 ms are considered to be normal. Corrected QT intervals >460 ms are considered abnormal and possibly consistent with the diagnosis of a long QT syndrome. Corrected QT intervals between 410 and 460 ms are in an undetermined zone, and may be seen in healthy individuals or patients with long QT syndrome. Genetic testing has recently become commercially available. With the use of genetic testing, 60% to 70% of patients who have an abnormal QT interval and syncope can be genotyped. The treatment of the long QT syndrome depends on the genotype that is present. β-Blockade has been the typical cornerstone of medical treatment. Patients with long QT syndrome are not allowed to participate in competitive situations, but are allowed to perform in recreational activities. Pacemakers and implantable defibrillators can be commonly used to treat these abnormalities. Patients and their families need to be aware of medicines that are known to

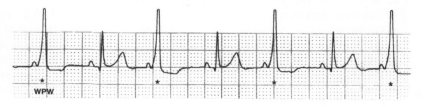

Figure 27.7 An electrocardiogram from a patient with Wolf-Parkinson-White syndrome (WPW) or ventricular pre-excitation. This demonstrates the classic findings in this abnormality. A short PR interval and a delta wave (early slurring of the QRS complex). Compare the normal beats with the starred (*) QRS complexes demonstrating Wolf-Parkinson-White pattern.

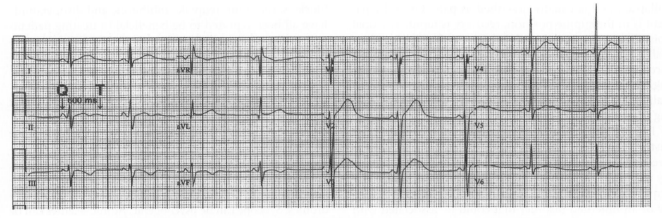

Figure 27.8 A 12-lead electrocardiogram in a patient with long QT syndrome. The QT interval is 600 ms. The T wave is humped or bifid in many leads. These findings are classic in symptomatic patients with long QT syndrome.

prolong the QT intervals and have to be avoided. Parents are advised to learn CPR, and some parents have purchased an automatic external defibrillator. Family members (such as parents and siblings) should be screened to see if they have the same abnormality on their EKG.

REVIEW EXERCISES

QUESTIONS

1. All the following statements are true concerning congenital complete heart block *except:*
a) It can be associated with maternal systemic lupus erythematosus.
b) It can be associated with complex congenital heart disease.
c) It is typically treated with a cardiac pacemaker.
d) The EKG typically demonstrates a prolonged PR interval.

Answer
The answer is d. Congenital complete heart block is extremely common in infants whose mothers have lupus erythematosus; recent studies have shown that as many as two thirds of infants of mothers with lupus have congenital complete heart block. Congenital heart block can also be associated with complex congenital heart disease, particularly L-TGA and a univentricular heart. Today, congenital heart block is typically treated using a pacemaker. The EKG of patients with congenital complete heart block usually shows a normal PR interval.

2. Sinus tachycardia can be associated with all of the following situations *except:*
a) Fever
b) Hemorrhage
c) Exercise
d) Breath holding
e) Anxiety

Answer
The answer is d. Sinus tachycardia is seen with any physiologic phenomenon that increases the heart rate, such as anemia, fever, exercise, and anxiety. It is not associated with breath holding.

3. A 6-week-old infant is brought to your office for a well-baby visit. Your nurse discovers a rapid heart rate. The EKG shows a regular, narrow QRS tachycardia with a rate of 260 beats/minute. Appropriate therapy for this problem could include all of the following *except:*
a) Intravenous administration of adenosine
b) Placing an examination glove filled with ice over the infant's forehead
c) Intravenous administration of verapamil
d) Application of gentle abdominal pressure to mimic a Valsalva maneuver

Answer
The answer is c. The infant in this example has SVT. Appropriate treatments include attempting to stimulate the diving reflex by placing an examination glove filled with ice over the infant's forehead. The powerful diving reflex may terminate the tachycardia. The gentle application of abdominal pressure mimicking a Valsalva maneuver may halt the tachycardia. The intravenous administration of adenosine is a safe and sometimes diagnostic procedure for SVT. However, verapamil should be administered only intravenously with extreme care; in most infants, verapamil is a dangerous medication that should be given under controlled circumstances in the hospital.

4. A 10-year-old boy presents to your office with a history of frequent near-syncopal episodes. He is alert during your examination. The blood pressure is normal and the heart rate is 42 beats/minute and regular. His EKG reveals a ventricular rate of 42/minute and an atrial rate of 90/minute. The *most* appropriate diagnosis is:

a) Atrial flutter with variable conduction
b) Sinus bradycardia
c) Complete heart block
d) Junctional tachycardia

Answer

The answer is c. A patient with a ventricular rate of 42/minute and atrial rate of 90/minute is not in 2 to 1 type heart block. The correct answer is complete heart block. The atrial rate is too slow for atrial flutter. In sinus bradycardia, the atrial and ventricular rate are slow and *equal*. In junctional tachycardia, the ventricular rate is equal to or faster than the atrial rate.

5. In an evaluation of PVCs, the finding that is commonly associated with a benign prognosis is:
a) PVCs that disappear with exercise
b) Ventricular couplet (two consecutive PVCs)
c) Ventricular tachycardia
d) Multiform PVCs (PVC with more than one morphology)

Answer

The answer is a. PVCs that disappear with exercise tend to be benign. Children and adolescents frequently have unifocal PVCs at rest that disappear with exercise and are completely normal. Ventricular couplet is not a normal finding, and ventricular tachycardia is potentially a very serious rhythm, as are multiform PVCs.

6. The *most* common cause of syncope in childhood is:
a) Tachycardias associated with Wolff-Parkinson-White syndrome
b) Long QT syndrome
c) Breath-holding spells
d) Hypertrophic cardiomyopathy
e) Neurocardiogenic syncope

Answer

The answer is e. The most common type of syncope in childhood is neurocardiogenic syncope. Breath-holding spells are unlikely to cause syncope. Hypertrophic cardiomyopathy is a rare cause of syncope, as is a long QT syndrome. Tachycardias associated with Wolff-Parkinson-White syndrome are also a rare cause of syncope.

7. A 10-year-old boy presents for an evaluation of syncope that he experienced while playing basketball. His paternal uncle drowned at the age of 9 years. His physical examination findings are normal. Of the following, the *most* likely cause of this patient's syncope is:
a) Severe aortic stenosis
b) Long QT syndrome
c) Seizure disorder
d) Fluid depletion
e) Hypoglycemia

Answer

The answer is b. Presence of syncope during exertion in a 10-year-old boy is a cause for concern. This type of

syncope is a particular cause for concern when a family history of drowning is elicited because this is so commonly associated with long QT syndrome. It is not known why water stimulates ventricular tachycardia with long QT syndrome, but a family history of drowning is extremely common. The physical examination findings are not normal in severe aortic stenosis; normally, a grade 4–5/6 loud, systolic murmur is heard. A seizure disorder is possible, but the patient has no history of tonic-clonic movements. Fluid depletion and hypoglycemia are also possible, although these would not explain the family history of drowning.

8. In which of the following clinical situations would a cardiology referral be recommended?
a) Lightheadedness after movement from a supine to an upright position
b) Febrile seizure
c) Syncope during exercise
d) Syncope during hair brushing

Answer

The answer is c. Syncope during exercise is always a cause for concern and requires a more detailed cardiovascular examination than is included in a routine pediatric checkup. Lightheadedness during movement from a supine to an upright posture is extremely common and a normal phenomenon. Febrile seizures also are extremely common and do not require a cardiac evaluation. Syncope associated with straining in the bathroom or hair brushing is not an indication for a cardiac referral.

9. Appropriate therapy for patients who have neurocardiogenic or vasovagal syncope includes:
a) β-Blockers
b) Increased intake of fluids and sodium
c) Mineralocorticoids
d) All of the above

Answer

The answer is d. The frontline therapy for patients who have neurocardiogenic or vasovagal syncope is an increased intake of fluids and salt. However, β-blockers and mineralocorticoids also are effective. Therefore, all the choices are correct.

SUGGESTED READINGS

1. Behrman RE, Kligman RM, Jenson HB. Cardiac arrhythmias. In: Dubin A, ed. *Nelson textbook of pediatrics*, 17th ed. Philadelphia: Elsevier, Part XIX, Section 4, 2004:1554–1565.
2. DiVasta AD, Alexander ME. Fainting freshman and sinking sophomores; cardiovascular issues of the adolescent. *Curr Opin Pediatr* 2004;16:350–356.
3. Kaltman J, Shah M Evaluation of the child with an arrhythmia. *Pediatr Clin North Am* 2004;51:1537–1551.
4. Schwartz PJ, Moss AJ, Vincent GM, et al. Diagnostic criteria for the long QT syndrome: an update. *Circulation* 1993;88:782–784.
5. Stefanelli CB, Fischbach PS. Cardiac arrhythmias in children. *ACC Current J Rev* 2003;103–107.

Chapter 28

BOARD SIMULATION: Cardiology

Daniel J. Murphy Jr.

QUESTIONS

Case 1

While performing ultrasonography on a 31-week fetus, an obstetrician notes that the heart rate ranges from 62 to 66 beats/minute. The fetal growth appears normal, and no structural cardiac anomalies are identified. On echocardiography, the fetal atria appear to be contracting at 140 beats/minute, with a ventricular rate of 65 beats/minute.

1. Which of the following is the *next* step in the management of this infant?
a) Administer β-agonist drug therapy to the mother.
b) Assess the cardiac status of the infant following labor and delivery.
c) Counsel the parents that intrauterine fetal death is likely.
d) Perform amniocentesis to confirm lung maturity, and if the lungs are mature, perform an immediate cesarean section.
e) Repeat fetal echocardiography and ultrasonography in 1 week.

Answer

The answer is e. This fetus has complete (third-degree) AV block with a slow regular ventricular rate and no relationship between the atrial rate and ventricular rate. Congestive heart failure and intrauterine fetal demise are common when complete AV block accompanies structural heart disease. With normal anatomy, congestive heart failure and hydrops fetalis may develop, and close observation with serial ultrasonographic examinations is indicated. If signs of congestive heart failure develop, medical management is unlikely to be beneficial, and delivery is indicated.

Case 2

2. A 1-day-old term infant has dysmorphic features that include a low nasal bridge, flat occiput, clinodactyly of the fifth digits, wide spacing between the first and second toes, and hypotonia. He is cyanotic, and results of the lung and abdominal examinations are normal. No heart murmur is heard, and the pulses are normal. The likelihood that this infant has clinically significant congenital heart disease is *closest* to:
a) <20%
b) 20%–35%
c) 40%–55%
d) 60%–70%
e) 80%–95%

Answer

The answer is c. This infant has features suggestive of trisomy 21 (Down syndrome). The incidence of congenital heart disease in association with Down syndrome is approximately 50%. The presence of cyanosis could be secondary to a cardiac defect or mild persistent pulmonary hypertension. The absence of a heart murmur should not reassure the clinician, and echocardiography is indicated for any infant with Down syndrome.

Case 3

A 1-year-old child is brought to the emergency department because his parents thought his heart was "pounding" as they were putting him to bed. Electrocardiography reveals a heart rate of 300 beats/min that spontaneously converts to sinus rhythm at 100 beats/min. The parents estimate that the tachycardia lasted 20 minutes; the child was asymptomatic throughout.

3. Of the following, the *most* appropriate management of this child is:
a) Administration of a β-blocker
b) Administration of digoxin
c) Administration of procainamide
d) Administration of verapamil
e) Observation without drug therapy

Answer

The answer is e. This child likely has reentrant SVT through either the AV node or an accessory bypass tract. An electrocardiogram would be appropriate, and if it showed preexcitation (Wolff-Parkinson-White syndrome), a cardiology consultation would be indicated.

If the child presented in tachycardia, vagal maneuvers or intravenous adenosine could be used to restore sinus rhythm. Long-term drug therapy is generally not indicated for infrequent, brief, unsustained episodes of SVT.

Case 4

A 3-month-old boy has respiratory distress and lethargy. Findings include tachypnea, hepatomegaly, heart rate of 300 beats/min, and a narrow QRS complex consistent with supraventricular tachycardia (SVT).

4. Of the following, the *most* appropriate treatment for the patient at this time is:
a) Electric cardioversion
b) Intravenous verapamil
c) Oral digoxin
d) Oral verapamil
e) Parenteral digoxin

Answer

The answer is a. Of the choices presented, cardioversion is most appropriate. Intravenous verapamil is contraindicated in infants, and a prompt response is not obtained with oral drugs. Vagal maneuvers or the administration of intravenous adenosine would be appropriate options for prompt conversion to sinus rhythm.

Case 5

A 30-year-old woman who has active systemic lupus erythematosus is pregnant.

5. Of the following abnormalities of cardiac conduction, the one that is *most* likely to occur in her infant is:
a) Atrial flutter
b) First-degree heart block
c) SVT
d) Third-degree heart block
e) Ventricular tachycardia

Answer

The answer is d. Infants of mothers who have connective tissue disease with or without clinical symptoms, especially in the presence of anti-Ro (SS-A) or anti-La (SS-B) antibodies, are at significant risk for the development of conduction abnormalities, most commonly third-degree AV block. Close observation with fetal echocardiography is indicated. A neonatal lupus syndrome can develop that is characterized by dermatologic, hematologic, or cardiac abnormalities, or a combination thereof. The skin lesions and cytopenia resolve spontaneously, but the cardiac manifestations are permanent.

Case 6

A 5-year-old girl is very excited following a ride on a Ferris wheel. In the midst of her excitement, she suddenly loses consciousness and falls to the ground. Paramedics on the scene document ventricular tachycardia. The family history reveals a maternal uncle who died suddenly at 16 years of age.

6. Following treatment of the ventricular tachycardia, an electrocardiogram *most* likely will demonstrate:
a) Corrected QT interval of 0.52 seconds
b) P-wave axis of 30 degrees
c) PR interval of 0.81 seconds
d) QRS axis of −15 degrees
e) QRS interval of 0.12 seconds

Answer

The answer is a. This child most likely represents a case of long QT syndrome. A sudden loss of consciousness during activity without a prodrome is not suggestive of neurocardiogenic syncope (simple faint). Wolff-Parkinson-White syndrome (short PR interval) might cause SVT but would rarely result in a sudden loss of consciousness or ventricular tachycardia. Arrhythmogenic right ventricular dysplasia is a familial disorder that generally presents as ventricular tachycardia, syncope, or sudden death in adolescents or adults. The electrocardiographic findings are usually normal.

7. In addition to a prolonged QT interval, a person with Jervell and Lange-Neilsen syndrome is *most* likely to have:
a) Alopecia universalis
b) Cranial bruits
c) Hepatosplenomegaly
d) Rotary nystagmus
e) Sensorineural hearing loss

Answer

The answer is e. In addition to being associated with sensorineural hearing loss, long QT syndrome can be inherited in an autosomal-recessive or autosomal-dominant pattern with variable penetrance. The mutations cause abnormalities in cellular sodium or potassium channels.

8. The sport you are *most* likely to suggest that patients with long QT syndrome avoid is:
a) Bicycling
b) Bowling
c) Ice skating
d) Swimming
e) Tennis

Answer

The answer is d. In addition to swimming, patients are restricted from vigorous exercise, competitive sports, and high-risk occupations, such as flying. β-Blockade is the mainstay of therapy, along with the avoidance of medications that have the potential to prolong the QT interval further, including tricyclic antidepressants, erythromycin, and QT-prolonging antiarrhythmic drugs.

9. The upper limit of a normal corrected QT interval (QTc) is:
a) 0.40 second in boys
b) 0.40 second in girls

c) 0.46 second in boys
d) 0.46 second in girls
e) 0.46 second in boys and girls

Answer

The answer is e. The QTc is calculated according to the formula $QTc = QT/(R\text{-}R)^{1/2}$, with the R-R interval measured in seconds. The upper limit of normal is 0.46 second for boys and girls.

Case 7

A 16-year-old athlete has a syncopal episode immediately following a high school basketball game. The electrocardiogram reveals a QTc of 0.52 second.

10. Which of the following family members would you recommend *must* have a screening electrocardiogram?
a) All first-degree relatives
b) Brothers and male first cousins
c) Sisters and female cousins
d) Father and both grandfathers
e) Mother and both grandmothers

Answer

The answer is a. In most cases, long QT syndrome is inherited as an autosomal-dominant trait. Some mutations may be transmitted in an autosomal-recessive pattern. The condition is not gender specific.

Case 8

A 14-year-old girl falls during a race. She is unconscious and cyanotic and has no pulse, but she revives spontaneously within seconds. Both the patient and family histories are benign. Results of a physical examination, chest roentgenography, echocardiography, electroencephalography, and exercise electrocardiography during a treadmill stress test are normal.

11. Which of the following is the most appropriate *next* step in management?
a) Order a 30-day electrocardiographic event recorder.
b) Perform cardiac catheterization studies.
c) Perform 24-hour ambulatory electrocardiographic monitoring.
d) Perform tilt-table testing.
e) Reassure the family that cardiac causes have been excluded.

Answer

The answer is b. The most common cardiac causes of sudden death in adolescent athletes are hypertrophic cardiomyopathy (excluded by echocardiography), arrhythmogenic right ventricular dysplasia (strong family history, usually diagnosed by magnetic resonance imaging or at autopsy), and anomalies of the coronary arteries, most commonly of the origin of the left coronary artery from the right coronary artery. The origins of the coronary arteries can sometimes be confirmed by echocardiography, but catheterization

should be performed if any doubt remains. In this case, if the catheterization findings are normal, an electrophysiologic study and long-term event recording are indicated.

Case 9

A 4-year-old boy has had daily fevers for 10 days. During the first few days of fever, a diffuse rash developed that has since disappeared. Current findings include cracking of the lips, conjunctival erythema, diffuse lymphadenopathy, hemoglobin level of 12 g/dL, white blood cell count of 8700/mm^3, platelet count of 1.2 million per cubic millimeter, and aneurysms of the proximal right and left coronary arteries.

12. Of the following, the *best* therapy would be:
a) Dipyridamole (1 mg/kg per day)
b) Salicylate (2–5 mg/kg per day)
c) Salicylate (2–5 mg/kg per day) plus prednisone (2 mg/kg per day)
d) Salicylate (100 mg/kg per day)
e) Salicylate (100 mg/kg per day) plus dipyridamole (1 mg/kg per day)

Answer

The answer is d. This boy has Kawasaki disease with coronary artery aneurysms. Aspirin is given in antiinflammatory doses until the inflammation resolves. Thereafter, aspirin is continued in antiplatelet doses. Dipyridamole is rarely indicated. For patients with giant coronary artery aneurysms, warfarin (Coumadin) is given in addition to aspirin. Intravenous immune globulin is administered during the first 7 to 10 days of illness to prevent the development of coronary artery aneurysms. In this case, many practitioners would give intravenous immune globulin. Steroid administration is not indicated as primary therapy for Kawasaki disease, but the role of steroids is currently under investigation.

13. Which of the following statements regarding the epidemiology of Kawasaki disease is *true*?
a) Children of European ancestry are at greater risk than those of Asian ancestry.
b) Girls are affected more often than boys.
c) The incidence remains relatively constant from year to year.
d) Most cases occur in children younger than 5 years of age.
e) The prevalence is greater in summer than in winter.

Answer

The answer is d. The incidence of Kawasaki disease is greater in Asian populations. The disease is not seasonal, but occasional "epidemics" occur in different places from one year to the next. Eighty percent of patients are under 5 years of age, with boys affected more often than girls (male-to-female ratio of 1.5:1).

14. Which of the following is the earliest manifestation of Kawasaki syndrome?
a) Conjunctivitis
b) Fever
c) Lymphadenopathy
d) Maculopapular rash
e) Strawberry tongue

Answer

The answer is b. The disease may start with upper respiratory or gastrointestinal prodromal symptoms followed by an abrupt onset of high fever. The other features listed occur during the acute phase of the illness.

15. The most important factor in planning follow-up care for a child with Kawasaki syndrome is:
a) Age of the patient
b) Duration of the febrile illness
c) Presence or absence of arthritis
d) Presence or absence of coronary artery abnormalities
e) Severity of the original liver disease

Answer

The answer is d. The only permanent sequelae of Kawasaki disease are arterial aneurysms. Coronary artery aneurysms usually develop during the first 3 weeks of the illness. Complications include coronary thrombosis or stenosis and can occur acutely or during long-term follow-up. Patients without coronary artery involvement do not necessarily require long-term follow-up.

Case 10

A 10-year-old girl has had fever, joint pain, and fatigue for 10 days. She has also had symptoms of an upper respiratory tract infection several times during the past 2 months. Findings include normal joints, a grade 1/6 high-pitched decrescendo diastolic murmur at both the right third intercostal space and left lower sternal border, and a grade 2/6 high-pitched holosystolic murmur at the apex.

16. The *most* likely explanation for these findings is:
a) Acute rheumatic fever
b) Bicuspid aortic valve
c) Complete atrioventricular (AV) canal defect
d) Purulent pericarditis
e) Viral myocarditis

Answer

The answer is a. The patient has murmurs of aortic and mitral regurgitation (major) in addition to fever and arthralgia (minor). Evidence of a recent streptococcal infection (antistreptolysin O titer) should be sought to confirm the diagnosis before she is treated with anti-inflammatory drugs. If the history or other evidence suggests a congenital heart defect, blood cultures should be performed to diagnose infective endocarditis before she is treated with antibiotics.

Case 11

During the preschool physical examination of a 4-year-old child, you note a grade 2/6 high-pitched continuous murmur in the third right intercostal space while the patient is in the sitting position. The murmur is ablated by compressing the child's neck veins.

17. Of the following, the *most* likely diagnosis is:
a) Aortic stenosis and insufficiency
b) Arteriovenous malformation
c) Patent ductus arteriosus
d) Still murmur
e) Venous hum

Answer

The answer is e. The Still murmur is a systolic ejection murmur. Patent ductus arteriosus causes a continuous murmur at the upper left sternal border that is not altered by a change of position, head turning, or compression of the jugular veins. An arteriovenous malformation also produces a continuous murmur that is unaffected by any manipulation. Venous hums can be heard on the right or left and are most common in toddlers.

Case 12

Subacute bacterial endocarditis develops following extraction of a tooth in a 9-year-old boy with a bicuspid aortic valve.

18. The organism that *most* likely is causing this patient's endocarditis is:
a) *Candida albicans*
b) *Escherichia coli*
c) *Haemophilus influenzae*
d) *Staphylococcus aureus*
e) *Streptococcus mitis*

Answer

The answer is e. Viridans streptococci, including *S. mitis*, are the most common causative organisms of subacute bacterial endocarditis. Endocarditis caused by *E. coli* may be associated with manipulation of the gastrointestinal or genitourinary tract. Fungal species may also cause endocarditis, especially in patients who are being treated with broad-spectrum antibiotics, in whom an indwelling catheter has been placed, or who are receiving parenteral nutrition. *H. influenzae* rarely causes endocarditis, but cases caused by other *Haemophilus* species do occur. *S. aureus* is the most common cause of acute endocarditis.

19. Of the following, the procedure that requires antibiotic prophylaxis in a child with a prosthetic mitral valve is:
a) Cystoscopy
b) Dental cleaning
c) Tonsillectomy

d) Rigid bronchoscopy
e) Sigmoidoscopy

Answer
The answer is c. Tonsillectomy, adenoidectomy, and surgical procedures or biopsies involving the respiratory mucosa require antibiotic prophylaxis in selected patients. Among dental procedures, dental cleaning, the adjustment of orthodontic appliances, and simple fillings do not require prophylaxis, but extractions do. According to the recently revised guidelines, genitourinary and gastrointestinal procedures no longer require prophylactic antibiotics.

Case 13
Following an uncomplicated delivery, cyanosis develops in a 3.7-kg term infant during the first hour of life. The findings at 3 hours of age include cyanosis, heart rate of 140 beats/min, respiratory rate of 56 breaths/min, and no heart murmurs. The pulse oximetry reading in room air is 70% in the right hand and 75% in the foot; with a 100% fraction of inspired oxygen (FIO_2) via head hood, the oxygen saturation remains 70% in the hand but increases to 90% in the foot. The chest roentgenographic findings are normal.

20. These findings are *most* consistent with:
a) Primary pulmonary hypertension of the newborn
b) Pulmonary valve atresia
c) Transient tachypnea of the newborn
d) Transposition of the great arteries
e) Truncus arteriosus

Answer
The answer is d. In primary pulmonary hypertension, one would expect to see a lower oxygen saturation in the lower body (postductal). In pulmonary atresia, the administration of oxygen should not affect the arterial oxygen saturation. Patients with truncus arteriosus have complete mixing and the same saturation in the ascending aorta, pulmonary arteries, and descending aorta. The absence of a heart murmur is not helpful in excluding congenital heart disease.

21. Causes of acrocyanosis include all the following *except*:
a) Sepsis
b) Colic
c) Cold
d) Cardiogenic shock
e) Hypoglycemia

Answer
The answer is b. Acrocyanosis is common in infants and usually indicates poor perfusion of the extremities secondary to vasoconstriction. It must be distinguished from central cyanosis and arterial desaturation.

Case 14
A 6-week-old boy with known congestive cardiomyopathy weighs 4 kg. He takes only 12 oz of formula daily.

22. Of the following, the *most* likely consequence of decreased intake in this infant is:
a) Hypocalcemia
b) Hypoglycemia
c) Hypokalemia
d) Poor growth in length
e) Poor weight gain

Answer
The answer is e. Feeding difficulties in infants with congestive heart failure are most likely to result in poor weight gain.

23. The infant is being treated with furosemide and digoxin. Measurement of serum electrolyte concentrations reveals the following values: sodium, 131 mEq/L; potassium, 3.5 mEq/L; chloride, 90 mEq/L; bicarbonate, 38 mEq/L. The *most* likely cause of these findings is:
a) Congestive heart failure
b) Digoxin therapy
c) Furosemide therapy
d) Poor nutrition
e) Tachypnea

Answer
The answer is c. The boy has a hypochloremic metabolic alkalosis, which is commonly associated with the long-term administration of furosemide, especially when given two or three times daily. Congestive heart failure can be associated with hyponatremia.

24. Regarding digoxin,
a) The digitalizing dose is 10 μg/kg.
b) The maintenance dose is 5–10 μg/kg per day.
c) Levels should be monitored for therapeutic effect.
d) Hyperkalemia enhances digoxin toxicity.
e) Overdose is treated with hemodialysis.

Answer
The answer is b. When digitalization is required, the total digitalizing dose is 10 to 20 μg/kg orally in a preterm infant and 20 to 30 μg/kg orally in a term infant and older child. The intravenous dose is approximately 80% of the oral dose. Hypokalemia enhances digoxin toxicity. Digoxin is not dialyzable, and overdose is treated with digoxin antibodies.

25. Signs of digoxin toxicity include all the following *except*:
a) Short PR interval
b) Anorexia
c) Lethargy
d) Supraventricular arrhythmias
e) Ventricular arrhythmias

Answer
The answer is a. Digoxin toxicity prolongs the PR interval.

26. In an infant with a left-to-right shunt,
a) Oxygen can be deleterious.
b) Caloric needs are reduced.
c) Rales accompany congestive heart failure.
d) Afterload reduction is contraindicated.
e) Intravenous furosemide is ineffective.

Answer
The answer is a. Oxygen is a pulmonary vasodilator, and by decreasing the pulmonary vascular resistance, it can actually cause an increase in pulmonary blood flow, pulmonary edema, and a decrease in systemic output. Afterload reduction should improve the systemic flow and decrease the excessive pulmonary circulation. The increased pulmonary flow causes an increase in the work of breathing and an increase in caloric needs. Although infants with pulmonary edema frequently present with wheezing, rales usually suggest pneumonia. Diuretics can be helpful in reducing pulmonary edema.

Case 15
An 18-month-old boy treated 6 days ago with amoxicillin for otitis media returns today with a persistent daily fever of at least 39.8°C. The physical examination reveals a listless child with a maculopapular rash over the trunk, injected sclerae, and dry, fissured lips. The palms of his hands and fingertips are indurated and erythematous.

27. Of the following, the *most* likely diagnosis is:
a) Scarlet fever
b) Drug reaction
c) Juvenile rheumatoid arthritis
d) Kawasaki syndrome
e) Measles

Answer
The answer is d. The patient has had fever for more than 5 days in addition to: (a) oropharyngeal changes, (b) rash, (c) changes of the extremities, and (d) nonpurulent conjunctivitis. He does not yet have significant lymphadenopathy, but he meets the criteria for Kawasaki syndrome. Drug reaction (Stevens-Johnson syndrome) is always included in the differential diagnosis when symptoms develop after drug administration. Conjunctivitis and rash are features of measles; it would be appropriate to obtain an immunization history.

Case 16
A systolic ejection murmur is detected in a highly competitive 16-year-old high school athlete during a routine examination required before participation in sports.

The electrocardiogram demonstrates a sinus bradycardia (50 beats/min) and borderline left ventricular hypertrophy. Echocardiography reveals mildly enlarged left and right ventricles with a ventricular shortening fraction of 40% (normal, >28%).

28. Of the following, the *most* likely explanation for these findings is:
a) Autonomic dysfunction
b) Cardiovascular response to athletic training
c) Early evidence of dilated cardiomyopathy
d) Early evidence of hypertrophic cardiomyopathy
e) Myocarditis

Answer
The answer is b. These findings are fairly typical of the "athlete heart." The trained athlete has a resting bradycardia and mildly enlarged cardiac chambers. The fact that she is able to compete with her peers suggests that overall her cardiac function is normal. Any family history of cardiomyopathy should prompt further investigation and follow-up because many forms do not present until adolescence or young adulthood.

29. The *most* common cause of syncope in young children is:
a) Automonic dysfunction associated with prolonged standing
b) Breath-holding spells
c) Cataplexy
d) Panic attack associated with hyperventilation
e) Prolonged QT syndrome

Answer
The answer is b. The commonest form of syncope in childhood are the neurally mediated syncopes, which include reflex syncopes such as breath holding spells, and postural orthostatic tachycardia syndrome. Breath holding spells are most common in toddlers and manifest as reflex asystile followed by an anoxic seizure in response to a noxious stimulus. In adolescents, neurocardiogenic syncope is generally postural and associated with a prodrome such as dizzines, nausea and pallor. Cardiac causes of syncope, such as prolonged QT syndrome are more dangerous, but less common.

SUGGESTED READINGS

1. Ayoub E, Ahmed S. Update on complications of group A streptococcal infections. *Curr Probl Pediatr* 1997;27:90–99.
2. Burns JC, Mason WH, Glode MP, et al. Clinical and epidemiologic characteristics of patients referred for evaluation of possible Kawaski disease. *J Pediatr* 1991;118:680–686.
3. Ferrieri P, Gewitz MH, Gerber MA, et al. Unique features of infective endocarditis in childhood. *Pediatr* 2002;109:931–943.
4. Lue HC, Wu MH, Wang JK, et al. Long-term outcome of patients with rheumatic fever receiving benzathine penicillin G prophylaxis

every three weeks versus every four weeks. *J Pediatr* 1994;125: 812–816.

5. Martin JM, Neches WH, Wald ER. Infective endocarditis: 35 years of experience at a children's hospital. *Clin Infect Dis* 1997;24: 669–675.
6. McLeod, KA. Syncope in childhood. *Arch Dis Child* 2003;350–353.
7. Mori M, Imagawa T, Yasui K, et al. Predictors of coronary artery lesions after intravenous gamma-globulin treatment in Kawasaki disease. *J Pediatr* 2000;137:177–180.
8. Moss AJ, Schwartz, PJ, Crampton RS, et al. The long QT syndrome: a prospective international study. *Circulation* 1985;71:17.
9. Newburger JW, Takahashi M, Beiser AS, et al. A single intravenous infusion of gamma globulin as compared with four infusions in the treatment of acute Kawasaki syndrome. *N Engl J Med* 1991;324: 1633–1639.
10. Rowley AH, Shulman ST. Kawasaki syndrome. *Pediatr Clin North Am* 1999;46:313–325.
11. Villain E, Levy M, Kachaner J, et al. Prolonged QT interval in neonates: benign, transient, or prolonged risk of sudden death. *Am Heart J* 1992;124:194–197.
12. Vincent GM, Timothy KW, Leppert M, et al. The spectrum of symptoms and QT intervals in carriers of the gene for the long-QT syndrome. *N Engl J Med* 1992;327:846.
13. Wilson W, et al. Prevention of infective endocarditis: guidelines from the American Heart Association. *Circulation* 2007;116: 1736–1754.

Chapter 29

Allergic Disorders

Alton L. Melton Jr.

Allergic diseases affect approximately 20% to 30% of the pediatric population in the United States and are responsible for 15% to 25% of physician visits to pediatricians. Their prevalence has been increasing significantly throughout the developed world.

Symptoms of classical allergic disease and anaphylaxis result from the formation of antigen specific IgE by B lymphocytes under the direction of Th2 CD4+ helper T cells. These T cells secrete certain cytokines like interleukin 4 and interleukin 13 that promote IgE production. IgE is secreted and ultimately binds to high affinity receptors on the surface of mast cells and basophils, and to low-affinity receptors on eosinophils and other cells. Antigen binds to specific IgE on the mast cell surface causing activation of the cell. The mast cell degranulates, releasing vasoactive substances such as histamine, prostaglandin D2, proteases, proteoglycans, and other mediators of the "early phase" reaction. These mediators act immediately to produce vascular leakage, pruritus, edema, erythema and can progress to urticaria, itch, swelling, severe bronchospasm, and cardiovascular collapse. Mast cell activation also leads to production of "late-phase" mediators such as leukotrienes and cytokines, which are proinflammatory and can cause intense inflammation and target tissue hyperreactivity. Chronic inflammation can result from repeated or continuous allergen exposure.

ALLERGIC RHINOCONJUNCTIVITIS

This is the most common allergic disease, affecting 10% to 20% of US children. Symptoms include:

- Sneezing
- Clear rhinorrhea
- Congestion
- Nasal and eye itching
- Mucosal swelling
- Eye redness
- Conjunctival swelling
- Eyelid swelling
- Photophobia
- Tearing

Signs on physical exam include:

- Pale, boggy, swollen nasal turbinates that have a pale bluish tint
- Clear rhinorrhea
- Conjunctival injection and swelling
- Eyelid swelling
- Tearing
- Photophobia

A transverse nasal crease is often present. Multiple infraorbital folds (Dennie-Morgan lines) may also be present.

Allergic rhinoconjunctivitis (AR) can have either perennial or seasonal symptoms or elements of both. Perennial AR is characterized by year-round symptoms, usually because of chronic exposure to indoor allergens such as dust mite, animal danders, and mold spores. Chronic congestion is often the most prominent symptom. Reduction of exposure is vital to effective treatment. Dust mites reside in cloth items that are not laundered frequently, such as mattresses, carpeting, and stuffed animals. Plastic mattress encasing and bedroom carpet removal are the two most effective avoidance measures. For animals, pet elimination is greatly preferred, but frequent cat and dog washing may reduce pet allergenicity. Dehumidification and chlorine bleach cleaning are effective for indoor mold reduction.

Seasonal AR is usually caused by sensitivity to outdoor allergens such as pollens and mold spores. Allergy seasons and offending allergens are region and climate dependent. Throughout most of the United States, tree pollens cause signs and symptoms of intense nasal and eye itching, mucosal swelling, sneezing, eye redness, rhinorrhea, and tearing in the early spring (March through May). In the Northeast and Midwest, oak and birch are prevalent. In the Southeast, hickory and pecan are most prevalent. In the Southwest, red cedar is a particularly allergenic tree. Pine pollen rarely causes allergy. In the late spring (May through June) grass pollen allergy predominates. In the early fall (late August through October) ragweed is the major allergen.

AR is treated with avoidance, medical management, and allergen immunotherapy. Avoidance is best for indoor allergens. Mild or intermittent symptoms usually respond well to oral antihistamine given as needed with or without decongestant. Chronic perennial or seasonal AR is best treated with ongoing therapy, which can include:

- Topical nasal corticosteroids
- Antileukotriene agents
- Topical ocular or nasal antihistamines
- Topical nasal or ocular cromolyn

More severe cases may require topical ocular steroids or occasional courses of oral steroids. Prolonged use of topical decongestants, which can cause rhinitis medicamentosa, should be avoided. Allergen immunotherapy involves administration of the offending allergen, in escalating doses until the patient develops sufficient tolerance.

ANAPHYLAXIS

Anaphylaxis usually results from severe IgE mediated sensitization to substances that are either ingested or encountered systemically such as foods, medications, allergenic extracts, latex, and bee venom. Rapid onset of breathing difficulty and/or cardiovascular collapse can ensue, and this requires quick and decisive action for successful treatment and prevention of death. Early and frequent administration of epinephrine 1:1000, 0.01 mL/kg SQ up to 0.3 mL per dose, is the cornerstone of therapy. Use of an antihistamine, such as diphenhydramine 1 mg/kg given parenterally up to every 4 to 6 hours is also important. Many experts recommend adding a histamine 2 (H2) blockade, such as cimetidine (4 mg/kg parenterally). A corticosteroid (methylprednisolone 1–2 mg/kg) can be helpful in preventing a late-phase reaction and is also recommended. Supportive therapy with supplemental oxygen, aerosolized bronchodilators, supine positioning with elevation of the lower extremities, compression trousers, and intravenous fluid administration may be required if more severe or protracted signs and symptoms develop. In rapidly progressive severe reactions, intravenous vasopressors, intravascular colloidal solutions, intravenous aminophylline, and mechanical ventilation should be considered.

Anaphylactoid reactions, which are not IgE mediated, resemble anaphylaxis caused by direct mast cell degranulation. These have been observed most commonly with radiocontrast media and opiates. These reactions should be treated with similar medical management. Pretreatment with antihistamine and corticosteroid is effective in reducing severity for most cases of anaphylactoid reactions, but is *not* effective for IgE-mediated anaphylaxis as with latex or penicillin. Use of lower osmolality radiocontrast can reduce the risk of reaction in patients with a past history of reaction. There is no allergic cross- reaction between radiocontrast media and seafood.

Penicillin is the most frequently implicated medication and reactions are often caused by allergy to metabolites of the parent compound. There exists extensive cross-reactivity among the penicillins. Cephalosporins usually show about 20% cross-reactivity with penicillins, but this percentage is probably higher for true anaphylaxis. If penicillin is required, allergy skin testing cannot currently be performed, as the test reagent for the major metabolite was recalled and has been unavailable for several years. For patients with histories of anaphylaxis or other severe reactions, successful desensitization can be undertaken in intensive care settings if penicillin is needed. For those with milder histories, a closely supervised test dose challenge can be considered. Reliable testing is not yet available for other antibiotics.

High molecular weight biological medications are also frequent causes of anaphylaxis and include allergenic extracts for immunotherapy, insulin, chymopapain, and horse serum (snake bite antivenin). Latex allergy appears to be a frequent cause of intraoperative anaphylaxis in patients with spina bifida and congenital urogenital anomalies. Among cancer chemotherapeutic agents, cis-platinum is a frequent cause of anaphylaxis. Beta-blockers can make anaphylaxis extremely difficult to treat and may increase the likelihood of anaphylaxis.

Food anaphylaxis is more common in children than adults, and can be fatal, especially with severe peanut allergy. The most common allergenic foods in children are peanut, milk, egg, soybean, fish, and wheat. Shellfish and nuts are also common offenders. Keep in mind peanuts are legumes, not nuts. Complete dietary avoidance is necessary for true food allergy. Injectable epinephrine should be kept on hand at all times for emergency use.

STINGING INSECT ALLERGY

Allergenic reactions to insect stings affect approximately 1% to 5% of children with most manifesting as large local swelling, redness, pain, and itch at the site of the sting. Extremely large local reactions, distant cutaneous reactions, and systemic reactions with respiratory and/or cardiovascular compromise are much more serious problems that usually require some medical intervention.

Stinging insects include honeybees (Apis), Vespids (yellow jacket, white-faced hornet, yellow hornet), wasps (Polistes), and imported fire ants (Solenopsis). Bee venom contains many proteins that can act as potential allergens such as Phospholipase A, hyaluronidase, mellitin (Apis), and acid phosphatase (Vespids). There is extensive cross-reactivity of allergy among the Vespids, about 50% cross-reactivity between Vespids and wasps, and much less cross-reactivity between Vespids and honeybees. Yellow jackets are the most frequent cause of stings and reactions because of their aggressive nature. Allergy to stings is more likely with multiple sting exposures and very frequent stings. Progression from milder to more serious reactions is the exception rather than the rule in individual children with large local or distant cutaneous reactions without respiratory or cardiovascular involvement. Therefore, skin testing and immunotherapy are only recommended for children with histories of respiratory or cardiovascular reactions to stings. These children should have injectable epinephrine available at all times during the seasons at risk for stings. Immunotherapy is effective in the majority of cases and represents the only viable preventive treatment for bee sting allergy. Use of insect repellant, avoidance of bright clothing, perfumes, garbage cans, and careful examination of all outdoor food items are also important preventive measures.

URTICARIA

Urticaria or hives can result from allergic reactions, usually to ingestants such as foods or medicines or allergens encountered systemically. Contact urticaria has also been reported. Acute allergic urticaria of this type is usually short-lived and responds to elimination of the offending allergen and symptomatic treatment with oral antihistamines. Delayed-onset drug reactions like serum sickness can cause urticarial reactions that are more persistent, and usually require corticosteroid in addition to antihistamine for effective treatment.

Chronic urticaria represents a more difficult diagnostic challenge. Approximately 90% of urticaria lasting 6 weeks or more is idiopathic. Among the other 10% is a list of causes that includes allergy, vasculitis, lupus, chronic infection, parasitic infestation, hepatitis, chronic inflammation, lymphoma, and physical urticarias. Physical stimuli that can cause urticaria include exercise (heat or cholinergic urticaria), light pressure (dermographism), deep pressure, vibration, sunlight, water, and cold temperature. People with cold urticaria should avoid swimming or immersion, which can cause anaphylaxis upon body re-warming because of massive mast cell degranulation. *The cutaneous manifestation of mastocytosis called urticaria pigmentosa presents as reddish brown macules that urticate on stroking (Darier's sign).* Papular urticaria refers to large local reactions to biting (not stinging) insects. *Hereditary angioedema* is an autosomal dominant condition that causes nonpruritic episodic swelling, usually at sites of trauma, but that can occur anywhere, including the airways where it can be life threatening. *This is due to the absence of the complement regulatory protein C1 inhibitor.* Several variations have been described, including one in which the C1 inhibitor level is normal, but the protein is nonfunctional.

The diagnosis of urticaria depends on identification of the suspected trigger. For allergic urticaria, allergy skin testing and/or challenge testing is indicated. For cold urticaria, placement of an ice cube on the forearm for 10 minutes with observation thereafter is diagnostic. Cholinergic urticaria yields a positive methacholine skin test. Skin biopsy is recommended for urticaria pigmentosa, suspected vasculitis, and protracted cases of idiopathic urticaria. A serum tryptase level can help distinguish cutaneous mastocytosis from the more severe systemic form. Hereditary angioedema is best detected by a low C4 level, although quantitative and functional assays of C1 inhibitor can be helpful. For idiopathic urticaria a reasonable work up includes: CBC, differential count, sedimentation rate or CRP, urinalysis, blood chemistries, and possibly chest radiography, serology, antinuclear antibody, sinus CT scan, rheumatoid factor, stool for ova and parasites, and thyroid studies.

Classical antihistamines provide relief from pruritus and swelling in most cases of urticaria and these represent first line medical therapy for chronic urticaria. Diphenhydramine, hydroxyzine, and doxepin are especially effective. Newer nonsedating antihistamines may be helpful in many cases, in which side effects need to be avoided. Cyproheptadine is especially helpful for cold urticaria. Resistant cases and cases of urticaria pigmentosa often required combined H1 and H2 antihistamines. Vasculitic urticaria usually requires oral corticosteroids. Androgenic steroids like danazol can reduce frequency and severity of attacks of swelling in hereditary angioedema.

REVIEW EXERCISES

QUESTIONS

1. The stinging insect most likely to cause an anaphylactic reaction is:
a) Honeybee
b) Wasp
c) Yellow jacket
d) White faced hornet
e) Imported fire ant

Answer

The answer is c. Yellow jackets are aggressive and abundant and often sting without provocation. Honeybees are docile and almost require disturbance of the hive or actual physical contact to sting. Wasps and hornets build nests high above ground and are less frequently encountered than yellow jackets. Fire ants are restricted to the extreme Southern United States.

2. A 7 year-old girl presents with a history of episodic severe swelling at areas of trauma without pruritus. Her father has a similar history. The single best screening test for her conditions is:
a) C3 complement assay
b) C1 inhibitor level
c) CH50
d) C4 complement
e) Serum IgE concentration

Answer

The answer is d. Episodic severe swelling at areas of trauma without pruritus, but with autosomal dominant inheritance, suggests that this patient has hereditary angioedema (C1 inhibitor deficiency.) A functional defect in C1 inhibitor consumes C4 to some degree continuously, whereas C3 is usually spared. Variants of HAE do exist where measurable C1 inhibitor is detectable, but is nonfunctional. CH50 is usually normal unless there is massive reduction of C4 during an acute episode. This angioedema has nothing related to allergy or immediate hypersensitivity. Therefore, C4 is the best screening test.

3. A 9-year-old boy presents with bilateral eye swelling, itch, photophobia and frequent sneezing with runny nose in late April. He has had similar symptoms during the same time of year the last 2 years. He is relatively asymptomatic at other times. The most likely offending allergen is:
a) Oak tree pollen
b) Rye grass pollen
c) Dust mite
d) Ragweed pollen
e) Indoor mold spores

Answer

The answer is a. In most regions of the country, trees pollinate in early spring, often peaking in late April to early May. Grass pollinates predominantly in May and June, whereas ragweed pollinates in late summer and early fall. Indoor allergens like house dust mite and mold spores are more likely to cause perennial rather than seasonal symptoms.

4. Which of the following patients are candidates for bee venom skin testing and immunotherapy?
a) Immediate large local swelling at the sting site with redness and swelling of the entire extremity
b) Immediate large local reaction at the sting site with accompanying urticaria over the entire body
c) Moderate swelling at the site of the sting with development of diffuse urticaria and joint pain 5 days later
d) Immediate swelling at the site of the sting with wheezing in an asthmatic patient

Answer

The answer is d. In children under 16 years of age, the risk of subsequent anaphylaxis is relatively low for those who experience anything less than an immediate respiratory or cardiovascular reaction to an insect sting. Because of this, only those with these more severe reactions are candidates for bee venom testing and immunotherapy.

5. The single best avoidance measure for dust mite allergy is:
a) Plastic mattress encasing
b) Frequent vacuuming of carpets
c) Dehumidification of basement area
d) Spraying carpet with insecticide
e) Use of an electronic air cleaner

Answer

The answer is a. House dust mite concentrations are highest in mattresses, and the close proximity of respiratory organs to the source of dust mite exposure during sleeping makes the mattress the most important point of intervention. Carpet removal can also be effective, but standard vacuuming may actually stir up dust mite allergen. Dehumidification of basement areas is especially helpful for mold allergy. Insecticides may have inherent toxicity and are effective only for a short time. Air cleaners are less effective for house dust mite allergy than for other allergens, and less effective than mattress encasing and bedroom carpet removal.

6. Which of the following is *not* a common food allergen?
a) Egg
b) Milk
c) Peanut

d) Chocolate

e) Soybean

Answer

The answer is d. Egg, milk, peanut, and soybean are the four most common food allergens for children, probably because of their relative allergenicity and early and frequent exposure. Chocolate is an uncommon allergen, and reactions to chocolate ingestion are often traced to milk or peanut ingredients.

7. A 10 year-old girl comes for evaluation after an episode of urticaria and anaphylaxis after swimming. What is the single best test for diagnosis of her condition?

a) Methacholine skin test

b) C1 inhibitor level

c) Allergy skin testing

d) Skin biopsy

e) Ice cube test

Answer

The answer is e. Urticaria after swimming suggests cold urticaria. Methacholine skin test is best for cholinergic (heat) urticaria. C1 inhibitor level is not even the best screening test for hereditary angioedema. Cold urticarias rarely have an allergic component, if ever. Skin biopsy is usually indicated for vasculitis urticarias. An ice cube test will confirm the presence of cold urticaria.

8. A 6 month-old child presents with a persistent rash. On exam, several reddish brown macules are seen that urticate on stroking. The best diagnostic test for this patient is:

a) Skin biopsy

b) Serum IgE level

c) CBC, diff, sed rate

d) Methacholine skin test

e) C1 inhibitor function

Answer

The answer is a. Reddish brown macules that urticate on stroking (Darier's sign) are characteristic of urticaria pigmentosa, a sign of mastocytosis. Skin biopsy is recommended to confirm the diagnosis. This is not an immediate hypersensitivity condition, nor related to idiopathic or cholinergic urticaria, or hereditary angioedema.

9. Which of the following is *not* true regarding reactions to radiocontrast media?

a) Mast cell degranulation is involved.

b) Pretreatment with antihistamine reduces severity.

c) No cross-allergenicity to iodine or seafood exists.

d) Reactions are IgE mediated.

e) Reactions are more likely with high osmolarity radiocontrast.

Answer

The answer is d. Reactions to opiates or radiocontrast media (RCM) involve direct mast cell degranulation and do not involve IgE or the IgE receptor. Although

RCM contains iodine, the reactions are more closely related to the osmolarity rather than iodine content. Seafood allergy involves IgE-immediate hypersensitivity to specific seafood protein antigens, and has absolutely no relationship to RCM reactions. Because the amplification inherent in the IgE-mediated response is not present, pretreatment with antihistamines, steroids, and bronchodilators can reduce reaction severity of RCM reactions.

10. Which is *not* true regarding drug anaphylaxis?

a) Minor determinants are involved in a high percentage of penicillin reactions.

b) Penicillin is the most frequently implicated single drug.

c) Reliable skin testing is available for penicillins, macrolides, and sulfonamides.

d) Cephalosporins exhibit approximately 20% cross-reactivity with penicillin.

e) Horse serum in snake bite antivenin represents an important potential allergen.

Answer

The answer is c. Reliable skin testing was commercially available for penicillin, but not at present. No reliable testing is available for other antibiotics. Many severe penicillin reactions are mediated by metabolites of penicillin, including those called minor determinants. Penicillin is the most commonly implicated drug for allergic reactions, including anaphylaxis. Most sources quote a cross-reactivity of approximately 20% between penicillins and cephalosporins, although the true percentages may differ depending on the nature of the reaction. Horse serum contains potent allergenic proteins that were responsible for numerous reactions in the past. Snakebite antivenom remains one of the few therapeutic preparations where horse serum is still used.

SUGGESTED READINGS

1. Golden DBK. Insect sting allergy and venom immunotherapy: a model and a mystery. *J Allergy Clin Immunol* 2005;115:349–447.
2. Greenberger PA. Drug allergy. *J Allergy Clin Immunol* 2006;117:S464–470.
3. Gruchalla R. Antibiotic allergy. *N Engl J Med* 2006;354:6019.
4. Joint Task Force on Pediatric Parameters. The diagnosis and management of allergic rhinitis. *J Allergy Clin Immunol* 288;122:S3–84.
5. Kaplan AP. Chronic urticaria: Pathogenesis and treatment. *J Allergy Clin Immunol* 2004;114:465–474.
6. Kemp SF, Lockey RF. Anaphylaxis: a review of causes and mechanisms. *J Allergy Clin Immunol* 2002;110(3):341–348.
7. Lieberman P, Kemp SF, Oppenheimer J, et al. The diagnosis and management of anaphylaxis: an updated practice parameter. *J Allergy Clin Immunol* 2005;115:S-483–523.
8. Moffitt JE, Golden DBK, Reisman RE. Stinging insect hypersensitivity: a practice parameter update. *J Allergy Clin Immunol* 2004;114:869–886.
9. Sampson HA. Update on food allergy. *J Allergy Clin Immunol* 2004;113:805–819.
10. Scurlock AM, Lee LA, Burks AW. Food allergy in children. *Immunol Allergy Clin North Am* 2005;25:369–388.

Chapter 30

Asthma

Velma L. Paschall

ETIOLOGY AND EPIDEMIOLOGY

Asthma, a chronic inflammatory disease of the airways, is the most common chronic illness in children. It accounts for a large proportion of school days lost to illness and is the most frequent diagnosis for admission in hospitalized children. Between 5% and 15% of all children have asthma at some time during their childhood. In children younger than 10 years, approximately twice as many boys as girls are affected, and by 14 years of age, four times as many boys as girls have asthma. The male predominance begins to decrease after midadolescence, and by early adulthood the incidence among both sexes is approximately equal.

Although asthma prevalence rates have stabilized in the United States during the past few years, worldwide prevalence has increased. Risk factors for the development of childhood asthma, in addition to male sex, include:

- Atopy or family history of atopy
  - Parental history of asthma (especially maternal)
- Early viral respiratory infection
- Maternal smoking
- Prematurity
- Passive exposure to tobacco smoke
- Maternal age <20 years at the time of birth

Despite recent declines in rates of asthma-related hospitalization and asthma mortality in the United States, racial and ethnic minorities continue to be disproportionately affected with severe asthma. The rates of hospitalization for asthma and asthma-related deaths are three times higher in African Americans than white Americans based on data from The Center for Disease Control in 2005. Known risk factors for *fatal* asthma include:

- Previous nearly fatal episodes of asthma
- Hospitalization or care in an emergency department within the previous year
- History of psychosocial problems or psychiatric disease

- History of poor compliance with asthma medications
- Current use of or withdrawal from systemic corticosteroids
- Poor access to health care
- Exposure to tobacco smoke

The tendency to have asthma is inherited, and the mode of inheritance is polygenic and complex. The risk for the development of asthma in a child with one affected parent is 25%, and the risk increases to approximately 50% if both the parents have asthma. Environmental factors that may be important for the complete expression of the disease in a genetically predisposed child include:

- Viral respiratory infections during infancy
- Passive exposure to cigarette smoke
- Intensive exposure to environmental aeroallergens

PATHOPHYSIOLOGY

Asthma is an inflammatory disorder of the airways in which inflammation contributes to respiratory symptoms, limited airflow, and chronic disease. Immunohistopathology studies of biopsy specimens from the bronchi of asthmatic children reveal an inflammatory process manifested by denudation of the airway epithelium, goblet cell hyperplasia, mucous plugging, deposition of collagen beneath the basement membrane, mast cell activation, and infiltration by inflammatory cells consisting of neutrophils, eosinophils, and T-helper subset 2 (T_H2) lymphocytes.

The inflammatory process may be precipitated by one or more triggers (i.e., inhaled allergen, viral infection) that lead to the release of inflammatory mediators from the bronchial mast cells and also from macrophages, T lymphocytes, and epithelial cells. Both stored and newly synthesized mediators are released from the mucosal mast cells following activation. These mediators, which include histamine, leukotrienes C_4, D_4, and E_4, and platelet-activating factor, initiate bronchoconstriction and edema and direct the migration and activation of other inflammatory cells that cause injury (e.g., eosinophils, neutrophils) into the airways. Airway damage is manifested by denudation of the epithelium, hypersecretion of mucus, changes in mucociliary function, bronchospasm, and airway hyperresponsiveness. Bronchial hyperreactivity to viral infection, cold air, exercise, allergens, and environmental irritants is a major feature of asthma, and the level of airway hyperresponsiveness usually correlates with its clinical severity.

CLINICAL PRESENTATION

The clinical manifestations of asthma result from airway obstruction and inflammation. Acute exacerbations are most frequently precipitated by exertion or exposure to inhalant allergens or irritants. Exacerbations caused by viral respiratory infections tend to be slower in onset and worsen gradually. Symptoms of asthma include:

- Cough, usually dry but sometimes productive
- Wheezing
- Dyspnea
- Chest pain or tightness

Only one of these symptoms, such as cough, may be present, and patients may be symptom-free between exacerbations.

The physical findings vary depending on the severity and chronicity of disease. Signs that may be present during acute exacerbations include:

- Tachypnea
- Retractions, use of accessory muscles of respiration
- Cyanosis
- Pulsus paradoxus
- Hyperexpansion of the thorax

On auscultation of the chest, wheezing, crackles, rhonchi, a prolonged expiratory phase of respiration, and diminished breath sounds may be observed, although the chest findings may be completely normal between exacerbations and in children with mild disease. Digital clubbing occurs rarely, even in severe asthma; if present, it suggests a diagnosis of cystic fibrosis or another chronic obstructive lung disease, either alone or in combination with asthma.

DIAGNOSIS

A correct diagnosis of asthma is established by first obtaining a careful medical history and performing a focused physical examination. In children, a history of any of the following strongly suggests a diagnosis of asthma: cough (particularly cough that is worse at night), recurrent wheezing, recurrent difficulty breathing, and recurrent chest tightness. The pattern of symptoms is variable and may be perennial, seasonal, continual, or episodic. Diurnal variations are common, in which symptoms develop or worsen at night and interfere with sleep. Typically, symptoms are precipitated or worsened by one or more of the following factors:

- Viral respiratory infection
- Exercise
- Environmental irritants
- Inhalant allergens
- Changes in weather
- Cold air
- Expression of strong emotions (crying, laughing, anger)

Viral upper respiratory infections are the most common precipitants of asthma exacerbations in children <2 years, but as the children become older, sensitivity to aeroallergens increases, and exposure to environmental allergens plays a more important role.

The physical examination focuses on both the upper and lower respiratory tracts and also the skin. Signs of other atopic diseases, such as allergic rhinitis and eczema, are often present, even between asthma exacerbations when the chest examination findings are completely normal.

Pulmonary function tests, particularly spirometry, may be helpful in establishing a diagnosis of asthma by objectively determining the presence of an airflow obstruction and whether it is partially or completely reversible. Spirometry measures the forced vital capacity (FVC), forced expiratory volume in 1 second (FEV_1), and forced expiratory flow at 25%, 50%, 75%, and between 25% and 75% of the FVC (FEF_{25}, FEF_{50}, FEF_{75}, and FEF_{25-75}). Some children can perform reproducible spirometric maneuvers at the age of 4 years, and most can do so by 6 years of age. Measurements of lung function should be obtained both before and after bronchodilation, with improvements of 12% in the FEV_1 and 25% in the FEF_{25-75} considered clinically significant.

Although recurrent episodes of cough and wheezing in children are most frequently caused by asthma, other causes of airway obstruction must be considered in the differential diagnosis. A number of other disorders affecting the upper, middle, and lower respiratory tract that can be associated with cough or wheezing are listed in Table 30.1.

MANAGEMENT AND TREATMENT

The long-term goals of asthma therapy, established by the National Asthma Education and Prevention Program (NAEEP), are reduction of impairment and risks associated with asthma.

Reducing the impairment associated with asthma involves:

- Prevention of chronic and troublesome symptoms (e.g., coughing, shortness of breath at night, in the early morning, and after exertion)
- Infrequent use of inhaled short-acting beta$_2$-agonists for quick relief of symptoms (≤2 days per week)

TABLE 30.1

DIFFERENTIAL DIAGNOSIS OF INFANT AND CHILDHOOD ASTHMA

Upper Airway Disorders	Disorders Involving Large Airways	Disorders Involving Small Airways
Rhinitis (allergic, nonallergic, infectious)	Foreign body in trachea or esophagus	Viral bronchiolitis
Sinusitis	Vascular rings	Cystic fibrosis
Adenoidal or tonsillar hypertrophy	Laryngeal webs	Chronic aspiration
Foreign body	Tracheoesophageal fistula	Bronchopulmonary dysplasia
	Tracheostenosis, bronchostenosis, laryngomalacia, tracheomalacia	Heart disease
	Space-occupying lesions (enlarged lymph nodes, tumor)	Gastroesophageal reflux
	Vocal cord dysfunction	Bronchiectasis
		Foreign body
		Tumor

Modified from National Institutes of Health. NAEPP guidelines for the management and diagnosis of asthma. *National Asthma Education and Prevention Program.* NIH Pub No 02-5075, Bethesda, MD: 2002, NIH.

- Maintenance of near "normal" pulmonary function
- Maintenance of normal activity levels (including exercise and other physical activity and attendance at work or school)
- Meeting patients' and families' expectation of and satisfaction with asthma care

Reducing the risk associated with asthma includes:

- Prevention of recurrent exacerbations and minimizing the need for emergency department visits and hospitalizations
- Prevention of progressive loss of lung function; for children, prevention of reduced lung growth
- Provision of optimal pharmacotherapy with minimal or no adverse effects

Successful implementation of these goals begins with an assessment of the severity of a case of asthma. Whenever possible, evaluation of severity should be performed at the time of diagnosis and before initiation of treatment to determine the type of medication and appropriate dosage for a given patient. When a patient who is being seen for the first time has already initiated therapy, severity may be determined best by the minimum treatment required to maintain control. Asthma may be classified as intermittent, mild persistent, moderate persistent, or severe persistent based on patient's history, physical examination findings, and pulmonary function results (Tables 30.2, 30.3, and 30.4).

The current 2007 NAEPP guidelines for asthma management recommend initial pharmacologic treatment based on the classification of severity. Assessment of the level of asthma control should be performed on subsequent patient encounters to monitor and adjust therapy. Asthma control is assessed by impairment (daytime and nocturnal symptoms, interference with normal activities, need for rescue inhaled β_2-agonists, lung function measured by FEV_1 or peak expiratory flow rate, validated control questionnaires) as well as risk (number and severity of exacerbations per year, long-term loss of lung function, and adverse effects of treatment) (Tables 30.5, 30.6, and 30.7).

Therapy should be intensified if asthma is not adequately controlled, and if symptoms remain well controlled for several months, therapy can be stepped down to the least amount of medication needed to maintain control. The specific guidelines for pharmacotherapy used to achieve asthma control vary according to the patient's age and are shown in Tables 30.8, 30.9, and 30.10.

Pharmacotherapy

Pharmacologic therapy is used to prevent and control the symptoms of asthma, reduce the frequency and severity of exacerbations, and relieve the obstruction to the airflow. Asthma medications can be divided into two general classes: Those used for long-term control, taken daily on an extended basis to achieve and maintain control of persistent asthma, and those used for quick relief, taken to treat acute symptoms and exacerbations.

Medications used for long-term control include antiinflammatory agents, long-acting bronchodilators, and leukotriene modifiers. The most effective medications for long-term control are those that attenuate inflammation. Medications used for quick relief include short-acting β_2-agonists and anticholinergics. Inhaled short-acting β_2-agonists are the drugs of choice for treating acute symptoms of asthma and preventing exercise-induced bronchospasm. Despite their delayed onset of action, systemic corticosteroids are important in treating moderate to severe exacerbations because they help prevent the progression of symptoms, speed up recovery, and prevent early relapses.

TABLE 30.2

CLASSIFYING ASTHMA SEVERITY AND INITIATING TREATMENT IN YOUTHS ≥12 YEARS OF AGE AND ADULTS

Assessing severity and initiating treatment for patients who are not currently taking long-term control medications

Components of Severity		Classification of Asthma Severity ≥12 years of age			
		Intermittent	Persistent		
			Mild	Moderate	Severe
Impairment **Normal FEV$_1$/FVC:** 8–19 yr 85% 20–39 yr 80% 40–59 yr 75% 60–80 yr 70%	Symptoms	≤2 days/week	>2 days/week but not daily	Daily	Throughout the day
	Nighttime awakenings	≤2×/month	3–4×/month	>1×/week but not nightly	Often 7×/week
	Short-acting beta$_2$-agonist use for symptom control (not prevention of EIB)	≤2 days/week	>2 days/week but not daily, and not more than 1× on any day	Daily	Several times per day
	Interference with normal activity	None	Minor limitation	Some limitation	Extremely limited
	Lung function	• Normal FEV$_1$ between exacerbations • FEV$_1$ >80% predicted • FEV$_1$/FVC normal	• FEV$_1$ >80% predicted • FEV$_1$/FVC normal	• FEV$_1$ >60% but <80% predicted • FEV$_1$/FVC reduced 5%	• FEV$_1$ <60% predicted • FEV$_1$/FVC reduced >5%
Risk	Exacerbations requiring oral systematic corticosteroids	0–1/year (see note)	≥2/year (see note) ⟶		
		⟵ Consider severity and interval since last exacerbation. ⟶ Frequency and severity may fluctuate over time for patients in any severity category. Relative annual risk of exacerbations may be related to FEV$_1$.			
Recommended Step for Initiating Treatment **(See Table 30.8 for treatment steps.)**		Step 1	Step 2	Step 3	Step 4 or 5 and consider short course of oral systemic corticosteroids
		In 2–6 weeks, evaluate level of asthma control that is achieved and adjust therapy accordingly.			

Key: FEV$_1$, forced expiratory volume in 1 second; FVC, forced vital capacity; ICU, intensive care unit.

Notes:
- The stepwise approach is meant to assist, not replace, the clinical decisionmaking required to meet individual patient needs.
- Level of severity is determined by assessment of both impairment and risk. Assess impairment domain by patient's/caregiver's recall of previous 2–4 weeks and spirometry. Assign severity to the most severe category in which any feature occurs.
- At present, there are inadequate data to correspond frequencies of exacerbations with different levels of asthma severity. In general, more frequent and intense exacerbations (e.g., requiring urgent, unscheduled care, hospitalization, or ICU admission) indicate greater underlying disease severity. For treatment purposes, patients who had ≥2 exacerbations requiring oral systemic corticosteroids in the past year may be considered the same as patients who have persistent asthma, even in the absence of impairment levels consistent with persistent asthma.

The information in Table 30.2 is directly abstracted from the National Asthma Education and Prevention Program *Expert Panel Report 3: Guidelines for the Diagnosis and Management of Asthma.* National Institutes of Health, National Heart, Lung, and Blood Institute. August 2007. NIH publication 08-4051.

Corticosteroids

Corticosteroids are the most potent and consistently effective medications for the long-term control of asthma. They interfere with the inflammatory response by numerous mechanisms and clinically they have been shown to reduce the severity of symptoms, prevent exacerbations, improve lung function, decrease airway hyperresponsiveness, and may possibly prevent progression of airway remodeling.

Inhaled corticosteroids are the most effective long-term therapy for persistent asthma and in general are safe and well tolerated at recommended doses. Systemic effects can occur, especially at high doses, and occasionally at lower

TABLE 30.3

CLASSIFYING ASTHMA SEVERITY AND INITIATING TREATMENT IN CHILDREN 5–11 YEARS OF AGE

Assessing severity and initiating therapy in children who are not currently taking long-term control medication

Components of Severity		Intermittent	Mild	Moderate	Severe
			Persistent		
Impairment	Symptoms	≤2 days/week	>2 days/week but not daily	Daily	Throughout the day
	Nighttime awakenings	≤2×/month	3–4×/month	>1×/week but not nightly	Often 7×/week
	Short-acting beta$_2$-agonist use for symptom control (not prevention of EIB)	≤2 days/week	>2 days/week but not daily	Daily	Several times per day
	Interference with normal activity	None	Minor limitation	Some limitation	Extremely limited
	Lung function	• Normal FEV$_1$ between exacerbations • FEV$_1$ >80% predicted • FEV$_1$/FVC >85%	• FEV$_1$ = >80% predicted • FEV$_1$/FVC >80%	• FEV$_1$ = >60–80% predicted • FEV$_1$/FVC = 75–80%	• FEV$_1$ <60% predicted • FEV$_1$/FVC <75%
Risk	Exacerbations requiring oral systematic corticosteroids	0–1/year (see note)	≥2/year (see note) →		
		Consider severity and interval since last exacerbation. Frequency and severity may fluctuate over time for patients in any severity category. Relative annual risk of exacerbations may be related to FEV$_1$.			
Recommended Step for Initiating Therapy (See Table 30.9 for treatment steps.)		Step 1	Step 2	Step 3 medium-dose ICS option	Step 3, medium-dose ICS option, or step 4
				and consider short course of oral systemic corticosteroids	
		In 2–6 weeks, evaluate level of asthma control that is achieved and adjust therapy accordingly.			

Key: EIB, exercise-induced bronchospasm; FEV$_1$, forced expiratory volume in 1 second; FVC, forced vital capacity; ICS, inhaled corticosteroids.

Notes
• The stepwise approach is meant to assist, not replace, the clinical decisionmaking required to meet individual patient needs.
• Level of severity is determined by both impairment and risk. Assess impairment domain by patient's/caregiver's recall of the previous 2–4 weeks and spirometry. Assign severity to the most severe category in which any feature occurs.
• At present, there are inadequate data to correspond frequencies of exacerbations with different levels of asthma severity. In general, more frequent and intense exacerbations (e.g., requiring urgent, unscheduled care, hospitalization, or ICU admission) indicate greater underlying disease severity. For treatment purposes, patients who had ≥2 exacerbations requiring oral systemic corticosteroids in the past year may be considered the same as patients who have persistent asthma, even in the absence of impairment levels consistent with persistent asthma.

The information in Table 30.3 is directly abstracted from the National Asthma Education and Prevention Program *Expert Panel Report 3: Guidelines for the Diagnosis and Management of Asthma*. National Institutes of Health, National Heart, Lung, and Blood Institute. August 2007. NIH publication 08-4051.

TABLE 30.4

CLASSIFYING ASTHMA SEVERITY AND INITIATING TREATMENT IN CHILDREN 0–4 YEARS OF AGE

Assessing severity and initiating therapy in children who are not currently taking long-term control medication

		Classification of Asthma Severity (0–4 years of age)			
			Persistent		
Components of Severity		Intermittent	Mild	Moderate	Severe
Impairment	Symptoms	≤2 days/week	>2 days/week but not daily	Daily	Throughout the day
	Nighttime awakenings	0	1–2x/month	3–4x/month	>1x/week
	Short-acting beta₂-agonist use for symptom control (not prevention of EIB)	≤2 days/week	>2 days/week but not daily	Daily	Several times per day
	Interference with normal activity	None	Minor limitation	Some limitation	Extremely limited
Risk	Exacerbations requiring oral systemic corticosteroids	0–1/year	≥2 exacerbations in 6 months requiring oral systemic corticosteroids, or ≥4 wheezing episodes/1 year lasting >1 day AND risk factors for persistent asthma		
		←——— Consider severity and interval since last exacerbation. ———→ Frequency and severity may fluctuate over time. Exacerbations of any severity may occur in patients in any severity category.			
Recommended Step for Initiating Therapy (See Table 30.10 for treatment steps.)		Step 1	Step 2	Step 3 and consider short course of oral systemic corticosteroids	
		In 2–6 weeks, depending on severity, evaluate level of asthma control that is achieved. If no clear benefit is observed in 4–6 weeks, consider adjusting therapy or alternative diagnoses.			

Key: EIB, exercise-induced bronchospasm.

Notes

- The stepwise approach is meant to assist, not replace, the clinical decisionmaking required to meet individual patient needs.
- Level of severity is determined by both impairment and risk. Assess impairment domain by patient's/caregiver's recall of previous 2–4 weeks. Symptom assessment for longer periods should reflect a global assessment such as inquiring whether the patient's asthma is better or worse since the last visit. Assign severity to the most severe category in which any feature occurs.
- At present, there are inadequate data to correspond frequencies of exacerbations with different levels of asthma severity. For treatment purposes, patients who had ≥2 exacerbations requiring oral systemic corticosteroids in the past 6 months, or ≥4 wheezing episodes in the past year, and who have risk factors for persistent asthma may be considered the same as patients who have persistent asthma, even in the absence of impairment levels consistent with persistent asthma.

The information in Table 30.4 is directly abstracted from the National Asthma Education and Prevention Program *Expert Panel Report 3: Guidelines for the Diagnosis and Management of Asthma.* National Institutes of Health, National Heart, Lung, and Blood Institute. August 2007. NIH publication 08-4051.

doses in individual patients. Recent studies have not shown any significant effect on the long-term linear growth in children receiving long-term therapy with inhaled corticosteroids at low to medium doses. Rinsing the mouth and spitting following inhalation and using a spacer, significantly decreases local side effects and systemic absorption. Oral corticosteroids are occasionally indicated for long-term therapy in patients with severe persistent asthma who remain poorly controlled despite optimal medical management and pharmacotherapy. Alternate-day dosing with the lowest dose of oral corticos-

teroid that controls disease is recommended to minimize both short- and long-term side effects.

Cromolyn Sodium and Nedocromil

Cromolyn and nedocromil are chemically unrelated drugs with similar mild anti-inflammatory effects. Both inhibit the activation of inflammatory cells, release of mediators, recruitment of eosinophils into the airways, and early and late asthmatic responses to the allergen challenge. Although neither drug has any direct bronchodilating effect, both are effective in preventing exercise-induced bronchospasm

TABLE 30.5

ASSESSING ASTHMA CONTROL AND ADJUSTING THERAPY IN YOUTHS ≥12 YEARS OF AGE AND ADULTS

	Components of Control	Classification of Asthma Control (≥12 years of age)		
		Well Controlled	**Not Well Controlled**	**Very Poorly Controlled**
Impairment	Symptoms	≤2 days/week	>2 days/week	Throughout the day
	Nighttime awakenings	≤2×/month	1–3×/week	≥4×/week
	Interference with normal activity	None	Some limitation	Extremely limited
	Short-acting beta$_2$-agonist use for symptom control (not prevention of EIB)	≤2 days/week	>2 days/week	Several times per day
	FEV$_1$ or peak flow	>80% predicted/ personal best	60–80% predicted/ personal best	<60% predicted/ personal best
	Validated questionnaires ATAQ ACQ ACT	0 ≤0.75* ≥20	1–2 ≥1.5 16–19	3–4 N/A ≤15
Risk	Exacerbations requiring oral systemic corticosteroids	0–1/year	≥2/year (see note)	
		Consider severity and interval since last exacerbation		
	Progressive loss of lung function	Evaluation requires long-term followup care		
	Treatment-related adverse effects	Medication side effects can vary in intensity from none to very troublesome and worrisome. The level of intensity does not correlate to specific levels of control but should be considered in the overall assessment of risk.		
Recommended Action for Treatment (see Table 30.8 for treatment steps)		• Maintain current step. • Regular followups every 1–6 months to maintain control. • Consider step down if well controlled for at least 3 months.	• Step up 1 step and • Reevaluate in 2–6 weeks. • For side effects, consider alternative treatment options.	• Consider short course of oral systemic corticosteroids. • Step up 1–2 steps, and • Reevaluate in 2 weeks. • For side effects, consider alternative treatment options.

*ACQ values of 0.76–1.4 are indeterminate regarding well-controlled asthma.
Key: EIB, exercise-induced bronchospasm; ICU, intensive care unit.
Notes:
• The stepwise approach is meant to assist, not replace, the clinical decisionmaking required to meet individual patient needs.
• The level of control is based on the most severe impairment or risk category. Assess impairment domain by patient's recall of previous 2–4 weeks and by spirometry/or peak flow measures. Symptom assessment for longer periods should reflect a global assessment, such as inquiring whether the patient's asthma is better or worse since the last visit.
• At present, there are inadequate data to correspond frequencies of exacerbations with different levels of asthma control. In general, more frequent and intense exacerbations (e.g., requiring urgent, unscheduled care, hospitalization, or ICU admission) indicate poorer disease control. For treatment purposes, patients who had ≥2 exacerbations requiring oral systemic corticosteroids in the past year may be considered the same as patients who have not-well-controlled asthma, even in the absence of impairment levels consistent with not-well-controlled asthma.
• Validated Questionnaires for the impairment domain (the questionnaires do not assess lung function or the risk domain)
    ATAQ = Asthma Therapy Assessment Questionnaire© (See sample in "Component 1: Measures of Asthma Assessment and Monitoring.")
    ACQ = Asthma Control Questionnaire© (user package may be obtained at www.qoltech.co.uk or juniper@qoltech.co.uk)
    ACT = Asthma Control Test™ (See sample in "Component 1: Measures of Asthma Assessment and Monitoring.")
    Minimal Important Difference: 1.0 for the ATAQ; 0.5 for the ACQ; not determined for the ACT.
• Before step up in therapy:
    —Review adherence to medication, inhaler technique, environmental control, and comorbid conditions.
    —If an alternative treatment option was used in a step, discontinue and use the preferred treatment for that step.

The information in Table 30.5 is directly abstracted from the National Asthma Education and Prevention Program *Expert Panel Report 3: Guidelines for the Diagnosis and Management of Asthma*. National Institutes of Health, National Heart, Lung, and Blood Institute. August 2007. NIH publication 08-4051.

TABLE 30.6

ASSESSING ASTHMA CONTROL AND ADJUSTING THERAPY IN CHILDREN 5–11 YEARS OF AGE

	Components of Control	Classification of Asthma Control (5–11 years of age)		
		Well Controlled	**Not Well Controlled**	**Very Poorly Controlled**
Impairment	Symptoms	≤2 days/week but not more than once on each day	>2 days/week or multiple times on ≤2 days/week	Throughout the day
	Nighttime awakenings	≤1x/month	≥2x/month	≥2x/week
	Interference with normal activity	None	Some limitation	Extremely limited
	Short-acting beta$_2$-agonist use for symptom control (not prevention of EIB)	≤2 days/week	>2 days/week	Several times per day
	Lung function			
	• FEV$_1$ or peak flow	>80% predicted/personal best	60–80% predicted/personal best	<60% predicted/personal best
	• FEV$_1$/FVC	>80%	75–80%	<75%
Risk	Exacerbations requiring oral systemic corticosteroids	0–1/year	≥2/year (see note)	
		Consider severity and interval since last exacerbation		
	Reduction in lung growth	Evaluation requires long-term followup.		
	Treatment-related adverse effects	Medication side effects can vary in intensity from none to very troublesome and worrisome. The level of intensity does not correlate to specific levels of control but should be considered in the overall assessment of risk.		
Recommended Action for Treatment (See Table 30.9 for treatment steps.)		• Maintain current step. • Regular followup every 1–6 months. • Consider step down if well controlled for at least 3 months.	• Step up at least 1 step and • Reevaluate in 2–6 weeks. • For side effects: consider alternative treatment options.	• Consider short course of oral systemic corticosteroids, • Step up 1–2 steps, and • Reevaluate in 2 weeks. • For side effects, consider alternative treatment options.

Key: EIB, exercise-induced bronchospasm; FEV$_1$, forced expiratory volume in 1 second; FVC, forced vital capacity.
Notes:
• The stepwise approach is meant to assist, not replace, the clinical decisionmaking required to meet individual patient needs.
• The level of control is based on the most severe impairment or risk category. Assess impairment domain by patient's/caregiver's recall of previous 2–4 weeks and by spirometry/or peak flow measures. Symptom assessment for longer periods should reflect a global assessment such as inquiring whether the patient's asthma is better or worse since the last visit.
• At present, there are inadequate data to correspond frequencies of exacerbations with different levels of asthma control. In general, more frequent and intense exacerbations (e.g., requiring urgent, unscheduled care, hospitalization, or ICU admission) indicate poorer disease control. For treatment purposes, patients who had ≥2 exacerbations requiring oral systemic corticosteroids in the past year may be considered the same as patients who have persistent asthma, even in the absence of impairment levels consistent with persistent asthma.
• Before step up in therapy:
—Review adherence to medications, inhaler technique, environmental control, and comorbid conditions.
—If alternative treatment option was used in a step, discontinue it and use preferred treatment for that step.

The information in Table 30.6 is directly abstracted from the National Asthma Education and Prevention Program *Expert Panel Report 3: Guidelines for the Diagnosis and Management of Asthma*. National Institutes of Health, National Heart, Lung, and Blood Institute. August 2007. NIH publication 08-4051.

TABLE 30.7

ASSESSING ASTHMA CONTROL AND ADJUSTING THERAPY IN CHILDREN 0–4 YEARS OF AGE

Components of Control		Classification of Asthma Control (0–4 years of age)		
		Well Controlled	Not Well Controlled	Very Poorly Controlled
Impairment	Symptoms	≤2 days/week	>2 days/week	Throughout the day
	Nighttime awakenings	≤1x/month	>1x/month	>1x/week
	Interference with normal activity	None	Some limitation	Extremely limited
	Short-acting beta$_2$-agonist use for symptom control (not prevention of EIB)	≤2 days/week	>2 days/week	Several times per day
Risk	Exacerbations requiring oral systemic corticosteroids	0–1/year	2–3/year	>3/year
	Treatment-related adverse effects	Medication side effects can vary in intensity from none to very troublesome and worrisome. The level of intensity does not correlate to specific levels of control but should be considered in the overall assessment of risk.		
Recommended Action for Treatment (see Table 30.10 for treatment steps)		• Maintain current treatment. • Regular followup every 1–6 months. • Consider step down if well controlled for at least 3 months.	• Step up (1 step) and • Reevaluate in 2–6 weeks. • If no clear benefit in 4–6 weeks, consider alternative diagnoses or adjusting therapy. • For side effects, consider alternative treatment options.	• Consider short course of oral systemic corticosteroids. • Step up (1–2 steps), and • Reevaluate in 2 weeks. • If no clear benefit in 4–6 weeks, consider alternative diagnoses or adjusting therapy. • For side effects, consider alternative treatment options.

Key: EIB, exercise-induced bronchospasm.
Notes:
• The stepwise approach is meant to assist, not replace, the clinical decisionmaking required to meet individual patient needs.
• The level of control is based on the most severe impairment or risk category. Assess impairment domain by caregiver's recall of previous 2–4 weeks. Symptom assessment for longer periods should reflect a global assessment such as inquiring whether the patient's asthma is better or worse since the last visit.
• At present, there are inadequate data to correspond frequencies of exacerbations with different levels of asthma control. In general, more frequent and intense exacerbations (e.g., requiring urgent, unscheduled care, hospitalization, or ICU admission) indicate poorer disease control. For treatment purposes, patients who had ≥2 exacerbations requiring oral systemic corticosteroids in the past year may be considered the same as patients who have not-well-controlled asthma, even in the absence of impairment levels consistent with not-well-controlled asthma.
• Before step up in therapy:
  —Review adherence to medications, inhaler technique, and environmental control.
  —If alternative treatment option was used in a step, discontinue it and use preferred treatment for that step.

The information in Table 30.7 is directly abstracted from the National Asthma Education and Prevention Program *Expert Panel Report 3: Guidelines for the Diagnosis and Management of Asthma*. National Institutes of Health, National Heart, Lung, and Blood Institute. August 2007. NIH publication 08-4051.

when taken before exertion. Recent studies have shown these drugs to be less effective in controlling asthma than inhaled corticosteroids. Cromolyn and Nedocromil are still considered treatment options for mild persistent asthma in adults and children ≥5 years of age (cromolyn only for children 0–4 years) although both are less preferred than inhaled corticosteroids.

Long-Acting β$_2$-Agonists

Salmeterol and formoterol are long-acting β$_2$-agonists that are currently approved in the United States for use in children. The bronchodilator effect of both these drugs lasts at least 12 hours after a single dose. The onset of action of salmeterol, but not of formoterol, is slower than that of inhaled albuterol. These drugs are indicated for the

TABLE 30.8

STEPWISE APPROACH FOR MANAGING ASTHMA IN YOUTHS ≥12 YEARS OF AGE AND ADULTS

Intermittent Asthma	**Persistent Asthma: Daily Medication** Consult with asthma specialist if step 4 care or higher is required. Consider consultation at step 3.

						Step up if needed
Step 1 *Preferred:* SABA PRN	**Step 2** *Preferred:* Low-dose ICS *Alternative:* Cromolyn, LTRA, Nedocromil, or Theophylline	**Step 3** *Preferred:* Low-dose ICS + LABA OR Medium-dose ICS *Alternative:* Low-dose ICS + either LTRA Theophylline, or Zileuton	**Step 4** *Preferred:* Medium-dose ICS + LABA *Alternative:* Medium-dose ICS + either LTRA, Theophylline, or Zileuton	**Step 5** *Preferred:* High-dose ICS + LABA AND Consider Omalizumale for patients who have allergies	**Step 6** *Preferred:* High-dose ICS + LABA + oral corticosteroid AND Consider Omalizumale for patients who have allergies	(first, check adherence, environmental control, and comorbid conditions) *Assess control* Step down if possible (and asthma is well controlled at least 3 months)

Each step:	**Patient education, environmental control, and management of comorbidities.**
Steps 2–4:	Consider subcutaneous allergen immunotherapy for patients who have allergic asthma (see notes).

Quick-Relief Medication for All Patients

- SABA as needed for symptoms. Intensity of treatment depends on severity of symptoms: up to 3 treatments at 20-minute intervals as needed. Short course of oral systemic corticosteroids may be needed.
- Use of SABA >2 days a week for symptom relief (not prevention of EIB) generally indicates inadequate control and the need to step up treatment.

Key: **Alphabetical order is used when more than one treatment option is listed within either preferred or alternative therapy.**
EIB, exercise-induced bronchospasm; ICS, inhaled corticosteroid; LABA, long-acting inhaled beta$_2$-agonist; LTRA, leukotriene receptor antagonist; SABA, inhaled short-acting beta$_2$-agonist.
Notes:
- The stepwise approach is meant to assist, not replace, the clinical decisionmaking required to meet individual patient needs.
- If alternative treatment is used and response is inadequate, discontinue it and use the preferred treatment before stepping up.
- Zileuton is a less desirable alternative due to limited studies as adjunctive therapy and the need to monitor liver function. Theophylline requires monitoring of serum concentration levels.
- In step 6, before oral systemic corticosteroids are introduced, a trial of high-dose ICS + LABA + either LTRA, theophylline, or zileuton may be considered, although this approach has not been studied in clinical trials.
- Step 1, 2, and 3 preferred therapies are based on Evidence A; step 3 alternative therapy is based on Evidence A for LTRA, Evidence B for theophylline, and Evidence D for zileuton. Step 4 preferred therapy is based on Evidence B, and alternative therapy is based on Evidence B for LTRA and theophylline and Evidence D for zileuton. Step 5 preferred therapy is based on Evidence B. Step 6 preferred therapy is based on (EPR—2 1997) and Evidence B for omalizumab.
- Immunotherapy for steps 2–4 is based on Evidence B for house-dust mites, animal danders, and pollens; evidence is weak or lacking for molds and cockroaches. Evidence is strongest for immunotherapy with single allergens. The role of allergy in asthma is greater in children than in adults.
- Clinicians who administer immunotherapy or omalizumab should be prepared and equipped to identify and treat anaphylaxis that may occur.

The information in Table 30.8 is directly abstracted from the National Asthma Education and Prevention Program Expert Panel Report 3: Guidelines for the Diagnosis and Management of Asthma. National Institutes of Health, National Heart, Lung, and Blood Institute. August 2007. NIH publication 08-4051.

TABLE 30.9

STEPWISE APPROACH FOR MANAGING ASTHMA IN CHILDREN 5–11 YEARS OF AGE

Intermittent Asthma	**Persistent Asthma: Daily Medication** Consult with asthma specialist if step 4 care or higher is required. Consider consultation at step 3.

Step 1
Preferred:
SABA PRN

Step 2
Preferred:
Low-dose ICS
Alternative:
Cromolyn, LTRA, Nedocromil, or Theophylline

Step 3
Preferred:
EITHER:
Low-dose ICS + either LABA, LTRA, or Theophylline
OR
Medium-dose ICS

Step 4
Preferred:
Medium-dose ICS + LABA
Alternative:
Medium-dose ICS + either LTRA or Theophylline

Step 5
Preferred:
High-dose ICS + LABA
Alternative:
High-dose ICS + either LTRA or Theophylline

Step 6
Preferred:
High-dose ICS + LABA + oral corticosteroid
Alternative:
High-dose ICS + either LTRA or Theophylline + oral systemic corticosteroid

Step up if needed

(first, check adherence, inhaler technique, environmental control, and comorbid conditions)

Assess control

Step down if possible

(and asthma is well controlled at least 3 months

Each step: Patient education, environmental control, and management of comorbidities.

Steps 2–4: Consider subcutaneous allergen immunotherapy for patients who have allergic asthma (see notes).

Quick-Relief Medication for All Patients

- SABA as needed for symptoms. Intensity of treatment depends on severity of symptoms: up to 3 treatments at 20-minute intervals as needed. Short course of oral systemic corticosteroids may be needed.
- Caution: Increasing use of SABA or use >2 days a week for symptom relief (not prevention of EIB) generally indicates inadequate control and the need to step up treatment.

Key: **Alphabetical order is used when more than one treatment option is listed within either preferred or alternative therapy.** ICS, inhaled corticosteroid; LABA, inhaled long-acting beta$_2$-agonist, LTRA, leukotriene receptor antagonist; SABA, inhaled short-acting beta$_2$-agonist.
Notes:
- The stepwise approach is meant to assist, not replace, the clinical decisionmaking required to meet individual patient needs.
- If alternative treatment is used and response is inadequate, discontinue it and use the preferred treatment before stepping up.
- Theophylline is a less desirable alternative due to the need to monitor serum concentration levels.
- Step 1 and step 2 medications are based on Evidence A. Step 3 ICS + adjunctive therapy and ICS are based on Evidence B for efficacy of each treatment and extrapolation from comparator trials in older children and adults—comparator trials are not available for this age group; steps 4–6 are based on expert opinion and extrapolation from studies in older children and adults.
- Immunotherapy for steps 2–4 is based on Evidence B for house-dust mites, animal danders, and pollens; evidence is weak or lacking for molds and cockroaches. Evidence is strongest for immunotherapy with single allergens. The role of allergy in asthma is greater in children than in adults. Clinicians who administer immunotherapy should be prepared and equipped to identify and treat anaphylaxis that may occur.

The information in Table 30.9 is directly abstracted from the National Asthma Education and Prevention Program *Expert Panel Report 3: Guidelines for the Diagnosis and Management of Asthma.* National Institutes of Health, National Heart, Lung, and Blood Institute. August 2007. NIH publication 08-4051.

prevention of exercise-induced bronchospasm and the long-term prevention of symptoms, especially nocturnal symptoms, in combination with anti-inflammatory therapy. The 2007 NAEEP guidelines state that the combination of a low-dose inhaled corticosteroid plus an inhaled long-acting β$_2$-agonist is equivalent in terms of outcomes to use of a medium-dose inhaled corticosteroid in children ≥5 years of age and adults. For children <5 years of age who are not well controlled on a low-dose inhaled corticosteroid, increasing the dose of the inhaled corticosteroid is preferred over the addition of a long-acting β$_2$-agonist.

Methylxanthines

Theophylline, the principally used methylxanthine, provides mild to moderate bronchodilation and also has mild

TABLE 30.10

STEPWISE APPROACH FOR MANAGING ASTHMA IN CHILDREN 0–4 YEARS OF AGE

Intermittent Asthma	Persistent Asthma: Daily Medication
	Consult with asthma specialist if step 3 care or higher is required. Consider consultation at step 2.

Step 1
Preferred:
SABA PRN

Step 2
Preferred:
Low-dose ICS
Alternative:
Cromolyn or Montelukast

Step 3
Preferred:
Medium-dose ICS

Step 4
Preferred:
Medium-dose ICS + either LABA or Montelukast

Step 5
Preferred:
High-dose ICS + either LABA or Montelukast

Step 6
Preferred:
High-dose ICS + either LABA or Montelukast
Oral systemic corticosteroids

Step up if needed
(first, check adherence, inhaler technique, and environmental control)

Assess control

Step down if possible
(and asthma is well controlled at least 3 months

Patient Education and Environmental Control at Each Step

Quick-Relief Medication for All Patients

- SABA as needed for symptoms. Intensity of treatment depends on severity of symptoms.
- With viral respiratory infection. SABA q 4–6 hours up to 24 hours (longer with physician consult). Consider short course of oral systemic corticosteroids if exacerbation is severe or patient has history of previous severe exacerbations.
- Caution: Frequent use of SABA may indicate the need to step up treatment. See text for recommendations on initiating daily long-term-control therapy.

Key: **Alphabetical order is used when more than one treatment option is listed within either preferred or alternative therapy.**
ICS, inhaled corticosteroid; LABA, inhaled long-acting beta₂-agonist; SABA, inhaled short-acting beta₂-agonist.
Notes:
- The stepwise approach is meant to assist, not replace, the clinical decisionmaking required to meet individual patient needs.
- If alternative treatment is used and response is inadequate, discontinue it and use the preferred treatment before stepping up.
- If clear benefit is not observed within 4–6 weeks and patient/family medication technique and adherence are satisfactory, consider adjusting therapy or alternative diagnosis.
- Studies on children 0–4 years of age are limited. Step 2 preferred therapy is based on Evidence A. All other recommendations are based on expert opinion and extrapolation from studies in older children.

The information in Table 30.10 is directly abstracted from the National Asthma Education and Prevention Program *Expert Panel Report 3: Guidelines for the Diagnosis and Management of Asthma.* National Institutes of Health, National Heart, Lung, and Blood Institute. August 2007. NIH publication 08-4051.

---

anti-inflammatory effects. Sustained-release theophylline is primarily used as an adjunctive therapy in moderate or severe persistent asthma and is partially effective for controlling nocturnal asthma symptoms. Oral steroid-sparing effects of sustained-release theophylline have been demonstrated in children with moderate to severe persistent asthma, and it can be used as an alternative to inhaled medications if cost, side effects, or failure to adhere to a medication regimen are issues that prevent the use of inhaled drugs. Theophylline therapy can cause significant side effects and, therefore, is infrequently used in children currently.

Leukotriene Modifiers

Leukotriene modifiers are relatively new medications for the treatment of asthma and have the ability to target leukotrienes, a specific component of the inflammatory process in asthma. Three leukotriene modifiers (zafirlukast, zileuton, montelukast) are available in the United States, but only one, montelukast, is currently approved for use in very young children. Zafirlukast and montelukast are leukotriene receptor antagonists, and zileuton inhibits the enzyme 5-lipoxygenase to decrease the synthesis of leukotrienes. Leukotriene modifiers can protect against exercise-induced bronchospasm, and in chronic

TABLE 30.11

SUMMARY OF CONTROL MEASURES FOR ENVIRONMENTAL FACTORS THAT CAN MAKE ASTHMA WORSE

Allergens: Reduce or eliminate exposure to the allergen(s) to which the patient is sensitive, including

- Animal dander: Remove animal from house or, at a minimum, keep animal out of patient's bedroom and use a filter to seal or cover the air ducts that lead to the bedroom.
- House dust mites:
  - Essential: Encase mattress in an allergen-impermeable cover; encase pillow in an allergen-impermeable cover or wash it weekly; wash sheets and blankets on the patient's bed in hot water weekly (water temperature ≥54.44°C [130°F] is necessary for killing mites). Desirable: Reduce indoor humidity to <50%; remove carpets from the bedroom; avoid sleeping or lying on upholstered furniture; remove carpets that are laid on concrete.
- Cockroaches: Use poison bait or traps to control. Do not leave food or garbage exposed.
- Pollens (from trees, grass, or weeds) and outdoor molds: To avoid exposures, adults should stay indoors with windows closed during the season when they have problems with outdoor allergens, especially in the afternoon.
- Indoor mold: Fix all leaks and eliminate water sources associated with mold growth; clean moldy surfaces. Consider reducing indoor humidity to <50%.

Tobacco smoke: Advise patients and others at home who smoke to stop smoking or to smoke outside the home. Discuss ways to reduce exposure to other sources of tobacco smoke, such as day care providers and coworkers who smoke. *Indoor/outdoor pollutants and irritants:* Discuss ways to reduce exposures to the following:

- Wood-burning stoves or fireplaces
- Unvented stoves or heaters
- Other irritants (e.g., perfumes, cleaning agents, sprays)

From National Institutes of Health. NAEPP guidelines for the management and diagnosis of asthma. *National Asthma Education and Prevention Program*, NIH Pub No 02-5075. Bethesda, MD: 2002, NIH.

asthma improve the signs and symptoms, although their clinical effects are generally modest. They are taken orally and may be used as an alternative, although less preferred, to low-dose inhaled corticosteroids in children with mild persistent asthma.

Anti-IgE Therapy

Omalizumab, the first selective anti-immunoglobulin E (IgE) therapy, is a recombinant mouse humanized monoclonal antibody directed against human IgE. A multicenter study in children older than 6 years who were well controlled on inhaled corticosteroids showed that treatment with omalizumab allowed significant reductions in inhaled corticosteroid doses without worsening of their asthma. Omalizumab is given by subcutaneous injection every 2 or 4 weeks. It is currently indicated for adults and children 12 years of age or older, who have moderate to severe asthma that is inadequately controlled on inhaled corticosteroids and those who have evidence of specific allergic sensitivity by positive results for skin or blood tests.

Environmental Control

For the successful long-term management of asthma, it is crucial to identify and reduce exposure to environmental factors known to precipitate or exacerbate symptoms. Exposure to inhalant allergens to which a child is sensitive or to airborne irritants increases airway inflammation and symptoms, whereas significant reduction of such exposure reduces inflammation, symptoms, and the need

for medication. Recommended measures to control environmental factors that can exacerbate asthma are summarized in Table 30.11.

Asthma Education

Educating asthmatic children and their families about all aspects of the disease is an important component of overall management. The NAEPP advocates the following measures directed toward achieving this goal:

- Begin patient education at the time of diagnosis and integrate additional information into each step of asthma care.
- Involve all members of the health care team in educating patients and families.
- Teach and reinforce at every available opportunity basic facts about asthma and the role of medication. Patients should also be instructed in the use of inhalers and spacers, in self-monitoring, rescue medication, and methods of environmental control.
- Provide all patients with a written daily plan for self-management and an action plan for dealing with exacerbations.

PROGNOSIS

The prognosis for young children with asthma is generally quite good. Approximately 20% of infants who have wheezing associated with viral infections during the first year of life no longer wheeze by the time they are 3 years old. Approximately 50% of all asthmatic children are essentially free of symptoms 10 to 20 years later, but recurrence of symptoms during adulthood is common. The remission rate for children in whom mild asthma develops between the age of 2 years and puberty is approximately 50%, with severe disease developing in only 5%. Fewer than 20% of children with persistent wheezing during childhood become completely free of wheezing, and therefore persistent wheezing during childhood is an unfavorable prognostic sign.

Airway hyperreactivity may persist indefinitely in formerly asthmatic patients despite the complete absence of clinical signs and symptoms of asthma. Studies have demonstrated abnormal responsiveness in some of these patients for up to 20 years after their symptoms have completely resolved.

REVIEW EXERCISES

QUESTIONS

Case 1

A 1-year-old girl with recurrent wheezing is referred to your office for evaluation. She required inhaled albuterol three to four times a week during the last 3 months to treat her symptoms. The environmental history reveals that there are two dogs in the home and that both parents smoke.

1. Which of the following statements regarding the environmental factors in her home is *true?*
a) Placing a high-quality air filter in her bedroom will significantly reduce her exposure to dust mites.
b) She is likely to experience more frequent exacerbations of wheezing during the next year unless the dogs are removed from the home.
c) Continued exposure to passive cigarette smoke will increase her risk for having asthma later in childhood.
d) Encasing her mattress and pillow in allergen-impermeable covers is likely to result in less frequent wheezing, particularly at night.

Answer
The answer is c. Passive exposure to tobacco smoke is a risk factor for the development of asthma in children. It is unusual for children younger than 2 years to be clinically sensitive to inhalant allergens, such as dust mites, animal danders, and mold, although intense exposure to some inhalant allergens early in life may be a risk factor for the development of asthma later in childhood. It has not been proved that air filters significantly reduce the level of dust mites in bedrooms. However, encasing mattresses and pillows in allergen-impermeable covers and removing carpeting from bedrooms are effective measures for reducing exposure to dust mites.

2. The preferred therapy for the long-term management and control of her wheezing is:
a) Inhaled albuterol given three to four times daily
b) Sustained-release theophylline
c) A long-acting β_2-agonist given every 12 hours
d) Low-dose inhaled corticosteroid given by nebulization

Answer
The answer is d. The frequency of symptoms in this child is consistent with mild persistent asthma. The most appropriate long-term control medication for mild persistent asthma is an anti-inflammatory drug. A low-dose inhaled corticosteroid is the preferred therapy for this level of severity in children of all ages.

3. Alternative therapy for long-term management and control of her wheezing is:
a) Cromolyn
b) Theophylline
c) Montelukast
d) a and c

Answer
The answer is d. Cromolyn and montelukast are both alternatives to low-dose inhaled corticosteroids for treatment of mild persistent asthma in children 0 to 4 years of age.

Case 2

You are evaluating a 9-year-old girl for cough and wheezing that are usually responsive to inhaled albuterol. She typically has symptoms four or five times a week, and she wakes up at night because of coughing two to three times a month.

4. The level of asthma severity that *best* fits her symptoms is:
a) Moderate persistent
b) Mild intermittent
c) Severe persistent
d) Mild persistent

Answer
The answer is d. Patients with mild persistent asthma typically have symptoms more often than twice a week but less often than once a day. Nocturnal symptoms may occur more frequently than twice a month but not more often than once a week.

5. Which of the following should *not* be used as monotherapy for the long-term control of her symptoms?
a) Long-acting β_2-agonist
b) Low dose of an inhaled corticosteroid
c) Sustained-release theophylline
d) Leukotriene modifier

Answer
The answer is a. All are effective long-term control medications, but long-acting β_2-agonists should always

be used in combination with an anti-inflammatory asthma drug, not as monotherapy.

Case 3

The mother of one of your asthmatic patients is pregnant and concerned that her second child will also have asthma.

6. Which of the following does *not* increase the risk that her next child will have asthma?

a) The mother has a history of asthma.
b) The mother is a smoker.
c) The mother is past the age of 35 years.
d) The mother knows that her second child will be a boy.

Answer

The answer is c. A maternal age of less than 20 years at the time of birth is a risk factor for the development of asthma. Male sex, maternal smoking, and parental history of asthma are also risk factors for the development of childhood asthma.

SUGGESTED READINGS

1. Agertoft L, Pedersen S. Effect of long-term treatment with inhaled budesonide on adult height in children with asthma. *N Engl J Med* 2000;343:1064–1069.
2. Childhood Asthma Management Program Research Group. Long-term effects of budesonide or nedocromil in children with asthma. *N Engl J Med* 2000;343:1054–1063.
3. Martinez FD, Wright AL, Taussig LM, et al. Asthma and wheezing in the first six years of life. *N Engl J Med* 1995;332:133–138.
4. National Asthma Education and Preventin Program (NAEEP). *Expert Panel Report 3: Guidelines for the Diagnosis and Management of Asthma*, Full Report 2007. Bethesda, MD: National Heart, Lung, and Blood Institute; August 2007, NIH Publication 07-4051.
5. Reed CE. The natural history of asthma. *J Allergy Clin Immunol* 2006;118:543–548.
6. Sears MR, Greene JM, Willan AR, et al. A longitudinal, population-based, cohort study of childhood asthma followed to adulthood. *N Engl J Med* 2003;349:1414–1422.
7. Yawn BP, Brennemen S.K, Allen-Ramey FC, et al. Assessment of asthma severity and asthma control in children. *Pediatrics* 2006; 118:322–329.

Chapter 31

BOARD SIMULATION: Airway and Pulmonary Disorders

Samiya Razvi

QUESTIONS

1. An infant is born at 32 weeks gestation by cesarean section to a 19-year-old primigravida mother who had no antenatal care and whose Group B Streptococcal (GBS) status is unknown. He weighs 1100 g at birth; Apgar scores are 6 and 9 at 1 and 5 minutes. He is placed on continuous positive airway pressure (CPAP) with supplemental oxygen ($FiO_2 = 0.5$).

At 12 hours of age, he is noted to have increased retractions, grunting, and mild cyanosis. His heart rate is 170/minute, pulses are well felt, respiratory rate is 54/minute, and blood pressure is 70/40. Breath sounds are diminished on auscultation but heard equally over both lung fields. No murmur is heard on cardiac examination.

A portable chest radiograph (CXR) shows ground glass opacities and diffuse haziness of both lung fields. The most likely diagnosis is:

a) Transient tachypnea of the newborn
b) Meconium aspiration syndrome
c) Congenital pneumonia with neonatal sepsis
d) Respiratory distress syndrome with surfactant deficiency
e) Congenital diaphragmatic hernia with cardiorespiratory compromise

Answer

The answer is d. The primary cause of *respiratory distress in the newborn* is inadequate surfactant, which serves to decrease alveolar surface tension. Inadequate surfactant results in diffuse alveolar atelectasis, decreased aeration, reduced lung compliance, edema, and cell injury. Clinically this is manifested as tachypnea, increased work of breathing with retractions, grunting, and cyanosis because of hypoxemia. Radiologically, the classic appearance is of low lung volumes, diffuse reticulogranular patterns, and air bronchograms on CXR. Management is aimed to prevent hypoxia and acidosis and includes surfactant replacement, optimizing fluid balance, reducing metabolic demands, and limiting lung injury because of barotrauma and oxygen while providing ventilatory support.

Transient tachypnea of the newborn is a self-limited disorder seen more often in near term or term infants, particularly those born by cesarean section. It represents transient pulmonary edema as a result of delayed absorption of pulmonary lung fluid by the pulmonary lymphatics. Infants are tachypneic with retractions, grunting within a few hours of delivery, and have a mild to moderate oxygen requirement. Symptoms typically last for 12 to 24 hours and rarely persist longer than 72 hours in severe cases.

Meconium aspiration syndrome (MAS) occurs because of acute or chronic hypoxia of the fetus with passage of meconium in utero. Gasping or initial breathing efforts of the fetus or newborn infant can result in aspiration of amniotic fluid contaminated by meconium. Meconium obstructs the airways and interferes with gas exchange resulting in severe respiratory distress. MAS occurs in about 8% to 15% of live births, rarely occurs prior to 37 weeks gestation but may occur in more than one third of post-term pregnancies. Prevention is by clearing the nose and oropharynx before the infant's chest is delivered. Next, the trachea should be intubated under direct vision before inspiratory efforts begin and meconium suctioned to clear the trachea as possible.

2. A 6-month-old term infant born without complications is seen at a routine visit for immunization. She is alert, interactive, pink, and well appearing. Her weight is at the 50th and length at the 25th percentile for age. She has audible inspiratory stridor without retractions or distress. Her lungs are clear on auscultation.

She is feeding well with occasional spit ups and is gaining weight. Her mother has noted this noisy breathing, which she calls "wheezing" since 2 weeks of age. The "wheezing" was louder a week ago when she had a cold and upper respiratory symptoms for a few days. There is family history of asthma in both parents and two older siblings. The investigation you would consider at this point is:

a) CXR to evaluate for hyperinflation, asthma
b) Upper GI study to screen for structural anomalies
c) Chest computed tomography (CT) scan for structural abnormalities
d) Bronchoscopy to evaluate the airways
e) No investigations now, continue to observe and monitor clinically

Answer

The answer is b. *Stridor* is an audible, coarse, grating sound with a classic crowing quality, caused by turbulent air flow during respiration as a direct result of narrowing of the airway. Factors that lead to increased airflow turbulence such as agitation, crying, and exertion result in an increase in stridor. Stridor may be decreased or even absent when the patient is breathing calmly at rest, or when asleep. The timing of stridor in the respiratory cycle can broadly help localize the site of location of airflow obstruction as shown in Table 31.1. Causes of stridor in infancy include:

- Laryngomalacia
- Tracheomalacia
- Subglottic stenosis
- Airway lesions such as webs, cysts, and hemangioma
- Vascular malformations such as "ring/sling" anomalies
- Vocal cord paralysis
- Infection: croup, epiglottitis, bacterial tracheitis
- Foreign body aspiration

The key/discerning features of these causes of noisy breathing in infants and children are summarized in Table 31.2.

The word *malacia* denotes an abnormal "softness of the tissues." *The most common cause of stridor in infants is laryngomalacia;* there is softness of the laryngeal cartilages and increased collapsibility of the larynx and supralaryngeal tissues into the glottis during inspiration leading to airway obstruction. Symptoms classically appear soon after birth, and increase in intensity as the infant grows and becomes increasingly active.

Although there are several possible causes of stridor, a careful history and physical examination help to differentiate those who need further evaluation and intervention from those who may safely be monitored clinically and observed. *A barium swallow and upper gastrointestinal study is useful to screen for vascular (ring/sling) anomalies* that can cause airway compromise seen as a filling defect in the barium column or indentation of the esophagus. Symptoms resolve with increasing age in the majority by

TABLE 31.1

TIMING OF STRIDOR AND ITS RELATION TO AIRWAY OBSTRUCTION

Phase of Respiration When Stridor Occurs	Location of Airway Obstruction	Features
Inspiration	Extrathoracic airway: Larynx, extrathoracic trachea	Extrathoracic airway subject to negative intrapleural pressures generated in inspiration and collapses
Expiration	Intrathoracic airway: Trachea, large bronchi	Intrathoracic airways subject to extramural positive pressures that compress airways during expiration
Biphasic: both inspiration and expiration	Suggestive of fixed airway obstruction at any site in trachea	Fixed obstruction causes constant airflow obstruction in both phases of respiration
Variable: changing	Suggestive of dynamic, changing airway obstruction	Lesions that cause varying obstruction of airway, e.g., airway polyps, hemangiomas

12 to 18 months of age and infants may be followed closely without intervention if feeding, growth, and development are normal. Severe cases of laryngomalacia may interfere with feeding and surgical interventions to trim the redundant supralaryngeal tissues may be indicated.

Asthma is associated with wheezing, an expiratory high pitched whistling sound indicative of small airways obstruction, and not stridor. Chest CT scan is not indicated here as there are no symptoms or signs of lower airway or parenchymal lung disease. Bronchoscopy is a definitive, diagnostic tool to examine the airways and airway dynamics but is invasive and requires sedation. It is not indicated at this point in an otherwise well, thriving infant with inspiratory stridor and typical presentation of laryngomalacia.

3. A healthy 10-year-old boy is active in sport and plays soccer. He has a history of wheezing with respiratory infections, especially in winter and fewer symptoms in summer. He has frequent sneezing, nasal congestion, and watering of eyes in spring and fall. He uses inhaled bronchodilators (Albuterol) with good symptom relief. His father notes that he coughs while running and playing soccer and is visibly short of breath. He coughs at night, but this does not awaken him from sleep. You decide to evaluate his symptoms with spirometry (pre- and postbronchodilator), which assesses:
a) Oxygenation and desaturation pre- and post-exercise
b) Diffusing capacity of the lungs for oxygen
c) Expiratory flow rates and volumes
d) Maximal minute ventilation and exercise capacity

TABLE 31.2

KEY DISCERNING FEATURES OF COMMON CAUSES OF "NOISY BREATHING" IN INFANTS AND CHILDREN

	Timing	Feature	Bronchoscopy	Diagnosis
Laryngomalacia	Inspiratory "Crowing"	Improves with age, ↑ with exertion ↑ supine, ↓ prone	Curled epiglottis ("omega") Prolapse of arytenoids	Clinical features Natural course Bronchoscopy
Tracheomalacia	Wheezing biphasic	Prematurity, Postsurgical inflammation ↑ agitation ↑ exertion	Anteroposterior dynamic collapse of trachea	Flexible bronchoscopy Airway fluoroscopy
Subglottic stenosis	Biphasic High-pitched	History of intubation, trauma	Narrowing of subglottis	Radiograph of airway Bronchoscopy
Vascular ring or sling	Inspiratory stridor Wheeze	Indentation of esophagus on barium swallow	May have dysphagia, reflux	Upper GI study (indentation of esophagus) CT imaging
Vocal cord palsy	Dysphonia Aphonia	Trauma CNS lesions Cardiac surgery	Immobile cords Unilateral or bilateral	Direct visualization by endoscopy

e) Total lung capacity, vital capacity, residual volume and air trapping secondary to small airway obstruction

Answer

The answer is c. Asthma is characterized by *expiratory airflow obstruction* with wheezing, a high-pitched whistling sound in expiration, cough indicative of airway inflammation, and often exercise-induced symptoms. A careful history of *symptom pattern and recurrence and treatment response* to inhaled β-agonists (which cause bronchodilatation) and/or anti-inflammatory medications (corticosteroids, leukotriene inhibitors) is consistent with the clinical diagnosis of asthma. Spirometry is an objective test for asthma and measures expiratory airflow rates and volumes on a forced expiratory maneuver that requires patient cooperation. Measurements are compared with population based norms for airflow rates, forced vital capacity (FVC), and forced expiratory volume in one second (FEV1) and are expressed as a percentage of predicted measures.

Typical patterns in the configuration of the flow volume loop and airflow indices on spirometry are seen in *obstructive diseases* (e.g., asthma, airway malacia or narrowing) and *restrictive diseases* (e.g., respiratory muscle weakness in muscular dystrophy, neuromuscular disease, and thoracic cage abnormalities such as kyphoscoliosis). Classic spirometry patterns shown in Figure 31.1 are summarized in Table 31.3. *Body plethysmography* measures lung volumes including total lung capacity and residual volumes. The *diffusing capacity* of the lungs for oxygen uptake is measured utilizing carbon monoxide, an inert gas. An *exercise test* assesses the cardiopulmonary responses to graded exercise in the laboratory, including the anaerobic threshold and whether there is ventilation limitation in an individual's response to the physiologic demands of exercise.

4. A 2-year-old boy is brought to the emergency room at midnight with difficulty breathing and respiratory distress. There are multiple sick contacts at home this past week. He has had nasal discharge, cough, and fever for

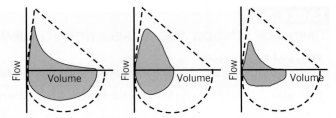

Figure 31.1 Spirometry and flow-volume patterns in obstructive, restrictive, and mixed pattern lung disease.

3 days. His cough increased this evening since he was put to bed. He appears anxious, tired and toxic. He is febrile (104°F), HR = 150/min, RR = 40/minute with lower intercostal and subcostal retractions. Pulse oximetry is 93% on oxygen via facemask at 6 L/minute. CXR shows ragged appearance of the tracheal air column. The best *first* step in managing this patient is to:
a) Obtain an urgent x-ray of the lateral soft tissues of neck and airway.
b) Obtain a chest CT scan with contrast.
c) Plan an urgent bronchoscopy.
d) Intubate the boy in a controlled manner.
e) Obtain a stat arterial blood gas.

Answer

The answer is d. The differential diagnoses for this clinical scenario and their key discerning features are given in Table 31.4. Clinical considerations include the age of the child, onset, progression and severity of respiratory distress, and assessment of airway compromise in determining appropriate management decisions.

In children with respiratory distress, particularly infants, there is a real danger of respiratory muscle fatigue and cardiorespiratory decompensation requiring intubation and ventilatory support. In an older child with a febrile, toxic illness, clues to airway compromise may be based on radiologic evidence (ragged air column), as in this case in addition to clinical signs.

TABLE 31.3

KEY SPIROMETRY FEATURES OF AIR FLOW PATTERNS IN LUNG DISEASE

	Obstructive	Restrictive	Mixed
Configuration of flow-volume loop	Concave	Normal but decreased volume	Both concave and decreased volume
FVC	↓	↓↓↓	↓↓
FEV1	↓↓↓	↓↓↓	↓↓
FEV1/FVC ratio	↓↓	Normal or ↑↑	↓↓
FEF 25%–75%	↓↓	Normal or ↑↑	Normal or ↓↓

FEF 25%–75%, forced expiratory flows between 25% and 75% of FVC; FEV1, forced expiratory volume in 1 second; FVC, forced vital capacity.

TABLE 31.4

KEY DISCERNING FEATURES OF A YOUNG CHILD WITH RESPIRATORY DISTRESS

	Age Group	Etiologic Agent	Radiographic Features	Treatment
Croup, Laryngotracheobronchitis (LTB)	Infancy to early childhood	Viral *Parainfluenza* type 1	"Steeple sign" on PA neck film	Cool mist Racemic epinephrine Corticosteroids
Epiglottitis	2–7 years	Group A Strep *S. aureus* *Haemophilus influenzae* type b	"Thumb sign" on lateral neck film	Secure airway Intubate Antibiotics
Bacterial tracheitis	Older children	*Staph aureus* Patients with Tracheostomy: gram-negatives	Subglottic narrowing Ragged air column	Secure airway Intubation Antibiotics Corticosteroids
Airway foreign body	Toddlers, any age		Persistent atelectasis Localized hyperinflation	Rigid bronchoscopy for removal

It is important *to avoid agitation* of the already anxious child, and defer any invasive, painful procedures or tests. If essential, testing should be performed in a controlled setting, in which the airway can be safely secured in the event of clinical deterioration or respiratory compromise. In acute respiratory distress, maintenance of a stable airway is a priority. Elective rather than emergency intubation is preferred, as this will cause least manipulation and trauma to the airway.

Epiglottitis in the postvaccination (*Haemophilus influenzae* type b) era can be caused by other bacterial pathogens including *Staphylococcal aureus* and *Streptococcus pyogenes*. *Laryngotracheobronchitis* (croup) is often preceded by a viral prodromal illness, and responds well to systemic corticosteroids administered either intramuscularly or orally. A number of viruses can cause laryngotracheobronchitis, but the most common are *parainfluenza viruses 1, 2, and 3*, with type 1 being more common than types 2 and 3. Other viral pathogens in croup include influenza A virus, influenza B virus, adenovirus, respiratory syncytial virus, and the rhinoviruses. *Retropharyngeal abscess* presents with drooling and stridor in a febrile, toxic child with significant airway compromise. There is a widening of the prevertebral soft tissues and edema on lateral soft tissue films of the neck, and surgical drainage of pus is often required. *Bacterial tracheitis* is a fulminating infection, with mucosal sloughing, pus, and pseudomembrane formation that can occlude the airway. *Staphylococcus aureus* is the most common cause of bacterial tracheitis, but tracheal aspirate cultures should be done to tailor antibiotic therapy accordingly.

5. A 12-year-old girl with trisomy 21 and asthma is on inhaled corticosteroids (Fluticasone) twice daily and is on immunotherapy for allergic rhinitis. She is not very physically active and has gained 15 lbs over the past year. She had been doing well in special education until recently. She has been irritable in class with a poor attention span and has not been learning well. Her parents admit that they have not been regular with her inhaled asthma medications and that she has a daily cough. She has always had snoring, but this has increased in recent months with restless sleep and frequent awakenings. Your priority in her management at this time is:
a) Refer her for a sleep study.
b) Increase inhaled asthma medication regimen including a long-acting β-agonist (LABA) for better control.
c) Refer her for screening and evaluation of attention deficit hyperactivity disorder (ADHD).
d) Perform nutrition counseling for weight gain.
e) Repeat skin testing for environmental triggers; intensify treatment for allergic rhinitis and nasal obstruction causing snoring.

Answer
The answer is a. *Primary snoring* is common in children because of adenoid and tonsillar enlargement in early childhood. Symptoms of *sleep disordered breathing* include:

- Observed pauses in breathing
- Choking and frequent awakenings resulting in poor sleep quality
- Difficulty in waking up in the morning

Children seldom experience daytime somnolence as compared to adults. Irritability, mood changes, learning problems and poor school performance are often indicators of disrupted and nonrefreshing sleep. Craniofacial malformations, hypotonia, and neurological disorders causing increased upper airway collapsibility in sleep are risk factors for obstructive sleep apnea (OSA). *The physiologic consequences of OSA are:*

- Nighttime hypoxemia
- Decreased ventilation resulting in hypercarbia
- Right heart strain over time

Overall there are significant adverse effects on growth and neurologic and cardiac function. A sleep study or *polysomnogram* is the gold standard and remains the study of choice. Treatment includes adenotonsillectomy. Noninvasive ventilation during sleep using either continuous positive airway pressure (CPAP) or bilevel positive airway pressure (BiPAP) using a nasal mask interface are also useful.

6. A 4-year-old girl who recently migrated to the United States from Southeast Asia has nasal discharge, dry cough, and intermittent fever for 3 days. She now presents with high fever of 103°F, decreased oral intake, abdominal pain, and weight loss. She is grunting and tachypneic with intercostal retractions. Breath sounds are diminished and harsh, tubular over the right chest with scattered crackles. There is no wheeze. Labs show a white blood cell count of 22,000 with shift to the left, ESR of 64 mm/hour and decreased serum sodium of 130 mEq/L. A PPD is placed, blood culture is drawn and CXR is done, which shows lobar consolidation of the entire right upper lobe of the lung. The most likely etiology/pathogen is:

a) *Mycoplasma pneumoniae*
b) Adenovirus
c) *Mycobacterium tuberculosis*
d) *Streptococcus pneumoniae*
e) Methicillin-resistant *Staphylococcus aureus* (MRSA)

Answer

The answer is d. This is a classic presentation of pneumococcal pneumonia with high fever, bacteremia, lobar involvement, high white blood cell count, and hyponatremia secondary to the syndrome of inappropriate antidiuretic hormone production. Additionally, there may be shaking chills or rigors and rusty sputum production. Classically, there is defervescence with parenteral antibiotic therapy and complete recovery is usual. Complications include pleural effusion, empyema, and abscess formation and rarely bronchopleural fistula formation. Clinical resolution may occur rapidly, but radiologic lag is recognized and CXRs may take up to 4 to 6 weeks for complete resolution.

Viruses cause the majority of community-acquired pneumonia in childhood and may be difficult to differentiate from bacterial pneumonia. A viral prodrome may be present; clinically patients may be tachypneic and more hypoxemic because of interstitial involvement. *Mycoplasma pneumoniae* causes atypical or walking pneumonia and patients may not appear as sick or debilitated. Cold agglutinins or antibodies against red cell antigens may be absent in about half the cases, and are not specific. *Mycobacterium tuberculosis* causes primary complex tuberculosis associated with fever, failure to thrive with radiological infiltrates, lymphadenopathy, and positive tuberculin skin test. Children with primary tuberculosis do *not* have cavitary disease and hence are not infectious to others. The usual source of tuberculous infection for a child is an adult contact, and family members must be screened thoroughly with tuberculin skin testing, CXR, and sputum cultures.

7. A 9-month-old white infant has had a daily cough since birth. His cough is worse with upper respiratory infections and is associated with wheezing. His cough has never really cleared. He is active, and feeds well and vigorously without choking. He does spit up frequently, but is playful and does not appear distressed. He has had colic since the neonatal period with abdominal bloating and frequent loose stools. His weight gain has been slow, and current weight is below the fifth percentile for age, whereas his length is at the 25th percentile. There is a family history of asthma and gastroesophageal reflux. The most likely clinical diagnosis at this point before further investigation is:

a) Mild persistent asthma
b) Cystic fibrosis
c) Gastroesophageal reflux with wheezing
d) Swallowing dysfunction with microaspiration
e) Bilateral vocal cord palsy, growth and developmental delay

Answer

The answer is b. *Cystic fibrosis* (CF) is the most common inherited disease in whites, affecting 1 in 3300 individuals; about 1 in 25 are carriers. The most common mutation is δ508 (deletion of phenylalanine at position 508). There are more than 1000 recognized genetic mutations that cause CF and a wide spectrum of disease severity. Therefore, it is essential for clinicians to maintain a high index of suspicion for CF because of the heterogeneity and variability of disease. Clinical features that should prompt screening for CF are:

- Chronic cough (or wheeze)
- Recurrent pneumonia
- Gastrointestinal symptoms of malabsorption
- Failure to thrive

Meconium ileus in the neonatal period is a hall mark of pancreatic insufficiency and CF. About 85% to 90% of patients with CF are pancreatic insufficient.

Newborn screening for CF tests for elevated levels of immunoreactive trypsinogen (IRT) followed by a mutation screening. The gold standard for diagnosis of CF is the sweat test; an elevated sweat chloride level is diagnostic. CF patients have viscous respiratory secretions, leading to airway obstruction, inflammation, and respiratory infections with a cascade of pathogens beginning in infancy. *Pseudomonas aeruginosa* colonizes CF lungs and is pathognomonic of the disease. By age 8 to 10 years almost 80% of patients are colonized with *Pseudomonas aeruginosa*. Pulmonary exacerbations of CF are characterized by increased cough and sputum production, decreased pulmonary function on spirometry, and weight loss. Management includes aggressive use of antibiotics by the parenteral or oral route in addition to inhaled antibiotics and chest physical therapy using mechanical percussion or vibratory vest devices to aid airway clearance.

8. A 12-year-old girl is hit by a car while rollerblading. She falls several feet and sustains multiple injuries, including closed head injury, facial trauma, bilateral rib, and pelvic and extremity fractures. She is transported by EMS to the nearest trauma center and is drowsy but arousable. Her heart rate is 140/minute and regular, respirations are 24/minute with pulse oximetry saturations of >94% on oxygen via face mask. Her initial blood pressure was low and she received parenteral fluids. A head CT scan is done, which is normal. On returning from CT scan, she is noted to have sudden duskiness of lips, respiratory distress, and cold, clammy extremities with poorly palpable pulses. Breath sounds are absent over the right hemithorax. Your first step in managing this child is:

a) Initiate 100% oxygen via a non-rebreather mask, start chest compressions, and draw up ionotropic drugs.
b) Intubate the patient and start mechanical ventilatory support.
c) Obtain an urgent CXR.
d) Begin immediate needle decompression of the right pleural cavity.
e) Call for an urgent surgical consult for chest tube placement.

Answer

The answer is d. Important considerations in a patient with trauma are assessment and stabilization of the airway particularly with facial and neck/cervical spine injury. Chest trauma with thoracic cage fractures leads to flail chest and ineffective ventilatory efforts. Rib fractures or penetrating chest wounds can lead to air leak resulting in pneumothorax and/or pneumomediastinum.

Tension pneumothorax is a true life-threatening emergency with rapid and severe cardiorespiratory decompensation. Clinical diagnosis is based on decreased or absent breath sounds with hyperresonance of the affected hemithorax, tracheal deviation to the opposite side, respiratory distress, hypotension, and shock resulting from decreased cardiac output. The first step in management of a rapidly decompensating patient with clinical signs of tension pneumothorax is emergency needle decompression of the pneumothorax. This can be followed by chest tube placement for continued drainage of the air leak. Supplemental oxygen, ventilatory and circulatory support, and fluid resuscitation can be instituted as indicated to further stabilize the patient.

Spontaneous pneumothorax can occur in the neonatal period in up to 1% of deliveries secondary to high negative intrapleural pressures generated with the first breaths following birth. Asymptomatic, small pneumothoraces can be managed expectantly; providing

100% inspired oxygen can aid in absorption of the pneumothorax by nitrogen washout. In older children, spontaneous pneumothorax can occur without an underlying cause, secondary to spontaneous rupture of an underlying bullous lung lesion or asthma. *Pneumomediastinum* can occur spontaneously, and is often asymptomatic. Subcutaneous emphysema may be noted with pneumomediastinum secondary to tracking of the air along the mediastinum and into the subcutaneous tissues of the neck. Management is often careful monitoring of cardiorespiratory status until spontaneous resolution occurs. Rarely, a large pneumomediastinum can cause impaired cardiac filling in diastole, pulsus paradoxus, and cardiac tamponade.

9. A 17-year-old league football player had an ankle fracture last year that prevented him from playing an entire season. He is anxious to get back on the team this year. He has a history of exercise-induced asthma and seasonal allergies, and uses Albuterol prior to exercise with benefit. He now reports shortness of breath when playing football and reduced exercise tolerance. He finds it extremely hard to breathe, and feels like his "chest is closing and he cannot catch a breath" within a few minutes of playing. He also reports palpitations and severe chest pain and has to stop playing until symptoms subside. He is very anxious, as this has affected his game and performance on the team. Of the conditions listed in the following, the most likely diagnosis at this time would be:

a) Inadequately controlled asthma that is exercise induced
b) Chronic sinusitis
c) Suboptimal/poor physical conditioning
d) Vocal cord dysfunction
e) Undiagnosed cardiac condition unmasked during exercise

Answer

The answer is d. *Vocal cord dysfunction* (VCD) occurs when the vocal cords close paradoxically in inspiration causing obstruction of airflow at the level of the glottis. This results in severe dyspnea, which patients describe as a sensation of their "throat closing" and being "unable to get a breath in." Symptoms are dramatic, often start within a few minutes of exertion and end abruptly, unlike exercise-induced bronchoconstriction, which typically occurs several minutes into moderate physical exertion. There may be associated inspiratory stridor, as the vocal cords are held classically in adduction. There is a posterior glottic chink, which allows airflow; hence, these patients are rarely hypoxemic. A clue to diagnosis is that dyspnea and shortness of breath brought on by exercise are not relieved by inhaled bronchodilators, as is the case with exercise-induced asthma.

Vocal cord dysfunction can occur in patients with asthma, and there may be considerable symptom overlap. A *careful history is needed* to distinguish between symptoms; notably inspiratory difficulty and stridor in VCD. The majority of patients with VCD are female and are usually high achievers. Airway outflow rates are normal on spirometry in VCD without asthma; there may be truncation of the inspiratory loop of the flow volume curve, indicating airflow obstruction during inspiration. It is important to diagnose VCD to avoid unnecessary medications (inhaled therapies and corticosteroids) as well as emergency invasive intervention such as intubation, as these patients often have a dramatic presentation and do not respond to usual asthma medications. Diagnosis is made by flexible nasopharyngoscopy and visualization of the vocal cords in the classic adducted position when the patient is symptomatic. Treatment involves behavioral modification, relaxation techniques, and alleviation of underlying anxiety if present.

10. An 18-year-old girl has had chronic cough since childhood, frequent ear and sinus infections, recurrent pneumonia, and asthma. She has had frequent antibiotic courses and hospitalizations for pneumonia. She uses an inhaler twice daily (combination inhaled corticosteroid and long-acting β-agonist), a leukotriene inhibitor daily at bedtime, and Albuterol as needed. Her daily cough is productive of yellowish-green sputum. She is able to tolerate moderate activity, but reports shortness of breath with exertion. She denies smoking or use of recreational drugs. Her CXR shows dextrocardia and increased lung markings with peribronchial thickening in both lower lobes of the lungs. The most likely diagnosis is:

a) Bronchiectasis with acute exacerbation
b) Acute asthma exacerbation
c) Cystic fibrosis
d) Kartagener syndrome
e) Common variable immune deficiency (CVID) with frequent infections

Answer

The answer is d. *Kartagener syndrome* is a triad of:

- Situs inversus ("mirror image" reversal of thoracic and abdominal organs)
- Chronic sinusitis
- Bronchiectasis

Bronchiectasis describes dilated, damaged airways that have lost their normal smooth tapering configuration as a result of infection, airway obstruction, mucus stasis,

and chronic inflammation. *Anatomic classification* includes saccular (or cystic) and cylindrical (or tubular) bronchiectasis. Common causes of bronchiectasis in children include:

- Cystic fibrosis
- Primary ciliary dysfunction
- Immune deficiency with recurrent infections
- Healed tuberculosis
- Allergic bronchopulmonary aspergillosis

Bronchial obstruction secondary to bronchial stenosis or narrowing or resulting from extrinsic compression because of enlarged lymph nodes can also result in mucus stasis, recurrent infection, and bronchiectasis.

Clinical manifestations include chronic, daily productive cough, failure to thrive secondary to repeated infection, digital clubbing caused by suppurative lung disease, and coarse wet crackles on auscultation of the chest. Radiologic findings include bronchial wall thickening and dilatation, honeycomb pattern, and mucus impaction of airways. *High-resolution chest CT scan* (HRCT) is the study of choice and delineates altered bronchial anatomy and distortion; bronchography using contrast media is no longer used. Management includes vigorous chest physical therapy of affected lobes for airway clearance of mucus, using chest clapping, postural drainage, or use of the mechanical percussor vest. Patients should receive regular care, including serial pulmonary function tests and sputum cultures, which can be used to guide antibiotic therapy. Rarely, surgical resection is indicated if recurrent episodes of pulmonary infection in localized disease in an affected lobe with bronchiectasis.

SUGGESTED READINGS

1. American Academy of Pediatrics. Clinical practice guideline: diagnosis and management of childhood obstructive sleep apnea syndrome. *Pediatrics* 2002;109(4):704–712.
2. Expert Panel Report 3 (EPR-3). *Guidelines for the diagnosis and management of asthma*. Summary Report 2007; http://nhlbi.nih.gov/guidelines/asthma/asthsumm.htm
3. Gibson RL, Burns JL, Ramsey BW. Pathophysiology and management of pulmonary infections in cystic fibrosis. *Am J Respir Crit Care Med* 2003;168(8):918–951.
4. Mueller GA, Eigen H. Pulmonary function testing in pediatric practice. *Pediatr Rev* 1994;15:403–411.
5. Weinberger M, Abu-Hasan M. Pseudo-asthma: when cough, wheezing, and dyspnea are not asthma. *Pediatrics* 2007;120(4):855–864.

Chapter 32

BOARD SIMULATION: Allergy and Immunology

Nicola M. Vogel

QUESTIONS

1. An 8-year-old girl has asthma and atopic dermatitis and documented skin test positive hypersensitivity to tree pollen and dust mites. Her parents ask you what the likelihood is that she will outgrow her asthma. What is the *best* response?

a) Fewer than 20% of children with asthma outgrow the symptoms by adulthood.

b) Children with asthma and multiple inhalant allergies are less likely to outgrow asthma than children with asthma alone.

c) Children with exercise-induced asthma rarely outgrow asthma.

d) Children with asthma and atopic dermatitis are more likely to outgrow asthma than children with asthma alone.

e) You cannot predict if she will outgrow asthma.

Answer

The answer is b. Children with asthma and atopy such as allergic rhinitis and atopic dermatitis have a poorer prognosis for persistent asthma. Other risk factors for persistence of asthma into adulthood include a maternal or paternal history of asthma, presence of childhood asthma with the onset of symptoms after the age of 2 years, and a history of multiple asthma exacerbations.

2. A 15-month-old female infant has been hospitalized for several serious infections caused by *Staphylococcus aureus*, including osteomyelitis, hepatic abscess, and pneumonia with pneumatocele formation. What is the *most* likely diagnosis?

a) Wiskott-Aldrich syndrome

b) Selective immunoglobulin A (IgA) deficiency

c) Leukocyte adhesion deficiency

d) Common variable immunodeficiency (CVID)

e) Chronic granulomatous disease (CGD)

Answer

The answer is e. Recurrent infection with bacteria of low virulence such as Staphylococcus aureus suggests a phagocytic abnormality. CGD is a phagocytic disorder, and occurs in roughly 1 in 250,000 live births in the United States. The X-linked form (70%) is more common then the autosomal recessive forms (30%). Neutrophils and monocytes are unable to destroy some types of bacteria and fungi after phagocytosis secondary to defects in oxidative metabolism required for the generation of superoxide and peroxide. Characteristic deep-seated granulomatous abscesses with catalase-positive bacteria and fungi occur in the lung, lymph nodes, skin, liver, and bones. Catalase-positive organisms cannot produce reduced oxygen metabolites such as hydrogen peroxide that would supply a reactive oxygen metabolite to facilitate destruction. Organisms that often cause infections in patients with CGD include *S. aureus*, *Serratia marcescens*, *Burkholderia cepacia*, *Nocardia* sp., and *Aspergillus* sp.

Wiskott-Aldrich syndrome is an X-linked recessive syndrome that is characterized by a triad of recurrent infections, eczema, and thrombocytopenia. Infections are often caused by encapsulated organisms such as *Streptococcus pneumoniae* and *Haemophilus influenza*. Atopic dermatitis and recurrent infections often develop during the first year of life. Selective IgA deficiency is the most common inherited immunodeficiency. Although patients with IgA deficiency are often asymptomatic, the clinical presentation can include recurrent sinopulmonary infections. Leukocyte adhesion deficiency is also associated with recurrent infections. Unlike CGD, abscess formation is unusual because the leukocytes in patients with this syndrome lack the ability to adhere to blood vessel walls and to migrate to the site of infection. CVID is an acquired hypogammaglobulinemia characterized by a deficiency of antibodies of several isotypes.

Similar to CGD, patients with CVID also present with recurrent infections. Unlike CGD, the onset of symptoms is often later in life and infections are often secondary to encapsulated organisms.

3. A 12-month-old female infant presents to your office for her first influenza and measles, mumps, and rubella (MMR) vaccinations. Her history is significant for a previous anaphylactic reaction to egg. What is the *best* option for this patient in your office?
a) Administer influenza and MMR vaccines.
b) Administer MMR vaccine but not influenza vaccine.
c) Administer influenza vaccine but not MMR vaccine.
d) Do not administer either vaccine.

Answer
The answer is b. Inactivated influenza vaccine is grown in the allantoic fluid of embryonated chicken eggs and contains egg proteins that may induce immediate hypersensitivity reactions in children with hypersensitivity to egg. In general, children with an anaphylactic reaction to egg should not receive the influenza vaccine because of the risk of a similar life-threatening reaction. Skin testing with egg and the vaccine can be done for patients who must receive the influenza vaccine. If the skin test result is positive, the vaccine is often administered by a desensitization procedure or graded dose challenge by trained personnel.

Although measles and mumps vaccines are grown in chicken embryo fibroblast tissue cultures, they do not contain significant amounts of egg protein. Children with hypersensitivity to egg are at low risk of anaphylactic reactions to the MMR vaccine. Most immediate hypersensitivity reactions after MMR immunization are likely secondary to other vaccine components such as gelatin or neomycin.

4. Immunotherapy is effective for IgE-mediated hypersensitivity to all of the following *except*:
a) Cat dander
b) Grass pollen
c) Ragweed pollen
d) House dust mites
e) Foods

Answer
The answer is e. Many studies have confirmed the effectiveness of immunotherapy with several inhalant allergens including pollens, molds, animal allergens, dust mites, and cockroaches for the treatment of conditions including allergic rhinitis and allergic asthma. Currently, immunotherapy is not standardized for the treatment of IgE-mediated food hypersensitivity. Although some studies have suggested a therapeutic role for immunotherapy and/or desensitization in food hypersensitivity, and alternative strategies to treat food allergic patients are being explored, these should be considered investigational. Currently, the safest available therapy for

food hypersensitivity is elimination of the food. Families must be educated about how to avoid accidental ingestions and how to recognize early symptoms of an allergic reaction.

5. An 18-year-old boy with a history of allergic rhinitis had wheezing, generalized urticaria, and documented hypotension after a honeybee sting 8 weeks ago. After referral to the local allergist for venom skin testing, the allergist recommended venom immunotherapy. Your patient wants to know what his chances are of having another life-threatening reaction in the next 5 years if he successfully completes venom immunotherapy. The *best* answer to his question is:
a) Venom immunotherapy will be approximately 95% effective in preventing a future systemic reaction.
b) Venom immunotherapy will be approximately 67% effective in preventing a future systemic reaction.
c) Because he has allergic rhinitis, venom immunotherapy will be <60% effective in preventing a future systemic reaction.
d) Because he had a severe anaphylactic reaction with hypotension, venom immunotherapy will be <40% effective in preventing a future systemic reaction.
e) You cannot predict how effective venom immunotherapy will be in reducing the chance of another life-threatening reaction.

Answer
The answer is a. Venom immunotherapy is >95% effective in preventing systemic reactions in patients sensitive to insect stings. Patients older than 16 years with a history of a severe anaphylactic reaction to a sting, including vascular or respiratory symptoms, are at high risk for anaphylaxis in the event of a subsequent sting. Skin testing and possibly immunotherapy are recommended. Patients who are younger than 16 years whose previous reaction included generalized cutaneous symptoms such as pruritus, flushing, or urticaria without vascular or respiratory symptoms are generally at low risk for future anaphylaxis and often do not need allergy skin testing or immunotherapy. If the reaction included involvement of other organ systems such as hypotension, bradycardia, wheezing, shortness of breath, or loss of consciousness, then skin testing and possibly immunotherapy are recommended. Current recommendations are to consider discontinuation of venom immunotherapy after 5 years. After immunotherapy is stopped, the chance of a systemic reaction is approximately 10% with each sting.

6. You are seeing a 10-year-old boy in the late spring who has a 4-week history of sneezing, nasal congestion, and rhinorrhea. You suspect he has allergic rhinitis. What medication would be *most* effective in controlling his nasal symptoms?
a. Oral leukotriene receptor antagonist
b. Intranasal corticosteroid

c. Intranasal antihistamine

d. Oral antihistamine

Answer

The answer is b. Medications for the management of allergic rhinitis include oral and intranasal antihistamines, oral leukotriene receptor antagonists, and intranasal corticosteroids. Guidelines from American Academy of Allergy, Asthma and Immunology recommend intranasal corticosteroids as first-line therapy. Oral antihistamines and oral leukotriene receptor antagonists improve symptoms of allergic rhinitis compared with placebo. However, comparison studies between intranasal corticosteroids and either oral antihistamines or oral leukotriene receptor antagonists demonstrate that intranasal corticosteroids are most effective for nasal symptoms. Intranasal corticosteroids are approved for use in patients as young as 2 years old.

7. You are seeing a 3-year-old girl and her 5-year-old brother for a well child check-up. Both have food allergies. Her mother asks you about the likelihood that they will outgrow their food allergies. What is the *best* response to her question?

a) Most children do not outgrow food allergies.

b) Children with egg allergy are not likely to outgrow the allergy.

c) Children with peanut and tree nut allergy are not likely to outgrow the allergy.

d) Children with milk and soy allergy are not likely to outgrow the allergy.

Answer

The answer is c. Sensitivity to several food allergens, including cow's milk, soy, egg, and wheat frequently resolves in late childhood. On the other hand, the persistence of allergies to peanut, tree nuts, fish, and shellfish beyond childhood is common. Approximately 85% of children with cow's milk allergy will have resolution of the allergy by 3 years of age, whereas only 20% of children with peanut allergy will have resolution of the allergy by 5 years of age. Children diagnosed with food allergy after 3 years of age are less likely to lose the sensitivity. Children who have one IgE-mediated food allergy are at increased risk of developing allergies to other foods and also inhalant allergens.

8. You are giving a lecture to a group of parents in your community about asthma and the risk factors for the development of asthma. Of the following, which is *not* a risk factor for the development of asthma in children?

a) Prematurity

b) History of hospitalization for respiratory syncytial virus (RSV).

c) Personal history of eczema or allergy to dust mites and cockroaches

d) Parental history of asthma

e) None of the above

Answer

The answer is e. Prematurity has been associated with the development of asthma. Follow-up studies of children with a history of hospitalization for respiratory infections such as RSV suggest that these children are predisposed to developing asthma. Family history of asthma and a personal history of atopic dermatitis or allergic rhinitis have also been associated with the development of asthma.

9. A 12-month-old infant was diagnosed with X-linked agammaglobulinemia (XLA), a recessive B-cell deficiency, after having had multiple sinopulmonary tract infections such as otitis media, sinusitis, and pneumonia. What is an appropriate treatment for him?

a) Plasmapheresis and broad-spectrum antibiotics

b) Intravenous immunoglobulin (IVIg) and broad spectrum antibiotics

c) Chemotherapy

d) Enzyme replacement therapy

Answer

The answer is b. Replacement therapy with IgG is the basis of therapy for patients with agammaglobulinemia, including XLA and autosomal recessive agammaglobulinemia, and also for patients with CVID. Clinical features of XLA include an absence of lymph nodes and tonsils, total absence or marked deficiency of serum Ig, an inability to produce antibodies, and very low or absent B cell counts. Because cellular immunity remains intact, viral, and fungal pathogens often do not produce serious infections. Replacement therapy with IgG is also an important for patients with combined immunodeficiency such as Wiskott-Aldrich syndrome, ataxia-telangiectasia and hyper-IgM syndrome. In patients with XLA, early diagnosis, treatment with broad-spectrum antibiotics, and replacement IgG therapy have been helpful in preventing severe acute bacterial infections and bronchiectasis. The gene responsible for XLA is a cytoplasmic tyrosine kinase called Bruton tyrosine kinase (Btk).

10. A 3-day-old infant is hospitalized with seizures. Subsequent evaluation demonstrates that she has hypocalcemia, and a chest x-ray demonstrates an abnormally shaped heart. What immunodeficiency should you suspect?

a) Ataxia-telangiectasia

b) X-linked hyper-IgM syndrome

c) DiGeorge syndrome

d) Severe combined immunodeficiency (SCID)

e) Leukocyte adhesion deficiency

Answer

The answer is c. DiGeorge syndrome is caused by embryonic dysmorphogenesis of the third and fourth branchial pouches and is associated with deletions in the chromosome 22q11. It is characterized by the absent or diminished thymus development, cardiovascular structural defects usually involving the aortic arch, facial dysmorphism, and hypoparathyroidism. Characteristic facial features include hypertelorism, shortened philtrum and low-set, abnormally shaped ears. The severity of immune impairment relates to the extent of thymic dysplasia. Treatment of patients with complete DiGeorge syndrome usually requires cellular reconstitution with thymus transplant, T-cell transplantation, or bone marrow transplant.

Ataxia-telangiectasia is characterized by a triad of cerebellar ataxia and oculocutaneous telangiectasias along with immunodeficiency. The X-linked hyper-IgM syndrome occurs when normal isotype switching from IgM to other Igs does not occur, and patients have elevated levels of IgM and low or absent levels of IgG, IgA, and IgE. Clinical features of SCID which generally present within the first few months of life include diarrhea and malabsorption, failure to thrive, and recurrent, persistent or severe bacterial, and viral or fungal infections.

11. A 17-year-old patient with documented latex allergy presents to a local emergency department with symptoms of anaphylaxis. What food *most likely* triggered his symptoms?
a) Cow's milk
b) Soy
c) Strawberries
d) Banana
e) Wheat

Answer

The answer is d. The symptoms of latex-fruit syndrome result from cross-reactivity between natural rubber latex proteins and fruit proteins. The most commonly reported cross-reactive foods include banana, avocado, kiwi, and chestnut. Factors that increase the risk for developing allergy to latex include a history of atopy, spina bifida, or frequent surgery, and frequent contact with latex products (such as healthcare workers).

12. A 14-year-old girl with persistent asthma has an elevated total serum IgE level >2000 ng/mL, a history of transient pulmonary infiltrates on chest radiographs, and now has proximal bronchiectasis on a computed tomograph (CT) scan. What test would *best* help diagnose her underlying disorder?
a) Skin test for *Aspergillus* species or *A. fumigatus*
b) Skin test for *Coccidioides immitis*
c) Sweat test
d) Lung biopsy for noncaseating granulomas
e) Sputum culture for *Histoplasma capsulatum*

Answer

The answer is a. Allergic bronchopulmonary aspergillosis (ABPA) complicates chronic pulmonary disease in approximately 10% of children with asthma or cystic fibrosis. Colonization with *A. fumigatus* produces an exaggerated IgG and IgE response, resulting in recurrent bronchospasm and bronchiectasis. ABPA should be considered in children with persistent asthma who have transient pulmonary infiltrates. Criteria for diagnosis include asthma, an elevated total serum IgE concentration >1000 ng/mL, positive skin test results to *Aspergillus* species or specific serum IgE and/or IgG to A. fumigatus, infiltrates on chest radiograph, and proximal bronchiectasis. The goal of the treatment of ABPA is to treat exacerbations to prevent or minimize bronchiectasis.

Sweat testing is useful for the diagnosis of cystic fibrosis. The prevalence of ABPA is higher in patients with cystic fibrosis than in patients with persistent asthma. A lung biopsy with noncaseating granulomas is suggestive of sarcoidosis. Sarcoidosis is a chronic multisystem disease characterized by noncaseating granulomatous lesions of almost any organ of the body. Lung findings include parenchymal infiltrates, miliary nodules, and hilar lymphadenopathy.

Sputum culture for *H. capsulatum* would be helpful in the diagnosis of histoplasmosis. Most immunocompetent patients with histoplasmosis are asymptomatic. The most common chest radiograph finding is a solitary pulmonary nodule, frequently with hilar and mediastinal lymphadenopathy. *C. immitis* is concentrated in arid areas of the southwest United States. In the acute infection, flu-like symptoms such as malaise, chills, and fever, and other symptoms such as chest pain, night sweats, and anorexia are common. Diagnosis of coccidioidomycosis is confirmed by the detection of double-contoured spherules with endospores characteristic of the fungus, *C. immitis*. Often this can be isolated from an excised pulmonary nodule, bronchoalveolar lavage, or gastric aspirates.

13. A 17-year-old boy has a history of an adverse reaction to radiocontrast media (RCM) 2 years ago that included diffuse pruritus and urticaria accompanied by hypotension. Which statement is *true* regarding his adverse reaction to RCM?
a) History of this type of reaction is an absolute contraindication to further administration of RCM.
b) He should avoid RCM and iodine, such as in iodine cleaning solutions and shellfish.
c) He should receive high-osmolar, ionic RCM for the next procedure.
d) He should receive antihistamines and prednisone prior to the next procedure with RCM.

Answer

The answer is d. RCM reactions are most likely mediated by a non-IgE mechanism. Mast cells mediate these anaphylactoid reactions likely by direct activation and degranulation by RCM. Systemic reactions to RCM are rapid in onset, with symptoms such as pruritus, urticaria, angioedema, hypotension, and syncope. Risk factors for RCM reactions include patients with asthma and allergic diseases, use of β-blockers, and a previous reaction to RCM. High-risk patients should receive prophylaxis with prednisone and antihistamines prior to administration of RCM, and the RCM should be low-osmolar and nonionic. With pretreatment and use of lower-osmolar agents, the risk of a reaction can be reduced to 1%.

14. An 8-year-old boy initiated a 10-day course of oral amoxicillin 12 days ago. Two days ago, he developed fever, malaise, arthralgia of multiple joints, and nausea and diarrhea. Today, he developed urticaria. By the Gell and Coombs classification of human hypersensitivity, what type of adverse reaction is he experiencing?
a) Type I
b) Type II
c) Type III
d) Type IV

Answer
The answer is c. There are four types of immunologic re-actions. Serum sickness is a classic example of a type III hypersensitivity reaction mediated by IgG or IgM anti-body–antigen complexes. Complexes can be deposited in various organs and activate the complement. In serum sickness, serum complement levels such as C3 and C4 are often decreased and the erythrocyte sedimentation rate is usually elevated. Less common symptoms include mild proteinuria, hemoglobinuria, and microscopic hematuria. Supportive treatment with analgesics and an-tihistamines is appropriate, and if symptoms are severe, corticosteroids may be used. Serum sickness cannot be prevented by desensitization with the offending agent or by pretreatment with corticosteroids.

Type I reactions are IgE-mediated immediate reactions that can progress to anaphylaxis. When IgE molecules at-tached to mast cells are cross-linked by antigen, the mast cells are degranulated and release mediators such as hist-amine. Type II reactions involve IgG or IgM antibody-mediated cytolysis. Examples include hemolytic anemia and Rh incompatibility. Type IV reactions are delayed hypersensitivity reactions. Examples include contact dermatitis and positive tuberculin skin testing during which the T cells react to the tuberculin antigen.

15. A 5-year-old boy with a history of severe asthma pre-sents to your clinic for a well child visit. He has been taking oral prednisone 30 mg daily for the past 15 days. He is otherwise healthy. When can he receive his MMR vaccination?
a) Today
b) 2 weeks after discontinuing oral steroids
c) 3 weeks after discontinuing oral steroids
d) 1 month after discontinuing oral steroids

Answer
The answer is d. Children on systemic steroid therapy can become immunosuppressed. The minimal amount of systemic steroids and duration of administration suf-ficient to cause immunosuppression in a healthy child

are not well defined. Current recommendations for administration of live virus vaccines to previously healthy children receiving steroid therapy are as follows:

- Children receiving low or moderate doses of systemic steroids daily or alternate days including <2 mg/kg/day of prednisone or equivalent, or <20 mg/day if weight is >10 kg, can receive live-virus vaccines.
- Children receiving high doses of systemic steroids given daily or alternate days for <14 days including >2 mg/kg/day of prednisone or equivalent, or >20 mg/kg/day if weight is >10 kg can receive live-virus vaccines immediately after completing steroids. Some experts would delay immunization for 2 weeks.
- Children receiving high doses of systemic steroids given daily or alternate days for more than 14 days should not receive live-virus vaccine until steroid therapy has been discontinued for at least 1 month.

16. You are seeing a 10-month-old boy with severe eczema who recently moved to your town. His mother mentions that he has had recurrent infections requiring antibiotics. She brought you paperwork from previous labs, and you notice he has low platelets. What is the *most likely* immunodeficiency?
a) X-linked hyper-IgM syndrome
b) Severe combined immunodeficiency
c) Wiskott-Aldrich syndrome (WAS)
d) Leukocyte adhesion deficiency
e) Chediak-Higashi syndrome

Answer
The answer is c. Wiskott-Aldrich Syndrome (WAS) is an X-linked recessive syndrome characterized by a triad of recurrent infections, eczema, and thrombocytopenia. Patients may have bruising and bleeding related to thrombocytopenia. Recurrent otitis media, sinopul-monary infections, and viral illnesses are common. Patients may have both B- and T-cell immunodeficien-cies. Western blot and flow cytometry analysis can help establish a diagnosis by determining the absence of WAS protein. Patients initially can be treated with splenectomy, antibiotics, and IgG replacement therapy, but the only curative therapy for WAS is bone marrow transplant.

The X-linked hyper-IgM syndrome occurs when nor-mal isotype switching from IgM to other Igs does not occur, and patients have elevated levels of IgM and low or absent levels of IgG, IgA, and IgE. Children with SCID have a profound combined defect in antibody and cell-mediated immunodeficiency, and are susceptible to bacte-rial, viral, and fungal infections. Patient with leukocyte adhesion deficiency have recurrent infections without ab-scess formation. The leukocytes of these patients lack the ability to adhere to blood vessel walls and migrate to the site of infection. Chediak-Higashi is an autosomal reces-sive disorder with recurrent infections and characteristic findings of partial oculocutaneous albinism along with giant lysosomal granules in neutrophils and other cells.

17. Which of the following has NOT been associated with an increase in asthma symptoms?
a) Exercise
b) Viral URI
c) Tobacco smoke
d) Aspirin
e) β-blockers
f) None of the above

Answer
The answer is f. Asthmatic patients may have a variety of triggers for respiratory symptoms including exercise, viral URI, weather changes, exposure to inhalant allergens, weather changes, exposure to tobacco smoke, aspirin or other NSAIDs, and β-blockers.

18. A 12-year-old patient with severe asthma was admitted to the hospital for an acute asthma exacerbation and has been treated with a variety of medications including albuterol over the past 24 hours. You are concerned that he might have symptoms related to albuterol toxicity. Which of the following is *not* a side effect of inhaled albuterol?
a) Muscle tremor
b) Hypotension
c) Hypokalemia
d) Tachycardia
e) Nervousness

Answer
The answer is b. The clinical manifestations of toxicity to inhaled β-adrenergic agonists include hypokalemia, tachycardia, palpitations, muscle tremors and muscle cramps, hypertension (not hypotension), headache, nervousness, and insomnia and dizziness.

19. Which of the following risk factors is *not* associated with an increased risk of a child dying from asthma?
a) One or more life-threatening episodes
b) Poor control of daily symptoms
c) Depression
d) Use of oral leukotriene receptor antagonist
e) Family dysfunction

Answer
The answer is d. The risk factors for a child at increased risk of dying from asthma include one or more life-threatening episodes, severe asthma requiring chronic corticosteroids, poor control of daily symptoms, abnormal FEV1, poor compliance, family dysfunction, depression, and atopy.

20. What is the *best* test for diagnosis of chronic granulomatous disease (CGD)?
a) Immunoglobulin levels
b) Nitroblue tetrazolium test
c) Absolute neutrophil count
d) Absolute T and B cell count
e) None of the above

Answer
The answer is b. CGD is characterized by defective intracellular killing of bacteria and fungi after phagocytosis secondary to defects in oxidative metabolism. Diagnosis can be established by measurement of phagocyte oxidase activity. In the nitroblue tetrazolium dye test (NBT), the yellow water-soluble tetrazolium dye is reduced to the blue insoluble forms in pigment by the superoxide anion generated from normal phagocytes. Phagocytes from patients with CGD cannot reduce NBT because they cannot produce superoxide anion. Patients can also be diagnosed by dihydrorhodamine reduction assay with flow cytometry, but the availability of this test is currently limited.

SUGGESTED READINGS

1. American Academy of Pediatrics. Active and passive immunization. In: Pickering LK, ed. *Red book: 2006 report of the committee on infectious diseases*, 27th ed. Elk Grove Village, IL: American Academy of Pediatrics, 2006:46–47.
2. American Academy of Pediatrics. Immunization in special clinical circumstances. In Pickering LK, Baker CJ, Long SS, McMillan JA, eds. *Red Book: 2006 Report of the Committee on Infectious Diseases*, 27th ed. Elk Grove Village, IL: American Academy of Pediatrics, 2006:76–77.
3. Bonilla FA, Bernstein IL, Khan DA, et al. Practice parameter for the diagnosis and management of primary immunodeficiency. *Ann Allergy, Asthma Immunol* 2005;94:S1–63.
4. Bonilla FA, Geha RS. Primary immunodeficiency diseases. *J Allergy Clin Immunol* 2003;111:S571–S581.
5. Boxer LA. Neutrophil abnormalities. *Pediatr Rev* 2003;24(2):52–61.
6. Buckley RH. Primary immunodeficiency diseases. In: Adkinson NF Jr, Yunginger JW, Busse WW, et al., eds. *Allergy: principles and practice*, 6th ed. Philadelphia: Mosby, 2003:1015–1042.
7. Chapman JA, Bernstein IL, Lee RE, et al. Food allergy: a practice parameter. *Ann Allergy Asthma Immunol* 2006;96:S1–68.
8. Gedalia A, Shetty AK. Chronic steroid and immunosuppressant therapy in children. *Pediatr Rev* 2004;25:425–434.
9. Golden DBK. Insect allergy. In: Adkinson NF Jr, Yunginger JW, Busse WW, et al., eds. *Allergy: principles and practice*, 6th ed. Philadelphia: Mosby, 2003:1475–1486.
10. Greenberger PA. Allergic bronchopulmonary aspergillosis. *J Allergy Clin Immunol* 2002;110(5):685–692.
11. Guill MF. Asthma update: epidemiology and pathophysiology. *Pediatr Rev* 2004;25(9):299–304.
12. Joint Task Force on Practice Parameters. Stinging insect hypersensitivity. A practice parameter update. *J Allergy Clin Immunol* 2004; 114:869–886.
13. Kelso JM. Adverse reactions to vaccines. In: Adkinson NF Jr, Yunginger JW, Busse WW, et al., eds. *Allergy: principles and practice*, 6th ed. Philadelphia: Mosby, 2003:1665–1678.
14. Kumar S, Mahalingam R. Anaphylactoid reactions to radiocontrast agents. *Pediatr Rev* 2001;22(10):356.
15. Li JT, Lockey RF, Bernstein IL, et al. Allergen immunotherapy: a practice parameter. *Ann Allergy Asthma Immunol* 2003;90:1–40.
16. Lieberman P, Kemp SF, Oppenheimer J, et al. The diagnosis and management of anaphylaxis: an updated practice parameter. *J Allergy Clin Immunol* 2005;115:S483–523.
17. Mahr TA, Sheth K. Update on allergic rhinitis. *Pediatr Rev* 2005; 26:278–282.

18. Moss MH, Gern JE, Lemanske RF Jr. Asthma in infancy and childhood. In: Adkinson NF Jr, Yunginger JW, Busse WW, et al., eds. *Allergy: principles and practice*, 6th ed. Philadelphia: Mosby, 2003:1225–1255.

19. National Institutes of Health, National Asthma Education and Prevention Program. *Expert panel report 3: guidelines for the diagnosis and management of asthma*. Bethesda, MD: 2007 [Accessed June 16, 2008]. NIH Publication No. 08-4051. Available from http://nhlbi.nih.gov/guidelines/asthma/asthgdln.pdf

20. Sampson HA. Update on food allergy. *J Allergy Clin Immunol* 2004:113(5):805–819.

21. Shearer WT, Fleisher TA. The immune system. In: Adkinson NF Jr, Yunginger JW, Busse WW, et al., eds. *Allergy: principles and practice*, 6th ed. Philadelphia: Mosby, 2003:1–14.

22. Sicherer SH, Leung DYM. Serum sickness. In: Behrman RE, Kliegman RM, Jenson HB, eds. *Nelson textbook of pediatrics*, 17th ed. Philadelphia: WB Saunders, 2004:782–783.

Chapter 33

Epilepsy and Anticonvulsant Therapy

Deepak K. Lachhwani and Elaine Wyllie

Epilepsy is a common disorder, affecting approximately 2% of the U.S. population. For every patient, two types of diagnosis are important: the *seizure type* and the *epilepsy syndrome*. The epilepsy syndrome diagnosis is based on seizure type as well as other features such as etiology, neurologic examination, age of onset, and the results of the electroencephalograph (EEG) and neuroimaging. The epilepsy syndrome diagnosis, therefore, is a more powerful tool than the seizure type alone as a basis for treatment and prognosis. Treatment modalities include antiepileptic medication, ketogenic diet, vagus nerve stimulation, and epilepsy surgery.

ETIOLOGY

The most likely etiologies vary with age. Neonatal asphyxia, congenital malformations, and inherited metabolic disorders tend to manifest with seizures in infancy and early childhood; trauma and neoplasms are important in childhood, adolescence, and adulthood; and vascular insults are a common etiology of seizures later in life. Idiopathic epilepsies most often start in childhood and adolescence and are believed to represent genetic disorders manifesting only as seizures. With the exception of the idiopathic syndrome of benign focal epilepsy of childhood, patients of any age with partial seizures or a focal abnormality indicated on EEG should be evaluated for the possibility of a cerebral structural lesion. Magnetic resonance imaging (MRI) is the test of choice in this setting.

CLASSIFICATION OF SEIZURES

Throughout this chapter, the terminology is that of the current classification system of the International League Against Epilepsy. In this classification, the primary division of seizures is that between partial and generalized seizure types. *Partial* seizures have an abnormal electrical activity on the EEG localized to a limited area of the cerebral cortex in one hemisphere, whereas *generalized* seizures begin diffusely. Partial seizures may evolve into secondarily generalized seizures when the epileptiform discharges begin on one side of the brain and spread to involve both hemispheres.

Partial seizures are further divided into simple or complex types primarily based on whether consciousness is preserved during the event. *Complex partial* seizures involve impairment of consciousness, defined by amnesia, but *simple partial* seizures do not. When the simple partial seizure is sensory in its presentation, it is called an aura. Simple partial seizures with focal jerking of a limb or one side of the face are called focal motor seizures, and when the motor activity moves sequentially through muscle groups it may be said to have a Jacksonian march. The patient remains awake and aware throughout a simple partial seizure, even if he or she is unresponsive during the event because of motor involvement of the face and throat or because of strong, distracting sensory stimuli. Even when these features are present, patients with simple partial seizures will remember an ictal event.

Complex partial (*psychomotor* or automotor) seizures, by definition, involve impairment of consciousness with postictal amnesia. They may be preceded by a simple partial seizure, such as an aura, which may be remembered afterward, but during the complex partial seizure, the patient has altered awareness and impaired responsiveness. Most patients with complex partial seizures also have automatisms; that is, stereotyped, repetitive, and semipurposeful motor activity. The automatisms may be gestural (including fumbling with nearby objects or picking at clothes or bedsheets), alimentary (chewing, swallowing, or lip smacking), mimicking (with facial expressions suggesting an emotion such as fear), verbal (yelling, laughing, or repetitive speech), or ambulatory (walking or running). Complex partial seizures may also involve loss of posture or abnormal face or limb movements, or autonomic phenomena. Afterward, there may be postictal confusion for minutes to hours, and this is a significant feature that distinguishes complex partial seizures from generalized absence attacks.

Generalized seizures include a wide variety of clinical types. *Generalized tonic-clonic* seizures or *grand mal* convulsions may involve several phases: a tonic phase, with sudden loss of consciousness, falling, involuntary crying-out, muscle stiffening, and altered breathing pattern; a clonic phase, with rhythmical muscle spasms and limb jerking, possible cheek or tongue biting with bleeding, foamy salivation, irregular breathing with possible cyanosis, and possible urinary or bowel incontinence; and a postictal phase, with deep hyperventilation, and gradual return of consciousness over several minutes. During the event, there may be vomiting or loss of bowel or bladder control and afterward there is temporary confusion or sleepiness. Primary generalized tonic-clonic seizures are not preceded by a simple or complex partial seizure.

Generalized *absence* seizures (*petit mal* attacks) have no warning or aura; they involve interruption of activity with loss of consciousness and amnesia, and there is no postictal confusion. Attacks are brief, rarely lasting longer than 20 seconds, and they typically occur many times a day in untreated patients. These features are useful in distinguishing between absence and complex partial seizures. In longer absence seizures, the patient may also have some loss of muscle tone, subtle myoclonic jerks, or automatisms. Because automatisms may occur in both, absence or complex partial seizures, they should not be used to differentiate the two seizure types.

Other types of generalized seizures include:

- *Myoclonic* seizures: sudden, quick jerks of the limbs, trunk, or head
- *Atonic (akinetic or astatic)* seizures: sudden loss of muscle tone, head drops, or falling seizures
- *Tonic* seizures: longer, steady contraction of muscle groups
- *Infantile* spasms: occur serially in clusters in affected infants
- *Atypical absence* seizures: prolonged staring spells, often with some motor phenomena

In some patients, two or more types of these generalized *minor motor* seizures occur together, often in the presence of mental retardation.

CLASSIFICATION OF EPILEPSIES

Epilepsy syndromes as well as seizures have been classified by the International League Against Epilepsy. With this classification, patients are grouped not just by the seizure type, but also by the presence of similar clinical, electrographic, radiographic, and pathologic findings. By this classification, certain types of epilepsy may include one or more different types of seizures.

Epilepsies are traditionally categorized in two basic ways: by etiology as either idiopathic (with no known cause) or symptomatic (with an identified underlying cause), and by type of seizure onset as either localization-related (with focal-onset seizures) or generalized (with diffuse-onset seizures). In patients with *idiopathic* epilepsy, the brain structure and neurologic examination are normal, a familial pattern may be present, and there is a typical age of onset. Idiopathic epilepsies probably are because of specific genetic abnormalities. In patients with epilepsy, there may be evidence of previous head trauma, metabolic disease, stroke, *symptomatic* tumor, or other brain insult, and the patient may have dementia, paresis, or sensory deficits. The onset of seizures in symptomatic epilepsy may be soon after brain injury or delayed by many years.

One form of idiopathic, generalized epilepsy is *childhood absence epilepsy (petit mal)*. This epilepsy typically has school-aged onset, involves absence and generalized tonic-clonic seizures (convulsions are present in approximately 50% of patients), and includes a characteristic electroencephalogram picture of a generalized *3-per-second spike-and-slow wave complexes especially during hyperventilation.* Patients typically have a good response to medication, and seizures usually remit spontaneously before early adulthood. Absence seizures alone are usually controlled with the administration of either ethosuximide or valproate alone, but valproate is the preferred choice if generalized tonic-clonic seizures are also present. The newer antiepileptic medication, lamotrigine, may also be proved effective in the treatment of childhood absence epilepsy.

Another form of idiopathic, generalized epilepsy is *juvenile myoclonic* epilepsy. This type of epilepsy has peak onset in adolescence, involves myoclonic and generalized tonic-clonic seizures on awakening, and records an electroencephalogram with generalized poly spikes. Patients typically have a good response to medication such as valproate or benzodiazepines, but the seizures do not remit spontaneously, and lifelong medication is generally needed. Juvenile myoclonic epilepsy is especially interesting from a scientific viewpoint because it is one of the first epilepsies in which a chromosomal abnormality has been identified. Valproate has been the drug of choice, but newer alternatives include lamotrigine and topiramate.

West syndrome is an epileptic syndrome that may be either idiopathic or symptomatic. Onset is in the first year of life, the seizure type is infantile spasms, and the EEG shows hypsarrhythmia. Mental retardation is part of the definition of West syndrome, but not all infants with infantile spasms and hypsarrhythmia have an impaired intellect. Infantile spasms may be flexor (salaam, jackknife, or head nodding), extensor, or mixed (with both flexor and extensor components). The mixed type is most common. Clustering of spasms is typical and should suggest this syndrome. Spasms typically occur when the infant is awake or upon awakening or during the drowsiness period just prior to sleep.

West syndrome may be idiopathic (40% of cases) or symptomatic. Underlying etiologies include perinatal events such as hypoxia-ischemia, infection, prematurity, or hemorrhage; genetic disorders such as tuberous sclerosis or Aicardi syndrome; malformations of cortical development; and inborn metabolic errors such as phenylketonuria. Important tests to identify an etiology include an MRI scan, a dilated eye examination, and a careful Wood lamp skin evaluation of the patient and his or her family, looking for neurocutaneous stigmata, and metabolic and genetic evaluations. Video-EEG, high-resolution MRI scan, and positron emission tomography (PET) may be appropriate in refractory cases to explore the possibility of a focal structural abnormality, for example, a focal malformation of cortical development. Patients with refractory infantile spasms because of focal structural lesions may be eligible candidates for epilepsy surgery.

Medical treatment options for infantile spasms include intramuscular adrenocorticotropic hormone (ACTH), 20 to 60 U/day, or prednisone, 2 mg/kg per day, used for 6 weeks and then weaned. Other options include valproate or benzodiazepine. The prognosis of West syndrome is better when there is no known etiology. Hrachovy, et al., (1988) reported that 38% of infants with idiopathic West syndrome had a normal outcome without mental retardation, compared with only 5% of those with the symptomatic form. Among children in both groups, the infantile spasms remitted or changed to different seizure types by 2 or 3 years of age. Additionally, the hypsarrhythmic electroencephalogram pattern resolved or changed to a different abnormal pattern by 5 or 6 years of age.

Lennox-Gastaut syndrome is another type of generalized epilepsy that may be either idiopathic or symptomatic. Onset is in infancy or childhood, and patients have multiple types of generalized seizures, including atonic or myoclonic attacks. Patients have mental retardation, and the electroencephalogram shows generalized slow spike and slow wave complexes and background slowing. A similar clinical picture may also be seen in children with an electroencephalogram picture of multifocal sharp waves from each hemisphere. Possible etiologies may include the same disorders as for West syndrome. The seizures are often intractable, and sometimes require treatment with two or more drugs. It is important to avoid polypharmacy whenever possible, so that patients are less likely to have additional cognitive deficits resulting from drug toxicity. The ketogenic diet or vagus nerve stimulation may be helpful to patients with Lennox-Gastaut syndrome and other types of refractory epilepsy.

Benign focal epilepsy with centrotemporal spikes is a common type of idiopathic, localization-related epilepsy. This epilepsy typically begins at 4 to 12 years of age, with peak onset between 8 and 10 years of age; involves infrequent partial motor seizures of the face and arm or nocturnal generalized tonic-clonic seizures (80% of patients have only nighttime convulsions). The electroencephalogram shows centrotemporal sharp waves that have a typical morphology and marked activation during sleep. In these children, the brain structure and neurologic examination are usually normal. These patients generally have a good response to antiepileptic medications such as carbamazepine or gabapentin. However, in most cases treatment with medication is not needed. Identification of this syndrome is important, because if a child fits neatly into this patient group, the family can be reassured that the patient will have spontaneous remission of his or her seizures by the age of 16 years.

Temporal lobe epilepsy is a form of symptomatic, localization-related epilepsy. Onset is usually in the school age or during teenage years, but may be earlier. Seizures are typically complex partial with automatisms, and the electroencephalogram shows temporal lobe sharp waves. In some cases, the seizures may be intractable despite treatment with maximum tolerated doses of antiepileptic medication. The rate of spontaneous remission is low. It is critical to exclude a structural lesion (e.g., tumor, malformation of cortical development, or hippocampal sclerosis) by performing an MRI scan. Many traditional and newer antiepileptic medications have been shown to be effective against partial seizures in temporal or extratemporal epilepsy, with carbamazepine usually considered a first-line choice. Patients with refractory temporal lobe epilepsy may be favorable candidates for epilepsy surgery. *Extratemporal epilepsy* is another form of symptomatic, localization-related epilepsy. Patients may have simple or complex partial seizures with symptoms reflecting the origin of onset, namely from the frontal, parietal, or occipital regions. Extratemporal epilepsy is similar to temporal lobe epilepsy in the age of onset, prognosis, and possibility of a structural lesion.

FEBRILE SEIZURES

Clinical Features

A simple febrile seizure is defined as a generalized seizure lasting <15 minutes, occurring only once in a 24-hour period, in a febrile child who does not have an intracranial infection. Although strictly not an epilepsy syndrome, this is the most common provoked seizure that afflicts children between 6 months and 5 years of age. It is estimated that approximately 3% of all children experience a febrile seizure at some point. Most children outgrow these seizures by 6 years of age and have a good long-term prognosis. The risk of developing epilepsy is low and no adverse effects on cognitive development are to be expected.

The only real risk is that of experiencing a *recurrence* of the febrile seizure. For children younger than 12 months at the time of experiencing their first febrile seizure, the risk of recurrence is approximately 50%. Children older than 12 months at the time of their first febrile seizure have a 30% risk of a second event. After two febrile seizures, there is a 50% chance of at least one more recurrence.

The risk of developing epilepsy is only marginally higher in otherwise healthy children with typical febrile seizures, when compared with the overall population. By 7 years of age, a little more than 1% of children with febrile seizures are expected to develop epilepsy; even after multiple febrile seizures the risk of developing epilepsy by 25 years of age increases only to 2.4%. It is evident that this compares favorably with the overall population risk of 1% of developing epilepsy.

Generalized Epilepsy with Febrile Seizures

Infrequently, children with febrile seizures early in life may subsequently manifest with other types of unprovoked seizures. These patients are loosely described as having generalized epilepsy with febrile seizures+ (GEFS Plus). Careful analyses of families with multiple affected individuals have improved the understanding of the clinical spectrum of GEFS+. It is a rare syndrome, which has been described in at least 21 family pedigrees so far, with an autosomal-dominant mode of inheritance.

In the mildest form of GEFS+, seizures associated with fever may persist beyond 6 years of age, only to remit by mid-adolescence. Other phenotypes include febrile seizures associated with different seizure types including absence seizures, myoclonic seizures, atonic seizures, or myoclonic astatic epilepsy. For obvious prognostic implication, in a child presenting with recurrent febrile seizures, the clinical quandary is whether they have typical febrile seizures or GEFS+. Until further advanced diagnostic testing becomes available, one must rely on careful family history. If the family history is suggestive of other individuals with febrile seizures beyond early childhood or febrile seizures along with other seizure types, then GEFS+ syndrome enters the differential diagnoses.

Treatment

In general, only first aid measures need to be implemented and no further intervention is required to treat febrile seizures. This is based largely on the understanding of the benign nature of febrile seizures and also because of lack of effective treatment agents without the inherent risk of some adverse effects. Of the available antiepileptic medications, data are available on the role of phenobarbital, valproate, carbamazepine, and phenytoin in the daily treatment of febrile seizures.

Carbamazepine and phenytoin have not been found to be effective in controlling recurrences. However, phenobarbital as well as valproic acid are two choices that are effective in reducing the rate of subsequent febrile seizures when used in monotherapy. The relatively unfavorable adverse-effect profiles of both these agents make them less preferred for daily therapy.

Intermittent therapy with antipyretic agents without anticonvulsants is ineffective in preventing febrile seizures. Use of a benzodiazepine such as diazepam, at the onset of fever is shown to reduce the risk of febrile seizures and may be recommended. Potential drawbacks include sedation and the risk of masking the signs of an evolving central nervous system. When counseling families, it should be reiterated that there is *no evidence to support:*

- That treatment of febrile seizures prevents future development of epilepsy
- That simple febrile seizures cause any structural damage
- That children with febrile seizures are at risk of cognitive decline

TREATMENT WITH ANTIEPILEPTIC MEDICATIONS

Once the diagnosis of epilepsy is confirmed, certain factors need to be considered when deciding whether to treat with antiepileptic medication. These include the seizure type, seizure frequency, time of seizure occurrence, predisposing factors to injury if a seizure were to occur, as well as psychosocial and social consequences of additional seizures. Taken together, this information must be weighed against the risk of antiepileptic medication–related adverse effects. If it is decided to treat with antiepileptic medication, then the next step is to select a drug effective for the patient's seizure type (Table 33.1). Currently, not all antiepileptic medications are labeled for use in pediatric patients and even fewer of these are labeled by the U.S. Food and Drug Administration (FDA) for use in epilepsy syndromes. Therefore, in many instances antiepileptic medications are used in an off-label manner on the basis of the efficacy demonstrated in clinical practice.

It may be said that the treatment of pediatric epileptic patients is just as much art as it is science. Although there are certain doses and serum concentrations that have more commonly been found to result in seizure control with no or minimal adverse effects, these values are not universally optimal for every individual. Therefore, it is helpful to think of antiepileptic drug treatment in terms of *common recommended doses* and *usual therapeutic ranges*. These serve as initial *target ranges* and act as reasonable starting points for the treatment of most patients. In general, there are certain principles that may be used when initiating and switching among antiepileptic medications. These principles are as follows:

- Start therapy at a low dose with one drug and titrate the doses up slowly to the commonly recommended dose or to a serum concentration in the lower end of the target range.
- If seizures persist, advance the dose as necessary until seizures cease or there are adverse effects, regardless of serum concentrations.
- If there are adverse effects, decrease the dose slightly to the maximum tolerated dosage, give the medication more frequently throughout the day, and observe for at least 1 month.
- If seizures persist despite maximum tolerated doses of one medication, switch over to another single drug. This is done by slowly increasing the dose of the added drug until it is at a therapeutic concentration, then gradually removing the first medication.
- Monotherapy is desired if at all possible; however, if repeated attempts with monotherapy at maximum tolerated doses have failed, then the use of two-drug combinations is warranted. Ideally, if poly therapy is initiated then one should attempt to use medications with different mechanisms of action, minimal drug–drug interaction potential, and dissimilar side effect profiles.
- In patients failing two or more medications because of lack of efficacy, consider epilepsy surgery, the ketogenic diet, or the vagal nerve stimulator.
- If for some reason these options are not suitable and all reasonable one- or two-drug regimens have failed, then return to the regimen that was most effective and best tolerated.

TABLE 33.1

EFFICACY OF ANTIEPILEPTIC MEDICATION

Seizure Type	Initial Choices	Alternatives
Complex partial (with or without generalization)	Carbamazepine, lamotrigine, oxcarbazepine	Felbamate, gabapentin, levetiracetam, phenobarbital, primidone, phenytoin, tiagabine, topiramate, zonisamide
Primary generalized tonic-clonic	Lamotrigine, valproate	Felbamate, phenobarbital, primidone, phenytoin, topiramate, zonisamide
Absence	Ethosuximide, lamotrigine, valproate	Clonazepam, topiramate, zonisamide
Tonic, myoclonic, or atonic	Lamotrigine, valproate	Clonazepam, felbamate, phenobarbital, primidone, topiramate, zonisamide
Benign focal epilepsy of childhood	Carbamazepine, gabapentin	Phenytoin, valproate
Infantile spasms	ACTH, prednisone, pyridoxine, vigabatrin	Clonazepam, lamotrigine, phenobarbital, primidone, tiagabine, topiramate, zonisamide
Juvenile myoclonic epilepsy	Valproate	Lamotrigine, topiramate, zonisamide
Lennox-Gastaut syndrome	Clonazepam, valproate	Felbamate, lamotrigine, phenobarbital, pyridoxine, topiramate, zonisamide

ACTH, adrenocorticotropic hormone.

When planning a dosage schedule, it is important to keep in mind the usual half-life of the medication. Drugs with long half-lives, such as phenobarbital (40–120 hours) or phenytoin (10–30 hours) may need to be given only once or twice a day. Drugs with shorter half-lives, such as carbamazepine (8–25 hours), primidone (6–12 hours), and valproate (6–18 hours), need to be given two or three times a day to sustain effective serum concentrations. Some drugs may need to be given more often during the day to reduce episodic dose-related side effects because of peak levels, even is the half-life is fairly long. Likewise, peak-related adverse effects are also more common with immediate-release dosage forms such as syrups and suspensions. Therefore, they may need to be administered more frequently than the same medication given as a tablet, capsule or sprinkle. Infants and young children tend to have greater clearance and shorter half-life of antiepileptic medications, so that once a day dosing is rarely appropriate.

Treatment with Specific Antiepileptic Medications

Carbamazepine (CBZ, Carbatrol, Tegretol) may be the best initial choice for simple or complex partial seizures. Often it is also effective against generalized tonic-clonic seizures. Unlike phenobarbital and phenytoin, it has minimum adverse effects on cognition at usual doses. Drawbacks include short half-life and the lack of an intravenous form. In addition, carbamazepine has an active metabolite (carbamazepine-10, 11-epoxide) that is not routinely measured. Accumulation of this metabolite can result in toxicity even when carbamazepine concentrations are normal. Adverse effects include *bone marrow suppression (with granulocytopenia)* and *hyponatremia* because of the syndrome of inappropriate secretion of antidiuretic hormone (SIADH). Carbamazepine needs to be increased gradually to avoid dose-related side effects such as ataxia, diplopia, and lethargy.

Ethosuximide (ESM, Zarontin) may be an effective initial drug for absence seizures in childhood absence epilepsy. However, valproate is more appropriate if generalized tonic-clonic seizures are also present. Advantages include few serious side effects (rare bone marrow suppression) and a long half-life. Disadvantages include gastrointestinal (GI) upset and a possibility of some cognitive effects.

Felbamate (FBM, Felbatol) has broad-spectrum efficacy against partial seizures, secondarily generalized tonic-clonic seizures, and the multiple generalized seizure types of Lennox-Gastaut syndrome. The drug is strikingly free of adverse effects on cognition and alertness. *The main concern about felbamate, however, is the risk for fatal aplastic anemia or hepatotoxicity.* Because of the risk of these complications, the FDA and the manufacturer have recommended that felbamate be used only for refractory seizures when the potential benefits clearly outweigh the risk. During felbamate therapy, it has been recommended that patients have screening laboratory testing (complete blood cell count and liver function tests) done every 2 weeks. Felbamate has many drug–drug interactions: It decreases the clearance of phenytoin, valproate, and carbamazepine epoxide, whereas its own clearance is increased by carbamazepine and phenytoin and decreased by valproate.

Gabapentin (GBP, Neurontin) is effective against partial and secondarily generalized tonic-clonic seizures. It has a low toxicity profile with minimal cognitive impairment. Adverse effects may include transient dizziness, lethargy, and ataxia, and weight gain may occur at higher doses. Children may exhibit paradoxical aggressive behaviors. Gabapentin is not bound to plasma proteins and it is excreted unmetabolized by the kidneys. Because of these favorable pharmacokinetic features, there are no drug–drug interactions and gabapentin is easily used as an add-on medication.

Lamotrigine (LTG, Lamictal) is effective against partial or secondarily generalized tonic-clonic seizures, absence seizures, and generalized seizure types, including those associated with Lennox-Gastaut syndrome. It has a low toxicity profile with minimal cognitive impairment. Adverse effects may include lethargy, ataxia, headache, and GI distress. However, the main concern with lamotrigine is *skin rash*, which may be severe and is estimated to occur in as many as 1 in 100 children. The risk for a serious dermatologic reaction (*Stevens-Johnson syndrome or toxic epidermal necrolysis*) appears greater if the patient is already on valproate, or if the lamotrigine is introduced quickly. Slow titration of the medication has been shown to decrease the risk of rash. If rash does occur in a pediatric patient, it is advised that the medication be discontinued. Lamotrigine's hepatic metabolism is markedly affected by other medications: induced by carbamazepine, phenytoin, and phenobarbital and inhibited by valproate. This requires that separate dosing schedules be used to start lamotrigine, depending on the baseline antiepileptic medication.

Levetiracetam (LEV, Keppra) is effective in the treatment of partial or secondary generalized seizures. Currently, there is little information regarding its efficacy in other seizure types. Levetiracetam has the advantage of being able to be introduced fairly rapidly without significant adverse effects. It also does not undergo hepatic metabolism nor is it significantly bound to plasma proteins; therefore, it does not interact with other medications. Although generally well tolerated, levetiracetam may cause somnolence, dizziness, asthenia, or headache. There have also been reports of worsening of behavior (depression, emotional lability, or aggression) with the use of this medication.

Oxcarbazepine (OXC, Trileptal) is a drug similar to carbamazepine, but it has the advantage that it does not undergo autoinduction. It is effective for the treatment of partial and secondary generalized seizures. Oxcarbazepine is a prodrug that is rapidly converted to its monohydroxy derivative (MHD), which is primarily responsible for the anticonvulsant effects of this medication. Overall, it has been shown to be well tolerated; however, it may be associated with dizziness, fatigue, nausea, and rarely hyponatremia (SIADH). In patients who develop a rash while receiving carbamazepine, only 25% to 30% experience a rash when switched to oxcarbazepine. It is important to realize that oxcarbazepine is a less potent inducer than carbamazepine, phenytoin, or phenobarbital. Therefore, if the decision to switch to oxcarbazepine is made, then the doses of any concurrent hepatically metabolized medications may need to be decreased to prevent toxicity.

Phenytoin/fosphenytoin (PHT, Dilantin/Cerebyx) is effective against partial or generalized tonic-clonic seizures. It is inexpensive and has a fairly long half-life. It can usually be given once or twice a day. Cosmetic side effects such as hirsutism and gum hypertrophy may occur. Subtle cognitive effects may also be noted. The average starting dose is 4 to 8 mg/kg per day or 300 mg/day for adults. Intravenous loading may be performed using phenytoin or fosphenytoin if needed to obtain an immediate serum concentration in the usual therapeutic range (10–20 mg/L). Fosphenytoin is a prodrug of phenytoin that is not associated with the extreme venous irritation (including infiltration) commonly found with intravenous phenytoin. It is preferred for patients with poor intravenous access or with uncontrolled, prolonged, or repetitive seizures.

Phenobarbital (PB) is effective in the treatment of partial or generalized tonic-clonic seizures. It is inexpensive, has a long half-life, and can be taken once a day. It is safe in regard to renal, hepatic, and bone marrow function, but a common side effect is sedation or impaired cognitive ability. Children may have significant hyperactivity or irritability. Because of these adverse effects, the drug is rarely the best initial choice outside the newborn and infancy age group. Because of the long half-life, it is important to wait for at least 2 weeks before beginning to assess the efficacy of the drug and its initial dosage. A serum concentration in the usual therapeutic range (15–40 mg/L) can be obtained very quickly with intravenous loading, but the inevitable side effect is somnolence.

Primidone (PRM, Mysoline) is an interesting drug because it is metabolized in the body into other active substances including phenobarbital. Therefore, it is important during primidone treatment to monitor the phenobarbital serum concentrations. Primidone is effective against partial and generalized tonic-clonic seizures. The main disadvantage is cognitive side effects.

Tiagabine (TGB, Gabitril) is effective for partial onset seizures. There are pilot data suggesting it may be effective for infantile spasms because it increases the brain's level of GABA in a manner similar to the medication, vigabatrin. Side effects of this medication include somnolence, dizziness, trembling, nervousness, and irritability. It may also rarely result in nonconvulsive status epilepticus.

Topiramate (TPM, Topamax) is effective for both partial and generalized seizure types. Although it is considered very efficacious, there are concerns over its cognitive side effects, namely psychomotor slowing, memory difficulties, confusion, and sedation. These effects are less when the medica-

tion is titrated slowly. Topiramate has also been associated with weight loss and paresthesias. In rare instances, kidney stones and reversible glaucoma occur. If these side effects are suspected, discontinuation of topiramate is advised.

Valproate (VPA, Depakene, Depakote) may be the best initial choice for some forms of primary generalized epilepsy, such as childhood absence epilepsy with absence and primary generalized tonic-clonic seizures. It may also have some efficacy against partial seizures, but this has been less well documented. A major advantage is valproate's lack of cognitive effects. Its disadvantages include its relatively short half-life and an association with:

- Cosmetic changes (weight gain and hair loss)
- Polycystic ovary disease
- Pancreatitis
- Rare but serious hepatotoxicity

Idiopathic hepatotoxicity has been found to be more common in patients receiving polytherapy and in those younger than 2 years. *Liver and hematologic function tests must be performed periodically during the treatment.*

Zonisamide (ZNS, Zonegran) is a medication that has been extensively used in Japan and has recently been approved in the United States for the treatment of partial seizures. However, it also has efficacy in generalized seizure types. Zonisamide and topiramate share many of the same adverse effects including; cognitive effects, weight loss, and kidney stones. Unlike topiramate, zonisamide can cause oligohidrosis and rarely reversible psychosis. The psychosis is unique, in that it may continue even after the medication cannot be detected in the patient's blood. However, it is important to remember that these symptoms are reversible. Because it is a sulfonamide, zonisamide should not be used in patients with a sulfa allergy.

Monitoring

Once antiepileptic treatment is initiated, it is important to monitor the patient for seizure control and drug side effects (Table 33.2). Periodic visits to the clinic and laboratory testing are appropriate. An occasional check of the serum drug concentrations is helpful in the evaluation of compliance or in the assessment of toxic side effects. However, serum concentrations play only a limited role in determining the appropriate dosage of medication. This decision is predominantly based on clinical factors. In patients taking carbamazepine, valproate, or primidone, it is appropriate to check hematologic and hepatic parameters periodically. The appropriate frequency for laboratory testing is controversial. Very frequent hematologic and hepatic testing is recommended during treatment with felbamate. Monitoring of renal function is recommended for gabapentin, topiramate, and levetiracetam. Serum sodium and blood cell counts should be checked for those receiving oxcarbazepine. For other antiepileptic medications, guidelines for monitoring are less well defined.

TABLE 33.2

ADVERSE EFFECTS OF ANTIEPILEPTIC MEDICATIONS

Medication	Adverse Effects
Carbamazepine	Lethargy, ataxia, diplopia, neutropenia, hyponatremia, rash
Ethosuximide	Gastrointestinal distress, lethargy, blood dyscrasias
Felbamate	Sedation, dizziness, ataxia, behavioral disturbances
Gabapentin	Headache, insomnia, weight loss, gastrointestinal distress, aplastic anemia, hepatotoxicity
Levetiracetam	Somnolence, dizziness, behavioral disturbances
Lamotrigine	Sedation, dizziness, lethargy, ataxia, headache, rash (including Stevens-Johnson syndrome and toxic epidermal necrolysis)
Oxcarbazepine	Somnolence, gastrointestinal distress, hyponatremia
Phenobarbital	Lethargy, ataxia, hyperactivity, cognitive difficulty
Phenytoin	Lethargy, ataxia, diplopia, gum hyperplasia, hirsutism, macrocytic anemia, osteomalacia, cerebellar dysfunction
Primidone	Lethargy, ataxia, diplopia, blood dyscrasias
Tiagabine	Somnolence, dizziness, trembling, nervousness and irritability, nonconvulsive status epilepticus
Topiramate	Dizziness, drowsiness, paresthesias, psychomotor and cognitive slowing, weight loss, nephrolithiasis, secondary glaucoma
Valproate	Gastrointestinal distress, tremor, weight gain, hair loss, polycystic ovary disease, thrombocytopenia, pancreatitis, hepatotoxicity
Zonisamide	Dizziness, drowsiness, weight loss, cognitive and psychomotor slowing, oligohidrosis, nephrolithiasis, psychosis, cross-sensitivity with sulfa medications

In patients in whom seizures are not controlled and the diagnosis is unclear, intensive monitoring with EEG should be considered. The intensive EEG evaluation may confirm that the problem is in fact epilepsy and not psychogenic seizures, or it may demonstrate that the events are nonepileptic. If careful medication trials have been unsuccessful, then an epilepsy surgery should be considered.

Drug–Drug Interactions

The most common effect of adding a second antiepileptic drug to the medication regimen is the alteration of drug metabolism. It is important to check for this possibility when medications are added or removed. Some drugs induce hepatic activity so that when added to a medication regimen they cause the serum concentration of the first drug to decrease, whereas some drugs inhibit metabolic enzymes so that their addition causes the serum concentration of the first drug to increase. For example, phenytoin metabolism may be accelerated by the addition of phenobarbital, primidone, or carbamazepine and carbamazepine metabolism may be accelerated by the addition of phenytoin, phenobarbital, or primidone. Another effect of adding a second medication is the alteration in protein binding. For example, the free fraction of phenytoin may be increased with the addition of valproate, as the two drugs compete for albumin binding sites. If hepatic enzymes can metabolize the additional free portion, then the total serum concentration may fall. If hepatic

enzymes are saturated, then the free fraction may remain increased even with unchanged total concentration, resulting in drug toxicity.

Similar interactions may occur with the addition of drugs other than antiepileptic medications. For example, *inhibition of phenytoin metabolism may occur with warfarin, chloramphenicol, propoxyphene, sulfamethoxazole, methylphenidate, or other drugs; and an important inhibitor of carbamazepine metabolism is erythromycin.* Antiepileptic medications that induce hepatic metabolism have the potential to reduce the concentrations of other medications used in other medical conditions. This may be particularly important in certain clinical populations. For example, in patients who undergo transplantations, immunosuppressant drugs used to prevent organ rejection may be significantly reduced and lead to organ rejection. In female patients, it is always important to check for any interaction that may occur between an antiepileptic medication and oral contraceptives.

EPILEPSY AND PREGNANCY

Women of childbearing age should receive counseling on several points about possible pregnancy. They should be aware that there is a small increase in risk to the fetus from exposure to medications taken by the mother, with two to three times increase in the rate of fetal malformation compared with the general population. A special concern is *neural tube defects,* reported to be increased in infants of mothers treated with valproate or carbamazepine. Not much is known about the newer antiepileptics and their effects in pregnancy. It has been suggested that prenatal vitamins with folate should be recommended for all epileptic women of childbearing age, to minimize this risk. In general, most specialists feel that prospective mothers should be treated throughout pregnancy with the drug that best controls their seizures. If possible, drug regimens should be simplified to minimize fetal exposure when pregnancy is anticipated. Medications should be maintained at the lowest dosage that gives seizure control. If feasible, prospective mothers could be considered for medication withdrawal; but if the seizures are uncontrolled, or if they have generalized tonic-clonic seizures, then it is likely that the risk of medication withdrawal to the fetus would be greater than that of medication exposure.

Pregnancy may increase, decrease, or not change the mother's seizure frequency. One concern is that during pregnancy, especially in the second trimester, the drug serum concentrations may decrease below the necessary level required for seizure control. Typically, monthly antiepileptic drug concentration monitoring is required to guide dosage increase. Because protein binding may be decreased during pregnancy, monitoring of free concentration is warranted for phenytoin and valproate. Within a few weeks of delivery, it is important to decrease the dosage as pharmacokinetics return to normal to prevent drug toxicity. Antiepileptic medications may result in increased risk for hemorrhagic disease in the newborn. To prevent this, it may be helpful to treat the mother with vitamin K_1, 20 mg/day, for 2 weeks prior to the delivery. Nursing mothers should be aware that antiepileptic medications are excreted in breast milk to varying degrees. In most cases the dosage to the nursing infant causes no problems, although the infant's serum level may not be negligible. Some infants may become lethargic because of the medication, in which case it may be necessary to change to formula feeding.

STATUS EPILEPTICUS

Status epilepticus has been described as epileptic seizures that are so frequently repeated or so prolonged as to create a fixed and lasting condition for 30 minutes or more. It may be convulsive, with generalized tonic-clonic seizures, or nonconvulsive, with absence, simple partial, or complex partial seizures. The most common etiology is antiepileptic drug withdrawal in patients with epilepsy, but other causes include an acute neurologic insult such as infarction, tumor, trauma, infection, anoxic encephalopathy, metabolic encephalopathy, alcohol withdrawal, or drug abuse. The acute mortality is 8% to 12%, and is usually related to the underlying etiology. Mortality is lower in individuals with epilepsy who have an exacerbation of seizures, and higher in patients with acute central nervous system injury. Death

may occur because of systemic effects of status epilepticus, including cardiovascular stress because of tonic contraction of skeletal muscles; metabolic changes including acidosis, hypoxia, hyperkalemia, hypoglycemia, or azotemia; anticonvulsant effects including myocardial depression, arrhythmia, or respiratory depression; rhabdomyolysis leading to myoglobinuria and renal failure; pulmonary edema; or autonomic dysfunction.

The management of status epilepticus can be considered in relation to the time from first physician contact. Within the first 5 minutes, the goal is to give attention to the airway, breathing, and circulation. A brief history and physical examination are performed, and blood is tested for antiepileptic drug levels, electrolytes, glucose, blood urea nitrogen, and drug screening. Between 6 and 9 minutes, and intravenous line is established with saline infusion, and glucose 1 to 2 mg/kg or 25 to 50 gm is given. Adults also receive thiamine 100 mg. Between 10 and 30 minutes, antiepileptic medications are given, depending on the patient's baseline regimen. Naïve patients may receive phenytoin 20 mg/kg, given intravenously more slowly than 25 mg/minute (for children) to 50 mg/minute (for adults) with electrocardiogram (EKG) recording and blood pressure monitoring. If needed, the patient may then receive lorazepam 2 to 8 mg (0.1 mg/kg for children) or diazepam 10 to 20 mg (0.3 mg/kg for children) intravenously. Alternatively, some feel that a benzodiazepine should be used first, with subsequent loading doses of phenytoin or other antiepileptic medication. Fosphenytoin (discussed in the subsequent text) is a safer alternative to phenytoin that may be used for patients with status epilepticus. If seizures persist, the patient may need elective intubation and injection of phenobarbital 10 mg/kg. If seizures still persist, then stat serum drug concentrations should be obtained and more phenytoin or phenobarbital should be given as indicated to bring the concentrations to high levels (phenytoin at 20–25 mg/L, phenobarbital at 40–45 mg/L or higher). If seizures continue for more than 1 hour despite these measures, the patient may need barbiturate coma with EEG monitoring and anesthesia.

Fosphenytoin is a new preparation available for intravenous or intramuscular use. The fosphenytoin molecule is much more soluble in water than phenytoin, and it does not require the propylene glycol solvent needed for phenytoin. Fosphenytoin, therefore, has fewer adverse effects than intravenous phenytoin, and does not cause tissue damage if extravasated. Fosphenytoin is administered in phenytoin equivalents (PEs) so that the milligram doses are the same as for phenytoin. It should be given faster than phenytoin, 150 mg PE/minute, to compensate for the time required for conversion to the phenytoin molecule. Other parenteral medications that have been used to treat status epilepticus include midazolam and intravenous valproate. For nonconvulsive status epilepticus, lorazepam, or intravenous valproate is effective.

REVIEW EXERCISES

QUESTIONS

1. A mother brings her 6-year-old daughter to your clinic and states that her academic performance has decreased during the last year. Her teacher notices her staring frequently throughout the day. Sometimes, she seems "off in her own world" and does not respond to questions. An electroencephalogram reveals a 3-Hz generalized spike-and-wave pattern that can be triggered by hyperventilation. What seizure type is this patient *most* likely to have?
a) Tonic-clonic
b) Myoclonic
c) Absence
d) Complex partial

Answer
The answer is c.

2. What antiepileptic medication would you recommend for this patient?
a) Phenobarbital
b) Carbamazepine
c) Ethosuximide
d) Valproate
e) Either c or d

Answer
The answer is e.

3. A 10-year-old boy has had complex partial seizures since the age of 7 years. He has failed treatment with carbamazepine, lamotrigine, and phenytoin. Four weeks ago, it was decided to add topiramate to his other current medication (carbamazepine). His mother informs your office that his school performance has declined and he appears "dull." What is the *most* likely cause and what should be done?
a) He is experiencing side effects of topiramate, which should be reduced or withdrawn.
b) He most likely has attention deficit disorder, and methylphenidate should be started.
c) The topiramate is affecting carbamazepine metabolism; as a result, new side effects have developed, and the carbamazepine should be reduced.

Answer
The answer is a.

4. A previously healthy 9-year-old boy is in your office with his mother, referred from the emergency department. At approximately 4:00 a.m. that day, the mother heard gurgling and thrashing noises. She went into the boy's bedroom and found him unconscious, with limb and body jerking and drooling that lasted for about a minute. Afterward, he was groggy and then went back to sleep. By the time he was seen in the emergency department, he had returned to baseline behavior, with normal neurologic examination findings and no fever or stiff neck. In your office, the boy states that he does not remember the event. An EEG performed later that day shows left centrotemporal sharp waves. What is the *most* likely diagnosis?
a) Juvenile myoclonic epilepsy
b) Benign focal epilepsy of childhood
c) Temporal lobe epilepsy secondary to a low-grade tumor

Answer
The answer is b.

5. What treatment would you recommend for the patient in the previous question?
a) Carbamazepine
b) Gabapentin
c) No antiepileptic drug at this point

Answer
The answer is c.

6. Etiologic causes that may lead to infantile spasms include:
a) Idiopathic
b) Genetic and metabolic
c) Focal brain malformations
d) All of the above

Answer
The answer is d.

7. A 2.5-year-old boy was brought to your office after experiencing his second febrile seizure. These episodes were 4 months apart and described as generalized tightening of the body followed by jerking involving all four extremities and lasting 3 to 5 minutes each time. The child was noted to have a fever of >38.88°C (102°F) on both occasions. At this time, your recommendation would be:
a) Further tests including EEG and MRI scan
b) Treatment with phenobarbital
c) Treatment with valproate
d) Education and counseling for the family

Answer
The answer is d.

8. Skin rash is an important concern for which of the following antiepileptic medications?
a) Topiramate
b) Gabapentin
c) Lamotrigine
d) Oxcarbazepine

Answer
The answer is c.

9. Adverse effects of topiramate include (more than one answer may be correct):
a) Cognitive difficulties
b) Nephrolithiasis

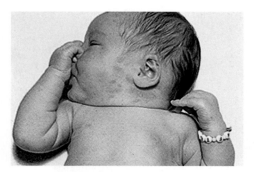

Figure 1.1

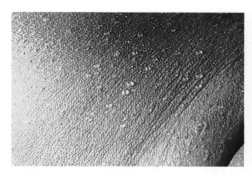

Figure 1.2

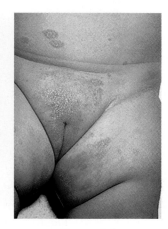

Figure 1.3

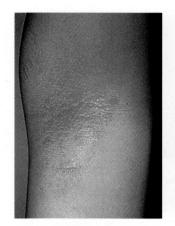

Figure 1.4

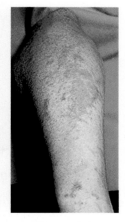

Figure 1.5

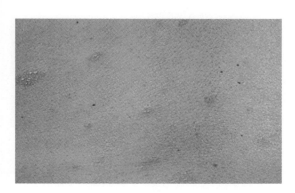

Figure 1.6

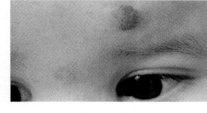

Figure 1.8

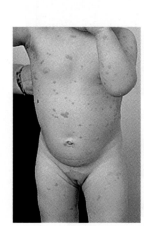

Figure 1.7

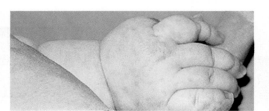

Figure 1.9

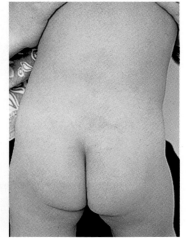

Figure 1.10

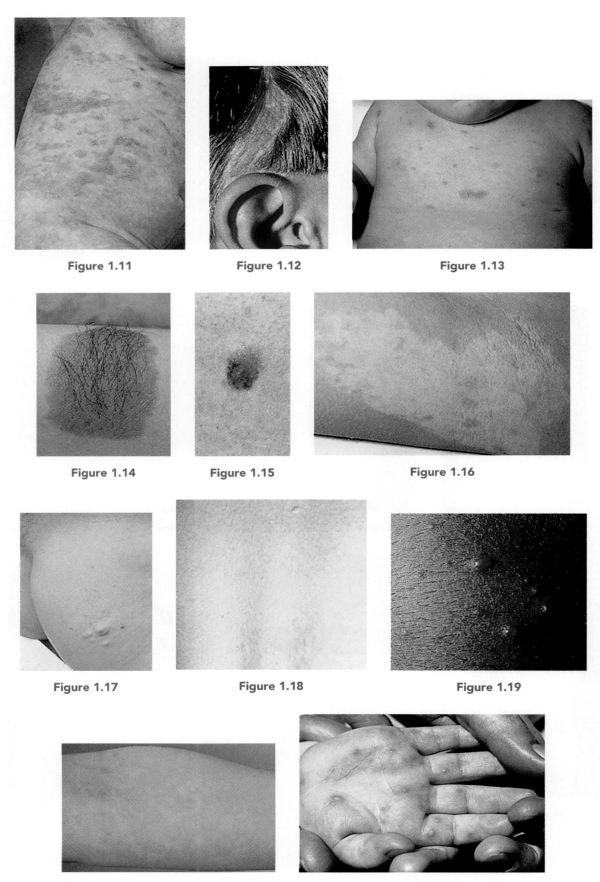

Figure 1.11

Figure 1.12

Figure 1.13

Figure 1.14

Figure 1.15

Figure 1.16

Figure 1.17

Figure 1.18

Figure 1.19

Figure 1.20

Figure 1.21

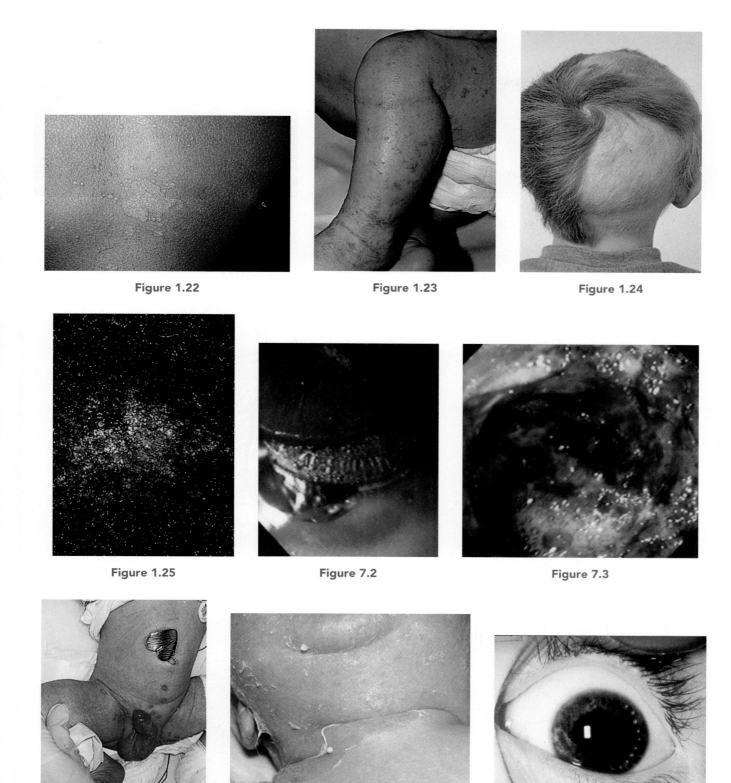

Figure 1.22

Figure 1.23

Figure 1.24

Figure 1.25

Figure 7.2

Figure 7.3

Figure 22.1

Figure 23.1

Figure 23.2

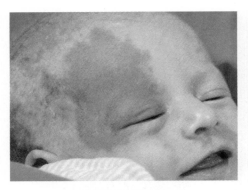

Figure 23.3

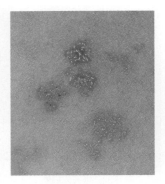

Figure 23.5

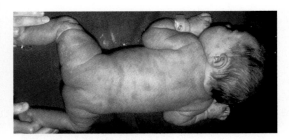

Figure 23.7

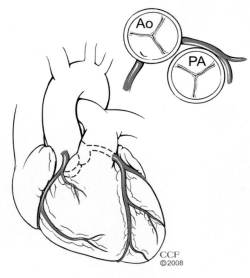

Figure 25.4

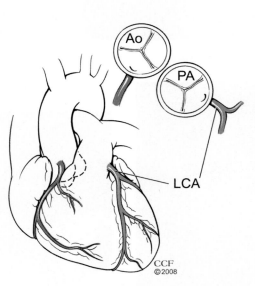

Figure 25.5

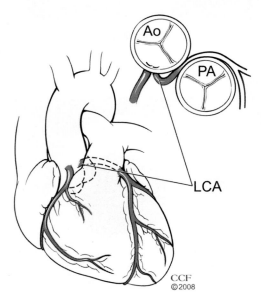

Figure 25.6

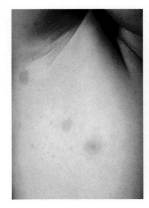

Figure 35.1

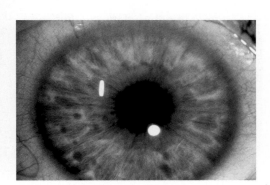

Figure 35.3

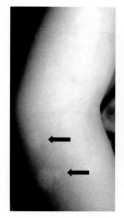

Figure 35.5

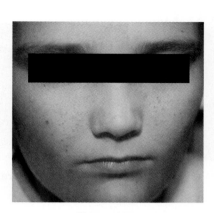

Figure 35.6

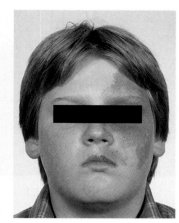

Figure 35.8

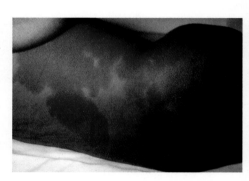

Figure 35.10

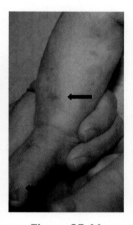

Figure 35.11

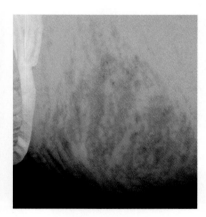

Figure 35.12

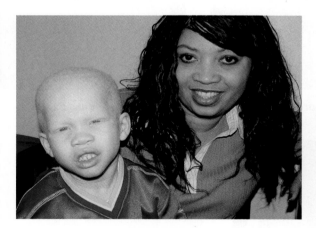

Figure 35.13

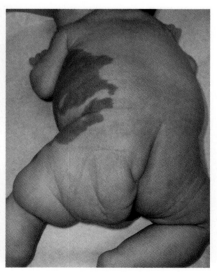

Figure 35.15

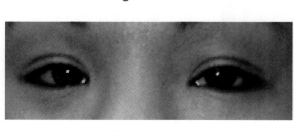

Figure 35.14

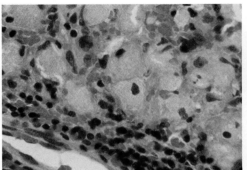

Figure 43.1

Figure 48.1

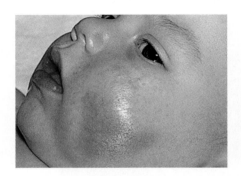

Figure 48.2

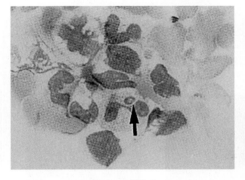

Figure 50.1

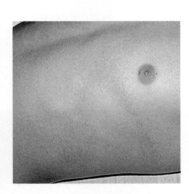

Figure 50.2

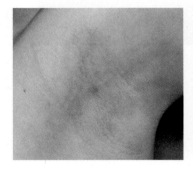

Figure 50.3

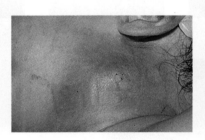

Figure 51.1

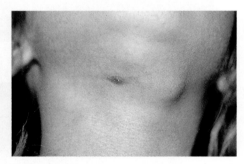

Figure 51.2

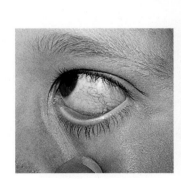

Figure 51.3

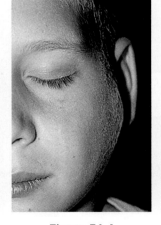

Figure 51.4

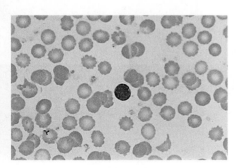

Figure 51.5

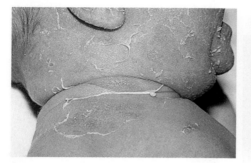

Figure 51.6

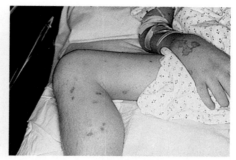

Figure 51.7

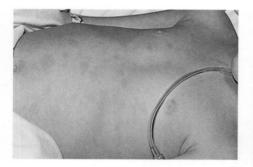

Figure 51.8

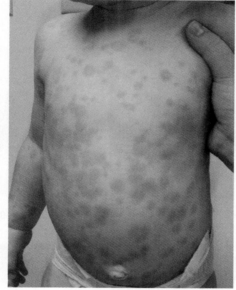

Figure 51.9

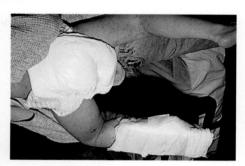

Figure 51.11

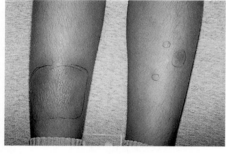

Figure 51.10

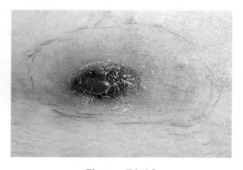

Figure 51.12

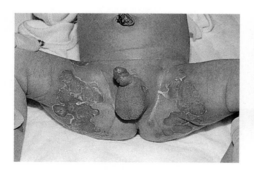

Figure 51.13

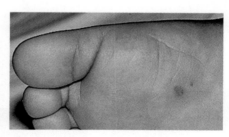

Figure 51.14

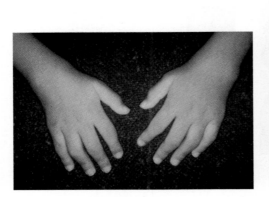

Figure 52.1

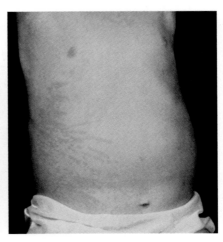

Figure 52.2

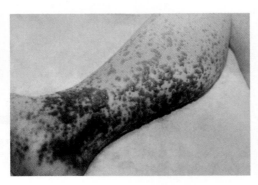

Figure 52.3

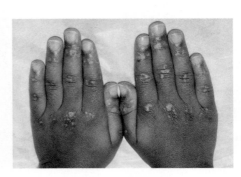

Figure 52.4

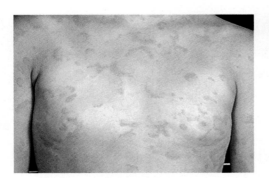

Figure 67.2

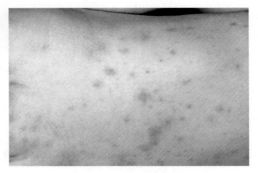

Figure 67.3

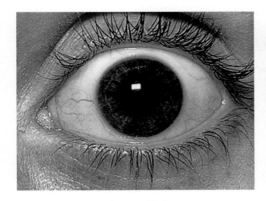

Figure 67.6

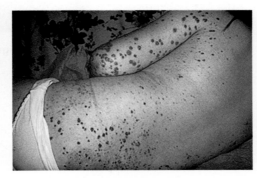

Figure 67.8

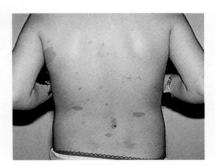

Figure 68.4

c) Hepatic failure

d) GI upset

Answer

The answer is a and b.

10. Significant antiepileptic medication interaction may be observed with which of the following combinations?

a) Levetiracetam and carbamazepine

b) Gabapentin and phenobarbital

c) Valproate and lamotrigine

d) Felbamate and oxcarbazepine

Answer

The answer is c.

SUGGESTED READINGS

1. Abdul M, Riviello JJ. Update on the newer antiepileptic drugs in child neurology: advances in treatment of pediatric epilepsy. *Curr Treat Options Neurol* 2007;9(6):395–403.
2. Aicardi J. Epilepsy in children. In: *International review of child neurology series*, 2nd ed. New York: Raven Press, 1994.
3. Azar NL, Abou-Khalil BW. Considerations in the choice of an antiepileptic drug in the treatment of epilepsy. *Semin Neurol* 2008;28(3):305–316.
4. Baulac S, Gourfinkel-An I, Nabbout R, et al. Fever, genes, and epilepsy. *Lancet Neurol* 2004;3(7):421–430.
5. Bourgeois B. New antiepileptic drug in children: which ones for which seizures? *Clin Neuropharmacol* 2000;23:119–132.
6. Camfield PR, Camfield CS, Gordon K, Dooley JM. If a first antiepileptic drug fails to control a child's epilepsy, what are the chances of success with the next drug? *J Pediatr* 1997;131(6):821–824.
7. Camfield PR, Camfield CS, Shapiro SH, et al. The first febrile seizure-antipyretic instruction plus either phenobarbital or placebo to prevent recurrence. *J Pediatr* 1980;97(1):16–21.
8. Commission on Classification and Terminology of the International League Against Epilepsy. Proposal for revised clinical and electroencephalographic classification of epileptic seizures. *Epilepsia* 1981;22:489.
9. Commission on Classification and Terminology of the International League Against Epilepsy. Proposal for classification of epilepsies and epileptic syndromes. *Epilepsia* 1985;26:268.
10. Ellenberg JH, Nelson KB. Febrile seizures and later intellectual performance. *Arch Neurol* 1978;35(1):17–21.
11. Farwell JR, Lee YJ, Hirtz DG, et al. Phenobarbital for febrile seizures: effects on intelligence and on seizure recurrence. *N Engl J Med* 1990;322(6):364–369.
12. Gerard F, Pereira S, Robaglia-Schlupp A, et al. Clinical and genetic analysis of a new multigenerational pedigree with GEFS+ (Generalized Epilepsy with Febrile Seizures Plus). *Epilepsia* 2002;43:581–586.
13. Malphrus AD, Wilfong AA. Use of the newer antiepileptic drugs in pediatric epilepsies. *Curr Treat Options Neurol* 2007;9(4):256–267.
14. Mamelle N, Mamelle JC, Plasse JC, et al. Prevention of recurrent febrile convulsions: a randomized therapeutic assay: sodium valproate, phenobarbital and placebo. *Neuropediatrics* 1984;15(1):37–42.
15. Marson AG, Kadir ZA, Chadwick DW, et al. New antiepileptic drugs: a systematic review of their efficacy and tolerability. *BMJ* 1996;313:1169–1174.
16. Mattson RH, Cramer JA, Collins JF, et al. Comparison of carbamazepine, phenobarbital, phenytoin, and primidone in partial and secondarily generalized tonic-clonic seizures. *N Engl J Med* 1985;313:145–151.
17. Mattson RH, Cramer JA, Collins JF, et al. A comparison of valproate with carbamazepine for the treatment of complex partial seizures and secondarily generalized tonic-clonic seizures in adults. *N Engl J Med* 1992;327:765–771.
18. Pellock J. Managing epilepsy syndromes with new antiepileptic drugs. *Pediatrics* 1999;104:1106–1116.
19. Rosman NP, Colton T, Labazzo J, et al. A controlled trial of diazepam administered during febrile illnesses to prevent recurrence of febrile seizures. *N Engl J Med* 1993;329(2):79–84.
20. Singh R, Scheffer IE, Crossland K, et al. Generalized epilepsy with febrile seizures plus: a common childhood-onset genetic epilepsy syndrome. *Ann Neurol* 1999;45:75–81.
21. Treiman DM, Meyers PD, Walton NY, et al. A comparison of four treatments for generalized convulsive status epilepticus. *N Engl J Med* 1998;339:792–798.
22. Verity CM, Greenwood R, Golding J. Long-term intellectual and behavioral outcomes of children with febrile convulsions. *N Engl J Med* 1998;338(24):1723–1728.
23. Vining EP, Mellitis ED, Dorsen MM, et al. Psychologic and behavioral effects of antiepileptic drugs in children: a double-blind comparison between phenobarbital and valproic acid. *Pediatrics* 1987;80(2):165–174.
24. Wallace SJ, Smith JA Successful prophylaxis against febrile convulsions with valproic acid or phenobarbitone. *BMJ* 1980;280(6211):353–354.
25. Wyllie E, ed. *The treatment of epilepsy: principles and practice*, 3rd ed. Baltimore: Lippincott Williams & Wilkins, 2001.
26. Zahn CA, Morrell MJ, Collins SD, et al. Management issues for women with epilepsy: a review of the literature. *Neurology* 1998;51:949–956.

Chapter 34

Nonepileptic Paroxysmal Disorders in Children

Ajay Gupta, Bruce H. Cohen, and Elaine Wyllie

APPROACH TO CHILDREN WITH PAROXYSMAL EVENTS

A variety of disorders in children present as paroxysmal events that may be confused with epileptic seizures. Careful considerations to several factors during clinical evaluation help in making the accurate diagnosis. A correct diagnosis is the vital step that leads to timely management of the underlying condition, which may have serious implications if the diagnosis is delayed or missed. A correct diagnosis also avoids unnecessary testing, costly investigations, and inappropriate treatment with antiepileptic drugs. Infrequently, nonepileptic paroxysmal events may coexist with epileptic seizures in children, and this should always be kept in the mind, especially in children with mental retardation or learning and development disabilities.

Clinical history and examination remains the cornerstone for correct diagnosis of such events. The following factors in the history and physical examination aid in determining the nature of events.

- Age of onset
- Description of spells (duration, frequency, symptoms during a spell, stereotypic or nonstereotypic)
- Course of the events (stable, improving, or worsening)
- Timing of occurrence (sleep or daytime in school or home or seen in multiple settings)
- Precipitating and relieving factors (relationship to meals, emotions, exercise, head injury, etc.)
- Family history (tics or movement disorders, epilepsy, migraine)
- Cognitive and behavior functioning (developmental delay, attention deficit hyperactivity disorder, pervasive developmental disorder)

- Through physical examination with special attention to neurologic exam, heart rate/rhythm, heart murmurs, orthostatic blood pressures, and abnormal posture or movements

Sometimes more extensive investigations may be required to make an accurate diagnosis. When the etiology of paroxysmal events remains undetermined or a possibility of epileptic seizures remains, video EEG monitoring may be necessary to clarify the diagnosis. Common nonepileptic paroxysmal events in children are discussed here.

BREATH-HOLDING SPELLS

Breath-holding spells are very common in pediatric practice; therefore, they are discussed separately. There are two types, cyanotic and pallid, with presumed different pathophysiologic mechanisms. Breath holding spells usually begin in the second half of the first year and are precipitated by frustration or anger. They rarely begin after the age of 2 years, although they may persist in some children until 6 years of age. Breath-holding spells may occur frequently once or several times in a week. A positive family history may be found in children with this disorder.

Cyanotic Spells

This is the more common type of breath-holding spell. The spell usually begins with uncontrolled crying that follows a seemingly trivial event, such as being reprimanded or sustaining a fall with a head bump. After few seconds of crying, the child holds his or her breath, and cyanosis develops. At times, consciousness may be lost. Tonic, clonic, or myoclonic movements may occur later in the attack, but are usually self-limited. These involuntary tonic or tonic-clonic movements are secondary to brain hypoxia and should not be treated with anticonvulsants. The interictal EEG is usually normal but may reveal slowing or suppression during the acute event. Aside from the safety issue of a possible fall during a breath-holding spell, these events are considered benign. In some instances, psychologic referral for behavior modification is required and may benefit both the parents and the child. In most instances, children outgrow breath-holding spells without sequelae or future behavioral problems. The pathophysiologic mechanism is not well understood, but correction of any underlying anemia has been shown to reduce the frequency of attacks, with reports suggesting iron therapy even without frank anemia can be helpful.

Pallid Spells

In the *pallid* type of spell, bradycardia or brief asystole causes a loss of consciousness soon after the attack begins. Again, the attack may be precipitated by a head bump that may be seemingly trivial. The child suddenly becomes pale and often loses consciousness. Clonic or myoclonic jerks may occur near or at the end of the attack. Most patients suspected of having this syndrome may undergo routine ECG and Holter monitoring to exclude any treatable cardiac condition or rhythm disorder. Children with pallid breath-holding spells are believed to have autonomic dysregulation caused by parasympathetic disturbance distinct from that found in cyanotic breath-holding. In severe cases, atropine or similar agents may be used to block the bradycardia associated with the syndrome.

GASTROINTESTINAL DISORDERS

Gastroesophageal Reflux (Sandifer Syndrome)

Gastroesophageal reflux in children, usually infants, sometimes presents with unusual posturing of the neck, torso, and arms. The posturing may be sustained (like dystonia) or intermittent. It may also present as apneic episodes with cyanosis and or pallor. This disorder is most often described in children with tone abnormalities and developmental disorders, but may occur in normal children. The diagnosis is confirmed with a pH probe test. Episodes usually resolve with treatment of gastroesophageal reflux.

Cyclic Vomiting

Cyclic vomiting is characterized by spontaneously recurrent bouts of severe emesis lasting minutes to many hours. In some cases the emesis can last for several days before relenting. The cycles of emesis occur every few weeks to months. The episodes may be precipitated by stress, infection, fasting, poor sleep, or mesntrual periods. No cause is apparent when the child is investigated during an acute episode. A diagnosis of viral gastritis or gastroenteritis is usually presumed during initial episodes before the correct diagnosis is recognized. The child is normal between episodes, and the examination findings raise no concerns. Cyclic vomiting is usually seen in young children. The syndrome has also been considered a migraine variant, as it has been shown occasionally to evolve into migraine headaches. In some children, the family history is also positive for migraine. If the patient has experienced many episodes over time, the physician may be able to make the diagnosis without the use of laboratory tests. Defects in intermediary metabolism (including but not limited to urea cycle disorders such as ornithine transcarbamylase deficiency in girls) and intracranial pathology may present with recurrent vomiting, and these should be considered in appropriate clinical scenarios. Acute episodes may require intravenous hydration, antiemetics, and mild sedation. Triptans may be used in the acute treatment when headache is a prominent symptom. Prophylactic treatment of cyclic vomiting may require antimigraine medications such as cyproheptadine, β-blockers, and tricyclic antidepressents. Topiramate, valproate, and calcium channel blockers, used widely in migraine prophylaxis, are other agents that have been anecdotally reported to be effective in cyclic vomiting.

SLEEP-RELATED EVENTS

Benign Neonatal Myoclonus

Benign neonatal myoclonus is a common condition seen in newborns and young infants. It is seen during sleep as rapid (myoclonic) movements involving one or more extremities or the torso in a random fashion. The movements occur as isolated events or in intermittent clusters that may continue during all stages of sleep. Attacks are usually a few minutes in duration, but in some infants movements may last for hours, intruding into sleep. Passive restraint of extremities does not stop the movements. EEG shows no epileptiform activity during the movements. The movements stop when the infant is woken up and are never seen in a fully awake and alert baby. No treatment is generally required. The movements typically disappear over several months. It is important to recognize this benign condition as it may lead to overaggressive investigation and treatment looking for seziures resulting from genetic or metabolic causes. Infants with this condition have had brain MRIs, cerebrospinal fluid examinations, skin and muscle biopsies, and admission to the intensive care unit with intravenous regimens of mulitple antiepileptic medications.

Head Banging (Jactatio Capitis or Rhythmic Movement Disorder)

This disorder is considered a form of parasomnia usually seen during the periods of transition from wakefulness to sleep or between different stages of sleep. Onset is usually in infancy. The child performs bizarre head and neck movements, such as head banging or rolling. Events may last from 15 to 30 minutes. Soon the child drifts off to sleep and the movements disappear. Episodes rarely recur in the same night during periods of sleep transition. The EEG is usually normal both during and between the episodes. Most children recover within few years after onset. Many parents have to repeatedly check the child at night when they wake up from the sounds of head banging. Parental reassurance is necessary. Measures to ensure safety (from fall or head banging against hard objects) of the child in his or her bed at night are important. Rarely, short-acting benzodiazpenes may be used half an hour before bedtime with good results.

Nightmares

Nightmares are behavior episodes that are believed to be associated with sleep dreams. They occur during REM sleep. Onset may be at any time, but is usually at around 2 to 5 years of age. Children may spontaneously wake up and be restless, crying, frightened, and sometimes have autonomic symptoms. They cling to the parents and generally calm down when reassured. Occasionally, incontinence may occur during a frightening episode, which may lead to a misdiagnosis of seizure. Most children are able to at least partially recall the dream. An EEG recorded during these events shows arousal from REM sleep. Most children improve over the course of few years. Episodes are generally infrequent and lead to no significant sleep disruption. Most children warrant no treatment. Counseling may help in older children with frequent episodes who are afraid to go to bed alone at night.

Night Terrors (Pavor Nocturnus)

Night terrors are considered to parasomnias that occur during the deep stages of non-REM sleep (stages III and IV). They usually begin around the age of 4 to 8 years, slightly later than the age of onset for nightmares. The child suddenly wakes up with inconsolable screaming, profuse sweating, agitation, tachycardia, and dilated pupils. The attack lasts for several minutes, and may even continue for as long as 15 to 20 minutes. It is often difficult to console or reason with the child during an episode. The child usually drifts back to sleep once the attack is over. Most children are not able to recall the episode the next morning. Attacks are usually isolated events a few nights a month, causing no regular sleep disruption. The usual course is that of improvement and subsequent disappearance of episodes.

The parents usually are very apprehensive, and may demand confirmation by video EEG for reassurance. No treatment is generally recommended.

Sleepwalking (Somnambulism)

Sleepwalking is an uncommon type of parasomnias that occurs during the deep stages of non-REM sleep (stages III and IV). The usual age of onset is 5 to 12 years. The child gets up from the bed, usually mumbling with a vacant look and open eyes, and then walks around in a trance before returning to bed. The usual time of occurrence is 2 to 4 hours after falling asleep. Sometimes bizarre activities such as eating, dressing, opening doors and windows, and touching objects are seen during an episode of somnambulism. The child rarely walks into objects. Most children sleepwalk close to their bed and the room in which they were sleeping. Episodes may last for several minutes, and never occur more than once in a night. Children are unable to recall the episodes the next morning. Serious accidents are rare in sleepwalking children. Violence is not described during typical events. Most children are able to be calmly redirected to their bed when parents find them during an episode. Complex partial seizures should be excluded before a diagnosis of sleepwalking is presumed. Treatment usually is not necessary if the child's safety can be ensured at night. Short-acting benzodiazepines are sometimes indicated for frequent or prolonged attacks of sonambulism.

Narcolepsy and Cataplexy

These are rare sleep disorders, but are important differential diagnoses in children who suddenly lose tone and posture. Narcolepsy is sudden intrusion of REM sleep during wakefulness, leading to excessive daytime sleepiness. Other symptom complexes in patients with narcolepsy include sleep paralysis (transient episodes of inability to move on awakening), hypnagogic hallucinations, and cataplexy. Cataplexy produces a sudden loss of tone with a drop to the ground in response to an unexpected touch or emotional stimulus, such as laughter. Children with narcolepsy and cataplexy may present with attention difficulties in school, irritability, and unexplained fatigue and falls. Consciousness is not lost during these brief attacks. Narcoleptics have short sleep latency as measured by standardized measurement of sleep latency tests (MSLT). MSLT will show REM sleep patterns on EEG recordings within 10 minutes of falling asleep. It is important to demonstrate normal sleep the night before an MLST with a polysomnogram (PSG), as primary sleep disorders such as sleep apnea syndrome can cause a narcoleptic picture, when in fact the patient is not sleeping at night and thus is excessively tired during the day. Narcolepsy is strongly associated with the HLA DQB1*0602 genotype, and is also associated with HLA DR2 and HLA DQ1, but narcolepsy is multifactorial and these tests are not diagnostic.

Narcolepsy may be treated with a stimulant drug, but behavioral management is also important as part of the comprehensive treatment plan.

MIGRAINE VARIANTS

Migrainous disorders are common in children. A relationship between migraine and epilepsy has been noted in some patients. Headaches mimicking migraines have been described in some children with mitochondrial disorders; therefore, caution is advised before a diagnosis of primary headache disorder is made in a child with new-onset headaches. A few types of migraines associated with abnormal movements or an altered state of awareness may be confused with seizures.

Acute Confusional Migraines

Acute confusional migraines begin with an acute alteration in consciousness, which may include varying degrees of lethargy, disorientation, agitation, and stupor. Fugue-like states are also described. Abnormal behaviors may be intermittent with somnolence, alternating with agitation and inappropriate motor hyperactivity. Episodes of acute confusional migraine typically last for a few hours, much longer than a complex partial seizure. These events may not be accompanied by any headache as in classic migraine. Patients frequently sleep for a few hours after an episode is over. When questioned later, patients are generally not able to completely recall the episode. Acute confusional migraine begins in childhood, after the age of 5 years, and may eventually evolve into typical migraine as the patient becomes older. A positive family history of migraine is usually present, and is very useful for making a diagnosis. The differential diagnosis includes a prolonged partial complex seizure, nonconvulsive status epilepticus, drug intoxication, and other etiologies that cause acute encephalopathy. If the diagnosis reamains unclear, a video EEG is helpful in distinguishing this disorder from a seizure. Acute episode is treated with ensuring safety, intravenous hydration, sedation (induce sleep), and control of emesis and pain (if headache is present). The role of tryptans is controversial: the management of acute confusional migraine. Prophylactic antimigraine therapy may be helpful in preventing frequent and prolonged attacks but no class I data are currently available.

Benign Paroxysmal Vertigo

Benign paroxysmal vertigo occurs in children between the ages of 1 and 4 years. It is also considered a precursor of migraine. A positive family history of migraine is often elicited. The attacks occur irregularly and are brief, lasting seconds to minutes. The episode begins suddenly with severe vertigo, and the child instantly spins or falls to the ground. True ataxia is not present, but the vertigo prevents sitting or standing during an episode. Nystagmus or torticollis may be seen, but examination and EEG reveal normal results between episodes. The level of alertness is normal. The diagnosis is usually made on clinical grounds. These attacks are quite frightening to the child. Parental reassurance is important. Treatment usually is not warranted. Medications such as meclizine occasionally have been used for brief periods in children with daily episodes.

Basilar Artery Migraines

Basilar artery migraines may also be confused with seizures. Basilar migraines are related to brainstem and cerebellar dysfunction in the vascular distribution of the basilar artery. Symptoms during an episode may include ataxia, nausea and emesis, dysarthria, hemiparesis, visual disturbances, and impairment of consciousness. Vertigo, tinnitus, and paresthesia are less common symptoms. The attacks last moments to hours and may be followed by severe occipital headaches. Acute treatment involves pain control, sedation, and antiemetic agents. The role of tryptans is still controversial. Prophylactic antimigraine therapy is usually warranted if repeated attacks are documented.

PAROXYSMAL MOVEMENT DISORDERS

A variety of involuntary movements occur in children that may be confused with epileptic seizures. Children with chronic central nervous system disorder may have epileptic seizures in addition to a movement disorder. All older children and adolescents with dystonia, myoclonus, athetosis, or chorea, with or without psychiatric symptoms, must be evaluated for Wilson disease. Wilson disease is a neurodegenative disorder of copper metabolism. If diagnosed and treated early, symptoms may be reversible.

Opsoclonus and Myoclonus Syndrome

Paroxysmal movements in infants and toddlers may be seen in paraneoplastic syndrome of opsoclonus and myoclonus that is *associated with neuroblastoma*. This disorder is also known as Kinsbourne encephalopathy. A previously normal child may also develop encephalopathy of varying severity soon after the onset of opsoclonus and myoclonus. Although the movements are usually persistent, at times they may become less pronounced and appear to be paroxysmal. A consultation for evaluation for neuroblastoma should be performed. Treatment involves aggressive tumor management for those patients with neuroblastoma. The use of high-dose glucocorticosteroids or IVIg can be helpful in some patients.

Jitteriness

Jitteriness is common in neonates and young infants and could be mistaken for clonic seizures. Episodes of jitteriness are characterized by sudden rapid tremulousness involving the whole or part of the body. Episodes are usually provoked by sudden noise or touch or crying. Infants remain alert during the episode. An easy bedside test to differentiate jitteriness from epileptic seizure is by passive flexion of the extremities, which usually results in disappearance of jitteriness (tremulousness) but not clonic jerks. No cause is usually apparent in a jittery infant with no perinatal risk factor and a normal exam. These infants improve over few months with eventual disappearance of jitteriness. However, jitteriness may occur secondary to hypoxic-ischemic insults, metabolic encephalopathies, hypoglycemia, hypocalcemia, drug intoxication or withdrawal, and intracranial hemorrhage. Treatment and prognosis in such infants depends upon the etiology. Seizures may be associated with jitteriness in infants with intracranial pathology.

Paroxysmal Infantile Torticollis

Paroxysmal torticollis usually appears in the first year and may come and go for months, with episodes lasting few minutes to several hours or even a day. The events are repetitive and occur without warning. The child tilts or turns the head to one side and resists attempts to straighten the neck. The child may be uncomfortable or irritable but is fully alert. Nystagmus does not occur in torticollis, as it does in benign paroxysmal vertigo and spasmus nutans. If the child is old enough to walk, a gait imbalance may be noted. The cause of this disorder is not known, but many children have a family history of similar events and migraine headaches. In some children, migraines eventually develop. These attacks may appear similar to the head tilt in Sandifer syndrome. Craniocervical and cervical dislocation should be eliminated, and further evaluation is required if the neurologic examination findings are not normal. If the head tilt is sustained, infantile torticollis is not the correct diagnosis. Treatment is usually not necessary because the problem generally disappears in the first few years of life. Acute treatment of episode with ibuprofen and/or paracetamol may be tried if child is in pain or has other symptoms of migraine.

Tics

Tics are sudden, repetitive, nonpurposeful or semipurposeful movements with a waxing and waning course, usually exacerabated by anxiety and stress. They typically disappear in sleep. Tics may be simple or complex, rhythmic or irregular, and motor or vocal. Common simple tics are facial twitches, head shaking, eye blinking, sniffling, throat clearing, and shoulder shrugging. More complex tics are facial distortions, swaying, touching, restless stereotypic movements, or jumping. Vocal tics are coughing, tongue clicking, and repeating words aloud (sometimes inappropriate words). Children may be able to briefly with hold a tic, but they are not under complete voluntary control.

Tourette syndrome is the most common condition in children in which chronic tics are seen. Many patients with Tourette syndrome have associated learning disabilities, hyperactivity, attention deficits, and compulsive and defiant behaviors. Acute tics, usually in association with other types of involuntary movements, may be seen in conditions such as postinfectious immune-mediated disorder (steptococcus A infection), brain hypoxia, and drug-related side effects. Medical options for the treatment of chronic tics includes clonidine, haloperidol, and pimozide. Use of stimulants such as methylphenidate for the treatment of attention deficit disorder has been reported to exacerbate tics in some children.

Stereotypies

Stereotypies are nonpurposeful, intermittent, and repetitive movements or behaviors usually seen in neurologically impaired children. They are commonly mistaken for seizures. Stereotypies reported in the literature are protean, but these behaviors are usually similar (stereotypic) in a given child. Reported movements include head shaking, head nodding, rocking movements, jumping, tongue thrusting, chewing, hyperventilation, hand shaking, and tonic postures, etc. These are often confused with seizures. The etiology of stereotypies is not known, but in general, these are considered to be self-stimulatory behaviors. No treatment is necessary. Stereotypies usually abate or improve over time. The prognosis is guarded in neurologically impaired children.

Paroxysmal Dyskinesias

Paroxysmal dyskinesias are characterized by repetitive episodes of dystonia or choreoathetosis or both. They may be categorized as familial or nonfamilial, and further categorized as primary or symptomatic. Finally, they are classified according to whether the abnormal movement is triggered by a normal movement (kinesigenic paroxysmal choreoathetosis) or not (nonkinesigenic paroxysmal choreoathetosis).

Kinesigenic paroxysmal dyskinesia usually presents in late childhood with unilateral (70%) or bilateral (30%) dystonic or choreoathetotic movements triggered by a movement or exercise. Alcohol and caffeine may precipitate episodes in some children. Multiple brief attacks may occur daily. The dyskinesias usually last for seconds. Consciousness is not impaired, and no postictal weakness or confusion develops. The child reports discomfort, spasm, a peculiar feeling, and sometimes the inablity to continue the ongoing activity or sport. Kinesiogenic dyskinesia has also been described secondary to hypoxic injury, hypoglycemia, and thyrotoxicosis. The scalp EEG during an episode does not show an epileptic pattern. Patients respond to low doses of anticonvulsants such as carbamazepine. Experience with other antiepileptic medications is not available. The family history may be suggestive of dominant or recessive inheritance.

Nonkinesigenic dyskinesia usually begins in infancy or early childhood. Episodes may be longer in duration and may last up to several minutes. An autosomal-dominant pattern of inheritance is usually noted. Episodes may not require any chronic treatment. Anticonvulsant treatment is generally unsuccesful. Other treatments used in anecdotal reports are benzodiazepines, baclofen, and dopamine-altering drugs.

Shudder Attacks

Shudder attacks are considered a streotypic behavior or movement that resembles shivering with a voluntary component. It is a form of stereotypy that is commonly recognized. The disorder may begin in infants as young as 4 months of age and last for a few years. The child suddenly develops body tremors with adduction of upper extremities and flexion at the elbows. No mental status changes are associated. Episodes last for a few seconds, may occur in a cluster, and usually are precipated by excitement or frustration. A family history of essential tremor is often identified in children with shudder attacks. Episodes may be confused with atypical absence or tonic seizures. No treatment is required or effective.

Spasmus Nutans

Spasmus nutans is a complex movement disorder that consists of the triad of head tilt, head titubation, and nystagmus. It usually begins in first few months of life. The events are intermittent and repetitive, and the child may be irritable but alert. The disorder is benign and self-limiting. In most children, it usually remits spontaneously within 1 or 2 years after onset, but rarely may last as long as 8 years. Minor EEG abnormalities have been reported in children with spasmus nutans but no ictal EEG patterns are recorded during episodes. Spasmus nutans must be diagnosed as a disorder of exclusion since many serious neurologic conditions can mimic spasmus nutans. Investigations are necessary to rule out congenital visual pathway tumors, oculomotor disorders associated with metabolic disorders of energy metabolism, and malformations of the optic apparatus. A careful history, neurologic examination, ophthalmology consultation, and magnetic resonance imaging of the brain are required. No treatment is necesssary in the idiopathic form, as it is a self-limiting condition and causes no impairment in child's development.

Medication Related Movement Disorders

A number of medications can cause movement disorders in children. In the case of a prescribed medication, the movements may come and go as the drug levels rise and fall. When a medication is taken by accident, the movements may appear suddenly, but only within an identified time frame. Theophylline may cause choreiform and dystonic movements. Other common medications known to produce abnormal movements include antiemetics, antihistamines, anticholinergics, tricyclic antidepressants, meperidine, high doses of phenytoin, and neuroleptics.

MISCELLANEOUS EVENTS DURING WAKEFULNESS

Staring Spells

Many parents seek a neurologic opinion when their child is reported to be daydreaming or has repetitive inattentive periods. School professionals are usually the first to point out these spells. Nonepileptic staring spells are confused with absence seizures or complex partial seizures. Staring spells are likely to be nonepileptic when reported by school personnel, they occur in a child with previously diagnosed attention deficit disorder, the description (onset, course, duration, frequency, event recall, interruption of activity) is vague, and when the child can be shaken out of it by a touch or call. The EEG is normal during and between episodes in children with nonepileptic staring spells. Rarely, the presence of coincidental benign focal epileptiform discharges of childhood in a scalp EEG may lead to an incorrect diagnosis of seizure disorder. Treatment requires evaluation for learning difficulities and attention deficit and hyperactivity disorder. Consideration of a sleep disorder should be made, and if the history is suggestive of such, a PSG ordered. Stimulant medications are the first-line treatment for improving attention span.

Benign Myoclonus

Myoclonic movements have been described in awake infants. Sometimes they may resemble infantile spasms (head drops with elevation of arms). Infants are usually healthy, with normal exam and no evidence of neurologic deterioration. The EEG is normal. Myoclonic episodes abate after a few months without treatment.

Stool-Withholding Activity

Children may have sudden interruption of ongoing behavior with motionless posture and lower trunk or hip flexion when experiencing discomfort from withholding stool. The withholding behavior is a way to prevent the painful passage of stool that is large and hard because of chronic constipation. Fecal incontinence may occur during or following an episode. The episodes may be mistaken for tonic seizures. Treatment requires evaluation for constipation and intensive bowel regimen and counseling.

Syncope (Fainting Spells)

Syncope is common in adolescents or older children. A good history is often sufficient to exclude epileptic seizures. Most children describe prodrome of few seconds before fainting. The prodromal symptoms are reported as lightheadedness, dizziness, sounds appearing distant, and blurring of vision. Soon the child may lose awareness for a few seconds. Unsupported falls are uncommon but may occur, leading to injury. A supine position quickly restores cerebral perfusion with recovery to full awareness. A few clonic jerks or incontinence may occur late in syncope, especially when it is prolonged. Syncope may be precipitated or caused by a variety of conditions. Cardiac disorders and rhythm disturbances must be considered in the differential diagnosis. Common precipitating factors for syncope (vasovagal syncope) are minor trauma such as a venipuncture, sudden emotional stress, or hot weather. Orthostatic syncope may follow prolonged standing or sudden change in posture. Several medications may cause orthostatic symptoms. Several measurements of blood pressures in supine and standing posture may help diagnose orthostasis. A tilt table test may be helpful in difficult cases. Reflex syncope may be seen with bouts of coughing, swallowing, defecation, or micturition. In resistant cases without a clear explanation of events, EKG or holtor monitoring and EEG may help to excluded serious conditions.

Masturbation

Infantile masturbation is a self-stimulatory developmental behavior that may be seen in normal infants and toddlers. However, more commonly this behavior is reported in children with developmental delay. Several behaviors may characterize infantile masturbation. Commonly reported episodes in girls include sitting or laying prone with legs held tightly together rubbing against an object or the ground. Sometimes rocking with legs straddling across the bars or a crib or playpen is noted. Episodes may last for several minutes, and the child may resume this behavior intermittently many times a day without any apparent reason. The child remains alert during episodes, and distraction usually aborts the episode. Parents are often embarrassed to learn the diagnosis, but their fears should be allayed by emphasizing the developmental nature of this activity and its gradual resolution over few months to a year. No treatment is warranted.

NONEPILEPTIC (PSYCHOLOGENIC) SEIZURES

In adults, nonepileptic seizures can be encountered as part of the clinical features of a number of psychiatric disorders, including conversion disorder, somatization disorder, factitious disorder with physical symptoms, malingering, and schizophrenia. Nonepileptic seizures may occur in children over the age of 8 years. In children and young adolescents, conversion disorder or somatization disorder is most likely. Less likely are the possibilities of child abuse and Münchhausen syndrome by proxy. When one of this group of diagnoses is suspected, the clinician must approach the patient and family in a gentle and nonjudgmental manner. To convince the patient and family that the diagnosis is accurate, expert advice from a psychologist or psychiatrist familiar with the disorder is needed. Reviewing the video EEG with the family, and demonstrating that the event is not accompanied by any ictal changes, is sometimes helpful. With proper diagnosis and counseling, the outcome—measured by the absence of nonepileptic seizures at 3 years—is much better in children than adults (80% vs. 40%). If the physician can explain the diagnosis as one that is both frequently encountered and treatable, the chance of a successful outcome is improved. Video EEG monitoring may be required to confirm the diagnosis. In some patients, nonepileptic seizures may coexist with epileptic seizures. Common features of nonepileptic seizures that help distinguish them from epileptic seizures are the following:

- Events precipitated by stress
- Gradual onset of events (minutes)
- Prolonged and waxing/waning events
- Arrhythmic/out-of-phase jerking
- Bilateral movements with preserved consciousness
- Lack of postictal confusion
- Shouted obscenities
- Movements not typical of true seizures (e.g., thrashing, pelvic thrusting, rolling, wild movements)

REVIEW EXERCISES

QUESTIONS

1. The role of EEG monitoring (as opposed to simple EEG) is to:
a) Diagnose epilepsy
b) Aid the clinician in distinguishing between seizures, nonepileptic seizures, sleep disorders, and other PNEDs
c) Distinguish between psychiatric illness and epilepsy
d) Distinguish between generalized seizures and partial seizures
e) All of the above

Answer

The answer is e.

2. Breath-holding spells are:

a) Associated with future psychiatric problems

b) Usually self-limited and should be addressed with supportive parental education, although iron therapy may be beneficial

c) Best treated with psychologic counseling

d) Occasionally associated with seizures, in which case anticonvulsant medication is required

e) A figment of the parents' imagination

Answer

The answer is b.

3. Migraine variants in children may include as part of the syndrome:

a. Acute confusional episodes

b. Acute vertigo that causes the child to fall to the ground and cry

c. Loss of ocular function (e.g., pupillary dilation and droopy eyelids)

d. Vomiting to the point of dehydration

e. All of the above

Answer

The answer is e.

4. Which of the following is a true statement concerning breath-holding spells?

a) They are most common in children 2 to 5 years of age.

b) Bradycardia is a common feature of the *cyanotic* type of breath-holding spell.

c) Loss of consciousness may be a feature.

d) Future behavioral problems are common sequelae.

Answer

The answer is c.

SUGGESTED READINGS

1. Alper K. Nonepileptic seizures. *Neurol Clin North Am* 1994;12:153–173.
2. Bickerstaff ER. Basilar artery and the migraine-epilepsy syndrome. *Proc R Soc Lond* 1961;55:167.
3. Brunt ER, van Weerden TW. Familial paroxysmal kinesigenic ataxia and continuous myokymia. *Brain* 1990;113:1361–1382.
4. Cohen BH. Headaches. In: Kliegman R, ed. *Practical strategies in pediatric diagnosis and therapy.* Philadelphia: Saunders, 1996:574–589.
5. Cohen BH. Headache as a symptom of neurologic disease. *Semin Neurol* 1995;2:144–150.
6. Deonna T, Martain D. Benign paroxysmal torticollis in infancy. *Arch Dis Child* 1981;56:956.
7. Donat JF, Wright FS. Episodic symptoms mistaken for seizures in the neurologically impaired child. *Neurology* 1990;40:156–157.
8. Dunn DW, Synder CH. Benign paroxysmal vertigo of childhood. *Am J Dis Child* 1976;130:1099.
9. Ehyai A, Fenichel GM. The natural history of acute confusional migraine. *Arch Neurol* 1978;35:368.
10. Fenichel GM. Migraine as a cause of benign paroxysmal vertigo of childhood. *J Pediatr* 1967;71:114.
11. Golden GS, French JH. Basilar artery migraine in young children. *Pediatrics* 1975;56:722.
12. Gordon N. Migraine, epilepsy, post-traumatic syndromes, and spreading depression. *Dev Med Child Neurol* 1989;31:682.
13. Goodenough DJ, Fariello RG, Annis BL, et al. Familial and acquired paroxysmal dyskinesias. *Arch Neurol* 1978;35:287.
14. Gumnit RJ. Psychogenic seizures. In: Wyllie E, ed. *The treatment of epilepsy: principles and practice.* Philadelphia: Lea & Febiger, 1993:692–696.
15. Kinast M, Erenberg G, Rothner AD. Paroxysmal choreoathetosis: report of five cases and review of the literature. *Pediatrics* 1980;65:74.
16. Kinsbourne M. Hiatus hernia with contortions of the neck. *Lancet* 1964;1:1058–1061.
17. Livingston S. Breath-holding spells in children: differentiation from epileptic attacks. *JAMA* 1970;212:2231.
18. Lombroso C, Lerman P. Breath-holding spells (cyanotic and pallid infantile syncope). *Pediatrics* 1967;39:563.
19. Metrick ME, Ritter FJ, Gates JR, et al. Nonepileptic events in children. *Epilepsia* 1991;32:322–328.
20. Nardocci N, Lamperti E, Rumi V, et al. Typical and atypical forms of paroxysmal choreoathetosis. *Dev Med Child Neurol* 1989;31:670.
21. Pellock JM. The differential diagnosis of epilepsy: nonepileptic paroxysmal disorders in children. In: Wyllie E, Gupta A, Lacchwani D. eds. *The treatment of epilepsy: principles and practice.* Philadelphia: Lippincott Williams & Wilkins, 2004.
22. Praeek N, Fleisher DR, Abell T. Cyclic vomiting syndrome: what a gastroenterologist needs to know. *Am J Gastroenterol* 2007;102:2832–2840.
23. Pranzatelli MR, Albin RL, Cohen BH. Acute dyskinesias in young asthmatics treated with theophylline. *Pediatr Neurol* 1991;7:216–219.
24. Pratt JL, Fleisher GR. Syncope in children and adolescents. *Pediatr Emerg Care* 1989;5:80–82.
25. Rothner AD. The migraine syndrome in children and adolescents. *Pediatr Neurol* 1986;2:121.
26. Saneto RP, Fitch JA, Cohen BH. Acute neurotoxicity of meperidine in an infant. *Pediatr Neurol* 1996;14:339–341.
27. Saneto RP, Fitch JA, Cohen BH. Paroxysmal events in children with mitochondrial cytopathies and epilepsy. *Ann Neurol* 2001;50:3[Suppl 1]:S101–S102.
28. Silbert PL, Gubbay SS. Familial cyanotic breath-holding spells. *J Paediatr Child Health* 1992;28:254–256.
29. So NK, Andermann F. Differential diagnosis. In: Engel J, Pedley TA, eds. *Differential diagnosis in epilepsy: a comprehensive textbook.* Philadelphia: Lippincott-Raven; 1998:791–797.
30. Swaiman WF, Frank Y. Seizure headaches in children. *Dev Med Child Neurol* 1978;20:580.
31. Vannasse M, Bedard P, Andermann F. Shuddering attacks in children: an early clinical manifestation of essential tremor. *Neurology* 1976;26:1027.
32. Vela-Bueno A, Soldatos CR. Episodic sleep disorders (parasomnias). *Semin Neurol* 1987;7:269–276.
33. Weinberg WA, Brumback RA. Primary disorder of vigilance: a novel explanation of inattentiveness, daydreaming, boredom, restlessness, and sleepiness. *J Pediatr* 1990;116:720–725.
34. Wolf DS, Singer HS. Pediatric movement disorder: an update. *Curr Opin Neurol* 2008;24:491–496.
35. Wyllie E, Friedman D, Luders H, et al. Outcome of psychogenic seizures in children and adolescents compared with adults. *Neurology* 1991;41:742–744.

Chapter 35

Neurocutaneous Syndromes

George E. Tiller

The neurocutaneous syndromes or phakomatoses (*phakos, Gr., a lentil, or lentil-shaped spot*) are a group of unrelated disorders characterized by congenital abnormalities of the skin and nervous system. Some are malformations or embryonic dysplasias and are associated with benign or malignant neoplasms. The most common neurocutaneous disorders include neurofibromatosis type 1 (NF1), tuberous sclerosis (TS), albinism, Sturge-Weber syndrome (SWS), and neurofibromatosis type 2 (NF2). Other less commonly encountered neurocutaneous syndromes include Waardenburg syndrome, incontinentia pigmenti, hypomelanosis of Ito, ataxia-telangiectasia, von Hippel-Lindau (vHL) syndrome, and Proteus syndrome.

PATHOPHYSIOLOGY

All the neurocutaneous syndromes mentioned in the preceding text (except for SWS) have a genetic basis. Those that are associated with neoplasms (NF1, NF2, TS, vHL) are caused by mutations in tumor-suppressor genes. Some of these disorders (albinism, TS, Waardenburg syndrome) display genetic heterogeneity, meaning that a single mutation in one of several genes is responsible for the disease in a particular family or individual.

MORE COMMON NEUROCUTANEOUS SYNDROMES

Neurofibromatosis Type 1

- Incidence: 1/3000
- Inheritance: autosomal dominant
- Features: neurofibromas, optic gliomas, *café au lait* spots, axillary and inguinal freckling, Lisch nodules, and osseous lesions

- Primary defect: neurofibromin, a tumor-suppressor gene on chromosome 17

NF1 is the most prevalent neurocutaneous syndrome, occurring once in every 3000 births. The clinical manifestations vary widely, and the condition may not be apparent in infancy. Additional stigmata may appear as the patient ages. The disorder is secondary to a defect in the gene neurofibromin (on chromosome 17). NF1 is inherited in an autosomal-dominant pattern. In approximately half the patients with NF1, a parent is similarly affected. In those with no family history of NF1, it is assumed that the patient's disease is the result of a spontaneous mutation; the disorder is then passed along to the patient's progeny in an autosomal-dominant manner.

A diagnosis of NF1 in children relies on fulfillment of at least two of the following seven clinical criteria:

1. Six or more *café au lait* macules >5 mm in diameter (prepubertal) or >1 cm in diameter (postpubertal) (Fig. 35.1)
2. Two or more neurofibromas of any type, or one plexiform neurofibroma
3. Freckling in the axillary or inguinal region (see Fig. 35.1)
4. Presence of an optic glioma (Fig. 35.2)
5. Two or more Lisch nodules (Fig. 35.3)
6. A distinctive osseous lesion such as sphenoid dysplasia or pseudoarthrosis
7. A first-degree relative diagnosed with NF1 on the basis of the preceding criteria

Café au lait spots are the most common clinical finding in children with NF1 (see Fig. 35.1). They are usually recognized in the first year of life and appear to "increase" in number, size, and darkness with age. The borders are generally smooth, and detection is enhanced by using a Wood's lamp. No correlation has been found between the number of spots and the severity of the disorder. Patients

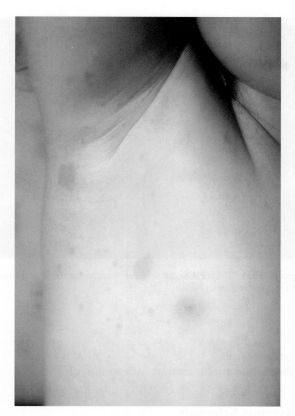

Figure 35.1 *Café au lait* macules and axillary freckling in a patient with neurofibromatosis type 1. (See color insert.)

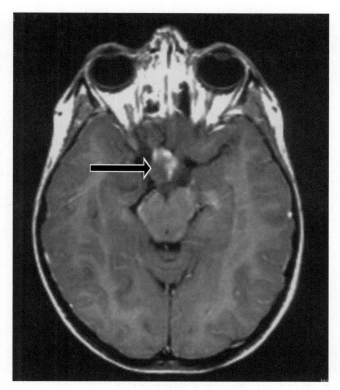

Figure 35.2 Optic glioma in a 9-year-old girl with NF1.

with NF1 may have axillary and inguinal freckling (see Fig. 35.1) and areas of hyperpigmentation over the plexiform neurofibromas.

Neurofibromas may develop on any nerve at any location in the body, externally or internally. Cutaneous neurofibromas are rare in infancy but become more common after puberty. Some patients have very few lesions, whereas others have hundreds of them. Neurofibromas rarely transform into neurofibrosarcomas. Plexiform neurofibromas are larger, soft, spongiform masses that may be congenital, may enlarge, and may cause cosmetic and functional problems.

Lisch nodules are pigmented hamartomas of the iris (see Fig. 35.3) that usually appear after school age. They are not a threat to vision. A slit-lamp examination is necessary to identify them. The incidence of optic nerve gliomas in patients with NF1 is 5% to 10%; they usually resorb over time, but may progress and require close follow-up.

The skeletal manifestations of NF1 include scoliosis, kyphosis, short stature, pseudoarthrosis, and pectus excavatum. Infants should be examined for pseudoarthrosis, and children entering adolescence should be closely observed for kyphoscoliosis.

The neurologic aspects of NF1 may include macrocephaly, hydrocephalus, skull defects, central nervous system (CNS) and peripheral nervous system tumors, mental retardation, learning disabilities, and epilepsy.

Patients with NF1 may also have vascular disorders. Renal artery stenosis with aneurysm formation may cause hypertension and pheochromocytoma, and cerebrovascular lesions may result in hemorrhage and stroke.

If a child is suspected of having NF1, a complete physical examination, including blood pressure measurement, formal funduscopic examination, and an assessment of visual acuity and visual fields, should be undertaken. Cutaneous lesions should be recorded. If cutaneous lesions enlarge rapidly, become painful, or develop in an

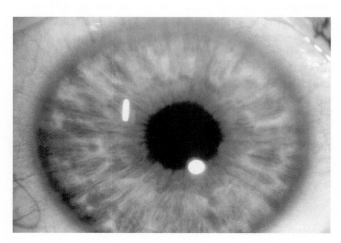

Figure 35.3 Pigmented hamartomas of the iris (Lisch nodules) in a patient with neurofibromatosis type 1. (See color insert.)

area that causes discomfort, such as the foot or waistline, the patient should be referred for removal of the lesions. If diminished visual acuity or a visual field cut is noted, magnetic resonance imaging (MRI) with orbital views performed with and without contrast is indicated. Many children have benign macrocephaly. Patients should be followed up yearly, and they and their parents should be questioned concerning development or change in any of the neurologic symptoms. Because the incidence of learning disabilities in children with NF1 is very high (35%), early intervention should be considered in an effort to identify and remediate any learning difficulties.

Genetic counseling is necessary in all instances. When NF1 is identified in a child, the parents should undergo a cutaneous examination and a slit-lamp examination. If NF1 is recognized in either of them, that parent should be followed up yearly. As the pediatric patient reaches maturity and enters the reproductive years, genetic counseling is again indicated. DNA testing for NF1 is not 100% sensitive, and therefore is not routinely utilized.

Neurofibromatosis Type 2

- Frequency: 1/35,000
- Inheritance: autosomal dominant
- Features: late onset (approximately 22 years), acoustic neuromas (cranial nerve [CN] VIII), schwannomas, gliomas, meningiomas, neurofibromas, cataracts, and few *café au lait* spots
- Complications: hearing loss, tinnitus, and visual loss
- Primary defect: schwannomin (a.k.a. *merlin*) gene on chromosome 22

NF2, initially thought to be the "central" form of NF1, is now recognized as a separate disorder. It is secondary to an abnormality in the schwannomin gene (on chromosome 22). Patients usually present in early to middle adult life with hearing loss, at which time bilateral acoustic neuromas are identified (Fig. 35.4). Their children should undergo a thorough examination, including MRI of the head and spine and auditory evoked potentials. NF2 is more aggressive if presenting in childhood, and most pediatric patients have acoustic neuromas and spinal cord tumors at the initial evaluation. Patients with NF2 must be evaluated and followed up by a geneticist, and they require the lifelong services of neurologists, otologists, and neurosurgeons.

The diagnostic criteria for NF2 (only one criterion is required):

- *Bilateral* CN VIII mass on MRI with gadolinium
- Positive family history (parent, child, or sibling)

and either *unilateral* CN VIII mass *or* one of the following:

- Neurofibroma
- Meningioma
- Glioma

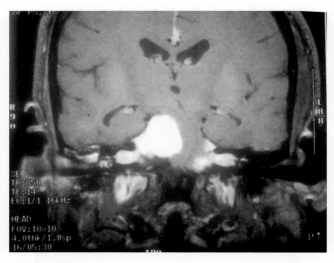

Figure 35.4 Bilateral acoustic neuromas (enhanced by gadolinium) in a patient with NF2.

- Schwannoma
- Posterior capsular cataract (at young age)

Tuberous Sclerosis

- Frequency: 1/25,000
- Inheritance: autosomal dominant
- Features: ash leaf spots, shagreen patches, *café au lait* spots, adenoma sebaceum, subungual fibromas; epilepsy, mental retardation, intracranial calcifications; cardiac rhabdomyoma; renal anomalies
- Primary defect: tuberin (chromosome 16), or hamartin (chromosome 9) mutations

TS is an autosomal-dominant condition that occurs in 1 in 25,000 live births; however, the spontaneous mutation rate is 60% to 70%. The disorder is caused by an abnormality in either the hamartin gene (on chromosome 9) or the tuberin gene (on chromosome 16). Characteristic manifestations include skin abnormalities, epilepsy, and mental retardation. Roach and Sparagana (2004) suggested that the features of this disorder can be classified as major or minor. The *major* features include:

- Facial angiofibromas or forehead plaques
- Nontraumatic ungual or periungual fibroma
- Hypomelanotic macules (more than three)
- Shagreen patch (connective tissue nevus)
- Multiple retinal nodular hamartomas
- Cortical tuber
- Subependymal nodule
- Subependymal giant cell astrocytoma
- Cardiac rhabdomyoma, single or multiple
- Lymphangiomyomatosis
- Renal angiomyolipoma

The *minor* features include:

- Multiple pits in dental enamel
- Hamartomatous rectal polyps
- Bone cysts
- Radial migration lines in cerebral white matter
- Gingival fibromas
- Nonrenal hamartomas
- Retinal achromic patch
- *Confetti* skin lesions
- Multiple renal cysts

The definitive diagnosis is based on the presence of either two major features or one major and two minor features. TS is "probable" in the presence of one major and one minor criteria.

The cutaneous manifestations of TS include hypopigmented macules or ash leaf spots (Fig. 35.5), adenoma sebaceum (fibrous lesions appearing in a butterfly distribution across the bridge of the nose and cheeks just before adolescence) (Fig. 35.6), subungual or periungual fibromas, and shagreen patches. Approximately 25% of patients with TS have a few *café au lait* spots. The earliest cutaneous manifestation is the hypopigmented macule or ash leaf spot, which can be seen in the newborn. It is easier to visualize when a Wood's ultraviolet lamp is used.

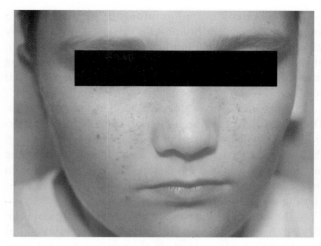

Figure 35.6 Characteristic appearance of adenoma sebaceum in a patient with tuberous sclerosis. (See color insert.)

Retinal hamartomas are difficult to visualize unless a dilated funduscopic examination is performed. These may be either opalescent plaques or calcified nodular plaques. They usually do not interfere with vision and do not change in size throughout life.

The CNS manifestations of TS include cortical hamartomas and subependymal nodules. The former are cortical, and the latter are most frequent along the ependymal surfaces of the ventricles (Fig. 35.7).

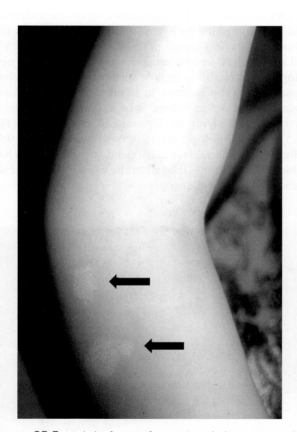

Figure 35.5 Ash leaf spot (forearm) and shagreen patches *(arrows)* in a patient with tuberous sclerosis. The appearance of ash leaf spots is enhanced by the ultraviolet light of the Wood's lamp. (See color insert.)

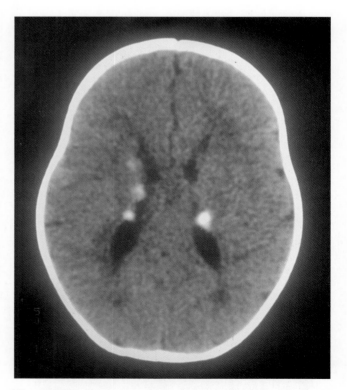

Figure 35.7 Computed tomogram from a patient with tuberous sclerosis, illustrating nodules (tubers) in the subependymal areas of the ventricles.

The most debilitating symptoms in patients with TS are seizures, especially *infantile spasms*. Approximately 25% of patients with infantile spasms have TS. However, any and all types of seizures may develop, including myoclonic, partial, complex partial, and generalized seizures.

Patients with TS may also have cardiac rhabdomyomas. These may be detected in utero or during the neonatal period. They tend to regress as the patient becomes older. Patients with TS may also have renal disorders, including angiomyolipomas and renal cysts. These lesions are often progressive and require periodic follow-up. Renal cell carcinoma may develop rarely.

In the asymptomatic patient with TS, no treatment is indicated. If developmental difficulties arise, special education should be instituted. If the patient has seizures, antiepileptic medication should be initiated. If the patient has symptoms of increased intracranial pressure, MRI is indicated. For all patients, genetic counseling should be sought, both at the time of diagnosis and later as they enter their reproductive years. As with all neurocutaneous syndromes, yearly surveillance is suggested.

Sturge-Weber Syndrome

- Frequency: uncommon
- Inheritance: sporadic

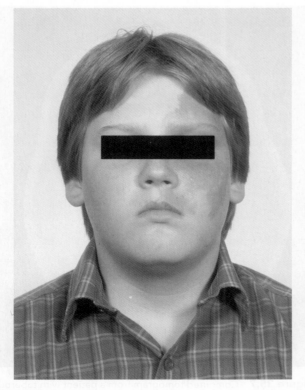

Figure 35.8 A port wine nevus, the most obvious manifestation of Sturge-Weber syndrome. (See color insert.)

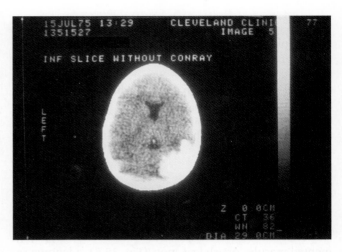

Figure 35.9 Computed tomogram from a patient with Sturge-Weber syndrome, illustrating a leptomeningeal angioma.

- Features: port wine stain CN V1 distribution (100%); seizures (75%); glaucoma (60%); port wine stain on extremities (50%); developmental delay (60%); leptomeningeal angiomas, and intracerebral calcifications
- Primary defect: unknown
- Note: 75% seizures <1 year; 60% glaucoma <1 year

SWS is a congenital malformation syndrome characterized by a facial port wine nevus (stain) (Fig. 35.8) in the distribution of the first branch of the trigeminal nerve (CN V1) and an ipsilateral leptomeningeal angioma. Associated neurologic manifestations include seizures, hemiparesis, and mental retardation. Seizures, in addition to hemiparesis and visual field cut, are considered to be secondary to changes in the cortex underlying the leptomeningeal angioma (Fig. 35.9). Ophthalmologic manifestations include visual field defects, glaucoma, and retinal detachment. SWS is not a heritable disorder, but is thought to be caused by a focal somatic event during embryogenesis.

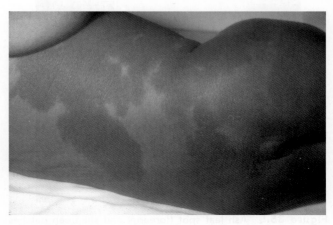

Figure 35.10 Torso of an infant with Klippel-Trenaunay-Weber syndrome. (See color insert.) Note incidental Mongolian spot over buttocks.

LESS COMMON NEUROCUTANEOUS SYNDROMES

Klippel-Trenaunay-Weber Syndrome

- Frequency: uncommon
- Inheritance: sporadic
- Features: port wine stain (sparing the face) (Fig. 35.10), hemangiomas, varicose veins, hemihypertrophy, normal intellect
- Complications: arteriovenous (AV) fistulae, congestive heart failure (CHF), cellulitis, and thrombocytopenia

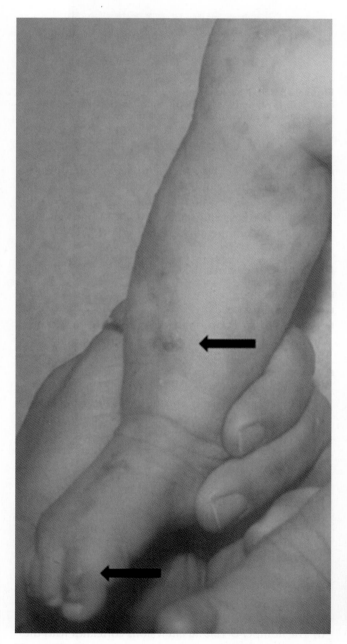

Figure 35.11 Vesicular *(arrows)* and verrucous (warty) lesions of stages 1 and 2 incontinentia pigmenti. (See color insert.)

- Primary defect: unknown; thought to be caused by a focal somatic event during embryogenesis.

Incontinentia Pigmenti

- Frequency: rare
- Inheritance: X-linked dominant (lethal in males)
- Features: skin changes such as (a) vesicular (Fig. 35.11), (b) papular, (c) hyperpigmentation (Fig. 35.12), (d) atrophy; alopecia; retinal abnormalities; nail/tooth anomalies; mental retardation
- Primary defect: κ beta-essential modulator (NEMO), a nuclear factor
- Note: swirled cutaneous pattern may be secondary to mosaicism or Lyonization

Hypomelanosis of Ito

- Incidence: 1/10,000
- Inheritance: sporadic
- Features: hypopigmented whorls, streaks, and patches; dental anomalies; colobomas, cataracts, limb anomalies, mental retardation, seizures, and neuronal migration anomalies
- Notes: a nonspecific marker for chromosomal mosaicism? genetically heterogeneous

Albinism

- Incidence: 1/20,000
- Inheritance: autosomal recessive (AR); X-linked recessive (XLR)

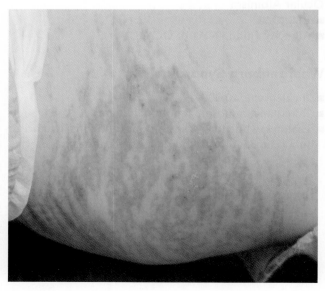

Figure 35.12 *Marble cake* swirled hyperpigmentation of stage 3 incontinentia pigmenti. (See color insert.)

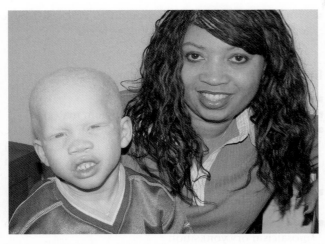

Figure 35.13 Four-year-old African-American boy (and his unaffected mother) with oculocutaneous albinism. (See color insert.)

- Features: decreased pigmentation of skin, hair, iris, and retina (Fig. 35.13); nystagmus; foveal hypoplasia; increased decussation of optic fibers
- Complications: decreased visual acuity, hearing loss, skin cancer
- Primary defects: genetically heterogeneous

Classification of Albinism
Oculocutaneous Albinism
- Tyrosinase negative: oculocutaneous albinism (OCA) 1A
- Tyrosinase deficient
  - OCA1B (yellow)
  - OCA1MP (minimal pigment)
  - OCA1TS (temperature-sensitive)
- Tyrosinase positive: OCA2

Ocular Albinism
- XLR: OA1
- AR: OA2 (mild OCA1 or OCA2?)

Waardenburg Syndrome
- Incidence: 1/40,000
- Inheritance: autosomal dominant, rare AR
- Features: white forelock, albinotic fundi, iris heterochromia (Fig. 35.14), leukoderma, cochlear deafness

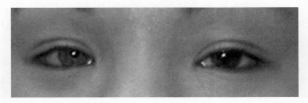

Figure 35.14 Iris heterochromia in an adult with Waardenburg syndrome. (See color insert.)

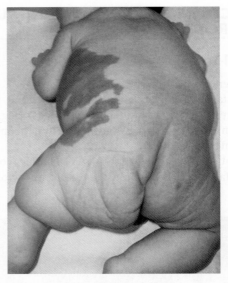

Figure 35.15 Newborn with Proteus syndrome. Note proximal limb girth asymmetry, asymmetric buttocks because of lymphangioma, and extensive truncal hemangioma. (See color insert.)

- Occasional: hypertelorism, cleft palate, neural tube defects, Hirschsprung disease
  - Primary defects: paired box gene 3 (PAX3), microphthalmia transcription factor (MITF), endothelin 3 (EDN3), endothelin-B receptor (EDNRB)

Proteus Syndrome
- Incidence: rare
- Inheritance: sporadic
- Features: disproportionate overgrowth of limbs, skull, and/or internal organs; lipomas; hemangiomas; lymphangiomas (Fig. 35.15)
- Occasional: CNS anomalies; developmental delay
  - Primary defect: some cases with PTEN mutations (allelic with Bannayan and Cowden syndromes); genetically heterogeneous vs. somatic origin of mutations?

REVIEW EXERCISES

QUESTIONS

1. Which of the following is a *true* statement regarding NF1?
a) It results from a congenital malformation.
b) It is inherited in an autosomal-dominant manner.
c) Lisch nodules are commonly present at birth.
d) The number of *café au lait* lesions correlates with the degree of involvement.

Answer

The answer is b. NF1 is an inherited disorder, not a congenital malformation. The disorder is secondary to a defect in the neurofibromin gene (on chromosome 17) and is inherited in an autosomal-dominant manner. Lisch nodules, which are pigmented hamartomas of the iris, are not present at birth, but become more frequent at school age. The number of *café au lait* lesions does not correlate with the severity of the disease process.

2. Which of the following is *not* a diagnostic criterion for NF1?

a) Axillary freckling

b) Two or more neurofibromas

c) Two or more *café au lait* macules more than 5 mm in diameter

d) A first-degree relative with NF1

Answer

The answer is c. The presence of axillary (and/or inguinal) freckling, presence of two or more neurofibromas, and a first-degree relative with NF1 are diagnostic criteria for NF1 in children. The presence of six *or more* café au lait macules is also a criterion.

3. Which of the following is a *true* statement concerning TS?

a) Infantile spasms are commonly seen in patients with TS.

b) The mode of inheritance of TS is AR.

c) Hypopigmented macules develop during adolescence.

d) The presence of seizures early in life is not a predictor of mental retardation.

Answer

The answer is a. Infantile spasms, frequently occurring in infants 4 to 12 months of age, are common in patients with TS. Approximately 25% of children with infantile spasms have TS, although their presence is not a diagnostic criterion. Patients with TS who have seizures, which are difficult to control, early in life are more likely to be mentally retarded. Hypopigmented macules are the earliest cutaneous manifestations of TS. Adenoma sebaceum commonly appears just before adolescence. Like that of NF1, the mode of inheritance of TS is autosomal dominant.

4. Which of the following is a *true* statement concerning SWS?

a) The port wine stain associated with this syndrome is commonly bilateral.

b) Ophthalmic and CNS manifestations always accompany the nevus.

c) Seizures are a common complication of the syndrome.

d) A chromosomal abnormality has been proved for this syndrome.

Answer

The answer is c. SWS results from a congenital malformation. Seizures are commonly associated with this syndrome and can be very difficult to control. The most characteristic feature is the port wine stain, which is characteristically located on the upper eyelid and forehead, and cheek. It is very rarely bilateral. The vascular marking may be present with or without ophthalmic or CNS abnormalities.

SUGGESTED READINGS

1. American Academy of Pediatrics www.aap.org/healthtopics/genetics.cfm. Under the "AAP Policy" heading, see *Health supervision of children with neurofibromatosis*, updated 2008.
2. Baser ME, R Evans DG, Gutmann DH. Neurofibromatosis 2. *Curr Opin Neurol* 2003;16:27–33.
3. Evans DG, Baser ME, et al. Management of the patient and family with neurofibromatosis 2: a consensus conference statement. *Br J Neurosurg* 2005;19:5–12.
4. Farrell CJ, Plotkin SR. Genetic causes of brain tumors: neurofibromatosis, tuberous sclerosis, von Hippel-Lindau, and other syndromes. *Neurol Clin* 2007;25(4):925–946, viii.
5. GeneReviews at GeneTests: Medical Genetics Information Resource. Seattle: University of Washington, 1993–2009. Available at www.genetests.org.
6. Jones KL. *Smith's recognizable patterns of human malformation*, 6th ed. Philadelphia: Elsevier-Saunders, 2005.
7. National Center for Biotechnology Information (NCBI). Genes and disease. Available at www.ncbi.nlm.nih.gov/books/bv.fcgi?rid=gnd&ref.
8. Nowak CB. The phakomatoses: dermatologic clues to neurologic anomalies. *Semin Pediatr Neurol* 2007;14(3):140–149.
9. Online Mendelian Inheritance in Man, OMIM (TM). Baltimore: McKusick-Nathans Institute for Genetic Medicine, Johns Hopkins University, and Bethesda, MD: National Center for Biotechnology Information, National Library of Medicine 2009. Available at http://www.ncbi.nlm.nih.gov/sites/entrez?db=omim.
10. Roach ES, Sparagana SP. Diagnosis of tuberous sclerosis complex. *J Child Neurol* 2004;19:643–649.
11. Tonsgard JH. Clinical manifestations and management of neurofibromatosis type 1. *Semin Pediatr Neurol* 2006; 3:2–7.

Chapter 36

Neuromuscular Disorders: Muscular Dystrophies and Congenital Myopathies

Neil R. Friedman

Childhood myopathies are a heterogeneous group of disorders primarily affecting skeletal muscles. They must be differentiated from primary neuropathic processes affecting other elements of the motor unit (anterior horn cell or peripheral nerve). Both typically present with weakness, but a number of distinguishing features may be identified (Table 36.1).

CLASSIFICATION

The childhood myopathies can be broadly classified into six major groups. The myasthenic syndromes, which involve disorders of the neuromuscular junction, are included in this classification scheme because their presentation is often similar to that of myopathies and they are frequently considered in the differential diagnosis:

- Muscular dystrophies
- Congenital myopathies
- Inflammatory myopathies
- Metabolic myopathies
- Channelopathies
- Myasthenic syndromes

This chapter deals with the two most common groups of pediatric neuromuscular diseases, muscular dystrophies and congenital myopathies.

MUSCULAR DYSTROPHIES

Muscular dystrophies are a group of genetically determined primary degenerative myopathies. Their distinguishing feature is the muscle pathology that shows dystrophic changes; these include variation in muscle fiber size, increased number of internal nuclei, increased amount of fat and connective tissue, and evidence of degeneration/regeneration (e.g., whorled fibers, split fibers, small and angulated fibers). The pattern of genetic inheritance and, more recently, the identification of specific proteins associated with the cytoskeletal framework have improved our understanding of the pathophysiology of these disorders and have made possible a better and more precise classification of the muscular dystrophies as a whole. The major proteins associated with this framework (Fig. 36.1) include dystrophin (a subsarcolemmal protein discovered in the late 1980s), dystrophin-associated glycoproteins (α-, β-, γ-, and δ-sarcoglycans and the dystroglycan complex), and merosin/laminin 2 (extracellular matrix protein). An absence or reduced amount of these proteins is associated with a number of different muscular dystrophies. A fifth sarcoglycan (ϵ-sarcoglycan) has been mapped to chromosome 7q21 and appears homologous to α-sarcoglycan. More recently, mutations in this gene has been associated with myoclonus-dystonia syndrome, but affected individuals have no signs or symptoms of muscle disease.

TABLE 36.1

DIFFERENTIATING A MYOPATHY FROM A NEUROPATHY

	Myopathy	Neuropathy
Weakness	Usually proximal > distal (e.g., iliopsoas, deltoid); with chronicity, distal musculature becomes involved	Tends to be distal predominantly, although some notable exceptions (e.g., SMA in anterior horn cell disease, congenital hypomyelinating neuropathy)
Reflexes	Present or minimally diminished early on; with chronicity, become reduced/absent	Absent or markedly diminished
Muscle bulk	Either disuse atrophy *without* fasciculations or pseudohypertrophy from fatty replacement of muscle	Atrophy associated *with* fasciculations
EMG/NCV	EMG is myopathic (i.e., decreased amplitude and duration, polyphasic motor unit potentials with increased recruitment). NCV normal	EMG is neuropathic (i.e., increased amplitude and duration, polyphasic motor unit potentials with fibrillations, fasciculations, or sharp waves). NCV reduced/slowed (demyelinating > axonal)
Sensory involvement	Absent	Usually present
Creatine kinase	Variable: normal, mildly, or markedly elevated	Usually normal or only mildly elevated

EMG, electromyography; NCV, nerve conduction velocity; SMA, spinal muscular atrophy.

Muscular dystrophies can be classified according to their mode of inheritance. An incomplete list of the more common muscular dystrophies appears in Table 36.2.

X-Linked Dystrophies

Duchenne Muscular Dystrophy and Becker Muscular Dystrophy

Duchenne muscular dystrophy (DMD) and Becker muscular dystrophy (BMD) are the prototype muscular dystrophies affecting 1 in 3500 and 1 in 30,000 liveborn male infants, respectively. They are also known as the Xp21 dystrophies because of the locus of the involved gene. The defective gene product is dystrophin (see Fig. 36.1). In DMD, dystrophin is essentially absent and its absence is associated with a severe phenotype; in BMD, the gene deletion or point mutation results in a reduction in the amount of dystrophin, or in the formation of a truncated protein, and a milder phenotype. Because the inheritance is X-linked–recessive, males are affected and

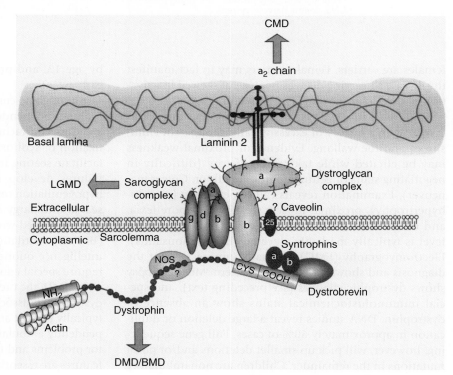

Figure 36.1 Diagrammatic association of the dystrophin-associated protein complex. BMD, Becker muscular dystrophy; CMD, congenital muscular dystrophy; CYS, cysteine; DMD, Duchenne muscular dystrophy; LGMD, limb-girdle muscular dystrophy; NOS, nitric oxide synthetase. (From Bonnemann CG, McNally EM, Kunkel LM. Beyond dystrophin: current progress in the muscular dystrophies. *Curr Opin Pediatr* 1996;8:569–582, with permission.)

TABLE 36.2

CLASSIFICATION OF MUSCULAR DYSTROPHIES

X-linked–recessive	Duchenne muscular dystrophy (dystrophin) (Xp21)
	Becker muscular dystrophy (dystrophin) (Xp21)
	Emery-Dreifuss muscular dystrophy (emerin) (Xq28)
Autosomal dominant	Limb-girdle muscular dystrophy (LGMD) (type 1)
	LGMD 1A (5q31)
	LGMD 1B (1q11-21)
	LGMD 1C (6q23)
	LGMD 1D (caveolin) (3p25)
	LGMD 1E (7q)
	Emery-Dreifuss muscular dystrophy (Lamin A/C) (1q21.3)
	Myotonic dystrophy (19q13)
	Facioscapulohumeral muscular dystrophy (4q35)
	Oculopharyngeal muscular dystrophy (14q11.2-q13)
	Bethlem myopathy (21q22.3 and 2q37)
Autosomal recessive	Congenital muscular dystrophy (CMD)
	Classic or *pure* CMD *(without* CNS involvement)
	Merosin-positive
	Merosin-negative (6q2)
	CMD *with* CNS involvement
	Fukuyama CMD (fukutin) (9q31-q33)
	Walker-Warburg syndrome (9q34)
	Muscle-eye-brain disease (1p3)
	Limb-girdle muscular dystrophy (type 2)
	LGMD 2A (calpain) (15q15)
	LGMD 2B (dysferlin) (2p13)
	LGMD 2C (γ-sarcoglycan) (13q12)
	LGMD 2D (α-sarcoglycan) (17q21)
	LGMD 2E (β-sarcoglycan) (4q12)
	LGMD 2F (δ-sarcoglycan) (5q33-34)
	LGMD 2G (telethonin) (17q11-12)
	LGMD 2H (e3-ubiquitin ligase) (9q31-34)
	LGMD 2I (fukutin related protein) (19q13)
	LGMD 2J (titin) (2q31)

Gene loci and gene products are within parentheses.
CNS, central nervous system.

females are carriers. Female carriers may in fact manifest the disease to varying degrees because of skewed inactivation of the X chromosome (Lyon hypothesis).

Children with DMD typically present after the age of 2 years with a history of excessive falling, apparent clumsiness, and toe walking. Evidence of proximal weakness may be elicited while taking the history (difficulty in negotiating stairs or getting up from the floor, Gower maneuver). Examination reveals calf hypertrophy (pseudohypertrophy), proximal muscle weakness, hyporeflexia, and the presence of a Gower sign. The creatine kinase level is typically markedly elevated (in the thousands). Electromyography (EMG) is usually unnecessary for the diagnosis and shows a myopathic pattern. Muscle biopsy shows dystrophic changes (see preceding text), and special immunohistochemical stains show an absence of dystrophin. DNA studies reveal a large deletion or duplication in approximately 60% of cases. Full gene sequencing, however, will pick up smaller deletions and/or point mutations in the remainder. Children are nonambulatory by age 13, and premature death typically occurs in the early twenties.

Although no cure is available, treatment is aimed at prolonging independent ambulation (orthoses or steroids), avoiding contractures, and providing early surgical stabilization of scoliosis to preserve respiratory function and facilitate seating in a wheelchair. Cardiac and respiratory failures develop during the teenage years. Nocturnal hypoventilation resulting in early morning headache, nausea, and lethargy secondary to hypercarbia can be effectively managed with nasal bilevel positive airway pressure (Bi-PAP) ventilation. Children with DMD often have an intelligence quotient that is lower than normal and may require special educational services.

In BMD, the preservation of a reduced or altered form of dystrophin is associated with a milder phenotype. Children typically present at a slightly later age and are usually independently ambulant beyond their 16th birthday. The motor problems and the clinical, biochemical, and pathologic features are essentially the same as in DMD. Staining of the muscle for dystrophin, however, shows some preservation of the protein, and gene deletion studies, when results are positive, may be able to predict the phenotype. If the mutation is associated with preservation of the *reading frame* sequence, BMD is typically predicted (with a few exceptions), whereas if the mutation involves the promoter region or disrupts the translational reading frame *(out of frame)*, a Duchenne phenotype is typical. In BMD, prolonged ambulation with orthoses may be possible, and life expectancy is longer. However, cardiomyopathy often develops earlier, and must be closely monitored.

Female siblings and mothers of affected children should be screened by determining the creatine kinase level to look for possible carrier status. However, if a deletion is found in the index case, this is a more sensitive and specific marker for screening family members. Approximately two thirds of mothers of children with DMD or BMD carry the deletion. The reasons why not all mothers carry the deletion or point mutation are the high frequency of spontaneous mutation of the gene (1 in 10,000 gametes) because of its large size (2.5 million base pairs, or approximately 1% of the X chromosome) and germline mosaicism. The presence of a deletion allows for prenatal diagnosis.

Emery-Dreifuss Muscular Dystrophy

Emery-Dreifuss muscular dystrophy (EDMD) is characterized by a triad of:

- Early contractures of the elbows and Achilles tendons
- A slowly progressive myopathy (humeroperoneal distribution)
- Cardiac involvement, including conduction block (atrial paralysis), which may result in sudden death, and ultimately cardiomyopathy.

It is inherited in either an X-linked–recessive manner, or autosomal dominant pattern (AD-EDMD). Rare autosomal-recessive forms have been described. The creatine kinase level may be mild to moderately elevated, and muscle biopsy shows nonspecific dystrophic changes. X-linked EDMD is caused by a mutation of the emerin gene at the Xq28 locus. Emerin is a nuclear membrane–associated protein, and the exact mechanism by which it causes muscular dystrophy is unknown. In contrast to the weakness of DMD/BMD, the weakness in EDMD is slowly progressive, and long-term survival often depends on the severity of cardiac involvement. The autosomal-dominant form of EDMD involves another nuclear membrane protein, lamin A/C encoded by the *LMNA* gene mapped to chromosome 1q21.3. The clinical phenotype is the same as in the X-linked–recessive forms of EDMD; however, cardiomyopathy may occur earlier and in the absence of a conduction defect. Certain mutations of the *LMNA* gene may result in *pure* or isolated cardiac involvement (so-called dilated cardiomyopathy 1A), with little or no skeletal muscle involvement, whereas others result in a limb-girdle phenotype (LGMD 1B), Charcot-Marie-Tooth phenotype or lipodystrophy.

Autosomal-Dominant Dystrophies

Myotonic Dystrophy

The clinical hallmark of myotonic dystrophy is myotonia (i.e., sustained muscle contraction). This is a multisystem disease with variable clinical expression. The congenital form presents during the newborn period with severe hypotonia, marked weakness (including facial diplegia), feeding difficulties, and respiratory failure. Myotonic dystrophy is an autosomal-dominant disorder of maternal transmission, and examination of the mother usually establishes the diagnosis (facial diplegia, percussion myotonia). Muscle biopsy may show little in terms of dystrophic change.

Myotonic dystrophy is part of a new group of genetic disorders known as *trinucleotide repeat disorders.* It is caused by an abnormal CTG triplet repeat expansion on chromosome 19 that encodes a protein kinase. The length of expansion of the trinucleotide predicts the severity of disease. Healthy individuals have five to 37 repeats. Mildly affected individuals have >50, and those with the severe congenital form have >2000 repeats. The inheritance is autosomal dominant and associated with the phenomenon of genetic anticipation (i.e., subsequent generations exhibit further increases in the number of trinucleotide repeats and more severe clinical expression). The mechanism by which the triplet repeat gives rise to myotonic dystrophy is unknown.

Unlike the weakness of most myopathies, that of myotonic dystrophy is relatively distal, affecting the hands and forearms especially. It is usually slowly progressive, but in the mildest forms, very little weakness may be noted. The patient typically exhibits ptosis, facial diplegia, and an inability to bury the eyelashes fully. The face tends to be slightly elongated, and the lower jaw is often slightly open because of weakness of the masseter muscle. Percussion myotonia of the tongue or thenar eminence may be elicited. Involvement of the diaphragm may result in respiratory weakness. The onset of the noncongenital form is during adolescence or adulthood. Nonmuscular involvement includes cataracts, frontal balding, testicular atrophy, diabetes, and heart disease (cardiomyopathy, conduction defects). EMG shows evidence of myotonia. DNA testing confirms the CTG expansion. Muscle biopsy is usually not necessary and tends to show dystrophic changes. Treatment is symptomatic: phenytoin, carbamazepine, or mexiletine for the myotonia, braces for the foot drop, and treatment of cardiac arrhythmias if they occur. Daytime somnolence (centrally mediated secondary to involvement of the reticular activating system) may occur and is often responsive to methylphenidate. Intellectual deficits are common. Depolarizing muscle relaxants should be avoided. The prognosis depends on the severity of the associated respiratory and cardiac problems.

Facioscapulohumeral Muscular Dystrophy

Facioscapulohumeral muscular dystrophy affects primarily the muscles of the face and shoulder girdle, with scapular winging being noted. The peroneal muscles may also be involved. This is an autosomal-dominant disorder, although sporadic cases occur. The gene, which has been mapped to chromosome 4q35, and its product remain unknown. The clinical (including intrafamilial) expression is variable; mild cases show only facial weakness, whereas more severe cases (approximately 20%) have significant generalized weakness that may result in loss of ambulation. The onset varies from early childhood to adulthood. The weakness tends to be slowly progressive. Sensorineural hearing loss and retinal telangiectasia may develop. The creatine kinase level is normal or mildly elevated. No specific treatment is available, although prednisone, creatine, and more recently albuterol have been tried.

Oculopharyngeal Muscular Dystrophy

Oculopharyngeal muscular dystrophy is a rare disorder in which the onset varies from adolescence to adulthood. The eye involvement includes ptosis and ophthalmoplegia. The pharyngeal involvement results in dysphagia. Facial weakness may occur. The presentation may be similar to that of myasthenia gravis, which should be excluded by an edrophonium (Tensilon) test. The gene locus has been mapped to 14q11-13 and encodes the protein PABP2 (poly(A) binding protein 2).

Bethlem Myopathy

In Bethlem myopathy (BM), muscle weakness involves the proximal muscle groups and is slowly progressive. The face is spared. It is allelic to Ullrich congenital muscular dystrophy (UCMD)—an autosomal recessive entity. In addition to the weakness, atrophy and early multiple joint contractures occur (long finger flexors, elbows, and ankles). Respiratory involvement is uncommon. Intelligence is normal. The onset is usually in the first two decades of life, but adult onset may occur. Life expectancy is not affected. Both intrafamilial and interfamilial variations in clinical expression have been noted. Creatine kinase may be normal or mildly elevated. BM and UCMD are due to mutations in the collagen VI gene (COL6A1, COL6A2, and COL6A3 subunits), which encodes the extracellular matrix component of collagen VI.

Autosomal-Recessive Dystrophies

Congenital Muscular Dystrophies

This group of autosomal-recessive conditions is subdivided into two major types (Table 36.3):

- Syndromic congenital muscular dystrophy (CMD *with* marked central nervous system (CNS) involvement)
- Nonsyndromic congenital muscular dystrophy (typically *without* significant CNS involvement—includes merosin negative and positive forms).

Defining features include weakness, which may be manifested as severe hypotonia during the neonatal period (floppy infant syndrome) or as delayed motor milestones with proximal weakness during infancy and early childhood. Muscle biopsy findings are variable, but specimens may show marked dystrophic changes with prominent fatty tissue replacement or mild myopathic features. The EMG pattern is myopathic, and the creatine kinase levels may be normal or moderately elevated. An associated arthrogryposis (fixed flexion deformities of the extremities) with hip dislocation is often present at birth. In cases with an early onset, respiratory failure and feeding difficulties may occur. The weakness may be static or slowly progressive, but function may vary in the classic form. More than nine genes have been identified to date.

The classic, *pure* or occidental form of CMD may be further divided into merosin-positive and -negative types depending on the presence or absence of the laminin 2 chain (see Fig. 36.1) known as *merosin*. Although clinical evidence of CNS dysfunction is usually lacking, white matter changes may be present on brain magnetic resonance imaging (MRI). More recently, children with cortical dysplasias have been described in the merosin-negative group. Additionally, merosin-negative children tend to be more severely affected clinically and are less likely to achieve independent ambulation than merosin-positive children. The merosin-negative *CMD* gene has been mapped to chromosome 6q2 and encodes LAMA2 (laminin α_2 chain of merosin).

TABLE 36.3
CLASSIFICATION OF THE CONGENITAL MUSCULAR DYSTROPHIES

Name	Brain Involvement	Gene Symbol	Location	Protein
Merosin deficient	White matter hypodensity	LAMA2	6q	Laminin-alpha2
Fukuyama	Mental retardation and structural changes	FKTN	9q	Fukutin
Muscle-eye-brain disease	MR and structural changes	POMGnT1 (FKRP)	1p	POMGnT1
Walker-Warburg syndrome	Structural changes	POMT1	9q	POMT1
MDC1C	Variable	FKRP	19	FKRP
MDC1D	MR and structural changes	LARGE	22q	LARGE
RSMD1	None	SEPN1	1p	Selenoprotein-1
Integrin at deficiency	None	ITGA7	12q	Integrin alpha 7
Ullrich disease	None	COL6A1, A2, A3	2 and 21q	Collagen VI

Of the merosin-negative forms of CMD, the most common is probably Ullrich congenital muscular dystrophy (UCMD). It forms part of a spectrum with Bethlem myopathy (see the preceding). It tends to be more severe than Bethlem myopathy, and is characterized by early-onset weakness at birth, hypotonia, proximal joint contractures, and striking hyperlaxity of the hands. Other features include prominent calcanei and early and severe respiratory involvement. Although some children do acquire the ability to ambulate independently, with time and disease progression, many children lose this ability, whereas many children never acquire the ability to walk. Scoliosis may occur. UCMD results from mutations in the collagen VI gene (*COL6A1*, *COL6A2*, and *COL6A3* subunits), which encodes the extracellular matrix component of collagen VI.

In children with CMD *plus* CNS involvement, the so-called "syndromic" CMD, the prognosis is significantly worse, with more severe motoric delay, mental retardation, multiorgan involvement, and often early demise. The prototype is Fukuyama CMD, which is highly prevalent in Japan and is associated with cortical migrational defects, seizures, severe developmental delay, marked motor delay, and early death. The gene has been mapped to chromosome 9q31-33 and encodes the protein fukutin. In the Walker-Warburg syndrome (chromosome 9q34), the cortical dysgenesis is typically more severe; lissencephaly (type II) or Dandy-Walker malformation with hydrocephalus is frequently seen. Ocular anomalies of varying types occur. The biochemical defect in this group of disorders is caused by disruption of alpha dystroglycan—either because of errors in glycosylation (Fukuyama CMD) or O-mannosylation (Walker-Warburg syndrome and muscle-eye-brain disease).

Limb-Girdle Muscular Dystrophies

The limb-girdle muscular dystrophies (LGMDs) are a heterogeneous group of disorders that are inherited as either an autosomal-dominant (type 1) or -recessive (type 2) trait. They are characterized by proximal muscle weakness (shoulder and pelvic girdle), sparing of the face and extraocular muscles, muscle wasting, and variable elevations in the creatine kinase levels (which may also be normal). The onset is typically during the first two decades of life. The EMG pattern is myopathic, and muscle biopsy shows features consistent with a dystrophy. Weakness is progressive, but the rate of progression is highly variable.

The pathophysiology of the autosomal-recessive group of LGMDs is intriguing. LGMD 2A, also known as *calpainopathy* from its gene product calpain 3 (a muscle-specific calcium-dependent protease), is novel in that it is the first enzyme deficiency known to cause a muscular dystrophy. The precise mechanism is unknown. LGMD 2B, known as *dysferlinopathy* after its gene product, is interesting in that it has recently been shown to be allelic with Miyoshi myopathy, a distal form of muscular dystrophy. LGMDs 2C through 2F are caused by mutations in genes encoding the sarcoglycans (Fig. 36.1), structural proteins intricately involved in maintaining the integrity of the muscle membrane. Collectively, they are referred to as *sarcoglycanopathies;* as a group, they tend to be more severe than the other forms of LGMD. LGMD 2C, formerly known as *severe childhood autosomal-recessive muscular dystrophy* (SCARMD), tends to present relatively early with a severe phenotype resembling that of DMD. A reduction in one of the sarcoglycans often disrupts the entire complex, with diminished histochemical staining of the other three proteins; hence, all four proteins should be evaluated when one is reduced, to assess which one is most severely reduced and represents the primary deficit. An antibody to α-sarcoglycan is usually used to screen the complex. Because the recessive forms of LGMD tend to be more severe clinically than the dominant forms, they usually present earlier, during childhood. However, they may occasionally be associated with a milder phenotype and a more protracted course, and the phenotype-genotype correlation is not as predictable as in DMD. Cardiac involvement does occur but is less common than in DMD or BMD.

One important feature of the autosomal-dominant LGMD 1B is a strong association with cardiac involvement (cardiac arrhythmias and cardiomyopathy); this may present early, with little in the way of muscle weakness to suggest a myopathy. It is associated with mutations of the *LMNA* gene. Other mutations of the same gene give rise to a variety of phenotypes, including autosomal-dominant EDMD (see preceding text).

CONGENITAL MYOPATHIES

Congenital myopathies are a heterogeneous group of disorders of variable inheritance. They may present with hypotonia and weakness during the neonatal period (*floppy infant syndrome*), or with weakness and motor delay during infancy and childhood. Although they were initially thought of as a *benign* group of disorders that tend to be nonprogressive and change little over time, it is now well recognized that they vary widely in clinical presentation and severity. The weakness may be progressive in certain instances and the severity such that early demise occurs. It is also now well recognized that muscle weakness may appear in adulthood for the first time. Specific structural and pathologic features noted on the muscle biopsy specimen determine the unique characteristics. Specific clinical findings in some of the congenital myopathies may provide a clue to the diagnosis (e.g., ophthalmoplegia and ptosis in myotubular myopathy, facial features and prominent respiratory and feeding difficulties in nemaline rod myopathy, and arthrogryposis in fiber-type disproportion). The creatine kinase level is typically normal or may be mildly elevated. The EMG shows nonspecific myopathic features, but findings are normal in approximately one third of the cases. The definitive diagnosis rests on the muscle biopsy

TABLE 36.4

COMMON FORMS OF CONGENITAL MYOPATHY

Central core myopathy
Minicore/multicore myopathy
Nemaline rod myopathy
Centronuclear/myotubular myopathy
Fiber-type disproportion

because routine genetic testing is not yet available for most forms. Both histochemistry *and* electron microscopy studies should be performed on the muscle specimen to evaluate for ultrastructural changes. Additional testing for cardiac, respiratory (diaphragm weakness, nocturnal sleep hypoventilation), and orthopaedic (scoliosis, skeletal deformities) involvement may be necessary. Malignant hyperthermia is a potential anesthetic risk, especially in central core myopathy, nemaline rod myopathy, and minicore myopathy, but caution should be exercised in all forms of congenital myopathy.

A number of congenital myopathies are well recognized and established clinically and morphologically (Table 36.4). However, others are extremely rare and the subject of only one or two case reports. This latter group includes such entities as zebra body myopathy, broad A band myopathy, and trilaminar myopathy. Only the more common congenital myopathies are described in the following sections.

Central Core Myopathy

Central core myopathy may be sporadic or inherited as an autosomal-dominant trait. Linkage analysis in certain families maps the gene locus to 19q13.1, which is also the region for the malignant hyperthermia gene. Susceptibility to malignant hyperthermia is therefore a potential risk. Mutations in the ryanodine receptor occur in both conditions. The condition may present at birth with mild neonatal hypotonia, or later during infancy with delayed motor milestones. Clinically, the weakness varies markedly. It may be proximal or generalized and is usually associated with hypotonia and diminished reflexes. Skeletal abnormalities, which are rare, include clubfoot, scoliosis, and dislocated hip. Sparing of the facial, ocular, and pharyngeal muscles is typical. Muscle biopsy shows cores in the center of type I muscle fibers, and a predominance of type I fibers may be noted.

Minicore Myopathy

The inheritance pattern of minicore myopathy is variable. Most cases are sporadic. The gene locus is not yet known. Minicore myopathy is also known as *multicore myopathy*. Muscle biopsy shows multiple, well-circumscribed, oval cores in both type I and type II muscle fibers. The cores are deficient in adenosine triphosphatase and oxidative enzyme activity. Type I fibers usually predominate. Clinically, the weakness is typically greater in the upper extremity, with a proximal-to-distal gradient noted, and tends to be mild to moderate. Mild facial weakness may be present. Dilated cardiomyopathy and conduction disturbances may occur. Diaphragmatic involvement may cause nocturnal hypoventilation. The cardiac and respiratory involvement may be out of proportion to the degree of weakness. Scoliosis may occur. Malignant hyperthermia is a risk.

Nemaline Rod Myopathy

Nemaline rod myopathy occurs in both autosomal-recessive and autosomal-dominant forms. Five different gene loci have been identified to date. This includes three autosomal-dominant forms namely 1q42, which encodes ACTA 1 (α-actin, skeletal); lq21-23, which encodes TPM3 (α-tropomyosin$_{slow}$); and 9pl3 encoding TPM2 (β-tropomyosin). The recessive forms include loci at chromosome 2q21-22, which encodes NEM2 (nebulin) in some European families, and 9ql3 encoding TNNT1 (slow troponin T). Three main clinical presentations occur:

- A severe neonatal form that usually results in death at birth
- A *classic* neonatal or early childhood form (most common)
- An adult-onset form

The early forms present with hypotonia and weakness, usually in a proximal-to-distal gradient but sometimes generalized. Prominent respiratory difficulties (secondary to diaphragmatic involvement) and swallowing difficulties occur and are usually disproportionate to the weakness. The characteristic phenotype includes an elongated, narrow face; facial diplegia; and a high, arched palate, with the lower jaw usually open. Skeletal deformities such as clubfoot and scoliosis may occur. Cardiomyopathy is more common in the late-onset form. Nocturnal hypoventilation resulting from diaphragmatic weakness may cause early morning headache, lethargy, nausea, and decreased appetite secondary to carbon dioxide retention. The adult-onset form is less common, and atrophy is prominent. Red-staining rod-like structures (nemaline rods) are demonstrated by trichrome stain and are also seen on electron microscopy. They are generally more numerous in type I fibers.

Centronuclear/Myotubular Myopathy

Centronuclear/myotubular myopathy occurs in sporadic, X-linked, autosomal-dominant, and autosomal-recessive forms. Facial diplegia, ptosis, and external ophthalmoplegia are often present and help differentiate this condition from other forms of congenital myopathy. The X-linked form tends to be more severe, with prominent respiratory involvement and usually early demise. Long-term ventilatory support is often required. Cardiac involvement may be prominent. The gene locus (MTM1) maps to chromosome Xq28 and encodes a tyrosine phosphatase protein, myotubularin. The autosomal forms tend to present later, during childhood, adolescence, or even adulthood. Excessive, prominent central nuclei are present on muscle biopsy specimens, in addition to immature muscle fibers resembling myotubules. In the X-linked–recessive form, the muscle fibers express both vimentin and desmin.

Congenital Fiber-Type Disproportion

The inheritance of congenital fiber-type disproportion appears variable, with sporadic, autosomal-recessive, and autosomal-dominant forms described. The condition may present at birth with the floppy infant syndrome, or later in life with delayed motor milestones. The weakness is of variable severity. Associated features include multiple joint contractures (arthrogryposis), torticollis, congenital dislocation of the hip, foot deformities (pes cavus and pes planus), and scoliosis. A more severe form, with prominent respiratory weakness and failure and early demise, has been described. Muscle biopsy shows a predominance of type I muscle fibers (>80%); these are also smaller (>12%) than the type II muscle fibers, which may be hypertrophic.

REVIEW EXERCISES

QUESTIONS

1. The following are all inherited as an X–linked–recessive trait *except*:
a) DMD
b) BMD
c) EDMD
d) Myotonic dystrophy

Answer
The answer is d. Myotonic dystrophy is a trinucleotide repeat disorder resulting from an expansion of a CTG triplet repeat on chromosome 19. The inheritance is autosomal dominant with genetic anticipation (i.e., subsequent generations have a further increased number of trinucleotide repeats with more severe clinical expression).

2. The risk that a daughter of a female carrier of BMD is a carrier is:
a) 33%
b) 50%
c) 75%
d) 100%

Answer
The answer is b. DMD and BMD are X-linked–recessive conditions. A female carrier has one affected allele and one normal allele at the Xp21 gene locus. A daughter inherits one X chromosome from her father and therefore

has a 50% chance of inheriting the affected allele from her mother.

3. In DMD, the proportion of dystrophin in muscle is approximately:
a) 0%
b) 25%
c) 50%
d) 100%

Answer
The answer is a. DMD is differentiated from BMD by an *absence* of dystrophin. In BMD, the amount of dystrophin is reduced or the protein is truncated, but it is present at levels 10% or more of those seen in normal controls.

4. Ophthalmoplegia and ptosis are commonly seen in:
a) DMD
b) Myotubular myopathy
c) CMD
d) LGMD
e) Congenital fiber-type disproportion

Answer
The answer is b. Hallmarks of myotubular myopathy are ptosis and ophthalmoplegia, which allow this congenital myopathy to be differentiated from other types. In DMD, LGMD, and CMD, sparing of the facial and ocular muscles is typical. Fiber-type disproportion is usually associated with skeletal abnormalities (arthrogryposis, scoliosis, foot deformities, congenital hip dislocation) and torticollis.

5. Cardiac involvement occurs in which of the following?
a) Myotonic dystrophy
b) LGMD
c) EDMD
d) Minicore myopathy
e) All of the above

Answer
The answer is e. Myotonic dystrophy is associated with conduction defects and cardiomyopathy. LGMD may be associated with cardiomyopathy, although not as universally as DMD and BMD. LGMD 1B (autosomal-dominant) is different in this regard in that it is frequently associated with heart disease, even when muscle disease is minimal. Conduction abnormalities, and ultimately cardiomyopathy, are key features of both the X-linked and autosomal-dominant forms of EDMD. In minicore myopathy, a congenital myopathy, the cardiac involvement is often disproportionate to the muscle weakness.

6. Malignant hyperthermia is a potential anesthetic risk in:
a) Central core myopathy
b) Nemaline rod myopathy
c) Minicore myopathy
d) All of the above

Answer
The answer is d. In all the congenital myopathies, malignant hyperthermia is theoretically a risk, but the central core, nemaline rod, and minicore myopathies are most strongly associated with a risk for malignant hyperthermia. Central core myopathy maps to the same region on chromosome 19q13 as the malignant hyperthermia gene.

SUGGESTED READINGS

1. Bonnemann CG, McNally EM, Kunkel LM Beyond dystrophin: current progress in the muscular dystrophies. *CurrOpin Pediatr* 1996;8:569.
2. Dubowitz V. *Muscle disorders in childhood,* 2nd ed. Philadelphia: Saunders, 1995.
3. Kirschner J, Bonnemann CG. The congenital and limb-girdle muscular dystrophies. *Arch Neurol* 2004;61:189–199.
4. Laval SH, Bushby KMD. Limb-girdle muscular dystrophies - from genetics to molecular pathology. *Neuropathol Appl Neurobiol* 2004;30:91–105.
5. Mathews KD. Muscular dystrophy overview: genetics and diagnosis. *Neurol Clin N Am* 2003;21:795–816.
6. Muntoni F, Voit T. The congenital muscular dystrophies in 2004: a century of exciting progress. *Neuromuscul Disord* 2004;14:635–649.
7. Neuromuscular disorders: gene location. *Neuromuscul Disord* 2005;15:89–114.
8. Riggs JE, Bodensteiner JB, Schochet SS. Congenital myopathies/dystrophies. *Neurol Clin North Am* 2003;21:779–794.
9. Zatz M, de Paula F, Starling A, et al. The 10 autosomal recessive limb-girdle muscular dystrophies. *Neuromuscul Disord* 2003;13:532–544.

Chapter 37

BOARD SIMULATION: Neurology

Bruce H. Cohen

QUESTIONS

1. A 4-year-old boy is being evaluated for developmental delay. His parents describe him as a very slow feeder who often choked on his bottle. He did not stand until he was 18 months old and took his first steps at 24 months of age. He is now beginning to place two words together and has a vocabulary of 50 words. His examination is significant for moderate hypotonia and obesity. His mother states he has a voracious appetite. Which of the following laboratory tests would *most* likely confirm the diagnosis?
a) Routine chromosome testing
b) Fluorescence in situ hybridization (FISH) study for subtelomeric rearrangements
c) FISH testing of the 15q11.2-q13 region
d) *MECP2* gene sequencing
e) Lactic acid level

Answer
The answer is c. This child has Prader-Willi Syndrome (PWS). Infants with PWS are often hypotonic and may have difficulty gaining weight because of slow feeding. Their neurocognitive development is slow and most children ultimately do not achieve normal intelligence. Obesity caused by uncontrolled hunger is frequent. These children are often growth hormone deficient and have hypogonadism. The FISH test of the 15q11.2-q13 region detects most children with PWS. However, a specific methylation DNA test does exist that detects those children who inherit the condition as a result of parental disomy, and should be obtained in those children who fit the clinical phenotype for PWS but have normal FISH evaluations. Routine chromosomal testing will be normal in PWS, and although it is not "wrong" to order this test as part of the evaluation of a syndromic developmentally delayed child, it is not the best answer. Deletions

and rearrangements in the subtelomeric regions of the chromosomes are associated with syndromic mental retardation but again, is not a test that detects PWS. Mutations in the *MECP2* gene are the cause of Rett syndrome. Elevated lactic acid levels are indicative of many different disorders and are not helpful or specific in detecting PWS.

2. A 4-year-old boy is being evaluated for unilateral blindness due to an optic glioma. On examination, a dozen *café au hit* macules measuring >1.5 cm in diameter and freckling in the axilla and inguinal regions are noted. It is noted that his father also has dozens of *café au hit* macules as well as freckling in the axilla and inguinal regions. His mother's examination is normal. The risk for each subsequent child of this couple to have the same disorder is:
a) One fourth because the disorder is autosomal dominant
b) Half because the disorder is autosomal dominant
c) One fourth because the disorder is autosomal recessive
d) Half because the disorder is autosomal recessive
e) There is a minimal risk because the mother is normal

Answer

The answer is b. This child has NF1, which is an autosomal-dominant disorder. The incidence of NF1 is approximately 1 in 4000 individuals, and this incidence does not vary across ethnic groups. Mutations in the *NF1* gene located on the 17th chromosome are responsible for the disease, but there is no one specific mutation that causes the disease; dozens of mutations have been described. Approximately one half of affected individuals inherit the gene from an affected parent, whereas the other half develops the mutation as a result of a spontaneous mutation. Regardless, if one parent has the mutation, the risk with each pregnancy is half, as this is an autosomal-dominant disorder.

3. A 7-year-old girl is being evaluated for repetitive episodes of vomiting, which have required eight prior hospitalizations for intravenous rehydration. Her examination in your office is normal. She had a brother who died at 3 days of life, and the coroner ruled that the death was a result of sudden infant death syndrome. The *most* likely laboratory abnormalities that would be noted during the next exacerbation would be:
a) Elevated blood ammonia level with low blood urea nitrogen (BUN) levels
b) Elevated blood and cerebrospinal fluid (CSF) glycine levels
c) Low CSF glucose with normal blood glucose
d) Normal blood glucose level with no urine ketones
e) Elevated blood glucose level with no urine ketones

Answer

The answer is a. This girl is affected with the X-linked disorder *ornithine transcarbamylase deficiency*. This enzyme is one of the urea acid cycle enzymes. In boys, the defect is lethal at an early age, but because girls have two X chromosomes, the relative deficiency of this enzyme can present as intermittent hyperammonemia, with vomiting as a key feature, especially during viral illnesses. It is important to remember that "BUN" means simply "urea level" and the BUN will be low in all urea acid cycle defects and in the organic acidurias, which inhibit the urea acid cycle. (If you see a dehydrated and ill-appearing child with a BUN of 0, 1, 2, or 3, think of ordering an ammonia level test.) Elevated glycine levels can occur in nonketotic hyperglycinemia, which usually presents as a catastrophic seizure disorder in infancy. Low CSF glucose in the context of an acellular CSF occurring in an infant with seizures is a clue for glucose transport disorder.

4. Which of the following clinical features is *not* part of the migraine spectrum in children?
a) Headache
b) Transient visual loss
c) Abdominal pain, cramping, and vomiting
d) Olfactory hallucinations
e) Relief of symptoms with sleep

Answer

The answer is d. Olfactory hallucinations are most often caused by seizures originating in the lower portion of the frontal lobes. Children will describe the event as a horrible smell, like a skunk or burnt rubber. Such a symptom should indicate to the physician a structural abnormality in the brain and warrants MRI testing. The other symptoms are among the most common features of pediatric migraine, which is reported to occur in approximately 5% of all children.

5. An 8-year-old boy was playing with friends when it was noted that he was lying unconscious. Neighbors called 9-1-1 and he began to return to consciousness when the ambulance squad arrived. No shaking movements were noted by the adults at the scene and the playmates offered no clues as to what happened, except to say that he was fine one minute and found lying on the ground the next. His neurologic examination was normal, as were magnetic resonance imaging (MRI) of the brain and an electroencephalograph (EEG). Because of the severe nature of the event, it was decided to treat him with an anticonvulsant. Over the next year there were four similar events, all occurring while seemingly having a good time playing with other children. His anticonvulsant levels were normal. Apart from falling asleep in school, which has resulted in poor progress at school, he was a normal and well-adjusted child. His mother reports that he is in bed promptly by 8:30 p.m. and sleeps until she awakens him at 6:30 a.m. Which of the following would be the next *best* step in the evaluation?

a) Prolonged (96-hour) EEG
b) Psychology referral
c) Social service evaluation
d) Polysomnogram (PSG) and multiple sleep latency test (MSLT)
e) Urine and blood toxin screening

Answer

The answer is d. This boy is affected with both narcolepsy (the sudden onset of sleep at inappropriate times) and cataplexy (sudden onset of sleep initiated by laughter, fear, or surprise). Simple narcolepsy occurs in approximately 1:1000 individuals, although cataplexy is a rare form of the illness. Individuals with narcolepsy often have other sleep disorders, such as hypnagogic hallucinations—vivid, realistic, and often frightening dreams; and sleep paralysis—temporary inability to move, which occurs upon awakening from sleep. The polysomnogram (sleep study) offers an analysis of the efficiency of sleep, to make sure the child does not have sleep apnea or other sleep disorders. The MSLT provides a systematic analysis of how quickly the child falls asleep after a "good night's sleep." Treatment with psychostimulants is often effective. Sleep disorders in children are underdiagnosed and can only be evaluated and treated if they are considered in the differential diagnosis.

6. An 8-year-old girl is being evaluated for her poor performance at school. Her teachers wish to hold her back. On examination she is clearly distractible and inattentive. Her weight is less than the third percentile for age, although her height is at the 50th percentile. She has very little muscle bulk and her facial muscles are especially thin. Her father has a similar appearance and was not able to finish high school because of academic issues but has maintained full-time employment as a cashier at the airport bookshop. The father is affected by what he calls *hand cramps*, which occur whenever he grips an object tightly. Which of the following would *best* explain the child's medical condition?

a) Attention deficit disorder without hyperactivity
b) Attention deficit disorder with hyperactivity
c) Central core disease
d) Myotonic dystrophy
e) Poor nutrition

Answer

The answer is d. Myotonic dystrophy is an autosomal-dominant disorder that is caused by a trinucleotide repeat, meaning that the condition can worsen with successive generations. Individuals with this condition have very poor muscle bulk and have a thin *hatchet-like* face. Cognitive delays are common, but not universal, and it is not uncommon for older family members to have

escaped diagnosis. The myopathy is also variable, but a common feature is myotonia—an abnormal sustained contraction of muscle groups when the muscle is contracted. This causes difficultly releasing the handgrip when shaking hands or turning a doorknob. Early balding, cataracts, diabetes mellitus, hypothyroidism, and cardiac conduction defects can also be part of this condition. Central core disease is another autosomal-dominant muscle disease that causes thin facies and mild weakness, but intelligence is normal. Although attention deficits are often part of myotonic dystrophy, the family history and abnormal neurologic examination should clue the doctor into thinking further than the obvious presenting complaint. Despite the fact that the child is *underweight*, there is nothing in the history to suggest malnutrition.

7. An infant is born at term to a 35-year-old woman. The pregnancy was perfectly normal and the child was monitored during labor with a normal tracing. The delivery was normal, and the child was nondysmorphic with a normal birth weight, length, and head circumference. The child had poor respiratory effort and hypotonia that did not improve with bagging, and the infant required endotracheal intubation. Arterial blood gases were normal and an emergency head ultrasonography was normal. Aside from the hypotonia, the child looked alert and attentive. After examining the infant and drawing blood for necessary laboratory tests, you went to talk with the parents, who were obviously upset by the events. Upon entering the room you noted that the mother was sobbing and shaking because she was so upset, and also that she had a very thin face and difficulty relaxing her hand after you had shaken it, so that your hand remained "stuck" in her grip. The *most* likely explanation of the situation is:

a) Neonatal sepsis
b) Prader-Willi syndrome (PWS)
c) Birth anoxia
d) Leigh syndrome
e) Myotonic dystrophy

Answer

The answer is e. Infants of women with myotonic dystrophy who also are affected by disease (the 50% that inherit the gene defect) can present in the delivery room with severe hypotonia, to the point that intubation and ventilation are required. The only treatment is supportive care and over time the infant will likely gain enough strength to be self-sufficient. Sepsis should be considered in this situation. There are infants with PWS who are profoundly hypotonic at birth, but the mother's examination in this scenario suggests myotonic dystrophy. There is no suggestion that birth anoxia plays any role in this case. Leigh syndrome, which does not present in the delivery room, is a progressive disorder marked by seemingly normal development followed by stepwise neurologic decline and respiratory failure resulting from disorders of energy metabolism.

8. A 4-month-old infant girl is brought in by her parents with the chief complaint of lethargy. She is a breast-fed infant and until a week ago was a good feeder, but has become increasingly disinterested in feeding. Her mother noted that constipation has also developed over the last few days and even use of a glycerin suppository was not effective. On examination, the child has normal vital signs, although she seems to be using her abdominal muscles to assist in breathing. She seems very alert and attentive, but has a distinctly weak cry when you draw her blood sample. Her abdomen is distended and bowel sounds are absent. Her pupils do not react to light, she is hypotonic and muscle stretch reflexes are absent. Her illness is *most* likely a result of:
a) Spinal muscular atrophy (Werdnig-Hoffman syndrome)
b) Infantile botulism
c) Sepsis
d) Intussusception
e) Nonaccidental trauma

Answer

The answer is b. This clinical picture is most consistent with infantile botulism. Ingestion of the botulinum spore (found in honey or the dirt of certain regions) can result in this illness. Approximately 90% of reported cases in the United States are from California, Utah, and southeast Pennsylvania, likely because of high concentrations of *Clostridium botulinum* spores in the soil of these regions. This disorder usually presents before the first birthday in a previously healthy child. Subacute weakness and constipation are the key features, with a preserved mental status. Although the child may appear lethargic, she is in fact quite alert but simply too weak to move because the toxin affects the neuromuscular junction. Treatment is supportive, although botulinum immune globulin has been used to shorten the course of the illness. The presentation of the weakness in spinal muscular atrophy is more chronic and the constipation is not a key feature, but this is a good thought and should be kept in mind. Also, the papillary light reflex is normal in spinal muscular atrophy but not in infantile botulism. This case is not the typical clinical presentation of sepsis or nonaccidental trauma. Infants with intussusception may have altered mental status but they are not hypotonic.

9. A 17-year-old girl had a brief loss of consciousness after striking her head on the cement, when she fell off a motor scooter while not wearing a helmet. The computed tomograph (CT) scan of the brain taken at the time of the accident was normal and she was observed overnight in the hospital. On the morning of hospital discharge she was upset because she learned that she was

grounded for 3 months for disobeying her parent's rule not to ride her boyfriend's motor scooter. Three weeks later she is complaining of headaches, difficulty concentrating in school, and feeling dizzy all the time. Her neurologic examination is normal. Which of the following offers the *best* explanation for her situation?
a) Delayed subdural hemorrhage
b) Trauma-triggered migraine disorder
c) Postconcussive syndrome
d) Conversion disorder
e) Partial complex seizures

Answer

The answer is c. This scenario is most consistent with a postconcussive syndrome. The pathophysiology of this disorder, which tends to follow relatively mild head trauma and concussions, is not understood. Within a few weeks of the injury, and after an apparent recovery, the child develops headaches, difficulty in concentrating, poor memory, and dizziness, along with other somatic complaints that have no clear etiology. The MRI/CT scan and EEG are normal in this syndrome, although these tests are not needed to diagnose or evaluate for postconcussive syndrome. Treatment is supportive care. The use of antidepressant medication is sometimes helpful, as are psychostimulant medications. Although the educational program must be adjusted to meet the ability of the patient, the patient should not be allowed to either stop schooling or be kept at home during the recovery. A complete recovery occurs in weeks to months. Although there may be a psychological component to the illness, it is not a primary psychiatric condition. Delayed subdural hemorrhages are rare in children, but it is often not practical not to evaluate for this possibility given how poorly functional these children may be during the presenting days of the syndrome. Trauma-triggered migraine is a disorder in which the migraine, with a distinct beginning and end, is triggered by a very mild head trauma, such as bumping against a wall. Because of the social history surrounding the accident and the punishment, it is difficult to sort out what could be a conversion disorder in this case. Finally, seizures can occur after head injury, but there is nothing about the history to suggest that the patient is having epileptic events.

10. A 6-year-old girl presents to the emergency department with a 5-hour history of progressive gait ataxia. She has been febrile for 2 days with an illness that included headache, runny nose, and a mild rash, but her mother thought she was improving. Her examination is significant for a temperature of 38.44°C (101.2°F), extreme irritability that makes it difficult to judge the presence of true meningismus, and gait ataxia. The nursing staff has already placed an intravenous catheter and obtained a complete blood count, comprehensive chemistry panel, and blood cultures. Which of the following outlines the *best* sequence of evaluation and treatment for this child?

a) Lumbar puncture (LP), CT scan of the brain, antibiotics/antiviral agent
b) CT scan of the brain, LP, antibiotics/antiviral agent
c) Antibiotics/antiviral agent, LP, CT scan of the brain
d) Antibiotics/antiviral agent, CT scan of the brain, LP
e) LP, antibiotics/antiviral agent, CT scan of the brain

Answer

The answer is d. This child likely has meningitis or encephalitis, although it is not possible to tell from the history whether this is a benign viral meningitis, a harmful bacterial or herpes meningitis/encephalitis, or a postviral ataxia syndrome that can follow, for example, varicella. Other less common possibilities include a mass-occupying lesion (bacterial, tumor, blood). This is a common scenario in which the clinician is faced with the decision to err on the side of having a correct and firm infectious diagnosis with a small chance of causing harm to the patient (choice e), or err on the side of possibly or probably losing a chance of a firm diagnosis but guaranteeing earliest treatment of a potentially life-threatening illness in which time is of the essence and not proceeding with a procedure that has possible deleterious effects (the correct choice d). Time is a critically important component to the decision and it is clear that administering antibiotics takes little time, as does performing an LP under emergency situations such as this case. Performing a CT scan on an irritable child can be time consuming. However, the most likely disease this child has will be best treated with antibiotics and antiviral therapy, so once that is initiated, the next step is to evaluate for mass lesions and/or increased intracranial pressure prior to performing a test (the LP) that could cause harm if there is elevated intracranial pressure. Choice c will correctly initiate treatment but places the risk in front of the test that will evaluate the possibility of that risk. Choices a and b are not correct because there would never be reason to delay antibiotics until *after* an LP.

11. A previously well, 15-month-old boy with a decreased sensorium is brought into the emergency department by his parents. The parents had gone out for dinner the evening before leaving the child with a babysitter, a high school senior who recently moved next door. The child threw a tantrum and was crying when the parents left home. After returning home later that evening, the parents noted that the child had a fitful night's sleep. When they woke him up that morning he started crying and refused breakfast. He was put back to sleep for another hour and when the parents tried to wake him up, he did not behave normally and so they brought him to the emergency room. His vital signs showed a respiratory rate of 48/minute, heart rate of 150/minute, a blood pressure of 140/98, and a temperature of 37.88°C (100.2°F). Rales were heard in both lung fields and some pink froth was found in the posterior pharynx. His neurologic examination was significant for being very lethargic. The nursing staff has placed an intravenous catheter and obtained a complete blood count, comprehensive chemistry panel, and blood cultures. Which of the following evaluations will *most* likely yield an answer for this child's condition?

a) Antibiotic/antiviral therapy, CT scan of the brain, LP
b) Funduscopic examination, CT scan of the brain
c) Renal ultrasonography, BUN, serum creatinine
d) Chest x-ray, arterial blood gas, bronchoscopy
e) Toxin screening, aspiration of stomach contents

Answer

The answer is b. The clinician should recognize this as a case of nonaccidental trauma, specifically shaken baby syndrome. The other answers include tests that may be performed as part of the early evaluation of this child but are simply distracters. Although evaluation of the optic fundi is *part* of the neurologic examination, it is often omitted because it can be cumbersome, the equipment may not be functioning, and so on. However, this will take less than a minute and lead the doctor immediately to the correct diagnosis, which can be confirmed with a brain CT scan. Retinal hemorrhage in this age group is both relatively sensitive and specific for shaken baby syndrome. The history suggests that this healthy child may not have been well when the parents returned home. The vital signs are not specific but the increased respiratory rate, heart rate, and blood pressure can be seen in any disorder that injures the central nervous system. The respiratory rate, pulmonary examination, and finding of pink froth in the pharynx indicate the presence of neurogenic pulmonary edema. This finding should be sought for every child with altered mental status and should be part of the examination repertoire of every pediatrician. The CT scan will likely show cerebral edema, loss of the gray/white matter interface, and subarachnoid and subdural blood. Although shaken baby syndrome may be part of a more chronic abuse situation, and certainly this child should have a total body radiograph and evaluation for blunt trauma to the abdomen, it can be seen in isolation, in which case the perpetrator may be an inexperienced parent, babysitter, or older sibling.

12. A 17-year-old young woman presents with a 3-month history of intermittent severe headaches. There have been five discrete instances. Although there is no precipitating event, all the headaches are similar: She feels nauseated and turns pale, which is followed by a pounding unilateral pain, photophobia, and phonophobia. The headache lasts for several hours, and she has noted that if she falls asleep she will wake up feeling better. On one occasion she vomited, and on two occasions she noted that her vision became blurred, once to the point that she could not see the chalkboard at school. Her mother noted that her speech seemed slurred with the last headache, so she went to the emergency department, where she was treated with meperidine (Demerol). She underwent an MRI of the brain, which was normal. Her medical history is unremarkable, although she has irregular menstrual cycles. Her mother and maternal aunt are affected with migraine. Apart from borderline obesity, her general physical and neurologic examinations are normal. She is a good student and is part of the school's swimming team. After the family leaves the room, you also obtain a history that she is sexually active with a boyfriend. She uses condoms as a method of birth control and has been compliant "most of the time." She does not smoke, drink alcohol, or take illicit drugs. You advise the patient about diet, exercise, and social issues. In terms of the headaches, you decide the *best* course of action will be to:

a) Prescribe daily sodium divalproate (Depakote).
b) Prescribe daily propranolol (Inderal).
c) Prescribe daily cyproheptadine (Periactin).
d) Prescribe one of the triptan medications as abortive therapy.
e) Prescribe daily topiramate (Topamax).

Answer

The answer is e. Topiramate is indicated for preventive treatment of migraine in patients older than 16 years, although it is often used in younger patients because of its side effect profile and relative efficacy. It may cause a minor amount of weight loss. Patients must be advised to ensure adequate fluid intake, as there is a risk of kidney stones. At higher dosages, which will not likely be needed in this patient, there may be a decreased ability to perspire, so patients would need to be warned about overheating with exercise, especially on warm days. Sodium divalproate is an effective prophylactic therapy for migraine, but carries with it a risk of birth defects if a child is conceived while the mother is taking the medication, as well as weight gain, thinning scalp hair, and tremor. Propranolol is also an effective prophylactic therapy for migraine, but at dosages needed to be effective there may be a significant degree of sedation and β-blockade, as well as associated weight gain, which makes it less desirable in adolescents. Cyproheptadine is free of serious side effects, but causes a significant increase in appetite and associated weight gain. This is an excellent choice for thin children of all ages as a prophylactic therapy for migraine, but is not accepted by patients if they are already fighting with impending obesity. Although the triptan groups of medications are excellent abortive medications, they should not be used in patients with complicated migraines—those with neurologic deficits during their attacks, such as slurred speech or visual loss. Finally, be aware that there are *herbal* and vitamin remedies that may be effective in some patients, such as riboflavin (vitamin B$_2$), magnesium salts, and coenzyme Q10. The combination of riboflavin, magnesium, and an herb (feverfew) is found in many health food stores and many patients have effective control with these medicines, although they have not found their way into *American medicine* yet.

13. A mother brings her 12-month-old daughter in for her well-child visit. You have seen this girl many times since you first met the family during a prenatal interview. As part of the general developmental screening, you learn that the child has just begun to babble and has begun to cruise around the furniture. You note that the head circumference falls at the 50th percentile, whereas it has always followed the 75th percentile curve. The child appears well and your examination is otherwise normal. When the child returns for her 15-month checkup, the mother tells you that there have been no gains in motor skills and in fact she is having more trouble ambulating. She is also not babbling. You note that her head has really not grown in the last few months. Because you take the head circumference measurements yourself, you feel the values are reliable. Diagnostic possibilities can be *best* evaluated with which of the following?

a) Routine chromosome testing
b) Referral to a developmental center for occupational and physical therapy
c) Referral to a developmental pediatrician
d) *MECP2* gene sequencing
e) Brain MRI

Answer

The answer is d. This is a classic presentation of Rett syndrome. Rett syndrome is an X-linked dominant disorder that occurs in girls (although boys may have the gene, if they do not die in utero, they present with a profound neonatal encephalopathy and early death). After a period of normal development for the first 6 to 18 months, girls stop obtaining milestones and lose any language function they may have acquired. They also experience a slowing in head growth resulting in *acquired microcephaly*, and when they do become ambulatory develop an ataxia. Difficult-to-control seizures, bruxism, and abnormal breathing patterns are common. The classic finding of a *hand washing* behavior may not manifest until they are 5 years old. This case is an excellent example as to why one doctor should follow up a patient through their *well-child visits*. In this case, the pediatrician has evaluated the child's development sequentially and is in the best position to identify that the development has not advanced normally. Furthermore, there is examiner-to-examiner variability in taking head circumference measurements, and this case outlines why only one individual (the primary care physician) should be obtaining and documenting head circumference measurements. The spectrum of severity in Rett syndrome is quite broad. Rett syndrome is the first human disease to be caused by defects in a protein involved in regulation of gene expression through its interaction with methylated DNA. During development many genes are expressed, that is, they are translated into proteins. This occurs in different tissues of the body at different times and at different rates. MECP2 involves one of the many biochemical switches needed to control the complex expression pattern of other genes by telling them when to turn off. The lack of properly functioning MECP2 protein will allow other genes to turn on or stay on at inappropriate stages in development. The MECP2 protein is likely involved in turning off (or *silencing*) several other genes.

This prevents the genes from making proteins when they are not needed. The MECP2 protein binds to DNA at regions called CpG islands, which frequently occur near the beginning of a gene. The protein then interacts with other proteins to form a complex that turns off the gene. It is not known which genes are targeted by MECP2, but such genes are probably important for the normal function of the central nervous system. As a result, the protein is unable to bind to DNA or turn off other genes. Genes that are normally regulated by MECP2 remain active and continue to make large amounts of proteins when they are not needed. This defect probably disrupts the normal functioning of nerve cells, leading to the signs and symptoms of Rett syndrome.

It is presumed that many neurodevelopmental disorders may have similar mechanisms. Most cases (99.5%) of Rett syndrome are new and not inherited. There is no one mutation that causes Rett syndrome and although there are *hot spots* in the gene that cause Rett syndrome, each patient may have a unique mutation on the gene. In addition, there may be many more mutations of MECP2 that cause Rett syndrome. The location of the mutation in the *MECP2* gene *may* account for the severity or kind of symptoms as different regions of genes affect the function or quantity of the proteins they produce. Variable and random X-inactivation may also explain some of the clinical variability.

There are four stages of Rett syndrome; this patient is in the first phase known as *early onset*. Between the ages of 1 and 4 years the girls enter a *rapid destructive phase* that is variable in its severity. The *plateau phase* begins between ages 2 and 10 years and may last for years or decades. Higher-functioning girls and women in this phase can form emotional relationships and although they are not verbal, they can be quite happy and function in a family or group home setting. The last phase is the *late deterioration,* which results in weakness and dystonia but without a decline in cognition.

Routine chromosome testing and brain MRI will not be helpful in diagnosing Rett syndrome, although these may be helpful in the general setting of evaluating for a possible neurogenetic disorder. Although referral to a developmental specialist and therapist is indicated, that alone will not result in a diagnosis.

14. An 8-year-old boy is brought into your office for evaluation of acne. His medical history is not remarkable. His family history is significant for a 2-year-old sister with mental retardation and seizures. His mother is healthy and little is known about the father's health, although he had a similar-appearing acneform pattern on his face. On examination you find what appears like acne around his nose, but not elsewhere on his body. He has several growths around his nail bed and several oval white macules on his trunk and limbs. Which of the following describe this patient's condition?
a) von Hippel-Lindau syndrome
b) Neurofibromatosis type 1 (NF1)
c) NF2
d) Tuberous sclerosis
e) Sturge-Weber syndrome

Answer
The answer is d. Tuberous sclerosis is an autosomal-dominant disorder, and although it can be inherited, almost 75% of cases are a result of a spontaneous mutation. There are now two genes known to cause tuberous sclerosis and both are available by commercial testing. The *TSC1* gene is located on chromosome 9q34 and the *TSC2* gene on chromosome 16p13. The list of clinical features is broad, and varies among patients. These include hamartomaceous lesions of the brain (tubers), benign brain tumors known as giant cell astrocytomas, and hamartomaceous lesions in the heart (atrial myxomas), kidneys (angiomyolipomas), skin, lungs, and eyes. Mental retardation, seizures, and autism may be seen as part of the condition but are often absent. Fibromas of the finger and toenails, pitted teeth, and dermatologic lesions are common. The facial adenoma sebaceum looks like acne. The hypomelanotic lesions are also known as ash leaf spots.

15. Parents who are new to your practice have adopted 4-year-old twins, a boy and a girl, from another country. Nothing is known about their biologic family but the new parents were told that the children were always healthy. Your first examination of the children revealed no abnormalities, although the children had not learned any English. Six months after the adoption the children had adapted beautifully and were now almost age-appropriate in their English language development. About a year later the parents bring in their son (now 5½ years old) because he has been toe walking and falling. On examination, his calves appear hypertrophied and he is not able to get up from a supine to standing position without using his hands to assist. You order a creatine kinase (CK) level test, which comes back as 8200 U/L (normal 20–220 U/L) and a subsequent muscle biopsy confirms the suspicion of Duchenne muscular dystrophy. Which of the following statements is the *most* accurate?

a) The twin sister will likely develop muscle symptoms some time soon.
b) The twin sister will likely develop muscle symptoms later in life.
c) The twin sister is an obligate carrier of the gene and will pass it on to her male children.
d) The twin sister has a 50% risk of carrying the gene and if so, will pass it on to her male children.
e) The twin sister has a 50% risk of carrying the gene and if so, will have a 50% risk of passing on the gene (and therefore the disease) to each son.

Answer

The answer is e. Duchenne muscular dystrophy is a recessive X-linked disorder caused by mutations at the Xp21 site, which encode for the protein dystrophin. The female twin (and all female siblings) has a 50% chance of inheriting the abnormal gene, but because she will only pass one copy of her two X chromosomes to her offspring, there is a 50% chance with each pregnancy of passing it on to an offspring. The disease is silent in female offspring because even if they inherit one abnormal copy of the gene, the second X chromosome can function to produce the protein. Therefore, the female twin does not develop the disease (so a and b are not correct). The female twin *is not* an obligate carrier of the gene, so answer c is not correct. Answer d is not correct because there is not a 100% chance of passing on the gene to each offspring.

16. A 3-year-old girl is being seen for an abnormal gait that has been noted for several months and seems to be getting worse. Her medical history is unremarkable. Her examination shows a normal mental status and perfectly normal gross and fine motor function in her hands. Her legs are somewhat spastic, and her gait is clumsy. When she runs, she tends to run on her toes. Deep tendon reflexes are normal in her arms, brisk at her knees, and demonstrate clonus at her ankles. The Babinski test result is positive. The sensory examination is simply not possible to interpret. The only findings on her general examination are a deep sacral dimple and tight heal cords. Which of the following tests, procedures, or consults would be *most* likely to provide a diagnostic answer?

a) Scoliosis series with special attention to the lumbosacral spine
b) Electromyogram (EMG) and nerve conduction velocity (NCV)
c) MRI of the brain
d) MRI of the spine
e) Physical therapy consult for muscle-stretching exercises

Answer

The answer is d. The key to neurologic diagnosis is to localize the lesion at a particular level in the nervous system and list the possible disorders that can affect that particular level. In this case, the patient's normal mental status and normal arm function suggests that there is not a global disorder involving the brain. (The one exception is discussed in the following.) The distinct difference between the arm function and the leg function suggests that the disorder is in the lower portion of the spinal cord, as opposed to the upper portion of the spinal cord. The only portion of the brain that could cause bilateral leg dysfunction without bilateral arm dysfunction or loss of cognitive abilities is a parasagittal lesion of the motor strip. However, given the unlikely development of a tumor in this area at this age, along with the physical finding of a deep sacral dimple, there is a higher likelihood of finding pathology in the lumbosacral region. An MRI of the spine, specifically of the lumbosacral spine, will most likely demonstrate the pathology, such as a tethered spinal cord, sacral lipoma with cord tethering, or another specific spinal dysraphism. Plain x-rays will only find bony lesions. An EMG/NCV may not be normal, but will not lead to a specific diagnosis. Although physical therapy may be needed, it is not prudent to ignore these physical findings and not seek a specific diagnosis.

17. A 15-year-old girl in your practice is brought in by her parents for a general health evaluation. Her parents are quite concerned because of recent events. Over the last 6 months, she has become increasingly oppositional and there have been two recent psychiatric hospitalizations for aggressive behavior. (She struck her parents and teacher.) She was started on risperidone with some improvement and visits a psychologist weekly. The parents also report a tremor that was first noticed about a year before but that has progressed. During the session, the patient appears withdrawn and angry. Her examination is significant for a tremor of her arms that is most apparent when she raises her arms at the shoulder joint. Which of the following tests will be *most* helpful in making the diagnosis?

a) Thyroid function tests
b) Slit-lamp examination of the cornea, levels of serum liver enzyme, serum cooper, and ceruloplasmin
c) Brain MRI
d) Polysomnogram and MSLT
e) Blood and urine porphyrin and porphobilinogen levels

Answer

The answer is b. This young woman has the classic adolescent-adult onset form of Wilson disease, a diagnosis to consider whenever someone of this age presents with psychiatric illness de novo and a movement disorder. This illness is caused by the liver's inability to release copper into the bile. There are more than 200 different mutations within the gene *ATP7B*, located on chromosome 13 that may cause this illness. Approximately 1 in 30,000 individuals has this illness. When presenting before adolescence, the most common affected organ is the liver. This gene encodes for the protein ceruloplasmin. Copper will accumulate in the liver, brain, as well as other organs. The most apparent outward sign is the presence of a Kayser-Fleischer ring, a rusty brown ring around the cornea that is best seen in a slit-lamp examination (see Fig. 67.8). Treatment with zinc acetate, which blocks absorption of copper from the intestine, or D-penicillamine and trientine hydrochloride, drugs that help remove copper from tissue, are lifesaving if the illness is detected before permanent damage is done to the brain or liver.

18. A 7-year-old girl presents to the emergency department with a 12-day history of progressive gait disturbance. At first, the weakness was barely noticeable but now she is having difficulty walking. She had a runny nose for 3 days before the weakness began, but no fever. Her examination shows normal strength in the arms and hips, but moderate weakness in her knees and profound weakness in her ankles. Deep tendon reflexes are absent throughout. A spine MRI is normal. The working diagnosis is acute inflammatory demyelinating polyradiculopathy (AIDP or Guillain-Barré syndrome) and an LP is performed. Which of the following CSF patterns is *most* consistent with this diagnosis?
a) Protein 20 per high-power field (hpf), white blood cells (WBC) 0 hpf, red blood cells (RBC) 0 hpf
b) Protein 20 hpf, WBC 160 hpf, RBC 0 hpf
c) Protein 20 hpf, WBC 0 hpf, RBC 60 hpf
d) Protein 60 hpf, WBC 10 hpf, RBC 0 hpf
e) Protein 60 hpf, WBC 160 hpf, RBC 0 hpf

Answer
The answer is d. The CSF in AIDP shows a rising protein level that is relatively acellular. Although the CSF may appear normal (answer a) during the first few days of the illness, the protein concentration 1 week after the onset of symptoms is clearly above normal.

19. A 17-year-old young man presents to the emergency room after he fainted briefly in the locker room following cross-country running practice. He had no falls or injuries during the run. He is complaining of back and leg pain. Vital signs were normal. A complete blood count and basic chemistry panel were normal. His urine analysis showed a specific gravity of 1.030, with the dipstick being positive for heme, yet the microscopic analysis did not show any RBCs. The lab did note that the urine was tea-colored. The next step in evaluating this patient would be:
a) MRI of the spine
b) CT scan of the abdomen
c) Test for blood creatine kinase (creatine phosphokinase [CPK]) level

d) CT scan of the brain
e) Make sure the lab performs a urine culture

Answer
The answer is c. This is a case of rhabdomyolysis, which may occur in the setting of heat stress and dehydration. In this case, there is no evidence of heat stroke or heat shock given the normal body temperature and normal vital signs. Muscle pain is often present with this diagnosis. The urine specific gravity suggests that the patient is relatively dehydrated. Both myoglobin and hemoglobin levels will make urine dipsticks positive for *heme*, but the microscopic analysis suggests that there is no blood in the urine. A CK will show elevated levels of the MM fraction, indicating skeletal muscle breakdown. The CK measurement may range from 500 U/L to 20,000 U/L and above. Treatment of uncomplicated rhabdomyolysis consists of rehydration and maintenance intravenous fluids and a close evaluation of electrolytes and urine output. Prevention requires adequate hydration during exercise. In patients with recurrent rhabdomyolysis, evaluation for a disorder of fatty acid oxidation or a glycogen storage disease is suggested.

20. A 3-year-old boy with mild developmental delays is being evaluated for recurring seizures. His first seizure was 3 months ago, which was described as left arm twitching lasting for 5 hours before it stopped spontaneously. A brain CT with and without contrast was normal and his EEG was also normal. Since that time his seizures have been both focal and focal with secondary generalization. He has been on four different anticonvulsants, none of which has been effective. He has been admitted twice with status epilepticus and is now being admitted for persistent left-sided seizures involving his arm and leg. His liver enzymes are 10 times the upper limit of normal. His unenhanced brain CT shows diffuse atrophy. Which of the following would be the most likely explanation for his illness?
a) Expanding brain tumor
b) Rasmussen encephalitis
c) Alpers-Huttenlocher syndrome
d) Amebic encephalitis
e) Lyme encephalitis

Answer
The answer is c. Alpers-Huttenlocher syndrome is one of many different allelic presentations for those with mutations in *POLG* (polymerase gamma), the gene that encodes for the mtDNA polymerase. The allelic frequency of mutations in this gene is as high as 2% of the Western European population, and over 150 distinct mutations have been identified in this gene associated with human disease. The spectrum of illness caused by mutations in this gene is under-recognized. In Alpers-Huttenlocher syndrome, the affected children may be

developmentally slow or normal. Although the age of onset can vary, seizures develop usually before age 7 years. These seizures are often difficult to control and status epilepticus and epilepsia partialis continua (focal seizures that will persist despite treatment) are common. The usual course will include cortical blindness, neuropathy, spasticity, dystonia, dementia and cortical atrophy. Death occurs 1 to 20 years after presentation. Liver failure will accompany the neurologic illness and often is the cause of death, but the use of valproate is associated with the rapid onset of liver necrosis. The spectrum and severity of diseases caused by this mutation is enormous, and not only involves the brain, peripheral nervous system and muscle, but also the heart, liver, pancreas, ovaries, and testicles. Psychiatric illness is common in adults with the less fulminate forms of the illness.

21. A developmentally normal 5-year-old girl is evaluated for a brief seizure that began in her left arm and quickly generalized. The seizure lasted 30 seconds and the child was in a postictal state for an hour before returning to normal. She was seen in the emergency department, where a CT of the head was done and was normal. An EEG revealed focal slowing over the right frontal region and an MRI showed focal pachygria of the right frontal lobe. She was treated with an anticonvulsant after her second seizure and has remained seizure-free for 3 years. The child did well at school but speech therapy was initiated by the school for articulation difficulties. The child failed her hearing screen at school and was found to have a mild–moderate sensorineural hearing loss. A repeat MRI did not show any changes. Which of the following should be considered?

a) No further evaluation is necessary
b) A genetics evaluation, and if no further issues are identified, testing is complete
c) Genetic testing for X-linked lissencephaly
d) Genetic testing for Fragile X syndrome
e) FISH testing of 22q11.2 (velocardiofacial syndrome)

Answer

The answer is e. This is a complete presentation of a child with velocardiofacial syndrome, which is associated with deletion at 22q11.2. This microdeletion syndrome involves a portion of the human genome with more than 30 genes within the region of deletion. This

syndrome has a huge array of presenting features in addition to the classic presentations that would include neonatal hypocalcemia, conotruncal cardiac defects, and immune disorders. Most of those affected are not dysmorphic and presentations with features restricted to the rare enormous array of described features are not unique. One under-recognized feature is that psychosis can be common (30%) in this disorder and up to one fourth eventually are diagnosed with schizophrenia. The combination of more than one syndromic feature should suggest to the physician to look for a named (or unidentified disorder). In this case the diagnosis could have been made by ordering the selected FISH test for 22q11.2. This case was actually diagnosed by recognizing the fact that a microdeletion disorder could be the underlying cause of her clinical features (but not recognizing the specific disorder), and ordering a comparative genomic hybridization chip (chromosomal microarray gene chip), which tests for over 100 known microdeletion disorders and screens for unknown microdeletion disorders. Answer b is partially correct in that a genetics consultation is always preferable, but incorrect in failing to recognize the importance of the clinical laboratory in the diagnosis of genetic disorders in those who have multiple congenital anomalies.

SUGGESTED READINGS

1. Evans OB, Vedanarayanan V. Guillain-Barré syndrome. *Pediatr Rev* 1997;18:10–16.
2. Haas RH, Parikh S, Falk MH, et al. The in-depth evaluation of suspected mitochondrial disease. *Mol Genet Metab* 2008;94:16–37.
3. Haas RH, Parikh S, Falk MJ, et al. Mitochondrial disease: a practical approach for primary care physicians. *Pediatrics* 2007;120(6):1326–1333.
4. Haslam RHA. Neurocutaneous syndromes. In: Behrman R, Kliegman R, Jenson H, eds. *Nelson textbook of pediatrics*, 17th ed. Philadelphia: Saunders, 2004:2015–2019.
5. Murphy KC, Scamble PJ, eds. Velo-cardio-facial syndrome: a model for understanding microdeletion disorders. New York: Cambridge University Press, 2005.
6. Parikh S, Cohen BH, Gupta A, et al. Metabolic testing in the pediatric epilepsy unit. *Pediatr Neurol* 2008;38:191–195.
7. Sarnat H. Neuromuscular disorders. In: Behrman R, Kliegman R, Jenson H, eds. *Nelson textbook of pediatrics*, 17th ed. Philadelphia: Saunders, 2004:2053–2082.
8. Segawa M, Nomura Y. Rett syndrome. *Curr Opin Neurol* 2005;18:97–104.
9. Wong L-J C, Naviaux RK, Brunetti-Pierri N, et al. Molecular and clinical genetics of mitochondrial diseases due to *POLG* mutations. *Hum Mutat* 2008;1020(29):E150–E172.

Chapter 38

Normal Child Growth and Development

Mark H. Deis and Roberta E. Bauer

Pediatricians at well-child visits are the first and most consistent screeners of development, and they along with parents monitor growth and gross motor, fine motor, problem-solving, language, and social skills of the child during the first 2 years of life. Knowledge of the functions expected at the time of the customarily scheduled immunization visits enables the pediatrician to estimate the age from an examination description of a typically developing child, or to refer children not achieving expected milestones for additional assessment. This chapter addresses normal growth and development of the child in regard to:

- Parameters of physical growth
- Gross motor milestones
- Fine motor milestones
- Speech and language milestones
- Cognitive and social-emotional milestones

PARAMETERS OF PHYSICAL GROWTH

Physical growth data (Table 38.1) are valuable for providing general trends. The head circumference should grow at an average of:

- 2.0 cm/month during the first 3 months of life
- 1.0 cm/month during months 3 through 6 of life
- 0.5 cm/month from months 6 through 12

The median head circumference for a 3-year-old child would be 50.8 cm. Lengths increase from approximately 50 to 87 cm from birth to the age of 2 years, and then approximately 7 cm a year. Doubling the 2-year-old height provides a reasonable estimate of adult height. *Weights double by 5 months of life, triple by 1 year, and quadruple by 2 years.*

Points to consider regarding physical growth are the following:

- Large or small heads warrant close assessment to detect treatable problems (hydrocephalus, metabolic disturbances or syndromes, anatomic problems, congenital infections) and monitor development.
- Large or small stature can be associated with a number of syndromes, including developmental delays (Soto syndrome and various chromosomal abnormalities).

Careful examination for dysmorphic features can yield diagnostic clues. One should become familiar with the linear growth patterns in various common childhood conditions that inhibit growth, in addition to the trends in growth of tissue types during childhood and adolescence. These patterns are shown in Figures 38.1 and 38.2.

GROSS MOTOR MILESTONES

Gross motor milestones are listed in Table 38.2.

Monitoring progress in motor development makes it possible to identify underlying muscle, peripheral nerve, anterior horn cell, spinal cord, or central nervous system injuries that present in the first 2 years of life with gross motor changes. *Findings that are a cause of concern include:*

- Rolling before 3 months
- Poor head control at 5 months
- Lack of sitting by 9 months
- Persistence of Moro reflex, asymmetric tonic neck reflex, and tonic labyrinthine reflex past 6 months
- Lack of development of protective supportive reactions (e.g., lack of parachute response by 12 months)
- Hand dominance before 18 months
- Inability to walk independently by 18 months

TABLE 38.1

AVERAGE VALUES FOR PHYSICAL GROWTH PARAMETERS IN THE FIRST 2 YEARS OF LIFE

	Head Circumference (cm)	Height (cm)	Weight (kg)
Birth	35	50.8	3–3.5
1 year	47	76	10
2 years	49	88	12–12.5

Rolling before 3 months may occur with hypertonicity. Poor head control in the pull-to-sit maneuver by 5 months may suggest muscle weakness or slowed progress of cephalic–caudal control over the body caused by injury or changes in the central nervous system. Likewise, persistence of primitive reflexes that should have been integrated may indicate a neuromotor disorder. Lack of independent sitting by 7 months or altered sitting in a W position may be caused by hip adductor spasticity or muscle hypotonia. Lack of emergence of an anterior protective response in sitting by 5 months, lateral protective responses in sitting by 7 months, or parachute protective responses by 12 months may indicate neuromotor disorders. The developmental sequence of locomotion beyond 1 year of age changes as improved balance and coordination allow a narrower base

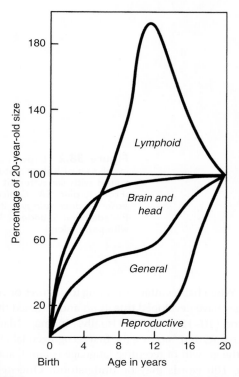

Figure 38.1 Growth patterns of various systems. (From Bickley LS, Hoekelman RA. *Bates's guide to physical examination and history taking*, 7th ed. Philadelphia: Lippincott Williams & Wilkins, 1999:621, with permission.)

of support in the gait. Likewise, time sequences of use of muscle groups allow more complex motor patterns. Running efficiently by 2 years is followed by jumping on two feet, balancing on one foot (36 months), and hopping (48 months), and skipping. *Early motor* control *should be symmetric with strong hand* dominance expected at 18 months or after. *Throwing a ball overhand is present by 23 months but catching requires more integration of eye–hand coordination and is present by 5 years.*

FINE MOTOR MILESTONES

Fine motor milestones are listed in Table 38.3.

Key issues in hand function include loss of obligatory fisting by 3 months, transferring a toy from one hand to the other across the midline by 6 months, and isolating the index finger, which allows pointing by 10 months. Fine motor functioning impacts both communication and self-care independence. Neat pincer function is expected for picking up small objects by 1 year and aids self-feeding; and at that age children can voluntarily release a cube into a cup. Building towers of 1-inch cube blocks improve with two blocks expected at 15 months, four blocks at 18 months, and six blocks at 2 years. By 15 months, children should drink from a cup, by 18 months use a spoon, and by 24 months remove simple clothing, potentially allowing early efforts at toileting. Early vertical, horizontal, and general circular scribbling can be imitated from the examiner's model at 2 years. A practical way to assess fine motor skills is to ask a child to copy a drawn figure:

- 3-year-old: circle
- 4-year-old: cross
- 4.5-year-old: square
- 5-year-old: triangle

Fine motor development may be sensitive to the same delaying factors as gross motor development. In general, the development of fine motor skills proceeds in a proximal-to-distal direction. In children with visual impairment, it may be more efficient to explore with the whole hand rather than just the index finger. Similarly, children with a lack of depth perception or visual acuity may have difficulty with stacking activities. As the use of tools becomes more complex, cognitive delays may be reflected in the fine motor function.

SPEECH AND LANGUAGE MILESTONES

Speech and language milestones are listed in Table 38.4.

Language development is one of the most important parameters of cognitive *and emotional* development. In infancy, language development is categorized as prespeech (birth–10 months); at this time, the skills needed to understand

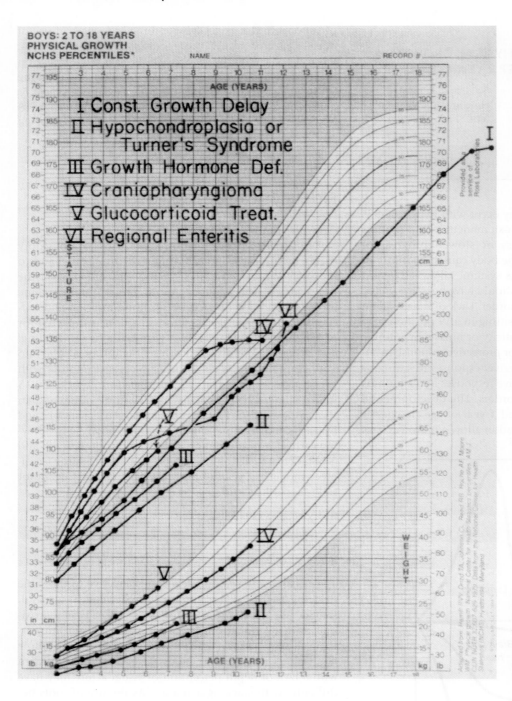

Figure 38.2 Growth patterns in children with short stature associated with six different causes. (From Kaplan SA. *Clinical pediatric endocrinology*, 2nd ed. Philadelphia: Saunders, 1990:51, with permission.)

language (receptive) are acquired by learning to localize sound. Expressive skills begin with cooing (vowel sounds) and differentiated crying when the baby is hungry, hurt, or in need of attention. At 3 months, babies begin vocalizing when they see an adult, and at 5 months, they take turns vocalizing with adults, quieting when the other speaks, and mimicking tone changes, although not actual words. At 6 months, babies add consonants (babbling), and when their parents respond to "mama" and "dada" with smiles and hugs, the baby eventually connects meaning to those sounds. When babies attach meaning to gestures or vocalizations, they have developed true *words* and initiated the naming period (10–18 months). Usually, "mama," "dada," the infant's name, and "no" are the first recognized labels. Once begun, the growth of receptive language is rapid, and by 12 months, 100 words may be understood. One-step commands associated with a gesture can be understood by the child at 1 year of age, and the need for a gesture is lost in a few months. The development of expressive skills progresses more slowly, with most children having at least one true

TABLE 38.2
GROSS MOTOR MILESTONES

Age	Gross Motor Skill	Mobility
Newborn	Moves symmetrically	Lies down
2 months	Lifts shoulders up in prone position	Head up in prone position
	Head bobs in supported sitting position	
3–4 months	Up on forearms in prone position	Puppy prop
	Rolls from front to back	Extended arms
	Steady head control while sitting	
	Bears weight on legs when standing	
5–6 months	Tripod sitting (propped by hands)	Rolls back to front
		Tripod sitting
	No head lag on pulling to sit from supine position	
	Sits with support	
7 months	Bounces in supported standing	Free sitting
	Supports weight in standing with assistance for balance	
	Feet to mouth	
	Commando crawls	
8 months	Gets to sitting position	Reaches
	Reaches with one hand from four-point kneeling from quad	
9 months	Sits without support	
11 months	Stands	
12 months	Independent steps	Steps
		Pulls to stand
	Creeps	Cruises
15 months	Walks well independently	
	Plays ball with examiner	
	Gives and takes a toy	
	Stoops to floor and recovers to standing position	
16 months	Creeps up stairs	
	Stoops and recovers	
	Walks backward	
18 months	Walks fast, seldom falls	
	Runs stiffly	
	Walks up stairs with one hand held	
	Pushes/pulls large objects	
	Throws ball while standing	
	Seats self in small chair	
	Climbs onto an adult chair	
24 months	Kicks ball	
	Jumps in place (both feet off floor)	
	Throws a ball overhand	
	Walks up stairs by placing both feet on same step	
36 months	Walks up stairs by alternating feet	
	Walks well on toes	
	Stands on one foot for 1–2 seconds	
	Broad jumps	
	Jumps from a step	
	Hops two or three times	
	Pedals tricycle	
4 years	Dresses without help	
	Walks up and down stairs by alternating feet	
	Balances on one foot for 3 seconds	
	Hops on one foot	
5 years	Tandem walks backward	
	Skips by alternating feet	
	Hops ten times	
6 years	Rides a bicycle	

TABLE 38.3
FINE MOTOR MILESTONES

Age	Fine Motor Function
Newborn	Hands tightly fisted
2 months	Holds rattle briefly if placed in hand
3 months	Hands *unfisted* most of time, bats at objects
4 months	Retains rattle
	Scratches and clutches at objects while supine
5 months	Transfers objects from hand to mouth to hand
	Palmar grasp of objects (thumb adducted)
6 months	*Transfers* objects from hand to hand across midline
	Reaches for objects
	Has radial palmar grasp of a cube
	Rakes at pellet with whole hand on contact
7 months	Radial palmar grasp of cube
	Pulls round peg out
8 months	Scissors grasp of pellet
	Holds cube in each hand
9 months	Inferior pincer grasp of pellet
	Feeds self with fingers
	Plays gesture games (pat-a-cake, wave bye-bye) in imitation
	Bangs two objects together
	Holds two objects at one time
10 months	Isolated *index* finger, pincer grasp pellet
12 months	Fine pincer grasp of raisin or pellet with fingertips
	Releases cube voluntarily into a cup
	Marks with crayon
	Drinks from a cup held by another individual
15 months	Plays ball with examiner
	Gives and takes a toy
	Drinks from a cup
	Scribbles with a crayon
	Puts cube into a cup
16 months	Releases pellet into container, cube into cup
	Tower of three cubes
	Imitates scribble
	Drinks from a cup
18 months	Tower of four cubes
	Imitates single stroke
	Spontaneous scribbling
	Turns two to three pages of a book at one time
	Feeds self with spoon
24 months	Tower of four to six cubes
	Train of cubes
	Turns single pages of a book
	Washes and dries hands
	Removes clothing
	Puts on a hat
	Feeds self with spoon and fork
36 months	Tower of eight cubes
	Imitates vertical stroke with crayon
	Copies a circle, imitates cross
	Imitates bridge of three cubes
	Puts on tee shirt, shorts
48 months	*Copies a cross*
	Draws an individual with two to four parts plus head
	Imitates gate of five cubes
60 months	Copies a square
	Draws an individual with six body parts
	Ties a knot in string
	Grabs a pencil maturely
	Prints letters
72 months	Writes name

word before their first birthday and most of their verbalization consisting of complicated multisyllabic consonant and vowel sounds with intonation changes, called *jargon*. By the end of the naming period, 18-month-old children use approximately 25 meaningful words spontaneously.

Pointing is also an important expressive modality. Infants begin pointing at objects and looking at adults expectantly in the hope of acquiring the objects (referred to as *protoimperative pointing*). Later, the infant may first point to an object and then point to an adult while vocalizing. Next, infants may point to an interesting object in an attempt to get an adult to focus attention on the same object. The object becomes a tool for gaining a parent's attention, and this desire/ability of infants to share interest in an object with a caregiver is a social action called *protodeclarative pointing*. It is frequently recognized by 14 months, should be present by 18 months, and is an important milestone in distinguishing social communicative intent. Finally, infants point at objects and vocalize questioningly to adults in an effort to learn labels; this phenomenon (referred to as *pointing for naming*) is a helpful strategy in extending expressive vocabularies. Pointing can also be used to demonstrate receptive language skills, and infants begin to take part in pointing games after they realize that individuals and objects have labels. Therefore, by year 1, we can expect fine motor development to allow isolated use of the index finger, and by 15 months we can see infants able to point to a body part or favorite toy. Beyond 18 months, we can use screening instruments to ask young children to indicate choices with pointing.

Beyond 18 months is the word combination period. Six to eight months after the emergence of true words, children start combining words. It may begin with combinations the child hears together frequently—"go bye-bye," "thank you," "all done"; however, these do not qualify as separate word phrases. True phrases begin to appear after a vocabulary of approximately 50 words has been acquired and should be present by 2 years. The beginning combinations are described as *telegraphic speech*. More sophisticated grammatic and syntactic structures evolve during the next years and are sensitive to environmental modeling in typically developing children.

The most common cause of language delay is cognitive delay, but hearing impairment, oral–motor incoordination (as in cerebral palsy), environmental deprivation, and autism spectrum disorder can all present with expressive language delay. It should be remembered that even children with complete hearing impairment coo and continue to vocalize, although with less tone variation and frequency than children who can hear. Hearing-impaired children also become expert at noting visual cues and may follow commands associated with gestures, so that it appears they have heard. Milder hearing losses may present as attentional problems or articulation difficulty. Difficulty in localizing sounds, or in some cases inattention, may suggest unilateral hearing loss.

Important language milestones are summarized in Table 38.5.

TABLE 38.4
SPEECH AND LANGUAGE MILESTONES

Age	Receptive	Expressive
1 month	Alerts to sound	Cries
2 months	Regards speaker	Social smile
		Coos
		Reciprocal vocalizations
4 months	Looks toward voice	Laughs out loud
6 months	Turns toward voice	Babbles "baba" "gaga" (consonant sounds)
		Imitates speech sounds
9 months	Associates meaning with words	"Mama/dada" inappropriate
	Orients to name	Waves good-bye
10 months	Comprehends "no"	
11 months	Looks for named caregiver	First word
12 months	Follows command with gesture	"Dada/mama" appropriate
		Says at least one specific word (in addition to "mama/dada")
		Points at desired object
14 months	Follows command without gesture	Names one object
		Says "no" meaningfully
		Protodeclarative pointing
15 months	Points to body part	Three to five words, jargon
		Follows simple commands
		Indicates some needs or desires by pointing
18 months	Points to three body parts	10–25 Words
	Points to self	Names picture on command
		Uses words for wants or needs
		Identifies one or more parts of the body
24 months	Two-step commands	50+ Words
	Understands "me/you"	Two- to three-word sentences (noun, verb)
	Points to six pictures	>50% intelligibility
		Refers to self by name
		Uses "I," "me," "mine"
36 months	Knows age and sex	Repeats six-syllable sentence
		Speaks in five- to eight-word sentences
		Names a playmate
		Knows simple adjectives (i.e., tired, hungry, thirsty)
		~75% Intelligibility
48 months	Counts to 4	Tells a story
		~100% Intelligibility
60 months	Counts to 10	Names four colors, repeats ten-syllable sentence

TABLE 38.5
SUMMARY OF IMPORTANT LANGUAGE MILESTONES

Age	Milestones
2 months	Smiles
6 months	Localizes sound and babbles
12 months	Uses "mama/dada" appropriately
	Follows a one-step command with gesture
	Has one true word
	Points to indicate need
14 months	Protodeclarative pointing
18 months	Points to three body parts
	Uses 10 to 25 words
2 years	Two-step commands
	Two-word sentences
	Fifty-word vocabulary
	Fifty percent intelligent speech

COGNITIVE AND SOCIAL–EMOTIONAL MILESTONES

Cognitive milestones are listed in Table 38.6, and social–emotional milestones in Table 38.7.

Cognitive processing depends on attention, information processing, and memory. It can be assessed by measures of comprehension, reasoning, and judgment. Standardized testing of intellectual abilities is available after infancy to measure the intelligence quotient (IQ) on the basis of verbal and nonverbal performance. During infancy, the attainment of language milestones and the emergence of problem-solving, play, and adaptive strategies are indicators of cognitive development. As children perceive how the world around them works, cognitive, social, emotional, and adaptive behavioral changes are closely intertwined during certain stages of development.

During the first months of life, the ways in which an infant seeks and takes in sensory information by sound,

TABLE 38.6
COGNITIVE MILESTONES

Age	Milestones
Term infant	Alerts to sound (bell or voice)
	Fixates on face or object and follows briefly
2 months	Follows an object through 180-degree arc
	Has facial response to a bell ring
4 months	Takes dangling ring to mouth or regards in hand
6 months	Transfers a ring across midline and regards by manipulating
	Mouthing to explore, still regardless of function (bell, cube)
10 months	Explores with index finger details of objects, bangs two objects together
	Uncovers toys hidden under cloth as child watches the hiding
12 months	Plays with toys appropriate to function (rings bell not mouths it)
	Explores bell mechanism with index finger
	Follows command associated with gesture (give me)
	Points to make needs known, at least one word
15 months	Points to one body part, dumps pellet after demonstration
	Places circle in a form board
18 months	Points to self, names a picture, 10–25 words, matches pairs of objects, symbolic play with doll
2 years	Sorts objects, uses words to make needs known
	Understands me/you, another, two-step commands
3 years	Pretends involving others in theme
4 years	Names four colors
	Asks questions (e.g., when? why? how?)
	Relates events
5 years	Prepares bowl of cereal
	Plays board or card games
	Defines words
	Counts five blocks
	Names all primary colors
6 years	Counts 10 objects
	Knows right from left
	Copies two-part figure

TABLE 38.7
SOCIAL AND EMOTIONAL MILESTONES

Age	Milestones
Full-term infant	Alerts to sound (bell or voice)
	Fixates on face or object and follows briefly
4 months	Laughs out loud, squeals
	Initiates social contact
8 months	Gaze monitoring
9–12 months	Stranger distress behaviors
10 months	Following a point, turns when name called
12 months	Pointing to request, bringing or giving behaviors
14 months	Pointing to comment
18 months	Feeds self with utensils, with spills
	Carries or hugs a doll
2 years	Pretend play (puts doll to bed, feeds doll, pours from teapot)
3 years	Names playmate, includes others in pretending
4 years	Displays cooperative play, interest in gender specific tasks

vision, and touch change. The newborn's focus on the face, changes in breathing or sucking pattern in response to novel sounds, and preference for nutritive or non-nutritive sucking of objects placed in the mouth indicate sensory awareness, even at this early stage. Infants generally follow a visual stimulus to the midline by 2 to 4 weeks of age, and past the midline by 8 weeks of age. Most infants begin to look at their own hands for at least several seconds by the age of 8 weeks. It is clearly abnormal for a baby to lack visual tracking by 4 months of age. As the motoric organization and coordination of infants improve, they assume a more active role in exploring the environment, visually orienting themselves to sources of sound, and placing their hands or objects in their mouths (by 5 months). With improving fine motor control, infants can hold an object in one hand while touching it with the other and *manipulating* it for further exploration by 6 months. Typical oral–motor play at 6 months consists of using a palmar grasp to obtain an object, transferring it to the opposite hand to regard it further, and then placing it in the mouth to finish the evaluation. Improved visual acuity allows the baby to discriminate strangers from familiar caregivers, with the potential for an emergence of *stranger anxiety* behaviors.

The lengthened attention span of the 9- or 10-month-old child allows a truer *inspection* of toys with use of the improving fine motor functions of an isolated index finger and inferior pincer grasp. The baby can now begin to compare two objects, each held in one hand, and combine toys to produce interesting results (bangs blocks on a table at 9 months or together at 10 months). The memory capacity to recall that objects still exist even when they are out of sight or touch can be demonstrated in the 9-month-old child who uncovers a toy hidden from view by a cloth. This object permanence function can be used to help parents understand the emerging separation *distress* behaviors their appropriately attached and developing 9- to 12-month-old child may demonstrate. When parents leave the room or stray from voice range, they are *out of sight but* no longer *out of mind* for their infant. Likewise, the baby's fascination with the fatiguing game of "drop the toy off the high chair, then grunt, and point for mom to pick it up" can be framed as a cognitive and communicative advance by 1 year of age.

Information from the treatment of children with autism spectrum leads us to attend more carefully to the development of *joint attention* in typically developing children. "Coordinating attention between an object and an individual in a social context" defines joint attention. It is measured by milestones such as gaze monitoring at 8 months. (Children and caregivers gazing into each other's eyes, who are interrupted when the mother looks away at the clock, for example, and the child also looks at the clock then looks back to the mother to see if she's focused on him again.) Next comes *following a point* at 10 months when the child demonstrates looking at the object or an individual the caregiver is directing attention to with a pointed finger. Protoimperative pointing (pointing at things desired) by the child, and *bringing* behaviors (physically handing objects of interest to caregivers but expecting them back) are expected at 1 year of age. By 14 to 15 months, children should be *pointing to comment* (protodeclarative) on interesting things they wish to share attention to with their caregivers. Studies link the development of shared attention to the development of verbal language within a year, but joint attention milestones also provide tools to measure social relatedness important for early identification of children with autism spectrum.

By 1 year of age, infants play with objects that they find interesting. Well beyond the oral–motor transferring and mouthing strategies, the baby tries out functional play, attempting to stack blocks, shaking a bell, or using objects as tools. The 1-year-old infant who only mouths or transfers and drops toys warrants concern for cognitive progress.

With advances in functional play come advances in the infant's understanding of causality. Young babies will repeat an action that causes an interesting result—4-month-old babies may shake a rattle again after it makes a noise. The emergence of deliberate behavior and intent in babies can be observed at 8 months when they use tools to obtain a desired object (pull an attached string to secure a ring) or when they use their improved mobility skills to move to get a toy. At 1 year, the use of tools in a manner specific to their function parallels the emergence of the use of true words—a dawn of the idea that sounds have a function. Likewise, the idea emerges that the babies have a sort of function themselves—they have an effect on those around them. One-year-old infants begin to smile and cry to produce effects that are goal-directed and intentional in those around them. They are said to have a concept of themselves and to have their own *will* that are demonstrable. They demonstrate some solitary play and begin forming different types of relationships with caregivers than with strangers. Fifteen-month-old children demonstrate pride in their own accomplishments and may clap for themselves. They may express behaviors suggesting that they feel shame or guilt or contempt. They may demonstrate symbolic play with themselves—sipping from an empty cup. By 19 months, children may be able to associate feelings with their verbal labels. They may use early pretend play with dolls—feeding the doll from a spoon. During the second year, whereas language expression is exploding, the development of inner language and thought is also thought to be emerging and may be cautiously inferred from play behaviors.

Past 24 months, children can begin to choose whether to demonstrate feelings or not, according to the reactions of those around them. The socialization process of modulating or masking emotions can be observed. The whole challenge of parenting a 2-year-old child is to shape the expression of emotion into adaptive ways to interact with others while allowing the child to retain an inner self and will. Two-year-old children are still interested in imitating others to please them—just not all the time. They engage in parallel play with peers, and more imaginary play evolves between 2 and 3 years.

Toilet Training

Bowel and bladder control typically evolves in the following order:

- Nocturnal bowel control
- Daytime bowel control
- Daytime control of voiding

Seventy-five percent of children are fully toilet trained by 3 years. Nocturnal enuresis occurs in up to 15% of 5-year-old children; it ceases in approximately 15% of involved children each year thereafter.

REVIEW EXERCISES

QUESTIONS

1. The skills of kicking a ball and jumping in place are gross motor milestones that occur at which age?
a) 15 months
b) 18 months
c) 24 months
d) 30 months

Answer
The answer is c.

2. A 4-year-old child should be able to:
a) Ride a bicycle
b) Hop on one foot
c) Skip by alternating the feet
d) Tandem walk backward

Answer
The answer is b.

3. The ability to *follow a point* occurs at what age?
a) 8 months
b) 10 months
c) 15 months
d) 18 months

Answer
The answer is b.

4. The ability to build a tower of three cubes occurs at what age?
a) 15 months
b) 16 months

c) 18 months
d) 24 months

Answer
The answer is b.

5. A vocabulary of 50 or more words and the ability to speak in two- and three-word sentences should be acquired by what age?
a) 15 months
b) 18 months
c) 24 months
d) 30 months

Answer
The answer is c.

SUGGESTED READINGS

1. Beker L, Cheng TL. Principles of growth assessment. *Pediatr Rev* 2006;27:196–198.
2. Colson ER, Dworkin PH. Toddler development. *Pediatr Rev* 1997;18:255–259.
3. Dawson P. Normal growth and revised growth charts. *Pediatr Rev* 2002;23:255–256.
4. Grizzle KL, Simms MD. Early language development and language learning disabilities. *Pediatr Rev* 2005;26:274–283.
5. Lord C. *Education of children with autism.* Washington, DC: National Academy of Science Press, 2001.
6. Oelberg DG. Consultation with the specialist: prenatal growth: the sum of maternal, placental, and fetal contributions. *Pediatr Rev* 2006;27:224–229.
7. Rosen DS. Physiologic growth and development during adolescence. *Pediatr Rev* 2004;25:194–200.
8. Sturner RA, Howard BJ. Preschool development part 1: communicative and motor aspects. *Pediatr Rev* 1997;18:291–301.
9. Sturner RA, Howard BJ. Preschool development part 2: psychosocial/behavioral development. *Pediatr Rev* 1997;18:327–336.

Chapter 39

Developmental Disabilities

Roberta E. Bauer and Mark H. Deis

The developmental disabilities reviewed in this chapter include:

- Mental retardation (MR)
- Cerebral palsy (CP)
- Myelomeningocele (MMC)
- Autism and pervasive developmental disorder
- Attention deficit hyperactivity disorder (ADHD)
- Fetal alcohol syndrome
- Learning disabilities/educational issues
- Language/speech delay

MENTAL RETARDATION

The features of MR are summarized in Table 39.1.

Etiology and Epidemiology

Standardized measures of intelligence assume that intelligence occurs along a Gaussian (bell-shaped) distribution curve. MR is defined as an intelligence quotient (IQ) that is more than two standard deviations below the mean for that age (i.e., an IQ of 70 seen in 3% of the population)

TABLE 39.1

SUMMARY OF MENTAL RETARDATION

- Diagnosis: IQ <70, onset before 18 years, in association with adaptive behavior disturbances
- Risk factors: growth disturbances, dysmorphologies, perinatal complications, head trauma, genetics
- Biomedical causes more likely to be found in more severely affected individuals
- Presentations
  - Neonatal: dysmorphia, metabolic instability, neurologic syndromes
  - 3–6 Months: colic, visual or hearing deficits, feeding problems, abnormal tone
  - 6–12 Months: motor delay, abnormal tone
  - 12–24 Months: motor delay, language delay
  - >24 Months: language delay, behavioral disturbance, problem-solving delay
- Effects in all spheres of function; global delays characterize mental retardation

IQ, intelligence quotient.

on a standardized IQ test. The diagnosis of MR requires poor performance both on standardized tests of intelligence and in daily adaptive behavior (must be significantly limited in adaptive functioning in at least two of the following: communication, self-care, social skills, self-direction, academic skills, work, leisure activities, health, and safety). Because of the requirement that affected individuals must meet both criteria, the overall prevalence of MR is 1% to 2%.

Several classification schema exist, but classification according to IQ scores is most often defined as:

- 70 to 85, borderline normal intelligence
- 50 to 70, mild MR
- 35 to 50, moderate MR
- 20 to 35, severe MR
- <20, profound MR

This classification scheme is slowly being replaced by a scheme on the basis of "Intensity of Needed Levels of Support" required by the child: intermittent, limited, extensive, or pervasive.

Intelligence is remarkably stable over time, so that an individual with an IQ of 60 can be expected to acquire new skills at a rate 60% of that of an individual with average intelligence. Common causes of MR may be:

- Metabolic
  - Lysosomal storage disease (includes the mucopolysaccharidoses, mucolipidoses, and oligosaccharidoses; organic acidemias and aminoacidemias)
  - Leukodystrophies
  - Any postnatal condition that can cause hyperbilirubinemia, hypoglycemia, or hypernatremia

- Chromosomal
  - Trisomies (13, 18, 21)
  - Fragile X syndrome
  - X-linked disorders
  - Translocations and deletions
- Infectious
  - Congenital TORCH (toxoplasmosis, rubella, cytomegalovirus, herpes simplex) infection
  - Perinatally acquired human immunodeficiency virus infection
  - Postnatally acquired meningitis and encephalitis
- Teratogenic
  - Alcohol, drugs, radiation, maternal phenylketonuria, and lead

Clinical Presentation

The most common presenting symptom of MR, when identified after the age of 2 years, is language delay. Before 18 months of age, the most common presenting feature is delayed achievement of gross motor milestones.

Gross motor delay does not predict MR, nor is gross motor delay seen in most children with MR. In most children with mild to moderate MR, the early motor milestones are normal. The issues are the following:

- Most parents and professionals are best at recalling gross motor milestones.
- Language skills are still rather rudimentary before 18 months.
- Accurate testing of cognition is extremely difficult during the first few years of life.

The age at which delay in cognitive development first becomes apparent usually correlates with the degree of MR:

- Identification before 2 years of age predicts severe or profound MR.
- Identification after 2 years of age predicts moderate to mild MR.
- Mild MR and borderline intelligence may not be recognized until a child enters school.

In children with structural anomalies, neurocutaneous or metabolic disorders, or syndromes associated with dysmorphic changes that are apparent prenatally or at birth, MR can be diagnosed very early, but only a small percentage of the total population of children with MR are affected by such conditions. Neurologic abnormalities are frequently associated with MR. Neonatal coma or intractable seizures are strongly related to abnormal developmental outcomes. Other neurologic signs are more common but less specific. Abnormal muscle tone, difficulty in feeding, seizures, and gross motor delays (*neurologic soft signs*) all serve as markers of developmental dysfunction. Abnormal muscle tone on evaluation warrants an assessment of other aspects of brain function, although muscle tone by itself is not believed to be directly related to cognition.

Diagnosis

There is no single gold standard for the medical evaluation for children with suspected or proven MR. Evaluation should be directed by patient history and physical examination, and a family pedigree. Possible considerations include the following:

- Audiologic, vision, and speech/autism screening should be done in all children suspected of having MR.
- Periodic screening for serum levels of lead and testing for anemia should be performed when indicated.
- Children with confirmed serum levels of lead between 10 and 20 μg/dL have been shown to score two to five points lower on standardized IQ testing when other variables are controlled.
- Dysmorphic children or children with a significant family history of developmental delay should undergo chromosomal studies (include testing for fragile X syndrome if most of the affected family members are male).
- The number of dysmorphologic features is not predictive of IQ unless neuroimaging shows abnormalities of the gray matter.
- Children with signs of motor delay and cognitive delay or failure to thrive may benefit from studies done to assess for inborn errors of amino acid or organic acid metabolism.
- Weakness or floppy muscle tone should suggest the possibility of muscular dystrophy, in which case a serum creatine phosphokinase or aldolase determination may be diagnostically helpful.
- Thyroid screening should be considered if indicated by growth changes or symptoms.
- Electroencephalography, computed tomography, and magnetic resonance imaging (MRI) are generally reserved for children with asymmetric findings on neurologic examination, weakness, seizures, abnormal head growth, blindness, deafness, or other changing impairments. However, MRI evaluations yield subtle findings of cerebral dysgenesis in children who present with MR or learning problems, even when their neurologic examination findings appear normal. Abnormalities of cerebral migration or subtle anatomic changes may have a genetic basis. In such cases, notification of the family is warranted, and the recommendations regarding imaging studies in children with MR may be changed, even when no imminent clinical action is taken based on the results of the studies.
- When considering laboratory and imaging evaluations for underlying etiologies of intellectual impairment, the following statistics are pertinent:
  - Specific etiology of mild mental retardation is identifiable in <50% of individuals. A definite genetic cause is found in about 5% of mild MR although familial clustering of individuals of MR is common.
  - Mothers who never completed high school are four times more likely to have children with mild MR than mothers who completed high school.
- A definite genetic cause can now be identified in about 50% of severely mentally retarded individuals. There are more than 500 chromosomal and non-chromosomal dysmorphic syndromes associated with intellectual impairment. These are updated and found listed at the National Institute of Health website at http://www.ncbi.nlm.nih.gov/omim.
- Down syndrome, Fragile X, and fetal alcohol spectrum disorder together account for about 1/3 of all identifiable causes of severe intellectual disabilities.
- Recurrence risk in families with one child with severe intellectual disability of *unknown* origin is 3% to 9%. Known origin risks vary with the cause.

Comorbidities

Neurobehavioral disturbances resulting from disordered neural functioning, although not unique to MR, are a frequent accompaniment. During infancy, these disturbances may present as excessive colic, inconsolability, disturbed interactional abilities, or disturbances in the sleep–wake cycle.

Strauss syndrome, which is characterized by attentional disturbance (either too short or perseverative), distractibility, impulsivity, and temper tantrums, may present in preschool children with MR. Although mildly retarded children may resemble those with *classic* hyperactivity, more significantly retarded children do not resemble children with ADHD clinically. Bruxism, rocking, or other perseverative motor behaviors and self-injurious or aggressive behaviors are characteristic of *expanded Strauss syndrome*. These are seen in more severely retarded children. However, it should be recalled that head banging, bruxism, and similar behaviors are seen in normal children also.

Secondary emotional problems may arise when children are unable to cope with familial, educational, or peer expectations.

Engaging in oppositional behaviors to avoid failure or frustration is also a common presentation of MR during the preschool and early elementary school years. Aggression, self-abusive behavior, and psychiatric disorders are a greater detriment to successful integration into the community than decreased cognitive functioning per se.

Speech, language, and hearing disorders, seizures, motor impairments and/or CP, sleep disorders, and visual disorders are also seen often in children with MR.

Prognosis

In most children with MR (i.e., 85%–90% of affected children), the condition is mild, and they can be expected to live independently, read at a fourth to sixth grade level, maintain a competitive semiskilled job, and be physically and psychologically capable of parenthood.

Children with moderate MR may require some degree of support and supervision as adults (usually in a supportive extended family setting or supervised group home).

They have academic skills that range from prekindergarten to third grade level.

Adult outcome cannot be predicted by IQ alone because it does not account for social adaptation and functioning (both of which have a tremendous effect).

CEREBRAL PALSY

The features of cerebral palsy (CP) are summarized in Table 39.2.

Etiology and Epidemiology

CP is defined as persistent impaired motor function or posture that is evident at birth or becomes evident during early infancy. It is not progressive (i.e., it is a static encephalopathy, although the clinical manifestations may evolve and/or change over the course of the child's lifetime) and usually not genetic, although it may be part of a genetic syndrome. If it is unclear whether a child's condition is nonprogressive, the child should not be given a diagnosis of CP. Gross or microscopic changes in the brain are found in <50% of affected patients. Also, although the definition of CP is defined as motor control problems, the white matter CNS injury is associated with more subtle gray matter effects that can impact learning and cognition in children with cerebral palsy.

The overall incidence in the general population is 2 to 3 in 1000 live births. The prevalence is 1.4 to 2.4/1000 children by early school age. The incidence in preterm infants is inversely proportional to their gestational age. Children born prematurely currently represent about one half of the children newly diagnosed with cerebral palsy.

Although the cause is unknown in most cases, risk factors include:

- Intraventricular hemorrhage into the germinal matrix/periventricular leukomalacia
- Apgar score of 3 or lower at 10 minutes
- Hypoxic-ischemic encephalopathy in very few cases
- Congenital brain malformations
- Chromosomal abnormalities and certain syndromes
- Intrauterine growth restriction
- Postnatal events (e.g., meningitis or brain trauma)
- Premature birth before 28 weeks
- Multiple gestations
- Fetal infections (cytomegalovirus, toxoplasmosis)
- Maternal chorioamnionitis or hypercoagulopathies

Clinical Presentation

Spastic diplegia presents initially with hypotonia, and delay in sitting, standing, and ambulating is typical. Six-month-old children who are floppy with brisk deep tendon reflexes in the lower extremities, fall backward when

---

TABLE 39.2

SUMMARY OF CEREBRAL PALSY

- Static central nervous system lesion affecting motor function, onset before 1 year
- Multiple causes of central nervous system injury before birth, at birth, during myelinization
- Most cases occur in term infants, but premature birth is a leading risk factor
- Must rule out progressive degenerative disorders or treatable lesions (tumor, hydrocephalus)
- Types defined by areas involved (hemiplegia, diplegia, quadriplegia) and by type of motor impairment or abnormal movement
- Presentation
  All types: delayed motor skills
  - Spastic types:
    Hypotonia that progresses at 6 months to hypertonia
    Increased deep tendon reflexes
    Sitting delayed by tight hip flexors, ambulation by tight hip adductors
  - Athetoid type: hypotonia that progresses to rigidity at 12–18 months
  - Atonic type: hypotonia associated with profound global delays
  - Ataxic type:
    Hypotonia with normal deep tendon reflexes but poor sitting
    Balance impairment, broad-based gait starting at approximately 18 months Intention tremors, usually after 2 years
- Comorbidities
  - Visual acuity problems or strabismus (75% spastic diplegia or quadriplegia)
  - High-frequency hearing impairment (70% athetoid, 30% other types)
  - Mental retardation (50% of all cases, highest rate with atonic type or quadriparesis)
  - Seizures (highest rate with hemiplegia)
  - Scoliosis or progressive orthopaedic contractures or deformations
  - Oral motor coordination problems (feeding, speech, drooling)
- Other issues (depression, attention deficit hyperactivity disorder, learning disabilities, reflux, obesity, feeding difficulties, and constipation)

attempting to sit, and stiffen from the top of the head down through the hips and knee to support their weight on tiptoe when attempting to stand, are likely to have spastic diplegia.

In children with spastic quadriplegia, all four extremities are affected with tightness and exaggerated reflexes, and the incidence of associated neurobehavioral problems, such as seizures, MR, strabismus, and oral motor dysfunctions, is higher. Spastic hemiparesis commonly becomes evident when asymmetries in tone or reflexes develop, usually after 4 months of age. Parents may note fisting on the affected side or early handedness. Late crawling or dragging one leg with an asymmetric push-off or support with the upper extremities may also be the presenting complaint. The full extent of spasticity and motor deficit may not be apparent until 3 years of age.

The child with athetoid CP may demonstrate hypertonicity very early, which then appears to resolve by 3 months of age. The motor milestones are delayed by *floppiness* in the presence of normal deep tendon reflexes. An obligatory asymmetric tonic neck response may be present. By 10 months of age, the child may use raking movements rather than the expected pincer grasp, but it is not until 12 to 18 months of age that involuntary dystonic posturing is manifested during voluntary attempts at movement. Around this age, the hypotonia evolves into rigid or cogwheel hypertonicity.

The ataxic type of CP presents with hypotonia of the trunk and extremities, but the deep tendon reflexes are normal. When ambulation is attempted, children lock their knees in hyperextension and use a broad-based gait to assist with balance. Walking is late, but it is rare to see head titubation or intention tremor during infancy.

Diagnosis

The diagnosis of CP is difficult to ascertain before 6 months for the following reasons:

- Most movement in normal infants at this age is under reflexive control, not cortical (volitional) control.
- Transient abnormalities in tone resulting from perinatal insults may resolve or at least change during the first year of life; for example, many children with eventual spastic diplegic CP are initially hypotonic for several months.

Tone, primitive reflexes, and deep tendon reflexes are the mainstays of physical diagnosis in CP.

During infancy, tone can be assessed by placing the infant in prone, supine, and suspended prone positions as well as in supported sitting and standing positions. Alternatively, one can assess the passive range of motion of the joints, or the active range of motion of the reflecting muscle groups (i.e., flexor/extensor, adductor/abductor). Newborns held in prone suspension should demonstrate flexor posturing of the trunk and extremities. By 6 weeks,

the head should be even with the body, and slightly less flexion of the arms and legs should be noted. If the head is hyperextended or the legs extend upward above the plane of the body, hypertonus is present. In vertical suspension, scissoring of the lower extremities after 2 months is also evidence of increased hip adductor tone.

Primitive reflexes can also provide clues to abnormal maturation of voluntary muscle control.

- The asymmetric tonic neck response should never be obligatory. (Roughly translated, this means that the response lasts for more than 30 seconds.) Persistent evidence of even a nonobligatory asymmetric tonic neck response beyond 6 months of age strongly suggests central nervous system (CNS) damage.
- Persistence of the Moro response beyond 6 months or absence of righting responses or parachute protective responses beyond 12 months strongly suggests abnormal maturation of the CNS voluntary movement pathways.

If a deep tendon reflex is increased or clonic, or if the area over which percussion can elicit a reflex is exaggerated, upper motor neuron injury is likely.

The classification of CP is based on the type of motor disorder, not on the cause. Four types are described, and a mix of the types is found in 20% of patients. The types are as follows:

- Spastic or *pyramidal* (65%)
- Dyskinetic or *extrapyramidal* (25%)
- Ataxic (5%)
- Hypotonic (5%)

In the *spastic or "pyramidal" type*, the upper motor neurons are involved. The characteristics are weakness, increased muscle tone, increased deep tendon reflexes, clonus, "clasp-knife" tightness or spasticity, extended and "scissored" (crossed) legs, and a tendency to develop contractures. This type may be further divided according to the areas of the body that are affected. In quadriplegia (also called *quadriparesis*), all four limbs are involved, whereas in diplegia both legs are involved primarily, with minimal arm involvement. The diplegic form is the most common; it is frequently seen after intraventricular hemorrhage or is associated with the development of periventricular leukomalacia. The incidence of both of these conditions (intraventricular hemorrhage and periventricular leukomalacia) is increased in association with a younger gestational age in premature infants. In hemiplegia, both limbs are involved on the same side.

The *dyskinetic or extrapyramidal type* causes abnormalities in muscle tone and consists of several subtypes: an athetotic form, chorea, dystonia, tremor, and rigidity. The athetotic form, the most common subtype in this category, involves impairment of volitional movements. Uncontrolled and purposeless movements are evident when the child is awake but disappear during sleep. Previously, the most frequent cause was hyperbilirubinemia/kernicterus, but at present it is hypoxic-ischemic encephalopathy (with resultant damage to the basal ganglia). The other subtypes are as follows:

- Chorea: rapid, irregular limb movements
- Dystonia: slow twisting of the proximal limbs, neck, and trunk
- Tremor: alternating contractions
- Rigidity: contractions in the flexor and extensor muscles

The ataxic type of CP is characterized by gait imbalance and incoordination. The most common cause is hydrocephalus or various genetic syndromes.

The hypotonic type may evolve into one of the three other types.

Comorbidities

MR is a comorbid factor in 50% to 60% of the cases. The incidence varies with the type of CP: 40% in patients with hemiplegia and 70% in those with quadriplegia. Of affected children, 15% have mild MR, 35% moderate MR, and 50% severe MR. *Hearing deficits* occur in 30% of cases of CP, mostly in children with the athetoid form, because of the association with hyperbilirubinemia. *Seizures* occur in 30% to 50% of cases, most commonly in hemiplegic children, least often in the athetoid form. *Drooling* is most common in children with involvement of the pseudobulbar system. Visual deficits, feeding and associated growth abnormalities, and behavioral and emotional disorders are also seen.

Treatment

Therapies to address the functional implications of difficulty with voluntary movement are the mainstays of treatment in CP. The goals of therapy are to:

- Establish mobility and prevent contractures by the use of orthoses and antispasticity treatments.
- Address communication problems in patients with dysarthria, dyspraxia, or central language disorders. (Manifestations of pseudobulbar palsy are often associated with athetoid or spastic forms of CP.)
- Correct visual deficits or strabismus (seen in as many as 75% of children with spastic types of CP).
- Control seizures.
- Obtain appropriate educational assistance for children with cognitive disorders.
- Prevent secondary emotional or health-related problems (failure to thrive or later obesity in nonambulators).

Multiple modalities are used to aid in the management of spasticity. These include serial casting techniques (which involve the use of casts to progressively stretch and increase the range of motion across a contracted joint), neurosurgical techniques (such as selective dorsal root rhizotomy, the more traditional approaches involving physical therapy), and orthopaedic interventions to lengthen or realign tendons. Each of these modalities requires ongoing follow-up and close communication among team members to optimize functional outcomes. Pumps placed intra-abdominally with a tunneled catheter can be used to deliver baclofen to the intrathecal space, and the injection of botulinum toxin into overactive muscle groups may also reduce spasticity. Other oral medications, such as baclofen, diazepam, lorazepam, clonazepam, and dantrolene may also provide benefit.

Pediatric anticipatory guidance can help families focus on fostering an independent, resilient young individual with good social skills and at the same time attend to the complicated medical and surgical aspects of addressing motor disability.

MYELOMENINGOCELE

The features of MMC are summarized in Table 39.3.

Spina Bifida Cystica (Spina Bifida Aperta)

Spina bifida cystica is what most physicians are referring to when they use the term MMC.

Etiology and Epidemiology

MMC occurs as a failure of fusion of the neural folds during embryologic development resulting in a defect of bone, meninges, and spinal cord. Clinically, it results in paralysis of the lower extremity, sensory loss, and neurogenic bowel and neurogenic bladder.

The risk for polygenically inherited recurrence is 2% to 4%. Gene markers have not yet been identified for familial

---

TABLE 39.3

SUMMARY OF MYELOMENINGOCELE

- Involves lack of fusion of the posterior bony arch(es) of various spinal cord segments, which may be accompanied by protrusion of a meningeal sac containing part of the spinal cord itself.
- Use of folic acid has been shown to reduce incidence and risk for recurrence of spina bifida greatly.
- Condition is generally detected by an abnormally elevated serum α-fetoprotein level *(tri-screen)* at 16 weeks, or by abnormalities on fetal ultrasonography.
- Most of the affected children (approximately 90%) have hydrocephalus, and nearly all require shunting; number of shunt infections/malfunctions greatly determines intellectual outcome.
- Other causes of morbidity are urologic problems (urinary tract infection, vesicoureteral reflux), seizures, skin breakdown, and orthopaedic problems (hip dislocation, scoliosis).
- Urosepsis is a common and occasionally fatal complication.
- Most of the skin defects in children are surgically treated within first 24 hours of life; in many cases, a ventriculoperitoneal shunt is placed at the same time if needed to treat hydrocephalus.

identification. *Folic acid at a dose of 400 µg/day* given to women before conception appears to reduce the risk for first occurrences. Doses of 4 mg/day (i.e., ten times the usual recommended dose) appear to reduce the risk for recurrent neural tube defects (NTDs) and are recommended for families in which a previous child has been affected. This intervention can assist only if started prior to conception because neural tube closure occurs between day 26 and day 30—prior to the time that pregnancy itself is confirmed in many cases. Aminopterin and valproic acid have been implicated as teratogens that may result in NTDs. Hot baths, febrile illnesses, or hot tubs/saunas during the first trimester also increase the risk of NTDs.

Clinical Presentation

At birth, defects in the ectodermal elements of skin, bone, spinal cord, and meninges cause clinical signs of lower motor neuron impairment (hypotonia, paralysis, sensory defects, possible contractures, and bony deformities such as clubfoot). Hydrocephalus may be clinically apparent or demonstrable on ultrasonography. An Arnold-Chiari type II malformation (ACII) is nearly always present (displacement of the medulla and crowding of the cerebellar tonsils into the foramen magnum, caused in part by a small posterior fossa) but is symptomatic in only one third of the children. Hydrocephalus may result and 90% of all children with meningomyelocele require a ventriculoperitoneal shunt. A smaller group with ACII (17%–37%) have central ventilatory dysfunction with associated stridor, dysphagia/aspiration, central apnea, or vocal cord paralysis as the clinical results of the Arnold-Chiari malformation. These related problems are the most common causes of premature death. Finally, associated bladder dysfunction may result in bladder distension, secondary ureteral distension, and potential renal dysfunction.

Diagnosis

Prenatal diagnosis is possible by screening for elevated maternal levels of α-fetoprotein on the pregnancy triple screen test between 16 and 18 weeks gestation or high resolution ultrasonography (which often demonstrates a dorsal protrusion in the lumbosacral region and sometimes a secondary hydrocephalus).

Treatment

Delivery room management is as follows:

- Immediate care of the newborn infant includes careful handling and preventing stool or urine from contaminating the affected area. Also, the baby is kept in a prone position with a sterile saline dressing over the defect to prevent drying or rupture of the sac.
- Prophylactic antibiotics are often administered to prevent meningitis.
- Elective delivery by cesarean section is desirable to prevent further nerve injury or exposure to bacterial flora.

Postnatal management is as follows:

- Closure of the NTD as soon as the child is clinically stabilized and able to tolerate the procedure decreases the risk of central nervous system infection (7% if closed within 48 hours vs. 37% if closed later).
- A multidisciplinary team consisting of neurosurgeons, orthopaedists, neurologists, urologists, gastroenterologists, nutritionists, therapists (physical, occupational, and speech), and orthotists treats these children.

The primary goals of long-term management are to address hydrocephalus and urologic problems (prevent urosepsis and manage bladder dystonia), correct orthopaedic defects, and provide mobility aids.

Neurologic Issues

More than 90% of children with a lesion at the lumbosacral level (or higher) have hydrocephalus, with or without ACII. Hydrocephalus may be present even if macrocephaly is not. If the lower cranial nerves are stretched, respiratory dysfunction may be seen, including paralysis of the vocal cords, apnea, aspiration, and hoarseness. Aqueductal stenosis is present in 40% of cases and is the other major cause of hydrocephalus. Seizures develop in 20% of children with MMC at some point during their life. Tethering of the cord is universal in older children with MMC as the lumbosacral cord fails to ascend. Adhesions resulting from previous surgical repair may restrict the cord further, preventing its normal ascent during growth.

Signs and symptoms of tethered cord include neurologic (loss of sensation), orthopaedic (back pain), and urologic (loss of control or changes in urodynamics) abnormalities, and may cause additional morbidity in the form of limb atrophy, paralysis, or incontinence.

Mobility

Prediction of mobility patterns requires multifactorial consideration. Patients with thoracic and high lumbar level neurosensory deficits will need a wheelchair for part or all of their mobility. Patients with mid-lumbar deficits (iliopsoas and quadriceps have grade 4–5 strength, whereas hamstrings, anterior tibialis, and gastrocs are less or absent) will achieve community ambulation with bracing. Those with lower lumbar deficits have the best chance of independent community ambulation with strong antigravity gluteal strength. Weight gain with adolescence or prolonged immobilization after fractures or scoliosis surgery increases the risk of losing hard-achieved ambulatory status. Cultivation of independent mobility with or without wheelchair is important for reasons more than motoric convenience. Children with self-produced locomotion have improved development of independence and self-competency. Mobility restriction can result in acquisition of passive, dependent behavior patterns: specifically a lack of initiative and curiosity that may ultimately be more disabling than the primary motor deficit.

Orthopaedic Problems (and Associated Levels of Lesions)

Lesions above the third lumbar segment (L3) lead to ankle weakness. With lesions of L4, the anterior tibial muscle is left active and pulls the foot into dorsiflexion and inversion. The most common knee deformity is knee flexion contracture (with involvement of L3 and higher). Lesions of L3 and L4 put the child at risk for hip dislocation. Up to 85% of children with MMC have some degree of foot deformity, and congenital clubfoot may occur and is difficult to treat. Hip range of motion is important to maintain because any hip flexion contracture >20 degrees will interfere with ambulation. Spinal deformities such as scoliosis, seen in 100% of cases involving the thoracic cord and 42% to 90% of cases involving lower spinal cord segments, are caused either by congenital bony abnormalities or instability of the spine. Scoliosis is progressive and is not halted by puberty or bracing in this population. Rapidly progressive scoliosis should prompt an evaluation for syringomyelia. Indeed, any worsening of function or loss of sensation should prompt an evaluation for tethering of the spinal cord. Congenital lumbar kyphosis is a finding unique to patients with MMC.

Urologic Problems

Abdominal ultrasonography will detect a distended or poorly emptying bladder (postvoid residual of >20 mL is significant in a full-term child) or the presence of hydronephrosis. Seventy-five percent of children with MMC have normal upper tracts, but repeat ultrasonography of the kidneys every 6 months for the first 3 years is recommended. Vesicoureteral reflux or high pressure transmitted from a dyssynergic bladder place the renal function at risk. Intermittent catheterization can be begun during the toddler years in anticipation of independent participation by some children at school-going age.

Gastrointestinal Concerns

The presence of the anocutaneous or the bulbocavernosus reflexes are associated with the greatest likelihood of achieving bowel continence because the intact sacral afferents that mediate these reflexes also support rectal sensation to allow sphincter control. This occurs in <25% of children with MMC. Most can achieve social continence with education in a planned timing of defecation daily with stimulation, suppositories, or enemas to assist with evacuation at predictable times. Such bowel programs should be begun between the ages of 2 and 5 years. Training for independence in toileting skills begins around 4 years of age and is usually the most delayed activity of daily living in this population of children.

Skin Breakdown

Skin breakdown is common over insensate areas particularly in children with MR, large heads, kyphoscoliosis, chronic soiling, or orthoses. Teaching children self-inspection and ensuring well-adjusted seating and orthoses coupled with good hygiene and nutrition help minimize these risks.

Other Concerns

Obesity risk is increased by lower lean body mass and decreased activity levels. Short stature is exacerbated by shortened spines and less growth of insensate limbs, renal insufficiency, chronic illness, early puberty with accelerated skeletal maturation, or nutritional compromise.

Children with MMC can have normal intelligence. Ten percent have IQs <70 with risk for MR increased by higher lesions, degree of hydrocephalus, and control of intracranial pressure (numbers of shunt revisions and infections). Hydrocephalus may predispose to learning disabilities particularly in visual-spatial-organizational cognitive functions. Math and writing are important areas to screen for assistance.

Latex allergy was first identified in this population of patients. Multiple surgeries, catheters, and enemas may have increased the exposure to latex protein antigens and up to 30% of children born before 1990 developed life-threatening allergies to latex exposure. Since that time, avoidance of latex containing materials has been advocated.

Spina Bifida Occulta

Spina bifida occulta is a very common condition, seen in 10% of the US population. It results from failure of fusion of the posterior bony arch, but an overt overlying skin defect is lacking. A fat pad, dermal sinus, hairy tufts, or dimples in the lower back (lumbosacral region) are frequently seen. The diagnosis is made by radiographic examination (spinal ultrasonography before 6 months, MRI thereafter).

Frequently, no morbidity is associated. Children may present with bowel/bladder dysfunction, including urinary tract infections and other neurologic abnormalities. A child with neurologic symptoms should be referred to a neurosurgeon. If the lesion is limited to L5, patients can engage in sports, and bracing and surgery are unnecessary.

AUTISM AND PERVASIVE DEVELOPMENTAL DISORDER

The features of the spectrum of autism disorders are summarized in Table 39.4.

TABLE 39.4

SUMMARY OF THE SPECTRUM OF AUTISM DISORDERS

- Definition: demonstration of: (a) qualitative impairment in social interaction, (b) qualitative impairment in verbal and nonverbal communication, and (c) restrictive repetitive stereotypic patterns of behavior interests and activities in a child. The child must display six or more of the 12 symptoms listed in DSM-IV and at least two of those must be from the "social interaction" category, with at least one each from the language and behavioral criteria as well. The onset of symptomatology must be before 3 years of age.
- Numerous medical conditions may present with an autistic type of picture and each should be ruled out based on clinical data or laboratory/radiologic/electroencephalographic data.
- The treatment of autistic children is multidisciplinary but intensive speech/language/communication therapy and measures to improve socialization skills are paramount.

Modified from data in DSM-IV. American Psychiatric Association. *Diagnostic and statistical manual of mental disorders*, 4th ed. Washington, DC: American Psychiatric Association, 2000:70–71.

Etiology and Epidemiology

2007 CDC data place the prevalence of autism spectrum disorders at 1 per 150 children in pediatric care (if you include all five diagnoses grouped under the umbrella of pervasive developmental disorder), and autism is the third most common developmental disability after MR and CP. A child is newly diagnosed with autism spectrum disorder every 20 seconds in a male-to-female ratio of 4:1.

Etiology is multifactorial, but genetics plays a large role. Some believe the cause is genetic in 95% of cases. The cause is likely polygenetic, with multiple genes on chromosomes X, 7p, 7q, 15q11-13, as well as others being implicated. Multiple theories on etiology exist, but none have been proven.

Clinical Presentation

The clinical features vary with the age of the patient at presentation. In infancy, sensory modulation disturbances (colic, irritability, insatiety) are apparent, in addition to:

- Failure to smile or cuddle, visually fixate on caregiver
- Delayed social and adaptive skills (*peek-a-boo*, imitation skills)
- Lack of protodeclarative pointing

The manifestations in preschool children include:

- Failure to progress in language development
- Echolalia
- Lack of communicative intent with sounds
- Fascinations with objects, water, light, or reflections
- Stereotypic motor behaviors
- Panic attacks associated with change, sounds, and particular sensations

Comorbidities include:

- Obsessive–compulsive tendencies
- Attention deficit disorder (ADD)/ADHD
- MR (seen in 70% of autistic children)
- Seizures
- Disordered modulation of sensory input
- Aggression directed at self or others
- Savant skills
- Sleep disturbance
- Feeding intolerance

Diagnosis

As defined in the *Diagnostic and Statistical Manual of Mental Disorders*, 4th edition (DSM-IV), this group of disorders falls under the broad heading of pervasive developmental disorder. Five diagnoses are included under this umbrella:

- Autistic disorder
- Asperger disorder
- Pervasive developmental disorder—not otherwise specified
- Rett syndrome
- Childhood disintegrative disorder

According to the DSM-IV criteria, the symptoms of these conditions fall into three categories, including the following:

- Qualitative impairment in social interaction
  - Marked impairment in the use of multiple nonverbal behaviors
  - Failure to develop peer relationships appropriate to developmental level
  - Lack of spontaneous seeking to share enjoyment, interests, or achievements with other individuals
  - Lack of social or emotional reciprocity
- Qualitative impairment in verbal and nonverbal communication
  - Delay in or total lack of development of spoken language
  - In individuals with adequate speech, marked impairment in the ability to initiate or sustain a conversation with others
  - Stereotyped and repetitive use of language or idiosyncratic language
  - Lack of varied, spontaneous make-believe play or social imitative play appropriate to developmental level
- Restrictive, repetitive, stereotypic patterns of behavior, interests, and activities
  - Encompassing preoccupation with one or more stereotypic and restricted patterns of interest that is abnormal in either intensity or focus
  - Apparently inflexible adherence to specific, nonfunctional routines or rituals
  - Stereotypic and repetitive motor mannerisms
  - Persistent preoccupation with parts of objects

A diagnosis of each of the five conditions listed in DSM-IV requires different numbers and types of the total of 12 symptoms. To meet the diagnostic criteria for autistic disorder, a child must display six of the 12 symptoms, including at least two from the *social interaction* category, and the symptoms should not be better accounted for by one of the other four diagnoses. The symptoms must appear before the age of 3 years. A diagnosis of pervasive developmental disorder is based on the presence of five or fewer of the 12 symptoms from two but not three of the symptom categories. Efforts to identify children prior to 3 years old are confounded by the current lack of validated measures of developmental social skills for example "peer relationships." The diagnosis of "provisional autism" is proposed if children under 3 have the four core symptoms of:

- Lack of spontaneous seeking to share enjoyment, interests with other people
- Lack of social and emotional reciprocity
- Marked impairment in the use of multiple nonverbal behaviors, such as eye gaze, facial expression, and gestures to regulate social interactions
- Delay in or total of the development of spoken language (not accompanied by an attempt to compensate through gesture or mime)

The young child can then be involved in language and social interaction intervention services and can be reassessed with the ADOS and/or ADIR at age 3.

A directed medical workup should be considered; in other words, if you suspect that a child has a condition that is causing autistic behavior, test for it.

The differential diagnosis includes hearing loss, specific language disorder, MR, elective mutism, dysarthria, seizures, and syndromes (fragile X syndrome, untreated phenylketonuria, tuberous sclerosis, neurofibromatosis, Lesch-Nyhan syndrome, Angelman syndrome, and Moebius sequence).

Treatment

Therapy for autism is tailored to meet the specific needs of each child, and is highly variable. Parents often elect to use a behavioral management program, along with traditional and complementary/alternative therapies. A coordinated educational plan with input from all care providers is vital to the child's success in school. A high teacher-to-student ratio is mandatory. Because of the variability of treatments used and lack of agreement on efficacy of the various treatment options, creating test questions in this area is difficult.

Pharmacologic Therapy

Medication can be a beneficial adjunctive therapy, especially when it is used to treat such comorbidities as mood disorder, seizures, uncooperativeness, self-abusive or disruptive behavior, or ADHD. The most widely used medications are the neuroleptics. They are administered for a wide variety of indications, including aggressive or stereotypic behavior.

ATTENTION DEFICIT HYPERACTIVITY DISORDER

The features of ADHD are summarized in Table 39.5.

Etiology and Epidemiology

The prevalence of these disorders is 8% to 10%, and the male-to-female ratio is 3:1 (but is variable between the different subtypes). They are common among first-degree relatives (some studies report an incidence of up to 50%). Various causes of subtle brain injury have been implicated as causal, and minor differences in brain structure have also been noted in affected children. Research is ongoing, but changes in the frontal lobe and frontal subcortical connections have been implicated. However, the cause appears to be largely genetic. It also may accompany specific syndromes, such as Fragile X, or may be seen following toxic intrauterine exposures. Comorbidity is very common, seen in 65% of affected children.

- Twenty percent also have a learning disability.
- Thirty percent to 50% also have a conduct disorder.
- Children with ADD are at higher risk for depression than those without.

No consistent relation between diet and ADHD has been found.

Clinical Presentation

DSM-IV classifies children with the disorder into three groups:

- Those who are inattentive (children who meet at least six of the nine criteria for inattentive behavior), the second most common subtype, and has a more equal male-female distribution

TABLE 39.5

SUMMARY OF ATTENTION DEFICIT HYPERACTIVITY DISORDER

- Essential criteria for diagnosis:
  - Impairment before the age of 7 years
  - Occurrence of symptoms in more than one setting
  - Clear evidence of *clinically significant impairment in social, academic, or occupational functioning*
  - Symptoms present for at least 6 months
- Male-to-female ratio in childhood is 3:1; in adolescents/adults, it is 1:1
- Incidence of comorbidities (learning disability, conduct disorder) is high
- Diagnosis should include a standardized questionnaire or interview with parents and teachers, and narrative comments from both
- Most children (80%) respond to one of the stimulant medications, which remain the drugs of first choice

■ Those who are hyperactive–impulsive (children who meet at least six of the nine criteria for hyperactive–impulsive behavior)
■ Those with a combined type (children who meet at least six of the nine inattentive and six of the nine hyperactive–impulsive behavior criteria)

In general, patients who are not hyperactive, in comparison with those who are hyperactive:

■ Often respond to lower doses of medication
■ Have a higher incidence of anxiety disorder
■ Are more likely to be placed in special education classes for children with *learning disability*

Patients who are hyperactive, in comparison with those who are not hyperactive:

■ Are predominantly male in a 3:1 ratio
■ Are more aggressive and antisocial and therefore have problems with peer relations
■ Exhibit more behavioral problems and less self-control
■ Are given a diagnosis earlier because of difficulties in several areas of functioning
■ Are more likely to be placed in special education classes for children with *behavior disorders*

Diagnosis

The condition is identified most often in the early elementary school years. ADHD is difficult to diagnose in the early years of life. Standardized questionnaires for caregivers or teachers are often helpful, but no one single test should be considered diagnostic. Samples must be obtained from both teachers and parents.

Some investigators use *broadband* tests, such as the comprehensive screening instruments of behavior, to assess for ADD/ADHD, but in general these are not nearly as specific or helpful as the *narrowband* instruments designed to assess attention alone. Screening instruments can also be used to generate a score by which a child's response to therapy can be gauged.

Continuous performance tests are used by some (Test of Vigilance and Attention [TOVA], Gordon Diagnostic Test, Conners Continuous Performance Test). In these tests, sequential visual stimuli are presented to the child on a computer screen, and the child must respond. The test generally lasts approximately 15 minutes. The computer then scores how many correct answers the child has given. The tests are often applied in research, but their diagnostic usefulness is limited because their sensitivity and specificity in distinguishing children with ADHD from those without, is relatively poor.

In children with relatively severe ADHD, the neurologic examination may reveal *soft signs*, such as mirror movements and problems with rapidly alternating movements. It should be understood that a child's behavior in the office or a single observation in the classroom is of no value in predicting the presence or absence of ADD/ADHD.

An electroencephalographic examination should be reserved for children in whom *absence seizures* are suspected clinically (sudden cessation of motor activity or speech associated with brief, rhythmic twitching of the eyelids or lips, or induction of a staring spell by 2–3 minutes of hyperventilation).

Differential Diagnosis

The differential diagnosis includes diseases that acutely affect CNS function, hyperthyroidism, absence seizures, hearing loss, visual loss/impairment, central auditory processing disorder, mood disorders (particularly depression), and anxiety disorder.

Treatment

General principles regarding stimulant medications include the following:

■ Children who do not respond to one medication may respond to another.
■ If medications are tried sequentially, the rate of positive benefit approaches 80%.
■ The dosage is not weight-dependent, so start low and increase as needed.
■ The most powerful effects are on observable social and classroom behaviors and on core symptoms of inattention, hyperactivity, and impulsivity.
■ Year-round dosing of stimulants does not lead to attenuation of the response, and drug holidays are unnecessary.
■ Medications may unmask or worsen tics; however, the symptoms of ADHD generally disrupt a child's life more than tics. Development of tics after initiation of a stimulant medication is most often a transient phenomenon, and is not an absolute contraindication to the use of stimulants.
■ The mode of action is primarily dopaminergic; however, stimulants also affect norepinephrine and serotonin levels in various areas of the brain.
■ Nearly all stimulant medications come in extended-release formulations, and show better efficacy than the short-acting preparations.
■ In February, 2006 the United States Food and Drug Administration placed a black box warning on the stimulants for cardiovascular risk, with special caution to be used in those children with underlying heart disease.
■ In August 2008, in response to controversy regarding the need for electrocardiograms prior to stimulant use, the AAP published a policy statement that a careful history for identified cardiac conditions or palpitations, syncope or seizures, and a careful family history for sudden death in children or young adults, or for hypertrophic cardiomyopathy or long QT syndrome, and a physical exam

with a careful cardiac exam is warranted. Routine ECG or cardiology consultation was *not* recommended at this time.

Examples of stimulant medications are as follows:

- Methylphenidate (Ritalin, Metadate, Methylin, Concerta), Focalin (dexmethylphenidate), and Daytrana.
  - Seventy percent of patients experience psychostimulant withdrawal 5 to 15 hours after the last dose when short-acting forms are used.
  - This phenomenon, known as *behavioral rebound*, is characterized by irritability, talkativeness, noncompliance, excitability, hyperactivity, and insomnia.
  - Behavioral rebound can be treated by giving a 5-mg dose when the patient returns home from school or by switching to a sustained-release preparation.
- Dextroamphetamine (Dexedrine), pemoline (Cylert), mixture of dextroamphetamine and amphetamine salts (Adderall). Lisdexamfetamine (Vyvanse) is the prodrug form of long-acting (Adderall).
- Pemoline is rarely used because of the risk for fatal hepatotoxicity.

The side effects of stimulant medications include *insomnia, decreased appetite, irritability or other mood changes, headache, and abdominal pain, which often occur transiently after the initiation of therapy.* No significant effect on adult weight or height has been shown. The most serious side effect is the appearance of motor tics, but a tic disorder develops in <1% of children with ADHD.

Atomoxetine (Strattera) is a nonstimulant medication with an indication for the treatment of ADD/ADHD. It selectively inhibits norepinephrine reuptake, but its exact mechanism of action is unknown. Side effects are similar to the stimulants, but also include nausea, risk of hepatic injury, and development of suicidal ideation.

Tricyclic antidepressants and bupropion are effective in many patients who fail to respond to stimulant medications (their mode of action is noradrenergic). The antihypertensive α_2-agonists (clonidine and guanfacine) may also be effective. Psychotherapy and behavior modification techniques are generally not as effective as treatment with medication alone, but they are helpful in the treatment of comorbid conditions, and in a recent large study, children treated with both medication and behavioral modification techniques showed a greater reduction in core symptoms than did those treated with either modality alone.

A behavior modification program with strong positive reinforcement should be carried out both in school and at home. An individualized education plan may help with school issues. Mapping of electric activity in the brain, visual training, elimination diets, and the administration of megavitamins and pine bark extract (Pycnogenol) have all been attempted as therapy, but none have proved efficacious.

Prognosis

ADHD remains a problem in approximately 40% of adults (3%–4% of the US adult population) who were affected as children, and is associated with a high rate of academic and work failure and psychiatric illness. In the adolescent and adult years, the male-to-female ratio approaches 1:1, likely because of identification of the disorder in inattentive girls and women.

The prognosis varies considerably and depends on coexisting conditions, cognitive strengths and weaknesses, the family environment, and the timing and type of intervention. Twenty percent of adolescents and adults who have persistent symptoms of ADHD function poorly at follow-up in regard to emotional, educational, and social adjustment; 60% have an intermediate outcome; and 20% do well. Children with comorbid conduct or mood disorders have a worse outcome than do their counterparts with ADHD alone. In general, the symptoms of most affected children regress with age (symptoms of hyperactivity and impulsivity improve most).

FETAL ALCOHOL SYNDROME

Etiology and Epidemiology

Fetal alcohol syndrome (FAS) has been redefined to better describe the spectrum of neurobehavioral phenotypes as well as the teratogenic effects on other organ systems.

The new guidelines are more detailed and require more expertise in aspects of the diagnostic criteria. There are five new categories in what is now defined as fetal alcohol spectrum disorder (FASD).

1. FAS with confirmed alcohol exposure
2. FAS without confirmed exposure
3. Partial FAS with confirmed exposure
4. Alcohol-related birth defects (AFBD)
5. Alcohol-related neurodevelopmental disorder (ARND)

FAS with confirmed maternal alcohol exposure criteria:

A. Confirmed maternal alcohol exposure
B. Evidence of characteristic facial anomalies (short palpebral fissures, flat upper lip, flattened philtrum, and midface)
C. Evidence of growth retardation shown by LBW, decelerating weight gain over time not caused by nutrition, disproportional low weight to height ratio
D. Evidence of CNS neurodevelopmental abnormalities as in decreased cranial size at birth, structural brain abnormalities (microcephaly, agenesis of corpus callosum, cerebellar hypoplasia), or neurologic hard or soft signs (poor fine motor, hearing loss, poor tandem gait, poor hand–eye coordination)

FAS without confirmed alcohol exposure is obviously that criteria B, C, and D are met but not confirmed alcohol exposure. Partial FAS criteria are confirmed maternal alcohol exposure with:

- Evidence of some component of facial anomalies
- C or D or E
- C and D
- E, which is evidence of a complex pattern of behavior or cognitive abnormalities that are inconsistent with developmental level and cannot be explained by family background or environment alone (learning difficulties, poor impulse control, social perception, poor capacity for abstraction, specific deficits in math, memory, attention, or judgment)

Alcohol-related birth defects (ARBD) must have confirmed alcohol exposure *and*

- Cardiac: ASD, VSD, tetralogy of Fallot
- Skeletal: Hypoplastic nails, clinodactyly, pectus, radioulnar synostosis, flexion contractures, scoliosis
- Renal: Aplastic, dysplastic, hypoplastic, horseshoe, hydronephrosis
- Ocular: Strabismus, refractive problems
- Auditory: Neurosensory or conductive loss

Alcohol-related neurodevelopmental disorder (ARND) is defined by having confirmed alcohol exposure *and* the presence of at least one (or both) of the following:

- Evidence of CNS neurodevelopmental abnormalities
- Evidence of complex pattern of behavioral or cognitive abnormalities

The alcohol-related birth defects may exist separately or may coexist with alcohol-related neurodevelopmental disorder. If they are both present, both should be diagnosed.

LEARNING DISABILITIES AND EDUCATIONAL ISSUES

Etiology and Epidemiology

Learning disabilities occur in 6% to 8% of all school-age children. Disorders of learning may appear throughout a school career because academic achievement is closely associated with language skills. Emotional disorders can manifest as academic or behavioral problems.

Some therapeutic drugs, when used on a long-term basis, can affect intellectual outcome. Anticonvulsants may have irreversible adverse effects on the behavior, intellectual outcome, and school performance of children. Phenobarbital impairs the performance of tasks requiring sustained concentration and attention. Phenytoin impairs the performance of tasks requiring motor speed and accuracy. In some studies, theophylline has been shown to cause problems in visual-spatial planning, concentration, and activity levels, but these findings have not been confirmed in other studies. Carbamazepine affects cognition, and valproate has a slight negative effect on cognition.

Clinical Presentation

The presenting complaints of children with learning disabilities include difficulty remembering verbal instructions, numbers, and personal information; poor reading recall; difficulty finding words; mispronunciation or omission of words when speaking; and poor coordination. These symptoms overlap with those of many other conditions and are not seen in all children with learning disabilities.

Problems encountered in content classes (e.g., social studies, history) may reflect reduced reading comprehension, impaired short-term memory, or a slow reading rate. Most children with an isolated learning disability experience a problem either in language/verbal skills or mathematics/performance skills, but not in both. *Children with difficulties in both areas are likely to have a more pervasive problem, such as MR or ADHD.*

It should be recognized that reversals (e.g., the letters *b* and *d*) in writing can be normal in children around 7 years of age.

Various medical problems may present as complaints about school performance:

- Petit mal seizures
- Tourette syndrome
- Visual problems
- Mild conductive hearing loss

Diagnosis

The diagnosis of learning disability requires:

- Normal intelligence
- A discrepancy between potential (measured by IQ tests) and academic achievement (usually a difference of two standard deviations between the two measures)
- Absence of sensory deficits (hearing or visual impairments)
- Absence of severe cultural or educational neglect

Specific criteria for the diagnosis and qualifications for services vary from state to state.

Learning disabilities cannot be diagnosed at an age younger than when such learning is expected (e.g., a 4-year-old child cannot be given a diagnosis of dyslexia). The family history may be valuable in evaluating a child with learning difficulties. Strong evidence indicates that learning disabilities arise from a dysfunction of specific brain regions and are hence heritable. A gene locus for reading disability has been identified on chromosome 6, and the recurrence rate for reading disabilities ranges from 35% to 45% in an affected family. *Learning disabilities are associated with specific genetic syndromes (Turner syndrome, fragile X syndrome, Klinefelter syndrome, and neurofibromatosis type 1).*

Comorbidities

ADHD is reported in approximately 40% of children in whom a learning disability has been identified.

Treatment

An individualized education plan must be developed for each child with a learning disability.

- This delineates the child's disabilities, remediation activities and goals, and describes how and when the child will be reassessed.
- The plan is developed by a team of professionals that typically includes the school psychologist in addition to the child's teachers and therapists.

Extracurricular activities can be very beneficial for a child's self-esteem.

Prognosis

The eventual prognosis of a learning-disabled child depends on the severity of the disability; the child's emotional state, self-esteem, and intelligence; and the availability of advocacy/supportive education and career counseling. Continual school failure can lead to depression, aggressive behavior, reduced motivation to complete school work, juvenile delinquency, and school dropout. Learning disabilities are usually not outgrown.

LANGUAGE/SPEECH DELAY

Etiology and Epidemiology

The causes of delayed language development include prematurity, nutritional deprivation, exposure to toxins (e.g., lead), iron deficiency, severe neglect, syndromes, and MR. An association has been noted between mild conductive hearing loss secondary to serous otitis media and speech and language delay in school-aged children.

Clinical Presentation

Words in which two consonant sounds are blended together (e.g., *stop*) are more difficult to say and may be omitted (e.g., *top*) or substituted (e.g., *dop*). Difficulty pronouncing the *r, s, l, sh,* and *th* sounds may persist until the age of 7 years. Disfluency occurs normally in preschool children during the attainment of language skills (at age 2–3 years), but stuttering represents a clinical disorder in older children (>5 years of age).

Diagnosis

The diagnostic evaluation of a child with language delay should include a careful history exploring risk factors and milestone achievements, a physical examination, standardized language testing to assess expressive and receptive language abilities, auditory testing, and an assessment of other developmental domains to search for the possibility of a more global or pervasive problem.

Language problems for which a diagnostic evaluation should be considered include:

- Diminished vocalization or failure to vary the pitch of the voice at 4 months
- Failure to turn toward sound or voice by 6 months of age
- Lack of babbling of consonant sounds at 9 months
- Lack of true words or gestures with meaning at 15 months
- Lack of protodeclarative pointing at 18 months
- Communicating needs at 2 years of age by pointing or grunting rather than by verbalization
- Speech <50% intelligible to strangers by 2 years
- Lack of two-word combinations by 2 years
- Articulate and advanced expressive skills relative to lack of understanding of speech (may be echolalia)

Treatment

The principal goals of speech therapy are to maximize pragmatic communication skills and minimize frustration for the child and parent. Children who stutter should be enrolled in therapy if the disfluency leads to psychologic upset.

Prognosis

The prognosis for a child with isolated language delay is generally good.

REVIEW EXERCISES

QUESTIONS

1. All of the following statements regarding MR are true *except*:
a) The diagnosis requires a performance on standard measures of intelligence two standard deviations or more below the mean, or poor functioning in two areas of daily living as assessed by standardized measures.
b) The cause is most commonly unknown.
c) In general, MR is generally more severe in children in whom the signs become apparent at an earlier age.
d) Most of the affected children have mild MR.
e) Treatment is geared toward maximizing adaptive functioning.

Answer
The answer is a. The diagnosis of MR requires both poor performance on standardized tests of intelligence and poor adaptive functioning, not either of them alone.

2. A 6-month-old infant is transferred to your practice and is brought in for his well-child visit. On physical examination, you note a definite increase in the muscle tone of the lower extremities, particularly the ham strings and hip adductors, and brisk bilateral patellar reflexes.

You have difficulty placing the child in a seated position, but he is able to hold a rattle in either hand. The child also has a high-pitched cry, and the history reveals delayed global developmental skills. The medical history would be expected to reveal which of the following?
a) Prematurity
b) Traumatic brain injury
c) Bacterial meningitis
d) Significant intracranial hemorrhage
e) Any of the above

Answer
The answer is e. The history is suggestive of CP. Given that the child has signs of spasticity in both lower extremities but is able to hold a rattle in both hands (a 4-month-old's skill), he most likely has the spastic diplegia type of CP. Recall that CP is a static encephalopathy resulting from previous brain injury and is not progressive. Therefore, the child must be monitored closely for further signs of deterioration because it is difficult to make the diagnosis definitively at this early age. Any of the historical factors listed could lead to such a presentation in this 6-month-old infant.

3. A 12-year-old boy afflicted with spina bifida presents to you with incontinence of stool and urine for the previous 2 months that seems to be worsening. He was previously continent for bowel movements, and he uses clean intermittent urethral catheterization four times a day to empty his bladder. He had two previous urinary tract infections in the remote past, had hydrocephalus at birth that required the placement of a ventriculoperitoneal shunt, and uses oxybutynin to manage bladder dystonia. He also states that his feet seem to have become "more arched" during the last several months. The next step in management should include the following:
a) Increase the frequency of clean intermittent catheterization to every 4 hours.
b) Institute a bowel management program to curb fecal incontinence.
c) Perform a brain MRI.
d) Perform a sacral spine MRI.
e) Perform urodynamic studies.

Answer
The answer is d. This child's symptoms most strongly suggest tethered cord syndrome, a common phenomenon in all children with spina bifida, especially during periods of rapid growth. An early onset of puberty is frequently seen in a child with brain injury or congenital malformation, so that he is likely now in puberty and growing at an accelerated rate. Signs and symptoms of tethered cord syndrome include neurologic, orthopaedic, and urologic abnormalities and may result in significant morbidity if unrecognized. The child should also be evaluated for the possibility of urinary tract infection because

urosepsis causes significant morbidity and even mortality in this population.

4. A new 4-year-old patient is referred to you for the evaluation of suspected developmental delays. Careful review of his developmental history reveals that his language skills have been delayed since approximately 9 months of age, his fine and gross motor skills are mildly delayed, and his social skills are grossly delayed. He has no history of developmental regression and displays no stereotypic motor activity or behavior. You suspect a pervasive developmental disorder condition. Review of the DSM-IV criteria reveals that the child meets five of the 12 criteria necessary for such a diagnosis. This child *most* closely fits the diagnostic criteria for:
a) Autistic disorder
b) Asperger disorder
c) Pervasive developmental disorder—not otherwise specified
d) Rett syndrome
e) Childhood disintegrative disorder

Answer
The answer is c. The child cannot have autistic disorder because he does not meet six of the necessary criteria. Asperger disorder is ruled out because he has a history of language delay. He does not have Rett syndrome because he lacks stereotypic hand movements, and the fact that he is male greatly lessens the incidence of the condition. He does not have childhood disintegrative disorder because he has no history of developmental regression.

5. A 9-year-old child in your practice who is currently in the third grade is brought in by his mother for evaluation because his academic performance has significantly declined this year. He previously achieved average to above-average grades in his course work but now is in danger of failing his language arts and science classes. He displayed clownish, immature behavior at home and school in the past, which seems to have worsened during this academic year. His medical history is notable for pressure equalization tube placement at the age of 2 years and again at 3 years for recurrent otitis media. His family history is unremarkable for MR and learning disabilities. The next step in management should include all of the following *except*:
a) Vision screening
b) Hearing screening
c) Evaluation by a psychologist
d) Initiation of a trial of stimulant medication
e) Complete physical and neurologic examination

Answer
The answer is d. This child should undergo a complete physical examination, including hearing and vision

screening, to rule out sensory deficits or other possible medical causes of his academic difficulties. Evaluation by a psychologist is required to rule out the possibility of ADD, learning disability, and other comorbid conditions. A trial of stimulant medications should be instituted only if the diagnosis of ADD (or ADHD) is confirmed.

SUGGESTED READINGS

1. American Psychiatric Association. *Diagnostic and statistical manual of mental disorders*, 4th ed. Washington, DC: American Psychiatric Association, 2000.
2. Batshaw ML, Pellegrino L, Roizen N. *Children with disabilities*, 6th ed. Baltimore: Brooks Publishing, 2007.
3. Byrd RS, School failure: assessment, intervention, and prevention in primary pediatric care. *Pediatr Rev* 2005;26:233–243.
4. Capin DM. Developmental learning disorders: clues to their diagnosis and management. *Pediatr Rev* 1996;17:284–290.
5. Dias MS, Skaggs DL. Neurosurgical management of myelomeningocele (spina bifida). *Pediatr Rev* 2005;26:50–60.
6. Fein D, Stevens M, Dunn M, et al. Subtypes of pervasive developmental disorder: clinical characteristics. *Child Neuropsychol* 1999; 5:1–23.
7. Feldman HM. Evaluation and management of language and speech disorders in preschool children. *Pediatr Rev* 2005;26:131–142.
8. Johnson CP. Recognition of autism before age 2 years. *Pediatr Rev* 2008;29:86–96.
9. Johnson CP, Walker OW. Mental retardation: management and prognosis. *Pediatr Rev* 2006;27:249–256.
10. Loock C, Conry J, Cook JL. Fetal alcohol spectrum disorder: Canadian guidelines for diagnosis. *CMAJ* 2005;172(5 suppl).
11. Shaywitz SE, Shaywitz BA. Dyslexia (specific reading disability). *Pediatr Rev* 2003;24:147–153.
12. Simms MD, Schum RL. Preschool children who have atypical patterns of development. *Pediatr Rev* 2000;21:147–158.
13. Stein MT, Perrin JM. Diagnosis and treatment of ADHD in school-age children in primary care settings: a synopsis of the AAP practice guidelines. *Pediatr Rev* 2003;24:92–98.
14. Walker OW, Johnson CP. Mental retardation: overview and diagnosis. *Pediatr Rev* 2006;27:204–212.
15. Wender E. Managing stimulant medication for attention-deficit/hyperactivity disorder. *Pediatr Rev* 2001;22:183–190.

Chapter 40

BOARD SIMULATION:
Development

Roberta E. Bauer and Mark H. Deis

QUESTIONS

1. An infant remains in a seated position when placed on your examination table by his mother. His body stiffens when you push him laterally with a gentle nudge on each shoulder. He falls backward without protecting himself when you gently push on his chest. When placed in a prone position, he immediately gets up on his hands and knees and rocks back and forth, but his mother reports that he does not yet crawl. When placed in a seated position, he picks up his mother's keys and immediately transfers them to his other hand. His mother puts a small piece of cereal in front of him, and he picks it up between the palmar aspect of his thumb and the anatomic lateral aspect of his index finger. He turns toward you when you speak, but his mother reports that he does not seem to know his name, nor has he used any expressive word approximations. He has been babbling for approximately

2 months. He clearly enjoys your efforts to amuse him and displays no stranger anxiety. This infant is performing closest to the development expected at:

a) 6 months
b) 7 months
c) 8 months
d) 9 months
e) This is not typical development for any age.

Answer
The answer is c.

2. While obtaining a toddler's history at her well-child visit, you note that she walks with an unsteady gait, taking as many as five steps at a time. Her mother reports that she has been walking for approximately 3 weeks. She also crawls quickly between objects in the room. She picks up raisins with a mature pincer grasp. Her mother tells you that they have recently installed safety locks on all the cabinets at home because the child is beginning to open the doors. When given a crayon, she first places its end in her mouth but then holds it in her fist and rubs it on paper, imitating you. She clearly responds to her name when called, and her mother believes that she is beginning to understand "no." Her mother is able to keep her occupied by having her play with a toy from which figurines pop up when buttons are pressed. She imitates you when you play *peek-a-boo* with her during the physical examination, although she was clearly apprehensive when you first came near her. She has been using "dada" and "mama" nonspecifically for approximately 1 month, and her mother believes that she is beginning to use these words appropriately. This toddler is performing closest to the development expected at:

a) 10 months
b) 11 months
c) 12 months
d) 13 months
e) This is not typical development for any age.

Answer
The answer is c.

3. A child is brought into your office for a well-child visit. He runs down the hallway and into the examination room, following his older sibling. He begins to climb up onto a chair in the room and screams in protest when his sibling pulls him down and sits there herself. His mother reports that without constant vigilance at home, he "invents new ways to cause trouble." He is able to climb up the stairs but has not yet tried to walk up them. He is beginning to throw balls and other objects overhand but cannot quite yet kick a ball. He is able to feed himself, although he is quite messy at it. He loves to scribble. His favorite toy is one in which a small plastic hammer is used to activate various cause-and-effect mechanisms. His mother estimates that he has a 15-word vocabulary, most of which consists of

labels of familiar objects. He can point to his hair, eyes, and mouth when asked to do so. He again screams in protest and points to crackers that his sister has removed from their mother's bag and has not yet shared with him. He also grunts and points to a familiar cartoon character painted on the wall, looking at his mother while doing so. His mother places him on her lap so you can examine him, and he cries at your approach. She asks him to remove his shoes, which he promptly does, throwing them to the floor. He then claps as you both cheer him. This child is performing closest to the development expected at:

a) 16 months
b) 18 months
c) 20 months
d) 22 months
e) This is not typical development for any age.

Answer
The answer is b.

4. A child is brought in for assessment before entering preschool. The physical examination findings, including growth parameters, are typical for her age. Her mother reports that she can dress and undress by herself and is able to help with simple tasks at home, such as preparing the dinner table. She is able to ascend and descend stairs by placing one foot on each step, and recently she began riding a bicycle with training wheels. You draw various figures for her in an attempt to have her imitate you, and she is able to copy a circle and a cross, but not a square. Her speech is completely understandable. She is also able to relate a personal event and can identify four colors. This child is performing closest to the development expected at:

a) 36 months
b) 42 months
c) 48 months
d) 54 months
e) This is not typical development for any age.

Answer
The answer is c.

Case for Questions 5–7
Amy is a 2-year-old girl who is brought to your office to be assessed for tantrums. She appears well, her physical assessment findings are normal, and her growth parameter values (height, weight, and head circumference) are in the 10th percentile. She has no stigmata of neurocutaneous diseases or syndromes. Her gross motor skills show her walking and running well, but she has a hard time walking backward when asked to, although you later see her doing it quite well when her brother chases her. She feeds herself with her fingers, can pick up her toys with her mother demonstrating, and lets her mother know what she wants by leading her to it or by pointing. She likes to play by herself and enjoys taking toys in and out of her toy box or her

mother's cupboards. She enjoys throwing your blocks, but you can get her to stack only two. She scribbles well and prolifically and does not show a clear preference for her left or right hand. She missed her visit with you at 18 months because she had her booster at the health department, but she always passed her screening tests up to 1 year of age. Her mother says she becomes frustrated easily and does not respond to having the tantrums ignored. Your nurse could not get her to wear earphones or cooperate with the hearing screening.

5. Appropriate next steps in assessment might include:
a) Hearing screening
b) Vision screening
c) Formal developmental testing of all areas of function
d) Notifying a child protection agency regarding an inappropriate response to tantrums
e) Neurology referral
f) Magnetic resonance imaging of the brain

Answer

The answer is a, b, *and* c. Amy is throwing temper tantrums, a normal issue at 2 years of age. Her mother has appropriately responded by trying to distract her and ignoring the behavior, but the strategies are not working because other frustrations are causing Amy's tantrums. Her communication skills are significantly delayed. At 2 years of age, she is not using language to communicate her needs and has to rely on leading and pointing. If these were the only clues, we might suspect just a language disorder. With delayed expressive language, we might be concerned about hearing impairment, poor environmental stimulation and exposure to language modeling, pervasive developmental disorder of childhood, or dyspraxia. However, the description tells us that she is putting things into and taking them out of a box repeatedly, the kind of repetitive play that interests a 10- to 12-month-old, who is newly discovering that objects still exist even when you cannot see them. She does not understand verbal commands even with demonstrations (your request to walk backward or your nurse's request to move her finger on the side where she hears the noise), and an assessment of her self-help skills shows her finger-feeding and scribbling abilities. We do not know whether she has any vision or hearing impairment, but we do know that her mother is describing delayed play, self-help, and language skills, and we need to be concerned about the global delays of MR. So, appropriate additional evaluations are a, b, and c. Notifying a child protection agency is not appropriate. Certainly if focal abnormalities were noted on the physical examination, if any questions arose of seizure activity, or if the history suggested a loss of milestones or degeneration, then a neurologic consult might be appropriate at this point, but Amy's physical and neurologic examination findings and growth parameters are normal. An imaging study would not change the therapy in any direct way at this point and is not immediately indicated.

6. The history provided suggests which developmental delays?
a) Gross motor
b) Fine motor
c) Receptive language
d) Expressive language
e) Cognitive
f) Self-help areas

Answer

The answer is b, c, d, e, *and* f. The history suggests delays in all areas except gross motor. Trisomy 21 is typically associated with a number of physical findings. A diagnosis of failure to thrive is not justified with normal growth parameters and absence of downward crossing of percentiles. High-frequency hearing loss may well present with expressive language delays, but in the absence of cognitive difficulties, it should not affect self-help and play skills so noticeably.

7. This history and physical examination findings are consistent with:
a) Trisomy 21
b) Mental retardation (MR)
c) Failure to thrive
d) High-frequency hearing loss secondary to birth injury

Answer

The answer is b. MR is defined by significantly impaired performance on IQ testing (two standard deviations below the mean for age) coupled with impaired adaptive behavior. Therefore, for a diagnosis to be made, a child must undergo formal psychometric testing to measure the IQ. Such testing becomes stable and quite reliable past the age of 6 years and is not available before the age of 2 years. Until formal testing is available, the diagnosis of global developmental delay is appropriate. Notably, most children with MR do *not* have chromosomal disorders. The more profound the developmental delay, the more likely it is that a medical diagnosis is associated with the developmental issue, such as static encephalopathy, an inborn error of metabolism, or a chromosomal abnormality. In children with normal growth and no stigmata of minor or major malformation, the yield of metabolic studies is low. A family history of fetal wastage or MR should prompt a consideration of a chromosomal aberration or fragile X syndrome. Infants who are small for their gestational age or have microcephaly should be evaluated for congenital infection or anatomic abnormalities of the brain. Seizures and hard neurologic signs of upper motor neuron damage should prompt an evaluation for central nervous system injury or suggest the presence of a degenerative process. Milder forms of global developmental delay are common in fetal alcohol syndrome and familial inheritance of cognitive disorders. Two-year-olds who are not yet talking always warrant further evaluation.

Case for Questions 8–12

Ben is brought in for his 6-month visit. He is visually alert, but his eyes tend to drift toward his nose when he is tired. He is hard to hold according to his mother and has always been a "spitty baby." The problem is worse when she tries to feed him solid food because it comes out before she can get him to swallow. He gags easily and had a full startle reaction when you dropped his chart accidentally. He has been growing poorly, presently at just below the 10th percentile for weight, although he started out at the 50th percentile. His head circumference is at the second percentile, and his length at the 10th. On pull-to-sit maneuver, his head lags behind his shoulders. He does not sit independently and tends to fall backward when he tries. When you support him in a sitting position, he holds his arms up beside his shoulders and holds his head upright but stiff. He bears weight in a supported standing position but does so on the tips of his toes, and he is arched from the tip of his head to his toes. In a prone position, he screams and cannot seem to get his arms forward to support himself. He is fisted most of the time and will not grasp your toys. His cry is different when he is hurt than when he is just fussy, but he cries a lot, and the cry is high-pitched and shrill. He does not seem to localize sounds, but his mother is sure that he can hear because he calms down when she sings to him, even if she is not holding him. His physical examination findings are abnormal for brisk deep tendon reflexes in all four extremities and sustained ankle clonus.

8. Historical features that might assist you include:
a) Prenatal history of drug or alcohol exposure
b) Perinatal history of prematurity, abruption, or asphyxia
c) Family history of progressive loss of strength and mobility
d) Multiple miscarriages and family members with congenital anomalies

Answer

The answer is b. Ben presents with significant motor delay at the young age of 6 months, although we would suspect that his 2- and 4-month examination findings were also abnormal. Children can certainly show some delay in controlling conjugate gaze during the early months of life, but by 6 months, inwardly turning eyes are a cause for concern until proved otherwise. Some of the same insults that produce esotropia also affect the acquisition of motor control. Classically, the child with upper motor neuron damage is floppy early in life, and the resting tone then increases with age. By 6 months, delayed loss of primitive reflexes (the persistent startle when you dropped your chart), delayed acquisition of voluntary control of the head and trunk, delayed acquisition of protective reactions that allow independent sitting at least with propping, and an increase in deep tendon reflexes strongly suggest central nervous system injury. This concern is further supported by the child's

high-pitched cry, fussiness, gastroesophageal reflux, hyperactive gag when solid foods are introduced, and relative microcephaly. *The history most suggestive of this presentation is b, a significantly asphyxiated or premature infant with massive periventricular leukomalacia or significant intraventricular hemorrhage.* A prenatal history of drug abuse might support the presentation if poor prenatal care and nutrition, poor blood pressure control, and bleeding early on were present to a degree that interfered with intrauterine growth. Family disorders associated with progressive loss of strength are more likely to be muscular dystrophies, which do not present with spasticity but rather with weakness; demyelinating diseases, such as multiple sclerosis, which are reportable in the newborn to 6-month age range; or heritable neuropathies, which present at later ages. Fetal wastage and anomalies are more likely in children who are dysmorphic or excessively small at birth; Ben had been growing normally. Cerebral palsy is frequently associated with ocular muscle problems, bony deformities such as a dislocated hip or scoliosis, seizure disorders, and sensory disturbances such as myopia and hearing impairment.

9. Additional assessments might appropriately include:
a) Multidisciplinary evaluation by a physical therapist and an occupational therapist and oral–motor assessment by a speech therapist or an occupational therapist
b) Ophthalmology
c) Neurology
d) Audiology
e) Orthopaedics
f) All of the above

Answer

The answer is f. All the additional assessments suggested in Question 9 might be appropriate.

10. The Denver Developmental Screening Examination is an appropriate tool to continuously assess this child's cognitive, language, and self-help functioning.
a) True
b) False

Answer

The answer is b. Ben is clearly experiencing motor delay, and at this point we strongly suspect an underlying diagnosis that categorically qualifies him for early intervention services; therefore, the Denver Developmental Screening Examination is *not* an appropriate screening tool for him. The norms were determined in children with normal motor ability to demonstrate their self-help and play behaviors and would not accurately reflect Ben's potential ability to understand and comprehend. He should undergo specialized testing of his cognitive abilities with motor-free assessments, if possible.

11. This child can be referred to early intervention service coordination in his community even before a full diagnosis has been made.
a) True
b) False

Answer
The answer is a.

12. This clinical picture is *most* consistent with:
a) Trisomy 15
b) MR
c) Cerebral palsy (spastic quadriparesis)
d) Pervasive developmental disorder of childhood

Answer
The answer is c.

Case for Questions 13 and 14
Cheryl is a 3-year-old girl whose development seemed appropriate until about 18 months of age, when she stopped making any progress in language skills. She walks, dresses, and feeds herself, and she is completely happy entertaining herself for hours by lining up her stuffed animals in rows and then rearranging them. She does not interact with other children, and when she is upset, she shrieks and waves her arms in a flapping motion. She is panic-stricken when there are changes in routine or when she visits a new place. Her articulation is perfect for words she hears and can repeat, but she does not answer any questions or point to body parts or even offer you consistent eye contact when you talk with her. She flinches when you touch her face to try to gain eye contact and retreats to a corner of the examination room, where she rocks back and forth and wrings her hands. She has not lost any of the abilities that she previously acquired, and her strength and balance continue to improve.

13. Historical information that might suggest a cause of this disorder includes:
a) Birth history of prematurity
b) Seizure disorder in family members
c) Multiple miscarriages and children with congenital anomalies
d) Divorce in the family at 1 year of age
e) None of the above

Answer
The answer is e. Cheryl's presentation is fairly classic for pervasive developmental disorder of childhood. Her use of language is clearly impaired. Her expressive language is delayed, and the qualitative aspects are even more disturbed, with no demonstration of communicative intent. She is echolalic, does not respond to questions, and does not use language to make her desires known. Her socialization skills are impaired, she fails to make eye contact, and she does not interact with peers or appropriately turn to adults for assistance. She exhibits a number of repetitive motor behaviors that are stereotypic and nonpurpose-

ful. Her manner of interacting with objects is rigid, and she does not adapt well to changes in her environment. The onset of her speech changes was before the age of 2 years. She demonstrates self-stimulatory behaviors and poor adaptive responses to interactions. Pervasive developmental disorder or autism is not associated with any of the historical factors listed, so the answer is e.

14. Diagnostic assessments that would assist in the treatment include:
a) Computed tomography of the head
b) Chromosomal analysis
c) Multidisciplinary assessment of language, cognitive, and attentional strengths and weaknesses
d) Formal audiologic testing

Answer
The answer is *c, possibly d, and to a lesser extent b.* Imaging of the head does not yield any intervention, and if the examination findings are nonfocal and the history is not suggestive of degenerative issues, such imaging is not cost-effective outside research settings. Abnormalities of chromosome 15 and to a lesser extent that of chromosomes 6 and 7 have been identified in groups of autistic children, but most researchers feel that it is too soon to say anything definitive about genetic causes of autism (barring recognizable disorders, such as fragile X syndrome).

Questions 15–24
Match the neuropsychologic evaluation instrument or developmental/behavioral assessment tool listed in the numbered column with its intended use from the lettered column. Answers from the lettered column may be used more than once.

a) Global development
b) Gross motor development
c) Fine motor development
d) Speech/language development
e) Global assessment of behavior
f) Attention
g) Cognitive/intellectual functioning
h) Academic achievement

15. *Kaufman Assessment Battery for Children,* 2nd ed.
Answer
The answer is h.

16. Conners' Rating Scales, Revised
Answer
The answer is f.

17. Parents' Evaluations of Developmental Status (PEDS)
Answer
The answer is a.

18. Wide Range Achievement Test, 4th ed. (WRAT-4)
Answer
The answer is h.

19. Peabody Picture Vocabulary Test, 4th ed. (PPVT-4)

Answer
The answer is d.

20. Child Behavior Checklist

Answer
The answer is e.

21. Ages and Stages Questionnaire

Answer
The answer is a.

22. ADD-H Comprehensive Teacher's Rating Scale (ACTeRS)

Answer
The answer is f.

23. Stanford-Binet Intelligence Test, 5th ed.

Answer
The answer is g.

24. Early Language Milestone Scale, 2nd ed. (ELM Scale-2)

Answer
The answer is d.

Explanations for Answers 15–24

Listed in the subsequent text are instruments that can be used to screen behavior or various streams of development.

Tests for Developmental Screening and Assessment

Developmental Assessment Batteries

These are *screening* tests. Children who fail them should be referred for a comprehensive evaluation to define areas of further weakness.

- Denver Developmental Screening Examination—Revised (Denver II) (motor, social, language)
- Revised Denver Prescreening Developmental Questionnaire (R-PDQ)
- Parents' Evaluation of Developmental Status (PEDS)
- Ages and Stages Questionnaire
- Bayley Scales of Infant Development II (BSID- II)
- Bayley Infant Neurodevelopmental Screen (BINS)
- Battelle Developmental Inventory Screening Tool, 2nd ed. (BDI-ST)
- Brigance Screens- II
- Child Development Inventories (formerly Minnesota Child Development Inventories)

The rest generally include *development* or *infant intelligence* in the title.

Evaluation of Language Functioning
- Peabody Picture Vocabulary Test, 4th ed. (PPVT-4)
- Early Language Milestone Scale, 2nd ed. (ELM Scale-2)

- MacArthur-Bates Communicative Development Inventories
- Expressive and Receptive One-Word Picture Vocabulary Tests (EOWPVT, ROWPVT)
- Clinical Evaluation of Language Fundamentals, 4th ed. (CELF-4)
- Communication and Symbolic Behavior Scales Developmental Profile (CSBS DP)
- Clinical Adaptive Text-Clinical Linguistic Auditory Milestone Scale (CAT-CLAMS, aka Capute Scales)

The rest mention *language, articulation,* or *syntax* in the title.

Evaluation of Behavioral/Adaptive Functioning
- Vineland Adaptive Behavior Scales, 2nd ed. (Vineland-II)
- Preschool Attainment Record
- Scales of Independent Behavior-Revised (SIB-R)
- Children's Apperception Test (social and personality development)

Assessment of Cognitive/Intellectual Functioning
- Wechsler Preschool and Primary Scale of Intelligence, Third Edition (WPPSI-III)
- Wechsler Intelligence Scale for Children, 4th ed. (WISC-IV) (produces full-scale, performance, and verbal IQ scores, standardized for ages 6 through 16; full subtest profile of scores more useful than full-scale IQ score alone; average, age-standardized subtest score on the WISC of 10)
- Stanford-Binet Intelligence Test, 5th ed.
- Leiter International Performance Scale, Revised (Leiter-R)

Assessment of Academic Achievement
- Wide Range Achievement Test, 4th ed. (WRAT-4)
- Woodcock-Johnson III Tests of Achievement
- Kaufman Assessment Battery for Children, 2nd ed. (KABC-II)
- Peabody Individual Achievement Test, Revised (PIAT-R)
- Wechsler Individual Achievement Test, 2nd ed. (WIAT-II)

Assessment of Attention/Concentration
- ADHD Rating Scale-IV (ADHD-IV)
- Child Attention Profile
- Vanderbilt ADHD Diagnostic Parent Rating Scale
- Vanderbilt ADHD Diagnostic Teacher Rating Scale
- SNAP-IV Rating Scale-Revised (SNAP-IV-R)
- ADD-H Comprehensive Teacher's Rating Scale (ACTeRS)
- ADD-H: Comprehensive Teacher's Rating Scale: Parent Form (ACTeRS)
- Conners' Rating Scales, Revised (CRS-R)
- Attention Deficit Disorders Evaluation Scale, 3rd ed. (ADDES-3)
- Test of Vigilance and Attention (TOVA)

Behavioral Assessment
- Behavior Assessment System for Children, 2nd ed. (BASC-2)

- Child Behavior Checklist (parent and teacher forms available)
- Eyberg Child Behavior Inventory
- Pediatric Symptom Checklist
- Childhood Depression Inventory

Autism Assessment

- Autism Diagnostic Observation Schedule (ADOS)
- Autism Diagnostic Interview, Revised (ADI-R)
- Modified Checklist for Autism in Toddlers (M-CHAT)
- Most other instruments include "autism" or "pervasive developmental disorder" in the title.
- Also note that the ADOS and ADI-R are diagnostic tools to be used after a child has failed a screening instrument or demonstrated convincing clinical symptoms, and the M-CHAT is a screening instrument. This distinction may be important on the Boards exam.

Visual-Motor/Visual-Perceptual Function

- Modified version of the Bender-Gestalt Test for Preschool and Primary School Children
- Developmental Test of Visual-Motor Integration (VMI)
- Goodenough-Harris Draw-a-Person Test

Motor Assessment

- Peabody Developmental Motor Scales, 2nd ed. (PDMS-2)

Questions 25–28

Match the federal law listed in the numbered column with its primary intent from the lettered column. Answers from the lettered column may be used more than once.

a) First revision of IDEA to address behavioral issues
b) Mandated the provision of "transition services for students in special education programming who are over 16 years of age"
c) Mandated that all students be taught in the "least restricted environment"
d) Mandated the use of individualized education plans (IEPs)

25. Public Law No. 94-142 (Education for All Handicapped Children Act of 1975)

Answer
The answer is c.

26. Public Law No. 99-457

Answer
The answer is d.

27. Public Law No. 101-476 (Individuals with Disabilities Education Act [IDEA])

Answer
The answer is b.

28. Public Law No. 105-17 (IDEA, Part C [1997 Amendments])

Answer
The answer is a.

Explanations for Answers 25–28
Although the salient points of these laws are difficult to distinguish, they make great matching questions.

Laws Governing Alternative Educational Placement

- Public Law No. 94-142 (Education for All Handicapped Children Act of 1975)
  - Mandates that all children between the ages of 5 and 21 years who have disabilities receive free, appropriate, and individualized education with a *continuum of alternative placements* and in the *least restrictive environment.*
  - When an individualized program is deemed necessary, it should be outlined in an IEP and provided in either
  - A regular classroom (i.e., *mainstream*), or
  - A resource room where the student receives short periods of individualized assistance to complete assignments from regular classes, or
  - A special self-contained classroom for children with similar problems where all work at a slower, individualized pace, or
  - A tutoring program, the most restrictive environment, for children so learning-disabled that they are unable to participate in any of the above alternative placements. Tutoring may take place outside the school.
- Public Law No. 99-457
  - Mandates the extension of services down to 3 years of age
  - Mandates the use of IEPs
  - Also mandates the use of individual family service plans (IFSPs), to ensure that the services provided meet the needs of the entire family and the child
  - If a child's development is identified to be delayed by either a physician or parent, on the basis of either observation or developmental screening, the child should be referred for a comprehensive, multidisciplinary, developmental evaluation. If the evaluation confirms the delay, *the child must be enrolled in services (early intervention if younger than 3 years old or school system–based programs if after 3 years of age). It is the physician's responsibility to be aware of this requirement.*
- Public Law No. 101-476 (IDEA)
  - A 1990 amendment to Public Law No. 94-142
  - Broadly interprets educational integration by mandating the inclusion of all children, regardless of handicap or special need, in the educational setting provided for nonhandicapped children of the same age
  - School districts must by law provide a full continuum of services.
  - The concept of integration, called *normalization,* has been shown to improve socialization skills.

- Most importantly, IDEA mandates that *transition services* be provided for all students in special education who are 16 years of age or older (e.g., help in finding postsecondary education, vocational training, employment, or independent living).
- Public Law No. 105-17 (IDEA, Part C [1997 Amendments])
  - Parent issues: Parents must be included as team members when any decision affecting a child's identification, evaluation, program, and placement is made.
  - IEP issues
    - The IEP team has to include a regular education teacher if the student has to receive services in regular education classes.
    - IEP teams must consider the following: behavioral interventions when behavior interferes with the students' or others' learning, need for instruction in English, students' communication needs, and need for assistive technology.
    - Once a student reaches the age of 14 years, the IEP must address transition needs focusing on the students' course of study.
- Evaluation and re-evaluation issues
  - Informed consent must be obtained from parents for all evaluations and re-evaluations for special education services.
  - A formal re-evaluation is not required if the IEP team determines that the existing information is sufficient for continued eligibility.
- Disability-related misbehavior
  - IEP teams must determine within 10 days of a suspension whether or not the misconduct was a manifestation of the student's disability.
  - Students who are suspended for more than 10 days or expelled must continue to receive the special education services and supports outlined in their IEP.
  - Schools are allowed to remove students to an alternative educational setting for not more than 45 days if they are in possession of, use, or sell illegal drugs, or if they carry a weapon to school or a school function.

Case for Questions 29 and 30

Mrs. Williams comes to you with her twin 7-year-old boys, Charlie and Joey, to discuss their sleep problems. The boys in general have a well-established routine before bedtime and go to bed at around 8 p.m. each evening. Charlie wakes up at least two to three times a week between 11 p.m. and 1 a.m. appearing "absolutely hysterical" and sweaty; it is difficult or even impossible to awaken him, and he seems unaware that his parents are present in the room with him. He generally falls asleep afterward and has no recall of these events in the morning. Joey frequently awakens between 3 and 6 a.m., also very frightened but coherent and conversant. He tells of very frightening, fanciful dreams, resists

going back to sleep in his own bed, and has full recall of these events in the morning.

29. Charlie is experiencing:
a) Nightmares
b) Night terrors

Answer
The answer is b.

30. Joey is experiencing:
a) Nightmares
b) Night terrors

Answer
The answer is a. Charlie's symptoms are most consistent with night terrors, which tend to occur in stage IV sleep, whereas Joey is having nightmares, which tend to occur in rapid eye movement sleep.

Questions 31 and 32

You are asked to look at a research performed on a new rapid-screening test for group A streptococcal pharyngitis. The test was administered to 1000 children with the following results:

True-positives = 50
False-positives = 300
True-negatives = 600
False-negatives = 50

31. The sensitivity of this screening test is *most* approximately:
a) 33.3%
b) 50%
c) 66.7%
d) 95%

Answer
The answer is b.

32. The specificity of this screening test is *most* approximately:
a) 33.3%
b) 50%
c) 66.7%
d) 95%

Answer
The answer is c.

Explanations for Answers 31 and 32

The concepts of sensitivity, specificity, the null hypothesis, and power of a test are important. You should be able to explain these concepts verbally and by their formulas.

Statistical Definitions

Sensitivity is the likelihood that a test result will be positive in the presence of a targeted disease.

Specificity is the likelihood that a test result will be negative when the disease is absent.

Said another way

Sensitivity = A/A + C		Specificity = D/B + D
	Disease Present	Disease Absent
Test positive	A	B
	True-positives	False-positives
Test negative	C	D
	False-negative	True-negative

The *positive predictive value of a test* indicates the proportion of children with a positive test result who actually have the condition being studied. The lower the prevalence of a disorder, the lower the positive predictive value. Sensitivity may be a better measure in conditions with a low prevalence.

The *negative predictive value of a test* indicates the proportion of children with a negative test result who actually do not have the condition being studied. The value is influenced by the frequency or prevalence of a condition; in conditions with a low prevalence, specificity may be a better measure.

The *prevalence rate* is the number of children in a population with a given disorder among the total number of children in the population at a given time.

The *incidence rate* indicates the risk that a disorder will develop—namely, the number of new cases of a disorder that develop within a period of time.

A *type I error* occurs when, after testing, it is assumed that a given condition differs from normal when in actuality it does not.

A *type II error* occurs when it is assumed that a condition does not differ from normal when in reality it does.

The *null hypothesis* refers to a formal statement indicating no difference between two or more groups. Typically, researchers attempt to disprove the null hypothesis.

The *power of a test* refers to the ability of the test to detect a difference between groups when such a difference really exists. In essence, the power of a test is the probability of not making a type II error.

Reliability refers to consistency or accuracy in measurement.

Validity indicates whether a test measures what it purports to measure.

Case for Questions 33–35

Tommy Johnson, a 9-year-old patient of yours, is brought in for an extended visit by his mother because of her concern about his "problems at school." He is in the third grade, and his teachers have noticed that Tommy is not keeping up with work in class and frequently does not hand in his homework. They describe him as fidgety in class, and he often pesters the children who sit near him, causing disruptions in class. His teachers in the first and second grades never found him difficult to discipline, but this year's teacher states that Tommy rarely responds to verbal reprimands or loss of classroom privileges, and that he is being sent to see the principal with increasing regularity. He is especially problematic whenever called on to speak aloud in class; on such occasions, he becomes clownish. Teasing by other children about this behavior has led to two rather serious fights on the playground. He has engaged in numerous shouting matches with other children at school, and his mother notes that he is also beginning to instigate bad behavior in his brothers at home. Academically, he is struggling in several content courses (language arts, social studies, and science) but is getting a solid grade of B in mathematics. He produced average work in the first and second grades, and Mrs. Johnson states that he seemed to learn to read as well as his two older brothers, who are also average students, and that he rarely asks her for help with his homework. When you ask Mrs. Johnson when she and his teachers first became concerned about Tommy, she answers, "this year."

Like his father, a professional baseball player, Tommy is an avid little leaguer. He is a catcher, and although he performed above age level in the past, just this year he seems to be "out in space" during some games and has therefore had less playing time. You have followed Tommy since birth and are surprised by these recent developments. His physical examination findings are completely normal. A careful review of his family, social, and medical history is largely unhelpful, except that his father dropped out of school at age 16 because the "teachers didn't understand him" and that he had a chance to break into minor league ball. You explain that you would like to get in touch with Tommy's teachers for additional information before formulating a plan. Mrs. Johnson thanks you for your time, and after dismissing Tommy to the waiting room, she adds that Mr. Johnson was recently found to have testicular cancer and may not play next season, although she doubts that Tommy knows this.

33. After collecting your thoughts, you sit down to generate a differential diagnosis. On the basis of the knowledge currently available, which of these diagnoses can nearly certainly be ruled out?
a) Depression
b) Language-based learning disability
c) Attention deficit hyperactivity disorder (ADHD)
d) Oppositional defiant disorder
e) Conduct disorder

Answer

The answer is c. Tommy's situation is clearly complex but not uncommon in children seen in a busy general pediatrics practice. His behavior may suggest any of the diagnoses listed in Question 33. However, it is clear that his behavior has become problematic only this year; therefore, ADHD can be ruled out because one of the key diagnostic criteria is that symptoms must appear before the age of 7 years. Learning disabilities are a definite possibility and may not appear until this age because in general terms children learn to read in the first and second grades and read to learn thereafter. Many children also try to cover up their academic difficulties with misbehavior. Depression is clearly a possibility; since irritability and combativeness are the presenting complaints of many children who are depressed. Oppositional defiant disorder is possible but less likely because Tommy's behaviors are generally not at a level to warrant this diagnosis. Conduct disorder is also possible but less likely because Tommy is not as physically aggressive or seemingly bent on hurting others as are most children with conduct disorder. Therefore, the answer is c.

34. On the following day, you contact Tommy's school and speak with the principal, his teachers, and the school psychologist. The teachers suspect ADHD and wonder if a trial of medication might not be helpful. On the basis of your concern about a possible learning disability, the school psychologist agrees to perform a multifactored evaluation (MFE), which includes intelligence and achievement testing, in addition to separate testing for ADHD. The overall intelligence quotient (IQ) is 95, with verbal IQ subscore of 85 and a performance IQ of 108. The WRAT is also done, with a word identification score of 80, spelling score of 87, and mathematics computation score of 95. Two separate instruments are used to screen for ADHD; however, the results of neither are suggestive. Appropriate interventions would include which of the following?
a) Formal audiologic evaluation
b) Further testing to evaluate language abilities
c) Tutoring in reading and language skills
d) Preferential seating near the front of the classroom
e) All of the above

Answer
The answer is e. A hearing and vision screening is always a good idea in any child who is having difficulty in school. Tommy's scores do not meet the requirements of most states for learning disability because his IQ and achievement scores do not differ by two standard deviations, but his language scores are consistently lower than his mathematics and overall academic scores. This discrepancy would account for the difficulties he is experiencing in content courses because these classes are largely language based. Because Tommy's scores do not meet diagnostic criteria for learning disability or MR, the school system is not required to provide him with additional services, such as tutoring. However, his language scores put him very close to the diagnosis of a specific language-based learning disability, and many schools make accommodations for such children, such as a Title 1 reading

program. The family may also choose to enroll him in private tutoring. If he had met the criteria for the diagnosis of learning disability, his remediation program would have had to be detailed in an IEP, which is drafted for children over 3 years of age who receive special education services through their school system. In general, it states what the child's specific problem areas are, what will be done to remediate them, and how and when the child will be re-evaluated. An IEP should not be confused with an IFSP, which is the document drafted for children under 3 years of age to detail the services that will be provided to them in an early intervention program. Seating near the front of the room should be considered for all children with academic difficulties to reduce distractions. It should also be recalled that the most common comorbidity in children with learning disabilities is ADHD, and because many children display behaviors that are clearly problematic but not quite diagnostic for a specific psychologic diagnosis, Tommy may display many of the behaviors consistent with ADHD and learning disabilities. So, the most appropriate answer is e.

35. For assistance with behavioral intervention, you refer Tommy and his parents to a trusted child psychologist. She learns that Tommy inadvertently saw a letter to his father from his oncologist and recognized the word "cancer." He has also overheard his parents discussing the diagnosis late at night on several occasions because he has been having difficulty falling asleep. He is worried that he may lose his father but has been afraid to discuss this fear with his parents. He feels badly about his behavior at school but states that "he can't help it." His faltering grades have left him feeling poorly about himself, but he denies any suicidal ideations. He also denies any wish to harm others, animals, or property. Which one of the following suggestions made by the psychologist does not surprise you?
a) Retaining Tommy in the third grade next year
b) Instituting individual therapy for suspected depression
c) Instituting family therapy to explore the issues surrounding Mr. Johnson's cancer diagnosis
d) Instituting a trial of antidepressant medication for suspected depression
e) Enrolling Tommy in additional extracurricular activities to boost his self-esteem

Answer
The answer is b. With regard to Question 35, grade retention is rarely thought to be beneficial for children with academic difficulties; development of an effective remediation program is believed to be best. Although one could consider a trial of medication for Tommy, implementation of the aforementioned plans for a trial period seems to be a more prudent recommendation at this point. The initiation of psychologic counseling to help Tommy cope with the news of his father's illness

and his school issues seems very appropriate at this time. Individual therapy is likely to be most effective because many of Tommy's issues may be related to a reactive depression caused by the news of his father's cancer, which may be of less concern to him once he understands it better. However, counseling his parents on how to communicate these issues to him and how to handle his behavior would also be of benefit. Finally, although enrolling children with learning disabilities/difficulties in extracurricular activities that allow them to experience success is often helpful, Tommy's parents have already done this with baseball, and so further time away from home is not likely to be beneficial. Therefore, the preferred answer is b.

SUGGESTED READINGS

1. Achenbach TM, Ruffle TM. The child behavior checklist and related forms for assessing behavioral emotional problems and competencies. *Pediatr Rev* 2000;21:265–271.
2. Braaten EB, Norman D. Intelligence (IQ) testing. *Pediatr Rev* 2006;27:403–408.
3. Evans OB, Vedanarayanan V. Guillain-Barré syndrome. *Pediatr Rev* 1997;18:10–16.
4. Glascoe FP. Early detection of developmental and behavioral problems. *Pediatr Rev* 2000;21:272–280.
5. Johnson CP. Using developmental and behavioral screening tests. *Pediatr Rev* 2000;21:255–256.
6. Liptak GS. The pediatrician's role in caring for the developmentally disabled child. *Pediatr Rev* 1996;17:203–210.
7. Schreiner MS, Field E, Ruddy R. Infant botulism: a review of 12 years' experience at the Children's Hospital of Philadelphia. *Pediatrics* 1991;87:159–165.

Chapter 41

Chromosomal Abnormalities

George E. Tiller

For more than 50 years, chromosomal abnormalities have been recognized as the basis of certain genetic syndromes. Initially, only aneuploidies (the presence of more or fewer than 46 chromosomes) could be detected. Now, with the availability of fluorescence in situ hybridization (FISH) and DNA methylation testing, microdeletions and uniparental disomy (UPD) can be documented. The advent of microarray-based analysis (comparative genomic hybridization, or CGH) takes resolution to an even finer level, and introduces the confounding phenomenon of copy number variation. We have learned that although we carry two copies of each autosomal gene, the normal process of imprinting fine tunes the expression of certain regions of many chromosomes by silencing one copy of certain genes by DNA methylation. Consequently, UPD (presumably caused by trisomic "rescue" after fertilization) may result in the silencing of both copies of a gene or contiguous group of genes, despite the normal complement of 46 intact chromosomes. Further refinements in cytogenetic techniques, in tandem with molecular genetics, are making it possible to unravel normal processes in human development and pathologic processes in the origin of cancer.

The objectives of this chapter are to help the reader to:

- Identify several indications of karyotyping.
- Describe the clinical features of the more common chromosomal anomalies.
- Appreciate the concepts of contiguous gene syndromes, imprinting, and UPD.

INCIDENCE OF CHROMOSOMAL DISORDERS

Chromosomal disorders are:

- Found in >7% of human conceptuses
- Responsible for >50% of miscarriages (trisomy 16 > 45, XO > others)
- Found in 1 in 200 liveborn infants

INDICATIONS FOR CHROMOSOMAL ANALYSIS

Neonatal Period and Infancy (0–3 Years)

- Phenotype of chromosomal anomaly (+21, +18, +13, XO)
- Multiple congenital anomalies
- Ambiguous genitalia
- Certain tumors (retinoblastoma, Wilms tumor)

Childhood (4–10 Years)

- Mental retardation (MR) and multiple congenital anomalies
- Phenotype of chromosomal anomaly (XO, XXY, XYY)

Adolescence (11–20 Years)

- Primary amenorrhea
- Abnormal stature

Adults (20> Years)

- Infertility with or without habitual abortion
- Familial chromosomal aberration
- Leukemia or certain tumors
- Pregnancy at advanced maternal age
- Pregnancy with risk for X-linked disorder

TYPES OF CHROMOSOMAL ABNORMALITIES

Numeric Changes

- Of sets: triploidy, tetraploidy (all lethal)
- Individual: trisomy, monosomy, sex chromosome aneuploidy
- Mosaicism

Structural Changes

- Deletions
- Duplications
- Translocations
- Inversions

Functional Changes

- Methylation defects (often caused by UPD)

EXAMPLES OF CHROMOSOMAL DISORDERS

Trisomy 21 (Down Syndrome)

- *Incidence:* 1 in 750 (most common recognizable cause of MR)
- *Growth and development:* May or may not be small-for-gestational-age; short stature, MR
- *Central nervous system (CNS):* Hypotonia, delayed motor skills, premature aging
- *Craniofacial:* Flat face and occiput, upward-slanting palpebral fissures, epicanthal folds, Brushfield spots, prominent tongue, small ears, depressed nasal bridge
- *Extremities:* Simian creases, clinodactyly, short fingers, increased space between the first and second toes, increased ulnar loops
- *Cardiac:* Congenital heart disease in >50% of patients, including ventricular septal defect, endocardial cushion defects (atrioventricular canal)
- *Abdominal:* Umbilical hernia, diastasis recti, duodenal obstruction
- *Skin/hair:* Thin hair
- *Remarks:* Increased risk of hypothyroidism, leukemia; all trisomies associated with advanced maternal age

Trisomy 13

- *Incidence:* 1 in 5000
- *Growth and development:* Small-for-gestational-age, intrauterine growth retardation, failure to thrive, severe MR
- *CNS:* Hypotonia, seizures, apnea, deafness, holoprosencephaly
- *Craniofacial:* Microcephaly, microphthalmia, colobomata, cleft lip and palate, abnormal ears
- *Extremities:* Polydactyly (Fig. 41.1), flexion deformities, clubfoot
- *Cardiac:* Ventricular septal defect, patent ductus arteriosus, atrial septal defect, coarctation of the aorta
- *Abdominal:* Umbilical hernia, omphalocele, single umbilical artery
- *Renal:* Polycystic kidneys
- *Skin/hair:* Occipital scalp defects (cutis aplasia), hemangiomas
- *Remarks:* Survival rate beyond the first year is <20%

Trisomy 18

- *Incidence:* 1 in 3000
- *Growth and development:* Small-for-gestational-age, intrauterine growth retardation, failure to thrive, severe MR
- *CNS:* Hypertonia

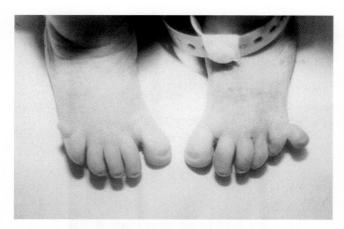

Figure 41.1 Newborn with trisomy 13. Note the postaxial poly-dactyly on left foot.

- *Craniofacial:* Prominent occiput; low-set, malformed ears; micrognathia; cleft lip and palate (Fig. 41.2)
- *Extremities:* Overlapping fingers, rocker-bottom feet, clubfoot (Fig. 41.3)
- *Cardiac:* Ventricular septal defect, patent ductus arteriosus, atrial septal defect
- *Abdominal:* Inguinal, umbilical hernias
- *Renal:* Various anomalies
- *Skin/hair:* Single flexion crease on digits
- *Remarks:* Survival rate beyond the first year is <10%

Turner Syndrome

- *Incidence:* 1 in 2500 liveborn girls
- *Growth and development:* Short stature, visual and spatial perceptive disabilities
- *CNS:* Hearing impairment
- *Craniofacial:* Short, webbed neck (Fig. 41.4); low posterior hairline, prominent ears

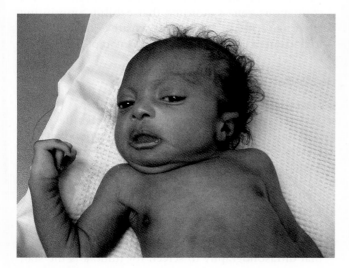

Figure 41.2 Six-week-old male infant with trisomy 18. Note the emaciated appearance, sloping forehead, and clenched fingers.

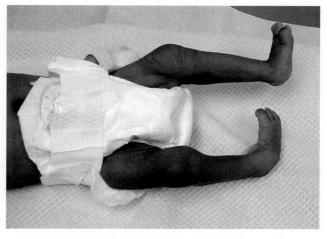

Figure 41.3 Six-week-old male infant with trisomy 18. Note the rocker-bottom feet.

- *Extremities:* Cubitus valgus (increased carrying angle at elbow)
- *Cardiac:* Coarctation of the aorta, hypoplastic left ventricle, aortic stenosis
- *Thorax:* Broad chest, widely spaced nipples
- *Renal:* Horseshoe kidney

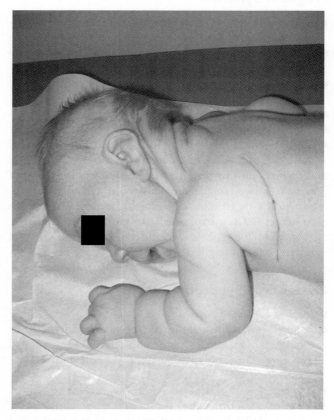

Figure 41.4 Infant with Turner syndrome. Note the remarkably excessive nuchal skin, puffy hand, and thoracotomy scar from coarctation repair.

- *Skin/hair:* Lymphedema in infancy, increased pigmented nevi
- *Genital:* Ovarian dysgenesis, primary amenorrhea, lack of secondary sexual characteristics, sterility, gonadoblastoma (if mosaic 45,X/46,XY)
- *Remarks:* 45,X in 50%; structural abnormality of X (ringX, isoX) in 25%; mosaicism in 25% (e.g., 45,X/46,XX; 45,X/46,XY); growth hormone and estrogen replacement therapies are well established

Klinefelter Syndrome

- *Incidence:* 1 in 800 (most common sex chromosome anomaly)
- *Growth and development:* Tall, thin; obese adults; mild developmental delay; expressive language disabilities
- *CNS:* Mild ataxia (some)
- *Extremities:* Long limbs
- *Abdominal/pelvic:* Female (eunuchoid) shape
- *Skin/hair:* Scant facial and pubic hair
- *Genital:* Hypogonadism, small penis, infertility
- *Remarks:* Increased gynecomastia, scoliosis; testosterone replacement therapy is well established; risk for breast cancer comparable with women

Fragile X Syndrome

- *Incidence:* 1 in 4000 males (second most common recognizable cause of MR)
- *Growth and development:* Autism, delayed and perseverative speech, echolalia, moderate to severe MR
- *Craniofacial:* Large, protruding ears; prognathism; long, narrow face; pale blue irides
- *Extremities:* Hyperextensible fingers, flat feet
- *Cardiac:* Mitral valve prolapse
- *Genital:* Macro-orchidism (only 40% of prepubertal patients); premature ovarian failure in carrier females
- *Remarks:* Learning disability or mild MR in one third of female carriers; fragile site marker on Xq27 is seen cytogenetically in 10% to 40% of cells; molecular methods to detect $(CCG)_n$ expansion are much more sensitive. More than 200 repeats is considered a full mutation and is diagnostic of fragile X syndrome

Prader-Willi Syndrome

- *Incidence:* 1 in 20,000
- *Features:* Small for gestational age, neonatal hypotonia, hypogonadism, small hands and feet, almond-shaped eyes (Fig. 41.5), polyphagia, obesity, short stature, skin-picking behavior, MR
- *Complications:* Pickwickian syndrome, diabetes mellitus
- *Remarks:* Deletions at chromosome 15q11 in 70% of patients, UPD in 25%; contiguous gene syndrome that exhibits imprinting; DNA methylation is the most

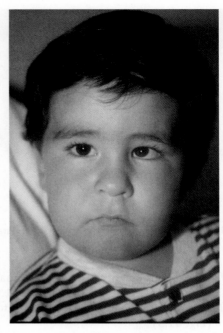

Figure 41.5 Five-year-old boy with Prader-Willi syndrome. Note the almond-shaped eyes, epicanthal folds, and incidental strabismus.

sensitive diagnostic test to document loss of *paternal* 15q11 component

Angelman Syndrome

- *Incidence:* 1 in 20,000
- *Features:* Microcephaly, broad mouth, large jaw, seizures, ataxia (*puppet-like* gait), inappropriate laughter, absent speech; autism
- *Remarks:* Deletions at chromosome 15q11 in 70% of patients, UPD in 7%, UBE3A gene mutations in 11%; contiguous gene syndrome that exhibits imprinting; DNA methylation is the most sensitive diagnostic test to document loss *of maternal* 15q11 component

Beckwith-Wiedemann Syndrome

- *Incidence:* 1 in 15,000
- *Features:* Large-for-gestational age, infantile hypoglycemia, macroglossia (large tongue), earlobe pits and creases, omphalocele, organomegaly, asymmetric limb length (Fig. 41.6)
- *Complications:* Increased risk for abdominal tumors (Wilms tumor, hepatoblastoma)
- *Remarks:* Methylation defects at chromosome 11p15 in 50% of patients, 20% because of UPD; contiguous gene syndrome that exhibits imprinting; serial abdominal ultrasonography to screen for tumors is the standard of care

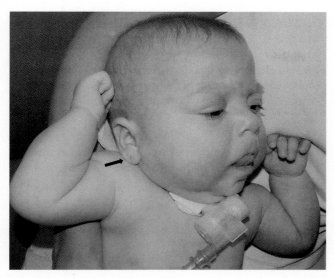

Figure 41.6 Infant with Beckwith-Wiedemann syndrome. Note the large tongue (necessitating tracheostomy), and earlobe creases (*arrow*).

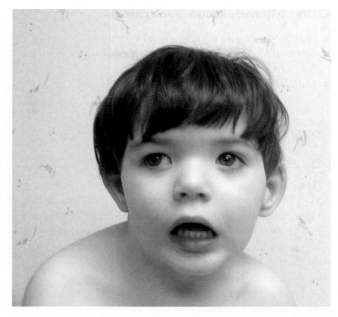

Figure 41.7 Three-year-old girl with cri du chat (5p-) syndrome. Note the hypertelorism, epicanthal folds, microcephaly, and downward-turned corners of mouth.

Williams Syndrome

- *Frequency:* 1 in 7500
- *Features:* Mild growth deficiency, variable MR, "cocktail party" personality, stellate irides, periorbital fullness, long philtrum, full lips, hoarse voice, supravalvular aortic stenosis
- *Complications:* Hypercalcemia, renal disease
- *Remarks:* Contiguous gene syndrome, including elastin gene on chromosome 7q 11; FISH is the preferred diagnostic test (>99% sensitivity)

Cri Du Chat Syndrome (5p-)

- *Incidence:* 1 in 20,000
- *Inheritance:* Sporadic (10% have parent with balanced translocation)
- *Growth and development:* Small-for-gestational-age, moderate to profound MR
- *Features:* weak, high-pitched "cat-like" cry; hypotonia, microcephaly, hypertelorism (**Fig. 41.7**), epicanthal folds, downward-slanting palpebral fissures, small jaw, low-set ears, congenital heart disease, inguinal hernias, profound speech impairment
- *Remarks:* Somewhat diminished life span; respond to infant stimulation

CATCH 22 Syndrome

- *Includes:* DiGeorge syndrome, Shprintzen (velocardiofacial) syndrome, isolated congenital heart disease (some)
- *Incidence:* 1 in 5000

- *Inheritance:* Most cases sporadic (10%–25% have normal parent with 22q deletion)
- *Features:* Cardiac defects (especially tetralogy of Fallot), abnormal facies, thymic hypoplasia (**Fig. 41.8**), cleft palate, hypocalcemia; developmental delay
- *Remarks:* Deletions at 22q11; FISH is the most sensitive diagnostic test; embryologic defect in DiGeorge syndrome is the underdevelopment of the fourth branchial arch and the third and fourth pharyngeal pouches

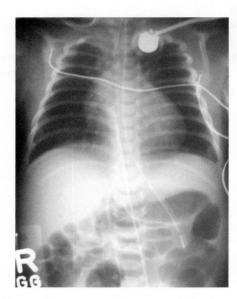

Figure 41.8 Newborn with DiGeorge syndrome. Note absence of thymic shadow.

Other Microdeletion Syndromes

- Smith-Magenis syndrome: 17p11 deletion
- Trichorhinophalangeal syndrome (Langer-Giedion): 8q24 deletion
- Miller-Dieker lissencephaly: 17p13 deletion

REVIEW EXERCISES

QUESTIONS

Case

1. An 11–year-old boy presents with a tall, thin stature. He is taller than either parent and is otherwise healthy, but a below-average student in school. Your differential diagnosis includes all of the following *except*:
a) Marfan syndrome
b) Klinefelter syndrome
c) Ehlers-Danlos syndrome
d) Beckwith-Wiedemann syndrome

Answer

The answer is d. Patients with any of the disorders listed except Beckwith-Wiedemann syndrome have a tall, thin stature. Patients with Beckwith-Wiedemann syndrome are more likely to be large and muscular.

2. Physical examination reveals hypogonadism, normal joint mobility, and no organomegaly. You elect to obtain a karyotype, which reveals 47,XXY in 20 of the 20 cells counted. What additional testing is indicated?
a) Echocardiography
b) Renal ultrasonography
c) Psychometric testing
d) None of the above

Answer

The answer is c. The incidence of major organ anomalies is not increased in Klinefelter syndrome. Psychometric testing may reveal a specific learning disability, which can be addressed to improve the patient's school performance.

3. What pharmacologic therapy might be considered at this time?
a) Methylphenidate
b) Testosterone
c) Follicle-stimulating hormone
d) Adrenocorticotropic hormone

Answer

The answer is b. If the boy is excessively tall, testosterone replacement therapy may be instituted at this age to initiate pubertal changes and close the epiphyseal growth plates.

4. What is the risk for recurrence in this patient?
a) 0%
b) 25%
c) 50%
d) 100%

Answer

The answer is a. All patients with Klinefelter syndrome are sterile. Testosterone therapy induces and maintains secondary sexual characteristics, but it does not cure infertility.

SUGGESTED READINGS

1. American Academy of Pediatrics http://www.aap.org/health-topics/genetics.cfm Under the "AAP Policy" heading, see Health Supervision of Children with Down syndrome (2001), Fragile X syndrome (1996), Turner syndrome (2003), and Williams syndrome (2001).
2. Chen C, Visootsak J, Dills S, Graham JM Jr. Prader-Willi syndrome: an update and review for the primary pediatrician. *Clin Pediatr* 2007;46(7):580–591.
3. GeneReviews at GeneTests: Medical Genetics Information Resource (database online). Copyright, University of Washington, Seattle. 1993–2008. Available at http://www.genetests.org
4. Jones KL. *Smith's recognizable patterns of human malformation*, 6th ed. Philadelphia: Elsevier-Saunders, 2005.
5. McDonald-McGinn DM, Kirschner R. The Philadelphia story: the 22q11.2 deletion: report on 250 patients. *Gen Couns* 1999;10: 11–24.
6. Moeschler JB, Shevell M. Clinical genetic evaluation of the child with mental retardation or developmental delays. *Pediatrics* 2006; 117:2304–2316.

Chapter 42

Dysmorphic Syndromes

George E. Tiller

Dysmorphology is the art and science of abnormal physical development. It is often subjective, and distinguishing between familial traits and true dysmorphic features is sometimes difficult. A recognizable pattern of human malformation is dubbed a *syndrome.* Some syndromes are associated with a single underlying genetic defect or chromosomal anomaly, others have a multifactorial basis (genetic plus environmental), and still others have no apparent genetic basis at all, being simply *birth defects.* Genetic disorders contribute significantly to morbidity and mortality at all ages. More than 3500 mendelian (single-gene) disorders have been catalogued. It has been estimated that 1% to 2% of newborns have significant birth defects. Although individually rare, genetically related disorders are responsible for one third of all pediatric hospital admissions. We must also appreciate that many genetic disorders are insidious in onset and may present to the clinician in a wide range of age groups.

A three-generation family history is an essential component of the evaluation of a possible genetic disorder. Questions about ethnicity and possible consanguinity are a routine part of this process. The family history is followed by a review of the patient's medical history and then by a careful, objective physical examination. Anthropometric graphs from appropriate texts can remove some of the subjectiveness involved in determining the disproportionality of body parts. Once a differential diagnosis has been constructed, specific testing can begin, if available. Genetic counseling is the last step in the clinical evaluation, once all the information available has been analyzed.

The objectives of this chapter are to help the reader:

- Distinguish different mechanisms underlying congenital anomalies
- Describe the clinical features and molecular basis (if known) of the more common *dysmorphic* syndromes

CATEGORIES OF CONGENITAL ANOMALIES

- *Malformation:* A morphologic defect resulting from an intrinsically abnormal developmental process. Causes may be chromosomal, genetic (a single gene), teratogenic, or idiopathic. Examples are cleft lip, cleft palate, congenital heart defects, and neural tube defects.
- *Deformation:* An abnormal form, shape, or position of a body part caused by mechanical forces. The cause is often uterine constraint. Examples are craniosynostosis and clubfoot.
- *Disruption:* Destruction of a previously normally forming body part. Causes include amniotic bands and vascular disruption. Examples are limb reduction defects and gastroschisis.
- *Dysplasia:* Abnormal organization or proliferation of cells into a tissue. Causes include some single-gene defects. Examples include ectodermal dysplasias and skeletal dysplasias.
- *Sequence:* A cascade effect resulting from a single embryologic event that may affect surrounding tissues. Examples include Pierre-Robin sequence, amnion rupture, oligohydramnios, and DiGeorge syndrome.

WHEN TO CONSIDER A DYSMORPHIC SYNDROME

Dysmorphic syndromes must be considered in the presence of:
- More than one anomaly present
- Phenotypic variation from parents and siblings
- Abnormal growth: prenatal (and sometimes postnatal) growth retardation (or overgrowth)
- Neurologic symptoms (e.g., seizures, mental retardation [MR], abnormal muscle tone, deafness, blindness, speech delay with or without motor delay)

331

EXAMPLES OF MORE "COMMON" GENETIC SYNDROMES

Achondroplasia

- *Frequency:* Most common nonlethal skeletal dysplasia (1 in 26,000)
- *Inheritance:* Autosomal dominant (80% new mutations)
- *Features:* Short-limbed dwarfism, macrocephaly with frontal bossing and saddle nose, infantile gibbus progressing to lumbar lordosis, trident hand, and tibial bowing **(Fig. 42.1)**
- *Complications:* Infantile hypotonia, apnea secondary to tight foramen magnum, ventriculomegaly, and cervical and lumbar spinal cord compression
- *Primary defect:* Fibroblast growth factor receptor 3

Marfan Syndrome

- *Frequency:* 1 in 10,000
- *Inheritance:* Autosomal dominant (>15% new mutations)
- *Features:* Tall, lanky habitus; dolichocephaly and high, arched palate; arachnodactyly, joint laxity; pectus deformity, scoliosis; myopia, ectopia lentis; mitral valve prolapse, aortic root dilatation; dural ectasias **(Figs. 42.2–42.4)**
- *Complications:* Joint instability, visual impairment, aortic insufficiency, aneurysmal rupture causing sudden death, spontaneous pneumothorax, and pulmonary blebs
- *Treatment:* Atenolol or other cardioselective β-blocker; losartan
- *Primary defect: Fibrillin,* a connective tissue protein

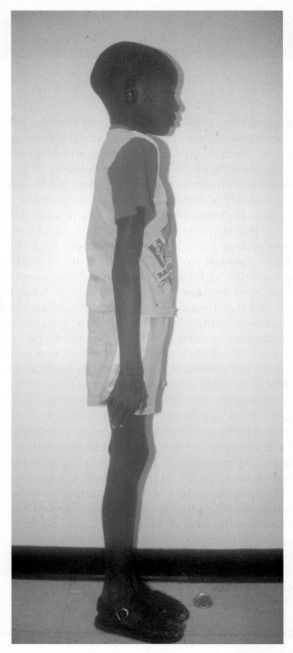

Figure 42.2 Nine-year-old boy with Marfan syndrome. Note the tall, thin stature.

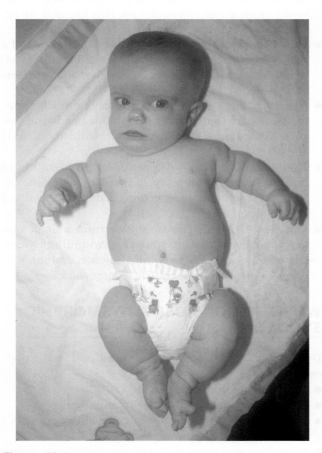

Figure 42.1 Six-month-old boy with achondroplasia. Note the macrocephaly, frontal bossing, upturned nares, and short limbs.

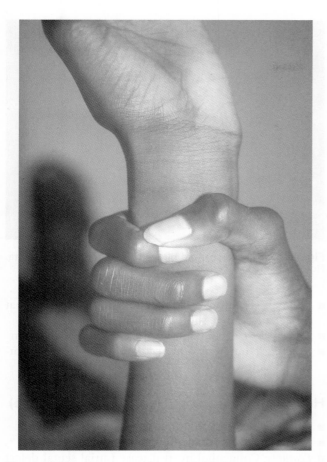

Figure 42.3 Nine-year-old boy with Marfan syndrome. Note the positive wrist sign.

Ehlers-Danlos Syndrome

- *Frequency:* 1 in 10,000
- *Inheritance:* Autosomal dominant (mostly), rarely autosomal recessive
- *Features:* Skin hyperelasticity (**Fig. 42.5**), poor wound healing, excessive bruising; joint laxity (**Fig. 42.6**), pectus deformity, and scoliosis
- *Complications:* Joint instability; aneurysmal rupture causing sudden death (type IV or *arterial* form only)
- *Primary defects:* Type III or V collagen; lysyl hydroxylase; others unknown
- *Remarks:* Ten known clinical types of Ehlers-Danlos syndrome, caused by defects in different genes and with varying severity

Osteogenesis Imperfecta

- *Frequency:* 1 in 20,000
- *Inheritance:* Autosomal dominant, rarely autosomal recessive
- *Features:* Vary from mild to lethal (perinatal); osteoporosis, bone fragility causing pathologic fractures (**Fig. 42.7**); dentinogenesis imperfecta (**Fig. 42.8**); Wormian bones in occiput; blue sclerae; hearing loss

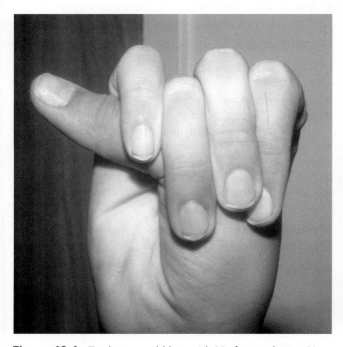

Figure 42.4 Twelve-year-old boy with Marfan syndrome. Note the positive thumb sign.

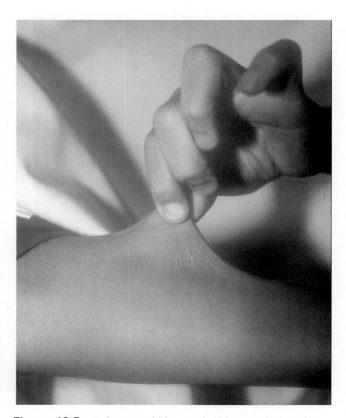

Figure 42.5 Eight-year-old boy with Ehlers-Danlos syndrome (type VIII). Note the skin hyperelasticity on the forearm.

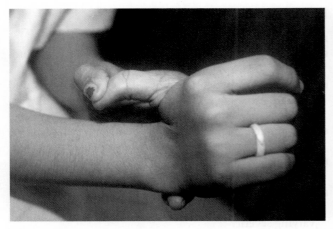

Figure 42.6 Eighteen-year-old woman with Ehlers-Danlos syndrome (type II). Note the joint hyperextensibility.

- *Complications:* Pulmonary hypoplasia, death (type II); scoliosis, progressive deformities (type III); short stature (type IV)
- *Primary defect:* Type I collagen

Anhydrotic Ectodermal Dysplasia

- *Frequency:* 1 in 10,000
- *Inheritance:* X-linked; female carriers mildly affected

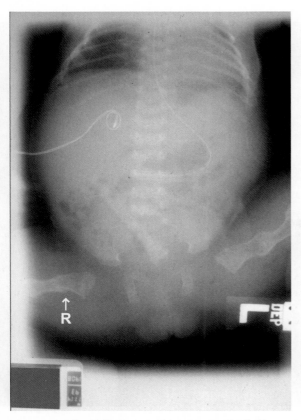

Figure 42.7 Radiograph of term newborn girl with osteogenesis imperfecta. Note the diffuse osteopenia, healed femoral fracture (L), and displaced acute femoral fracture (R).

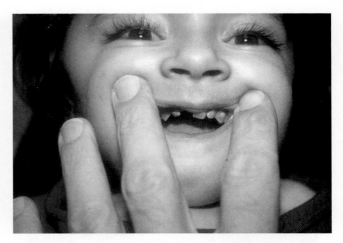

Figure 42.8 Five-year-old girl with osteogenesis imperfecta. Note the dentinogenesis imperfecta.

- *Features:* Hypotrichosis, hypodontia, anhydrosis, heat intolerance, atopy, short stature, and mild MR
- *Primary defect:* Ectodysplasin, a transmembrane protein
- *Remarks:* Numerous other ectodermal dysplasia disorders are known!

Holt-Oram Syndrome (Heart-Hand Syndrome)

- *Frequency:* 1 in 100,000
- *Inheritance:* Autosomal dominant, variable expression
- *Features:* Congenital heart disease (atrial septal defect > ventricular septal defect); finger-like or absent thumb (Fig. 42.9); radial hypoplasia
- *Primary defect:* TBX5 gene, a transcription factor

Thanatophoric Dysplasia

- *Frequency:* 1 in 50,000 (most common *lethal* skeletal dysplasia)
- *Inheritance:* Sporadic, dominant-acting mutation
- *Features:* Short-limbed dwarfism, curved long bones, narrow thorax, and flattened vertebrae (platyspondyly)
- *Complications:* Death resulting from pulmonary hypoplasia
- *Primary defect:* Fibroblast growth factor receptor 3 (allelic with achondroplasia)

Treacher-Collins Syndrome (Mandibulofacial Dysostosis)

- *Frequency:* 1 in 10,000
- *Inheritance:* Autosomal dominant
- *Features:* Malar and mandibular hypoplasia, external and middle ear anomalies, downward-slanting palpebral fissures (Figs. 42.10 and 42.11), eyelid colobomata, and cleft palate
- *Complications:* Feeding difficulties, conductive hearing loss, MR (5%), and congenital heart disease (10%)

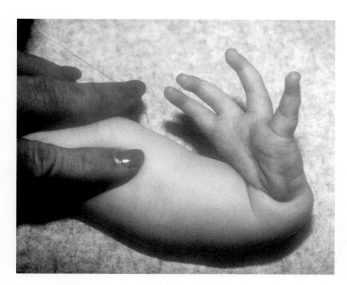

Figure 42.9 Three-month-old girl with Holt-Oram syndrome. Note the absence of thumb.

- *Primary defect:* TCOF1 (aka *treacle*), a nucleolar trafficking protein
- *Remarks:* Several features in common with Goldenhar syndrome, but anomalies in Treacher-Collins (TC) syndrome are usually symmetric, and TC syndrome is dominantly inherited

Goldenhar Syndrome (Facioauriculovertebral Spectrum)

- *Frequency:* 1 in 10,000
- *Inheritance:* Sporadic

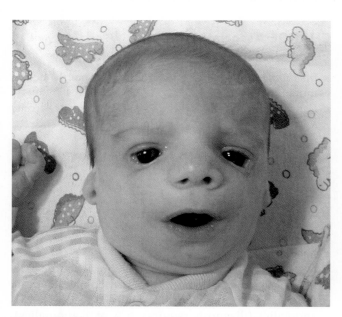

Figure 42.10 Three-week-old boy with Treacher-Collins syndrome. Note the downward-slanting palpebral fissures, malar hypoplasia, long philtrum, and dysplastic ears bilaterally.

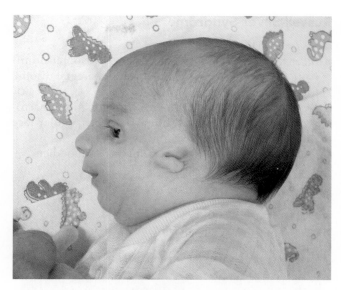

Figure 42.11 Three-week-old boy with Treacher-Collins syndrome. Note the micrognathia and low-set dysplastic ear.

- *Features:* Hemifacial microsomia (10%–30% bilateral), external and middle ear anomalies, macrostomia (larger mouth on affected side), micrognathia, epibulbar dermoids **(Fig. 42.12)**, colobomata, and cervical spine anomalies
- *Complications:* Feeding difficulties, conductive hearing loss, MR (10%), congenital heart disease (10%), and cleft palate (10%)
- *Cause:* Stapedial artery *disruption* possibly leading to first and second branchial arch hypoplasia
- *Remarks:* Several features in common with TC syndrome, but anomalies in TC syndrome are usually symmetric, and TC syndrome is dominantly inherited

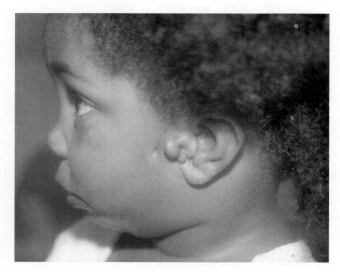

Figure 42.12 Four-year-old girl with Goldenhar syndrome. Note the micrognathia, epibulbar dermoid, preauricular skin tags, and low-set, posteriorly rotated ear. Opposite ear is normal in appearance.

Russell-Silver Syndrome

- *Frequency:* Uncommon
- *Inheritance:* Mostly sporadic; rarely autosomal dominant, autosomal recessive; maternal uniparental disomy for chromosome 7 (10%)
- *Features:* Prenatal/postnatal growth retardation, macrocephaly, large fontanelle, blue sclerae, triangular face (**Fig. 42.13**), and limb asymmetry
- *Complications:* Hypoglycemia in infants and toddlers

Noonan Syndrome

- *Frequency:* 1 in 2500
- *Inheritance:* Autosomal dominant

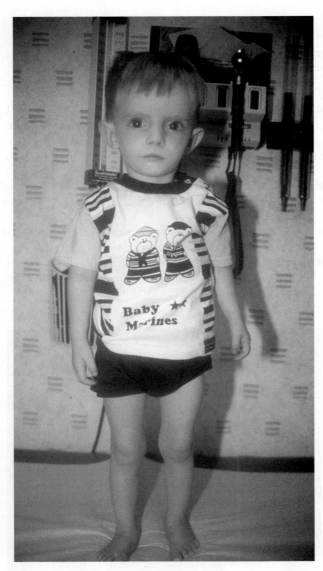

Figure 42.13   Three-year-old boy with Russell-Silver syndrome. Note the strikingly short stature, relative macrocephaly with broad forehead and triangular face. Asymmetry of limb length is not evident in this photograph.

- *Features:* Short stature, webbed neck, ptosis, pulmonic stenosis, mild MR, broad chest, vertebral anomalies, bleeding diathesis, and cryptorchidism
- *Primary defect:* Mutations in PTPN11 (50% of cases), a protein phosphatase, also in other genes (SOS1, RAF1, KRAS)
- *Remarks:* Often called *male Turner syndrome*, but chromosomes are normal and both males and females can be affected

Cornelia de Lange Syndrome

- *Frequency:* 1 in 25,000
- *Inheritance:* Sporadic; autosomal dominant-acting mutations
- *Features:* Prenatal and postnatal growth retardation, characteristic facies (synophrys, low anterior hairline, anteverted nares, maxillary prognathism, long philtrum, "carp" mouth), MR, cardiac defects, and upper limb anomalies
- *Primary defect:* "Nipped-B–like" gene, also called *delangin*

Rett Syndrome

- *Frequency:* 1 in 15,000
- *Inheritance:* X-linked dominant
- *Features:* Developmental arrest at 6 to 12 months, acquired microcephaly, epilepsy, loss of purposeful hand movements, autism, and growth failure
- *Primary defect:* MECP2 gene (methyl-CpG-binding protein)
- *Differential diagnosis:* Angelman syndrome

CHARGE Association

- *Frequency:* 1 in 15,000
- *Inheritance:* Sporadic; autosomal dominantly acting mutations
- *Features:* *C*oloboma, *H*eart anomalies, choanal *A*tresia, *R*etarded growth and development, *G*enital and *E*ar anomalies
- *Primary defect (some cases):* Chromodomain helicase DNA-binding protein 7 (CHD7)

VATER (VACTERL) Association

- *Frequency:* 1 in 8000
- *Inheritance:* Sporadic
- *Features:* *V*ertebral anomalies, *A*nal atresia, *C*ardiac defects, *T*racheo-esophageal fistula, *E*sophageal atresia (**Fig. 42.14**), *R*enal anomalies, *L*imb (especially radial) anomalies (diagnosis requires ≥ 3 of 7 anomalies); other anomalies may also be present

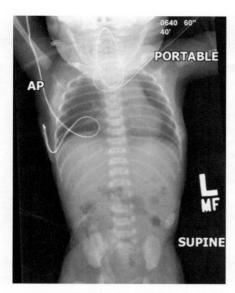

Figure 42.14 Chest radiograph of newborn with VATER association. Note the coiling of nasogastric tube due to T-E fistula with esophageal atresia. Vertebral defect is not evident.

- *Primary defect:* Unknown; increased incidence among infants of diabetic mothers

Klippel-Feil Anomaly

- *Frequency:* 1 in 40,000
- *Inheritance:* Sporadic; rarely autosomal dominant, autosomal recessive
- *Features:* Short, webbed neck; cervical vertebral fusion defects (**Fig. 42.15**); may be associated with hearing loss, laryngeal deformities, congenital heart disease, rib anomalies, upper limb defects, and genitourinary anomalies
- *Primary defect:* unknown; likely genetically heterogeneous
- *Differential diagnosis:* basal cell nevus syndrome, Wildervanck syndrome

Amyoplasia

- *Frequency:* 1 in 5000
- *Inheritance:* Sporadic
- *Features:* Multiple fixed joints, midline facial vascular markings, and normal intelligence
- *Primary defect:* Presumptive intrauterine insult to anterior horn cells innervating limbs
- *Remarks: Arthrogryposis* is a genetically heterogeneous feature; amyoplasia is a specific diagnosis within this group of disorders

Fetal Alcohol Syndrome

- *Frequency:* 1 in 1000 (uncertain); affecting only one third of infants born to mothers with chronic alcoholism

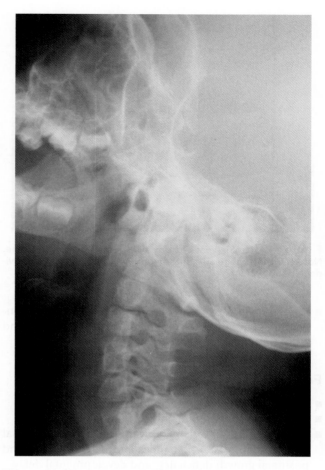

Figure 42.15 Lateral cervical spine film of a child with Klippel-Feil anomaly. Note the posterior fusion of C3-C4.

- *Inheritance:* (Environmental)
- *Features* (**Table 42.1**): Prenatal and postnatal growth deficiency; microcephaly, small palpebral fissures, long and smooth philtrum, thin upper lip; small distal phalanges and nails (**Fig. 42.16**); developmental delay, behavioral problems (irritability leading to hyperactivity), mild to moderate MR

TABLE 42.1

TEN MOST COMMON FINDINGS IN FETAL ALCOHOL SYNDROME

Microcephaly	Diminished intelligence quotient
Smooth philtrum	Retrognathia (small jaw)
Thin upper lip	Growth deficiency (prenatal, postnatal)
Hyperactivity	Eye anomalies (ptosis, strabismus)
Hypertonia	Finger anomalies (nail hypoplasia)

Adapted from Smitherman CH. The lasting impact of fetal alcohol syndrome and fetal alcohol effect on children and adolescents. *J Pediatr Health Care* 1994;8:121–126.

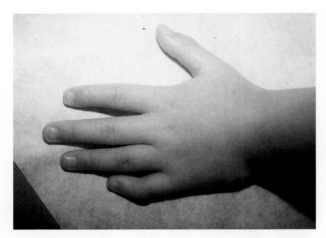

Figure 42.16 Six-year-old boy with fetal alcohol syndrome. Note the short, angulated fifth finger. Nail hypoplasia is not evident in this patient.

- *Complications:* Involvement of other organ systems (congenital heart disease, renal anomalies, cleft lip and palate, and cervical spinal anomalies)

Fetal Dilantin Syndrome

- *Frequency:* 10% of exposed fetuses
- *Inheritance:* (Environmental)
- *Features:* Hypertelorism, epicanthal folds, flat nasal bridge, small distal phalanges and nails; prenatal and postnatal growth deficiency, and developmental delay
- *Complications:* Involvement of other organ systems (congenital heart disease, renal anomalies, central nervous system anomalies); failure to thrive, and MR

Neural Tube Defects

- *Frequency:* 1 in 1000
- *Inheritance:* Usually sporadic
- *Features:* Variable, ranging from mild (spina bifida occulta) to severe (anencephaly)
- *Associations:* Isolated or part of syndrome or chromosomal anomaly
- *Recurrence:* Variable (3%–5% if an isolated malformation)
- *Prevention:* Folic acid supplementation before and throughout pregnancy

Cleft Lip and Palate

- *Frequency:* Cleft lip with or without cleft palate, 1 in 1000 births; isolated cleft palate, 1 in 2000 births
- *Causes:* Mendelian inheritance (autosomal dominant, autosomal recessive, X-linked); chromosomal (e.g., trisomies); environmental (phenytoin [Dilantin], amniotic bands); multifactorial (most cases); associated with syndrome (>150 possible); unknown

TABLE 42.2

RECURRENCE RISKS FOR ISOLATED CLEFTS

	Cleft Lip with or without Cleft Palate (%)	Cleft Palate (%)
General population	0.1	0.04
One affected sibling	3–7	2–5
One affected parent	2–4	3–7
One affected sibling and one affected parent	11–14	15–20
Two affected siblings	8–14	10–13

From Robinson A, Linden MG. *Clinical genetics handbook*, 2nd ed. Boston: Blackwell Science, 1993 (with permission).

- *Remarks:* Cleft palate without cleft lip more likely associated with other malformations; risk for recurrence (Table 42.2) dependent on etiology

A glossary of genetic terms is provided in Table 42.3.

REVIEW EXERCISES

QUESTIONS

1. A child is born with cleft lip and palate. What is the next appropriate step in the evaluation?
a) Head ultrasonography
b) Plastic surgery consultation
c) Careful physical examination
d) Karyotyping

Answer

The answer is c. The next appropriate step is a careful physical examination. To determine what consultations are appropriate, what tests are necessary, and what questions and answers should be shared with the family, one needs to survey the possibility of other birth defects. A thorough physical examination should precede any imaging studies and laboratory tests.

2. During the infant's circumcision procedure, hypospadias is noted. What is the next appropriate step in the evaluation?
a) Urology consultation
b) Renal ultrasonography
c) Family history and prenatal history
d) Karyotyping

Answer

The answer is c. Awkward situations can often be avoided by obtaining necessary information before surgical procedures are undertaken. A family history and prenatal history may alert the physician to other potential anomalies in an infant with cleft lip and palate or any other seemingly isolated birth defect.

TABLE 42.3

GLOSSARY OF GENETIC TERMS

Term	Definition
Allele	An alternative form of a gene at a given locus (i.e., mutant vs. normal)
Aneuploid	A chromosome number that is not a multiple of the haploid number; usually refers to an absence (monosomy) or extra copy (trisomy) of a single chromosome
Anticipation	Severity of a genetic disorder increased in subsequent generations, or age at onset decreased in subsequent generations
Autosome	Any of the 22 chromosomes other than the sex chromosomes (X or Y)
Carrier	A clinically unaffected individual who may have an affected offspring
Chorionic villus sampling	Procedure used to obtain fetal cells for prenatal diagnosis, performed at approximately 9–11 weeks of gestation
Chromosome	An ordered structure composed mainly of chromatin (DNA and associated proteins) that resides in the nucleus of eukaryotic cells
Codominant	Expression of both alleles in the heterozygote (e.g., AB blood type)
Compound heterozygote	An individual heterozygous for two different mutations at a given locus (e.g., hemoglobin SC disease, most inborn errors of metabolism)
Congenital	Present at birth; does *not* necessarily imply heritability (genetic)
Consanguinity	Relationship between two individuals by descent from a common ancestor
Contiguous gene syndrome	Condition caused by abnormalities (i.e., deletion) of two or more adjacent genes on a given chromosome
Diploid	Having two complete sets of homologous chromosomes (2N, or twice the haploid number), which is the case in all human cells (except egg, sperm, and non-nucleated red blood cells)
Dominant mutation	Produces an abnormal clinical phenotype (disorder) when a mutant allele is present in the heterozygous state (single copy)
Dysmorphology	Study of abnormal development
Fragile site	Gap or defect in a chromosome seen microscopically under special growth or staining conditions
Gene	Fundamental unit of heredity; a particular DNA sequence located on a particular chromosome that codes for a specific protein chain or has a specific regulatory function
Genetic heterogeneity	Similar phenotypes (clinical appearances) produced by different genotypes (mutant alleles at different loci)
Genome	Complete genetic information of an organism
Genotype	Genetic constitution of an individual cell or entire organism
Germ line (gonadal) mosaicism	Presence of two or more cell lines that differ in genetic makeup among germ cells; implies greater than background risk for recurrence of disorder
Heterozygous	Having two different alleles at a given genetic locus
Homozygous	Having identical alleles at a given genetic locus
Imprinting	Phenomenon whereby an allele at a given locus is altered or inactivated depending on whether it is inherited from the mother or the father
Locus	Site on a chromosome occupied by a gene
Lyonization	Normal, random inactivation of one X chromosome in each cell during early female embryonic development
Maternal inheritance	Pattern observed in mitochondrial disorders in which only mothers can pass on the disorder but the sons and daughters are equally affected
Meiosis	Type of cell division during gametogenesis in which the diploid chromosome number (2N) is reduced to the haploid number (N) in the sperm or ovum
Mitochondrial DNA	DNA distinct from nuclear (chromosomal) DNA that encodes some mitochondrial proteins, ribosomal RNA, and transfer RNAs
Mitosis	Type of cell division in somatic cells in which chromosome replication and division ensure a diploid (2N) complement of genetic material to each daughter cell
Mosaicism	Condition in which an individual harbors at least two genetically distinct cell lines as a result of a postzygotic (postfertilization) event in somatic cell division
Multifactorial inheritance	Determination of a phenotype by both genetic and nongenetic (environmental) factors (*polygenic* refers solely to multiple genetic factors)
Mutation	Permanent and heritable change in a gene
Penetrance	Clinical expression of a gene or mutation in a gene; if all individuals harboring a mutant gene have a recognizable phenotype (i.e., disease), trait completely penetrant; if only some individuals have the particular phenotype, trait incompletely penetrant
Phenotype	Observable characteristics (physical, physiologic, or biochemical) of a cell or organism
Pleiotropy	Multiple phenotypic events caused by a single gene, often seemingly unrelated
Polymorphism	Occurrence of two or more genetic forms, such as alleles of a gene
Proband	Index case that brings a family to medical attention
Recessive mutation	Produces an abnormal phenotype when a mutant gene is present in the homozygous state (two copies)
Recombination	Consequence of crossing over between homologous chromosomes during meiosis, leading to independent assortment of genes
Syndrome	Recognizable *pattern* of human malformation
Threshold	With respect to mitochondrial disorders, proportion of mutant mitochondria above which cell function is impaired
Translocation	Transfer of genetic material from one chromosome to a different (nonhomologous) chromosome (often reciprocal)
Trinucleotide repeat	Three-base repeat, such as $(CAG)_n$, usually polymorphic and sometimes prone to expansion, that may interfere with gene function
Uniparental disomy	Situation in which an individual carries both homologous chromosomes from the same parent
Variability	Differences in phenotype between individuals carrying the same mutant allele
Zygote	Diploid (2N) cell resulting from the fusion of haploid gametes (sperm and egg)

3. The family history is negative for similar birth defects or multiple miscarriages. The infant's mother reveals that she is epileptic. What medication(s) do you specifically need to ask about?
a) Phenobarbital
b) Phenytoin (Dilantin)
c) Carbamazepine (Tegretol)
d) Valproic acid

Answer

The answer is both b and d. Cleft lip and palate are associated with prenatal exposure to both phenytoin and valproate, and hypospadias is associated with prenatal exposure to valproate. Phenobarbital is considered the safest antiepileptic medication for expectant mothers, if effective.

4. What is the risk of this couple having another child with similar birth defects?
a) 10%–15%
b) 25%
c) 50%
d) 100%

Answer

The answer is a. If the mother is able to discontinue her medications successfully before the next conception, then the recurrence risk falls to 3% to 7% (one previously affected sibling). If not, the risk for having another child with fetal phenytoin or valproate embryopathy is 10% to 15%.

SUGGESTED READINGS

1. GeneReviews at GeneTests: Medical Genetics Information Resource (database online). Copyright, University of Washington, Seattle. 1993–2009. Available at http://www.genetests.org.
2. Jones KL. *Smith's recognizable patterns of human malformation,* 6th ed. Philadelphia: Elsevier-Saunders, 2005.
3. National Center for Biotechnology Information (NCBI). Genes and Disease. A growing series of short monographs describing >80 genetic disorders, arranged by organ system. Available at http://www.ncbi.nlm.nih.gov/books/bv.fcgi?rid=gnd&ref
4. Online Mendelian Inheritance in Man, OMIM (TM). McKusick-Nathans Institute for Genetic Medicine, Johns Hopkins University (Baltimore) and National Center for Biotechnology Information, National Library of Medicine, Bethesda, MD: 2009. Available at http://www.ncbi.nlm.nih.gov/sites/entrez?db=omim.
5. Reardon, W. *The bedside dysmorphologist.* New York: Oxford University Press, 2007.
6. Turnpenny P, Ellard S. *Emery's elements of medical genetics,* 13th ed. New York: Churchill Livingstone, 2007.
7. Westman JA. *Medical genetics for the modern clinician.* Baltimore: Lippincott Williams & Wilkins, 2005.
8. http://www.aap.org/healthtopics/genetics.cfm (American Academy of Pediatrics website) Under the "AAP Policy" heading, see Health Supervision of Children with Achondroplasia (2005) and Marfan syndrome (1996).

Chapter 43

Inborn Errors of Metabolism

George E. Tiller

Inborn errors of metabolism are last on everyone's list of differential diagnoses because of their individual rarity. They must always be considered in the evaluation of:

- An acutely ill neonate or infant
- Organomegaly
- Failure to thrive
- Mental retardation (MR)
- Developmental delay (especially a regression)

All states screen newborns for phenylketonuria, hypothyroidism, congenital adrenal hyperplasia, and galactosemia because these conditions are treatable and screening methods are inexpensive. Many states are adopting expanded metabolic screening, often including many untreatable disorders. *However, several disorders are still not currently detectable by newborn screening.*

The main objectives of this chapter are to help the reader:

- Understand the basis, selectivity, and shortcomings of neonatal metabolic screening
- Develop a general approach to the diagnosis of metabolic disease based on the use of readily available laboratory tests
- Appreciate the often critical nature of inborn errors of metabolism, and the components of initial management
- Become familiar with the features of a few representative inborn errors of metabolism

Selected disorders of inborn errors of metabolism are listed in Table 43.1.

PRINCIPLES OF NONSELECTIVE SCREENING OF NEWBORNS

Several important principles are critical in determining the disorders for which newborns should be screened for nonselectively. The disorder must be a heavy burden for the affected person to bear (i.e., be deadly, devastating). It

should be preventable and treatable, with a known inheritance pattern and pathogenesis. The methods of screening, diagnosis, and management must be practical and available to the general population, and genetic counseling must also be available. Finally, the benefit-to-cost ratio of nonselective screening must be high, as must be its sensitivity and specificity (no false-negative results and a low rate of false-positive results).

Newborn screening programs consists of five processes:

1. Newborn testing
2. Follow-up of abnormal screening results to facilitate timely diagnostic testing and management
3. Diagnostic testing
4. Genetic counseling and disease management
5. Continuous evaluation and improvement of the newborn screening system (Kaye et al., 2006).

Some diseases for which newborns can be screened are listed in Table 43.2.

The pitfalls of newborn screening include technical problems (e.g., mishandling and mislabeling of the sample, generation of false-positive and -negative results) and poor communication among the laboratory, primary care provider, family, and subspecialist. With some disorders, optimal testing entails a dietary prerequisite, which can contribute to invalid sampling and necessitate repeating studies.

Features of selected diseases detectable by screening are summarized in the following.

Disorders of Amino Acid Metabolism

Phenylketonuria

- *Incidence:* 1 in 15,000 (most common amino acid disorder)
- *Screening test:* Phenylalanine determination (dried blood spot)

TABLE 43.1

SELECTED EXAMPLES OF INBORN ERRORS OF METABOLISM

Amino Acidurias
Phenylketonuria
Homocystinuria
Tyrosinemia
Nonketotic hyperglycinemia
Carbohydrate disorders
Galactosemia
Fructose intolerance
Glycogen storage diseases
Lipidoses
Tay-Sachs disease
Gaucher disease
Metachromatic leukodystrophy
Purine metabolic disorders
Lesch-Nyhan syndrome (XLR)

Organic Acidurias
Methylmalonic aciduria
Propionic aciduria
Maple syrup urine disease
Transport disorders
Cystinuria
Cystinosis
Hypercholesterolemia (AD)
Lysosomal disorders
Mucopolysaccharidoses
  Hurler syndrome (MPS I)
  Hunter syndrome (MPS II; XLR)
I-cell disease (ML II)
Mitochondrial disorders
Leber hereditary optic neuropathy (MI)
MELAS (MI)

Urea Cycle Disorders
Ornithine transcarbamylase deficiency (XLR)
Arginosuccinate deficiency
Carbamyl phosphate synthetase deficiency
Peroxisomal disorders
Adrenoleukodystrophy (XLR)
Zellweger syndrome
Chondrodysplasia punctata
Metal metabolic disorders
Wilson disease
Menkes disease (XLR)
Hemochromatosis
Fatty acid oxidation defects
MCAD deficiency
Disorders of steroid metabolism
Smith-Lemli-Opitz syndrome
Congenital adrenal hyperplasia

Except for those disorders marked X-linked-recessive (XLR), autosomal dominant (AD), or mitochondrial (maternal) inheritance (MI), all the disorders listed in the table are inherited in an autosomal recessive pattern.
MCAD, medium-chain acyl coenzyme A dehydrogenase; MELAS, mitochondrial myopathy, encephalopathy, lactic acidosis, and stroke-like episodes.

TABLE 43.2

REPRESENTATIVE DISEASES FOR WHICH NEWBORNS CAN BE SCREENED

Disease	Incidence	Screening Test
Amino acid disorders		
■ Phenylketonuria	1/15,000	Phenylalanine
■ Tyrosinemia	1/100,000	Tyrosine, succinylacetone
■ Homocystinuria	1/100,000	Methionine
■ Nonketotic hyperglycinemia	1/75,000	Glycine
■ Maple syrup urine disease	1/100,000	Leucine, valine, isoleucine, alloisoleucine
Carbohydrate disorders		
■ Galactosemia	1/30,000	Galactose, gal-1-P transferase (GALT)
Organic acidemias		
■ Methylmalonic acidemia	1/100,000	C3, C4-DC
■ Propionic acidemia	1/100,000	C3
■ Isovaleric acidemia	1/100,000	C5
Fatty acid disorders		
■ SCAD	1/100,000	C4
■ MCAD	1/15,000	C6-C10
■ LCHAD	1/100,000	C14-OH, C16-OH
■ LCAD	1/100,000	C14, C16, C18
■ CPT deficiency	1/100,000	C16, C16:1,C18, C18:1
Other disorders		
■ Hypothyroidism	1/4500	T_4, TSH
■ Hemoglobinopathies (SS, SC, others)	1/400 US blacks	Hemoglobin electrophoresis
■ Biotinidase deficiency	1/60,000	Biotinidase
■ Congenital adrenal hyperplasia	1/10,000	17-Hydroxyprogesterone
■ Cystic fibrosis	1/3200 whites	Immunoreactive trypsinogen

State screening programs vary in methodologies employed, and therefore differ in the number of disorders that can be detected.
C3, a 3-carbon carboxylic acid; C4-DC, a 4-carbon dicarboxylic acid; C14-OH, a 14-carbon hydroxy-fatty acid; C16:1, a 16-carbon mono-unsaturated fatty acid; CPT, carnitine palmitoyl transferase; LCHAD, long-chain 3-hydroxyacyl-coenzyme A dehydrogenase; MCAD, medium-chain acyl-coenzyme A dehydrogenase; SCAD, small-chain acyl-coenzyme A dehydrogenase; T4, thyroxine; TSH, thyroid-stimulating hormone; VLCAD, very long-chain acyl-coenzyme A dehydrogenase.

- *Prerequisite:* Protein intake for longer than 24 hours
- *Diagnostic test:* Quantitative phenylalanine determination (plasma amino acid profile)
- *Clinical features:* Moderate to severe MR, autism, seizures, hypopigmentation, eczema
- *Primary defect:* Phenylalanine hydroxylase deficiency
- *Treatment:* Diet low in phenylalanine (low in protein; lifelong treatment optimal); tetrahydrobiopterin (BH_4) supplementation in mild cases
- *Remarks:* High phenylalanine levels and phenyl ketones are teratogenic. Untreated maternal phenylketonuria is associated with intrauterine growth retardation, microcephaly, MR, and structural birth defects

Homocystinuria
- *Incidence:* 1 in 100,000
- *Screening test:* Methionine determination (dried blood spot)
- *Prerequisite:* Protein intake for longer than 24 hours
- *Diagnostic test:* Measurement of methionine and homocystine levels in plasma (sent to laboratory on ice for amino acid profile)
- *Clinical features:* Tall stature, scoliosis, osteoporosis, mild MR, ectopia lentis, hypercoagulability, arterial and venous thrombi, stroke
- *Primary defect:* Cystathionine beta-synthetase deficiency (most common type)
- *Treatment:* Supplementation with betaine, folate, pyridoxine, or all three, depending on defect; aspirin for anticoagulation

DISORDERS OF CARBOHYDRATE METABOLISM

Galactosemia

- *Incidence:* 1 in 30,000
- *Screening test:* Galactose, galactose-1-phosphate uridyltransferase (GALT) determination
- *Prerequisite:* Galactose (lactose) intake
- *Diagnostic test:* GALT electrophoresis
- *Clinical features:* Neonatal nausea and vomiting, jaundice, hepatomegaly, hepatic dysfunction, cataracts, MR, death
- *Primary defect:* GALT deficiency
- *Treatment:* Galactose-free, lactose-free diet

CONGENITAL ADRENAL HYPERPLASIA

This is discussed in Chapter 16.

HYPOTHYROIDISM

This is discussed in Chapter 17.

DISORDERS OF FATTY ACID OXIDATION

Medium-Chain Acyl Coenzyme A Dehydrogenase (MCAD) Deficiency

- *Incidence:* 1 in 15,000
- *Screening test:* Acylcarnitine profile (plasma or dried blood spot)
- *Diagnostic test:* Repeated plasma acylcarnitine profile, DNA mutation testing
- *Clinical features:* Hypoglycemia without ketonuria; at risk for coma, sudden infant death syndrome
- *Primary defect:* MCAD deficiency
- *Treatment:* Carnitine supplementation; frequent feedings, avoid hypoglycemia

DISORDERS OF BIOTIN METABOLISM

Biotinidase Deficiency

- *Incidence:* 1 in 60,000
- *Screening test:* Enzyme assay from dried blood spot; increased plasma alanine, decreased carnitine also seen
- *Diagnostic test:* Repeat enzyme assay on fresh serum
- *Clinical features:* Hypotonia, seizures, rashes, alopecia
- *Primary defect:* Biotinidase deficiency, an enzyme that recycles biotin for multiple carboxylase enzyme reactions
- *Treatment:* Biotin supplementation

DISORDERS OF AMMONIA METABOLISM (UREA CYCLE)

Hyperammonemia may occur transiently in the newborn. It may also be associated with:

- Urea cycle disorders
- Organic acidemias
- Biotinidase deficiency
- Reye syndrome

Clinical features include progressive anorexia, lethargy, and vomiting that ultimately lead to coma. Hypothermia may also be a feature in the newborn period.

Treatment of urea cycle disorders includes:

- Preventing protein catabolism (high-calorie diet, arginine supplementation)
- Decreasing NH_3 load (protein restriction)
- Utilizing NH_3 scavengers (sodium benzoate, phenylacetate, and phenylbutyrate)

OTC Deficiency

- *Incidence:* 1 in 14,000 (most common urea cycle defect)
- *Inheritance:* X-linked recessive; carrier females may be symptomatic
- *Screening test:* Increased glutamine; decreased citrulline and arginine; increased urinary orotic acid

- *Diagnostic test:* Plasma amino acid profile, urine organic acid profile
- *Clinical features:* Hyperammonemia with resultant CNS depression and coma
- *Primary defect:* Ornithine transcarbamylase deficiency, the second enzyme in the urea cycle
- *Treatment:* Protein-restricted diet; citrulline supplementation; NH_3 scavengers

MITOCHONDRIAL DISORDERS

The mitochondria are the powerhouses of the cell, and the home of beta-oxidation of fatty acids, the tricarboxylic acid cycle, the electron transport chain, and parts of the urea cycle. Although many inborn errors of metabolism involve these pathways, the designation of *mitochondrial disorder* is reserved for those metabolic diseases that are caused by mutations in one of the 13 protein-coding genes or transfer ribonucleic acid (tRNAs) encoded by the mitochondrial genome. These disorders share a maternal inheritance pattern (in which all offspring are affected, and the disease cannot be passed on by males), and include MELAS (mitochondrial encephalopathy, lactic acidosis, and stroke-like episodes), MERRF (myoclonic epilepsy and ragged red fibers), Leber hereditary optic neuropathy, and some forms of Leigh syndrome. Suspicion of these disorders is based on mode of inheritance, family history, clinical findings, lactic acidosis, histologic findings on muscle biopsy, and mutation analysis of the mitochondrial genome. Treatment of this group of disorders is usually symptomatic, although some individuals respond to pharmacologic doses of cofactors and vitamins, such as coenzyme Q and riboflavin (B_2).

MELAS
- *Incidence:* 1 in 10,000
- *Inheritance:* Maternal (mitochondrial)
- *Screening test:* None routinely employed; elevated lactate; ragged red fibers on muscle biopsy; brain CT may reveal focal lucencies, basal ganglia calcifications
- *Diagnostic test:* Mitochondrial mutation analysis
- *Clinical features:* Onset by 2 to 15 years old; mitochondrial *M*yopathy, *E*ncephalopathy, *L*actic *A*cidosis, and *S*troke-like episodes; short stature; recurrent headache and vomiting; blindness; deafness; diabetes mellitus
- *Primary defect:* Mitochondrial leucine tRNA mutation (80%)
- *Treatment:* CoQ10 and carnitine supplementation of questionable benefit

LYSOSOMAL STORAGE DISORDERS

The lysosomal storage disorders are a group of approximately 30 disorders, each of which is due to deficiency of a specific acid hydrolase that resides in the lysosome. These enzymes are responsible for catabolizing and recycling a variety of macromolecules, including glycogen, mucopolysaccharides, sphingolipids, and glycoproteins.

Leukodystrophies

Gaucher Disease
- *Incidence:* 1 in 50,000 (~1/1000 Ashkenazi Jews)
- *Diagnostic test:* Glucocerebrosidase assay (leukocytes, skin)
- *Clinical features:* Variable, may include painless splenomegaly (Fig. 43.1), thrombocytopenia, excessive bleeding, bone pain, pathologic fractures, and mild to severe MR (types 2 and 3 only)
- *Primary defect:* β-glucosidase deficiency
- *Treatment:* Symptomatic; enzyme replacement therapy

Tay-Sachs Disease
- *Incidence:* 1 in 100,000 (1/3600 Ashkenazi Jews)
- *Diagnostic test:* Hexosaminidase A assay (serum, leukocytes, skin)
- *Clinical features:* Developmental regression, failure to thrive, cherry-red fovea, blindness, seizures, and death by age 2 years
- *Primary defect:* Hexosaminidase A deficiency
- *Treatment:* Symptomatic; carrier screening available

Mucopolysaccharidoses

Hurler Syndrome (MPS I)
- *Incidence:* 1 in 100,000
- *Screening test:* Quantitative urinary MPS
- *Diagnostic test:* Iduronidase assay (leukocytes, skin)
- *Clinical features:* Developmental regression, coarse features, and organomegaly (Fig. 43.2)

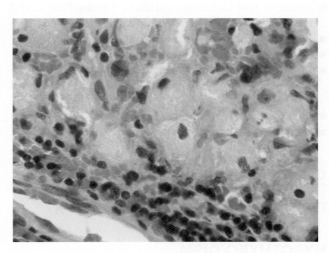

Figure 43.1   Gaucher cells in spleen of an affected child. Note the swollen appearance of cytoplasm, caused by storage of lipid (glucocerebroside). (See color insert.)

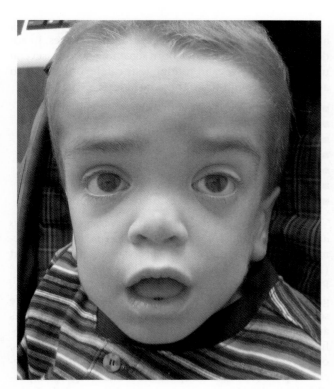

Figure 43.2 A 2-year-old boy with Hurler syndrome (mucopolysaccharidosis I [MPS I]), who received enzyme replacement therapy prior to bone marrow transplantation at 18 months. Note the large head and coarse facial features.

- *Primary defect:* Iduronidase deficiency
- *Treatment:* Symptomatic; stem cell therapy; enzyme replacement therapy

Hunter Syndrome (MPS II)

- *Incidence:* 1 in 100,000
- *Inheritance:* X-linked recessive (XLR)
- *Screening test:* Quantitative urinary MPS
- *Diagnostic test:* Iduronate sulfatase assay (leukocytes, skin)
- *Clinical features:* Developmental regression, coarse features, and organomegaly (Fig. 43.3)
- *Primary defect:* Iduronate sulfatase deficiency

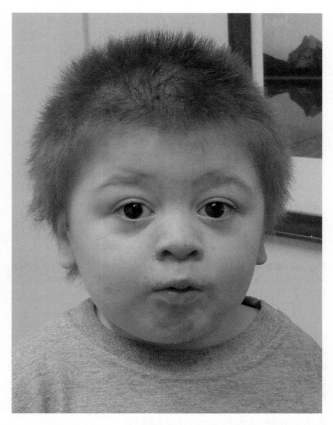

Figure 43.3 A 2-year-old boy with Hunter syndrome (mucopolysaccharidosis II [MPS II]). Note the large head, coarse hair, and coarse facial features.

- *Treatment:* Symptomatic; stem cell therapy; enzyme replacement therapy

The classification, modes of inheritance, and clinical features of mucopolysaccharidoses are summarized in Table 43.3.

PEROXISOMAL DISORDERS

The peroxisomal disorders are a group of metabolic conditions that result from defects in peroxisomal assembly or

TABLE 43.3
ABBREVIATED GUIDE TO THE MUCOPOLYSACCHARIDOSES

Type	Eponym	Inheritance	MR	Corneal Clouding	Hepatosplenomegaly
IH	Hurler	AR	++	+	+
IS	Scheie	AR	−	+	−
II	Hunter	XLR	++	−	+
III	Sanfilippo	AR	++	−	+/−
IV	Morquio	AR	−	+	+/−
VI	Maroteaux-Lamy	AR	−	+	+
VII	β-Glucuronidase	AR	++	+	+

AR, autosomal recessive; MR, mental retardation; XLR, X-linked recessive.

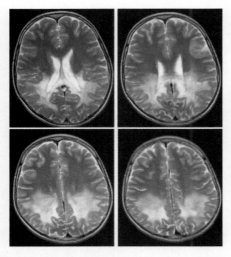

Figure 43.4 Brain MRI of a 9-year-old boy with X-linked adrenoleukodystrophy (ALD). Note the symmetric enhanced T-2 signal in the parieto-occipital region.

deficiency of a particular peroxisomal enzyme. These enzymes are responsible for oxidation of some very-long-chain fatty acids, degradation of hydrogen peroxide, and synthesis of certain lipids (e.g., plasmalogens), to name a few functions.

Adrenoleukodystrophy (ALD)

- *Incidence:* 1 in 50,000
- *Inheritance:* X-linked recessive (XLR)
- *Screening test:* Quantitative plasma very-long-chain fatty acid (VLCFA) profile
- *Diagnostic tests:* Combination of VLCFA profile and brain MRI
- *Clinical features:* Developmental regression, visual loss, white matter changes (Fig. 43.4), and adrenal dysfunction (late)
- *Primary defect:* Mutations in the ABCD1 gene, encoding a peroxisomal transporter protein
- *Treatment:* Symptomatic; stem cell therapy; Lorenzo's oil?

EVALUATION OF THE ACUTELY ILL NEONATE

The differential diagnosis in the nursery should be: (a) sepsis, (b) sepsis, (c) sepsis, and (d) metabolic disease. *Nonspecific symptoms* consistent with an inborn error of metabolism include respiratory distress, lethargy/poor feeding/hypotonia, seizures/apnea, vomiting, jaundice, and organomegaly. The *history* may include a normal course for 36 to 72 hours, parental consanguinity (most inborn errors of metabolism are inherited in an autosomal-recessive pattern), or a sibling who died of an unknown cause in the neonatal period. The *physical examination* findings are usually unremarkable, but organomegaly, neurologic symptoms, and cataracts are potential clues.

The *biochemical evaluation* need not be esoteric (at first), and helpful clues may be right in front of your eyes. In addition to expediting the newborn screening process, several useful, inexpensive, and routine tests can be ordered, with a quick turnaround time. These include:

- Complete blood count with differential and platelets
- Glucose
- Electrolytes
- Arterial blood gas or venous pH
- Ammonia (NH_3)
- Lactate/pyruvate
- Urinalysis for pH, ketones, and reducing substances

Inborn errors of metabolism may cause various combinations and degrees of metabolic acidosis, hypoglycemia, hyperammonemia, ketosis, leukopenia, and thrombocytopenia. The flowchart (Fig. 43.5) serves as a rudimentary diagnostic guide. Pending the results of plasma amino acid and urine organic acid determinations, glucose is almost always a safe source of energy for the sick neonate. Specific diagnoses are usually confirmed by amino acid or organic acid profiles and/or enzyme assays of leukocytes, skin fibroblasts, or a liver biopsy specimen. The diagnosis should be as specific as possible to afford optimal treatment regimens, possibly including dietary management with vitamin/cofactor supplementation, as well as specific drugs.

FACTORS IN SUCCESSFUL MANAGEMENT OF INBORN ERRORS OF METABOLISM

Although many inborn errors of metabolism are not currently treatable, factors critical to the successful management of those that are treatable include:

- Early detection
- Good compliance with treatment regimen
- Family education
- Financial and social support
- Early institution of treatment, periodic follow-up in a metabolic center
- Dietary treatment
- Anticipation of acute illnesses
- Pharmacologic treatment

DIETARY MANAGEMENT OF INBORN ERRORS OF METABOLISM

Recommended dietary regimens for the following disorders include:

- *Phenylketonuria:* Diet low in phenylalanine; protein restriction
- *Tyrosinemia:* Diet low in phenylalanine and tyrosine; protein restriction
- *Galactosemia:* Galactose-free diet (soy-based infant formulas contain sucrose rather than lactose)

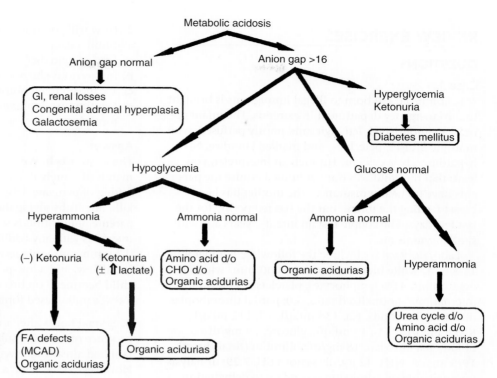

Figure 43.5 Flowchart for the evaluation of metabolic acidosis in the neonate. CHO, carbohydrate; d/o, disorder; FA, fatty acid; GI, gastrointestinal; MCAD, medium-chain acyl coenzyme A dehydrogenase deficiency.

- *Hereditary fructose intolerance:* Restriction of fruits, fruit juices, and products containing sucrose (table sugar) and high-fructose corn syrup
- *Urea cycle disorders (e.g., ornithine transcarbamylase deficiency):* Protein restriction
- *Maple syrup urine disease:* Branched-chain amino acid/protein restriction
- *MCAD deficiency:* Frequent feeding, high in carbohydrates; avoiding medium-chain triglycerides

- *Glycogen storage disease type I (von Gierke):* Supplement with corn starch to maintain normoglycemia

PHARMACOLOGIC MANAGEMENT OF INBORN ERRORS OF METABOLISM

The pharmacologic agents available for the management of certain disorders associated with inborn errors of metabolism are listed in Table 43.4.

TABLE 43.4

PHARMACOLOGIC AGENTS FOR DISORDERS OF INBORN ERRORS OF METABOLISM

Disorder	Agent
Phenylketonuria (mild)	Tetrahydrobiopterin (BH_4)
Homocystinuria	Betaine, pyridoxine (B_6), folate
Urea cycle disorders	Sodium benzoate, phenylacetate, phenylbutyrate, arginine
MSUD	Thiamine (B_1)
Methylmalonic acidemia	Carnitine, cobalamin (B_{12})
Propionic acidemia	Carnitine
Tyrosinemia	NTBC
Biotinidase deficiency	Biotin
MCAD deficiency	Carnitine
Cytochrome oxidase deficiency	Coenzyme Q, riboflavin (B_2)
Gaucher disease	Enzyme replacement therapy
Fabry disease	Enzyme replacement therapy
Hurler syndrome (MPS I)	Enzyme replacement therapy
Hunter syndrome (MPS II)	Enzyme replacement therapy

BH_4, tetrahydrobiopterin; MCAD, medium-chain acyl-coenzyme A dehydrogenase; MPS I, mucopolysaccharidosis I; MSUD, maple syrup urine disease; NTBC, 2-(2-nitro-4-trifluoromethyl-benzoyl)-1,3-cyclohexanedione.

REVIEW EXERCISES

QUESTIONS

Case 1

A 1-month-old girl born to illegal immigrants is brought to the emergency department in extremis. The infant appears malnourished, lethargic, and poorly perfused, with multiple bruises, petechiae, and marked jaundice. No hepatomegaly is evident. Through an interpreter, you learn that the child was born at home because the parents have no health insurance. The mother has been breast-feeding the infant, but she has fed poorly for the last few days. The couple lost an infant 2 years ago with similar symptoms.

Laboratory values include the following: hemoglobin, 11.9 g/dL; white blood cell count, 8000/mm^3 with 59% neutrophils, 41% lymphocytes; platelets, 79,000/mm^3; international normalized ratio, 3.0; partial thromboplastic time, 95 seconds; Na, 138 mEq/L; Cl, 112 mEq/L; K, 3.6 mEq/L; CO_2, 12 mEq/L; glucose, 79 mg/dL; blood urea nitrogen, 18 mg/dL; bilirubin (total/direct), 19/5 mg/dL; NH_3, 42 µg/dL; venous pH, 7.29; urinalysis unobtainable on admission secondary to dehydration.

1. Sepsis aside, what metabolic diseases are in your differential diagnosis?
a) Ornithine transcarbamylase deficiency
b) Phenylketonuria
c) Galactosemia
d) Methylmalonic aciduria

Answer

The answer is c. This infant is presenting with hepatic dysfunction in the newborn period. Ornithine transcarbamylase deficiency is excluded because it is an X-linked disorder, the patient is female, and the ammonia level is normal. Phenylketonuria has an insidious onset and does not present with hepatic dysfunction. Methylmalonic aciduria usually presents in the newborn period, but with mild hypoglycemia, a more profound metabolic acidosis, and an increased anion gap.

2. What additional laboratory tests do you want to obtain?
a) Urine organic acid profile
b) Plasma amino acid profile
c) Newborn screening card
d) Complete urinalysis
e) All of the above

Answer

The answer is e. Practically speaking, you may have a strong hunch for a particular diagnosis, but your patient has a life-threatening illness, and cost is no object. You may not have the luxury of time to order laboratory tests sequentially, and the tests listed are not unreasonable in this setting.

3. How will you nourish this infant while waiting for additional data?
a) Low-protein diet
b) Intravenous glucose only
c) Total parenteral nutrition
d) Continuous nasogastric feeding of a cow's milk formula

Answer

The answer is b. We often forget that the caloric demands of acutely ill patients are increased. Except in the setting of pyruvate dehydrogenase deficiency, you cannot kill patients by giving them intravenous glucose. Total parenteral nutrition is seldom a good choice because it interferes with any additional metabolic testing. Because the serum ammonia level is normal, a urea cycle disorder is unlikely, and a low-protein diet is not indicated. The child became ill on breast milk, so that continuing with a cow's milk–based formula is not recommended.

4. Several hours after admission, urinalysis reveals the presence of reducing substances and ketones, but the infant had already received intravenous ampicillin. However, 3 days later, a newborn screen reveals "an abnormality." What confirmatory test is likely indicated?
a) Plasma amino acid profile
b) Red blood cell GALT electrophoresis
c) Acylcarnitine profile
d) Pi Typing for α_1-antitrypsin deficiency

Answer

The answer is b. A plasma amino acid profile would aid in the diagnosis of tyrosinemia, but hypoglycemia, hypokalemia, and hepatomegaly are usually additional presenting features of this disorder. An acylcarnitine profile is not indicated because no evidence suggests a fatty acid oxidation defect, such as MCAD deficiency (the hypoglycemia is not marked, and ketones were eventually demonstrated in the urine). Although α_1-antitrypsin deficiency could present in this fashion, no newborn screening test includes any markers to suggest this diagnosis. GALT electrophoresis (from red blood cells) is the diagnostic test of choice for galactosemia. It distinguishes patients with classic galactosemia (GG), such as the infant described, from heterozygous asymptomatic carriers (NG) and persons with mild variants, such as Duarte galactosemia compound heterozygosity (DG).

Case 2

A 3-year-old boy is referred to you because of a plateau in his development. Motor milestones were met at an appropriate age, but speech development was slightly delayed. In the past 6 months, neither his expressive language nor his fine motor skills have progressed. The child has been healthy and has had no hospitalizations except for an inguinal hernia repair at the age of 2 years. On examination, he is of average height and weight, with an increased head circumference. His facial features are slightly coarse, with mild synophrys (mono-brow) and mild gingival hypertrophy. The corneas are clear. His liver edge is 2 cm below the right costal margin. No focal neurologic deficits are noted.

5. Into which general category of metabolic disease does this description *most* likely fit?
a) Leukodystrophy
b) Organic aciduria
c) Glycogen storage disease
d) MPS

Answer

The answer is d. The insidious onset of clinical signs and symptoms is suggestive of a storage disorder. The general good health of the patient speaks against an organic aciduria. The coarse facial features are not consistent with a leukodystrophy. The developmental arrest is not consistent with a glycogen storage disease. This patient has an MPS. The age at onset and male sex make Hunter syndrome (MPS II, XLR) and Sanfilippo syndrome (MPS III) the most likely diseases.

6. What screening test(s) will be helpful in arriving at the proper diagnosis?
a) Liver ultrasonography
b) Quantitative urine mucopolysaccharides
c) Mitochondrial DNA mutation testing
d) Plasma amino acid profile

Answer

The answer is b. Liver ultrasonography will not yield any specific findings in this disease. The absence of muscle weakness, seizures, and visual or hearing disturbances makes a mitochondrial disorder very unlikely. Aminoacidopathies do not present with coarsening of facial features and hepatomegaly. A quantitative urine mucopolysaccharide screening is indicated. A mere spot test is inadequate, and the evaluation should include electrophoresis to separate individual glycosaminoglycans (mucopolysaccharides). Differential elevations of individual macromolecules aid in determining which enzyme assays of leukocytes or cultured skin fibroblasts to perform for a definitive biochemical diagnosis.

7. What organ systems are likely to be involved in this condition?
a) Central nervous system (CNS)
b) Cardiac
c) Gastrointestinal
d) Skeletal
e) All of the above

Answer

The answer is e. Because almost all tissues contain glycosaminoglycans, the mucopolysaccharidoses present as multisystem diseases. Although a few mucopolysaccharidoses spare the CNS, most involve the CNS, cardiac valves, liver, and skeletal system *(dysostosis multiplex)*. An astute radiologist can often aid in refining the differential diagnosis. Bone marrow transplantation is effective in treating some of these disorders, and enzyme replacement therapy is being developed for additional disorders. The key management issue is to make the diagnosis before the CNS is irreparably damaged.

SUGGESTED READINGS

1. American Academy of Pediatrics. http://www.aap.org/health topics/genetics.cfm. Under the "AAP Policy" heading, see articles on congenital adrenal hyperplasia (2000) and hypothyroidism (2006).
2. American College of Medical Genetics. http://www.acmg.net.
3. Baumgartner MR, Saudubray JM. Peroxisomal disorders. *Semin Neonatol* 2002;7(1):85–94.
4. Chakrapani A, Cleary MA, Wraith JE. Detection of inborn errors of metabolism in the newborn. *Arch Dis Child* 2001;84:F205–F210.
5. GeneReviews at GeneTests: Medical Genetics Information Resource (database online). Copyright, University of Washington, Seattle. 1993–2009. Available at http://www.genetests.org.
6. Hoffmann GF, Nyhan WL, Zschocke J, et al., eds. *Inherited metabolic diseases*. New York: Lippincott Williams & Wilkins, 2002.
7. Kaye CI, Accurso F, La Franchi S, et al. Newborn screening fact sheets. *Pediatrics* 2006;118(3):e934–e963. Available online at http://aappolicy.aappublications.org/cgi/content/full/pediatrics; 118/3/e934.
8. Online Mendelian Inheritance in Man, OMIM (TM). McKusick-Nathans Institute for Genetic Medicine, Johns Hopkins University (Baltimore, MD) and National Center for Biotechnology Information, National Library of Medicine, Bethesda, MD: 2009. Available at http://www.ncbi.nlm.nih.gov/sites/entrez?db=omim.
9. Summar ML, Tuchman M. Proceedings of a consensus conference for the management of patients with urea cycle disorders. *J Pediatr* 2001;138:S6–S10.
10. Zschocke J, Hoffman GF. *Vademecum metabolicum: manual of metabolic paediatrics*, 2nd ed. Leck, Germany: CPI Books, 2004.

Chapter 44

Adolescent Development and Tanner Staging

Ajuah Davis

NORMAL PUBERTAL DEVELOPMENT

Puberty is the period of transition from sexual immaturity to potential fertility, during which secondary sexual characteristics develop. It begins with decreasing sensitivity of the hypothalamic-pituitary-gonadal (HPG) axis and increasing pulsatile release of gonadotropin-releasing hormone (GnRH), and the gonadotropins luteinizing hormone (LH), and follicle-stimulating hormone (FSH). The hormonal changes begin years before the physical changes are noted. *Breast development is the first sign of puberty in girls. In boys, puberty is heralded by an increase in testicular size* to a volume of 4 cc or a length >2.5 cm in the long axis. Pubertal events usually follow a sequence, with a mean age at onset of 11.2 years in girls and 11.6 years in boys. However, the onset of puberty in healthy children varies widely.

Tanner staging is used to correlate pubertal events and their typical ages at presentation (Tables 44.1 and 44.2). Along with height velocity, it provides a good measure of growth and physical maturation. Peak height velocity occurs early in girls, at Tanner stage II/III. In boys, it is a late pubertal event, occurring at Tanner stage IV. The appearance of acne occurs in late puberty in both boys and girls, as does the growth of axillary hair in girls and of axillary and facial hair in boys. Most girls experience menarche at the age of 12.8 ± 1.0 year, when they are at Tanner stage III/IV.

Two extreme variations of normal development are premature thelarche and premature adrenarche. *Premature thelarche* is characterized by early breast development without other signs of puberty. It occurs most often within the first 2 years of life, with a second peak noted after the age of 6 years. *Premature adrenarche*, characterized by the early development of pubic hair, usually occurs between the ages of 6 and 8 years. These conditions are not associated with other pubertal changes. No height acceleration or advancement in the bone age takes place. Follow-up of these patients is indicated every 4 to 6 months to confirm the benign, nonprogressive nature of their condition. In some cases, what was initially thought to be a benign condition evolves into precocious puberty. Pubertal gynecomastia is another normal variant that occurs in as many as 75% of boys during the teenage years. The problem typically resolves within 2 years, but in cases of prolonged or excessive breast development surgery is indicated. Some pathologic conditions can also be associated with gynecomastia.

The onset of puberty before the age of 8 years in girls and 9 years in boys is unusual and deserves evaluation. If puberty is caused by reactivation of the HPG axis, the condition is called *central precocious puberty*. The hormonal interactions are normal, but the timing is early. Central precocious puberty is five times more common in girls than in boys, and in most cases no cause is identified. In boys, neurological causes are seen in >60% of cases, so that a thorough search for central nervous system (CNS) pathology is especially important.

When puberty is not mediated by pituitary gonadotropin secretion, it is called *peripheral precocious puberty*. The source of the sex hormones may be exogenous or endogenous, gonadal or extragonadal. Maturation may be incomplete, with only one type of secondary sexual characteristic developing early. In some children the pubertal development can be contrasexual (characteristics of the opposite sex develop).

TABLE 44.1
MEAN AGES FOR TANNER STAGES IN U.S. GIRLS

Tanner Stage	Age (years) ± SD	Description
II: Breast development	11.2 ± 1.1	Elevation of breast and papilla, enlargement of areola
Pubic hair	11.6 ± 1.2	Sparse, long, lightly pigmented hair
III: Breast development	12.0 ± 1.0	Further enlargement of breast and areola
Pubic hair	11.8 ± 1.0	Darker, coarser, and spread over pubes
IV: Breast development	12.4 ± 0.8	Projection of areola and papilla to form a secondary mound
Pubic hair	12.4 ± 0.9	Adult in type but covers a smaller area
V: Breast development	14.0 ± 1.2	Mature stage, projection of papilla only
Pubic hair	14.0 ± 1.3	Adult in quantity and type, inverse triangle

SD, standard deviation.

PRECOCIOUS PUBERTY

When a girl younger than 8 years or a boy younger than 9 years presents with one or more of the features of breast development, growth of pubic hair, accelerated linear growth, menstruation, or acne development, an evaluation for possible precocious puberty is warranted. The goals of the evaluation are to:

- Document whether precocious puberty is taking place
- Differentiate central from peripheral precocious puberty
- Identify and appropriately treat the cause of the precocious puberty

The diagnosis of precocious puberty should be established by the physical examination. The normal variants, premature thelarche and premature adrenarche, usually can be distinguished on the basis of the examination and confirmed by careful medical follow-up.

The differential diagnosis for precocious puberty includes the following.

Central Precocious Puberty

- Idiopathic
- CNS lesions
  - Hypothalamic hamartoma
  - Tumors (neurofibroma, craniopharyngioma)
  - Malformations (septo-optic dysplasia, hydrocephalus, arachnoid cyst)
  - Infection (brain abscess, meningitis)
  - Trauma (surgery, irradiation, injury)
- States of peripheral precocious puberty

Peripheral Precocious Puberty

- Congenital adrenal hyperplasia
- Ovarian cysts
- Autonomous (McCune-Albright syndrome, testotoxicosis)
- Exogenous hormones
- Severe primary hypothyroidism
- Adrenal or gonadal tumors

TABLE 44.2
MEAN AGES FOR TANNER STAGES IN U.S. BOYS

Tanner Stage	Age (years) ± SD	Description
II: Genital development	11.6 ± 1.1	Testicular volume 4 cc, scrotal thinning
Pubic hair	13.4 ± 1.1	Sparse, long, lightly pigmented hair at base of penis
III: Genital development	12.9 ± 0.8	Growth of penis in length and breadth; further testicular, scrotal growth
Pubic hair	13.9 ± 1.0	Darker, coarser, and spread over pubes
IV: Genital development	13.8 ± 1.2	Penis, testes enlarged further
Pubic hair	14.4 ± 1.1	Adult in type but covers a smaller area
V: Genital development	14.9 ± 0.8	Penis of adult size and shape, testicular volume 20 cc
Pubic hair	15.2 ± 1.1	Adult in quantity and type, inverse triangle, spread onto medial thighs

SD, standard deviation.

The pubertal changes, and their duration and progression, should be determined. Slowly progressive or minimal physical changes are often benign in nature, whereas multiple changes in the same child are of concern. An assessment of the patient's general health, medications, and nutrition is required. It is important to obtain previous heights so that the patient's growth pattern can be determined. An increase in the growth velocity is seen during puberty. Prior to puberty the child's growth rate is approximately 2.5 in. or 6 cm per year. Any type of CNS dysfunction can cause central precocious puberty. A history of CNS trauma or infection, headaches, and visual changes should be elicited. Precocious puberty may develop in survivors of childhood cancers and CNS tumors as a result of their treatment. The age at onset of puberty in other family members should be noted because children often follow family patterns. The physician should also inquire about possible exposure to exogenous hormones.

During the physical examination, the physician should pay particular attention to Tanner staging and the presence of other pubertal changes, such as acne, adult body odor, and axillary hair. The skin should be carefully inspected for pigmented lesions (McCune-Albright syndrome or neurofibromatosis). A neurologic assessment should be performed. The ophthalmologic examination should include funduscopic and visual field evaluations.

The development of true breast tissue versus fatty tissue is assessed by palpation with the child in a supine position. In addition to the development of pubic hair, the color of the vaginal mucosa should be noted in girls. Visual inspection is adequate to assess the presence of estrogen stimulation. A glistening red appearance is consistent with a non–estrogen-stimulated mucosa, whereas a pinkish mucosa is suggestive of estrogen stimulation.

A bone age roentgenogram for skeletal maturation should be obtained immediately. *In children with precocious puberty, the bone age is usually advanced,* but advancement in the bone age may not be apparent if the pubertal changes have occurred rapidly. *Children with premature thelarche or adrenarche do not have an advanced bone age.* In many children with central precocious puberty, physical maturation progresses more rapidly than the normal pattern. A skeletal survey should be requested in suspected cases of McCune-Albright syndrome to look for polyostotic fibrous dysplasia.

Because of the episodic nature of gonadotropin secretion, random LH and FSH levels may not be elevated. A GnRH stimulation test should be performed to determine whether the gonadotropin response is consistent with maturation of the HPG axis. Children with central precocious puberty exhibit a brisk rise in FSH levels, and an even greater rise in LH levels. Prepubertal children or those with peripheral precocious puberty do not show a rise in LH and FSH levels. Measurement of the plasma estradiol or testosterone level can support the suspected diagnosis.

Additional laboratory testing to consider includes: measurement of thyroxine (T_4) and thyroid-stimulating hormone (TSH), dehydroepiandrosterone sulfate (DHEA-S), and 17-hydroxyprogesterone. Primary hypothyroidism is a rare cause of central precocious puberty. It is usually diagnosed on the basis of the symptoms of hypothyroidism, the most notable being arrested growth. In these cases, testicular enlargement and breast development are seen with little or no accompanying pubic hair. The plasma DHEA-S concentration is a useful marker for adrenarche (level appropriate for Tanner stage) and the presence of adrenal tumors (level extremely elevated). Late-onset congenital adrenal hyperplasia may be the cause of central precocious puberty when androgenic changes (i.e., body hair, body odor, acne) predominate.

Pelvic ultrasonography may be helpful in defining large ovarian cysts or neoplasms and can also assess the development of the uterus and ovaries. Ovarian cysts are the most common tumors associated with precocious puberty and are usually self-limited. Other ovarian tumors are infrequent and can be associated with masculinization. The chance of finding CNS pathology is greatest in younger children and boys. High-resolution magnetic resonance imaging (MRI) should be performed in girls younger than 5 years and for all boys with central precocious puberty. Specific imaging of the adrenals or gonads is warranted when a tumor is strongly suspected.

Treatment and Prognosis

For pituitary gonadotropins to produce and secrete LH and FSH, they must be stimulated by a pulse of GnRH every 90 to 120 minutes. Less frequent or, surprisingly, more frequent pulses of GnRH suppress the pituitary secretion of LH and FSH. A GnRH agonist binds to and causes continuous stimulation of the GnRH receptors on the gonadotrophs. With continuous stimulation, the gonadotrophs act as if they are receiving very frequent pulses of GnRH and stop secreting LH and FSH. The process is reversible on discontinuation of the GnRH agonist. These properties make GnRH agonists useful in the treatment of central precocious puberty when an underlying pathology is not found.

CNS tumors should be resected if possible and chemotherapy or radiation therapy, or both should be instituted as indicated. The *exception* to this rule is a hypothalamic hamartoma. This nonmalignant tumor acts as accessory hypothalamic tissue and can be treated successfully with a GnRH agonist.

Peripheral precocious puberty is treated by management of the underlying condition. Congenital adrenal hyperplasia is treated with physiologic glucocorticoid replacement to suppress excessive adrenal androgen secretion. Hypothyroidism requires thyroid replacement. Large ovarian cysts or ovarian tumors are resected. Adrenal and testicular tumors are also resected. For patients with

McCune-Albright syndrome and other conditions associated with autonomous gonadal steroid production, various agents are used to block puberty. Ketoconazole blocks androgen production; aromatase inhibitors such as testolactone and anastrazole block conversion of androgens to estrogens and spironolactone acts as an antiandrogen.

The importance of treating precocious puberty lies in the aspects of the psychosocial outcome. Affected children are usually bigger than their age-matched peers and are treated according to their size, not according to their age and developmental stage. Increased height velocity secondary to increased gonadal steroid secretion ultimately leads to premature epiphyseal fusion and the paradox of tall stature in childhood but short adult height. An additional consideration in girls is their social and psychological adaptation to early menstruation.

DELAYED PUBERTY

Delayed puberty is encountered more commonly in boys than girls. It is defined as a lack of secondary sexual characteristics by the age of 14 years in boys or 13 years in girls. The children are frequently smaller than their peers, and the difference is exaggerated when their classmates enter the pubertal growth spurt. Although some children are not particularly bothered, others are psychologically and socially devastated. Lack of progression through the stages of puberty within 4.5 to 5 years after its onset may also require evaluation.

The differential diagnosis for delayed puberty should include:

- Constitutional growth delay
- Hypopituitarism—idiopathic or acquired
  - Multiple pituitary trophic hormone deficiencies
  - Kallmann syndrome
- Chronic illness, malnutrition
- Hypothyroidism
- Hyperprolactinemia
- Turner syndrome
- Klinefelter syndrome
- Gonadal failure
- Miscellaneous disorders

Again, the history and physical examination are the most important steps in the evaluation. Recommendations for the evaluation are as mentioned in the section on precocious puberty. In many children, one or both parents have a history of delayed puberty. The physician should elicit a history of trauma or medical injury, look for eating disorders, and evaluate the nutritional status. *A history of anosmia in the patient or other family members suggests Kallmann syndrome.* This condition is associated with gonadotropin deficiency; the male-female ratio is 5:1. Rigorous physical training may also delay physical matura-

tion. Acquired hypothyroidism is usually associated with other signs of thyroid dysfunction when it is seen in the setting of delayed puberty. Children with hypopituitarism can have isolated gonadotropin deficiency or they may be missing several pituitary hormones.

The presence of dysmorphic features and body measurements should lead the examiner to consider diagnoses such as Turner syndrome, Klinefelter syndrome, and other chromosomal abnormalities. Karyotype determinations should be considered in all short girls without a diagnosis and in suspected cases of Klinefelter syndrome. A presumptive diagnosis often can be formed on the basis of the history and physical findings.

The bone age roentgenogram provides critical information because in most children with delayed puberty, the delay of growth and development is constitutional. In these children, the onset of puberty correlates better with bone age than with chronological age. Random LH and FSH levels are helpful in narrowing the differential diagnosis only if they are elevated. A GnRH stimulation test may be reassuring in cases in which the diagnosis of constitutional growth delay is not readily evident. In patients with cryptorchidism or very small testes, a human chorionic gonadotropin stimulation test can assess testicular responsiveness.

CNS tumors (or their prior treatment) can affect gonadotropin secretion and the secretion of other pituitary hormones. The T_4, TSH, and prolactin levels should be measured to detect abnormalities. Additional chemistries (metabolic panel, complete blood cell count) may also help direct the evaluation in selected cases. CNS imaging is performed in cases of suspected intracranial pathology.

Treatment and Prognosis

Underlying medical disorders are treated appropriately. Congenital or acquired gonadotropin deficiency secondary to CNS lesions requires replacement therapy with gonadal steroids at the normal age for the onset of puberty. Constitutional growth delay is treated with reassurance and follow-up. In cases where physical immaturity causes significant psychological maladjustment, a short course of hormones can be considered. Low-dose testosterone (50 mg intramuscularly every 28 days) or conjugated estrogen (0.3 mg daily) is used. Low-dose oxandrolone (1.25–2.5 mg daily) has also been used as an oral alternative to testosterone injections.

Careful monitoring of the progression of sexual maturation and growth is necessary. Secondary sexual characteristics usually become evident 1 to 2 months after the initiation of therapy. Hormone replacement can cause a worsening of acne, rapid weight gain, gynecomastia, liver dysfunction, and early closure of the growth plates. Low-dose therapy, however, is not usually associated with side effects.

REVIEW EXERCISES

QUESTIONS

Case 1

Breast development has been noted in a 6-year-and-10-month-old African-American girl. She began to grow rapidly and use deodorant more than a year ago. She has two loose teeth and several secondary teeth. She denies headaches or visual problems. Her past medical history is unremarkable. Her mother is 5 ft 4 in. tall and experienced menarche at the age of 10 years. Her father is 5 ft 3 in. tall.

The physical examination findings are as follows: height, 126.0 cm (90th percentile); weight, 28.8 kg (95th percentile); blood pressure, 120/70 mm Hg. The fundi are sharp bilaterally. She does not have a goiter. The left breast has 5 cm of palpable tissue, and mounding of the areola is noted on the right breast. Sparse straight pubic hairs are seen on the mons. Clitoromegaly is absent. The vaginal mucosa is pink without discharge. The patient has several axillary hairs and mild body odor. Her bone age is 6 years and 10 months.

1. Which of the following statements is *true*?
a) This child's precocious puberty most likely has a pathologic cause.
b) This patient has benign premature adrenarche.
c) This patient has Tanner stage II breast development.
d) Children with central precocious puberty usually have an advanced bone age.

Answer

The answer is d. On the basis of the history and examination findings, this patient has precocious puberty. Pubertal changes are considered precocious in a girl 8 years of age or younger and in a boy 9 years of age or younger. Central precocious puberty is more common in girls than boys, and approximately 95% of cases are idiopathic. Tanner stage IV breast development is characterized by areolar mounding. Early activation of the HPG axis leads to prolonged exposure to pubertal levels of the sex hormones and early skeletal maturation. This advancement in bone age may not be seen if the hormonal changes are recent.

2. The *best* treatment plan for this patient is:
a) Referral to an endocrinologist
b) Repeat examination in 4 to 6 months
c) Check LH and FSH levels
d) Treatment with an androgen-blocking agent

Answer

The answer is a. This patient has Tanner stage III/IV breast development and early Tanner stage II pubic hair. Such findings are more typically seen in a girl older than 11 years and should prompt additional investigation sooner rather than later. An advanced bone age may not

be evident if the pubertal changes have occurred rapidly. She does not have any physical signs that suggest adrenal or other pathology, so this is most likely a case of idiopathic central precocious puberty. A referral should be made to an endocrinologist to confirm the diagnosis and start treatment.

Case 2

A 2-year-and-8-month-old African-American boy is referred for evaluation of precocious puberty. His mother has noted pubic hair. He does not have acne or body odor. His past medical history is unremarkable and he takes no medications. His father is 5 ft 9 in. tall. His mother is 5 ft 3 in. tall and experienced menarche at the age of 13 years. He has a healthy 5-month-old sister. Prior to referral, random LH, FSH, and DHEA-S levels were checked and reported normal. His bone age was 6 years.

The physical examination findings are as follows: height 91.5 cm (35th percentile) and weight 13.5 kg (40th percentile). He is a well-appearing child with notable findings only on his pubertal examination. He has light hair on his upper lip. Pubic hair is in Tanner stage II; the testicular volume is 3 cc.

3. Which of the following conditions is *most* likely in this child?
a) Congenital adrenal hyperplasia
b) A hypothalamic hamartoma
c) Central precocious puberty
d) Benign premature adrenarche

Answer

The answer is a. Androgenic changes such as body odor, body hair, and acne are seen in congenital adrenal hyperplasia. These physical changes are associated with an advanced bone age. A hypothalamic hamartoma is a unique CNS lesion that acts as an accessory hypothalamus. This tumor stimulates pulsatile release of LH and FSH from the pituitary gland. Testicular enlargement is the first sign of puberty in boys and occurs with activation of the HPG axis. This child has prepubertal sized testes and normal LH and FSH levels so his problem is peripheral. The advanced bone age is not consistent with benign premature adrenarche.

4. Further testing confirms your suspected diagnosis. The next step in his evaluation and treatment should be:
a) A head MRI
b) A GnRH stimulation test
c) Low-dose testosterone therapy
d) Glucocorticoid replacement therapy

Answer

The answer is d. This child has a form of peripheral precocious puberty, which is treated by management of the underlying medical problem. In this case it is congenital adrenal hyperplasia. Central precocious puberty is not present since there is no testicular enlargement; the GnRH stimulation test is not indicated and is expected to be normal. A head MRI is essential in any boy or young child with central precocious puberty to look for CNS pathology. Testosterone therapy has no place in the treatment of precocious puberty.

5. Which of the following statements *best* describes his follow-up?
a) Early testosterone treatment will prevent adult short stature.
b) He should begin taking a GnRH agonist to delay further development.
c) A pituitary MRI is the next step in his evaluation.
d) He requires suppression of adrenal androgens.

Answer
The answer is d. Supplemental testosterone is used in some cases of delayed puberty; it has no role in this child's condition. This case does not illustrate any features of central precocious puberty. A GnRH agonist and pituitary MRI are not indicated. Treatment of congenital adrenal hyperplasia is suppression of excess adrenal androgen production. This is best accomplished with glucocorticoid replacement.

Case 3
A 6-year-and-7-month-old girl is referred for evaluation of precocious puberty. She has underarm odor and was noted to have pubic hair during a routine physical examination. She denies having headaches and has no history of head injury. She takes no medications, and her past medical history is unremarkable. Her father is 5 ft 7 in. tall and had normal pubertal development. He is African American. Her mother is 5 ft 1½ in. tall. She is white and experienced menarche at the age of 11 years. The maternal grandmother experienced menarche at the age of 9 years.

The physical examination findings are as follows: height, 113.6 cm (10th percentile); weight, 17.3 kg (5th percentile); blood pressure, 84/52 mm Hg. She has a palpable breast bud on the left side. One or two dark pubic hairs are present. The vaginal mucosa is red without discharge. Downy axillary hair and body odor are noted.

6. The patient's bone age is 5 years and 9 months. Which of the following statements is *true*?
a) She should be re-examined every 4 to 6 months.
b) She should begin taking a GnRH agonist to delay further development.
c) A GnRH test will show high LH and FSH levels.
d) No further evaluation is needed.

Answer
The answer is a. The fact that the bone age is not advanced indicates minimal hormonal exposure up to this time. The patient should be re-examined at regular intervals to confirm that she has a benign condition. This

patient would be expected to have a flat LH and FSH response during a GnRH stimulation test, which would be consistent with the normal bone age and physical findings. GnRH agonist therapy is not indicated if the HPG axis has not been activated. If her pubertal development progresses rapidly, future testing will show an advancing bone age and laboratory values consistent with puberty. All children with precocious puberty require follow-up to confirm their clinical diagnosis.

7. This clinical case is *most* like benign premature thelarche in the following way:
a) It is associated with Tanner stage II pubic hair.
b) It commonly occurs during the first 2 years of life.
c) Skeletal maturation is appropriate for chronological age.
d) They are both associated with early menses.

Answer
The answer is c. Benign premature thelarche is not associated with other physical signs of puberty or with an early occurrence of true puberty. Most patients present before the age of 2 years. This child has very early signs of puberty. The presence of pubic hair differs from premature thelarche. A bone age measurement, which is consistent with the chronological age, is one of the hallmarks of benign premature thelarche.

Case 4
A 14-year-and-4-month-old boy is referred for delayed puberty and short stature. He reports headaches during school hours but denies any other physical complaints. His past medical history is unremarkable. The father is 6 ft 3 in. tall, and his pubertal development was late. The mother is 5 ft 3 in. tall and experienced menarche at the age of 14 years.

The physical examination findings are as follows: height, 154.2 cm (<10th percentile); weight, 38.3 kg (3rd percentile); blood pressure, 110/62 mm Hg. His testicular volume is 4 cc. Pubic hair is in early Tanner stage II. He does not have acne. Axillary hair is present. The examination findings are otherwise unremarkable.

8. The best initial step in the assessment of delayed puberty is to obtain:
a) Measurement of serum gonadotropins
b) Measurement of estradiol or testosterone
c) Karyotype
d) Previous growth data and assessment of sexual maturity

Answer
The answer is d. The classic patient with constitutional growth delay has a family history notable for delayed puberty. The typical child has short stature and a late pubertal growth spurt. Initial evaluation includes family history, assessment of prior growth rate and Tanner staging. The bone age is delayed. Laboratory testing may not be diagnostic, which makes the history and follow-up

important. A karyotype should be obtained if the examination suggests a chromosomal abnormality.

9. The following problem should be considered in this patient's differential diagnosis:
a) Congenital adrenal hyperplasia
b) Hypothalamic hamartoma
c) Constitutional growth delay
d) Testotoxicosis

Answer

The answer is c. This child has a family history of pubertal delay. If his bone age is delayed, this finding will support the diagnosis of constitutional growth delay. He should be followed up to ascertain normal pubertal progression. The other conditions listed are associated with precocious puberty.

10. This boy can be expected to have the following finding:
a) Unilateral breast development
b) Pulsatile secretion of LH and FSH
c) A chromosomal abnormality
d) A pituitary tumor

Answer

The answer is b. An increase in testicular volume is the first sign of puberty in boys and occurs with activation of the HPG axis. This boy's physical exam shows signs of early pubertal changes. He will have pulsatile release of LH and FSH and should progress through the Tanner

stages over the next 2 to 4 years. If his puberty does not proceed as expected he may have an underlying abnormality such as a tumor or genetic problem. These secondary causes of delayed puberty are not always evident on initial evaluation. Male breast development is most often seen at Tanner stage II/III and can be unilateral or bilateral. It typically resolves in 18 to 24 months.

SUGGESTED READINGS

1. Kappy MS, Ganong CS. Advances in the treatment of precocious puberty. *Adv Pediatr* 1994;41:223–261.
2. Kletter GA, Kelch RP. Disorders of puberty in boys. *Endocrinol Metab Clin North Am* 1993;22:455–477.
3. Marshall WA, Tanner JM. Variations in the pattern of pubertal changes in boys. *Arch Dis Child* 1970;45:13–23.
4. Marshall WA, Tanner JM. Variations in the pattern of pubertal changes in girls. *Arch Dis Child* 1969;44:291–303.
5. Neinstein LS, Kaufman FR. Abnormal growth and development. In: Neinstein LS, ed. *Adolescent health care*, 4th ed. Philadelphia: Lippincott Williams & Wilkins, 2002:197–229.
6. Neinstein LS, Kaufman FR. Normal physical growth and development. In: Neinstein LS, ed. *Adolescent health care*, 4th ed. Philadelphia: Lippincott Williams & Wilkins, 2002:3–51.
7. Rosenfield RL. Puberty in the female and its disorders. In: Sperling MA, ed. *Pediatric endocrinology*, 2nd ed. Philadelphia: Saunders, 2002:455–518.
8. Styne DM. The testes: disorders of sexual differentiation and puberty in the male. In: Sperling MA, ed. *Pediatric endocrinology*, 2nd ed. Philadelphia: Saunders, 2002:565–628.
9. Tanner JM, Whitehouse RH. Clinical longitudinal standards for height, weight, height velocity, weight velocity, and stages of puberty. *Arch Dis Child* 1976;51(3):170–179.

Chapter 45

Sexually Transmitted Diseases

Ellen S. Rome

Sexually transmitted diseases (STDs) remain common in adolescents, with one in every four sexually active teens between the ages of 13 and 19 years being infected annually. This chapter reviews the evaluation, diagnosis, and management of the more common STDs in adolescence, including *Chlamydia trachomatis* infection, *Neisseria gonorrhoeae* infection, herpes simplex, syphilis, chancroid, and *Trichomonas vaginalis* infection. The recognition and management of physiologic leukorrhea, yeast vaginitis, and bacterial vaginosis are also reviewed because the presentation of each of these entities can be confused with those of the aforementioned STDs. Recent advances in testing strategies are discussed, including urine screening with DNA probes (nucleic acid amplification tests [NAATs], which have been found to be more sensitive than the previously used ligase chain reaction [LCR] and polymerase chain reaction [PCR]) and the appropriate use of culture versus other modalities.

STD rates are highest in the 15- to 24-year-old age group for a variety of reasons. Biologic factors include the prominent exocervix of adolescent girls, which involutes with age. During adolescence, this accessible transition zone serves as a magnet for STD organisms. Adolescents also have lower levels of protective antibodies because of a lesser degree of cumulative exposure to disease. Sperm can carry disease to the upper genital tract. Retrograde menstruation, which occurs in 25% of healthy women, spreads the infection to the fallopian tubes and contiguous areas.

Behavioral factors also increase the prevalence of STDs in adolescents, especially because risky behaviors in teenagers tend to be interrelated and clustered. The earlier teens begin sexual activity, the less likely they are to use a condom and the more likely they are to have multiple partners. In some cultures, it is normative for girls to date boys or young men much older than they are, so that condom negotiation is made difficult by the age and power

differential. The use of alcohol or drugs also decreases the use of condoms. Furthermore, the adolescent mindset contributes to the acquisition of STDs; the personal sense of invulnerability of early to middle adolescence coincides with the concrete thought processes that impede an adolescent's ability to see the consequences of behavior. The lack of education or awareness regarding STDs, the perceived lack of access to contraceptive services, fear of pelvic examination, and fear of disclosure to parents or other adults can serve as barriers to care and increase the risk for adolescent STD acquisition. Legally, with limited exceptions, all teens in the United States may consent to the confidential diagnosis and treatment of STDs. Moreover, teens can receive medical care for STDs without parental consent or knowledge, and adolescents may consent to human immunodeficiency virus (HIV) testing without parental consent in many states. Unfortunately, the lack of awareness among many teens and even healthcare providers of the adolescent and the adolescent's right to confidential care for STDs further blocks access to care.

After confidentiality has been established, the primary care clinician should ask all teens the HEADS questions: *h*ome (Who lives at home? What happens when someone argues at home?); *e*ducation (grades this year compared with those last year, grade level; recognizing that a slide in grades is a risk factor for various risk behaviors, including sexual activity); *a*ctivities; *d*rugs (including cigarettes and alcohol); *d*epression/suicide; *s*ex. The method of motivational interviewing allows for behavioral interventions to occur nonjudgmentally as questions are asked of the teen, helping them to shape healthier responses and finding motivation to change risk behavior patterns. Questions can move from less threatening to more invasive, allowing the teen to gain comfort and be empowered to make healthy choices using motivational interviewing. For example, when asking a teen who has admitted to having sex in the past, the clinician can ask, "What methods of contraception did you use?" If she answers condoms, the clinician can ask if she uses them sometimes, most of the time, or all the time. The clinician can then move on to asking what second method of contraception she uses, and if this question is met with an inquisitive look, the clinician can remind the teen that condoms are only 85% effective at pregnancy prevention with typical teen usage, so that means that "15 out of every shots will find their mark." The clinician can then discuss with the teen which second method the teen wishes to use if she has heterosexual sexual relations in the future. Adolescents should be asked about number of lifetime partners, and whether they have engaged in oral sex or anal sex, with motivational interviewing used to educate without having to step onto a soapbox, in a way that seems relevant to a specific teen's life. For those girls who are younger, it is easy to ask questions about the menstrual cycle first: when the last menstrual period occurred; whether they have experienced dysmenorrhea and vaginal itching, discharge, or odor; whether they have noted any changes in their cycle. Girls and boys should be asked if they have ever had anyone do anything to them sexually that made them uncomfortable; careful phrasing can make it "safe" to answer questions about sexual abuse for the teen who has been in a coercive situation where she or he may have been put at risk but may not self define it as "abuse." Teens should also be asked about sexual preference ("Are you attracted to guys, girls, or both?"); nonjudgmental phrasing can open doors for harm reduction in adolescents experimenting sexually in both same sex and opposite sex relationships. Boys should be asked about penile discharge, dysuria, and lesions and should be taught to perform a testicular self-examination.

Traditionally, the pelvic examination has been used to:

- Screen all sexually active teens for an abnormal result of the Papanicolaou (Pap) test and for STDs
- Determine the stage of a pregnancy
- Evaluate a patient with abdominal or pelvic pain
- Evaluate a patient with vaginitis or vaginal discharge (although urine screening and self-applied vaginal swabs may change this indication)
- Evaluate an adolescent with menstrual irregularity or evidence of androgen excess
- Perform a routine Pap test in patients older than 18 years

The question of who requires a pelvic examination continues to evolve. All sexually active teens require screening for STDs 3 to 6 months after acquiring each new partner; urine nucleic acid amplification strategies may be utilized for screening, with excellent sensitivity and specificity. With the ACOG recommendations of 2003, a pelvic examination should be first performed 3 years after coitarche, then annually in sexually active young people. For those who have not yet initiated sexual activity, the 2003 ACOG guidelines recommend a first pelvic at age 21 years, not at

18 years. Of note, adolescents tend not to differentiate the Pap smear from the pelvic examination; therefore, a teenager who underwent a pelvic examination in an emergency department setting, in which Pap smears are not performed, may not realize that the test was not done.

NEWER DEVELOPMENTS IN SCREENING FOR SEXUALLY TRANSMITTED DISEASE

Culture remains the gold standard for STD testing and must be used in cases of sexual abuse. In contrast to the older detection tests, amplified DNA testing does not require the presence of viable organisms or even large amounts of DNA to detect disease. If the question of the Pap smear is set aside, urine screening can improve the detection of STDs in settings in which pelvic examinations cannot be performed easily (e.g., schools, juvenile detention centers, shelters for the homeless, mobile crisis vans, and some pediatric clinics not set up for gynecologic services). Even beauty parlors and sporting event centers have been mentioned as possible sites where teens congregate and could be screened! Urine screening costs less than obtaining cervical specimens; in a hypothetical cohort of 100,000 young women, urine screening in asymptomatic women reduces the cost of preventing a case of pelvic inflammatory disease (PID) by 50%.

Self-obtained vaginal swabs have been used to detect infection with *N. gonorrhoeae* (found in 5.3% of asymptomatic girls), *C. trachomatis* (17.8%), and *T. vaginalis* (12.9%); this study did not compare pelvic examination with vaginal swabs, so some infections may have been missed. Adolescents, when asked to follow relatively simple printed instructions, successfully obtained their own vaginal introitus specimens for PCR testing for *C. trachomatis*; the sensitivity was 100% in a direct comparison with clinician-obtained cervical specimens. Urine culture for *T. vaginalis* infection has been found to yield poor results, and it may be easier for a patient to deliver a swab than urine to a laboratory. Vaginal infections with *T. vaginalis*, bacterial vaginosis, and vulvovaginal candidiasis can be diagnosed easily without a speculum, with no significant advantage noted for provider-obtained vaginal and cervical samples.

NEWER DEVELOPMENTS IN TREATMENT OF SEXUALLY TRANSMITTED DISEASES

Patient-delivered partner therapy (PDPT) or expedited partner therapy (EPT) have been identified as viable options for partner treatment among heterosexual persons with chlamydia and *N. gonorrhoeae*. Currently, EPT is not recommended for males having sex with males or in patients with syphilis. Limited data exist for female trichomoniasis partner management; among women with trichomoniasis, PDPT outcomes were similar to standard partner referral with less associated expense. Some states, such as California, have legally embraced PDPT or EPT, whereas others have prosecuted clinicians trying to treat partners without seeing them. The Centers for Disease Control and Prevention has a tool to assist programs in each state to understand the legal issues for using EPT; this information is available at http://www.cdc.gov/std/ept/legal/default.htm

NONGONOCOCCAL URETHRITIS

Epidemiology

Nongonococcal urethritis is caused by *C. trachomatis* in 23% to 35% of cases. Other pathogens include *Ureaplasma urealyticum*, *Mycoplasma genitalium*, *T. vaginalis*, and herpes simplex virus (HSV).

Presentation

Most boys infected with *C. trachomatis*, *N. gonorrhoeae*, and other pathogens are asymptomatic. Complications in men can include epididymitis and Reiter syndrome.

Diagnosis

The added sensitivity of urine DNA testing eliminates the need to screen boys with urethral swab, so that urine or penile discharge is sufficient for testing. The argument can now be made that all sexually active males should be screened annually for STD by urine testing. Certainly all boys with dysuria, discharge, or known STD exposure should be screened. Prescreening for leukocyte esterase with dipstick can also identify asymptomatic boys whose urine should definitely be tested. Further studies are required to determine the cost-effectiveness of screening all sexually active boys versus only those who test positive for leukocyte esterase with urine dipstick.

Treatment

According to the U.S. Centers for Disease Control and Prevention (CDC) 2006 guidelines for the treatment of STDs, first-line treatment consists of 1 g of azithromycin orally or 100 mg of doxycycline twice a day orally for 7 days. Alternative regimens include 500 mg of erythromycin base orally four times a day for 7 days, 800 mg of erythromycin ethylsuccinate orally four times a day for 7 days, or 300 mg of ofloxacin orally twice a day for 7 days or levofloxacin 500 mg orally once daily for 7 days. For those teens and young adults who have been compliant with recommended dosing and in whom re-exposure to

infection has been excluded, recurrent and persistent urethritis can be treated with 2 g of metronidazole orally as a single dose or tinidazole 2 grams orally as a single dose. Alternative regimens include 500 mg of erythromycin base orally four times a day for 7 days, or 800 mg of erythromycin ethylsuccinate orally four times a day for 7 days.

CHLAMYDIA TRACHOMATIS INFECTION

Epidemiology

In the United States, four million new cases of *Chlamydia* infection occur annually, with one million cases in the 15- to 19-year-old age group. The prevalence ranges from 5% to 15% in asymptomatic sexually active adolescents and young adults, 20% to 30% in adolescents and young adults seen in STD clinics, 40% to 50% in symptomatic patients, and 15% to 50% in patients with simultaneous *N. gonorrhoeae* infection.

Presentation

Most patients are asymptomatic. Boys may present with nongonococcal urethritis, epididymitis, conjunctivitis, Reiter syndrome, rectal infection, or proctitis. Girls may present with cervicitis, salpingitis (PID), urethritis, endometritis (postpartum and following abortion), *Fitz-Hugh-Curtis syndrome (perihepatis associated with PID)*, premature rupture of membranes, or premature labor.

Diagnosis

In cases that do not involve sexual abuse, DNA tests, or nucleic acid amplification strategies, of a cervical swab or a urine specimen are now commonly used in many centers. Cell culture, the gold standard for cases of sexual abuse, involves identification of characteristic intracytoplasmic inclusions with fluorescent antibody stain after 48 to 72 hours of growth. Culture is labor intensive, expensive, has low sensitivity (80%–90%), is technician dependent, and only detects live organisms. Enzyme immunoassays (EIAs) have sensitivities of 63% and 68.6% to 85%, respectively. A new qualitative dual-amplified EIA for the detection of chlamydial specific lipopolysaccharide antigens are now available and have a sensitivity of 85.7% to 95% and a specificity of 98.2% to 99%. Used on vaginal specimens, this test is less expensive than NAATs.

DNA probes can allow for single swab detection of both *C. trachomatis* and *N. gonorrhoeae*. Biro et al. found that nucleic acid-based assays (GenProbe PACE 2) had a specificity of 96% and a sensitivity of 72%. NAATs are highly sensitive and specific for the detection of *C. trachomatis* in both urine and endocervical specimens. These tests can also be used for self-collected or clinician-collected vaginal swabs, although this is not yet approved by the U.S. Food and Drug Administration. The NAAT, which uses endocervical or urine specimens, tends to be the preferred test for screening.

Treatment

Cervicitis, urethritis, and asymptomatic infection are treated with 1 g of azithromycin orally as a single dose or 100 mg of doxycycline orally twice a day for 7 days. Alternative regimens include 500 mg of erythromycin base orally four times daily for 7 days, 800 mg of erythromycin ethylsuccinate orally four times daily for 7 days, or 300 mg of ofloxacin orally twice daily for 7 days, or levofloxacin 500 mg orally once daily for 7 days. One third of the patients show resistance to ofloxacin in major cities. Azithromycin is ideal because of its single-dose regimen and minimal gastrointestinal side effects. Test of cure is no longer deemed necessary according to the CDC 2006 guidelines for the treatment of STDs, but testing for reinfection 4 weeks after initial screening may be indicated in adolescent patients in particular.

NEISSERIA GONORRHOEAE INFECTION

Epidemiology

The number of cases of gonorrhea reported to the CDC has decreased from one million annually to an estimated 400,000, at an estimated annual cost of $288 million per year.

Presentation

Girls and women often have asymptomatic infections. Symptomatic women may present with dysuria, dysmenorrhea, and dyspareunia with pain often beginning within 7 days of menses, lower abdominal pain, vaginal discharge, or a change in menstrual pattern. Perianal infection in men or women may present as proctitis, tenesmus, pruritus, or rectal bleeding. Pharyngeal infections can present as patchy erythema, exudates, and cervical lymphadenopathy with or without vesicopustular lesions on the soft palate and tonsils. Inflamed Bartholin glands present as pain and swelling of the labia minora, and inflamed Skene glands may present with periurethral pain or swelling. Men may present with urethritis, dysuria, or discharge, or they may be asymptomatic.

Diagnosis

The diagnosis is as discussed in the diagnosis section for *C. trachomatis*. As stated, NAATs are ideal for screening in an office-based setting, with culture reserved for cases of potential abuse.

TABLE 45.1

TREATMENT REGIMENS FOR *NEISSERIA GONORRHOEAE* INFECTION

Uncomplicated gonococcal infections of the cervix, urethra, and rectum
    Cefixime 400 mg orally in a single dose
    Ceftriaxone 125 mg IM in a single dose
    Ciprofloxacin 500 mg orally in a single dose
    Ofloxacin 400 mg orally in a single dose
    plus
    Levofloxacin 250 mg orally in a single dose
    Azithromycin 1 g orally as a single dose, or
    Doxycycline 100 mg orally twice daily for 7 days
Disseminated gonococcal infection
    Ceftriaxone 1 g IM or IV every 24 hours
    Alternative regimens
    Cefotaxime 1 g IV every 8 hours
    Ceftizoxime 1 g IV every 8 hours
    Ciprofloxacin 500 mg IV every 12 hours
    Ofloxacin 400 mg IV every 12 hours
    Levofloxacin 250 mg IV every 24 hours
    Spectinomycin 2 g IM every 12 hours
    Treatment should be continued until 24–48 hours after initial clinical improvement, then changed to oral therapy to complete a 1-week course of antibiotic with
    Cefixime 400 mg orally twice daily
    Ciprofloxacin 500 mg orally twice daily
    Ofloxacin 400 mg orally twice daily
    Levofloxacin 500 mg orally once daily

IM, intramuscularly; IV, intravenously.
Adapted from the 2006 Centers for Disease Control and Prevention guidelines for the treatment of sexually transmitted diseases.

Treatment

The treatment regimens for uncomplicated and disseminated gonorrhea are outlined in Table 45.1. Of note, a patient should be treated for *Chlamydia* infection when gonorrhea is suspected or diagnosed. Resistance to fluoroquinolones has been shown in larger cities.

PELVIC INFLAMMATORY DISEASE

Epidemiology

PID affects one out of every eight sexually active 15-year-old girls, with one million cases of PID in the United States annually. Traditionally, *N. gonorrhoeae*, by a direct cytotoxic effect, was thought to be the major causative organism in PID. Infection with *N. gonorrhoeae* at the endocervix is found in 33% to 81% of patients with PID, but the endocervical bacteria may not be the same as the pelvic bacteria found during laparoscopy in cases of PID. In two thirds to three fourths of patients with gonorrheal PID, symptoms appear within 7 days of menses. The etiology in most cases of PID is now considered to be *polymicrobial*, with *N. gonorrhoeae* accounting for 25% to 50% of cases, *C. trachomatis* for 25% to 43%, mixed anaerobic/aerobic organisms for 25% to 60%, and an unclear role for genital mycoplasmata. Anaerobic organisms may include *Peptostreptococcus* and *Bacteroides* species. Aerobic pathogens may include *Gardnerella vaginalis*, streptococci, *Escherichia coli*, and *Haemophilus influenzae*.

Risk factors for PID include low levels of protective antibody, the prominent exocervix, sperm as vectors of infection, retrograde menstruation, and douching, which shifts the pH of vaginal flora and may mechanically push infection to the upper genital tract. During menses, the cervical os is slightly more permissive of infection because of the loss of the cervical mucus plug, and because menstrual blood can serve as an excellent culture medium.

Diagnosis

The diagnosis of PID is problematic because even asymptomatic infection can cause serious sequelae, such as substantial tubal destruction. The gold standard for diagnosis is laparoscopy, but this procedure entails surgical risk, requires special expertise, and adds to the cost. The CDC 2006 guidelines for the treatment of STDs simplify the definition of PID from the classic triad of abdominal pain, cervical motion tenderness, and adnexal tenderness to now only two criteria: *uterine/adnexal tenderness and cervical motion tenderness*. Additional supportive criteria consist of any of the following *soft* signs: oral temperature above 38.3°C (101°F), abnormal cervical or vaginal discharge, elevated erythrocyte sedimentation rate or C-reactive protein level, and positive result of testing for cervical infection with *N. gonorrhoeae* or *C. trachomatis*.

The *laboratory evaluation* should include a complete blood cell count with differential, erythrocyte sedimentation rate, testing for gonorrhea and for *Chlamydia* infection, urine β-human chorionic gonadotropin, and rapid plasma reagin (RPR) testing for syphilis, with HIV testing considered. Urine culture should be considered if symptoms suggest cystitis or pyelonephritis. Ultrasonography can be useful when a bimanual examination is difficult or a mass is suspected. The differential diagnosis includes ectopic pregnancy and appendicitis (both of which are surgical emergencies and must be excluded as diagnostic possibilities), ruptured ovarian cyst, endometriosis, and normal pelvis.

Treatment

The various regimens are outlined in Table 45.2.

SYPHILIS

Epidemiology

In the United States, 40,000 individuals are infected with syphilis annually, with congenital syphilis occurring in

TABLE 45.2

TREATMENT FOR PELVIC INFLAMMATORY DISEASE

Parenteral regimen A
 Cefotetan 2 g IV every 12 hours
 or
 Cefoxitin 2 g IV every 6 hours
 plus
 Doxycycline 100 mg PO or IV every 12 hours
Parenteral regimen B
 Clindamycin 900 mg IV every 8 hours
 plus
 Gentamicin loading dose IV/IM (2 mg/kg of body weight), then maintenance dose (1.5 mg/kg) every 8 hours
Alternative parenteral regimens
 ■ Ofloxacin 400 mg IV every 12 hours + metronidazole 500 mg PO/IV every 8 hours
 ■ Ampicillin/sulbactam 3 g IV every 6 hours + doxycycline 100 mg PO/IV every 12 hours
 ■ Ciprofloxacin 200 mg IV every 12 hours + doxycycline 100 mg PO/IV every 12 hours + metronidazole 500 mg IV every 8 hours

IM, intramuscularly; IV, intravenously; PO, orally.
Adapted from the 2006 Centers for Disease Control and Prevention guidelines for the treatment of sexually transmitted diseases.

one of every 10,000 pregnancies. Caused by infection with the spirochete *Treponema pallidum*, syphilis develops in one third of exposed individuals.

Presentation

Syphilis can present in any of its five stages: incubation and the primary, secondary, latent, and tertiary stages. The incubation period lasts 10 to 90 days (average, 3 weeks) and is symptom free. During the primary stage of syphilis, nontender inguinal adenopathy develops (Table 45.3), plus a hard, painless chancre teeming with spirochetes at the site of entry. Untreated, this lesion clears spontaneously in 3 to 6 weeks. Secondary syphilis develops 2 weeks to 6 months after the appearance of the primary lesion. Systemic symptoms include fever, weight loss, headache, myalgia, and sore throat. A nonpruritic macular rash that classically does not spare the palms and soles is

TABLE 45.3

DIFFERENTIAL DIAGNOSIS OF GENITAL ULCERS AND NODES

Disease	Ulcer	Lymphadenopathy
Syphilis	Painless chancre	Painless nodes
Chancroid	Painful ulcer	Tender nodes
Herpes simplex virus infection	Painful vesicle or ulcer	Tender nodes

the hallmark of secondary syphilis and is the feature that often brings patients to the clinic for diagnosis and treatment. The latent stage of syphilis is without symptoms, but the patient is serologically positive. Tertiary syphilis is rarely seen in adolescents but occurs in 30% of untreated individuals who have syphilis for a 10- to 20-year period.

Diagnosis

The nontreponemal tests include the RPR test, Venereal Disease Research Laboratory (VDRL) test, and automated reagin test (ART). The RPR test result usually becomes positive 7 days after the initial chancre appears. A positive RPR or nontreponemal test result is then confirmed by a direct treponemal test, the fluorescent treponemal antibody absorption (FTA-ABS) test or the microhemagglutination assay for antibody to *Treponema pallidum* (MHA-TP). The results of these tests remain positive after treatment; therefore, the nontreponemal test results are tracked serially to ensure adequate treatment and should show a fourfold decline. False-positive RPR test results can be seen in infections with Epstein-Barr virus, hepatitis B virus, HSV, *Mycoplasma, Mycobacteria*, and pneumococci; they are also associated with systemic lupus erythematosus, Hashimoto thyroiditis, primary biliary cirrhosis, autoimmune hemolytic anemia, and pregnancy. The prozone effect consists of false-negative results early in primary syphilis and late in latent syphilis when the titer is very high.

Treatment

Parenteral penicillin G remains the treatment of choice, with 2.4 million units of benzathine penicillin G given intramuscularly as a single dose. During treatment, the *Jarisch-Herxheimer reaction* can occur, consisting of fever, hypotension, myalgia, headache, and tachypnea secondary to the rapid destruction of a large number of spirochetes.

CHANCROID

Epidemiology

The United States has recently seen a resurgence of chancroid. Caused by infection with *Haemophilus ducreyi*, a fastidious gram-negative bacillus, chancroid is also the most frequent form of sexually acquired genital ulceration in Africa. Although more cases occur in uncircumcised men, more advanced disease is seen in men who are circumcised. The male-to-female ratio is 10:1.

Diagnosis

Patients have multiple purulent ulcers with ragged edges and tender inguinal adenopathy. The definitive diagnosis is by culture on special media (sensitivity of only 80%).

Treatment

One gram of azithromycin orally as a single dose, 250 mg of ceftriaxone intramuscularly as a single dose, 500 mg of ciprofloxacin orally twice daily for 3 days, and 500 mg of erythromycin base orally four times daily for 7 days all adequately treat chancroid. Patients should be tested for HIV infection at the time of diagnosis and for HIV infection and syphilis 3 months after diagnosis because coinfection rates are high.

HERPES SIMPLEX VIRUS INFECTION

Epidemiology

Most genital herpes infections are caused by HSV-2, and most oral herpes infections are caused by HSV-1. An estimated 30 million Americans are infected with HSV-2, and 200,000 new cases are identified each year.

Presentation

Most patients with HSV infection are asymptomatic. Symptomatic patients have painful vesicles on the genitalia or in the surrounding areas. Other symptoms may include dysuria, vaginal discharge, pruritus (locally), and proctitis; patients with primary infection may have fever, myalgias, tender inguinal adenopathy, headaches, abdominal pain, and aseptic meningitis. Herpetic whitlow can also be found. Recurrent infection may be accompanied by prodromal symptoms, such as tingling or burning locally.

Diagnosis

The definitive diagnosis is by viral culture and typing; a specimen is obtained by unroofing a vesicle and rubbing a sterile swab vigorously over the base, then placing it immediately in viral transport media. Direct fluorescent antibody testing provides a sensitive and specific diagnosis. The sensitivity of a Tzanck test preparation is only 30% to 50%, whereas PCR testing has 75% sensitivity and 100% specificity. A positive result of PCR may not indicate infectivity because it detects viral DNA rather than only replicative virus.

Treatment

Recommended treatment regimens for initial and recurrent HSV infections appear in Table 45.4. The newer agents, valacyclovir and famciclovir, have improved oral bioavailability, but they are quite expensive. Use of daily suppressive valacyclovir at a dose of 500 mg per day decreases the rate of HSV2 transmission in discordant heterosexual couples (where one partner has HSV2 and the other does not). This schedule should be considered as part of a treatment strategy to prevent transmission for use with individuals having sex with

TABLE 45.4

TREATMENT RECOMMENDATIONS FOR HERPES SIMPLEX VIRUS INFECTION

Initial infection
　Acyclovir 400 mg orally three times daily for 7–10 days
　Acyclovir 200 mg orally five times a day for 7–10 days
　Famciclovir 250 mg orally three times daily for 7–10 days
　Valacyclovir 1 g orally twice daily for 7–10 days
Recurrent infection
　Episodic infections:
　　Acyclovir 400 mg orally three times daily for 5 days
　　Acyclovir 800 mg orally three times a day for 2 days
　　Acyclovir 800 mg orally twice daily for 5 days
　　Famciclovir 1 g orally twice a day for 1 day
　　Famciclovir 125 mg orally twice daily for 5 days
　　Valacyclovir 500 mg orally twice daily for 3 days
　　Valacyclovir 1 g orally a day for 5 days
　Daily suppressive therapy:
　　Acyclovir 400 mg orally twice daily
　　Famciclovir 250 mg orally twice daily
　　Valacyclovir 250 mg orally twice daily
　　Valacyclovir 500 mg orally once a day
　　Valacyclovir 1 g orally once a day

multiple partners (including males having sex with males) and in those patients with HIV who are symptomatic.

LYMPHOGRANULOMA VENEREUM

Epidemiology

Caused by three serotypes (L-1, L-2, and L-3) of *C. trachomatis*, lymphogranuloma venereum has been detected in cluster cases in various regions of the United States.

Diagnosis

With an incubation period of 3 days to 3 weeks, the primary lesion consists of usually one papule, vesicle, or pustule, 2 to 10 mm in size, which may be elevated, and round or oval. Initially, the patient may or may not notice a transient ulcer, which can be superficial or deep. The lesion itself may be firm, may or may not be tender, but tender lymphadenopathy usually is present, often unilaterally, which can be loculate or suppurative. Patients tend to present with tender, enlarged inguinal adenopathy and/or with rectal strictures. Diagnosis is made by isolation of the organism, immunofluorescence of inclusion bodies in leukocytes of a lymph node aspirate, or serologic testing.

Treatment

Doxycycline 100 mg orally twice a days for 21 days will eradicate the infection. Alternative treatments include erythromycin base 500 mg orally four times a day for 21 days.

TRICHOMONAS VAGINALIS INFECTION

Presentation

Patients present with a bubbly, malodorous, yellow/gray/green/white discharge with or without dysuria, postcoital bleeding, and dyspareunia. The incubation period is 4 to 20 days. With a prevalence of 7% to 33% in sexually active adolescents and young adults, the infection is usually sexually acquired. On physical examination, the patient may have a friable "strawberry cervix" and a frothy discharge.

Diagnosis

Trichomonads can be seen on wet preparation or Pap smear (although the latter method may yield some false-positives). The pH of the vaginal discharge is at least 4.5.

Treatment

A single 2-g dose of metronidazole treats *T. vaginalis* infection in both the patient and the partner. A newer treatment option involves use of tinidazole 2 g; tinidazole is equivalent, or superior, to metronidazole in achieving parasitologic cure and resolution of symptoms.

BACTERIAL VAGINOSIS

Epidemiology

Nonspecific vaginitis, G. vaginalis infection, and *nonspecific vaginosis* are all synonyms for the alteration in normal vaginal flora that occurs more commonly in sexually active women. Risk factors include the use of an intrauterine device, prior STD, smoking, low socioeconomic status, non-white ethnicity, and an uncircumcised partner. The prevalence is 4% to 25% of college students, 10% to 25% of pregnant women, and 33% to 37% of individuals treated at STD clinics.

Presentation

Girls and women present with a fishy, malodorous discharge or an irregular menses.

Diagnosis

Three of the following four criteria are required to make the diagnosis:

- Gray to white homogenous discharge that may adhere to the vaginal wall
- pH of 4.5 or higher

- Positive "whiff" test result (odor of "dead fish" when discharge comes in contact with sperm or potassium hydroxide)
- Presence of *clue cells* on wet preparation (constituting 20% of cells visualized)

Treatment

A 2-g oral dose of metronidazole provides adequate treatment for bacterial vaginosis, although some treatment failures have been documented with this schedule. Other options include 500 mg of metronidazole orally twice daily for 7 days, insertion of a 5-g applicator containing 2% clindamycin cream intravaginally before going to bed for 7 nights, insertion of a 5-g applicator containing 0.75% metronidazole gel intravaginally twice daily for 5 days, or 300 mg of clindamycin orally twice daily for 7 days.

The differential diagnosis may include physiologic leukorrhea, the normal vaginal discharge that begins in early puberty. This is caused by a rise in estrogen levels, which leads to a thickening of the vaginal mucosa and increased numbers of superficial cells containing glycogen. Colonizing lactobacilli use the glycogen to produce lactic acid and acetic acid, thereby changing the vaginal pH to between 3.5 and 5.0. Physiologic leukorrhea is the normal desquamation of epithelial cells secondary to the effect of estrogen, and it usually begins 6 to 12 months before menses. If it is profuse or bothersome to the patient, wearing cotton crotch underwear and loose clothing and practicing good local hygiene or sitz baths will help. The major causes of vaginitis in teens include disruption of the normal vaginal flora secondary to coital microtrauma, treatment with antibiotics, tight jeans and underwear, and STDs. Yeast vaginitis can present as a discharge resembling cottage cheese with or without local pruritus or inflammation. Hyphae can be seen on potassium hydroxide preparation in 80% to 90% of symptomatic patients, or on a positive culture grown on Biggy agar media. Intravaginal imidazoles are usually given as treatment.

HUMAN PAPILLOMAVIRUS INFECTION

Epidemiology

Highly prevalent in adolescent and young adult women, human papillomavirus (HPV) can be acquired perinatally or through sexual abuse, by skin-to-skin contact, and by sexual intercourse. Recurrent respiratory papillomatosis occurs rarely from vertical transmission from mother to newborn and is usually caused by HPV types 6 and 11. Genital warts occur in 1.4 million adolescents and adults in the 15- to 49-year-old age group annually, with a study by Koutsky estimating that 10% to 20% of individuals in this age-group display molecular evidence of genital HPV infection. The data show that 60% of 15- to 49-year-old men and women, or 81 million people, have been infected previously with HPV as evidenced by antibody positivity, with 15% currently infected. Of this latter group, 10% (14 million) have subclinical infection and are positive for HPV DNA or RNA only, 4% (5 million) have abnormal cytology, and 1% (1.4 million) have genital warts. Types 16, 18, 21, 33, and 35 have been associated with squamous vulvar intraepithelial neoplasia. Most often asymptomatic, rarely warts can be perceived as uncomfortable or pruritic.

The natural progression of HPV has been studied well by Moscicki et al., who followed up a longitudinal cohort of 618 HPV-positive young women of ages 13 to 21 years. With cytology, colposcopy, and HPV DNA testing occurring at 4-month intervals, regression rates were high (defined as three negative tests for HPV DNA by 30 months of follow-up). The regression rate for women with low-risk HPV types was 90%; for high-risk types, it was 75%. Only 22% developed LSIL during the 60 months of follow-up. If a high-risk type was detected on three to four of the preceding visits, the odds of developing HSIL was 14:1 when compared with women who were negative for high-risk types. However, 88% of women persistently positive for high-risk HPV did *not* develop HSIL during the study period.

Diagnosis

Younger children older than 3 years with HPV need to be evaluated for the possibility of sexual abuse. Adolescents can be easily assessed using liquid-based cytology with HPV DNA testing. Because of the transient nature of most HPV infections in adolescents, with the vast majority of low-grade lesions regressing, the risk of HSIL is low even in those adolescents with high-risk HPV types. The American Cancer Society recommends a first Pap smear 3 to 5 years after initial exposure to HPV, or by 3 years after initiating sexual activity. Screening should then be done annually as part of preventive care. The evaluation of the patient with an abnormal result of the Pap test is shown in Table 45.5.

Treatment

No treatment currently available eliminates HPV, so therapy is aimed at destruction of affected tissue, with the goal of removing warts. Without treatment, genital warts may resolve spontaneously. Treatment options depend on the child's or adolescent's symptoms, the extent of the disease, and the clinician's experience with the use of topical agents or other modalities such as laser. Laser ablation should be used in cases of extensive disease. Imiquimod (85%) trichloroacetic acid (TCA) or bichloracetic acid (BCA, 80%–90%) can be used. Cryotherapy, surgical removal with excision, curettage, or electrosurgery, and intralesional interferon are other available options. Podophyllin resin works as an antimitotic agent that causes tissue necrosis; it can have hematologic and central nervous system toxicity, as well as gastrointestinal symptoms, making it less popular

TABLE 45.5

THE EVALUATION OF THE PATIENT WITH AN ABNORMAL RESULT OF THE PAPANICOLAOU SMEAR

Abnormal Lesion	Intervention
ASCUS (atypical squamous cells of undetermined significance)	HPV DNA testing: if high-risk HPV found, repeat Pap test in 3 months. If progresses to LSIL: colposcopy Otherwise: repeat Pap test every 3–6 months
LSIL	Colposcopy: if negative for CIN, repeat Pap test every 6 months
HSIL	Colposcopy with endocervical assessment: if CIN 1 identified, diagnostic excisional procedure recommended. Follow-up with colposcopy and cytology every 4–6 months.

CIN, cervical intraepithelial neoplasia; HPV, human papillomavirus; HSIL, high-grade squamous intraepithelial lesions; LSIL, low-grade squamous intraepithelial lesions; Pap, Papanicolaou.

among prescribers and patients alike. If used, it needs to be washed off after 4 hours. The topical agents such as TCA and BCA also cause local irritation and pain where applied, with weekly office-based treatment used until the lesions are gone (which can take 6 to 8 weeks). Podofilox 0.5% solution or gel can be applied twice daily for 3 days, then not used for 4 days, with the cycle repeated for up to 4 weeks. Imiquimod is an imidazoquinolin heterocyclic amine that serves as a local immune enhancer by stimulating local production of interferon and other cytokines. It inhibits HPV replication directly and also enhances cell-mediated immune response against HPV. It can be applied nightly, three times a week, for up to 16 weeks. The area is then washed with soap and water 6 to 10 hours after application. Advantages include self-application and potentially lower recurrence rates. It is expensive, can cause local burning, itching, pain, and can take 4 months to be effective.

Prevention

Since its FDA approval in June 2006, over 20 million doses of the currently available HPV vaccine have been distributed in the United States alone. Made of the major capsid protein of the genital HPV, this vaccine consists of virus-like particle (VLP) subunit vaccines. It is highly immunogenic and safe, with vaccine adverse event reporting system (VAERS) running at 6%, lower than the anticipated 7% seen with most vaccines. It induces a strong cell-mediated and humoral response, with best immunity seen when administered in early adolescence, or by age 14 years. FDA approved for girls ages 9 to 26 years, the HPV vaccine is administered in the same schedule as hepatitis B vaccines, or at time 0, 2 months later, and 6 months after the initial shot (or 4 months after

#2). The American Academy of Pediatrics recommends beginning HPV vaccination at ages 11 to 12 years, or at Tanner stage 2. This vaccine has provided a window of opportunity to open doors of communication between parents and children, and clinicians, parents, and children, over development of a healthy sexuality, values clarification, and other hot topics. Most parents welcome the discussion along with words to tackle tough issues with their children. All parents, and many clinicians, can benefit from more education on this topic, as many adults do not wish to see their children as potential sexual beings until long after their child has engaged in risk-taking behavior. The young age of administration, endorsed not just by the AAP but also by the American College of Obstetrics and Gynecology, along with the American Academy of Family Practice, has given us a means of prevention of sexually transmitted infections by having families—and clinicians—initiate counseling on prevention ideally long before it is "necessary."

CONCLUSION

STDs are common in adolescents, and with the exception of HIV and HSV infections, they are entirely treatable. The best strategy for dealing with STDs remains primary prevention, ideally by abstinence, and if not, by the proper use of condoms. Primary prevention also includes vaccination, with the HPV vaccine already commercially available and HSV vaccination on the horizon. Secondary prevention includes early recognition of STD with provision of appropriate treatment; tertiary prevention involves the treatment of sequelae. Urine NAAT or DNA amplification testing serves as secondary prevention by detecting *N. gonorrhoeae* and *Chlamydia* infections while they remain asymptomatic, before PID or its sequelae have developed (tertiary prevention). Newer research will continue to focus on prevention while methods of recognition and treatment are further refined.

REVIEW EXERCISES

QUESTIONS

1. Appropriate treatment for PID in an adolescent includes:
a) Cefoxitin intravenously (IV) and azithromycin IV
b) Cefoxitin IV and doxycycline orally
c) Cefixime (Suprax) orally and azithromycin orally
d) Ceftriaxone intramuscularly and azithromycin orally
e) Cefixime (Suprax) orally, azithromycin orally, and metronidazole (Flagyl) orally

Answer
The answer is b. This answer is in accordance with the CDC 2006 guidelines for the treatment of STDs. The first regimen listed consists of 2 g of cefoxitin IV every 6 hours

combined with 100 mg of doxycycline orally or IV every 12 hours. Doxycycline is very sclerotic and painful when delivered IV, so the oral route is preferred. An alternative to cefoxitin is 2 g of cefotetan IV every 12 hours. Azithromycin has been tested as a treatment for adolescents; because adolescent girls are at the start of their reproductive cycles, the efficacy of azithromycin should be established before it is recommended for adolescents. Oral cefixime has shown efficacy against *N. gonorrhoeae* in cervical infections but has not proved useful in PID.

2. A 15-year-old boy comes in with a penile discharge. Appropriate management includes:
a) Urine testing for *N. gonorrhoeae* (GC) and *C. trachomatis* (CT) only
b) Urine testing for GC/CT and treatment with cefixime and azithromycin
c) Urethral swab only
d) Urine testing for GC/CT and treatment with 2 gm of azithromycin
e) Either b or d

Answer
The answer is e. In a symptomatic boy, coverage for *N. gonorrhoeae* and *C. trachomatis* infections is indicated. The former is adequately covered with 400 mg of cefixime, and 1 g of azithromycin covers the latter. The sensitivity and specificity of urine PCR/LCR/TMA (transcription-mediated amplification) are excellent, and adolescent boys are spared an unwelcome and unpleasant urethral swab. Either urine DNA probe or urethral swab for DNA probe is adequate to test for gonorrhea and *Chlamydia* infection. In a symptomatic patient, testing alone is insufficient as a public health measure because the teenager is likely to continue to spread the disease until the test results are available and the treatment is begun.

3. Risk factors for the acquisition of STDs in adolescents include all of the following *except:*
a) High rates of protective antibody in this population
b) Prominent exocervix in adolescent girls
c) Retrograde menstruation
d) Older partner
e) Use of alcohol or drugs

Answer
The answer is a. Risk factors for STDs in adolescents are both biologic and psychosocial. Biologic factors include the following: a prominent exocervix, which involutes with age; low levels of protective antibodies because of less cumulative exposure to disease; carriage of infection by sperm up to the fallopian tubes or upper genital tract; and retrograde menstruation, which occurs in 25% of healthy women. Behavioral factors include the following: sex with multiple partners and lower rates of condom use in younger patients; clouded judgment regarding sexual

activity and condom use as a consequence of exposure to alcohol and drugs; older men with greater cumulative exposure to disease having sex with adolescent girls, who are unable to refuse or negotiate safer sex; and the personal sense of invulnerability that is part of the adolescent mindset.

4. A 15-year-old girl comes into the office with a white vaginal discharge that is foul-smelling. She has been sexually active in the past and has no history of prior STD. Clue cells are visible on wet preparation, no yeast is seen on potassium hydroxide preparation, and the pH is 4.5. The *most* likely diagnosis is:
a) *T. vaginalis* infection
b) *C. trachomatis* infection
c) Physiologic leukorrhea
d) Bacterial vaginosis
e) *N. gonorrhoeae* infection

Answer
The answer is d. Bacterial vaginosis (nonspecific vaginitis, *G. vaginalis* infection) is the result of an alteration in normal vaginal flora that occurs more often in sexually active girls and women. Patients present with a malodorous discharge that smells like "dead fish" when mixed with potassium hydroxide or sperm (positive "whiff" test result). Three of the following four criteria are required for the diagnosis:

- Thin, homogenous white discharge
- Presence of clue cells on wet preparation
- pH of 4.5 or higher
- Positive "whiff" test result

Even with likely bacterial vaginosis, sexually active girls presenting with a discharge should also have urine testing by nucleic acid amplification strategy (NAAT) for *N. gonorrhoeae* and *Chlamydia* trachomatis.

5. A pelvic examination should be performed on any adolescent girl for each reason provided in the subsequent text *except:*
a) Screening for cervical cancer with the Pap smear
b) Determining the stage of a pregnancy
c) Evaluating pelvic pain
d) Before initiating treatment with oral contraceptives
e) Evaluating vaginitis in a patient with lower quadrant pain

Answer
The answer is d. Pelvic examinations can be used to stage a pregnancy, screen for STDs and HPV infection by DNA probe and for cervical cancer by Pap smear, determine the cause of abdominal or pelvic pain, and evaluate for vaginitis. However, an argument can be made to use urine screening with nucleic acid amplification test and perform Pap smears just once a year after the initiation of sexual activity. Traditionally used to

screen for vaginitis, patient-obtained vaginal swabs can also be used to screen for *T. vaginalis* infection when a pelvic examination cannot be performed. According to the American College of Obstetricians and Gynecologists and the Northern American Society for Pediatric and Adolescent Gynecology, a pelvic examination is not absolutely necessary before oral contraceptives are begun. However, if an individual has ever been sexually active, a follow-up visit for STD screening is indicated if not performed on the same day as the pill start. As per ACOG recommendations, a first PAP smear should occur 3 years after first sexual activity or by age 21 years (whichever comes first).

SUGGESTED READINGS

1. ACOG Practice Bulletin No.45. Cervical cytology screening. *Obstet Gynecol* 2003;102:417.
2. Alan Guttmacher Institute. Sexually transmitted diseases in the United States. *Facts in brief,* New York: Alan Guttmacher Institute, 1993.
3. Biro FM, Reising SF, Doughman JA, et al. A comparison of diagnostic methods in adolescent girls with and without symptoms of *Chlamydial* urogenital infection. *Pediatrics* 1994;93:476.
4. Blake DR, Duggan A, Quinn T, et al. Evaluation of vaginal infections in adolescent women: can it be done without a speculum? *Pediatrics* 1998;102:939–944.
5. Centers for Disease Control and Prevention. Sexually transmitted diseases treatment guidelines. *MMWR* 2006;55, RR-11:1–94.
6. Cerin A, Grillner L, Persson E. *Chlamydia* test monitoring during therapy. *Int J STD AIDS* 1991;2:176–179.
7. Donovan P. *Testing positive: sexually transmitted disease and the public health response.* New York: Alan Guttmacher Institute, 1993.
8. Emans SJ, Laufer MR, Goldstein DP. *Pediatric and adolescent gynecology,* 4th ed. Philadelphia: Lippincott Williams & Wilkins, 1998: 457–504.
9. Flood JM, Sarafian SK, Bolan GA, et al. Multistrain outbreak of chancroid in San Francisco 1989–1991. *J Infect Dis* 1993;167: 1106–1111.
10. Forna F, Gulmezogla AM. Interventions for treating trichomoniasis in women. *Cochrane Database Syst Rev* 2003;2:CD000218.
11. Goldenring JM, Cohen E. Getting into adolescent heads. *Contemp Pediatr* 1988;5:75–94.
12. Hatcher RA, Trussell J, Stewart F, et al. *Contraceptive technology,* 16th ed. New York: Irvington Publishers, 1994:77–106.
13. Jessor R, Jessor SL. *Problem behavior and psychosocial development: a longitudinal study of youth.* New York: Academic Press, 1977.
14. Joffe A. Amplified DNA testing for sexually transmitted diseases: new opportunities and new questions. *Arch Pediatr Adolesc Med* 1999;153:111–112.
15. Kane ML, Rosen DS. Sexually transmitted infections in adolescents: practical issues in the office setting. *Adolesc Med* 2004;15:409–421.
16. Kissinger Mohammed H, Richardson-Alston G, et al. Patient-delivered partner treatment. *Sex Transm Dis* 2006;33:445–450.
17. Koutsky LA, Galloway DA, Holmes KK. Epidemiology of genital human papillomavirus infection. *Epidemiol Rev* 1988;10:122.
18. Lawing LF, Hedges SR, Schwebke JR. Detection of *Trichomonas* in vaginal and urine specimens from women by culture and PCR. *J Clin Microbiol* 2000;38:3585–3588.
19. Moscicki AB. Genital HPV infections in children and adolescents. *Obstet Gynecol Clin North Am* 1996;23:675.
20. Polaneczky M, Quigley C, Polloack L, et al. Use of self-collected vaginal specimens for detection of *Chlamydia trachomatis* infection. *Obstet Gynecol* 1998;91:375–378.
21. Rome ES. Pelvic inflammatory disease in the adolescent. *Curr Opin Pediatr* 1994;6:383–387.
22. Rome ES. Pelvic inflammatory disease: the importance of aggressive treatment in the adolescent. *Cleve Clin J Med* 1998;65: 369–376.
23. Rome ES. Sexually transmitted diseases in the adolescent. Part II: syphilis, chancroid, and herpes. *Female Patient* 1998;23:67–73.
24. Shafer MB, Pantell RH, Schachter J. Is the routine pelvic examination needed with the advent of urine-based screening for sexually transmitted diseases? *Arch Pediatr Adolesc Med* 1999;153:119–125.
25. Smith K, Harrington K, Wingood G, et al. Self-obtained vaginal swabs for the diagnosis of treatable sexually transmitted diseases in adolescent girls. *Arch Pediatr Adolesc Med* 2001;155:676–679.
26. Spigarelli MG, Biro FM. Sexually transmitted disease testing: evaluation of diagnostic tests and methods. *Adolesc Med* 2004;15: 287–299.
27. Sung L, MacDonald NE. Gonorrhea: a pediatric perspective. *Pediatr Rev* 1998;19:13–16.
28. Tjiong MY, Out TA, Ter Schegget J, et al. Epidemiologic and mucosal immunologic aspects of HPV infection and HPV-related cervical carcinoma in the lower female genital tract: a review. *Int J Gynecol Cancer* 2001;11:9.
29. Washington AE, Katz P. Cost and payment source for pelvic inflammatory disease. Trends and projections, 1983 through 2000. *JAMA* 1991;266:2565.
30. Wilson J. Treatment of genital warts: what's the evidence? *Int J STD AIDS* 2002;13:216.
31. Zimet GD, Mays RM, Fortenberry JD. Vaccines against sexually transmitted infections: promise and problems of the magic bullets for prevention and control. *Sex Transm Dis* 2000;27:49.

Chapter 46

Amenorrhea

Karen S. Vargo

The evaluation of amenorrhea in the adolescent requires a basic understanding of pubertal development, including the role of the hypothalamic-pituatary-ovarian (HPO) axis and its effect on the menstrual cycle. The differential diagnosis for primary and secondary amenorrhea are very similar except for a few genetic conditions that only cause primary amenorrhea.

Both primary and secondary amenorrhea can be assessed in a similar manner. Begin with a complete history and physical examination, followed by a step-by-step laboratory evaluation. If a methodical approach is utilized, the pediatrician can diagnose and manage most cases of amenorrhea. The practitioner should be sensitive to the effect amenorrhea can have on an adolescent's body image and sexual identity.

DEFINITION OF AMENORRHEA

Primary amenorrhea is defined as:

- Absence of menarche by the age of 15 years in the presence of otherwise normal growth and development
- Absence of menarche and other signs of puberty, such as the development of breasts and pubic hair by the age of 13 years
- Failure of menarche to occur within 5 years after the beginning of breast development if that occurs before age 10 years

Secondary amenorrhea is defined as:

- The absence of menses for longer than 3 months in a female patient with well-established menstruation

PHYSIOLOGY OF THE MENSTRUAL CYCLE

The HPO axis is directly responsible for regulating the menstrual cycle (Fig. 46.1). Gonadotropin-releasing hormone (GnRH) from the hypothalamus stimulates the release of follicle-stimulating hormone (FSH) and luteinizing hormone (LH) from the pituitary. FSH and LH influence the ovarian production of estrogen and progesterone, which in turn have both a positive and negative feedback effect on the pituitary and the hypothalamus.

PHASES OF THE MENSTRUAL CYCLE

The menstrual cycle can be broken down into three phases (Fig. 46.2).

Follicular Phase

During the menses, low ovarian levels of estrogen stimulate the production of FSH. Final maturation of the follicle occurs under the stimulation of FSH. As the ovarian production of estrogen increases, the rising estrogen levels have a negative effect on FSH and a positive effect on LH. During the second half of this phase, estrogen stimulates growth of the endometrium.

Ovulatory Phase

The surge in LH secondary to positive estrogen feedback results in ovulation. As LH levels peak, estrogen levels fall.

Luteal Phase

This phase corresponds to the lifespan of the corpus luteum, which secretes progesterone and estrogen. Under the influence of these hormones, the endometrium becomes thicker and more vascular. Plasma levels of LH and FSH decline. If fertilization does not occur, the corpus luteum involutes within 14 days and estrogen and progesterone levels fall. With a fall in the levels of these hormones, the endometrium becomes necrotic and sloughs off in the process known as *menstruation*.

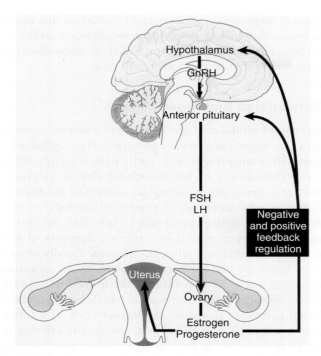

Figure 46.1   The hypothalamic-pituitary-ovarian axis. FSH, follicle-stimulating hormone; GnRH, gonadotropin-releasing hormone; LH, luteinizing hormone.

MENARCHE AND THE ADOLESCENT MENSTRUAL CYCLE

Menarche occurs at a mean age of 12.5 years, with a range of 9 to 16 years. In most cases it occurs 1 year after the peak growth velocity and 2 years after the development of breast buds. By menarche, most girls have completed 75% of their pubertal development and achieved 90% of their growth potential. Early menstrual cycles are anovulatory. Ovulation usually begins within 1 to 2 years after menarche and reflects synchronization and maturation of the HPO axis. A normal menstrual period lasts from 2 to 7 days, with an average blood loss between 30 and 40 mL. Cycle lengths can vary between 21 to 45 days but are usually constant for a given individual.

ETIOLOGY OF AMENORRHEA

In considering the etiology of amenorrhea (Table 46.1), it is helpful to think about where along the HPO axis the problem exists. Try to differentiate a central problem at the level of the hypothalamus or pituitary from an ovarian problem or an end-organ problem. The classification of *hypogonadotropic hypogonadism* refers to low FSH and LH levels seen in conditions affecting the hypothalmus and the pituatary. *Hypergonadotropic hypogonadism* refers to to high FSH and LH levels seen in conditions affecting the ovary. In *eugonadotropic* conditions FSH and LH levels are normal.

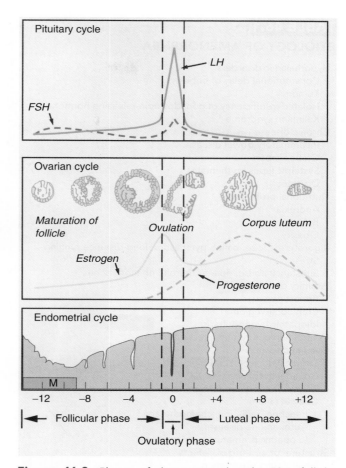

Figure 46.2   Phases of the menstrual cycle. FSH, follicle-stimulating hormone; LH, luteinizing hormone.

Hypothalamic Disorders

Any condition associated with a deficiency of GnRH can cause amenorrhea. Constitutional delay of puberty is a common etiology of primary amenorrhea. This condition may be associated with short stature and a family history of delayed puberty or delayed menarche in an older sibling or parent. Other conditions that cause GnRH deficiency include hypothalamic tumors, isolated GnRH insufficiency, and Kallmann syndrome (GnRH deficiency and anosmia). Any type of chronic disease, such as inflammatory bowel disease, cystic fibrosis, systemic lupus erythematosus, and diabetes; nutritional problems (e.g., anorexia, bulimia, obesity), rigorous exercise, stress, and substance abuse can also result in GnRH deficiency.

Pituitary Disorders

Pituitary disorders that can cause amenorrhea include tumors such as prolactinomas and craniopharyngiomas. Other causes are idiopathic hypopituitarism and a history of central nervous system infection.

TABLE 46.1
ETIOLOGY OF AMENORRHEA

Hypothalamic disorders
  Constitutional delay of puberty
  Tumors
  Isolated insufficiency of gonadotropin-releasing hormone
  Kallmann syndrome
Chronic disease
  Inflammatory bowel disease
  Cystic fibrosis
  Systemic lupus erythematosis
  Diabetes
Nutritional problems
  Anorexia
  Bulimia
  Obesity
Rigorous exercise: ballet, gymnastics, long-distance running
  Stress
  Substance abuse: opiates, heroin, phenothiazines
Pituitary disorders
  Prolactinoma
  Craniopharyngioma
  Idiopathic hypopituitarism
Central nervous system infection
Ovarian disorders
  Turner syndrome (45,X0)
  Gonadal dysgenesis (46,XX)
  Polycystic ovary syndrome
  Ovarian failure
    Infection, radiation, chemotherapy
    Autoimmune disease
    Idiopathic premature ovarian failure
Structural or end-organ defects
  Genital tract obstruction
  Imperforate hymen
  Transverse vaginal septum
  Asherman syndrome: ablation of uterine lining secondary to
    trauma or infection.
  Mullerian agenesis (46,XX): partial or total vaginal agenesis
  Androgen insensitivity syndrome (46,XY)
Other causes
  Pregnancy
  Hormonal contraception
  Endocrinopathies
  Diabetes mellitus
  Thyroid disease: hyperfunction or hypofunction
  Adrenal disease

Ovarian Disorders

Turner syndrome is one of the most common chromosomal disorders in humans and one of the most frequent causes of primary amenorrhea. It is characterized by a 45,XO karyotype, although up to 50% of affected persons may exhibit mosaicism (46,XX/45,XO). Some of the stigmata of Turner syndrome include short stature, webbed neck, shield chest, and streak ovaries.

Female gonadal dysgenesis is characterized by a 46,XX karyotype and streak ovaries.

Gonadal dysgenesis with a variety of other abnormal karyotypes such as XY or XXY may also occur. They are a rare cause of amenorrhea. Other ovarian conditions that result in amenorrhea include polycystic ovary syndrome and ovarian failure secondary to infection, radiation, chemotherapy, autoimmune disease, or an idiopathic cause.

Structural or End-organ Defects

Any sort of genital tract obstruction can result in amenorrhea. An imperforate hymen or a transverse vaginal septum will often present with cyclic pain resulting from the accumualtion of blood behind the obstruction. Asherman syndrome is iatrogenic scarring of the uterine lining, usually secondary to trauma sustained during a dilation and curettage procedure or infection. Mullerian agenesis refers to partial or complete agenesis of the vagina. The uterus and fallopian tubes are usually absent or rudimentary and the karyotype is 46,XX. In complete androgen insensitivity syndrome, the individual appears phenotypically female with normal female breasts and external genitalia. However, the vagina ends in a blind pouch and pubic hair is absent or sparse. The karyotye is 46,XY and inguinal or intra-abdominal testes are present. Because of the risk of malignancy, the testes should be removed after breast development and adult stature have been achieved.

Other Causes

Pregnancy should always be considered in both primary and secondary amenorrhea. Other considerations include hormonal contraception and endocrinopathies such as diabetes, thyroid disease, and adrenal disease.

EVALUATION OF AMENORRHEA

History

Begin the evaluation of primary and secondary amenorrhea with a detailed history of the patient's growth and development (Table 46.2). In the case of primary amenorrhea, specifically inquire about the age at thelarche (development of breast buds), adrenarche (growth of pubic hair), and the growth spurt. Important details of the menstrual history include the age at menarche, frequency and duration of menses, presence of dysmenorrhea, and breast changes associated with menses. Inquire about a history of chronic disease or a serious childhood illness, such as a central nervous system infection. The family history should include the ages of puberty and menarche for parents and siblings. Inquire about a history of psychiatric illness, environmental stress, medications, and drug abuse. Has the patient experienced a recent weight change? Take a detailed dietary history and ask about body image to explore the possibility of an eating disorder. Extreme exercise habits and participation in

TABLE 46.2

EVALUATION OF AMENORRHEA: HISTORY

Pubertal growth and development
Menstrual history
Past medical history
    Childhood illness
    Chronic disease
Family history
    Ages of parental growth and development
    Mother and sisters' age at menarche
Environmental stress
Psychiatric illness
Medications
Substance abuse
Diet
Exercise habits
Sexual history
History of androgen excess
Galactorrhea

competitive sports can cause amenorrhea in the female athlete. Obtain a sexual history regarding past and present sexual activity. Inquire about signs of androgen excess or virilization, such as acne and hirsutism. Also ask about galactorrhea associated with conditions causing hyperprolactinemia.

Physical Examination

Begin with the patient's vital signs. Look for evidence of hypothermia, bradycardia, tachycardia, or blood pressure abnormalities often seen in conditions such as eating disorders or thyroid disease (Table 46.3). Plot out the height, weight, and body mass index on growth charts. Assess the patient's overall body habitus and rate the sexual maturity of her breasts and pubic hair. Look for signs of androgen excess, such as acne or hirsutism, which are commonly seen in polycystic ovary syndrome. The absence of axillary and pubic hair in an otherwise physically mature female patient may indicate complete androgen insensitivity. Carefully palpate the thyroid gland to assess for hypertrophy or nodules. Check the abdomen for masses or pregnancy and the groin for inguinal testes.

TABLE 46.3

EVALUATION OF AMENORRHEA: PHYSICAL EXAMINATION

Vital signs: blood pressure, pulse
Growth charts: height and weight percentiles
Sexual maturity rating: Tanner stage of breasts and pubic hair
Body habitus
Signs of hirsutism or androgen excess
Careful palpation of thyroid, abdomen, and groin
Galactorrhea
Neurologic examination: cranial nerves, visual fields
Pelvic examination: external and internal exam

Perform a thorough neurologic examination, including an assessment of the cranial nerves and visual fields, to look for signs of a pituitary tumor or Kallmann syndrome. Perform a careful breast examination and check for the presence of galactorrhea.

Finally, a thorough genital examination is indicated to check for clitoromegaly and assess the presence and patency of the vagina. A speculum examination is recommended to evaluate the vaginal canal and verify the presence of a cervix. An examination with a single digit or a Q-tip may be used to assess vaginal patency in a virginal patient. A bimanual examination should be performed to check for the presence of a uterus and ovaries. If an internal exam is not possible, an ultrasound should be obtained to confirm the presence or absence of a uterus.

Evaluation of Amenorrhea with Delayed Puberty

Begin the evaluation with a detailed patient history (Table 46.2). Pay particular attention to past growth and development, previous medical problems or a history of systemic disease. Enquire about the age of puberty and menarche of other family members and ask about the patient's dietary history and exercise habits (Fig. 46.3). Complete a thorough physical examination, specifically addressing the items listed in Table 46.3. The initial laboratory evaluation (Table 46.4) includes a complete blood cell count and a determination of the erythrocyte sedimentation rate to rule out the possibility of a systemic illness such as Crohn disease. Thyroid function studies and a prolactin level should also be checked. Bone age measurement is indicated to evaluate for constitutional delay of puberty. A bone age more than one standard deviation below the chronologic age with otherwise normal laboratory and examination findings is consistent with constitutional delay of puberty. If all the above values are normal, measure the FSH and LH levels to help differentiate a hypothalamic or pituatary problem from an ovarian problem. In the case of *hypergonadotropic hypogonadism* (elevated LH level >40 IU/L and FSH level >30 IU/L), obtain a karyotype to differentiate gonadal dysgenesis from ovarian failure. If the LH and FSH levels are low or normal, consider magnetic resonance imaging (MRI) of the head to rule out a central lesion. Review the history and physical examination for clues of a chronic disease, an eating disorder, excessive exercise, stress, or drug use. All of these conditions can cause delayed puberty and amenorrhea.

Evaluation of Amenorrhea with Normal Pubertal Development

Obtain a detailed history and perform a thorough physical examination (Fig. 46.4). If the genital or pelvic examination reveals an absent vagina or blind vaginal pouch,

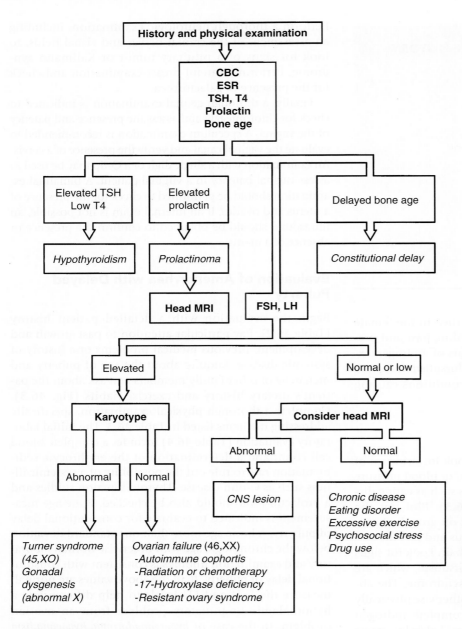

Figure 46.3 Amenorrhea with delayed puberty. CBC, complete blood count; CNS, central nervous system; ESR, erythrocyte sedimentation rate; FSH, follicle-stimulating hormone; LH, luteinizing hormone; MRI, magnetic resonance imaging; TSH, thyroid-stimulating hormone. (Adapted from Pletcher JR, Slap JB. Menstrual disorders. *Pediatr Clin North Amer* 1999;46(3): 513, WB Saunders Co.)

TABLE 46.4

EVALUATION OF AMENORRHEA: LABORATORY STUDIES

Pregnancy test
Complete blood cell count with differential
Sedimentation rate
Thyroid function tests
Prolactin
Follicle-stimulating hormone (FSH) and luteinizing hormone (LH)
Karyotype
Testosterone
Dehydroepiandrosterone sulfate (DHEA-S)
17-Hydroxyprogesterone
Fasting glucose
Fasting insulin
Bone age
Pelvic ultrasound
Pelvic/abdominal CT scan or MRI

proceed with ultrasonography and karyotyping to differentiate partial or complete vaginal agenesis (46,XX) from androgen insensitivity syndrome (46,XY). A testosterone level could also be utilized to differentiate these two disorders. In androgen insensitivity syndrome the testosterone levels are in the normal to high male range. In vaginal agenesis the testosterone levels are in the normal female range.

If the physical examination findings are normal, a pregnancy test is the next step in the evaluation and should never be overlooked. Once the possibility of pregnancy has been eliminated, measure a thyroid-stimulating hormone (TSH) level to rule out thyroid disease and a prolactin level to rule out a prolactinoma. If these results are normal, proceed with a progesterone challenge (medroxyprogesterone acetate 10 mg orally × 10 days). Withdrawal bleeding indicates adequate estrogen stimula-

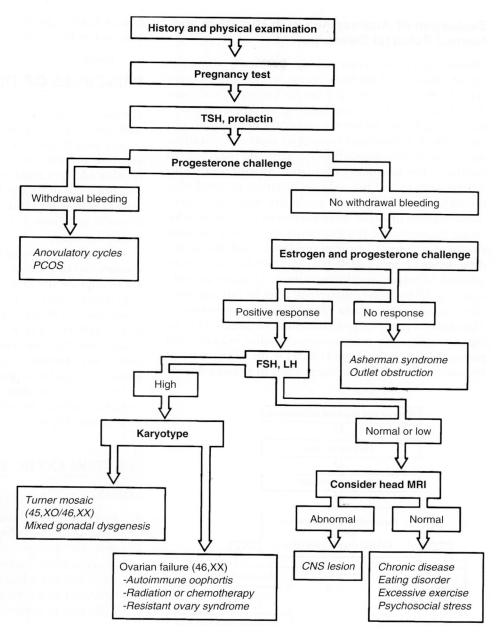

Figure 46.4 Amenorrhea with normal pubertal development. CNS, central nervous system; FSH, follicle-stimulating hormone; LH, luteinizing hormone; MRI, magnetic resonance imaging; TSH, thyroid-stimulating hormone; PCOS, polycystic ovarian syndrome. (Adapted from Pletcher JR, Slap JB. Menstrual disorders. *Pediatr Clin North Amer* 1999;46(3): 514, WB Saunders Co.)

tion of the endometrium. In this case, amenorrhea is most likely secondary to anovulatory cycles, as in polycystic ovary syndrome. If no withdrawal bleeding occurs, proceed with an estrogen and progesterone challenge (conjugated estrogen 0.625–1.25 mg daily × 21 days, with the addition of medroxyprogesterone acetate 10 mg daily for the last 5 days). If this produces no withdrawl bleeding, consider damage to the lining of the uterus, as in Asherman syndrome, or a previously overlooked outlet obstruction, such as a transverse vaginal septum. If a withdrawal bleed occurs after an estrogen and progesterone challenge, obtain FSH and LH levels to differentiate a central problem in the hypothalmus or pituatary from a problem at the level of the ovary. High levels of

FSH and LH *(hypergonadotropic hypogonadism)* indicate ovarian dysfunction. Proceed with a karyotype to differentiate Turner mosaicism or mixed gonadal dysgenesis from ovarian failure. Patients with Turner mosaicism (46,XX/ 45,XO) may have very small ovaries that involute over time. However, they may produce enough estrogen to stimulate the development of breasts and other secondary sexual characteristics. A 46,XX karyotype suggests ovarian failure. If the FSH and LH levels are normal or low *(hypogonadotropic hypogonadism),* consider an MRI of the head to rule out a central nervous system lesion. Review the history and physical examination findings for signs of a chronic disease, eating disorder, excessive exercise, stress, or substance abuse.

Evaluation of Amenorrhea with Hirsutism and Normal Pubertal Development

Obtain a detailed history, asking specifically about the recent onset of hirsutism, acne, or weight changes (Fig. 46.5). Inquire about a family history of androgen disorders, infertility, early balding, cardiovascular disease, or diabetes. Perform a physical examination, observing body habitus and looking for signs of virilization, such as acne, hirsutism, clitoromegaly, and male pattern baldness. The laboratory evaluation should begin with a pregnancy test. If the result is negative, proceed with measurement of the TSH, prolactin, and FSH levels. Abnormalities in any of these hormones may cause an increase in androgens. If these values are normal, measure the free and total testosterone levels and the dehydroepiandrosterone sulfate (DHEA-S) level to rule out an adrenal androgen–producing tumor. Measure an early morning 17-hydroxyprogesterone level to rule out nonclassic adrenal hyperplasia. If normal values are obtained, administer a progesterone challenge. Withdrawal bleeding in response to a progesterone challenge indicates that polycystic ovary syndrome (PCOS) is the likely cause of the amenorrhea. If the patient is obese or shows evidence

of acanthosis nigricans, consider obtaining a fasting glucose and an insulin level.

PRINCIPLES OF TREATMENT

The goals of treatment for amenorrhea are to identify and treat the underlying problem, restore ovulatory cycles, correct unopposed estrogen stimulation with cyclic progesterone or oral contraceptives, and when necessary, provide estrogen replacement therapy. Diseases such as constitutional delay can be treated with reassurance and regular follow-up. Structural abnormalities such as an imperforate hymen or transverse vaginal septum require corrective surgery.

PCOS can be managed with a combination of lifestyle changes and medication. The goals of treatment for PCOS are to regulate the menstrual cycle, prevent endometrial hyperplasia, manage hirsutism, improve acne, and decrease the risk of diabetes mellitus. Studies demonstrate that weight reduction and exercise can improve insulin resistance and decrease serum androgens. A combination of oral contraceptives, antiandrogens, insulin-sensitizing agents, and lipid-lowering agents may also be indicated.

Other endocrine abnormalities, such as ovarian failure, congenital adrenal hyperplasia, and Turner syndrome, are best managed by referral to an endocrinologist.

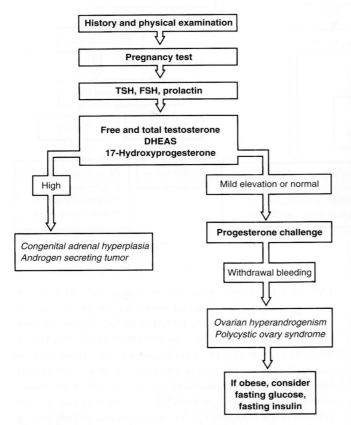

Figure 46.5 Amenorrhea with hirsutism and normal pubertal development. DHEAS, dehydroepiandrosterone sulfate FSH, follicle-stimulating hormone; TSH, thyroid-stimulating hormone. (Adapted from Pletcher JR, Slap JB. Menstrual disorders. *Pediatr Clin North Amer* 1999;46(3):514, WB Saunders Co.)

REVIEW EXERCISES

QUESTIONS

1. Evaluation for primary amenorrhea is indicated for:
a) Absence of menarche by the age of 15 years in the presence of normal pubertal growth and development
b) Absence of menarche and absence of breast development and pubic hair by the age of 13 years
c) Failure of menarche to occur within 5 years after the beginning of pubertal development
d) All of the above

Answer
The answer is d. All the listed scenarios require an evaluation for primary amenorrhea. Secondary amenorrhea is defined as the absence of menses for longer than 3 months in a female patient with established menstruation.

2. The study result most likely to be abnormal in constitutional delay of puberty is:
a) Bone age
b) TSH level
c) Erythrocyte sedimentation rate
d) Prolactin level

Answer
The answer is a. Constitutional delay of puberty is characterized by delayed menarche, short stature, negative

findings on a review of systems, and normal physical examination findings. There is often a family history of constitutional delay of puberty in parents or siblings. Laboratory studies including the complete blood cell count, erythrocyte sedimentation rate, results of thyroid function studies, and prolactin level, are all normal. The bone age is often delayed 2 to 4 years in comparison with the chronologic age. This is a diagnosis of exclusion and must be treated with reassurance.

3. The most important initial study in the evaluation of amenorrhea is:
a) LH level
b) Progesterone challenge
c) Pregnancy test
d) Prolactin level

Answer
The answer is c. A pregnancy test is the most important initial laboratory study in the evaluation of a patient with primary or secondary amenorrhea and normal pubertal development.

4. A 14-year-old presents to your office for an evaluation of primary amenorrhea. On examination, you note that she is below the fifth percentile for height and weight. She shows no signs of pubertal development. The physical examination reveals a webbed neck, widely spaced nipples, low hairline, and short fifth metacarpals. Based on your examination, you suspect a diagnosis of:
a) Congenital adrenal hyperplasia
b) Polycystic ovary syndrome
c) Turner syndrome
d) Hypothyroidism

Answer
The answer is c. Turner syndrome is characterized by a 45,XO karyotype. Manifestations include short stature, shield chest, widely spaced nipples, webbed neck, streak ovaries, hypoestrogenemia, sexual immaturity, and amenorrhea. A vagina and uterus are present but immature. Patients with Turner mosaicism (45,XO/46,XX) may show varying manifestations of Turner syndrome, depending on the amount of functioning ovarian cortical tissue present. Patients with polycystic ovary syndrome usually have secondary amenorrhea and signs of hyperandrogenism, such as acne or hirsutism. Congenital adrenal hyperplasia and hypothyroidism can present as primary amenorrhea, but these patients lack the characteristic stigmata of Turner syndrome.

5. The test that would confirm this diagnosis is:
a) LH level
b) Karyotype
c) TSH level
d) Bone age

Answer
The answer is b. The test that would confirm the diagnosis of Turner syndrome is a karyotype.

6. A 15-year-old female runner presents with a 12-month history of secondary amenorrhea. The patient states that in an effort to improve her athletic performance, she lost 20 lb by "eating more healthy." The examination reveals a very thin girl with a height at the 50th percentile. Her weight has fallen from the 25th percentile 1 year ago to <5%. The study result most likely to be abnormal is:
a) Prolactin level
b) Magnetic resonance imaging of the head
c) TSH level
d) Bone density

Answer
The answer is d. The patient described here is most likely exhibiting the female athlete triad of amenorrhea, disordered eating, and osteoporosis. The study most likely to be abnormal in this condition is the bone density. The female athlete triad is more frequently seen in girls who participate in activities such as ballet, gymnastics, and long-distance running, where lean body mass and endurance training are emphasized. The exact mechanism of the condition is unclear, but it appears to affect the hypothalamus and pituitary and result in a state of hypoestrogenism. In girls with secondary amenorrhea, a decrease in strenuous exercise, even without weight gain, can lead to a resumption of normal menses.

7. A 16-year-old female presents for evaluation of primary amenorrhea. History is unremarkable and physical exam reveals a young woman who is at the 50% for height and weight, and Tanner 5 for breasts and pubic hair. External genitalia are normal but attempts at performing a digital exam or introducing a Q-tip into the vagina are unsuccessful. The next step in evaluation of this patient would include:
a) Progesterone challenge
b) MRI of the head
c) Ultrasound of the pelvis
d) Testosterone level

Answer
The answer is c. This patient appears to have an absent vagina or a blind vaginal pouch. Vaginal or mullerian agenesis is also known as Mayer-Rokitansky-Kuster-Hauser syndrome. This condition is caused by a lack of mullerian development of unknown etiology. It is a relatively common cause of primary amenorrhea and occurs in 1 in 4000 female births. Usually there is an associated absence of the uterus and fallopian tubes, but occasionally the uterus can be normal. Ovaries are not mullerian structures and therefore ovarian function is normal. The differential diagnosis includes androgen insensitivity

syndrome, a low lying transverse vaginal septum, or an inperforate hymen. The next step in evaluation of this patient should include imaging studies such as an ultrasound or an MRI to help clarify the defect. In some cases testosterone levels and a karyotype may help to differentiate mullerian agenesis from androgen insensitivity.

8. A 17-year-old obese female presents with a long-standing history of irregular menses and a 4-month history of amenorrhea. She denies any other change in her overall health. Physical exam reveals a teenager who is at the 25% for height and well over the 100% for weight. She has evidence of hirsutism, truncal obesity, and acanthosis nigracans. A pregnancy test is negative. TSH, FSH, prolactin, DHEA-S, and 17-hydroxyprogesterone levels are all within normal limits. Free and total testosterone levels are mildly elevated. Withdrawl bleeding occurs in response to a progesterone challenge. The leading diagnosis in this patient is:
a) Congenital adrenal hyperplasia
b) Polycystic ovary syndrome
c) Autoimmune oophoritis
d) Androgen secreting tumor

Answer
The answer is b. This patient most likely suffers from polycystic ovary syndrome. This is a common disorder that accounts for a high percentage of cases of amenorrhea. The exact etiology of PCOS is unknown but there appears to be a strong genetic component. The current revised 2003 Rotterdam criteria require that two of the three following conditions be present in order to make the diagnosis of PCOS:

- Amenorrhea or oligomenrrhea
- Elevated serum androgen levels or clincal evidence of hyperandrogenism such as hirsutism or acne
- Polycystic ovaries on ultrasound

Other causes of menstrual irregularities and hyperandrogenism need to be excluded.

Based on these criteria, there is controversy whether a female without clinical or laboratory evidence of hyperandrogensim should be included in the diagnosis of PCOS.

The ovaries are responsible for the majority of the excess androgen production in PCOS, although adrenal androgens may play a small role. Markedly elevated serum androgen levels or the rapid onset of virilizing symptoms should prompt investigation to rule out an androgen secreting tumor of the ovary or the adrenal gland.

Clinically this condition is often characterized by obesity, hirsutism and acne. Adolescents with PCOS are at higher risk for Type 2 diabetes and the metabolic syndrome (insulin resistance, hyperlipidemia, and hypertension). PCOS can be treated with a combination of lifestyle modifications and medication.

9. Additional lab studies that may be indicated in this patient include:
a) Fasting glucose
b) Fasting insulin
c) Fasting lipids
d) All of the above

Answer
The answer is d. The presence of acanthosis nigricans in this patient should prompt further evaluation for insulin resistance and Type II diabetes. Acanthosis nigricans refers to a brownish gray discoloration of the skin usually involving the neck, axilla, groin, and beneath the breasts. The cause of acanthosis nigracans is not known, but it is highly correlated with insulin resistance and hyperinsulinemia in women with hyperandrogenism. This patient should also be screened for hyperlipidemia frequently seen in females with PCOS.

SUGGESTED READINGS

1. Emans SJ, Laufer M. *Pediatric and adolescent gynecology.* Philadelphia: Lippincott Williams & Wilkins, 1998.
2. Ehrmann DA. Polycystic ovary syndrome. *NEJM* 2005;352:1223–1236.
3. Mitan LA, Slap G. Adolescent menstrual disorders. *Med Clin North Amer* 2000;84:851–868.
4. Moran C, Azziz R. The role of the adrenal cortex in polycystic ovary syndrome. *Obstet Gynecol Clin North Am* 2001;28:63–75.
5. O'Brien RF, Emans SJ. Polycystic ovary syndrome in adolescents. *J Pediatr Adolesc Gynecol* 2008;21:119–128
6. Pletcher Jr, Slap GB. Menstrual disorders: amenorrhea. *Pediatr Clin North Am* 1999;46:505–518.
7. Polaneczky MM, Slap G. Menstrual disorders in the adolescent: amenorrhea. *Pediatr Rev* 1992;13:43–48.
8. Practice Committee of the American Society for Reproductive Medicine. Current evaluation of amenorrhea. *Fertil Steril* 2006;86:S148–155.
9. Prose CC, Ford CA. Evaluating amenorrhea: the pediatrician's role. *Contemp Pediatr* 1998;15:83–110.
10. Shangold M, Rebar RW, Wentz A, et al. Evaluation and management of menstrual dysfunction in athletes. *JAMA* 1990;263:1665–1669.
11. Speroff L. *Clinical gynecologic endocrinology and infertility.* Philadelphia: Lippincott Williams & Wilkins, 2005.

Chapter 47

Inherited Immunodeficiency Disorders

Alton L. Melton Jr.

Inherited immunodeficiency disorders represent defects in normal immune function that usually result in an increased susceptibility to infection. Many of the disorders have been traced to specific genetic mutations, in which the defective proteins have been identified. Although rare, these diseases have taught us much about normal and abnormal immune function.

Immunodeficiency is suspected in patients with unusual features of infections. These include an unusual frequency of infections (e.g., >10 bacterial ear infections per year), multiple sites of infection, unusual organisms causing infections, unusual severity of infections, and unusual manifestations or sites of infection (e.g., fungal osteomyelitis). In addition, many immunodeficiency disorders are coinherited with associated clinical disorders. Finally, the disruption of normal immune function can result in symptoms of autoimmune disease or malignancy because of a lack of proper immune surveillance.

The normal immune system consists of a complex network of cells, cytokines, and receptors, the purpose of which is to recognize foreign organisms or altered cells and eliminate them before they cause harm. B lymphocytes and T lymphocytes comprise the specific immune system. These cells have special receptors (immunoglobulin for B cells, T-cell receptors for T cells) that recognize specific peptide sequences on foreign proteins. This specific binding activates the cells to secrete factors that exert their own effects, and in turn activate the phagocytes and complement proteins that comprise the nonspecific immune system. The nonspecific immune system requires direction and activation by the specific immune system so that phagocytes and complement can carry out phagocytosis and cell lysis. Immune deficiencies have been described in each of the following four categories: B-cell or antibody deficiencies, T-cell or cell-mediated immunodeficiencies, phagocytic cell disorders, and complement protein deficiencies. Of these disorders of immunodeficiency, B-cell or immunoglobulin deficiencies are the most often encountered, and complement protein deficiencies are the least commonly encountered.

B-CELL OR IMMUNOGLOBULIN DEFICIENCIES

B lymphocytes produce immunoglobulins that serve as cell surface receptors and are also secreted into the systemic circulation. Secreted immunoglobulin performs several functions: neutralization (binding to an infectious agent to prevent mucosal penetration), opsonization (binding to an infectious agent to make phagocytosis more effective), complement fixation by immunoglobulin M (IgM) and IgG (activation of the complement protein cascade to cause cytolysis and enhance opsonization), and antibody-directed cell killing by phagocytes (via immunoglobulin receptors on phagocytes).

The five classes of immunoglobulin are IgG, IgM, IgA, IgD, and IgE. IgG has the highest concentration in the serum and provides protection from septicemia and deep tissue infections. IgG is the only immunoglobulin that crosses the placenta, so that newborns have relatively high levels of IgG. IgM is less efficiently produced than other immunoglobulin types, but it is the antibody produced during the primary immune response when an antigen is encountered for the first time. IgM can activate complement, as can IgG. IgM can combine into a pentameric structure, connected by the J chain. IgA is the major secretory antibody and often exists as a dimer in secretions. The dimer is connected by a J chain. Secretory IgA is protected by secretory component derived from mucosal epithelial cells, and in turn it protects the mucosal surfaces of the respiratory and gastrointestinal tracts from invading organisms. IgD is present in very small quantities, and its role in the immune response is unclear. IgE is present in the lowest concentration and is responsible for allergic diseases.

Deficiencies of immunoglobulin result in recurrent sinopulmonary infections by high-grade encapsulated bacteria, usually extracellular pathogens. Intracellular pathogens, such as viruses and fungi, cause few problems *with the exception of enteroviruses.* Striking growth retardation is usually absent, and such children generally survive to adulthood if treated appropriately.

Specific B-cell deficiencies include *X-linked agammaglobulinemia,* otherwise known as *Bruton's agammaglobulinemia.* In this *X-linked* disease, recurrent severe pyogenic infections involve the respiratory tract, skin, bloodstream, meninges, and deep tissues. The disorder usually presents at 4 to 8 months of age, after placentally acquired IgG has dissipated. Levels of all immunoglobulin types are low in this disease, and very few B cells can be identified in the bloodstream. Persons with the disease are at high risk for the development of a persistent meningoencephalitis caused by enteroviruses, including echovirus, coxsackievirus, and poliovirus. The lymphoid tissues of children with X-linked agammaglobulinemia are often sparse or absent because cortical follicles are lacking. The defect has been traced to the gene for a specific tyrosine kinase, named *btk* or *Bruton tyrosine kinase.* This disease is treated with regular intravenous (IV) administration of gamma globulin, which replaces IgG. These children should avoid daycare settings in which enterovirus transmission is common.

Common variable immunodeficiency results in a similar defect in antibody function but generally presents later in life, some even in adulthood. The usual inheritance pattern is reported to be autosomal recessive. The infections are similar to those associated with X-linked agammaglobulinemia, but the frequency and severity are more variable. The disease probably represents many different gene defects, and some element of immune dysregulation may be present in many of the patients. For this reason, the risk for the development of autoimmune diseases, such as hemolytic anemia, alopecia areata, arthritis, and pernicious anemia, is elevated. Common variable immunodeficiency is also treated with IV infusions of immunoglobulin. These must be given with caution to patients lacking IgA because cases have been reported in which IgG or IgE antibodies are directed against IgA, creating a risk for transfusion reactions or anaphylaxis during the administration of immunoglobulin containing trace amounts of IgA. Some defect in cellular immunity may also be present.

Selective IgA deficiency is the *most common inherited immunodeficiency,* affecting approximately 1 in 700 to 1000 persons. Most patients with low levels of IgA are asymptomatic. However, those with IgA levels <10 mg/dL are usually symptomatic and have recurrent infections. Chronic sinopulmonary infections caused by pyogenic bacteria may develop but are usually much less severe than those in X-linked agammaglobulinemia or common variable immunodeficiency. Systemic infections are rare in this setting. About 15% of patients with a selective absence of IgA have an associated lack of the IgG2 and IgG4 subclasses. Patients with IgA deficiency are at high risk for the development of anti-IgA antibodies, which can cause transfusion reactions. This disease is *not* amenable to replacement therapy with gamma globulin because IV immunoglobulin preparations contain only trace amounts of IgA.

IgG subclass deficiency may occur with deficiency in specific antibody production. It is known that IgG comprises four subclasses, of which IgG1 and IgG3 best respond to protein-based antigens (e.g., tetanus and diphtheria toxoid) and IgG2 and IgG4 best respond to polysaccharide-based antigens (e.g., components of the pneumococcal cell wall). Nevertheless, the overlap in function is considerable. Patients with immunodeficiency and recurrent sinopulmonary infections with low levels of IgG subclasses usually lack specific antibody titers to immunogens such as diphtheria and tetanus toxoid and pneumococcal antigens. The significance of an isolated low level of an IgG subclass without an absence of specific antibody responses is unclear. Those who do lack a response to immunogens benefit from IV immunoglobulin therapy. *Some patients with recurrent infections have impaired antibody response to immunogens, despite normal immunoglobulin levels and IgG subclasses.*

In *X-linked hyper-IgM syndrome,* normal isotype switching from a primary IgM response to a more efficient secondary IgG, IgA, or IgE response does not take place. As a result, IgM levels are elevated and levels of IgG, IgA, and IgE are low or absent. This disease has been traced to a defect in a protein on T-helper lymphocytes called *CD40 ligand.* Interaction between a CD40 molecule on the B cell and the CD40 ligand on the helper T cell signals the B cell to switch from producing IgM to producing other immunoglobulins. The deficiency leads to persistently inefficient antibody production and some cases may be caused by congenital rubella infection. Patients respond well to IV immunoglobulin therapy, showing a subsequent reduction of their elevated IgM levels. Because the defect is actually in the T lymphocyte, mild or later-onset infections with protozoa, viruses, or fungi may develop, notably sclerosing cholangitis with *Cryptosporidium.*

Transient hypogammaglobulinemia of infancy presents with low IgG concentration associated with recurrent respiratory infections often beginning in the first or second year of life. This typically resolves by age 4 to 6 years, and most have normal specific antibody responses. This likely represents a simple maturation delay.

DISORDERS OF T LYMPHOCYTES OR CELL-MEDIATED IMMUNITY

T lymphocytes perform numerous functions in the immune system. T helper cells generate factors that enhance the B cell production of immunoglobulin. T cytotoxic cells directly kill cells infected by intracellular pathogens, such as viruses or fungi. T cells also reject incompatible and grafted material and act as an immune surveillance system against malignant transformation. T lymphocytes are a major source of cytokines, which activate phagocytes and other elements of the immune system.

Cell-mediated immunodeficiency usually results in recurrent infections with intracellular pathogens that are often opportunistic in nature, such as viruses, fungi, and protozoa. Diarrhea and gastrointestinal infections are common and lead to chronic growth retardation and wasting. Because of their association with chronic infection and a lack of immune surveillance against malignancy, these diseases are not compatible with a long lifespan. In many of the disorders, a combination of defects in both T- and B-lymphocyte function causes both cell-mediated and antibody immunodeficiency. Vaccines, especially those containing live viruses, should not be administered to severely affected children. In addition, transfusion of nonirradiated blood containing donor lymphocytes carries a risk for fatal graft vs. host disease. The disorders usually present very early in life, generally within the first 3 months.

DiGeorge syndrome is caused by embryonic dysmorphogenesis of the third and fourth branchial pouches. This results in absence or hypoplasia of the thymus gland and parathyroid glands; the aortic arch and heart are also affected structurally. Patients present with:

- *Neonatal hypocalcemia* secondary to a lack of parathyroid glands
- *Congenital heart disease* (usually an aortic arch anomaly such as interrupted aortic arch, truncus arteriosis, or right-sided aortic arch)
- Early *infection, especially mucocutaneous candidiasis*

The clinical severity varies depending on the amount of thymic tissue present. Although the deficiency involves almost entirely T lymphocytes, mild B-cell functional impairment with inefficient antibody production may be present. In many patients, the disorder has been traced to a deletion on *chromosome 22*. Patients with severe DiGeorge anomalies should undergo some form of immune reconstitution, such as bone marrow, stem cell, or possibly fetal thymus transplantation. Most patients have a partial variant that often requires careful observation but usually no specific therapy.

Most other cell-mediated immune disorders involve a combination of antibody and cell-mediated immunodeficiency. The most impressive example is *severe combined immunodeficiency*. This designation actually comprises several different diseases, now characterized on the basis of their cell profiles and specific gene defects. Those with low T-cell numbers, but normal B-cell numbers (T − B + SCID) include the X-linked (most common), Janus kinase 3 deficiency, and IL7 receptor deficiency; T-B-SCID is seen with adenosine deaminase deficiency (ADA), and deficiency of recombinase activating genes RAG1 and RAG2; an isolated defect in CD8 cells is seen in ZAP 70 deficiency.

Key features of these disorders include:

- These all result in a profound lack of both cell-mediated immunity and antibody function.
- Children are susceptible to virtually all infectious agents, with early intractable diarrhea, candidiasis, cytomegalovirus infection, and *P. carinii* pneumonia. As maternal IgG wanes, severe bacterial infections can develop.
- Patients have lymphopenia, marked thymic hypoplasia, and hypogammaglobulinemia.
- Graft versus host disease and malignancy are risks.
- Most patients die within the first 2 years of life of the sequelae of infections barring strict isolation or immune reconstitution.

The X-linked form has been traced to a defect in the γ chain of the interleukin 2 receptor that is common to several cytokine receptors. *Adenosine deaminase deficiency* has been traced to a defect in the purine salvage pathway enzyme system. This was the first genetic disease to be treated with a trial of somatic gene replacement therapy, but is usually treated with ADA replacement. Patients with severe combined immunodeficiency require bone marrow transplantation for long-term survival. Patients with adenosine deaminase deficiency can also be treated with adenosine deaminase replacement therapy.

Wiskott-Aldrich syndrome is an *X-linked disease* characterized by a partial but significant deficiency in both the antibody and cell-mediated immune compartments. It produces a predictable triad of:

- Eczema
- Severe thrombocytopenic purpura
- Recurrent infections of all types

Splenectomy is often necessary to manage the thrombocytopenia. Patients are at high risk for *lymphoreticular malignancies*. They respond poorly to polysaccharide antigens and appear to be susceptible to infections such as varicella. An absence of blood group antibodies (isohemagglutinins) is a classic feature of this disease.

Ataxia-telangiectasia is an *autosomal-recessive* disorder of chromosomal repair. Mutations in immunoglobulin and T-cell receptor genes are not repaired, and progressive loss of immune function results. The clinical manifestations include:

- Progressive cerebellar ataxia
- Oculocutaneous telangiectasia
- Recurrent infections

These usually begin as recurrent sinopulmonary infections; a progressive development of infections of all types follows. The disorder is associated with a *very high incidence of lymphoreticular malignancy* in the second and third decades of life. *Deficient IgA and IgE levels* are often seen initially, with progressive loss of other immunoglobulin types and cell-mediated immune responses.

The *hyper-IgE syndrome* produces a clinical picture of:

- Recurrent skin abscesses
- Dental abnormalities
- Sinopulmonary infections, often with staphylococci
- Chronic dermatitis and coarse facies

The IgE level is usually markedly elevated; poor specific antibody responses and a partial T-lymphocyte deficiency are other possible features, but are less consistently seen. The gene defect for this disorder has not yet been found.

At present, no specific treatment is available for diseases such as Wiskott-Aldrich syndrome, ataxia-telangiectasia, and hyper-IgE syndrome other than possible bone marrow or stem cell transplantation. Because the deficiencies are only partial, pretransplant chemotherapy is necessary and often risky.

PHAGOCYTE DISORDERS

Phagocytes, like neutrophils, macrophages, monocytes, and tissue-specific macrophage-like cells, perform many immune functions at the direction of the specific immune system. Phagocytes exhibit chemotaxis (directed migration toward areas of inflammation), adherence to blood vessel walls, extravasation into inflamed tissue, enzymatic digestion, and oxidative degradation of bacteria. In patients with defects of phagocyte function, neutrophil counts are often greatly elevated or greatly depressed, depending on the specific disorder. These diseases tend to be associated with recurrent infections of the respiratory tract, skin, and deep tissues. Abscesses can form in any of these sites. Infections are usually caused by staphylococci, but the organisms may vary depending on the disease. Recurrent oral ulcerations and perirectal abscesses are common.

Chronic granulomatous disease is the best-known entity in this category. *X-linked* and *autosomal-recessive forms* have been described that result from genetic defects in the cytochrome P-450 system or in cytosolic accessory proteins of the NADPH (reduced nicotinamide adenine dinucleotide phosphate) oxidase system. The defects impair the oxidative metabolism required for superoxide and peroxide generation. The result is an inability to kill engulfed cells that produce catalase, such as *Staphylococcus aureus* and many other seemingly unrelated bacteria and fungi. *Recurrent skin and deep tissue abscesses, occasional osteomyelitis caused by unusual organisms, pneumonias (often associated with pneumatoceles and air-fluid levels), and septicemia are common.*

Almost all patients exhibit significant adenopathy and hepatosplenomegaly with generalized granuloma formation in these organs. The levels of white blood cells are usually elevated in the bloodstream and at sites of infection. The most frequently used diagnostic tool is the *nitroblue tetrazolium dye reduction test (NBT)*. Other measures of oxidative burst, such as superoxide generation, can substitute for the nitroblue tetrazolium dye reduction test. Antibiotic prophylaxis with trimethoprim/sulfamethazole can reduce frequency of infections, but the treatment of choice is recombinant interferon gamma, which improves immune function and prevents early death.

The *Chédiak-Higashi syndrome* is characterized by defective granulocyte function and recurrent infections, mainly with staphylococci. It is associated with partial oculocutaneous albinism. Usually large granules are evident in the cytoplasm of neutrophils on the blood smear. Chédiak-Higashi syndrome occasionally manifests a life-threatening proliferative phase.

Leukocyte adhesion deficiency (LAD1) is associated with recurrent infections, especially with staphylococci. However, pus rarely forms at the sites of infection because the leukocytes are unable to adhere to blood vessel walls or migrate to areas of inflammation as a consequence of lacking a specific adhesion molecule of neutrophils (CD18b or LFA-1). An interesting associated clinical finding is a *history of delayed separation of the umbilical cord*. An LAD2 has been described, that results from defective production of Sialyl-Lewis-X, preventing initial attachment to endothelial cells through binding to E-selectin adhesion molecules.

COMPLEMENT DEFICIENCY DISORDERS

The complement system comprises a series of serum proteins with numerous effects in the immune system. It exists as a cascade of proteins involving various amplification and regulatory steps. It can be divided into three components:

- The classical pathway, including C1, C2, C4, and C3
- The alternative pathway factors B, D, P, and C3
- The membrane attack complex, with components C5, C6, C7, C8, and C9

The classical pathway is activated by immune complexes and is likely involved in their processing and disposal before they cause tissue injury. The alternative pathway is activated by bacterial components and probably assists in bacterial killing. The membrane attack complex can be activated through either the classical or alternative pathway and results in cytolysis. In addition, functions of opsonization from component C3b and chemotaxis from component C5a enhance phagocytic cell activity. Other components (C3a, C4a, and C5a) can cause mast cell degranulation with vascular leakage.

Defects in the classical pathway components—namely, C1, C2, and C4—tend to cause immune complex–like diseases associated with autoimmune or lupus-like symptoms and an increased risk for sinopulmonary infections. Defects in the alternative pathway and C3 cause recurrent pyogenic infections, including septicemias similar to those seen in the immunoglobulin deficiencies. *Deficiencies of the membrane attack complex proteins, especially C5, C6, C7, and C8, are associated with recurrent and severe* Neisseria gonorrhoeae *and* Neisseria meningitidis *infections.* Of all the complement defects, C2 deficiency is the most common. Regulatory proteins are involved in complement function, and deficiency of the C1 inhibitor causes hereditary angioedema. Deficiency of the decay accelerating factor causes paroxysmal nocturnal hemoglobinuria. No specific treatments are directed at the complement deficiency disorders in general.

DIAGNOSIS AND TREATMENT OF INHERITED IMMUNODEFICIENCIES

To diagnose an immunodeficiency, a careful history, family history, physical examination, as well as a knowledge of the quantitative and qualitative functions of each of the component parts is required. In cases of immunoglobulin deficiency, quantitative measurements of immunoglobulins, IgG subclasses, and antibody titers against immunogens such as diphtheria and tetanus toxoid and pneumococci, both before and after immunization, provide valuable information. In cases of defects of cell-mediated immunity, delayed hypersensitivity skin testing can be performed in patients >24 months of age. Other helpful tests include a determination of T-cell numbers and subsets and an assessment of the response to T-cell mitogens and antigens. An absolute neutrophil count can be obtained in assessment of phagocyte defects. In most but not all cases, the neutrophil count is either elevated or greatly depressed. Specific tests for neutrophil chemotaxis and superoxide generation, the nitroblue tetrazolium dye reduction test, and measurements of leukocyte adhesion molecules by flow cytometry can help to pinpoint specific diseases. In complement disorders, the total serum hemolytic complement (CH_{50}) test can detect disorders of proteins in the cascade from C1 through C9. Alternative pathway complement assays are available from specialized laboratories. Assays for C3 and C4 are readily available in most laboratories, and tests for other specific components are available in specialized laboratories.

In the treatment of an immunodeficiency, a common sense approach is used to identify the site and cause of infection. Efforts to determine the responsible organism and site of infection must be much more aggressive than in immunologically normal children. Surgical intervention for drainage of infections, biopsy, or culture is often necessary. Appropriate and aggressive antibiotic therapy is essential, and broader-spectrum coverage should be considered until identification of the infecting organism is made. In severe combined immunodeficiency and T-cell defects, prophy-

laxis for *Pneumocystis* infection is required. In partial B-cell defects and phagocyte defects, prophylactic antibiotics may be of value. Avoidance of live virus vaccines in patients with cell-mediated immunodeficiencies is important. Patients with Bruton's agamma-globulinemia should avoid potential enterovirus infections. Close monitoring for signs of associated diseases, such as autoimmune disease and malignancies, is essential. Blood products given to patients with T-cell and combined immunodeficiencies must be irradiated and free of cytomegalovirus to reduce the risk for transmission of infection and potentially fatal graft versus host disease. Continuous blood product administration is required for igA deficient and CVID patients, due to risk of anti-IgA reactions. Many disorders can be corrected only by reconstituting normal immune function with bone marrow or stem cell transplantation. Finally, it should be kept in mind that most recurrent symptoms of viral upper respiratory tract infection more likely represent common allergic disease or frequent exposure, as in day care, and not necessarily immune deficiency.

REVIEW EXERCISES

QUESTIONS

1. A 1-year-old boy presents with recurrent otitis media, pneumonia, and sinusitis. The physical examination reveals bilateral otitis media, but no cervical nodes are palpable and the tonsils are not visible. This picture is most compatible with a diagnosis of:
a) Selective IgA deficiency
b) Chronic granulomatous disease
c) DiGeorge syndrome
d) X-linked agammaglobulinemia
e) C2 complement deficiency

Answer

The answer is d. In X-linked agammaglobulinemia, all immunoglobulin types are absent. The disease presents during the second 6 months of life with recurrent sinopulmonary infections and septicemia. Because no B lymphocytes are produced, lymph node follicles do not develop, and affected children have few palpable nodes and little tonsillar tissue despite recurrent infections. Selective IgA deficiency is milder and may be asymptomatic. Normal lymphoid follicles are present. C2 deficiency is associated with lupus-like disorders and recurrent infections. DiGeorge syndrome affects cell-mediated immunity and usually presents at or soon after birth. Opportunistic infections with diarrhea, wasting, and growth failure may be present. Endocrine and cardiac anomalies are also inherited. Chronic granulomatous disease is a phagocyte disorder characterized by frequent abscesses, pneumonia, and lymph node infection. The lymph nodes are usually greatly enlarged.

2. The triad of eczema, thrombocytopenia, and recurrent infections is characteristic of:
a) Chédiak-Higashi syndrome
b) Wiskott-Aldrich syndrome
c) Common variable hypogammaglobulinemia
d) Hyper-IgE syndrome
e) Adenosine deaminase deficiency

Answer

The answer is **b.** Wiskott-Aldrich syndrome is a combined immunodeficiency with X-linked inheritance. The clinical presentation includes eczema, thrombocytopenia, and recurrent infections. In Chédiak-Higashi syndrome, granulocyte abnormalities result in recurrent infections. Partial oculocutaneous albinism may be present. Patients with common variable hypogammaglobulinemia usually have recurrent bacterial infections and sometimes autoimmune disease. Patients with hyper-IgE syndrome have coarse facial features, dental abnormalities, recurrent abscesses, and pneumonias. Adenosine deaminase deficiency is a form of severe combined immunodeficiency associated with some bony abnormalities and recurrent infections.

3. A 2-year-old boy presents with a history of protracted lymphadenitis, cavitary pneumonia, and organomegaly. The single best test to diagnose his immunodeficiency is:
a) CH_{50}
b) Quantitative immunoglobulin measurement
c) Isohemagglutinin titers
d) Delayed hypersensitivity skin testing
e) Nitroblue tetrazolium dye reduction test

Answer

The answer is **e.** The clinical picture of lymphadenitis, organomegaly, and cavitary pneumonia (presumably with *S. aureus*) is characteristic of a phagocyte disorder, such as chronic granulomatous disease. The nitroblue tetrazolium test screens for oxidative capacity, which is lacking in chronic granulomatous disease. The CH_{50} screens for complement deficiencies. Isohemagglutinins are antibodies that are often decreased in Wiskott-Aldrich syndrome. Delayed hypersensitivity testing screens for cell-mediated immunodeficiency. Quantitative measurements of immunoglobulins are decreased in antibody deficiencies.

4. Infusions of interferon γ are especially helpful for patients with:
a) Hyper-IgM syndrome
b) Ataxia-telangiectasia
c) Chronic granulomatous disease
d) Severe combined immunodeficiency
e) Leukocyte adherence deficiency

Answer

The answer is **c.** Interferon γ has become the treatment of choice for chronic granulomatous disease; it improves

granulocyte function. Hyper-IgM syndrome is treated with IV immunoglobulin. Severe combined immunodeficiency requires immune reconstitution, as does ataxia-telangiectasia. Leukocyte adherence deficiency may require immune reconstitution or prophylactic antibiotic therapy.

5. The best screening test for immunodeficiency in a patient after her second episode of meningococcal meningitis is:
a) Quantitative immunoglobulin measurement
b) CH_{50}
c) Determination of T-cell subsets
d) Determination of IgG subclasses
e) Nitroblue tetrazolium dye reduction test

Answer

The answer is **b.** Recurrent *Neisseria* infections are characteristic of a deficiency of C5 through C9, detected by the CH_{50}. Quantitative immunoglobulins screen for antibody deficiency, as do IgG subclasses to an extent. T-cell subsets are used in evaluating cell-mediated immunity, and the nitroblue tetrazolium dye reduction test screens for chronic granulomatous disease.

6. Your patient requires a blood transfusion. In which condition must the blood be irradiated?
a) Chronic granulomatous disease
b) DiGeorge syndrome
c) X-linked agammaglobulinemia
d) Selective IgA deficiency
e) C3 deficiency

Answer

The answer is **b.** Patients with defects in cell-mediated immunity, such as severe combined immunodeficiency and DiGeorge syndrome, are at risk for graft versus host disease when they receive nonirradiated blood products containing immunoreactive T cells from unmatched donors. Defects of immunoglobulin function, phagocyte function, or complement components are not associated with such a risk. Patients with selective IgA deficiency may have anti-IgA antibodies, which can cause transfusion reactions. Irradiation of the blood does not prevent such a reaction.

SUGGESTED READINGS

1. Bonilla F, Bernstein IL, Khan DA, et al. Practice parameter for the diagnosis and management of primary immunodeficiency. *Ann Allergy Asthma Immunol* 2005;94:S1–63.
2. Bonilla FA, Geha RS. Primary immunodeficiency disease. *J Allergy Clin Immunol* 2003;111:S571–581.
3. Buckley RH. Primary immunodeficiency diseases due to defects in lymphocytes. *NEJM* 2000;343:1313.
4. Fischer A. Human primary immunodeficiency diseases: a perspective. *Nat Immunol* 2004;5:23–30.

Chapter 48

Infectious Diseases, Part I

Camille Sabella and Johanna Goldfarb

This chapter addresses the following pediatric infections:

- Gastrointestinal infections
- Skin, soft-tissue, bone, and joint infections
- Central nervous system (CNS) infections
- Pneumonia

GASTROINTESTINAL INFECTIONS

Bacterial, viral, and parasitic agents cause gastrointestinal infections in infants and children that range from mild and self-limited conditions to severe and life-threatening. Differentiating among the many pathogens that cause infectious gastroenteritis relies on an understanding of the epidemiology and clinical manifestations of the disease caused by each of them. This chapter focuses on the epidemiologic and clinical features of the most common infections, in addition to therapeutic considerations.

Bacterial Infections

Salmonella Infection

Nontyphoidal *Salmonella* infections are most commonly acquired by ingesting contaminated foods, milk, or water (Table 48.1). Poultry, pork products, eggs, and dairy products are the foods most likely to be contaminated. Infected reptiles, including pet turtles and iguanas, are increasingly being recognized as important sources of infection for infants and children. Although person-to-person transmission occurs with household exposure, *transmission and outbreaks in child care centers are uncommon.* The incubation period for nontyphoidal *Salmonella* infection is 6 hours to 4 days, and the incidence of infection is the highest among children <5 years.

Humans are the only known reservoir of *Salmonella typhi*, which is the cause of enteric or typhoid fever. Infection is acquired by ingesting foods or water contaminated by human feces. Most cases of enteric fever in the United States are related to travel to foreign areas in which *S. typhi* infection is endemic.

Clinical presentations of *Salmonella* infections include:

- Acute asymptomatic infection
- Acute gastroenteritis/enterocolitis
- Bacteremia with or without focal infection
- Enteric fever
- Asymptomatic chronic carrier state

Because of the large number of organisms (10^5–10^6) required to cause symptomatic disease, asymptomatic infection is likely more common than symptomatic disease. Acute gastroenteritis usually manifests with nausea, vomiting, cramping abdominal pain, nonbloody diarrhea, and fever. Bloody diarrhea can occur if an invasive serotype is responsible for the infection. Symptoms resolve within 2 to 7 days in most cases. Bacteremia is most common in infants <1 month and may be present in a patient without gastrointestinal symptoms. Focal complications such as osteomyelitis and meningitis occur in approximately 10% of bacteremic children. *Salmonella* osteomyelitis is most common in children with hemoglobinopathies, whereas meningitis occurs almost exclusively in neonates.

Enteric fever is caused by *S. typhi* or *S. paratyphi*. Manifestations include nonspecific symptoms, high fever, abdominal pain, hepatosplenomegaly, altered mentation, lymphadenopathy, relative bradycardia, and erythematous rash on the anterior chest wall (rose spots). Laboratory features include anemia, leukopenia, and elevated transaminase levels.

Asymptomatic chronic carriage is not uncommon following *Salmonella* gastrointestinal infection, and antimicrobial therapy can prolong the time during which the organism is excreted.

TABLE 48.1

CHARACTERISTICS OF NONTYPHOIDAL *SALMONELLA* VERSUS *SHIGELLA* INFECTIONS

	Salmonella	Shigella
Peak age	<12 months	1–4 years
Major mode of transmission	Food-borne Reptiles	Person to person
Inoculum size needed to cause disease	10^5–10^6 May be lower in infants and children	10–100
Importance in CCC outbreaks	Not as important Need to exclude from CCC until asymptomatic	Important Need to exclude from CCC until negative stool culture
Carrier state	Yes	No
Site of infection; invasiveness	Small intestine; rarely invasive	Colon; may be invasive
Stool characteristics	Watery stools Stools rarely bloody	Stools frequently bloody Mucous stools
Extraintestinal manifestations	Bacteremia Osteomyelitis (children with hemoglobinopathies) Meningitis (neonates)	Seizures Reactive arthritis Reiter syndrome
Antimicrobial therapy	Recommended for certain groups (see Table 48.2)	Recommended (see text)

CCC, child care center.

Antimicrobial therapy is *not* recommended for otherwise healthy children with gastroenteritis (Table 48.2). Patients with gastroenteritis who are at high risk and should be treated with antimicrobial therapy include infants <3 months, immunocompromised patients, children with hemoglobinopathies, and those with gastrointestinal dysfunction. Patients with bacteremia, osteomyelitis, meningitis, or enteric fever should also be treated with antimicrobial agents. The choice of antimicrobial therapy should be based on the susceptibility patterns and severity of infection. Cefotaxime or ceftriaxone is appropriate initial therapy for invasive infections or severe gastroenteritis in a high-risk patient. Ampicillin or trimethoprim/sulfamethoxazole can be utilized for susceptible strains.

Prevention

Since nontyphoidal *Salmonella* infections are not commonly transmitted in childcare centers, children with *Salmonella* infection who attend such centers can be read-

TABLE 48.2

SALMONELLA INFECTIONS THAT WARRANT ANTIMICROBIAL THERAPY

Gastroenteritis in patients at high risk for bacteremia/suppurative infections
  Infants <3 months old
  Immunocompromised individuals
  Children with hemoglobinopathies
  Children with gastrointestinal dysfunction
Bacteremia
Meningitis
Osteomyelitis or other suppurative infection
Enteric fever (infection with *S. typhi* or *S. paratyphi*)

mitted when they are asymptomatic. Stool cultures negative for *Salmonella* are not required for re-entry to a child care center, and contacts need not be tested unless they are symptomatic.

For child care attendees or staff who develop *S typhi* infections, contacts should be cultured and excluded if infected, until they have three negative stool samples (for children <5 years of age), or until they are asymptomatic (for those 5 years of age or older).

Shigella Infection

Because humans are the principal hosts, person-to-person transmission by fecal–oral spread accounts for most cases of shigellosis (Table 48.1). A small inoculum of organisms (10^2) can cause symptomatic disease and the incubation period is from 12 to 48 hours. Although *Shigella* infections are uncommon in the first year of life, they are important causes of outbreaks of infection in child care centers. Chronic carrier states are thought to be very rare among healthy children. *Shigella sonnei* is the most common serotype causing infection in the United States.

The clinical presentation of *Shigella* gastroenteritis varies from mild or no symptoms to severe symptoms. Infections with *S. sonnei* usually result in watery diarrhea. Infection with other species of *Shigella* may reflect the major virulent factor of these organisms, which is invasiveness. The classic picture of invasive *Shigella* gastroenteritis includes an abrupt onset of high fever, cramping abdominal pain, and early watery diarrhea that is followed by the development of mucous diarrhea with or without blood, associated with urgency and tenesmus. Approximately 50% of patients with invasive infection have bloody diarrhea, and symptoms may continue for a week or longer if specific antimicrobial therapy is not administered.

Extraintestinal manifestations of *Shigella* infections include:

■ Seizures
■ Hemolytic uremic syndrome
■ Septicemia
■ Reactive arthritis/Reiter syndrome
■ Toxic encephalopathy (ekiri syndrome)

Seizures are the most common extraintestinal manifestation, occurring in 10% to 45% of hospitalized children with shigellosis. They are generalized, brief, and benign, often appearing before the onset of diarrhea. Bacteremia and sepsis are rare complications of infection and usually occur in neonates and immunocompromised or malnourished patients.

Antimicrobial therapy for *Shigella* results in symptomatic improvement and prompt eradication of the organism from feces. Treatment is recommended for patients with severe symptoms, dysentery, and underlying conditions. Although most infections caused by *S. sonnei* are self-limited and may not require antimicrobial therapy, treatment is often given to prevent the spread of the organism. Since a significant percentage of *Shigella* strains in the United States are now resistant to ampicillin and trimethoprim/sulfamethoxazole, antimicrobial susceptibility testing of isolates is recommended. Third-generation cephalosporins, such as cefotaxime and ceftriaxone, and azithromycin, are effective alternatives.

Children who become infected with *Shigella* while attending child care centers should be treated with an appropriate antimicrobial agent and excluded from the center until they are asymptomatic and stool cultures test negative for *Shigella*. Stool specimens should be obtained from all symptomatic contacts and cultured; if the cultures are positive for *Shigella*, the children should be excluded from the center until they are asymptomatic and stool cultures are negative for the organisms.

Diarrheal Illness Caused by Escherichia coli

Several diarrhea-producing strains of *E. coli* have been identified. Three of the most important are described briefly.

Enterotoxigenic Escherichia coli

Transmission is most often from contaminated water and food, including dairy, meat, and seafood products. These organisms account for a significant percentage of cases of diarrhea in the developing world and are *the most common cause of traveler's diarrhea.* Enterotoxin-mediated disease is manifested as watery diarrhea and abdominal cramps. Antimicrobial therapy is usually not indicated.

Shiga Toxin–Producing Escherichia coli (formerly known as enterohemorrhagic Escherichia coli)

Transmission is from contaminated foods and by person-to-person contact. Undercooked and contaminated ground beef and unpasteurized milk have served as important transmission vehicles, although a wide variety of foods (salami, raw vegetables), water, petting zoos, and person-to-person transmission have been implicated in outbreaks. A small inoculum of organisms can cause significant illness, which tends to occur during the summer and is most likely to affect children between the ages of 2 and 10 years. The prototype organism is *E. coli* O157:H7, which can be identified in the laboratory by its inability to ferment sorbitol. This organism elaborates a shiga-like toxin, which causes invasive gastroenteritis characterized by bloody diarrhea. *The major complication of infection is hemolytic uremic syndrome, which occurs in 5% to 10% of individuals infected with* E. coli *O157:H7; most cases of hemolytic uremic syndrome in the United States are caused by this organism.* Antimicrobial therapy for these infections is generally *not* indicated because they have not been shown to be effective and *may* increase the incidence of hemolytic uremic syndrome. Children infected with this organism should be excluded from child care centers until they are asymptomatic and two consecutive stool cultures are negative for the organisms.

Enteropathogenic Escherichia coli

These organisms have been associated with outbreaks of infection in nurseries for newborns and child care centers. They cause either epidemic or sporadic disease, mainly in neonates and children <2 years of age, which is characterized by severe, dehydrating watery diarrhea.

Campylobacter Infection

Campylobacter jejuni organisms account for most cases of *Campylobacter* infection. Along with *Salmonella* species, they are the major cause of food-borne illness in the United States. Transmission is mainly from ingested untreated water and contaminated foods, including poultry, meats, and unpasteurized milk. Domestic and wild young animals, including chicken, turkeys, and many farm animals, serve as reservoirs of infection. Person-to-person spread is a much less frequent mode of transmission, and transmission in child care settings is uncommon. The incidence of infection is the highest in children <5 years, and the incubation period usually is from 1 to 7 days.

C. jejuni causes enteritis that mainly involves the terminal ileum and colon. Symptoms range widely, from mild diarrhea to severe inflammatory diarrhea. Fever, abdominal pain, vomiting, generalized malaise, headache, and dehydration are not uncommon. In most cases, the course is self-limited, but the illness can be protracted and severe. Without treatment, fecal shedding occurs for 2 to 3 weeks in most cases. Asymptomatic chronic carriage of the organism is uncommon. Bacteremia and sepsis are very rare complications of *C. jejuni* infection. *Campylobacter fetus* has been associated with neonatal bacteremia and meningitis.

Immunoreactive complications can occur following C. jejuni *infection; these include Guillain-Barré syndrome, reactive arthritis, and Reiter syndrome.*

When given early during an infection, appropriate antimicrobial therapy shortens the duration of illness and eradicates the organism within 2 to 3 days. The need for antimicrobial therapy in most cases of gastroenteritis is controversial. Treatment should be considered for patients with severe gastrointestinal or systemic symptoms and for those who are immunocompromised. Erythromycin or azithromycin can be used to treat *Campylobacter* infection.

Children with *Campylobacter* gastroenteritis should be excluded from child care settings until they are asymptomatic. It is not necessary to culture stool specimens from asymptomatic contacts.

Yersinia Infection

Yersinia enterocolitica and *Yersinia pseudotuberculosis* can cause food-borne illness in children and adolescents. Domestic and wild animals serve as major reservoirs, and transmission occurs most commonly when uncooked pork products, unpasteurized milk, and untreated water are ingested; raw pork intestines (chitterlings) are implicated occasionally. Children aged 5 to 15 years are at the highest risk for infection, which tends to occur in cooler climates and during the winter months.

Yersinia organisms can cause acute diarrheal illness in children and adolescents, manifested with fever, diarrhea (which may be bloody), colicky abdominal pain, and vomiting. *Occasionally, an intense suppurative mesenteric adenitis develops that causes acute abdominal pain and tenderness in the right lower abdominal quadrant, mimicking acute appendicitis.* This condition is most common in older children and adolescents. Individuals with *iron overload states*, including those being treated with deferoxamine, are more susceptible to severe infection and complications such as sepsis and cardiac involvement. Reactive arthritis, Reiter syndrome, and erythema nodosum have been described as complications of *Yersinia* infection.

Patients who are at risk for severe disease and those with severe infection should be treated with antibiotics. Aminoglycosides, cefotaxime, and trimethoprim/sulfamethoxazole are active against these organisms.

Clostridium difficile Infection

C. difficile, through the actions of its elaborated toxins A and B, can cause colitis in patients who are receiving or have recently received antimicrobial therapy for other infections. It is the most common organism that causes antibiotic-related diarrhea. Nosocomial transmission has been documented. Any antibiotic can be implicated, but cephalosporins and clindamycin are most often associated with antibiotic-related diarrhea.

Gastrointestinal symptoms may be mild or severe. Bloody or nonbloody diarrhea with fever, nausea, vomiting, abdominal pain, and leukocytosis are common manifestations.

The presence of pseudomembranes or plaques in the colon is diagnostic. The organism or its toxins can be demonstrated in the stool and are helpful in making the diagnosis. *Many neonates, infants, and young children normally harbor the organism and its toxins in the gastrointestinal tract. Therefore, testing for these toxins in infants is not recommended, as a positive result may not explain the etiology of the symptoms.*

The treatment of infection should include discontinuing antimicrobial agents when it is safe to do so and administering antimicrobial therapy with specific action against the organism. Metronidazole (given orally or intravenously) and vancomycin (only when administered orally) are equally effective in eradicating the infection. Vancomycin should not be given as the first-line agent because its use is associated with the development of resistant organisms in the gastrointestinal tract. Infection can recur in up to 40% of cases, but usually responds to a repeated course of the same treatment.

Washing with water and soap appears to be a more effective method of eliminating spores from contaminated hands than with alcohol-containing products, and is the recommended method of hand hygiene for this organism.

Viral Gastroenteritis

Viral agents are responsible for most cases of acute gastroenteritis in infants and children. When compared with bacterial causes of gastroenteritis, viral causes are more likely to be associated with vomiting, a shorter duration of illness, an absence of fecal blood and leukocytes, and seasonal epidemics. The most common viral agents, with an emphasis on epidemiology, are discussed briefly.

Rotavirus Infection

Rotavirus infections are the most common cause of acute gastroenteritis in infants and young children, accounting for 15% to 35% of cases. Rotaviruses show a striking tendency to cause illness during the winter in temperate climates. The highest incidence of infection is in infants aged 6 to 36 months. Almost all the children are infected by their third birthday. Asymptomatic infection, especially in older children and adults, is common. Person-to-person spread is the most frequent mode of transmission, and rotaviruses are an important cause of nosocomial gastroenteritis and gastroenteritis in children attending child care centers. Fomites may also serve as a mechanism of transmission.

The incubation period is 2 to 4 days, and the clinical features include vomiting, diarrhea, and fever. Dehydration and electrolyte imbalance may develop. Bloody stools or fecal leukocytes are noted in 10% to 15% of infants. Infection can be severe and life threatening in immunocompromised and malnourished patients.

Enzyme immunoassays and latex agglutination assays are utilized to detect rotavirus antigens in the stool.

Infection with Caliciviruses (including Noroviruses [formerly Norwalk-like viruses])
Caliciviruses are transmitted by person-to-person spread and the ingestion of contaminated food and water. Shellfish and water sources have been identified in outbreaks. Outbreaks in closed populations, such as child care centers and cruise ships, have recently been documented. Sporadic and epidemic infection with these agents has been documented in all age groups.

The incubation period is 12 to 72 hours, and a brief illness manifested by vomiting, diarrhea, fever, headache, and abdominal cramps is usual.

Astrovirus Infection
Astroviruses are transmitted from person to person. The incidence of infection appears to be the highest in children <4 years, and infection tends to occur during the winter. Self-limited acute gastrointestinal symptoms are common.

Enteric Adenovirus Infection
Adenovirus serotypes 40 and 41 are associated with acute gastroenteritis in infants and children and are spread by the fecal–oral route. The median age of affected children is 12 to 24 months; no seasonal predilection has been noted. Although self-limited vomiting and diarrhea are the most common manifestations, dehydration requiring hospitalization is not infrequent; these agents are probably second only to rotaviruses in causing diarrheal illness requiring hospitalization.

Gastroenteritis Caused by Parasites

Giardia lamblia Infection
G. lamblia infection is the most common protozoal illness in the United States. The organisms infect the proximal small intestine and biliary tract and exist in trophozoite and cyst forms. The cyst form is most commonly isolated from stools and is the infective form.

The organism is acquired through the fecal–oral route, either by person-to-person transmission or by the ingestion of contaminated water or food. Outbreaks caused by contaminated water supplies and outbreaks in child care centers have been documented. Asymptomatic infection is common, and as many as 20% of children attending day care centers may harbor the organism without signs of infection.

The clinical spectrum of symptomatic giardiasis is broad; acute gastrointestinal symptoms with diarrhea and abdominal pain may occur, and a subacute or chronic illness manifested with chronic abdominal pain, weight loss or failure to thrive, malabsorption, and abdominal distension has also been well described. Peripheral eosinophilia is rare. Children with immunodeficiencies are more susceptible to infection and have a higher rate of chronic diarrhea and recurrent infection. *Children with hypogammaglobulinemia and those infected with human immunodeficiency virus (HIV) are most susceptible,* although children with immunoglobulin A- or T-cell deficiency and cystic fibrosis may also be at increased risk for chronic and recurrent infection.

The diagnosis can be made by demonstrating the presence of trophozoites or cysts in the stool with direct microscopic examination or by a commercially available immunofluorescent assay or enzyme immunoassay. The sensitivity of direct smear examination of three stool specimens is approximately 95%, whereas the sensitivity of immunofluorescent assay or enzyme immunoassay of one stool specimen is 70% to 80%. A commercially available string test of duodenal aspirates is more sensitive than tests of stool specimens, and a duodenal biopsy is occasionally required to make the diagnosis.

Metronidazole is the drug of choice for the treatment of giardiasis. Nitazoxanide, tinidazole, furazolidone, and albendazole are also effective therapies for giardiasis. Infection recurs in 10% to 20% of patients; most respond to a second course. Immunocompromised patients may require repeated or prolonged courses of treatment. Treatment of asymptomatic individuals is not recommended.

Children attending day care centers in whom G. *lamblia* infection is diagnosed must be excluded until they are asymptomatic. *Excluding carriers and culturing specimens from asymptomatic individuals are not recommended.*

Cryptosporidium Infection
Cryptosporidium species are protozoa that cause diarrheal illness in normal and immunocompromised hosts. The proximal small intestine is most commonly affected, but the entire bowel may be involved in patients infected with HIV. Transmission of the organism is by person-to-person spread, ingestion of contaminated water, or close contact with farm livestock. Large-scale community outbreaks have been caused by contaminated water supplies and swimming pools, as have smaller outbreaks in child care centers. Groups at high risk include children attending day care centers, farmers and animal handlers, travelers to foreign countries, and individuals with T-cell immunodeficiencies. Children aged 6 to 24 months appear to be at highest risk for infection.

Cryptosporidiosis in healthy children can result in asymptomatic infection or a self-limited, nonbloody, watery diarrhea associated with vomiting, abdominal pain, and fever. In immunodeficient individuals, including those infected with HIV, unremitting and profuse diarrhea may develop and cause malabsorption, weight loss, and malnutrition, in addition to disseminated infection and cholangitis.

Oocytes can be visualized in stool by means of a modified acid-fast stain after obtaining appropriate concentration of the stool sample. Commercially available antigen detection assays can also be used to identify oocytes.

Nitazoxanide oral suspension has been licensed for the treatment of diarrhea caused by cryptosporidiosis in children 12 months of age and older.

Amebiasis

Entamoeba histolytica frequently causes intestinal infection in the developing world. Amebiasis is the third most common parasitic infection causing death, after malaria and schistosomiasis. The organism is ingested during its cystic stage, and the trophozoite causes invasive disease in the colon.

The cysts are most frequently transmitted through the fecal–oral route. The organism is more frequently found in developing countries and areas with poor sanitation, where as many as 50% of the population may be infected. Asymptomatic carriers of cysts are common.

Asymptomatic infection is most common; approximately 10% of the world's population is infected. Invasive infection can result in amebic dysentery or extraintestinal amebiasis.

Amebic dysentery presents as severe, bloody, inflammatory diarrhea that is associated with severe abdominal pain and fever and less frequently with abdominal distension and dehydration. Intussusception, perforation, and strictures are known complications. *Liver abscess* is the most common extraintestinal manifestation of amebiasis, occurring in 1% to 7% of children with invasive disease, in whom it causes high fever, abdominal distension, irritability, tachypnea, and hepatomegaly. Right upper quadrant pain is less common in children than in adults. Rupture of an abscess into the abdomen or chest is associated with a high mortality rate.

The identification of amebic cysts or trophozoites in stool samples is diagnostic, but it may be necessary to obtain several stool samples. Serologic assays may be useful in patients with liver involvement. Radiographic studies such as ultrasonography or computed tomography scan may be helpful in identifying liver abscess.

The treatment of amebiasis depends on the extent of involvement. Asymptomatic individuals who excrete the organism should be treated with an intraluminal agent, such as iodoquinol or paromomycin, or diloxanide. Patients with diarrheal illness, dysentery, or extraintestinal disease should be treated with metronidazole followed by an intraluminal agent.

SKIN, SOFT TISSUE, BONE, AND JOINT INFECTIONS

Skin and Soft Tissue Infections

The most common infections of the skin and soft tissues in infants and children, along with their microbial etiologic agents, are listed in Table 48.3.

Group A β-hemolytic streptococci and *Staphylococcus aureus* are responsible for most skin infections and are associated with significant systemic manifestations and serious sequelae.

Complications of group A β-hemolytic streptococci skin infection include necrotizing fasciitis, scarlet fever, toxic

TABLE 48.3

BACTERIOLOGIC ETIOLOGY OF COMMON SKIN AND SOFT TISSUE INFECTIONS

Infection	Etiologic Agent
Impetigo	Group A streptococci
	Staphylococcus aureus
Bullous impetigo	*S. aureus*
Erysipelas	Group A streptococci
Periorbital and buccal cellulitis	*Haemophilus influenzae* Type b (before *H. influenzae* Type b vaccine era)
	S. aureus
	Streptococcus pneumoniae
Human bites	Anaerobes (*Eikenella* sp.)
	Oral streptococci, *S. aureus*
Ecthyma gangrenosum	*Pseudomonas aeruginosa*
Burns	*S. aureus*
	P. aeruginosa
	Enterobacteriaceae
Water-contaminated wounds	*P. aeruginosa*
	Aeromonas species
Surgical wounds	*S. aureus*
	Coagulase-negative staphylococci
Necrotizing fasciitis	Group A streptococci
	Anaerobes
	S. aureus

shock syndrome, and glomerulonephritis. Scarlet fever and toxic shock syndrome secondary to *S. aureus* infection are well described.

Recently, "community-associated" strains of methicillin-resistant *S. aureus* (CA-MRSA) have emerged as important pathogens causing skin and soft tissue infections in otherwise normal hosts. These strains are distinct epidemiologically from healthcare-associated strains of MRSA, which cause infection in individuals who have risk factors related to hospitalization. Infections caused by CA-MRSA have mainly included local skin abscesses (boils), and locally invasive skin and soft tissue infections. However, these strains have been implicated in many other infections, including bone and joint infections, severe and complicated pneumonias, and sepsis. Unlike healthcare-associated MRSA, CA-MRSA remain susceptible to many non–β-lactam antibiotics, including trimethoprim-sulfamethoxazole, clindamycin, and tetracyclines. However, these strains may exhibit inducible clindamycin resistance, which may have therapeutic considerations. Testing strains for inducible clindamycin resistance can be accomplished in the laboratory by the double disk diffusion test (D-test), which should be undertaken whenever the strain shows in vitro resistance to erythromycin and susceptibility to clindamycin.

Important principles of management of CA-MRSA infections include:

■ Making an increased effort to obtain specimen for culture
■ Draining purulent collections

- Providing thorough wound care
- Making plans for reassessment of wounds following initial management
- Being familiar with local susceptibility trends

Draining purulent collections and careful follow-up of skin and soft tissue infections caused by strains of CA-MRSA appear to be more important than the choice of antimicrobial agent. Selection of an appropriate agent, however, should take into account the prevalence of these strains in a community, site of infection, severity of infection, and results of in vitro testing. Vancomycin should be used empirically for severe infections when these strains are suspected, until results of susceptibility testing are available. Appropriate oral agents for less severe skin and soft tissue infections and when outpatient management is warranted may include clindamycin or trimethoprim-sulfamethoxazole.

Periorbital (preseptal) cellulitis (Fig. 48.1) may be secondary to trauma or hematogenous spread of an organism, or may represent direct extension from the paranasal sinuses. The bacterial agent involved is related to how the condition is acquired. *S. aureus* organisms and group A streptococci are the most likely agents following trauma. *Haemophilus influenzae* Type b (HIB) was by far the most common agent involved in hematogenous spread in the pre-HIB vaccine era but has now been replaced by pneumococci. Pneumococci are also the most likely agents when periorbital cellulitis occurs as a complication of paranasal sinusitis.

Orbital (postseptal) cellulitis most commonly develops as a result of ethmoid sinusitis. The clinical manifestations may be identical to those of periorbital cellulitis, but the findings of *proptosis* and *ophthalmoplegia* are suggestive of an orbital rather than a periorbital process. Imaging studies (usually computed tomography) are indicated whenever the possibility of an orbital process arises that may reveal a subperiosteal abscess. The pathogens that commonly cause

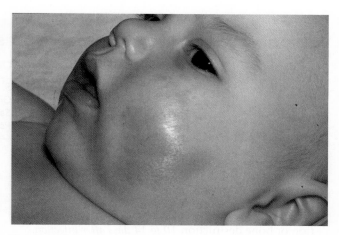

Figure 48.2 Buccal cellulitis in a fully vaccinated infant. *Streptococcus pneumoniae* was isolated from the blood of this infant. (See color insert.)

sinusitis (*Streptococcus pneumoniae, H. influenzae, Moraxella catarrhalis*) are often implicated in orbital cellulitis, but organisms that cause chronic sinusitis such as *S. aureus* and anaerobes should also be considered.

Buccal cellulitis (Fig. 48.2) most commonly results from hematogenous spread. Traditionally, HIB has been the organism most frequently implicated, and often has a characteristic bluish hue appearance, but pneumococci are the more likely culprits in the post-HIB vaccine era.

Osteomyelitis

Osteomyelitis can develop because of hematogenous spread, direct inoculation during trauma or surgery, or local invasion. The clinical features and microbiology vary according to the route of acquisition.

In infants and children, hematogenous spread is most common. Clinical features include fever, limitation of movement in the involved area, localized swelling, erythema, and point tenderness. Neonates may present with pseudoparalysis; multiple bones may be involved, and septic arthritis is often an accompanying feature because the epiphyseal-metaphyseal junction is within the joint capsule.

The microbial etiology of acute hematogenous osteomyelitis is summarized in Table 48.4. *S. aureus* is by far the most common cause of acute osteomyelitis in infants and children. HIB, formerly an important cause of bone and joint infections in children <2 years, is now rare. In children with sickle cell disease, *Salmonella* is the most common cause of osteomyelitis. *Serratia* and *Aspergillus* may be etiologic agents in patients with chronic granulomatous disease.

Laboratory features of acute osteomyelitis include positive blood cultures in about 50% of cases and an elevated erythrocyte sedimentation rate, which can be used to gauge the response to therapy. Direct bone aspirates prior to antibiotics can more often identify the pathogen and may be indicated if there is an abscess present, and also if medical

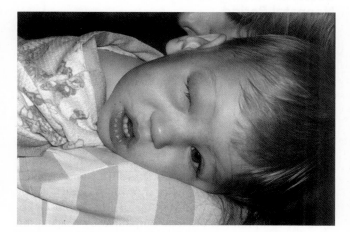

Figure 48.1 Periorbital cellulitis, characterized by swelling and erythema of the right eyelid. (See color insert.)

TABLE 48.4

MICROBIAL ETIOLOGY OF ACUTE OSTEOMYELITIS

Neonate	Infant	Older Child
Group B streptococci	S. aureus	S. aureus
S. aureus	Group A streptococci	Group A streptococci
Escherichia coli	Streptococcus pneumoniae	Salmonella species (children with hemoglobinopathies)
Candida species	Haemophilus influenzae Type b	Pseudomonas aeruginosa (children with puncture wound osteochondritis)

therapy fails to control infection. Radiographic studies helpful in the diagnosis of osteomyelitis include the following:

- Plain films of the affected area reveal periosteal elevation or bone destruction *10 to 14 days after infection.*
- Magnetic resonance imaging, which has emerged as a very sensitive and specific study, is the best imaging modality to detect subperiosteal abscesses and differentiate bone from soft-tissue infection. It is particularly useful for vertebral and pelvic osteomyelitis
- ^{99m}Tc bone scan can augment magnetic resonance imaging, and can be considered when multiple foci of infection are suspected.

Intravenous antimicrobial therapy is indicated, at least initially, for acute hematogenous osteomyelitis. In infants beyond the neonatal period and in older children, the course can be completed with oral therapy provided the patient has shown a complete clinical response, the organism has been recovered and is known to be susceptible to an agent with good bone penetration, the patient can tolerate oral antibiotics, and the parents are deemed reliable. The total duration of therapy is usually 4 to 8 weeks. The utility of serum bactericidal titers is controversial. Surgical intervention is often helpful and may be required to drain purulent subperiosteal material.

Puncture wound osteomyelitis most often arises after a foreign object has penetrated, usually through the soles of sneakers, the sole of a foot. Cellulitis develops in approximately 10% to 15% of cases and evolves into osteochondritis in 10% to 20% of these. Children aged 8 to 13 years appear to be at highest risk and present with pain, erythema, and local tenderness at the site of the wound. Fever is usually absent. The most common microbial agent in these circumstances is *Pseudomonas aeruginosa.* Management must include surgical debridement of necrotic bone and cartilage. A 14-day course of antipseudomonal therapy is effective for eradicating the infection, provided adequate debridement is performed.

Septic Arthritis

The clinical manifestations of septic arthritis include fever, an inability to walk, or a limp. Decreased mobility of the joint, erythema, and swelling are common. Large joints are most often affected. Neonates may have few signs of systemic illness, and multiple joints may be involved with accompanying osteomyelitis.

The microbial etiology of septic arthritis is similar to that of osteomyelitis. *Neisseria gonorrhoeae* is an important cause of septic arthritis in adolescents. In cases of *N. gonorrhoeae* infection, a *tenosynovitis-dermatitis syndrome* may occur in which smaller joints such as the wrist, hand, and fingers may be involved; alternatively, a *suppurative arthritis* may occur, in which a monoarticular arthritis of a large joint, such as the knee, is often involved.

Blood cultures are positive for bacteria in 30% to 40% of cases of septic arthritis, and joint aspirates maybe helpful in differentiating infectious from rheumatic causes of arthritis.

The management of septic arthritis includes appropriate specific antimicrobial therapy for at least 3 weeks and consideration of surgical intervention. Septic arthritis of the hip joint is an orthopaedic emergency requiring surgical drainage. Surgical drainage is also indicated for joint infections that do not respond to medical treatment, and for most neonatal cases of septic arthritis.

In the newborn, infection in the femur rapidly can expand into the joint, requiring consideration of this diagnosis early for proper management.

CENTRAL NERVOUS SYSTEM INFECTIONS

Bacterial Meningitis Beyond the Neonatal Period

Despite the dramatic decline in the incidence of HIB and pneumococcal disease since the introduction of HIB and pneumococcal conjugate vaccines, bacterial meningitis remains an important infection in infants and children.

Epidemiology and Etiology

Neisseria meningitidis and *S. pneumoniae are* the most common bacterial agents causing sepsis and meningitis in children older than 3 months. *N. meningitidis* meningitis may occur with or without evidence of sepsis. The term *meningococcemia* refers to the clinical syndrome in which septic shock is present with or without meningitis. Rapid hemodynamic compromise, often accompanied by coagulation disturbances and purpura, may develop despite early and appropriate therapy. The mortality and morbidity rates associated with meningococcemia are significant. *N. meningitidis* meningitis without sepsis responds promptly to antimicrobial therapy, and these children have a good prognosis. *Children who have terminal complement deficiencies are at risk for recurrent and severe infections with Neisseriae. Thus, children with meningococcal disease should be screened for this deficiency.*

The risk of household contacts of children with *N. meningitidis* meningitis for the development of meningitis is significantly greater (1000-fold) than the general risk of the community. Adult and child care contacts serve as important sources of infection for young children. The risk of invasive HIB disease is increased among unimmunized household contacts younger than 4 years of age, and probably among nursery and child care center contacts. Pneumococcal meningitis most often occurs sporadically.

Clinical Manifestations

The presenting features of meningitis vary according to the age of the child affected. Infants may display only fever and irritability. Headaches, nuchal rigidity, and photophobia are more common in older children. Focal neurologic signs and cranial nerve abnormalities are occasionally seen. Seizures occur in approximately 30% of children with meningitis. *If seizures occur at presentation or within the first 3 days of diagnosis, they are of no prognostic significance.* If they occur after the fourth day of therapy, they are associated with significant complications of meningitis, such as infarction or subdural empyema.

Diagnosis

Blood cultures are positive in approximately 90% of cases of pneumococcal or meningococcal meningitis. Lumbar puncture remains the most important diagnostic test (Table 48.5). Test results that show >1000 white blood cells/mm^3 with a predominance of neutrophils, a low cerebrospinal fluid (CSF) level of glucose (<40 mg/dL), and a high level of protein (>100 mg/dL) are typical. The Gram stain result is positive in 80% of cases, and the CSF culture serves as the gold standard for identifying the organism, provided the patient has not been previously treated with antibiotics.

Treatment

The initial therapy for proven or suspected cases of bacterial meningitis must include antibiotics that penetrate the CSF and are effective against meningococci and pneumococci, including penicillin and cephalosporin-resistant strains of pneumococci. *The combination of ceftriaxone or cefotaxime with vancomycin is recommended initially.* Once the organism has been isolated and the susceptibilities are known, the regimen can be adjusted. Vancomycin can be discontinued if meningococci are isolated or if a susceptible pneumococcal strain is found. The role of corticosteroids in the management of meningitis caused by *N. meningitidis* or *S. pneumoniae* is controversial.

Prognosis and Complications

The overall mortality rate for pneumococcal meningitis is 10% to 15%; the rate is 3% to 5% for meningococcal meningitis. Long-term sequelae occur in approximately 30% of patients with pneumococcal meningitis and 10% of those with meningococcal meningitis. Sensorineural hearing loss is the most common sequela. The syndrome of inappropriate secretion of antidiuretic hormone (SIADH) occurs frequently during the course of bacterial meningitis, but dehydration is more likely to be present at presentation and should be treated. Subdural effusions are usually benign and more often seen in pneumococcal than in meningococcal meningitis. Subdural empyema, infarction, and persistent seizures may occur.

TABLE 48.5

TYPICAL CEREBROSPINAL FLUID FINDINGS IN MENINGITIS OF DIFFERENT CAUSES

CSF Characteristic	Bacterial Infection	Partially Treated Bacterial Infection	Tuberculosis (see also Chapter 49)	Viral Infection	Brain Abscess
Cells (No/mm^3)	20–5000	20–5000	<1000	<1000	<500
Differential	Neutrophil predominance	Neutrophils	Lymphocytes	Neutrophils early; may persist or shift to lymphocytes	Neutrophils or lymphocytes
Glucose	Low	Low	Low	Normal	Normal
Protein	High (>80 mg/dL)	High (>80 mg/dL)	High	Mildly elevated	High
Gram stain	Positive in 90%	May be negative	Negative	Negative	Negative
Bacterial culture	Positive	May be negative	Negative	Negative	Negative

These CSF findings represent general rather than absolute guidelines.
CSF, cerebrospinal fluid.

Prevention

- Antimicrobial prophylaxis is recommended for all household, child care center, nursery school contacts, and anyone who has had intimate exposure to an index case of invasive meningococcal disease. Prophylaxis is generally not indicated for schoolroom and hospital contacts who have not been exposed to oral secretions of the index case.
- For invasive HIB disease, prophylaxis is indicated for households with at least one contact <4 years of age *who is unimmunized or incompletely immunized.* Prophylaxis is also recommended for nursery and child care center contacts when two or more cases of HIB invasive disease have occurred within 60 days and there are unimmunized or incompletely immunized children in the center.
- Rifampin is the prophylactic agent of choice for most children. Patients with meningococcal or HIB invasive disease who are treated with ceftriaxone or cefotaxime do *not* need to receive rifampin prophylaxis, as these agents are effective in eliminating colonization.
- No prophylaxis is recommended for the contacts of patients with pneumococcal meningitis.

Aseptic Meningitis

Aseptic meningitis can be caused by a wide variety of viruses, bacteria, fungi, mycoplasmata, and parasites, and it can be a feature of systemic illnesses, such as Behçet syndrome and Kawasaki syndrome. Viruses are by far the most common agents causing aseptic meningitis.

Enteroviruses account for most cases of viral meningitis. During the summer in temperate climates, these viruses often cause illness with mild, self-limited meningeal symptoms. Fever, headache, photophobia, vomiting, abdominal pain, and meningeal signs are common features. A rash may also be present, which may be macular, maculopapular, petechial, vesicular, or urticarial. When a petechial rash is present, differentiation from meningococcal disease becomes especially important. Examination of the CSF of a patient with enteroviral meningitis reveals a pleocytosis of 100 to 1000 cells, a normal or slightly elevated protein level, and a normal glucose level. A predominance of neutrophils is frequently seen early in the infection. This may persist, but usually the neutrophils are replaced by lymphocytes during the illness. Other viruses causing meningitis include Epstein-Barr virus (EBV), adenovirus, arbovirus, herpes simplex virus 2 (HSV-2), lymphocytic choriomeningitis virus, and West Nile virus. EBV and respiratory viruses may cause meningitis in young children without the other classic manifestations of infectious mononucleosis or respiratory symptoms. Arboviruses, which are borne by mosquitoes, cause acute encephalitis more often than meningitis. HSV-2 can cause meningitis, most often in adolescents with a primary herpes genital infection. Lymphocytic choriomeningitis is associated with exposure to rodents. West Nile virus, which is borne by mosquitoes, can cause a nonspecific febrile illness, which may include meningoencephalitis.

The diagnosis of enteroviral meningitis can be confirmed by isolating the virus in the CSF, rectum, or nasopharynx. Polymerase chain reaction is more sensitive and rapid than the earlier diagnostic methods. Serology is often performed on acute and convalescent titers to implicate other viral agents. Most often, no agent is identified in children with presumed viral meningitis.

Encephalitis

Encephalitis differs from meningitis in that the brain parenchyma is directly involved. Organisms can invade the brain directly, or the involvement may represent an immunologically mediated process that occurs following infection. Clinical features can include an altered mental status, seizures, hemiparesis, cranial nerve defects, ataxia, focal motor signs, and behavioral disturbances. Nuchal rigidity is usually not as pronounced as in meningitis. The term *meningoencephalitis* is used when the distinction is not clear.

Viral agents account for most cases of encephalitis. Those most often encountered include the following:

- Enteroviruses (most common cause, seasonal predilection)
- HSV-1 (most common cause of sporadic disease)
- Arboviruses (mosquito-borne)
- HSV-2 (cause of infection in neonates)
- EBV
- Respiratory viruses
- Varicella-zoster virus
- West Nile virus

Bacterial agents of encephalitis include *Bartonella henselae* (cat scratch disease), *Bordetella pertussis*, *Borrelia burgdorferi*, and spirochetes.

Fungi, mycoplasmata, rickettsiae, amebae, and parasites (*Plasmodium, Toxoplasma*) can also cause encephalitis.

The tests utilized to diagnose encephalitis include computed tomography scan, magnetic resonance imaging, and electroencephalography. *Focal involvement of the temporal lobes on these studies in a child with seizures, focal neurologic symptoms, or an altered mental status should raise the suspicion of the presence of HSV-1 encephalitis.* The CSF findings in viral encephalitis are similar to those in viral meningitis. A lymphocytic pleocytosis, *significantly elevated protein level*, and normal glucose level in a *hemorrhagic spinal fluid* are hallmarks of HSV-1 encephalitis. Polymerase chain reaction testing of the CSF for HSV-1, when performed by an experienced laboratory, is significantly more sensitive than viral culture and appears to be specific for the virus.

Intravenously administered acyclovir is the treatment of choice for a child with a confirmed or suspected case of HSV-1 encephalitis.

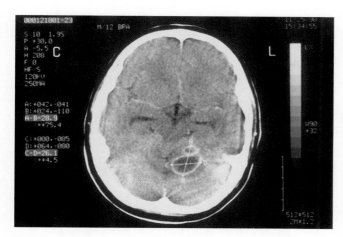

Figure 48.3 Computed tomogram of a child with an abscess in the left cerebellar hemisphere caused by direct extension of a middle ear and mastoid infection.

Brain Abscess

Brain abscesses in infants and children are most often:

- Caused by direct spread from adjacent structures, such as the mastoids, sinuses, and orbit **(Fig. 48.3)**
- Associated with congenital (usually cyanotic) heart disease
- Caused by hematogenous spread
- A complication of meningitis (in neonates)

Fever, irritability, vomiting, malaise, and focal neurologic signs are the major clinical manifestations. The CSF is typically sterile with a mild to moderate neutrophilic pleocytosis, elevated protein level, normal glucose level, and elevated opening pressure, but typically lumbar puncture is avoided when a brain abscess is suspected.

Brain abscesses are generally *polymicrobial.* Viridans streptococci, including organisms of the *Streptococcus milleri* group, anaerobic streptococci, and gram-negative aerobes, are the most common causes. Gram-negative organisms, especially *Citrobacter species,* are well-known causes of brain abscesses in *neonates.*

Imaging studies of the brain, such as computed tomography scan and magnetic resonance imaging, are diagnostic.

The need for surgical intervention is controversial. Broad-spectrum antibiotics, such as the combination of a third-generation cephalosporin (ceftriaxone or cefotaxime) and metronidazole, should be instituted.

PNEUMONIA

Pneumonia can result from invasion of the lung by a wide variety of infectious agents. Pneumonia in children can be classified according to etiology (viral, bacterial, or atypical), anatomic distribution (lobar or interstitial), affected age group, or clinical severity of infection.

Infants who are ill-appearing with an acute presentation and a lobar infiltrate on chest radiography are more likely to have bacterial pneumonia. Children who are well appearing with an indolent course and patchy or interstitial infiltrates are more likely to have viral pneumonia or pneumonia caused by an atypical organism. Infants and children who are immunocompromised are susceptible to a wide variety of common bacterial, viral, and atypical organisms, and they are also susceptible to much less common causes of pneumonia, such as *Pneumocystis jiroveci (carinii)* and other fungal agents.

Bacterial Pneumonia

Except for the newborn, in whom group B streptococci are the most common cause of bacterial pneumonia, *S. pneumoniae* is the most common cause of bacterial pneumonia in infants and children. HIB, formerly an important cause of bacterial pneumonia in infants, is now rare. *S. aureus,* including CA-MRSA strains, have emerged as important causes of bacterial pneumonia. *Streptococcus pyogenes* is an occasional cause of bacterial pneumonia.

Streptococcus pneumoniae

The pneumococcus accounts for >90% of cases of childhood bacterial pneumonia. Secondary infection with *S. pneumoniae* frequently follows a viral upper respiratory tract infection. Infants often are ill-appearing, with high fever, tachypnea, grunting respirations, flaring of the alae nasi, and tachycardia. Older children and adolescents often present abruptly with a shaking chill followed by high fever. Respiratory distress, restlessness, cough, and delirium may ensue. Children with lower lobe involvement may present with abdominal pain. The physical examination findings may be unrevealing, especially in young infants, whereas specific evidence of consolidation is more apparent in older children. Laboratory features consistent with pneumococcal pneumonia include an elevated white blood cell count, and rarely a low white blood cell count. Lobar consolidation **(Fig. 48.4)** is the most common radiographic finding,

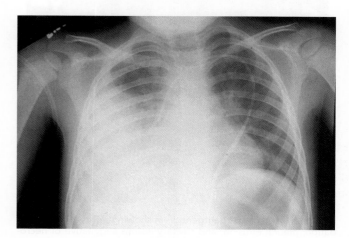

Figure 48.4 Chest roentgenogram of a child who presented with high fever and respiratory distress showing multilobar consolidation. *Streptococcus pneumoniae* was recovered from the child's bloodstream.

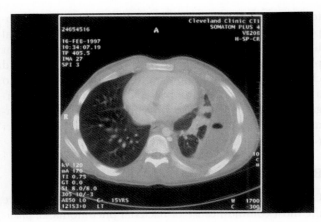

Figure 48.5 Computed tomogram showing a large, left-sided parapneumonic empyema in a child with pneumococcal pneumonia. Note multiple air-fluid levels within the fluid-filled collection.

although a diffuse pattern may be seen in young infants. Parapneumonic effusions and empyema (Fig. 48.5) are well-known complications of pneumococcal pneumonia. Pneumococci have also been associated with necrotizing pneumonia. Penicillins and cephalosporins remain active against most strains of *S. pneumoniae*. Cefuroxime, cefotaxime, or ceftriaxone is commonly utilized empirically to treat pneumonia in infants and children. These agents appear to be effective clinically, even for penicillin and cephalosporin-resistant strains of pneumococci.

Staphylococcus aureus

Staphylococcal pneumonia is a progressive and life-threatening infection that can complicate viral pneumonia, especially following an influenza infection. Staphylococcal pneumonia is associated with a high incidence of necrotizing cavitary pneumonia (Fig. 48.6), parapneumonic

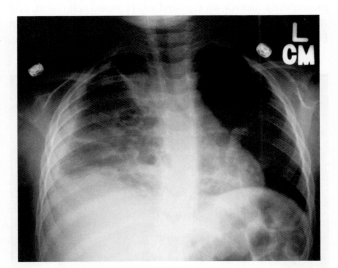

Figure 48.6 Chest roentgenogram showing right-sided consolidation, pleural effusion, and cavitary lesions suggestive of necrotizing pneumonia. This child's blood culture grew *Streptococcus pneumoniae* but this radiographic appearance is also consistent with pneumonia caused by *Staphylococcus aureus*.

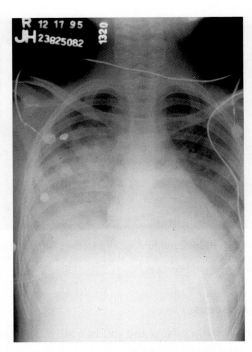

Figure 48.7 Chest roentgenogram of a child showing lobar consolidation and pleural effusion. Culture of the pleural fluid grew *Staphylococcus aureus*, and a respiratory viral panel revealed influenza.

effusions, and empyema (Fig. 48.7). Young infants appear to be more susceptible than older children, and the clinical features may be similar to those of pneumococcal pneumonia. Chest radiography not uncommonly reveals lobar or multilobar involvement. *Pneumatoceles and pyopneumothorax are common in cases of staphylococcal pneumonia.*

Viral Pneumonia

Viral agents are responsible for most cases of pneumonia in infants and preschool children. The peak incidence of viral pneumonia is among children 2- to 3-years old. In general, viral pneumonia is associated with less severe clinical features and low-grade fever, although more severe infection and respiratory failure can certainly occur, even in healthy children. Etiologic agents include:

- Respiratory syncytial virus
- Adenovirus
- Influenza virus
- Parainfluenza virus

Cough, fever, wheezing, and upper respiratory tract symptoms are common presenting features. Chest radiography commonly reveals patchy, diffuse perihilar infiltrates with hyperinflation. Therapy is supportive in most cases. The use of ribavirin for respiratory syncytial virus infection in infants at high risk for severe disease can be considered; its benefit is controversial and limited.

Mycoplasma Pneumonia

The most common cause of pneumonia in school-age children is M. pneumoniae, *and the peak incidence of* Mycoplasma pneumonia *is in children aged 10 to 15 years.* Infection before 3 to 4 years of age appears to be rare. Although the course of *Mycoplasma* infection varies greatly, the clinical onset is gradual and characterized by cough, which may be present for 1 to 2 weeks before other symptoms develop, and sore throat. Most cases resolve spontaneously within 3 to 4 weeks. Characteristically, the radiographic features are more severe than would be suggested by the generally healthy appearance of the child or adolescent; bilateral lower lobe interstitial infiltrates are most common. Lobar infiltrates, hilar adenopathy, and pleural effusions may be present during the course of the illness. Other manifestations of *Mycoplasma* infection, such as pharyngitis, rash (erythema multiforme), arthralgias or arthritis, and hemolysis, may be present in conjunction with pneumonia and may serve as clues to the diagnosis. The definitive diagnosis often relies on specific serologic testing. Antimicrobial therapy for *Mycoplasma* pneumonia with erythromycin or azithromycin modestly shortens the duration of illness.

Chlamydophila (formerly *Chlamydia*) *pneumoniae* Infection

C. pneumoniae is increasingly being recognized as a cause of pneumonia in children. Approximately 50% of adults have antibodies to this agent. A preceding pharyngitis, hoarseness, productive cough, and bronchospasm appear to be the common features of infection with *C. pneumoniae*. Commercially available serologic testing for *C. pneumoniae* is fraught with difficulty, and results should be interpreted with caution.

A macrolide, such as erythromycin, azithromycin, or clarithromycin are recommended for treatment.

Pneumocystis jiroveci (*carinii*) Pneumonia

P. jiroveci, a ubiquitous fungus, is known for causing severe, life-threatening pneumonia in immunocompromised patients. Most cases in infants and children occur in those with HIV infection or malignancy; *P. jiroveci* pneumonia remains one of the most common acquired immunodeficiency syndrome (AIDS)–defining illnesses in HIV-infected infants. HIV-infected infants most often present with respiratory distress, cough, low-grade fever, and cyanosis between 3 to 6 months. Hypoxemia is common at any age. Chest radiography can reveal any pattern; bilateral interstitial perihilar infiltrates are most common (Fig. 48.8). The definitive diagnosis is often made by demonstrating the organism in bronchoalveolar washings or lung biopsy specimens. High-dose trimethoprim/sulfamethoxazole is the drug of choice for the treatment of *P. jiroveci* pneumonia. Corticosteroids have been shown to be of benefit for HIV-infected patients with moderate to severe *P. jiroveci* pneumonia.

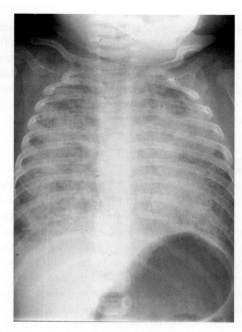

Figure 48.8 Chest roentgenogram showing severe, bilateral, diffuse interstitial and nodular infiltrates in a 6-month-old infant who presented with fever and severe respiratory distress. *Pneumocystis jiroveci (carinii)* was recovered from the bronchoalveolar lavage fluid, and further testing revealed human immunodeficiency virus infection.

REVIEW EXERCISES

QUESTIONS

1. A 3-year-old girl presents with a 2-day history of cramping abdominal pain and watery diarrhea. A brief generalized seizure develops, and she is hospitalized. During the next 24 hours, her diarrhea becomes profuse and bloody. The *most* likely agent causing this girl's gastroenteritis is:

a) *E. coli* O157:H7
b) *C. jejuni*
c) *Salmonella species*
d) *S. sonnei*

Answer

The answer is d. Seizures are a common extraintestinal manifestation of *Shigella* infection. Seizures that are characteristically brief, generalized, and self-limited develop in approximately 10% to 45% of hospitalized children with *Shigella* infection. They frequently occur before the onset of diarrhea and may be the presenting feature of shigellosis. The underlying cause of the seizures is not well understood. Simple febrile convulsions or electrolyte abnormalities can explain some but not most seizures. Other occasional neurologic findings in children with shigellosis include headaches, confusion, and hallucinations.

2. Fever, cramping abdominal pain, and bloody diarrhea develop in a 5-year-old boy. The day before the onset of symptoms, he had attended a picnic, where he ingested undercooked chicken. Of the following agents, the one *most* likely to be causing this boy's symptoms is:
a) *C. jejuni*
b) *S. sonnei*
c) *Y. enterocolitica*
d) *G. lamblia*

Answer
The answer is a. *Campylobacter* and *Salmonella* infections are the most common food-borne illnesses in the United States. Incompletely cooked poultry, unpasteurized dairy products, and untreated water serve as major vehicles of transmission of *C. jejuni*. Fever, cramping abdominal pain, and bloody diarrhea can be caused by any of the agents listed in the question, with the exception of *G. lamblia*, which causes a watery, nonbloody diarrhea that may be chronic and manifest with abdominal pain and malabsorption. Therefore, the history of epidemiologic factors becomes important in delineating the cause of infection. Person-to-person transmission of *S. sonnei* is more frequent than food-borne transmission. Uncooked pork products can serve as an important vehicle of transmission of *Y. enterocolitica*.

3. The *most* common etiologic agent causing acute osteomyelitis in a 2-year-old child is:
a) Group A streptococci
b) HIB
c) *S. pneumoniae*
d) *S. aureus*
e) *P. aeruginosa*

Answer
The answer is d. *S. aureus* is by far the most common cause of acute hematogenous osteomyelitis in children of any age, except in the neonatal period, when group B streptococci are also significant agents. Group A streptococci and *S. pneumoniae* are rare causes of acute osteomyelitis. HIB infection, even in the pre-HIB vaccine era, was less common than *S. aureus* infection, even in infants <2 years. *P. aeruginosa* causes puncture wound osteochondritis. This is most commonly seen in older children, in whom cellulitis and osteochondritis can develop following a puncture wound through a tennis shoe.

Case for Questions 4 and 5
High fever, lethargy, and listlessness develop in a 9-month-old child who attends a child care center. He experiences a 5-minute generalized tonic-clonic seizure. CSF analysis reveals:

- 10,000 White blood cells with 90% neutrophils and 10% lymphocytes
- Protein 130 mg/dL
- Glucose 5 mg/dL

4. Of the following, the *most* likely etiologic agent is:
a) HSV-1
b) *S. pneumoniae*
c) *Mycobacterium tuberculosis*
d) *E. coli*
e) *Cryptococcus neoformans*

Answer
The answer is b. This child has bacterial meningitis, given the number of white blood cells, predominance of neutrophils, elevated CSF protein level, and low CSF glucose level. The causes of bacterial meningitis beyond the neonatal period include *S. pneumoniae* and *N. meningitidis*. *E. coli* is a very uncommon cause of meningitis beyond the neonatal period; *M. tuberculosis*, *C. neoformans*, and HSV-1 do not cause this CSF picture.

5. Culture of the CSF reveals *N. meningitidis*. Which of the following statements is *true*?
a) Meningococcal vaccine should be given to all contacts at the child care center.
b) The occurrence of a seizure at the onset of this child's symptoms suggests a poor prognosis.
c) The overall prognosis for a child who has meningococcal meningitis is better than that for a child who has meningococcemia without meningitis.
d) Rifampin prophylaxis should be given to family contacts of this child but not to the child care contacts.

Answer
The answer is c. Meningococcemia is an acute, life-threatening complication of meningococcal bacteremia. It often manifests with fever, a rapidly progressing petechial or purpuric rash, and hemodynamic instability; the *absence* of meningitis is a poor prognostic sign, indicating fulminant sepsis. Children with meningococcal meningitis generally have a good prognosis. The routine prophylaxis of contacts with meningococcal vaccine is not indicated, but it has been used to control outbreaks of infections with serotypes included in the vaccine. Rifampin prophylaxis is indicated for household, child care, and nursery school contacts of index cases. The occurrence of seizures as the initial presentation of bacterial meningitis is common and is *not* of prognostic significance. Seizures that occur during the course of therapy for bacterial meningitis indicate a complication such as brain abscess, infarct, or subdural empyema.

6. A 9-year-old boy presents with a 10-day history of sore throat, dry cough, and fever. On physical examination, the child is well-appearing. He has a temperature of 39.2°C (102.56°F), a respiratory rate of 28 breaths/minutes, and scattered rales bilaterally. A chest radiograph reveals bilateral basilar interstitial infiltrates. The *most* likely agent of this boy's illness is:
a) *M. tuberculosis*
b) *M. pneumoniae*
c) *S. pneumoniae*
d) Group A streptococci

Answer

The answer is b. *M. pneumoniae* is the most common cause of pneumonia in school-age children, accounting for up to 20% of cases. Many, if not most infections, are asymptomatic or mildly symptomatic. The clinical features range from mild to severe. A subacute course with a dry cough and pharyngitis is common. Although the radiographic findings vary widely, bilateral basilar interstitial infiltrates are a frequent finding, and the radiographic appearance of the infiltrate(s) is often significantly worse than the appearance of the child.

7. A 6 month-old-male infant develops bacterial meningitis. CSF grows *H. influenzae* type b. He is treated with 14 days of intravenously administered Ceftriaxone. There is a healthy 2-year-old fully immunized sibling at home and two healthy parents. Neither the infant nor the 2-year-old sibling attends a child care center. Which is a true statement regarding antibiotic prophylaxis for this infant and his contacts?
a) Rifampin prophylaxis should be given to the parents and the 2-year-old sibling.
b) The infant should receive rifampin prophylaxis at the completion of his ceftriaxone course.
c) Rifampin prophylaxis should be provided only for the 2-year-old sibling.
d) No antibiotic prophylaxis is required in this scenario.

Answer

The answer is d. Unimmunized or incompletely immunized contacts <4 years of age are at increased risk of invasive HIB disease when in close contact with a child who has invasive HIB disease. Thus, prophylaxis is recommended for those households with at least one contact who is <4 years of age who is unimmunized or incompletely immunized. Prophylaxis is also recommended for:

■ Households with a child <12 months of age who has not received the primary HIB series
■ Households with a contact who is an immunocompromised child, regardless of the child's HIB immunization status
■ For nursery school and child care center contacts when two or more cases of HIB invasive disease are identified within 60 days and unimmunized or partially immunized children are attending

For the index case, no prophylaxis is required when they have been treated with ceftriaxone or cefotaxime, since these agents are effective in eliminating colonization.

SUGGESTED READINGS

1. American Academy of Pediatrics. *Shigella* infections. In: Pickering LK, Baker CJ, Long SS, McMillan JA, eds. *Red book: 2006 Report of the Committee on Infectious Diseases*, 27th ed. Elk Grove Village, IL: American Academy of Pediatrics, 2006:589–591.
2. American Academy of Pediatrics. Children in out-of-home child care. In: Pickering LK, Baker CJ, Long SS, McMillan JA, eds. *Red book: 2006 Report of the Committee on Infectious Diseases*, 27th ed. Elk Grove Village, IL: American Academy of Pediatrics, 2006: 130–145.
3. American Academy of Pediatrics. *Haemophilus influenzae* infections. In: Pickering LK, Baker CJ, Long SS, McMillan JA, eds. *Red book: 2006 Report of the Committee on Infectious Diseases*, 27th ed. Elk Grove Village, IL: American Academy of Pediatrics, 2006: 310–318.
4. American Academy of Pediatrics. Meningococcal infections. In: Pickering LK, Baker CJ, Long SS, McMillan JA, eds. *Red book: 2006 Report of the Committee on Infectious Diseases*, 27th ed. Elk Grove Village, IL: American Academy of Pediatrics, 2006: 452–460.
5. Bass ES, Pappano DA, Humiston SG. Rotavirus. *Pediatr Rev* 2007; 28:183–191.
6. Burnett MW, Bass JW, Cook BA. Etiology of osteomyelitis complicating sickle cell disease. *Pediatrics* 1998;101:296–297.
7. Centers for Disease Control and Prevention. Diagnosis and management of food-borne illnesses—a primer for physicians. *MMWR Morb Mortal Wkly Rep* 2001;50:RR-2.
8. Durbin WJ, Stille C. Pneumonia. *Pediatr Rev* 2008;29:147–160.
9. Gorwitz RJ. A review of community-associated methicillin-resistant *Staphylococcus aureus* skin and soft tissue infection. *Pediatr Infect Dis J* 2008;27:1–7.
10. Jacobs RF, Adelman L, Sack CM, et al. Management of *Pseudomonas* osteochondritis complicating puncture wounds of the foot. *Pediatrics* 1982;69:432–435.
11. Kaplan SL. Osteomyelitis in children. *Infect Dis Clin North Am* 2005;19:787–797.
12. Kirsch EA, Barton P, Kitchen L, et al. Pathophysiology, treatment and outcome of meningococcemia: a review and recent experience. *Pediatr Infect Dis J* 1996; 15:967–979.
13. Lewis P, Glaser CA. Encephalitis. *Pediatr Rev* 2005;26:353–363.
14. Mancini AJ Bacterial skin infections in children: the common and the not so common. *Pediatr Ann* 2000;29:26–35.
15. Muzumdar H, Arens R, Adam HM. Pleural fluid. *Pediatr Rev* 2007; 28:462–464.
16. Negrini B, Kelleher KF, Wald ER. Cerebrospinal fluid findings in aseptic versus bacterial meningitis. *Pediatrics* 2000; 105: 316–319.
17. Prober CG. The role of steroids in the management of children with bacterial meningitis. *Pediatrics* 1995;95:29–31.
18. Safdar N, Said A, Gangnon RE, Maki DG. Risk of hemolytic uremic syndrome after antibiotic treatment of *Escherichia coli* O157:H7 enteritis. A meta-analysis. *JAMA* 2002;288:996–1001.
19. Schuchat A, Robinson K, Wenger JD, et al. Bacterial meningitis in the United States in 1995. *NEJM* 1997;337:970–976.
20. Schultz KD, Fan L, Pinsky J, et al. The changing face of pleural empyemas in children: epidemiology and management. *Pediatrics* 2004;113:1735–1740.
21. Wald ER. Periorbital and orbital infections. *Pediatr Rev* 2004; 25:312–319.
22. Wong CS, Lelacic S, Habeeb RL, et al. The risk of the hemolytic-uremic syndrome after antibiotic treatment of *Escherichia coli* O157:H7 infections. *NEJM* 2000;342:1930–1936.
23. Zaoutis T, Klein I. Enteroviral infections. *Pediatr Rev* 1998;19: 183–191.

Chapter 49

Infectious Diseases, Part II

Camille Sabella and Johanna Goldfarb

This chapter includes discussions of selected viral, fungal, and mycobacterial infections.

VIRAL INFECTIONS

Human Parvovirus Infection

Human parvovirus (HPV) is a small DNA virus that replicates in human precursor red blood cells.

Primary infection most commonly occurs in school-aged children (5 to 15 years old) in the late winter and spring. At least 60% of adults are seropositive and immune to infection. Transmission is by respiratory spread and rarely by transfusion of blood from an acutely infected person. Vertical transmission during pregnancy is also possible. The secondary attack rate is approximately 50% with household contact and 20% to 30% with school exposure.

Most infections with HPV are asymptomatic. *Erythema infectiosum (slapped cheek or fifth disease) is the most recognizable form of infection.* This is characterized by an intensely erythematous rash on the cheeks, with mild systemic signs of illness developing approximately 1 week after a mild prodrome of fever, headache, and myalgias. A systemic, lace-like maculopapular rash, which may be pruritic, may also appear on the trunk and extremities (see Fig. 1.20). The rash is often evanescent for weeks, changing with varying temperature and exposure to sunlight.

The appearance of the rash in erythema infectiosum signifies an immune response to the infection. *Therefore, children with the rash are not contagious, and may attend school or child care centers.*

Other manifestations of HPV infection include:

- Arthritis
- Transient aplastic crisis in children with hemolytic anemia
- Chronic bone marrow infection in immunodeficient persons

- Fetal hydrops
- Papulopurpuric gloves-and-socks syndrome

Transient aplastic crisis occurs in persons who depend on rapid red cell production and whose hemoglobin levels are low, such as those who have hemolytic anemia associated with sickle cell disease. The aplastic crisis typically lasts 7 to 10 days, and children may require red blood cell transfusions to prevent or treat congestive heart failure. Children with aplastic crisis are highly contagious, and should be placed in droplet isolation when hospitalized.

Chronic bone marrow failure can develop in an immunodeficient child, resulting in severe anemia and, at times, thrombocytopenia and neutropenia. Intravenous immunoglobulin therapy may be effective.

The papulopurpuric gloves-and-socks syndrome is an atypical rash that can occur during parvovirus B19 infection. Its characteristics include a painful and pruritic papular, petechial and purpuric rash occurring symmetrically on the distal extremities. The rash may be accompanied by fever and perioral lesions. These manifestations occur during the period of viremia, and thus patients with this syndrome should be considered contagious.

Fetal hydrops is a potential consequence of maternal infection during pregnancy. The risk of fetal death associated with parvovirus B19 maternal infection is 2% to 6% and appears to be highest when maternal infection occurs in the first half of pregnancy.

Human Herpesvirus 6 Infection

Human herpesvirus 6 (HHV-6) is a ubiquitous herpesvirus that is the cause of exanthem subitum (roseola). Like all herpesviruses, HHV-6 causes a primary infection and then establishes latency. The distribution of HHV-6 is worldwide and nonseasonal, and primary infection most often occurs in children between the ages of 6 months and

2 years. Almost all children are seropositive for the virus by the age of 2 years. Transmission is thought to be from asymptomatic salivary shedding.

Classic roseola develops in approximately 20% of children infected with HHV-6. It is characterized by a high fever that lasts for 3 to 7 days, often associated with toxicity, followed by an erythematous maculopapular rash. HHV-6 also is a very common cause of *febrile illness without rash* or localizing signs in children aged 6 to 18 months. Other clinical features of HHV-6 infection include:

- Cervical and occipital adenopathy
- Respiratory symptoms and otitis media
- Gastrointestinal symptoms
- Bulging fontanelle
- Febrile seizures

Febrile seizures are thought to occur in approximately 15% of children who have a primary infection with HHV-6. Reactivation of the virus in immunocompromised persons may result in hepatitis, pneumonitis, and encephalitis.

Human Immunodeficiency Virus Infection in Children

Perinatal Transmission

Most cases of human immunodeficiency virus (HIV) infection in children are the result of perinatal transmission. The overall transmission rate from an infected mother to her infant if neither the mother nor the infant is treated with antiretroviral therapy ranges from 14% to 27% in developed countries. Transmission can occur:

- In utero (30% of cases)
- At the time of delivery (70% of cases)
- Postpartum (rarely)

Transmission in utero is associated with early onset of disease in the infant and decreased survival. By definition, infants infected in utero have a blood culture positive for HIV or evidence of HIV DNA on polymerase chain reaction (PCR) testing within 7 days of birth. A large maternal viral load and a low count of $CD4^+$ lymphocytes in the mother are risk factors for in utero transmission; primary infection during pregnancy carries the highest risk.

Peripartum transmission accounts for most cases of infection. The clinical course of these infants is much more variable. By definition, they do not have evidence of HIV on blood culture or PCR testing within the first 7 days of life. Risk factors for peripartum transmission include advanced maternal disease (large viral load, low count of $CD4^+$ lymphocytes), prolonged rupture of membranes, obstetric complications, and first-born twin.

Postpartum transmission occurs mainly through breastfeeding, mostly by mothers with acute seroconversion. Breastfeeding remains the recommended method of feeding in developing countries, whereas in the United States, breastfeeding is contraindicated if the mother is infected, given the availability of safe alternatives and the risk for transmission.

The *perinatal transmission of HIV can be reduced by two thirds* when the pregnant mother is treated with oral zidovudine beginning in the second trimester of pregnancy and intravenous zidovudine during delivery, and the infant is treated with oral zidovudine for the first 6 weeks of life. The transmission rate can be reduced further when mothers are treated more aggressively with antiretroviral agents during pregnancy. Other approaches utilizing shorter duration of antiretroviral agents in the mother at the time of delivery, using nevirapine therapy alone or in combination with other antiretroviral agents in the mother, and a single dose of nevirapine in the infant at birth, offer some benefit, but are less effective than the three-part zidovudine regimen or combination antiretroviral therapy during pregnancy. Cesarean delivery prior to rupture of membranes in mothers receiving zidovudine decreases the risk of perinatal transmission (2%), as compared to mothers on zidovudine therapy undergoing vaginal delivery (7%). However, the additional benefits of cesarean delivery in mothers who have low HIV viral loads (<1000/mL) are unknown and may not outweigh the added risk of an operative delivery for the infected woman. In the developing world, postpartum antiretroviral therapy for the mother is being evaluated to prevent breastfeeding transmission of infection.

Diagnosis

HIV infection is difficult to diagnose in young infants because maternal antibodies may persist until 18 months of age. Therefore, tests that reveal the presence of HIV antibodies are *not* useful for infants. *The detection of HIV DNA by PCR is the most reliable test for diagnosing HIV infection in a young infant.* Almost all infected infants will have a positive HIV DNA by the time they are 1 month of age. Antibody tests, such as enzyme immunoassay and Western blot, are reliable in older children (>18 months) unless they are severely malnourished or hypogammaglobulinemic and unable to mount an antibody response. Two tests should be done to confirm the diagnosis. The use of other modalities of diagnosis of HIV infection in infants and children, such as culture and detection of p24 antigen, are not recommended.

Clinical Features

The clinical features of HIV infection in children include:

- Failure to thrive
- Recurrent invasive bacterial infections
- Chronic lymphadenopathy
- Parotitis
- Recurrent diarrhea
- Oral candidiasis
- Hepatosplenomegaly
- Opportunistic infections

- Central nervous system disease, including developmental delay
- Lymphoid interstitial pneumonitis

Common opportunistic infections in children infected with HIV include:

- *Pneumocystis* pneumonia (PCP)
- Candidiasis of the lower respiratory tract or esophagus
- Chronic diarrhea secondary to cryptosporidiosis or isosporiasis
- Cytomegalovirus disease and retinitis
- Severe herpes simplex virus and varicella-zoster virus infections
- Invasive fungal infections
- Mycobacterial infections

PCP is one of the most common serious opportunistic infection in HIV-infected infants and children. It generally develops between 3 and 6 months of life and may be the presenting manifestation of HIV infection. An acute presentation, in which tachypnea and oxygen desaturation lead to respiratory failure, is not uncommon in these infants. Mortality from PCP infection in HIV-infected infants is high despite specific therapy. Trimethoprim/sulfamethoxazole is the drug of choice for the treatment of PCP in infants and children.

General Care of the Child Infected with Human Immunodeficiency Virus

Children with HIV infection should be allowed and encouraged to attend school. The physician and family are not required to reveal the diagnosis to the school or teachers, unless the child has a behavioral issue such as biting or is an infant in diapers. All schools should implement routine infection control procedures for managing exposure to blood or blood-containing fluids, regardless of the source of the blood. Schools should notify all parents when contagious diseases such as varicella and measles are reported in a school.

Most routine childhood vaccines should be administered to HIV-infected children at the appropriate age. Measles-mumps-rubella vaccine should be administered at 12 months of age unless the child has severe immunosuppression, defined as a low percentage (<15%) of CD4$^+$ lymphocytes. The second dose of measles-mumps-rubella vaccine should be administered as soon as 4 weeks after the first dose rather than waiting until school entry. Varicella vaccine should be administered for the HIV-infected child who is asymptomatic or mildly symptomatic and whose percentage of CD4$^+$ lymphocytes is normal.

Prevention of Opportunistic Infections

PCP prophylaxis with trimethoprim/sulfamethoxazole is recommended for all infants with suspected or proven HIV infection:

- Prophylaxis should be initiated at 4 to 6 weeks of age for all HIV-exposed infants until the diagnosis is excluded.

- Children 1 to 5 years infected with HIV should continue PCP prophylaxis unless the count and percentage of CD4$^+$ lymphocytes is greater than 500 cells/μL or >15%, respectively.
- Children 5 years and older, who are infected with HIV, should continue PCP prophylaxis unless the count and percentage of CD4$^+$ lymphocytes is >200 cells/μL or >15%.

Tuberculosis prophylaxis should be utilized for HIV-infected persons whose tuberculin skin test results are positive without evidence of active disease. Varicella-zoster immunoglobulin (or intravenous immune globulin) should be given to an HIV-infected child who is exposed to varicella. Immune globulin is indicated for the HIV-infected child who is exposed to measles, regardless of immunization status.

Antiretroviral Therapy

Antiretroviral therapy is indicated for most HIV-infected children. Recommendations regarding antiretroviral therapy are rapidly changing. In general, treatment is indicated for children who are symptomatic, have evidence of immunosuppression, or are <12 months of age. Treatment should consist of at least three antiretroviral agents, which is more effective than monotherapy. A protease inhibitor or a non-nucleoside reverse transcriptase inhibitor should be part of the regimen whenever possible. The desired goal of therapy is to decrease the viral load in the blood to undetectable levels.

FUNGAL INFECTIONS

Infections Caused by Dimorphic Pathogenic Fungi

Histoplasma, Blastomyces, and *Coccidioides* can cause localized and disseminated disease in normal and immunocompromised hosts, but most frequently cause asymptomatic infection. *Sporothrix schenckii* causes lymphocutaneous and cutaneous disease, usually without systemic signs and symptoms. The epidemiology and major clinical features of the dimorphic pathogenic fungi are summarized in **Table 49.1**.

Histoplasma capsulatum infection is endemic in the Ohio, Mississippi, and Missouri river valleys, and the skin test results of more than 50% of persons living in areas of endemicity are positive for the organism. *H. capsulatum* can be found in caves, attics, old buildings, and animal roosts. Person-to-person or animal-to-human transmission does not occur.

Ninety-five percent of infections are asymptomatic. Symptomatic infection may present with pulmonary, cutaneous, or disseminated disease. Most pulmonary disease is mild and brief and may be accompanied by hilar adenopathy and a mediastinal mass. More severe disease can develop, and may be accompanied by erythema nodosum,

TABLE 49.1

EPIDEMIOLOGY AND CLINICAL FEATURES OF DIMORPHIC PATHOGENIC FUNGI

Organism	Epidemiology	Clinical Features of Symptomatic Infection
Histoplasma capsulatum	Ohio and Mississippi river valleys; bat or bird droppings; caves	Acute influenza-like pulmonary illness Hilar adenopathy, mediastinal mass Disseminated disease in infants: fever, hepatosplenomegaly, adenopathy, pancytopenia
Blastomyces dermatitidis	Southeastern and central states; Uncommon in children	Acute pneumonia Cutaneous and bone involvement Chronic forms common
Coccidioides immitis	Southwestern United States	Acute pneumonia Disseminated disease with meningitis Bone and cutaneous involvement Hypersensitivity reactions (erythema nodosum, arthralgias/arthritis)
Sporothrix schenckii	Missouri and Mississippi river valleys. Rosebushes, barberry, grass species. Disease of gardeners, farmers	Lymphocutaneous or cutaneous disease Papule at inoculation site Ulcers and nodules along lymphatic chain. Satellite lesions

hepatosplenomegaly, and migratory arthritis. Disseminated disease may be acute, subacute, or chronic and most commonly involves the liver, spleen, lymph nodes, adrenal glands, and bone marrow. Eighty percent of cases of disseminated disease occur in immunosuppressed hosts, especially patients with malignancy and HIV infection. An acute form of histoplasmosis, most common in infants, manifests as overwhelming infection associated with high fever, hepatosplenomegaly, lymphadenopathy, pneumonia, and pancytopenia.

The diagnosis can be established histologically by demonstrating the organism or culturing it from peripheral blood, bone marrow aspirates, or bronchoalveolar lavage fluid. Immunodiffusion and complement fixation serologic techniques are often utilized for diagnostic purposes.

Patients with chronic pulmonary involvement, disseminated disease, or complications of infection are treated with antifungal therapy. Amphotericin B remains the most frequently utilized agent for initial therapy.

Coccidioides immitis can be found in the soil in the southwestern United States, including New Mexico, Arizona, and the central valley of California, regions where infection is endemic. The organism is acquired most often by inhalation. Person-to-person transmission does not occur.

Sixty percent of infections are asymptomatic. Most symptomatic infections manifest as pulmonary or disseminated disease. Pulmonary disease can range from mild flu-like illness to severe pneumonia that generally presents with fever, cough, and chest pain. A transient maculopapular skin rash occurs early in the infection in about half of symptomatic children. Hypersensitivity reactions, especially erythema nodosum, arthritis, and arthralgias, may develop during the course of the infection. Pulmonary infiltrates with perihilar adenopathy and pleural effusions

are common radiographic findings. Disseminated disease may develop a few weeks to a few months after the initial infection. The risk of disseminated disease is significantly higher in infants, Filipinos, African Americans, Hispanics, and immunocompromised persons. Meningitis is the most important feature of disseminated disease, and is associated with significant morbidity and mortality. *Coccidioides* meningitis can be acute or indolent, and may mimic tuberculous meningitis. Examination of the spinal fluid reveals a mononuclear pleocytosis with decreased levels of glucose and elevated levels of protein.

The diagnosis usually relies on serologic assays of blood and spinal fluid and on histopathology from infected body fluid sites.

Antifungal therapy is reserved for persons who have severe pulmonary and disseminated infection or who are at increased risk for disseminated disease. Amphotericin B is the drug of choice for serious infections not involving the central nervous system. Fluconazole is recommended for CNS infections, and is utilized for suppressive therapy, because recurrence of meningitis is not uncommon.

Opportunistic Fungal Infections

Candida species are dimorphic yeast organisms that not uncommonly colonize the mouth and the gastrointestinal and genitourinary tracts of humans. Their ability to cause disease depends on the host's ability to deal with them. The organisms are common causes of nosocomial infections, especially in:

- Premature neonates
- Children with malignancies or in whom central venous catheters have been placed
- Organ transplant recipients
- Persons with immunodeficiency syndromes

Manifestations of infection are both local and disseminated.

Cryptococcus neoformans is an encapsulated budding yeast that can be found in avian habitats, especially pigeon roosting sites. This yeast causes disease almost exclusively in immunocompromised patients. A subacute or chronic meningitis is the most common manifestation of infection in children. Headaches, mental status changes, vomiting, and meningeal signs are common. Cerebrospinal fluid (CSF) examination reveals a lymphocytic pleocytosis with an increased protein level, decreased glucose level, and elevated opening pressures. India ink examination may demonstrate the capsule of the organism, and aids in the diagnosis. Latex particle agglutination in specimens of serum and CSF fluid is more sensitive and specific diagnostically. A combination of amphotericin B and flucytosine is used to treat cryptococcal meningitis.

Aspergillus species are found in air, soil, water, and decaying vegetation. They can cause hypersensitivity reactions and both noninvasive and invasive disease. Allergic bronchopulmonary aspergillosis occurs in atopic children with a history of asthma and cystic fibrosis. Wheezing, pulmonary infiltrates, eosinophilia, elevated levels of immunoglobulin E (IgE) and IgG antibodies to *A. fumigatus*, and elevated IgE concentrations are characteristic.

Predisposing factors for invasive aspergillosis include:

- Corticosteroid therapy
- Neutropenia
- Cytotoxic chemotherapy
- Acute organ rejection

Invasive pulmonary aspergillosis is an acute life-threatening infection characterized by invasion of blood vessels, infarction, necrosis, and hematogenous dissemination to the brain, heart, liver, and other organs. Sinusitis, ocular infection, and endocarditis are other manifestations of invasive *Aspergillus* infection.

The mucormycoses are a group of opportunistic fungal infections associated with vessel invasion, tissue necrosis, and thrombosis. The organisms are easily isolated from soil and commonly found on fruit and bread mold. Infection is limited to children with risk factors, including poorly controlled diabetes with acidosis, malignancy, neutropenia, uremia, and burns. Rhinocerebral disease is the most common form in children and manifests with pain, facial swelling and tenderness, proptosis, and altered mental status. Rhinocerebral disease is seen mainly in children with diabetic ketoacidosis and is associated with a high mortality rate. Cranial nerve involvement and cavernous sinus thrombosis are not uncommon. Treatment involves surgical resection of the involved tissue, correction of the metabolic abnormalities, and administration of amphotericin B.

MYCOBACTERIAL DISEASE IN CHILDREN

Tuberculosis

Epidemiology

Mycobacterium tuberculosis, an acid-fast bacillus, is the usual etiologic agent of tuberculosis. Tuberculosis, although rare in the United States, can cause devastating infection, especially in infants and young children. Foreign-born and homeless persons, residents of correctional facilities, first-generation immigrants from high-risk countries, and people living in urban, low-income areas have the highest rates of infection. The organism is transmitted when droplet nuclei produced by an adult or postpubertal adolescent with cavitary, pulmonary disease are inhaled. Children with pulmonary tuberculosis are *not* usually contagious because the organism burden is small, they do not have cavitary disease, and cough is minimal or nonexistent. Therefore, for every child in whom tuberculosis is diagnosed, a contagious adult contact must be sought vigorously.

The development of a positive result of a tuberculin skin test, which normally occurs between 2 and 12 weeks after initial infection, indicates likely *infection* in an individual. A person with a positive tuberculin skin test result who has no physical findings of disease and normal findings on a chest radiograph has *latent tuberculous infection*. Tuberculosis *disease* is defined by the presence of pulmonary or extrapulmonary manifestations of *M. tuberculosis* in a person with infection.

Clinical Manifestations

Most infected children are asymptomatic. The interval between infection and disease may be several weeks to many years. *Infants and postpubertal adolescents with recent exposure to infectious adults are at highest risk for progression to disease.* Other persons at high risk for progression to disease include recent skin test converters and those who are immunodeficient or who are receiving immunosuppressive therapy.

Early disease (1–6 months after infection) in children can present with lymphadenopathy and pulmonary or extrapulmonary manifestations. Hilar, mediastinal, cervical, and supraclavicular lymph nodes may be involved. Pulmonary findings may include lobar or segmental involvement, pleural effusion, or miliary disease (Fig. 49.1). Extrapulmonary disease includes miliary tuberculosis and meningitis. Late disease (months to years after infection) represents reactivation of latent infection and may involve the middle ear, mastoids, bones, joints, and skin.

Meningitis and miliary tuberculosis are especially common in infants and young children. *Tuberculous meningitis* is most commonly characterized by a gradual onset during 2 to 3 weeks. Fever, listlessness, and irritability are common initially. These are followed by nuchal rigidity, signs of increased intracranial pressure, cranial nerve palsies

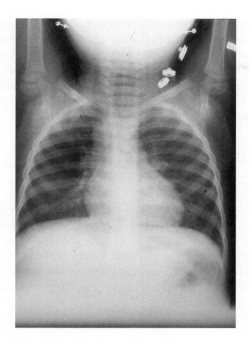

Figure 49.1 Miliary tuberculosis in an infant.

(especially of nerves III, VI, and VII), and seizures. Without therapy, neurologic progression to altered consciousness and posturing occurs. The CSF findings most commonly include:

- White blood cells 50 to 500/mm³ (neutrophils early, lymphocyte predominance later)
- Hypoglycorrhachia
- Elevated protein level

Diagnosis

Tuberculin skin testing is utilized to screen for tuberculosis infection in asymptomatic persons. The 5-tuberculin unit Mantoux intradermal skin test is the *only* recommended skin test and should be placed and interpreted by well-trained professionals. The American Academy of Pediatrics recommends that *only infants, children, and adolescents with factors that put them at high risk for tuberculosis be tested on a regular basis.* These include:

- Children infected with HIV or living with an HIV-infected person: annual testing
- Incarcerated adolescents: annual testing

Children at highest risk for tuberculosis should undergo immediate tuberculin skin testing. These include:

- Children who have contact with persons having confirmed or suspected active tuberculosis
- Children with clinical or radiographic features of tuberculosis
- Immigrants from regions of endemicity
- Children returning from areas of endemicity

The size of the induration produced by a skin test, in addition to the specific epidemiologic and clinical factors of the patient being tested, determine how the test result is interpreted:

- *An induration of 15 mm or larger is considered a positive test result in children who are 4 years of age or older, and have no risk factors for tuberculosis.*
- An induration of 10 mm or larger is considered a positive test result in children who are younger than 4 years or have any chronic conditions, or whose exposure to tuberculosis disease is deemed to be increased. This includes children born in or travel to high-prevalence areas, or who are exposed to adults who are at high risk for tuberculosis.
- An induration of 5 mm or larger is considered a positive result in children who:
  - Have been in close contact with individuals who have had or suspected to have had tuberculosis
  - Have clinical or radiographic evidence of tuberculosis disease
  - Are immunocompromised (including those with HIV infection)

Because approximately 10% of healthy children with culture-confirmed tuberculosis do not react to the tuberculin skin test, a negative test result never rules out tuberculosis. *Previous vaccination with Bacillus Calmette-Guérin (BCG) vaccine should never be a contraindication to skin testing.* The interpretation of skin test results in children previously vaccinated with BCG vaccine should be the same as in those who have not received BCG vaccine. Over time, positive skin test reactions diminish after BCG unless there has been TB infection, as the vaccine does not prevent infection, but only modifies the course.

Children who have a positive tuberculin skin test result should be evaluated with a complete physical examination and chest radiography. Children who are well, have normal physical examination findings, and negative findings on chest radiography are considered to have *latent tuberculous infection*. In children suspected of having clinical or radiographic features of tuberculous disease, appropriate cultures and smears should be taken from suspected sources of infection. Early morning gastric aspirates provide the best chance of recovery of *M. tuberculosis* organisms in the young child with or suspected of having pulmonary tuberculosis. Pleural fluid, sputum, and CSF fluid can be cultured for *M. tuberculosis* as the clinical situation warrants.

Prophylaxis and Treatment

Children who are found to have latent tuberculosis infection and have never been treated with antituberculosis therapy should be given isoniazid prophylaxis for 9 months (12 months if coinfected with HIV). This effectively prevents progression to disease.

TABLE 49.2

ADVERSE EFFECTS AND DRUG INTERACTIONS OF COMMONLY UTILIZED ANTITUBERCULOUS AGENTS

Drug	Adverse Effects/Drug Interactions
Isoniazid	Hepatitis (rare in children)
	Peripheral neuritis (from inhibition of pyridoxine metabolism)
	Increases serum phenytoin levels
Rifampin	Orange discoloration of body fluids
	Influenza-like reaction
	Hepatitis (especially in combination with isoniazid)
	Decreases serum levels of cyclosporine, digoxin, and theophylline
Pyrazinamide	Hyperuricemia
	Hepatotoxicity
Streptomycin	Vestibular and auditory toxicity
	Renal toxicity
Ethambutol	Optic neuritis
	Gastrointestinal toxicity

The treatment of tuberculosis disease should be based on knowledge of the resistance patterns of the organism in the geographic area where the infection occurred. In general, three or four antituberculosis medications should be used initially to treat the disease. When drug resistance is suspected, four drugs should be used initially. Isoniazid, rifampin, pyrazinamide, ethambutol, and streptomycin are the drugs most commonly utilized for the treatment of tuberculosis. Ethambutol is less frequently utilized in infants and young children because it can cause a reversible optic neuritis. Monitoring children for optic neuritis requires monthly tests for visual acuity, visual fields, and red-green color discrimination, which is difficult if not impossible in young children. The adverse effects of the commonly utilized antituberculosis agents are listed in Table 49.2.

Infection with Nontuberculous Mycobacteria

Cervical lymphadenitis is the most common clinical feature of nontuberculous mycobacterial infection in healthy children. *Mycobacterium avium* complex and *Mycobacterium scrofulaceum* are the species most often causing lymphadenitis. These infections most frequently occur in toddlers and are characterized by a subacute or chronic presentation. The insidious onset of a painless, firm, unilateral cervical adenitis is typical. Unlike tuberculosis, these infections are most common in children who live in rural areas and have no risk factors for tuberculosis. Tuberculin skin testing not infrequently reveals reactions of <10 mm. Treatment for these infections should consist of *complete excision of the lymph node*.

Disseminated infection with nontuberculous mycobacteria occurs almost exclusively in immunocompromised persons. Persons with altered cell-mediated immunity,

including those with HIV infection, are at greatest risk. *M. avium* complex organisms are the nontuberculous mycobacteria most commonly isolated from these patients. Features of disseminated infection include fever, weight loss, diarrhea, and night sweats. Disseminated infection caused by *M. avium* complex requires therapy with multiple drugs.

REVIEW EXERCISES

QUESTIONS

1. A 10-month-old infant is seen in your office with a history of fever up to 39.44°C (103°F) for the past 3 days. The child is playful, and the physical examination findings are unremarkable except for fever. No ill contacts are in the home and she does not attend a child care center. Of the following, the *most* likely virus causing this child's fever is:
a) Parvovirus
b) HHV-6
c) Herpes simplex virus
d) Epstein-Barr virus (EBV)
e) Cytomegalovirus

Answer

The answer is b. Of the choices listed, HHV-6 is the most likely etiologic agent. Although HHV-6 is the etiologic agent of exanthem subitum (roseola), the virus is also a very common cause of fever in infants without a rash. In a study from Rochester, New York, HHV-6 was isolated from 14% of febrile infants <2 years presenting to an emergency department. Parvovirus is uncommon in young infants and generally does not cause high fever. Herpes simplex virus is a very uncommon cause of fever without a source. EBV and cytomegalovirus may produce febrile illness without other findings in infants and children but are statistically less common than HHV-6.

2. A 30-year-old teacher calls your office seeking advice. She is 10 weeks pregnant, and an outbreak of *slapped cheek* disease has occurred in her school, with some of the cases in her classroom. Which of the following would be the *best* advice to this teacher?
a) Advise her that the risk to the fetus is low.
b) Recommend ultrasonography to look for hydrops fetalis in the beginning of her third trimester.
c) Recommend referral to a high-risk obstetric service to follow serial ultrasonograms and prepare for *in utero* transfusions.
d) Recommend that she take a leave of absence from work until the outbreak is over.

Answer

The answer is a. Infection with HPV can result in erythema infectiosum, also called *slapped cheek disease* because of the characteristic rash it produces. School-age children are at greatest risk for infection with this organism. HPV has also been associated with the development of nonimmune hydrops fetalis when it infects pregnant women. However, the risk for hydrops fetalis is estimated to be low given that >50% of women are seropositive for HPV before pregnancy, the transmission rate to susceptible contacts is 30% to 50%, and the estimated risk for fetal loss once infection occurs is 2% to 6%. Children with erythema infectiosum are not contagious at the time the rash appears, and asymptomatic infection is very common. For all these reasons, excluding pregnant women from the workplace where HPV is prevalent is *not* recommended.

3. A 6-month-old infant born to a woman with HIV infection is seen in your office with a 3-day history of upper respiratory infection symptoms and cough. A high fever has developed today, and on examination she is mildly tachypneic but has no other focal findings. Chest radiograph reveals a fine, diffuse infiltrate. Appropriate interventions at this point would include all of the following *except:*

a) Obtaining a nasopharyngeal swab and performing direct fluorescent antibody testing for respiratory syncytial virus, adenovirus, parainfluenza virus, and influenza virus

b) Obtaining a blood culture from the infant and commencing ceftriaxone therapy

c) Administering high-dose intravenous trimethoprim/sulfamethoxazole to the infant

d) Sending a sample of the infant's serum for HIV antibody testing

Answer

The answer is d. For a 6-month-old infant born to an HIV-infected mother and presenting with fever and a diffuse pneumonitis, PCP should certainly be included in the differential diagnosis, and because of the potential severity and mortality of this infection, empiric high-dose trimethoprim/sulfamethoxazole therapy (trimethoprim component 20 mg/kg/day) is indicated. Viral agents, including respiratory syncytial virus, influenza virus, parainfluenza virus, and adenovirus, may cause fever and a diffuse pneumonitis in healthy and immunocompromised persons. It is important to include bacterial pneumonia in the differential diagnosis of any ill infant with pneumonia. In addition, HIV-infected infants frequently become infected with bacterial pathogens such as *Streptococcus pneumoniae* and *Haemophilus influenzae*. Therefore, therapy with ceftriaxone after appropriate blood cultures have been obtained is warranted. Serologic testing for HIV antibodies is not appropriate in this infant, whose mother is known to be infected with HIV, because placentally transferred maternal antibodies will be present. HIV infection can be diagnosed in the infant by utilizing nucleic acid detection assays (PCR DNA).

4. A 3-year-old boy has had swollen lymph nodes in the left anterior cervical chain for several weeks. He has had low-grade fever but no other significant illness. He lives in a suburban area, is not in child care, and has no known exposure to anyone with tuberculosis. The induration of his purified protein derivative test measures 9 mm. His chest radiographic findings are normal. The *best* therapy for this child is:

a) Course of isoniazid, rifampin, and pyrazinamide

b) Biopsy of the node mass for culture

c) Course of clarithromycin and rifampin

d) Excision of the lymph node

Answer

The answer is d. Lymphadenitis caused by nontuberculous mycobacteria is the most likely diagnosis in this child, who has a subacute cervical lymphadenitis, a purified protein derivative test induration measuring 9 mm, a chest radiograph negative for lymphadenitis, and no risk factors for tuberculosis. The best course of action when a patient has adenitis caused by nontuberculous mycobacteria is complete excision of the node. Biopsy of the lymph node may be complicated by fistulous tract formation and is not recommended. Medical therapy with antituberculous therapy is generally not effective; although many species of nontuberculous mycobacteria are susceptible in vitro to clarithromycin and rifampin, these agents are of limited clinical use for this problem.

5. A 3-year-old Filipino girl from Arizona presents with a 3-week. history of headaches, increasing confusion, and fever. Her past medical history is unremarkable. Examination of her spinal fluid reveals 52 lymphocytes/mm^3, a protein level of 90 mg/dL, and a glucose level of 35 mg/dL. The organism *most* likely to cause this clinical picture is:

a) *C. immitis*

b) *H. capsulatum*

c) *S. schenckii*

d) *C. neoformans*

Answer

The answer is a. The spinal fluid findings reveal lymphocytic meningitis, which can be fungal or tuberculous. The epidemiologic clues to the diagnosis include the following: this girl is from Arizona, where *C. immitis* infection is endemic; she is a Filipino, so that her risk for disseminated disease with *C. immitis* is greatly increased, and she is previously healthy. *C. neoformans* can cause a similar clinical picture, but infection with this agent occurs almost exclusively in immunocompromised persons.

SUGGESTED READINGS

1. American Academy of Pediatrics. Human Immunodeficiency Virus Infection. In: Pickering LK, Baker CJ, Long SS, McMillan JA, eds. *Red book: 2006Report of the Committee on Infectious Diseases*, 27th ed. Elk Grove Village, IL: American Academy of Pediatrics, 2006:378–401.
2. American Academy of Pediatrics. Tuberculosis. In: Pickering LK, Baker CJ, Long SS, McMillan JA, eds. *Red book: 2006Report of the Committee on Infectious Diseases*, 27th ed. Elk Grove Village, IL: American Academy of Pediatrics, 2006:678–698.
3. American Academy of Pediatrics. Targeted tuberculin skin testing and treatment of latent tuberculosis infection in children and adolescents. *Pediatrics* 2004;114:S1175–S1201.
4. Caserta MT, Mock DJ, Dewhurst S. Human herpesvirus 6. *Clin Infect Dis* 2001;33:829–833.
5. Connor EM, Sperling RS, Gelber R, et al. Reduction of maternal–infant transmission of human immunodeficiency virus type 1 with zidovudine treatment. *NEJM* 1994;331:1173–1180.
6. European Collaborative Study. Mother-to-child transmission of HIV infection in the era of highly active antiretroviral therapy. *Clin Infect Dis* 2005;40:458–465.
7. Hall CB, Long CE, Schnabel KC. Human herpesvirus 6 infection in children. *NEJM* 1994;331:432–438.
8. Loeffler AM. Treatment options for nontuberculous mycobacterial adenitis in children. *Pediatr Infect Dis J* 2004;23:957–958.
9. Pruksananonda P, Hall CB, Insel RA, et al. Primary human herpesvirus 6 infection in young children. *N EnglJ Med* 1992;326: 1445–1450.
10. Stevens DA. Coccidioidomycosis. *NEJM* 1995;332:1077–1082.
11. Wolinsky E. Mycobacterial diseases other than tuberculosis. *Clin Infect Dis* 1992;15:1–12.
12. Young NS, Brown KE. Parvovirus B19. *NEJM* 2004;350:586–597.
13. Zerr DM, Meier AS, Selke SS, et al. A population–based study of primary human herpesvirus 6 infection. *NEJM* 2005;352: 768–776.

Chapter 50

Infectious Diseases, Part III

Lara Danziger-Isakov and Camille Sabella

This chapter includes discussions of selected tick-borne, zoonotic, and parasitic infections.

TICK-BORNE AND ZOONOTIC INFECTIONS

Rocky Mountain Spotted Fever

Rocky Mountain spotted fever (RMSF), caused by *Rickettsia rickettsii*, is the most prevalent rickettsial disease in the United States. It is most common in the southeastern and south central regions of the United States. Ticks, wild animals, and dogs serve as reservoirs of infection, and a tick bite is the usual mode of transmission. Children younger than 15 years account for two thirds of cases, and the disease is most common in spring and summer.

R. rickettsii causes a vasculitis that clinically manifests with fever, headache, rash, myalgias, and changes in mental status. *The rash can be maculopapular or petechial and usually begins peripherally on the wrist and ankle and spreads centripetally.* The palms and soles are commonly involved. Leukopenia, thrombocytopenia, anemia, elevated levels of aminotransferases and bilirubin, and hyponatremia are common laboratory findings.

A definitive diagnosis often cannot be made until the second week of illness because serologic assays are not sensitive early in the course of the disease. Fluorescent or peroxidase-tagged antibody tests of specimens from skin lesions can provide a rapid and highly specific diagnosis.

The differential diagnosis of RMSF includes:

- Meningococcemia
- Ehrlichiosis
- Atypical measles
- Enteroviral infection
- Henoch-Schönlein purpura
- Leptospirosis

Because the diagnosis often cannot be confirmed until the second week of the illness, a high index of suspicion and presumptive therapy is required. The institution of antimicrobial therapy within 6 days of the onset of illness is associated with low mortality. *Doxycycline is the treatment of choice for children of any age;* although the tetracyclines are generally contraindicated in children <8 years of age, doxycycline is recommended for the treatment of RMSF, regardless of age, given the effectiveness of this therapy, the low adverse effect profile even in young children, and the lack of effective alternative antimicrobials. Severe morbidity and mortality from cardiac failure, vascular collapse, and renal failure can occur and are usually related to a delayed diagnosis.

Ehrlichiosis

Human monocytic ehrlichiosis is caused by *Ehrlichia chaffeensis;* human granulocytic ehrlichiosis is caused by *Anaplasma* (formerly *Ehrlichia*) *phagocytophila* and *Ehrlichia ewingii.* Both forms of ehrlichiosis are transmitted by a tick bite; known reservoirs include the white-tailed deer and white-footed mouse. *E. chaffeensis* infections occur mainly in the southeastern and south central regions of the United States; most cases of human granulocytic ehrlichiosis have occurred in Wisconsin, Minnesota, Connecticut, and New York. The infections generally develop in spring and summer, and adults appear to be at greatest risk, although infection with *E. chaffeensis* is common in children. Immunocompromised individuals appear to be at greatest risk for severe infection.

The clinical features of the two types of human *Ehrlichia* infection are similar and also quite similar to the clinical features of RMSF. Rash is less common in ehrlichiosis, whereas anemia, leukopenia, and thrombocytopenia are more common in ehrlichiosis than in RMSF.

The identification of intraleukocytic inclusions (morulae) in peripheral blood monocytes (Fig. 50.1) or granulocytes and acute and convalescent serologic titers are used to confirm the diagnosis.

Doxycycline is the drug of choice for the treatment of Ehrlichiosis in children of any age.

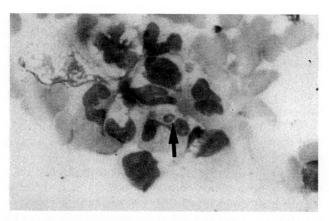

Figure 50.1 Peripheral blood smear showing an intraleukocytic inclusion (morula), characteristic of *Ehrlichia* infection. (See color insert.)

Tularemia

The etiologic agent of tularemia is *Francisella tularensis*, a small gram-negative coccobacillus. Important reservoirs of infection include rabbits, hares, and ticks. The most important route of transmission is a tick bite, but transmission can also result from direct contact with infected animals, aerosolization of the organism, or ingestion of contaminated water or meat. Infection is most common in the central states of Arkansas, Missouri, Tennessee, and Texas between the months of April and September.

The ulceroglandular form is the most common form of infection and is characterized by fever, regional lymphadenopathy, and skin lesions, usually an ulcer or papule at the site of inoculation. Pharyngitis, myalgias, vomiting, and hepatosplenomegaly may be present. Other forms of disease may also occur (glandular, pneumonic, oculoglandular), depending on the portal of entry of the organism.

A history of exposure to the organism *(tick bite, close contact with rabbits)* along with the characteristic clinical picture should lead the examiner to suspect tularemia. Serologic testing may be helpful diagnostically.

Streptomycin is the drug of choice, with gentamicin an effective alternative.

Leptospirosis

Leptospira organisms are spirochetes found in many wild and domestic mammals, including dogs, rats, and livestock. Transmission to humans results from contact with water and soil infected with the organism or from direct contact with infected animals. *Contaminated farm ponds and animal slaughterhouses* are settings in which transmission occurs.

Subclinical infection is most common, but clinical illness can manifest in either an anicteric (milder) or icteric (severe) form. Anicteric disease accounts for 90% of cases and presents with an abrupt onset of fever, headache, myalgia, and subconjunctival suffusion; a second phase of disease often follows, characterized by fever, rash, uveitis, and meningitis. The organism can be recovered from the blood and spinal fluid in the first phase of illness, and from the urine in the second phase. Icteric leptospirosis, also known as *Weil syndrome*, occurs in 10% of cases and is characterized by severe illness with liver and renal failure, hemorrhage, and myocarditis.

Special laboratory techniques are required to recover the organism. Serologic assays are utilized in confirming the diagnosis.

Most cases are self-limited. Patients with severe disease requiring hospitalization should be treated with intravenous penicillin. Amoxicillin and doxycycline (for children 8 years of age and older) are alternative therapies for patients with mild disease.

Lyme Disease

Borrelia burgdorferi is the etiologic agent of Lyme disease. Infected ticks serve as the vectors of transmission. Reservoirs include the white-footed mouse, birds, lizards, and deer. In the United States, most cases of Lyme disease are seen in the northeastern states, upper Midwest (Minnesota and Wisconsin), and northern California. Most cases occur between April and October.

The clinical manifestations can be categorized as:

- *Early localized disease*, occurring 3 days to 4 weeks after a tick bite
- *Early disseminated disease*, developing 4 weeks to 8 weeks after infection
- *Late disease*, occurring 2 months to several years after infection

In *early localized disease*, erythema migrans (Figs. 50.2, 50.3) develops at the site of the tick bite, which may or may not be recalled. Erythema migrans begins as an erythematous papule that expands to become an annular lesion measuring 3 to 15 cm, often with central clearing but occa-

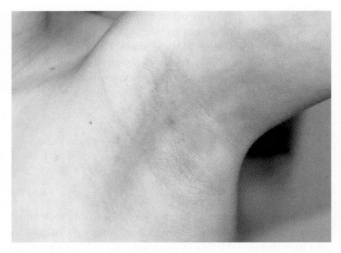

Figure 50.3 Annular lesion of erythema migrans in the axilla of a 12-year-old boy who presented with fever and this rash following a camping trip to eastern Pennsylvania. Note the presence of a small vesicle at the center of the lesion. (See color insert.)

sionally with a vesicular center. Multiple small lesions may also be present. Biopsy of the lesion with special culture media often reveals the organism. The lesion is frequently confused with ringworm, a spider bite, or nummular eczema. Nonspecific symptoms, such as fever, malaise, and arthralgias, may be present at this stage. Antibodies to *B. burgdorferi* are consistently absent at this stage of infection and remain so in persons who receive treatment at this stage. Although most untreated persons recover completely without further disease, late manifestations of Lyme disease develop in approximately 20% of untreated cases.

Features of *early disseminated disease* include:

- Multiple circular lesions
- Flu-like illness
- Neuritis (seventh cranial nerve palsy)
- Aseptic meningitis
- Carditis

Meningitis develops in a small percentage of untreated persons and manifests as headache, photophobia, and neck stiffness. The CSF fluid is aseptic with a lymphocytic pleocytosis, mildly elevated protein level, and normal glucose level. The diagnosis can be confirmed by demonstrating the intrathecal production of specific antibodies. *Seventh cranial nerve palsy* is more common than meningitis and is self-limited. Treatment does not alter the course of the neuritis but prevents late complications of infection. *Carditis* is quite uncommon, occurring in <5% of infected persons, and usually manifests as a transient alternating heart block.

Lyme *arthritis* is by far the most frequent manifestation of *late disease*. Lyme arthritis is characterized by involvement of the knee in >90% of cases and may be monoarticular or pauciarticular. The course may be chronic and intermittently flaring. Encephalopathy and polyneuropathies occur very rarely.

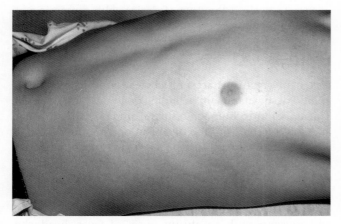

Figure 50.2 Erythema migrans in an adolescent with Lyme disease. Note the annular lesion with central clearing, characteristic of the rash. (See color insert.)

Early in the course of infection the diagnosis can be made clinically based on the appearance of the characteristic rash in a patient from an area in which Lyme disease is endemic. Routine serologic tests are *not* indicated in children with typical symptoms. Serologic tests can be helpful in diagnosing later stages of Lyme disease when the appropriate clinical features are present. This should be accomplished using an enzyme immunoassay and *confirmed* by Western immunoblot testing. When serologic tests are considered, only reference laboratories should be utilized. Serologic studies are not recommended for children with nonspecific symptoms whose probability of having Lyme disease is low, because these tests can be nonspecific.

The treatment recommendations for children with Lyme disease are summarized in **Table 50.1**. When children are treated according to these recommendations, the outcome is excellent. Prolonged (beyond the periods specified in Table 50.1) or repeated courses of antimicrobial therapy for Lyme disease are *not* indicated. Chemoprophylaxis following a tick bite, even for people living in areas of endemicity, is not routinely recommended.

Rat Bite Fever

Rat bite fever is caused by *Streptobacillus moniliformis* (more common in the United States) or *Spirillum minus*, which live in the upper respiratory tract of rodents. Rats are the most common source of infection, but other rodents, including mice, squirrels, and gerbils, can serve as additional reservoirs.

Symptoms of rat bite fever include abrupt onset of fever, myalgias, emesis, and headache. A maculopapular or petechial rash on the extremities is common; however, the bite site commonly heals quickly and is no longer visible at presentation. Migratory polyarthritis occurs in about 50% of patients, whereas pneumonia, endocarditis, and meningitis are rare. Without specific treatment, a relapsing course of symptoms can occur for several weeks. The diagnosis requires clinical suspicion. Recovery of *S. moniliformis* from the blood requires enriched culture media and prolonged incubation for up to 3 weeks.

Treatment with penicillin G for 7 to 10 days is recommended. Doxycycline or streptomycin can be substituted for penicillin-allergic patients. Therapy for 4 weeks with high-dose intravenous penicillin G is suggested for endocarditis.

Plague

The etiologic agent of plague is *Yersinia pestis*, a gram-negative coccobacillus. Plague manifests in several forms, including bubonic (most common), septicemic, or pneumonic forms. Uncommon presentations include meningeal, ocular, pharyngeal, or gastrointestinal plague. All presentations include fever and malaise. Buboes (painful lymph node swelling) commonly develop in the inguinal, axillary, and cervical regions. Infections most commonly occur in the western United States, including New Mexico, Arizona, California, and Colorado during the summers after mild winters or wet springs.

Y. pestis is spread from rodents by fleas through bites or by direct contact with infected animals. Pneumonic plague results from inhalation or infected respiratory droplets. The diagnosis of plague is confirmed by isolation of *Y. pestis* from blood, bubo aspirate, or other specimen. Rapid diagnosis by PCR testing is available is some public health laboratories. Serologic testing can be confirmatory with fourfold rise is antibody titer 4 weeks to several months after infection.

Streptomycin is the treatment of choice in children; Gentamicin is an alternative. Doxycycline is an alternative (children ≥8 years of age). Surgical drainage of buboes may be required.

TABLE 50.1

TREATMENT OF LYME DISEASE IN CHILDREN

Stage of Illness	Treatment Recommendations
Early localized disease	
≥8 years old	Doxycycline 100 mg orally twice a day for 14–21 days
All ages	Amoxicillin 50 mg/kg/day (maximum 1.5 g/day) for 14–21 days, *OR* Cefuroxime 30 mg/kg/day (maximum 1000 mg/day) for 14–21 days
Early disseminated and late disease	
Multiple erythema migrans	Same oral regimen as for early localized disease but for 21 days
Meningitis	Ceftriaxone 75–100 mg/kg (maximum 2 g/day) IV for 14–28 days, *or* Penicillin G 300,000 U/kg/day (maximum 20 million U/day) IV for 14–28 days
Isolated facial palsy	Same oral regimen as for early localized disease but for 21–28 days
Carditis	Same as for meningitis
Arthritis	Same oral regimen as for early localized disease but for 28 days
Persistent or recurrent arthritis	Ceftriaxone 75 mg/kg IV or IM for 14–21 days, *or* Penicillin G 300,000 U/kg/day IV for 14–28 days, *or* same oral regimen as for early disease

IM, intramuscular; IV, intravenous.

PARASITIC INFECTIONS

Protozoa

Discussions on important protozoal infections, including Giardiasis, *Entamoeba histolytica*, and *Cryptosporidium* infections can be found in Chapter 48. A discussion on *Toxoplasma* infections can be found in Chapter 22. A discussion of *Trichomonas* infection is found in Chapter 45.

Malaria (*Plasmodium* Infections)

The four important species that cause human infections include *P. falciparum*, *P. vivax*, *P. ovale*, and *P. malariae*. Malaria is endemic throughout the tropical areas of the world and is acquired from the bite of the female *Anopheles* mosquito. Most reported malaria cases in the United States are acquired in areas of the world in which malaria is endemic. This risk of acquiring malaria is highest among travelers to sub-Saharan Africa, intermediate among travelers to the Indian subcontinent, and relatively low in most of Southeast Asia and Latin America.

The classic clinical manifestations of malaria include paroxysms of high fever, chills, headache, rigors, nausea, vomiting, diarrhea, abdominal pain, malaise, myalgias, and arthralgias. Pallor and jaundice, secondary to hemolysis, may also be apparent. Common laboratory abnormalities include a normochromic hemolytic anemia secondary to hemolysis, thrombocytopenia, and hypoglycemia.

Features of *P falciparum* infection include a nonspecific influenza-like illness, potentially rapidly fatal course, and drug resistance. Infection with this species is associated with:

- Hyperparasitemia (>5%)
- Cerebral malaria (altered mental status, seizures)
- Severe anemia secondary to hemolysis

- Respiratory failure
- Renal failure
- Metabolic acidosis
- Hypoglycemia
- Vascular collapse and shock

Feature of infection with *P. vivax* and *P. ovale* include:

- Anemia
- Hypersplenism
- Relapse

Relapse after infection with these species is secondary to a latent hepatic stage, and may occur many years after the primary infection.

Infection with *P. malariae* is associated with chronic asymptomatic parasitemia and nephrotic syndrome.

Definitive diagnosis of malaria relies on the identification of parasites on stained blood films. The *thick* smear should be performed to find parasites that may be present in small numbers. A *thin* smear should be performed to identify the specific species causing the infection and to estimate the degree of parasitemia. Identification of the specific species causing the infection is important in guiding therapy.

Antimalarial therapy should take into account the severity of infection, the likelihood of chloroquine-resistant infections, and the infecting species. Severe malaria is defined by a parasitemia of $> 5\%$ of red blood cells, or signs of end-organ involvement. Patients who exhibit signs of severe malaria should be managed in an intensive care unit and treated with parenteral antimalarial therapy. For specific treatment recommendations (Table 50.2).

Travelers to malaria-endemic regions should receive chemoprophylaxis. Appropriate chemoprophylaxis for malaria should be determined by the traveler's risk of acquiring malaria and the risk of exposure to chloroquine-

TABLE 50.2

TREATMENT OF MALARIA

Clinical Scenario	Drugs of Choice	Comments
Severe malaria requiring parenteral therapy	Quinidine or quinine	Need to monitor continuous blood pressure, ECG, and glucose
P falciparum acquired in areas areas of chloroquine-resistance	Atovaquone/Proguanil, or Quinine sulfate plus doxycycline, or plus tetracycline, or plus clindamycin	Tetracyclines are contraindicated in children <8 years of age and in pregnancy
P vivax acquired in areas of chloroquine-resistance	Quinine sulfate plus doxycycline OR Mefloquine	Tetracyclines are contraindicated in children <8 years of age and in pregnancy
All *Plasmodium* species except chloroquine-resistant *P falciparum* and *P. vivax*	Chloroquine phosphate	
Prevention of relapse: *P. vivax* and *P. ovale* only	Primaquine phosphate	May cause hemolytic anemia, especially in patients with G-6-PD deficiency; thus patients should be screened for G-6-PD deficiency before treatment

Adapted from: American Academy of Pediatrics. Drugs for parasitic infections. In: Pickering LK, Baker CJ, Long SS, McMillan JA, eds. *Red Book: 2006 Report of the Committee on Infectious Diseases*, 27th ed. Elk Grove Village, IL: American Academy of Pediatrics, 2006:803–809.

resistant infections. Travelers to areas in which chloroquine-resistant malaria has not been reported should be prophylaxed with chloroquine. This drug is well tolerated, and the main adverse effects include gastrointestinal disturbances, headache, dizziness, and blurred vision. For travelers for areas in which chloroquine-resistant strains have been reported, prophylaxis with atovaquone/proguanil or Mefloquine should be used. Mefloquine is contraindicated in patients with depression or a history of depression, people with anxiety disorders, psychosis, and other major psychiatric disturbances, and individuals with a history of cardiac conduction abnormalities.

Babesiosis

Babesia microti are intraerythrocytic protozoa spread by ticks. Although most infections are asymptomatic, symptomatic cases include fever, malaise, myalgias, arthralgias, and headache. Mild splenomegaly, hepatomegaly, and conjunctival injection can also occur. Symptoms and severe illness are more likely in *asplenic and immunocompromised patients.*

The same tick, *Ixodes scapularis*, which transmits the agents of Lyme disease and Ehrlichiosis, can spread *B. microti* from the white-footed deer mouse to humans. Most infections occur in from late spring though the fall. Stains of thick and thin blood smears identify the organisms. Concurrent infection with *B. burgdorferi* (Lyme disease) should be considered.

Babesiosis can be treated with a combination of antimicrobials including clindamycin plus oral quinine or atovaquone plus azithromycin. Exchange blood transfusions with severe illness or high levels of parasitemia (≥10% of blood cells) may be utilized.

Intestinal Nematodes (Roundworms)

Ascaris lumbricoides Infections

Ascariasis is the most prevalent helminthic infection of humans. In the United States, infection occurs as an imported infection from tropical countries, in internationally adopted children and in the southeastern United States. Knowledge of the life cycle is important, as the clinical manifestations are attributed to the migration of adult worms and larvae. The life cycle begins with ingestion of infective eggs from soil. Larvae hatch in the small intestine, invade the mucosa and are transported to the liver and the lungs. The larvae then ascend to the trachea, are swallowed, and then *migrate* to the small intestine, where they mature into adult worms and lay infective eggs.

During the larval migratory phase, a *pneumonitis* may develop, characterized by cough, dyspnea, wheezing, and mild hemoptysis (Löffler syndrome). Fever, peripheral eosinophilia, and a pulmonary infiltrate may be present, especially with moderate to heavy infections. Complications from heavy worm burden in the small intestine include

epigastric pain and abdominal discomfort. *Acute intestinal obstruction* and perforation can also occur. Cholangitis, hepatitis, and pancreatitis can also complicate migration. Chronic infection can be associated with *malnutrition.*

The diagnosis can be established by finding characteristic ova on microscopic examination of the stool. Albendazole or mebendazole are recommended for treatment of symptomatic and asymptomatic individuals.

Hookworm (Necator americanus) Infections

N. americanus is the most prevalent species of hookworm in the Western hemisphere. Although most infections seen in the United States are imported from developing countries, acquisition in the rural southern United States occurs. Hookworm infection continues to be a leading cause of *iron-deficiency anemia* in the developing world.

Hookworm eggs are deposited in moist stool and progress to infectious larvae. These infectious larvae can then penetrate the skin of humans to initiate infection. They enter the circulation and migrate to the pulmonary circulation and eventually swallowed and travel to the small intestine. In the small intestine, the adult worms attach to the mucosa and begin to feed. Eggs are deposited into the lumen after adult worms mate and can be found in the feces.

Clinical manifestations of hookworm infection include:

- Intensely pruritic dermatitis at the site of hookworm entry
- *Hypochromic microcytic anemia* associated with pallor, dyspnea on exertion and fatigue
- Hypoproteinemia and edema
- Physical growth delay, neurodevelopmental delays secondary to chronic infection

The diagnosis is made by demonstrating hookworm eggs under microscopic examination of the stool.

Albendazole, mebendazole, and pyrantel pamoate are treatment options for hookworm infections.

Trichuris Trichiura (Whipworm)

Whipworm has worldwide distribution, but in the United States is found in rural areas of the southeast. Fertilized eggs are ingested and their larvae penetrate mucosal cells of the cecum or colon. The host inflammatory response is thought to play a major role in the pathogenesis of this infection.

Although most infections are asymptomatic, the major clinical entities associated with whipworm infections include:

- *Dysentery syndrome*, characterized by an acute bloody diarrhea with mucus. Trichuris, unlike Ascaris and hookworm, is commonly associated with diarrhea.
- Chronic colitis, which can mimic inflammatory bowel disease and lead to physical growth retardation.
- *Rectal prolapse* resulting from chronic infection with heavy infestation.

The diagnosis is made by finding *Trichuris* eggs on direct examination of the stool.

Albendazole and mebendazole are the commonly recommended treatment of whipworm infections.

Enterobius Vermicularis (Pinworms)

Enterobius infections are common in children, and high rates of transmission can be found among child care and school attendees. Clustering of infection within families is common. Eggs are transmitted by fecal–oral route, and this may occur via contaminated hands or fomites. Pinworm eggs are ingested, hatch, and eventually develop into mature adults in the cecum. Adult worms live in the colon and migrate out at night onto the perianal skin to lay eggs. Most eggs remain on the skin but can contaminate fingers and environmental surfaces.

The major clinical manifestations include *pruritus ani* and *pruritus vulvae*. This can lead to intense itching causing to excoriation of the area, and can lead to bacterial superinfection.

The diagnosis is most frequently made by visualizing adult worms in the perineal region (best examined 2–3 hours after the child is asleep), or by using transparent tape on the perianal skin to collect and visualize eggs that may be present. The tape is applied to a glass slide and examined microscopically. This should be done when the patient first awakens. Examination of the stool for ova and parasites is unrevealing given the small number of ova present in stool. Eosinophilia is unusual with pinworm infection.

Mebendazole, albendazole, and pyrantel pamoate are all effective in treatment of pinworm infection. These agents can be given as single dose therapy and repeated in 2 weeks.

Tissue Nematodes

Trichinella Spiralis

Infection with this organism occurs mainly through the ingestion of *raw or undercooked pork*, horse meat, and wild carnivores. Most infections in the United States can be traced to eating undercooked or raw pork. After ingestion of the infective larvae, they are released from the stomach into the small intestine, where the adults mature. After mating, newborn larvae are released into the systemic circulation and eventually enter striated muscle cells (tissue phase).

One to two weeks after ingestion of the infected meat, a gastroenteritis illness may develop. Typical features of the tissue phase, occurring 2 to 8 weeks after ingestion, include fever, myalgias, bilateral periorbital edema, and conjunctival and subungual hemorrhages. Invasion of the heart muscle can lead to myocarditis. A history of ingesting undercooked meat and illness in others who at the same meat is helpful in making the diagnosis. Laboratory features include a slightly elevated total white blood cell count, and eosinophilia, which can approach 70%. Elevated serum levels of creatine kinase and lactate dehydrogenase also occur.

The diagnosis is suggested by the dietary history and clinical and laboratory features. Skeletal muscle biopsy, as early as two weeks after infection, shows the characteristic encapsulated larvae. Serologic tests can also be helpful in confirming the diagnosis.

Mebendazole or albendazole, along with a corticosteroid are recommended for the treatment of *trichinella* infections.

Visceral Larva Migrans

Cases of visceral larva migrans in the United States are caused most commonly by the dog roundworm, *Toxocara canis*, and less commonly by the cat roundworm, *Toxocara cati*.

Ingestion of the embryonated eggs of these species commonly occurs in children <5 years of age, who are playing in sandboxes and playgrounds that are contaminated with dog and cat feces (pica). After the ingestion, larvae hatch in the small intestine, penetrate the intestinal wall, and migrate through the body, invading all organs. Visceral larva migrans is thought to represent a hypersensitivity reaction to dead and dying larvae.

The clinical manifestations include:

- Fever
- Hepatosplenomegaly
- Malaise
- Lower respiratory symptoms (bronchospasm mimicking asthma)
- Significant peripheral eosinophilia
- Leukocytosis
- Hypergammaglobulinemia

Pneumonia, encephalitis, and myocarditis also have been described. Ocular invasion, usually in the form of endophthalmitis or retinal granulomas (ocular larva migrans) appears to be a distinct clinical syndrome, without systemic manifestations.

The diagnosis can be confirmed with the use of serologic testing (enzyme immunoassay). *Hypereosinophilia, hypergammaglobulinemia*, and an elevated isohemagglutinin titer to the A and B blood group antigens, provides presumptive evidence of infection.

Albendazole and mebendazole are the recommended drugs for treatment of visceral larva migrans. These may not be effective for ocular larva migrans; surgery and/or corticosteroids may be required.

Tapeworm Infections

Cysticercosis

Human cysticercosis is caused by the larvae (*Cysticercus cellulosae*) of the pork tapeworm (*Taenia solium*). This infection is acquired by the ingestion of eggs of the pork tapeworm, which can occur via autoinfection or by fecal–oral contact with a person harboring the adult tapeworm. Humans are the obligate definitive host. Most cases in the United States are imported from Latin America or

Asia, but acquisition in this country has been reported from tapeworm carriers who are in the intestinal stage of the infection. After ingestion of the pork tapeworm, its metacestode migrates from the intestine and has a marked proclivity for the central nervous system.

The most common and serious manifestations of cysticercosis result from the presence of cysts in the brain (*neurocysticercosis*). The most common manifestations in infants and children are seizures, which are the result from the host inflammatory response. These may result from solitary or multiple parenchymal lesions, usually surrounded by edema and inflammation.

The diagnosis of neurocysticercosis is made by the demonstration of central nervous system lesions on computed tomography or magnetic resonance imaging studies. Serologic diagnosis from serum and CSF specimens is helpful.

Albendazole and praziquantel are the drugs used for treatment of neurocysticercosis. Therapy is recommended for nonenhancing or multiple cysticerci, often with the coadministration of corticosteroids.

REVIEW EXERCISES

QUESTIONS

1. Fever, headache, severe myalgias, and a dark rash on the hands and arms develop in a 12-year-old boy during a 5-day period after his return from a trip to North Carolina. On physical examination, he is febrile at 39°C (102.2°F) and has meningismus and a petechial rash on his upper extremities bilaterally. Laboratory findings reveal a white blood cell count of 3000/mm^3, platelet count of 90,000/mm^3, and serum sodium concentration of 129 mEq/L. Which is *true* concerning the diagnosis in this child?

a) Serum serologic testing performed early in the course of the illness is not likely to demonstrate evidence of this infection.

b) Ceftriaxone is effective therapy.

c) Bone marrow examination is required to reveal the cause.

d) Supportive therapy without antibiotics is the mainstay of management.

Answer

The answer is a. Fever, myalgias, meningismus, and a petechial rash developing over a 5-day period in a child with a recent history of travel to the southeastern United States are likely to be manifestations of RMSF, caused by *R. rickettsii*. The differential diagnosis must take into account the possibility of meningococcemia, an acute life-threatening infection. The time course in this patient is more consistent with the diagnosis of RMSF; meningococcemia is more likely than RMSF to

progress over a 12- to 24-hour period. The results of serum serologic testing performed early in the course of the illness are likely to be negative in patients with RMSF; they are often not positive until the second week of the illness. Therefore, therapy must be instituted based on a high index of suspicion. The outcome depends on the prompt institution of antimicrobial therapy (within 6 days of the illness). The drug of choice for children of all ages is doxycycline. Ceftriaxone maybe added if the diagnosis of meningococcemia is suspected, but this agent has no activity against *R. rickettsii*.

Questions 2–6

Match each of the clinical features with the most likely parasitic infection.

2. Rectal prolapse and dysentery

3. Iron deficiency anemia

4. Wheezing, eosinophilia and hypergammaglobulinemia

5. Acute intestinal obstruction

6. Fever, myalgias, periorbital edema, conjunctival and subungual hemorrhages

a) *Necator americanus*
b) *Toxocara canis*
c) *Trichuris trichiura*
d) *Trichinella spiralis*
e) *Ascaris lumbricoides*

Answers

2. The answer is c. Rectal prolapse and dysentery are most likely to occur with whipworm (*Trichuris trichiura*).

3. The answer is a. Hookworm infections (*N. americanus*) continue to be a leading cause of iron deficiency anemia worldwide.

4. The answer is b. Wheezing, eosinophilia, and hypergammaglobulinemia are most characteristic of visceral larva migrans, which is most commonly caused by *Toxocara canis*.

5. The answer is e. Acute intestinal obstruction can occur from a heavy infestation of *Ascaris lumbricoides*.

6. The answer is d. These features are most consistent with the tissue phase of trichinosis, caused by *Trichinella spiralis*.

7. During a camping trip in the Rocky Mountains, a 15-year-old boy reports that he scraped his leg. During the rest of the trip, the group camped in tents, hiked established trails, and waded across several steams. He now presents with fever, headache, nonpurulent conjunctivitis, and myalgias. He appears to be jaundiced. All of the following are indicated *except*:

a) Evaluation of liver enzymes
b) Hepatitis A immunoglobulin

c) Intravenous penicillin
d) Electrocardiogram

Answer

The answer is b. The symptoms presented including fever, myalgia, headache, and nonpurulent conjunctivitis are consistent with leptospirosis, for which intravenous penicillin is the recommended therapy. With the presence of jaundice, evaluation of liver enzyme levels is suggested. Weil syndrome, which is a severe manifestation of leptospirosis, includes jaundice and renal dysfunction. Cardiac arrhythmias and hemorrhagic pneumonitis can also occur. With jaundice, hepatitis A should be considered, but therapy is supportive and hepatitis A immunoglobulin is used for postexposure prophylaxis.

8. What is the most common route of tularemia transmission?
a) Aerosol inhalation
b) Direct animal exposure
c) Tick bite
d) Contaminated water

Answer

The answer is c. Inhalation of aerosols, ingestion of contaminated water, and direct animal exposure all transmit *Francisella tularensis*, but tick bites are the most common method of transmission. Diagnosis relies on history of exposure, clinical presentation, and serology.

9. Five days after being bitten by a pet mouse, a 7-year-old child develops abrupt onset of fever, chills, maculopapular rash on the extremities, muscle pain, and vomiting. You suspect rat bite fever. Blood culture will *most likely* grow:
a) *Pasteurella multocida*
b) Group A streptococcus
c) *Streptobacillus moniliformis*
d) *Eikenella corrodens*

Answer

The answer is c. *Streptobacillus moniliformis* is the most common cause of rat bite fever in the United States. The etiologic agent in Asia is *Spirillum minus*.

SUGGESTED READINGS

1. American Academy of Pediatrics. Ehrlichia and anaplasma infections. In: Pickering LK, Baker CJ, Long SS, McMillan JA, eds. *Red Book 2006 Report of the Committee on Infectious Diseases*, 27th ed. Elk Grove Village, IL: American Academy of Pediatrics, 2006:281–284.
2. American Academy of Pediatrics. Tapeworm diseases. In: Pickering LK, Baker CJ, Long SS, McMillan JA, eds. *Red Book 2006 Report of the Committee on Infectious Diseases*, 27th ed. Elk Grove Village, IL: American Academy of Pediatrics, 2006:644–646.
3. American Academy of Pediatrics. Lyme disease. In: Pickering LK, Baker CJ, Long SS, McMillan JA, eds. *Red Book 2006 Report of the Committee on Infectious Diseases*, 27th ed. Elk Grove Village, IL: American Academy of Pediatrics, 2006:428–433.
4. Arnold DH, Spiro DM. Visual diagnosis: a 5-year-old child who has a facial palsy and rash. *Pediatr Rev* 2007;28:465–469.
5. Gerber MA, Zemel LS, Shapiro ED. Lyme arthritis in children: clinical epidemiology and long-term outcomes. *Pediatrics* 1998;102:905–908.
6. Griffith KS, Lewis LS, Mali S, Parise ME. Treatment of malaria in the United States. A systematic review. *JAMA* 2007;297:2264–2277.
7. Jacobs RF, Schutze GE. Ehrlichiosis in children. *J Pediatr* 1997;131:184–192.
8. Razzaq S, Schutze GE. Rocky mountain spotted fever: a physician's challenge. *Pediatr Rev* 2005;26:125–130.
9. Wormser GP. Early Lyme disease. *NEJM* 2006;354:2794–2801.

Chapter 51

BOARD SIMULATION:
Infectious Diseases

Camille Sabella

QUESTIONS

1. Two days before delivering a term infant, the 20-year-old mother develops chickenpox. The *most* appropriate management plan is to:
a) Administer intravenous acyclovir to the infant at birth.
b) Administer both acyclovir and varicella-zoster immune globulin (Ig) to the infant at birth.
c) Administer varicella-zoster Ig to the infant at birth.
d) Administer varicella-zoster Ig to both the mother and the infant.
e) Administer varicella-zoster Ig to the infant if varicella develops.

Answer

The **answer is c.** Varicella-zoster Ig is given to *prevent* or modify the course of varicella in *susceptible* individuals at risk for severe varicella infection. This includes neonates of mothers in whom varicella develops between 5 days before and 2 days after delivery. Neonates born within this time frame are at high risk for severe infection because they acquire the virus transplacentally, without the benefit of protective maternal antibody. Other individuals who are candidates for receiving varicella-zoster Ig when they have a significant exposure include:

- Susceptible immunocompromised individuals
- Hospitalized premature infants (≥28 weeks gestation) whose mothers lack a reliable history of varicella or serologic evidence of protection against varicella
- Hospitalized premature infants who had <28 weeks of gestation or weigh 1000 g or less at birth
- Susceptible pregnant women

Varicella-zoster Ig should be given as soon as possible after the exposure and within 96 hours of the exposure to be effective. It is not effective for the treatment of established infection. If varicella zoster Ig is not available, intravenous Ig can be substituted.

Acyclovir is an antiviral agent used to *treat* varicella in immunocompromised patients and occasionally in healthy individuals who may be at increased risk for complications of varicella) Acyclovir may be used for postexposure prophylaxis for immunocompromised patients when varicella zoster Ig or Ig are not available, or when >96 hours have elapsed since exposure, although data regarding the effectiveness of this practice are scant.

Questions 2–6
From the list of viruses, choose the one *most* likely to be involved in each of the clinical scenarios.
a) Parvovirus B19
b) Measles
c) Epstein-Barr virus (EBV)
d) Rubella virus
e) Human herpes virus 6

2. A 13-year-old in whom a confluent rash develops during inadvertent treatment with ampicillin

3. A school-aged child with a lace-like reticular rash on the extremities

4. An adolescent with a discrete maculopapular rash beginning on the face and with tender postauricular and postoccipital adenopathy

5. An infant with a maculopapular rash following 3 to 5 days of high fever

6. A child with a croup-like cough, high fever, and confluent maculopapular rash

Answers
2. The **answer is c.** A rash develops in approximately 80% to 90% of individuals with infectious mononucleosis caused by EBV or CMV who are inadvertently treated with ampicillin. The reason is unclear.

3. The **answer is a.** Parvovirus B19 is the cause of erythema infectiosum, also known as *slapped cheek* or *fifth*

disease. An intense erythematous rash develops on the cheeks along with a systemic, lace-like eruption on the trunk and extremities (see Fig. 1.20). The eruption may be pruritic and is often evanescent.

4. The answer is d. Rubella, mostly an illness of adolescents and young adults in the postvaccine era, generally causes asymptomatic infection. The classic features, when present, include a discrete, often pinpoint rash that begins on the face and spreads to the trunk. Postauricular and postoccipital tender adenopathy is said to be most characteristic of rubella.

5. The answer is e. Classic roseola is characterized by 3 to 5 days of high fever, often associated with toxicity, followed by defervescence and the appearance of a maculopapular rash. Human herpes virus 6 is the etiologic agent of roseola; it is also a common cause of febrile illness without rash in infants and children.

6. The answer is b. Measles is characterized by a prodrome manifesting with fever, cough, coryza, conjunctivitis, and Koplik spots, the pathognomonic feature of measles. A rash, accompanied by high fever, follows the prodrome. The respiratory symptoms of measles, especially the cough, are striking. The rash typically begins on the neck, head, and face and spreads to the trunk and extremities. As the rash spreads, it becomes confluent.

7. *Mycoplasma pneumoniae* is associated with which of the following?
a) Laryngotracheitis
b) Erythema multiforme
c) Pharyngitis
d) Pneumonia
e) All of the above

Answer
The answer is e. *M. pneumoniae* is associated with many clinical manifestations. Atypical pneumonia in school-aged children and adolescents is the most important of these. *Indeed,* M. pneumoniae *is the most common cause of pneumonia in school-aged children.* Pharyngitis as an isolated finding is rare but is common in conjunction with pneumonia. Approximately 2% to 4% of cases of croup are caused by this organism. *M. pneumoniae* and herpes simplex virus are the most common infectious agents of erythema multiforme/Stevens-Johnson syndrome. *M. pneumoniae* is also associated with bullous myringitis and otitis media, hemolytic anemia, and common gastrointestinal symptoms. Neurologic manifestations of infection with this organism include aseptic meningitis, encephalitis, Guillain-Barré syndrome, and transverse myelitis.

8. A 5-week-old infant presents with a 5-day history of tachypnea and dry cough. The mother notes that the infant had drainage from both eyes 2 weeks before the onset of symptoms. Physical examination reveals an afebrile, well-appearing infant who is mildly tachypneic

and has rales bilaterally. Chest radiography reveals hyperexpanded lungs with bilateral interstitial infiltrates. The *most* likely etiologic agent is:
a) Group B streptococci
b) *Chlamydia trachomatis*
c) *Staphylococcus aureus*
d) *Streptococcus pneumoniae*
e) *Chlamyophila* (formerly Chlamydia) *pneumoniae*

Answer
The answer is b. Pneumonia develops in approximately 10% to 20% of infants born to women with *C. trachomatis* infection. The illness usually presents in infants between 3 and 12 weeks of age, and 30% to 50% of them have a history of conjunctivitis. The clinical onset is insidious, with persistent cough, tachypnea, and rales as common clinical features. Fever is characteristically absent. Peripheral eosinophilia is common. Chest radiography reveals hyperinflation and interstitial infiltrates. Erythromycin for 14 days is the standard treatment for infants with *Chlamydia* pneumonia and conjunctivitis.

Chamydophila (formerly *Chlamydia*) *pneumoniae* does not cause pneumonia in young infants. The initial illness develops during the school age years and is associated with asymptomatic infection, pharyngitis, and atypical pneumonia. Pneumonia associated with group B streptococci most commonly accompanies early-onset disease and is uncommon in late-onset disease. *S. pneumoniae* and *S. aureus* cause in young infants severe, febrile pneumonia that is associated with an acute onset, toxicity, and focal infiltrates.

9. A 1-year-old previously healthy boy presents with a 6-day history of fever and swelling on the right side of the neck. Physical examination reveals an erythematous, tender, 4 × 4-cm fluctuant lymph node at the angle of the mandible. The *most* likely etiologic agent causing the adenitis is:
a) Group B streptococci
b) *Mycobacterium avium* complex
c) *Bartonella henselae*
d) *S. aureus*
e) *Mycobacterium tuberculosis*

Answer
The answer is d. This infant has acute pyogenic cervical adenitis, which in most cases is caused by *S. aureus*, *S. pyogenes*, or anaerobic organisms. The adenitis is generally unilateral and occurs in children between the ages of 1 and 4 years. Infections with *S. aureus* can be difficult to distinguish from those with *S. pyogenes*, but in general, staphylococcal adenitis is more indolent although more likely to become suppurative (Fig. 51.1). Overall, 25% to 40% of infections with *S. aureus* become suppurative and require surgical drainage. Mycobacterial adenitis usually manifests as subacute or chronic lymphadenitis and is very rarely associated with fluctuance. *B. henselae* is the causative agent of cat scratch adenitis,

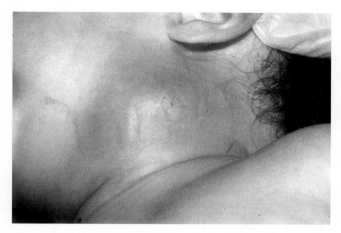

Figure 51.1 Suppurative adenitis in an infant. The purulent material drained from this infant grew *Staphylococcus aureus*. (See color insert.)

which characteristically has a subacute presentation. Group B streptococci can cause an adenitis-cellulitis syndrome, almost exclusively in neonates.

Questions 10–11

A 7-year-old child presents with a 4-week history of an enlarged, mildly tender submandibular lymph node. On physical examination, he is afebrile, nontoxic, and has a 4 × 4-cm mildly tender, nonfluctuant submandibular lymph node.

10. Appropriate management at this point would include:
a) Incision and drainage of the lymph node
b) Removal of the lymph node
c) Complete blood cell count and chest radiography
d) Placement of a double-strength (250-TU [tuberculin unit]) tuberculin skin test

Answer

The answer is c. This child has subacute lymphadenopathy. Potential causes include:

- Cat scratch disease
- *M. tuberculosis* infection
- Nontuberculous mycobacterial infection
- Actinomycosis
- Toxoplasmosis
- Malignancy

Of the choices given, a complete blood cell count and chest radiography are reasonable given that malignancy and tuberculosis are included in the differential diagnosis. Incision and drainage of the lymph node are indicated if the node is fluctuant. Removal of the node is appropriate if the diagnosis of nontuberculous mycobacterial infection is thought likely and other causes have been excluded. A double-strength tuberculin skin test should never be utilized to assess previous exposure to tuberculosis or nontuberculous mycobacteria; a standard 5-TU skin test should be applied. Appropriate management before any invasive procedures are undertaken includes eliciting

a detailed history, including tuberculosis and kitten exposures, and placing a 5-TU tuberculin test.

Further history reveals that the family has recently obtained a kitten with which the child has had close contact. The patient has no history of exposure to tuberculosis, and the result of a 5-TU tuberculin skin test is negative. On closer physical examination, you note a papule on the child's face medial to the enlarged lymph node.

11. Appropriate management at this point would include:
a) Incision and drainage of the lymph node
b) Skin test with cat scratch disease antigen
c) Therapeutic trial with azithromycin
d) No active intervention

Answer

The answer is d. This child most likely has cat scratch adenitis. Ninety percent of patients report exposure to cats or kittens, and 75% have a history of a cat bite or scratch. *B. henselae* is the organism that causes cat scratch disease, and confirmation of infection can be documented with commercially available serologic testing. A cat scratch skin test, which utilizes antigen derived from human sera, is not recommended. Subacute tender regional lymphadenopathy, most commonly involving the axillae and face, is the most common clinical finding. A macule or papule at the inoculation site is found in 60% of cases (**Fig. 51.2**). Systemic symptoms, such as fever, are found in <35% of cases. Atypical clinical manifestations of cat scratch disease include:

- Parinaud oculoglandular syndrome, which includes:
  - Conjunctival granuloma (**Fig. 51.3**)
  - Preauricular adenopathy (**Fig. 51.4**)
- Encephalitis and encephalopathy
- Neuroretinitis
- Hepatosplenic disease

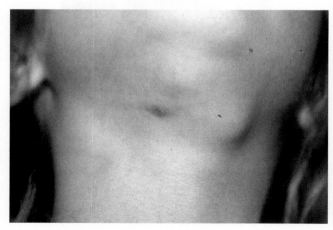

Figure 51.2 A child with cat scratch adenitis. Note the papular lesion, representing the site of the bite or scratch from a kitten. (See color insert.)

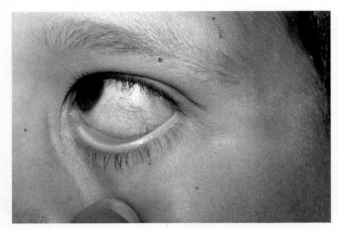

Figure 51.3 The conjunctival granuloma of Parinaud oculoglandular syndrome, a manifestation of cat scratch disease. (See color insert.)

The typical course of cat scratch adenitis is benign and self-limited. Therefore, antimicrobial therapy is not indicated in most cases. Antimicrobial therapy is commonly used for severe atypical disease, such as encephalitis, although no controlled trials have assessed the efficacy of such therapy.

Questions 12–13

A 6-year-old girl with nephrotic syndrome presents with abdominal pain and fever. She is taking prednisone 30 mg/day. She has no diarrhea or vomiting. Her abdominal pain has gradually worsened during the day and is now severe. On physical examination, she has a temperature of 38.4°C (101°F), pulse rate of 140/minute, respira-

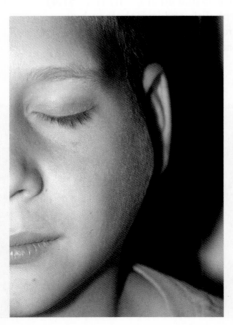

Figure 51.4 The preauricular lymphadenopathy of Parinaud oculoglandular syndrome, a manifestation of cat scratch disease. (See color insert.)

tory rate of 40/minute, and blood pressure of 90/60 mm Hg. She is ill-appearing and apprehensive. Her abdomen is distended, with guarding and rigidity. Bowel sounds are absent.

- White blood cell (WBC) count = 14,000/mm^3
- Hemoglobin = 9.0 g/dL
- Platelet count = normal
- Serum sodium = 130 mmol/L
- Blood urea nitrogen = 23 mg/dL
- Creatinine = 0.8 mg/dL

12. The *most* likely diagnosis is:
a) Acute appendicitis
b) Bacterial gastroenteritis
c) Spontaneous peritonitis
d) Bacterial pneumonia
e) Intussusception

Answer

The answer is c. The history and clinical features are most consistent with primary spontaneous peritonitis. This entity is extremely rare in *healthy* children; it occurs in children with underlying ascites resulting from nephrotic syndrome, liver disease, or rheumatic disorders. Children receiving corticosteroid therapy, which may mask the clinical features of peritonitis, are at highest risk. The organisms most commonly reach the peritoneum by hematogenous spread. Paracentesis is the procedure of choice to confirm the diagnosis; a large number of polymorphonuclear cells (>250/μL), a protein level >1 g/dL, a glucose level <50 mg/dL, and the presence of only gram-positive organisms with Gram staining are features that favor a diagnosis of primary peritonitis.

13. Paracentesis confirms the presence of spontaneous bacterial peritonitis. Of the following, the *most* appropriate antibiotic regimen for this child is to administer:
a) Ampicillin
b) Gentamicin and metronidazole
c) Nafcillin
d) Ceftriaxone
e) Clindamycin

Answer

The answer is d. *E. coli* and *S. pneumoniae* are the most common causes of primary peritonitis. Other, less common organisms include group A streptococci and *Klebsiella pneumoniae*. Anaerobes are *not* commonly isolated from the peritoneal fluid of patients with primary peritonitis, as they are present in secondary peritonitis. Therefore, antimicrobial therapy should include coverage against pneumococci and other streptococci in addition to coverage against gram-negative aerobes. Because a large percentage of *E. coli* organisms produce β-lactamases, ampicillin monotherapy is not adequate for initial therapy. The aminoglycosides provide good coverage against gram-negative aerobes but not against pneumococci. Metronidazole is not required for initial therapy because anaerobes are not common pathogens in primary peritonitis. Nafcillin and clindamycin have no activity against gram-negative organisms. Ceftriaxone provides excellent activity against gram-negative aerobes and *S. pneumoniae* and should be sufficient even for penicillin-resistant strains of pneumococci.

14. Which of the following is a *true* statement regarding the treatment of acute otitis media (AOM) in infants and children?

a) Amoxicillin has the best activity of any oral β-lactam in treating nonsusceptible strains of *S. pneumoniae*.

b) Clindamycin is an appropriate choice for initial empiric therapy.

c) High dosages of amoxicillin are recommended to overcome resistance caused by β-lactamase–producing organisms.

d) The advantage of amoxicillin–clavulanate over amoxicillin is improved activity against nonsusceptible strains of *S. pneumoniae*.

e) Macrolide antibiotics, such as azithromycin and clarithromycin, are considered first-line agents.

Answer

The answer is a. Appropriate antimicrobial therapy for AOM must take into account the pathogens involved and their resistance patterns. The three most common causes of AOM are *S. pneumoniae*, nontypable *H. influenzae*, and *M. catarrhalis*. *H. influenzae* and *M. catarrhalis* induce β-lactamases as their mechanism of resistance, which cannot be overcome by increasing the dosage of a β-lactam antibiotic agent. In contrast, resistance by the pneumococcus is mediated by altered penicillin-binding proteins, which is a stepwise process that can be overcome by increasing the dosage of β-lactams. On the basis of in vitro activity and achievable concentrations in the middle ear, amoxicillin is the most active of the oral β-lactams for the treatment of nonsusceptible strains of *S. pneumoniae*. The addition of clavulanate to amoxicillin adds a β-lactamase inhibitor to counter the effects of β-lactamases produced by *H. influenzae* and *M. catarrhalis*, but provides no added activity against *S. pneumoniae*. Although clindamycin has activity against *S. pneumoniae* and has been utilized to treat resistant pneumococcal infections, it does not have activity against *H. influenzae* and *M. catarrhalis*, and is therefore not recommended as initial empiric therapy. The macrolide antibiotics should not be used as first-line therapy for AOM, given the increasing rates of resistance against these agents, which is as high as 30% for strains of *S. pneumoniae*. These agents should be utilized as alternatives in patients who have severe allergies to β-lactam agents.

15. A 1-month-old girl presents with a 1-week history of upper respiratory symptoms, cough, recurrent episodes of gagging, and post-tussive emesis. On further questioning, the mother informs you that the infant often turns blue during the episodes of coughing and gagging. Physical examination findings are normal except for conjunctival hemorrhage. Complete blood cell count shows a WBC count of 38,000/mm³ with 85% small lymphocytes and a platelet count of 670,000/mm³. Which of the following is the *most* likely cause of the infant's symptoms?

a) Group B streptococcal pneumonia

b) Cystic fibrosis

c) *Bordetella pertussis* infection

d) EBV infection

e) Cytomegalovirus (CMV) infection

Answer

The answer is c. *B. pertussis* infection in young infants is associated with many of the features described in the case study. In neonates with pertussis, the classic paroxysmal cough may not be apparent, and the catarrhal stage is frequently absent or brief. These infants often present with feeding difficulties, recurrent episodes of gagging, apnea, bradycardia, and cyanosis. Apnea can follow episodes of coughing and gagging or can occur spontaneously during the course of the illness. Post-tussive emesis is very common at all ages. Laboratory features of pertussis include a leukocytosis with absolute lymphocytosis, the degree of which parallels the severity of the illness. The lymphocytosis consists of small T and B lymphocytes (Fig. 51.5) rather than the atypical-appearing lymphocytes of infectious mononucleosis. Thrombocytosis is common in children with pertussis infection. The differential diagnosis of pertussis includes:

- Adenovirus infection
- *Bordetella parapertussis* infection
- Viral bronchiolitis
- Cystic fibrosis
- Bacterial pneumonia

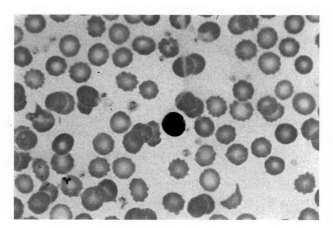

Figure 51.5 Blood smear of a child with *Bordetella pertussis* infection. The lymphocytosis of pertussis is characterized by normal small lymphocytes, whereas large atypical lymphocytes accompany infectious mononucleosis of viral causes. (See color insert.)

16. A 12-year-old boy presents with a 2-week history of fever, sore throat, anterior and posterior cervical lymphadenopathy, and splenomegaly. You suspect infectious mononucleosis. Which of the following statements is *true* regarding infectious mononucleosis?
a) The presence of atypical lymphocytes is specific for EBV and not seen with other causes of infectious mononucleosis, such as CMV.
b) Heterophil-positive mononucleosis occurs with EBV infection but not with CMV infection.
c) Older children and adolescents are more often asymptomatic than younger children.
d) The presence of antibodies against Epstein-Barr nuclear antigen is indicative of acute infection.

Answer
The answer is b. Heterophil antibodies are produced in EBV infection but not infectious mononucleosis syndromes with other causes, such as CMV or *Toxoplasma*, and in human immunodeficiency virus infection. The rapid spot tests (monospot slide tests) are highly sensitive and specific for EBV infection in older children. However, the antibodies may be absent in young children with EBV infection, and the diagnosis may require specific EBV serology. Absolute lymphocytosis with atypical lymphocytosis is not specific for EBV infection; it can be seen in infectious mononucleosis with other causes. Children <2 years are most commonly asymptomatic. Children, in comparison with adolescents, more frequently have nonspecific symptoms, such as fever, rash, abdominal pain, and upper respiratory symptoms. Older children and adolescents have more classic, mononucleosis-like symptoms. Antibodies to the nuclear antigen of EBV are produced 4 weeks after acute infection, are indicative of past infection, and persist for life. Immunoglobulin M (IgM) antibodies to the viral capsid antigen are produced early in the course of infection, are indicative of acute infection, and last for weeks to months. IgG antibodies to the viral capsid antigen are produced at the time of acute infection and last for life. Antibodies to the early antigen are produced acutely, disappear, and can reappear spontaneously.

17. Which of the following is *true* concerning the complications of infectious mononucleosis?
a) Severe thrombocytopenia occurs in approximately 50% of patients.
b) Cranial nerve palsies and encephalitis are the most common neurologic complications.
c) Corticosteroids are indicated for patients with neurologic or hematologic complications.
d) A clinically apparent hepatitis is evident in most patients.

Answer
The answer is b. Facial nerve palsies and encephalitis are the most common neurologic complications of infectious mononucleosis. Others include Guillain-Barré syndrome

and transverse myelitis. *Mild* thrombocytopenia occurs in up to 50% of patients with infectious mononucleosis. Mild autoimmune hemolytic anemia and granulocytopenia can also occur. Although mild subclinical hepatitis is common in infectious mononucleosis, severe hepatitis and liver failure are extremely rare and are seen in patients with X-linked lymphoproliferative disorder. Corticosteroid therapy for patients with infectious mononucleosis is indicated only in cases of severe airway obstruction secondary to tonsillar hypertrophy.

18. The organism responsible for the infection of the infant in **Figure 51.6** is *most* likely to be recovered from which of the following?
a) Nasopharynx
b) Blood
c) Urine
d) Skin lesion
e) Cerebrospinal fluid (CSF)

Answer
The answer is a. This infant has staphylococcal scalded skin syndrome (SSSS), a toxin-mediated process caused by circulating exfoliative toxins of *S. aureus*. The organism is very rarely recovered from the blood or bullous lesions because it is the *toxin* elaborated by the organism that is responsible for the epidermolysis. The organism most commonly is found in the nasopharynx, conjunctivae, umbilicus, or at the site of previous trauma or surgery, such as circumcision. SSSS is most common in infants and children <5 years. Malaise, fever, and tender skin are the first signs of infection, followed by diffuse erythema, a wrinkled appearance of the skin, circumoral erythema, and flaccid blisters. Facial edema and perioral crusting are common. Desquamation of the skin occurs 2 to 5 days after the onset of the erythema, representing cleavage of the stratum granulosum layer of the epidermis. The *Nikolsky sign* is separation of the epidermis by gentle shear force. The absence of a strawberry tongue in SSSS can help in differentiating this entity from systemic

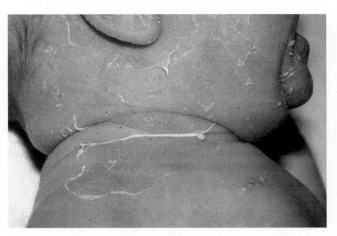

Figure 51.6 Rash in infant in question 18. See explanation of question 18 for details. (See color insert.)

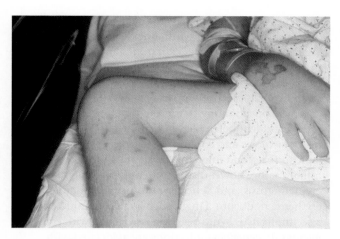

Figure 51.7 Nonblanching rash in the boy in question 19. See explanation of question 19 for details. (See color insert.)

skin infections caused by group A streptococci. Infants with SSSS generally appear well except for irritability likely caused by skin tenderness. Treatment with systemic antistaphylococcal antibiotics is indicated.

19. Of the following, the *most* appropriate initial antibiotic regimen for the 12-year-old boy (**Fig. 51.7**), who presented with a history of acute fever and nonblanching skin rash, is:
a) Nafcillin
b) Clindamycin
c) Doxycycline
d) Cefotaxime
e) No antibiotics because this illness likely has a viral cause

Answer
The answer is d. This boy has fever and a petechial rash, which may be caused by a wide variety of viral, bacterial, and rickettsial organisms, in addition to noninfectious entities. Although viruses (especially enteroviruses) are the leading causes of fever and petechial rashes in children, bacterial infections presenting in this manner are associated with the rapid development of septic shock. This is especially the case with infection caused by *N. meningitidis*, which accounts for approximately 10% of cases of fever and petechial rash in children. Because of the acute, life-threatening nature of meningococcemia, the prompt institution of systemic antibiotic therapy and aggressive fluid management are imperative in every pediatric febrile illness associated with a petechial rash until a bacterial infection has been excluded. Cefotaxime or ceftriaxone provide broad coverage against bacterial causes of sepsis, including meningococci, pneumococci, and *H. influenzae* Type b.

Poor prognostic factors in children presenting with fever and petechial rash who have meningococcemia include:

■ Hypotension
■ Development of petechial lesions within 12 hours of presentation

■ Peripheral WBC count of 10,000/mm^3 or less
■ Absence of meningitis

The absence of meningitis indicates a fulminant septic shock process and is associated with a high mortality rate, whereas children with meningococcal meningitis without evidence of shock have a good overall prognosis.

Because rickettsial infections can cause petechial rashes, doxycycline can be added to the regimen when these infections are considered based on epidemiologic factors and the clinical findings (see Chapter 50).

20. The *most* likely agent causing pneumonia and the rash in the patient in **Figure 51.8** is:
a) *M. pneumoniae*
b) Measles virus
c) EBV
d) *C. pneumoniae*
e) *S. pneumoniae*

Answer
The answer is a. This exanthem consists of wheal-like crops of lesions with areas of central clearing, most consistent with erythema multiforme (**Fig. 51.9**). As the name implies, the skin manifestations of erythema multiforme are variable, ranging from macular to urticarial to vesicobullous lesions. The center of the lesion may be clear, vesicular, purpuric, or necrotic. A wide spectrum of disease is associated with erythema multiforme, ranging from skin involvement alone (erythema multiforme minor) to a severe systemic form in which the mucous membranes are involved along with the skin (erythema multiforme major, or Stevens-Johnson syndrome). Erythema multiforme can be etiologically classified as follows:

■ Drug-induced
■ Idiopathic
■ Infectious or postinfectious

Antimicrobials and anticonvulsants are the most commonly implicated agents in drug-induced erythema

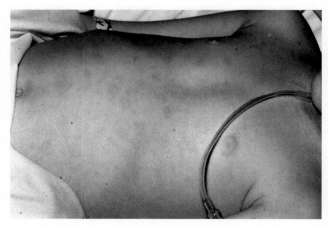

Figure 51.8 Rash in patient in question 20. See explanation of question 20 for details. (See color insert.)

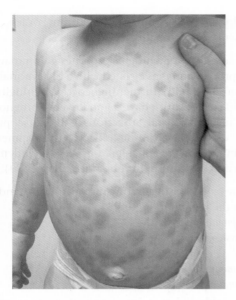

Figure 51.9 Erythema multiforme rash in a child. Note the wheal-like crops of lesions with areas of central clearing. (See color insert).

multiforme. Although many viral, bacterial, and fungal organisms have been associated, the major infectious causes of erythema multiforme appear to be *M. pneumoniae* and herpes simplex virus.

21. Of the following, which is *most* closely associated with the lesions shown in **Figure 51.10**?

a) *Pseudomonas aeruginosa* infection
b) Kawasaki disease
c) Lyme disease
d) Inflammatory bowel disease
e) Parvovirus B19 infection

Answer

The answer is d. These painful, indurated, erythematous/violaceous lesions are most characteristic of *erythema nodosum*, an inflammatory reaction to a variety of agents and conditions. The lesions are characteristically located on the shins, often in a symmetric distribution, but may also be seen on the upper extremities and other areas of the lower extremities. A wide variety of precipitating infections, agents, and systemic illnesses are implicated. Streptococcal infections are now believed to be the most common precipitating factor, but other infections implicated include tuberculosis, fungal infections such as histoplasmosis and coccidioidomycosis, yersiniosis, leptospirosis, and tularemia. Systemic illnesses, especially inflammatory bowel disease, sarcoidosis, systemic lupus erythematosus, and Behçet syndrome, may manifest as erythema nodosum. Drugs, such as sulfonamides, are also implicated. Lyme disease is associated with *erythema migrans*. *P. aeruginosa* infections are associated with *ecthyma gangrenosum*. Parvovirus B19 infection and Kawasaki syndrome are not associated with erythema nodosum.

22. Of the following, the bacterial organism *most* likely complicating the infection shown in **Figure 51.11** is:

a) *Streptococcus pyogenes*
b) *H. influenzae* Type b
c) *S. pneumoniae*
d) *Staphylococcus epidermidis*

Answer

The answer is a. Bacterial superinfection is the most common complication of varicella in otherwise healthy children. Group A streptococci (*S. pyogenes*) and *S. aureus* are the most common agents complicating varicella. In general, group A streptococci, in comparison with *S. aureus*, cause more acute infection that progresses more rapidly and is associated with the development of necrotizing fasciitis, myositis, and subcutaneous abscesses. Systemic antimicrobial agents active against group A streptococci and *S. aureus* should be administered pending the results of culture. Incision and drainage are required for pyogenic collections.

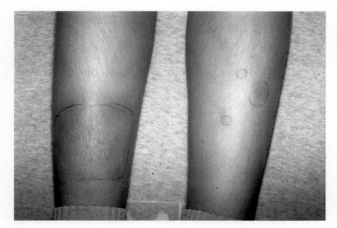

Figure 51.10 Lesions in patient in question 21. See explanation of question 21 for details. (See color insert.)

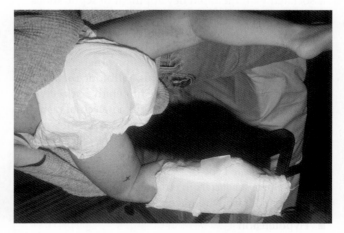

Figure 51.11 Infection in patient in question 22. See explanation of question 22 for details. (See color insert.)

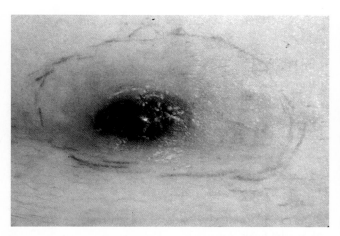

Figure 51.12 Skin lesion in patient in question 23. See explanation of question 23 for details. (See color insert.)

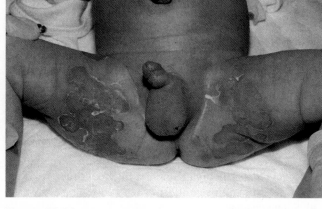

Figure 51.13 Skin lesions in infant in question 24. See explanation of question 24 for details. (See color insert.)

Other complications of varicella in otherwise healthy children are rare but include cerebellar ataxia, encephalitis, Reye syndrome, pneumonia, hepatitis, and myocarditis.

23. A 14-year-old girl undergoing chemotherapy for acute myelocytic leukemia presents with fever, neutropenia, and a skin lesion **(Fig. 51.12)**. The agent *most* likely causing this lesion is:
a) *Listeria monocytogenes*
b) *S. aureus*
c) *S. pyogenes*
d) *P. aeruginosa*

Answer
The answer is d. The history of the patient and the appearance of the lesion are most consistent with the diagnosis of *ecthyma gangrenosum,* which typically is a round, necrotic ulcer with gray or black eschar. The lesion represents invasion of the organism into the small arteries or veins. *The presence of this lesion in an immunocompromised patient most commonly signifies* P. aeruginosa *sepsis. Pseudomonas* bacteremia in children with cancer is frequently accompanied by cellulitis or ecthyma gangrenosum. The organism can usually be recovered from the blood and the lesion. Ecthyma gangrenosum has been associated less commonly with infection caused by other gram-negative organisms such as *S. aureus, Candida,* and *Aspergillus.*

24. The *most* likely diagnosis in the child shown in **Figure 51.13** is:
a) Streptococcal scarlet fever
b) Bullous impetigo
c) Necrotizing fasciitis
d) Infection with herpes simplex virus 2

Answer
The answer is b. This localized skin infection is most consistent with bullous impetigo, an infection in infants and young children. The impetigo commonly begins in the perineal area, especially in neonates and infants. The

lesions may be found on the extremities in older children. Bullae are filled with clear to yellowish fluid and rupture easily. Unlike the lesions of SSSS, these lesions typically are localized, rarely becoming widespread in young infants. The Nikolsky sign is typically absent; no intradermal separation of adjacent skin takes place in bullous impetigo. Systemic manifestations are rare. *Like SSSS, bullous impetigo is caused by* S. aureus *exclusively; however, the organism is commonly recovered from the fluid contained within the bullous lesions, whereas it is not in SSSS.* Localized lesions may be treated with topical mupirocin, but more widespread involvement usually requires systemic antistaphylococcal therapy.

25. Five days after being bitten by a wild mouse, a 7-year-old child has an abrupt onset of fever, chills, maculopapular rash on the extremities, muscle pain, and vomiting. You suspect rat bite fever. Blood culture will *most* likely grow:
a) *Pasteurella multocida*
b) Group A streptococcus
c) *Streptobacillus moniliformis*
d) *Eikenella corrodens*

Answer
The answer is c. Rat bite fever is a zoonotic illness most commonly transmitted by bites of rats, squirrels, and mice. Transmission can also occur from ingestion of contaminated food or milk products and by direct contact with an infected animal. The most common organism associated with rat bite fever in the United States is *S. moniliformis. Spirillum minus* is also a cause of rat bite fever but is more common in Asia. The clinical manifestations of rat bite fever include:

■ Incubation period of 3 to 21 days
■ Abrupt onset of fever and chills
■ Rash on the extremities, which may be maculopapular or petechial

- Nonspecific symptoms such as muscle pain, vomiting, headache, and adenopathy
- Nonsuppurative migratory polyarthritis that follows symptoms in 50% of patients

S. moniliformis is a fastidious organism but can be isolated from the blood, joint fluid, or material from the bite lesion. *S. minus* can be visualized by dark-field microscopy in wet mounts of blood or exudates of lesion. Penicillin is the drug of choice for the treatment of rat bite fever, caused by either organism.

26. A 5-year-old girl with sickle cell disease develops osteomyelitis. The organism *most* likely to cause osteomyelitis in this child is:
a) *S. pneumoniae*
b) *S. aureus*
c) *Bacteroides fragilis*
d) *Salmonella* sp.
e) *S. pyogenes*

Answer
The answer is d. Patients with sickle cell disease are at risk for infection with encapsulated organisms. Sepsis, pneumonia, and osteomyelitis are three of the more common infections occurring in these patients. Although the most common cause of sepsis and pneumonia in these patients is *S. pneumoniae,* the most common cause of osteomyelitis in these patients is *Salmonella.* A recent review has shown that *Salmonella* is the most common cause of osteomyelitis. *S. aureus,* the most common cause of hematogenous osteomyelitis in healthy children, is the second most common cause in patients with sickle cell disease. Prior to 1982, *Salmonella* was seven times as common as *S. aureus* in causing osteomyelitis in these patients. Since 1982 however, *Salmonella* infections are slightly more common than *S. aureus* infection. Overall, the ratio of osteomyelitis caused by *Salmonella* compared with those caused by *S. aureus* is 2.2:1.

27. A 3-year-old boy with sickle cell disease is admitted to the hospital with high fever, tachypnea, and subcostal retractions. Chest radiography demonstrates a left lower lobe infiltrate. The *most* likely organism causing these findings is:
a) *L. monocytogenes*
b) *C. pneumoniae*
c) *Salmonella* sp.
d) *Pneumocystis jiroveci (carinii)*
e) *S. pneumoniae*

Answer
The answer is e. Children with sickle cell disease have functional asplenia and are at high risk for infection with encapsulated organisms. Sepsis, meningitis, pneumonia, and osteomyelitis are commonly encountered in children with sickle cell disease. *S. pneumoniae* is the most common cause of sepsis and pneumonia in patients with sickle cell anemia. *Salmonella* is the most common cause of osteomyelitis in these patients.

L. monocytogenes is not an encapsulated organism and does not commonly cause infections in patients with sickle cell disease. *C. pneumoniae* is a rare cause of pneumonia in toddlers. *P. jiroveci (carinii)* is not a common cause of pneumonia in patients with sickle cell disease.

Questions 28–30
Match each of the clinical findings with the diseases from the choices listed in the subsequent text.

28. Migratory arthritis, erythema marginatum, and chorea

29. Toxin-mediated manifestation of group A streptococcal infection

30. Strawberry tongue and sandpapery rash
a) Scarlet fever
b) Rheumatic fever
c) Both a and b
d) Neither a nor b

Answers
28. The answer is b.
29. The answer is a.
30. The answer is a.

Migratory arthritis, erythema marginatum (see Fig. 67.2), and chorea are three of the five *major* criteria for rheumatic fever according to the revised Jones definition. The other two *major* criteria are carditis and subcutaneous nodules. Although the exact pathogenesis of rheumatic fever is yet to be defined, it is thought to be an abnormal immune response to group A streptococci, not a toxin-mediated response. Rheumatic fever is a nonsuppurative complication of group A streptococcal upper respiratory infection; it does not complicate group A streptococcal skin infections. In contrast, the other nonsuppurative complication of group A streptococcal infection, glomerulonephritis, can follow either streptococcal pharyngitis or skin infection.

Scarlet fever is caused by one of the three pyrogenic toxins of group A streptococci; it may accompany streptococcal pharyngitis or follow a skin infection with group A streptococci. The exanthem of scarlet fever is an erythematous, punctuate, or papular rash that has the texture of sandpaper. The rash is generalized but most intense in the axillae and perineal area. Areas of hyperpigmentation may be apparent in the folds of the antecubital fossae (Pastia lines). The face usually appears flushed, and circumoral pallor is common. A strawberry tongue is frequently present in scarlet fever and can be used to distinguish streptococcal scarlet fever from staphylococcal skin infection.

Questions 31–37
Match the following antimicrobial agents with the *most* likely adverse effect listed in subsequent text:

31. Rifampin

32. Isoniazid

33. Pyrazinamide

34. Ethambutol

35. Methicillin

36. Ceftriaxone

37. Chloramphenicol
a) Optic neuritis
b) Interstitial nephritis
c) Peripheral neuritis
d) Hyperuricemia
e) Biliary sludging
f) Aplastic anemia
g) Staining of contact lenses

Answers

31. The answer is g. Rifampin is associated with a range of adverse effects, including nausea, flu-like symptoms, hepatitis, orange discoloration of bodily secretions, staining of contact lenses, and interference with oral contraceptives.

32. The answer is c. Isoniazid causes peripheral neuritis and seizures related to the inhibition of pyridoxine metabolism. It is also associated with hepatitis and a mild elevation of serum liver chemistries. These adverse effects are rare in children.

33. The answer is d. Pyrazinamide is associated with arthralgias secondary to the inhibition of uric acid excretion and with hepatitis. These are rare side effects in children.

34. The answer is a. In addition to gastrointestinal disturbances, ethambutol causes a reversible optic neuritis that may result in an alteration of visual acuity, visual fields, or red-green discrimination. Because the patient's cooperation is necessary to test for these abnormalities, ethambutol may not be appropriate for young children, although a risk:benefit assessment may be required.

35. The answer is b. Methicillin, and less commonly other antistaphylococcal penicillins, are known to cause interstitial nephritis. This manifests with fever, rash, decreased urine output, a rise in the serum creatinine level, and urinary or peripheral eosinophilia. The process is reversible.

36. The answer is e. Ceftriaxone is excreted to a great extent into the biliary tract and is known to cause biliary sludging. This appears to be of no clinical significance.

37. The answer is f. Chloramphenicol has long been known for its tendency to cause two forms of aplastic anemia. The more common form is reversible and dose-dependent. The rarer form is an idiosyncratic reaction and is not reversible.

38. A 9-month-old boy presents with a 24-hour history of high fever, irritability, and decreased oral intake. On

physical examination, he is toxic appearing and has a bulging anterior fontanelle. Examination of his CSF obtained from a lumbar puncture reveals a WBC count of 2100/mm^3 with 98% polymorphonuclear cells, a protein level of 200 mg/dL and a glucose level of 10 mg/dL. Gram stain reveals gram-positive diplococci. Of the following, the *most* appropriate initial antimicrobial regimen for this child would be the administration of:
a) Vancomycin
b) Ceftriaxone
c) Ampicillin and ceftriaxone
d) Vancomycin and cefotaxime
e) Ampicillin

Answer

The answer is d. This infant has bacterial meningitis, as evidenced by his clinical history and results of his cerebrospinal examination. On the basis of the Gram stain, the most likely responsible organism is *S. pneumoniae*, although the possibility of *N. meningitidis* cannot be totally excluded based on Gram staining alone. Therefore, empiric therapy for bacterial meningitis in this setting needs to include coverage against both *S. pneumoniae* and *N. meningitidis*. *N. meningitidis* continues to be susceptible to β-lactam antibiotics; therefore, either ampicillin or a third-generation cephalosporin, such as ceftriaxone or cefotaxime, would be effective therapy. Vancomycin does not have activity against meningococcus. Penicillin-nonsusceptible strains of *S. pneumoniae* are now prevalent, accounting for approximately 40% of strains in the United States. In addition, approximately 10% to 15% of *S. pneumoniae* strains are fully or intermediately resistant to ceftriaxone or cefotaxime. Although β-lactam antibiotics, when given in appropriate doses, continue to be effective in treating non-meningeal infections caused by penicillin-nonsusceptible strains, adequate levels to treat meningitis may not be achieved. Therefore, initial therapy for children with meningitis caused by *S. pneumoniae* must include vancomycin in addition to a third-generation cephalosporin, such as ceftriaxone or cefotaxime, until the results of susceptibility testing are known. If the organism is found to be susceptible to ceftriaxone/cefotaxime, vancomycin can be discontinued. In cases in which the pneumococcus is found to be nonsusceptible to penicillin and ceftriaxone/cefotaxime, the ideal regimen is not clear, although many experts continue to utilize both vancomycin and ceftriaxone/cefotaxime, given the erratic CSF penetration of vancomycin and the vast experience in utilizing ceftriaxone and cefotaxime. Agents such as meropenem, rifampin, and chloramphenicol also warrant consideration in these difficult clinical settings.

39. An 8-week-old infant presents with a 2-day history of dry cough and nasal congestion. Physical examination reveals a well-appearing afebrile infant with a respiratory rate of 50/minute. Mild subcostal retractions are present, and auscultation reveals rhonchi and rales bilaterally. A chest radiograph reveals hyperinflation and diffuse interstitial markings. Of the following, the *least* likely to cause this clinical picture in the infant is:

a) Respiratory syncytial virus (RSV)
b) *C. trachomatis*
c) CMV
d) Group B streptococci
e) *Ureaplasma urealyticum*

Answer

The answer is d. This question addresses the *afebrile pneumonia syndrome*, which occurs in infants between the ages of 4 and 12 weeks. The infants are characteristically afebrile and well appearing. They often present with mild respiratory distress, cough, and congestion. Rales and rhonchi are frequent findings on auscultation. The chest radiographic findings are nonspecific; hyperinflation and diffuse infiltrates may be present. The differential diagnosis of the *afebrile pneumonia syndrome* includes:

- *C. trachomatis* infection (25%)
- *U. urealyticum* infection (20%)
- CMV infection (20%)
- *P. jiroveci (carinii)* infection (20%)
- Infection with viral agents, including RSV and adenovirus

A history of conjunctivitis in the infant or a history of maternal *Chlamydia* infection can be an important clue to *C. trachomatis* infection. It is important to note that they are generally healthy infants without any evidence of immunosuppression. Therefore, CMV and *P. jiroveci* infections in these infants are benign, self-limited illnesses.

40. Productive cough, high fever, and respiratory distress develop in a previously healthy 2-year-old boy 2 days following mild cold symptoms. Physical findings reveal an ill-appearing child with a temperature of 39.5°C (103.1°F) and respiratory rate of 60/minute. He has decreased breath sounds in the left base and nasal flaring. A chest radiograph reveals a large left lower lobe infiltrate. Of the following, the *best* course of action is to intravenously administer:

a) Cefotaxime
b) Erythromycin
c) Cefoxitin
d) Ceftazidime
e) Nafcillin

Answer

The answer is a. This child has moderate to severe respiratory distress and a lobar pneumonia. Therefore, a bacterial process is more likely than a viral process. An atypical process, such as that seen with *M. pneumoniae*, is unlikely, given the age of the child, the acuteness of onset, and the severity of illness. The most likely etiologic agent in this case is *S. pneumoniae*, by far the most com-

mon cause of bacterial pneumonia in infants and young children. Other bacterial causes include *S. aureus* and *H. influenzae*. The third-generation cephalosporins—namely, cefotaxime and ceftriaxone—are very active against pneumococci, including most penicillin-resistant strains. These antibiotics also are clinically effective for pneumonia caused by strains of pneumococci that are resistant to them because of the high serum levels that can be achieved, which overcome in vitro resistance. Erythromycin and nafcillin may be active against some strains of pneumococci but are less active than cefotaxime or ceftriaxone and have poor activity against penicillin-resistant strains. Ceftazidime and cefoxitin have poor activity against pneumococci.

Given the increasing incidence of pneumonia caused by community-associated methicillin-resistant strains of *S. aureus*, empiric therapy against this organism may be warranted in some areas of the country, depending on the local prevalence and susceptibility patterns of such infections. The addition of vancomycin or clindamycin would be appropriate empiric coverage for such infections in ill-appearing infants and children.

41. Right lower quadrant pain and fever develop in a 12-year-old boy. Appendicitis is suspected, and he undergoes appendectomy. Mesenteric adenitis is found at the time of surgery, and pathology shows a normal appendix. The pathogen *most* likely to mimic acute appendicitis is:

a) *Vibrio cholerae*
b) *Clostridium difficile*
c) CMV
d) *Yersinia enterocolitica*

Answer

The answer is d. *Y. enterocolitica* is a cause of acute diarrheal illness in children and adolescents. These organisms are known to produce an intense suppurative mesenteric adenitis, manifested clinically as severe abdominal pain and right lower quadrant tenderness that closely mimic acute appendicitis.

42. Which of the following organisms is *least* likely to be transmitted in a child care center?

a) *Shigella sonnei*
b) *Salmonella* sp.
c) *G. lamblia*
d) Rotavirus
e) Hepatitis A virus

Answer

The answer is b. Enteric pathogens that are commonly transmitted from person to person are important causes of outbreaks in child care settings (Table 51.1). *Salmonella* and *Campylobacter* species, which are more likely acquired from food-borne or animal sources (reptiles), are less commonly transmitted in child care settings.

TABLE 51.1

ENTERIC ORGANISMS COMMONLY TRANSMITTED IN CHILD CARE CENTERS

Bacteria	Viruses	Parasites
Shigella species	Rotavirus	*Giardia lamblia*
Escherichia coli 0157:H7	Hepatitis A virus	*Cryptosporidium parvum*
	Enteric adenoviruses	
	Astroviruses	

Many of the organisms frequently transmitted in child care centers can be spread directly from person to person or indirectly from fomites and food handlers.

43. A 16-year-old girl presents with fever and bilateral ankle pain and swelling. On physical examination, she has bilateral arthritis of the ankles, pustular lesions of the distal extremities, and necrotic lesions on the palms and soles. The diagnostic study *most* likely to reveal the diagnosis in this patient is:
a) Blood culture
b) Aspiration of the ankle joint
c) Cervical culture
d) Culture of the pustular lesion
e) Antistreptolysin O titer

Answer

The answer is c. This adolescent presents with septic arthritis of the ankles along with pustular lesions of the distal extremities and necrotic lesions on the soles and palms (Fig. 51.14), features characteristic of disseminated gonococcal infection. Women are commonly affected, and symptoms classically begin 1 to 4 weeks after infection. The most common manifestations include:

- Arthritis
- Tenosynovitis
- Dermatitis
- Endocarditis (rare)

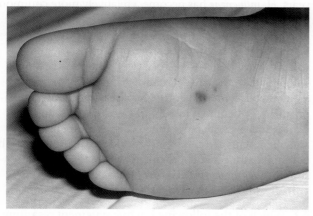

Figure 51.14 Necrotic lesions on the sole of an adolescent girl with disseminated gonococcal infection. (See color insert.)

- Osteomyelitis (rare)
- Meningitis (rare)

The arthritis of disseminated gonococcal infection can be monoarticular or polyarticular. It may involve the joints of the wrists, hands, and fingers (tenosynovitis–dermatitis syndrome) or the large joints, such as the knees and ankles (suppurative arthritis syndrome). Some overlap between these two syndromes may occur. The skin lesions usually begin as painful discrete macules that progress to pustules or petechiae and become necrotic. Necrotic pustules on an erythematous base may be found over the extremities, including the palms and soles.

The cervical cultures of patients with disseminated gonococcal infection are positive for *N. gonorrhoeae* in 80% to 90% of cases. In contrast, blood cultures are positive for the organism in 30% to 40% of cases, whereas cultures from the synovial fluid and skin lesions are infrequently positive.

44. Which of the following is a *true* statement regarding the currently available meningococcal vaccines?
a) They are protective against all serotypes of meningococcal disease that cause human infection.
b) They are live attenuated vaccines.
c) Children with asplenia should receive a meningococcal vaccine.
d) The vaccines can replace postexposure chemoprophylaxis with rifampin.

Answer

The answer is c. Two meningococcal vaccines are currently available in the United States (also see Chapter 2). The capsular polysaccharide vaccine (MPSV4) has been available for many years. More recently, a polysaccharide-protein conjugated vaccine (MCV4) has become available. Therefore, neither is a live vaccine. Both available meningococcal vaccines contain serogroups A, C, Y, and W135. However, neither vaccine is effective against serotype B, which is a significant cause of disease in infants. Both vaccines are approved for children 2 years of age and longer. In general, MCV4 is preferred over MPSV4 because it is a conjugate vaccine and elicits brisker and more long-lasting responses. Conjugate meningococcal vaccine is indicated for:

- All children and adolescents at 11 to 12 years of age, or at 15 years of age for those not vaccinated earlier.
- College freshmen planning to live in dormitories.
- Individuals who have anatomical and functional asplenia
- Individuals with deficiencies of terminal complement and properdin
- Children and adolescents infected with human immunodeficiency virus
- Travelers to areas where meningococcal disease is endemic
- Military recruits

In addition, meningococcal vaccine can be used to control outbreaks of meningococcal disease when the strain causing the outbreak is one of the serotypes contained in the vaccine.

Because these vaccines are not currently licensed for use in children <2 years, do not contain protection against serotype B, and because immediate protection is not possible with vaccination, they cannot be used to replace postexposure chemoprophylaxis with rifampin in children having close exposure to individuals with invasive meningococcal infection.

45. Which of the following is a *true* statement concerning viral laryngotracheitis?
a) The most common cause is RSV.
b) Children aged 3 to 6 years are at highest risk for viral laryngotracheitis.
c) Racemic epinephrine is of benefit for children with mild or moderate symptoms.
d) Corticosteroid therapy for viral laryngotracheitis is contraindicated.

Answer
The answer is c. The parainfluenza viruses account for most cases of viral croup. RSV, adenovirus, influenza virus, and measles virus are responsible for the rest of the cases. Children between the ages of 6 months and 2 years are at highest risk for viral laryngotracheitis, whereas children with epiglottitis more commonly present at a later age (3–7 years). Children with mild to moderate croup may benefit from aerosolized racemic epinephrine, which offers transient relief. Repeated treatments with racemic epinephrine may be required, and children must be observed for the possibility of recurrent stridor 2 to 3 hours after the administration of racemic epinephrine. Corticosteroids appear to be of benefit in children with moderate or severe croup.

46. Of the following, the animal *most* likely to harbor rabies is:
a) Skunk
b) Squirrel
c) Rabbit
d) Rat

Answer
The answer is a. Animals that should be regarded as rabid unless the geographic area is known to be entirely free of rabies, including skunks, bats, raccoons, foxes, and other carnivores. Most rodents, including squirrels, hamsters, rats, and guinea pigs, are almost never rabid. Likewise, rabbits and hares are almost never rabid. Dogs, cats, and ferrets should be regarded as possibly rabid; these animals should be observed for 10 days for signs of rabies if they are available. If the animals are rabid or suspected of being rabid, then postexposure prophylaxis is indicated. Decision regarding the need for rabies postexposure prophylaxis following animal bites or exposures should be made in conjunction with local public

health officials. See Chapter 2 for more detailed recommendations regarding rabies postexposure prophylaxis.

47. Regarding hepatitis B serology, in which of the following situations would a patient test positive for antibody to hepatitis B surface antigen (anti-HBs)?
a) Acute hepatitis B virus (HBV) infection
b) Carrier state of HBV
c) Chronic HBV infection
d) After vaccination

Answer
The answer is d. *Hepatitis B surface antigen* represents acute or chronic HBV infection.

Hepatitis B early antigen is not found in healthy carriers; it indicates active HBV infection, correlates with HBV replication, and assesses the infectiousness of a patient. *HBV DNA* indicates that DNA replication is occurring.

Antibody to hepatitis B surface antigen (anti-HBs) indicates previous hepatitis B infection, exposure, or vaccination (i.e., clinical recovery from HBV infection and/or immunity); it is not present in active, chronic infection or in the carrier state.

Antibody to hepatitis B core antigen (anti-HBc) indicates active HBV infection, either acute (IgM) or chronic.

48. Which of the following is a *true* statement regarding the etiology of AOM in infants and children?
a) Viral pathogens are rarely found in the middle ear of children with AOM.
b) Even when actively sought, no etiologic agent is found in approximately 50% of cases.
c) AOM caused by S. pneumoniae is less likely to remit spontaneously than when the infection is caused by *H. influenzae*.
d) A larger percentage of *H. influenzae* isolates produce β-lactamases than *M. catarrhalis* isolates.

Answer
The answer is c. S. pneumoniae, H. influenzae, and *M. catarrhalis* continue to be the leading bacterial pathogens isolated from children with AOM. In recent years, *H. influenzae* has become a relatively more common cause and has now likely surpassed S. pneumoniae as the leading bacterial cause of AOM. Infection with S. pneumoniae is the least likely of the three organisms to remit spontaneously (15%–20% of cases), whereas infections with *H. influenzae* and *M. catarrhalis* are likely to remit spontaneously in 50% and 80% of cases, respectively. An organism is identified in 80% of cases of AOM, and viruses such as RSV, parainfluenza virus, influenza virus, and adenovirus are commonly found as copathogens with bacterial pathogens. Approximately 40% to 50% of strains of *H. influenzae* elaborate β-lactamase, whereas virtually all strains of *M. catarrhalis* produce β-lactamase.

49. Which of the following is a *true* statement regarding the acute complications of infection with RSV?
a) Apnea is a rare complication of RSV disease.

b) Serious bacterial infection rarely complicates RSV disease.

c) Lower respiratory tract disease and respiratory failure are more common with reinfection than with primary infection.

d) Immunocompromised children are at low risk for severe RSV disease.

Answer

The answer is b. Many studies have documented that secondary serious bacterial infection rarely complicates RSV disease. However, apnea is not an uncommon clinical feature of RSV infection, especially in very young and preterm infants. The risk of developing lower respiratory tract disease and respiratory failure is significantly greater during a primary infection than a recurrent infection. Although it is common to have repeated infections with RSV throughout one's life, infection is generally milder and localized to the upper respiratory tract with subsequent infection. Children who are at high risk of developing severe or complicated RSV disease include:

- Preterm infants and children with chronic lung disease
- Individuals with congenital heart disease (especially hemodynamically significant cyanotic disease)
- Immunocompromised individuals

50. A 7-year-old boy who has a history of congenital hydrocephalus has a ventriculoperitoneal shunt, presents with lethargy, headaches, and low-grade fever. Examination of the CSF from the shunt reveals cloudy fluid. Three weeks prior to his presentation, he underwent elective revision of the ventriculoperitoneal shunt. You suspect bacterial infection of the ventriculoperitoneal shunt. Of the following, the organism *most* likely to cause this infection in this child is:

a) Coagulase-negative staphylococcus
b) *S. pneumoniae*
c) *N. meningitidis*
d) *Escherichia coli*
e) *P. aeruginosa*

Answer

The answer is a. Coagulase-negative staphylococci are the most common cause of ventriculoperitoneal shunt infections. Other skin flora such as *Propionibacterium acnes*, *Bacillus* sp., and *S. aureus* can cause these infections. Gram-negative bacteria account for approximately 20% of these infections. Fungal isolates such as *Candida* sp. are occasionally encountered. The clinical manifestations of ventriculoperitoneal infections are variable, ranging from a total lack of systemic symptoms to severe signs of increased intracranial pressure, high fever, and meningismus. Abdominal symptoms may predominate, especially if distal obstruction is present. Management includes the combination of systemic antibiotics and temporary removal of the shunt catheter.

Questions 51–56
Match the following clinical scenarios with the *most* likely agents of bioterrorism.

51. Respiratory distress followed by shock; widened mediastinum

52. Flaccid paralysis

53. Painful regional lymphadenopathy

54. Vesicular rash

55. Painful papular ulceration and regional cervical lymphadenopathy

56. Painless ulceration; black eschar
a) Bubonic plague, *Yersinia pestis*
b) Inhalation anthrax
c) Cutaneous anthrax
d) Botulism
e) Smallpox
f) Tularemia

Answers
51. The answer is b. The manifestations of inhalation anthrax include a prodrome of fever, sweats, cough, progressing to dyspnea, hypoxia, and fulminant shock, which is associated with a hemorrhagic mediastinal lymphadenitis. A *widened mediastinum* is the classic chest radiographic finding.

52. The answer is d. Botulism, caused by *Clostridium botulinum*, is characterized by an acute symmetrical descending flaccid paralysis. Cranial nerve involvement always occurs in botulism. Foodborne, wound, and infant botulism are the three naturally occurring forms of the infection.

53. The answer is a. Painful lymphadenopathy is most characteristic of bubonic plague, caused by *Yersinia pestis*. The manifestations of the naturally occurring form of this infection include an acute onset of fever and painful swollen regional lymphadenopathy. It is important to realize however, that other forms of this infection occur (pneumonic plague, septicemic form, meningeal form, pharyngeal form), and that the presentation of bioterrorism-related plague is most likely to be the pneumonic form. This form is characterized by cough, fever, dyspnea, and hemoptysis.

54. The answer is e. The manifestations of smallpox includes a prodromal period of high fever, malaise, headache, and abdominal pain, followed by lesions on the mouth and pharynx, and the typical vesicular rash, which begins on the face and progresses to involve the extremities, including lesions on the palms and soles.

55. The answer is f. Tularemia, caused by *Francisella tularensis*, has several forms, including the ulceroglandular form (most common), characterized by a painful popular lesion at the entry site with concomitant painful regional lymphadenopathy. Other forms include a glandular syndrome (regional lymphadenopathy without ulcer), oculoglandular syndrome, oropharyngeal syndrome, and typhoidal syndrome (fever, hepatosplenomegaly).

56. The answer is c. Cutaneous anthrax is characterized by a pruritic papule or vesicle that enlarges and form a painless central black eschar, often surrounded by edema and regional lymphadenopathy.

SUGGESTED READINGS

1. Aebi C, Ahmed A, Ramilo O. Bacterial complications of primary varicella in children. *Clin Infect Dis* 1996;23:698–705.
2. American Academy of Pediatrics. Varicella-zoster infections. In: Pickering LK, Baker CJ, Long SS, McMillan JA, eds. *Red book: 2006 Report of the Committee on Infectious Diseases,* 27th ed. Elk Grove Village, IL: American Academy of Pediatrics, 2006:711–725.
3. American Academy of Pediatrics. Children in out-of-home child care. In: Pickering LK, Baker CJ, Long SS, McMillan JA, eds. *Red book: 2006 Report of the Committee on Infectious Diseases,* 27th ed. Elk Grove Village, IL: American Academy of Pediatrics, 2006:130–145.
4. Balbi HJ. Chloramphenicol: a review. *Pediatr Rev* 2004;25:284–288.
5. Caldararo S. Measles. *Pediatr Rev* 2007;28:352–354.
6. Casey JR, Pichichero ME. Changes in frequency and pathogens causing acute otitis media in 1995–2003. *Pediatr Infect Dis J* 2004; 23:824–828.
7. Cimolai N. *Mycoplasma pneumoniae* respiratory infection. *Pediatr Rev* 1998;19:327–332.
8. Durbin WJ. Pneumococcal infections. *Pediatr Rev* 2004;25:418–424.
9. Florin TA, Zaoutis TE, Zaoutis LB. Beyond cat scratch disease: widening spectrum of Bartonella henselae infection. *Pediatrics* 2008;121:e1413–e1425.
10. Friedman AM. Evaluation and management of lymphadenopathy in children. *Pediatr Rev* 2008;29:53–59.
11. Hammerschlag MR. *Chlamydia trachomatis* and *Chlamydia pneumoniae* infections in children and adolescents. *Pediatr Rev* 2004;25: 43–51.
12. Kirsch EA, Barton P, Kitchen L, et al. Pathophysiology, treatment, and outcome of meningococcemia: a review and recent experience. *Pediatr Infect Dis J* 1996;15:967–979.
13. Mancini AJ. Bacterial skin infections in children: the common and the not so common. *Pediatr Ann* 2000;29:26–35.
14. Peter J, Ray CG. Infectious mononucleosis. *Pediatr Rev* 1998; 19:276–279.
15. Peters TR, Edwards KM. Cervical lymphadenopathy and adenitis. *Pediatr Rev* 2000;21:399–404.
16. Sabella C, Goldfarb J. Principles of selection and use of antimicrobial agents. *Sem Pediatr Infect Dis* 1999;10:3–13.
17. Seigel RM, Bien JP. Acute otitis media in children: a continuing story. *Pediatr Rev* 2004;25:187–193.
18. Stagno S, Brasfield DM, Brown MB, et al. Infant pneumonitis associated with cytomegalovirus, *Chlamydia, Pneumocystis,* and *Ureaplasma:* a prospective study. *Pediatrics* 1981;68:322–329.

Chapter 52

Rheumatic Disorders

Philip J. Hashkes

JUVENILE RHEUMATOID ARTHRITIS AND OTHER CHRONIC ARTHRITIDES OF CHILDHOOD

Epidemiology and Etiology

The term *juvenile rheumatoid arthritis* (JRA) describes the condition of chronic arthritis of unknown cause in children <16 years and includes several subgroups (Table 52.1). JRA is the most common chronic rheumatic disease in childhood with an estimated *incidence* of 1:10,000 children per year and an estimated *prevalence* of 1:1000. The gender ratio and age of onset differ for each subtype. JRA rarely presents before 6 months of age. Other chronic arthritides in children, not included under the term JRA, include psoriatic arthritis and spondyloarthropathies. The latter is also termed enthesitis-related arthritis (inflammation at the point of attachment of tendon to bone) or HLA-B27–related arthritides. There is a new method of classification for all types of chronic arthritis in childhood of

TABLE 52.1

CHARACTERISTIC FEATURES OF SUBGROUPS OF CHILDHOOD CHRONIC ARTHRITIS

	Polyarticular JRA		Pauciarticular JRA	Systemic-onset JRA	Enthesitis-related[a]
	RF−	RF+			
Relative frequency	25%–30%	5%–10%	40%–50%	10%–20%	Unknown
Age at onset	Childhood (mode 2–5 years)	Adolescence	Early childhood (mode 1–4 years)	Any age	Late childhood (>8 years)
Sex (Female/male)	3:1	3:1	5:1	1:1	1:7
No. of joints involved in first 6 months	5 or more	5 or more	4 or less	Variable	Variable
Uveitis	5%–10%	Rare	25%–35%	Rare	15%–25%[b]
RF	No	Yes	No	No	No
ANA positivity	40%–50%	40%–50%	50%–75%	<10%	<10% (HLA-B27 ~90%)
Prognosis	Good–moderate	Poor	Excellent (good–moderate if becomes polyarticular, as in approximately 1/3 of cases; or, if with severe uveitis)	Good (pauci) to poor (poly)	Moderate

[a]Formerly called pauciarticular type II, spondyloarthropathy.
[b]Acute uveitis.
ANA, antinuclear antibody; JRA, juvenile rheumatoid arthritis; RF, rheumatoid factor.

unknown cause, under the umbrella term of juvenile idiopathic arthritis (JIA). This term is currently used more often by pediatric rheumatologists than JRA and has more scientific validity. However, since board questions relate to JRA, the term JRA was chosen for this chapter.

The causes of JRA are still unknown. However, genetic associations have been identified. Several human leukocyte antigen (HLA) genes have been associated with pauciarticular JRA and uveitis in young females with a positive antinuclear antibody (ANA). HLA-DR4 is associated with polyarticular JRA, particularly in rheumatoid factor (RF) and anticyclic citrullinated peptide (CCP) antibody positive polyarthritis found primarily in adolescent girls. Antibodies and cellular immune reactivity to type II collagen have also been found in children with JRA. Although several infectious agents have been reported as triggers, none have been consistently implicated in JRA. Polymorphisms of genes associated with macrophage as well as T- and B-cell activity are associated with an increased risk of developing JRA or a more severe clinical course.

Pathology

JRA is an autoimmune disorder that targets the synovial tissue of the joints. Examination of the synovial membrane shows villous hypertrophy and hyperplasia of the synovial lining that results in an increased secretion of joint fluid. Edema, hyperemia, vascular endothelial hyperplasia, and lymphocyte infiltration are seen. The inflammatory process,

termed *pannus*, can eventually result in the erosion and destruction of articular cartilage and bone. *Rheumatoid nodules* are the consequence of small blood vessel vasculitis with a central area of necrosis and granulation. The *rash* of systemic-onset JRA is a result of neutrophil infiltration and perivasculitis. Inflammatory infiltrates may also be present in the liver and tissues such as pericardium, pleura, and peritoneum. The number of white blood cells, primarily polymorphonuclear leukocytes, in joint fluid varies from mild inflammation (5000/mm^3) to purulent (>100,000/mm^3). The severity of synovial leukocytosis does not correlate with the clinical course or outcome.

Clinical Presentation

JRA is classified into three subgroups according to the pattern of onset: pauciarticular, polyarticular, and systemic. The clinical manifestations vary among subgroups.

The *arthritis* of JRA is defined by the following:

- Age at onset of less than 16 years
- The presence of arthritis defined as articular swelling and effusion (Fig. 52.1), or the presence of two of the following findings in joints (even in the absence of swelling): warmth, limitation of motion, and tenderness or pain on motion
- Duration of arthritis of at least 6 weeks
- Exclusion of other causes of arthritis

Other symptoms may include pain and morning stiffness, or stiffness after a nap or prolonged sitting. Children

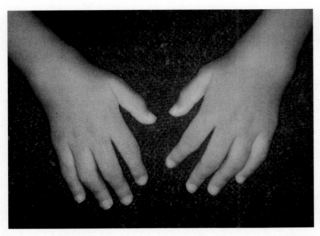

Figure 52.1 Polyarticular juvenile rheumatoid arthritis in a young child with swelling in proximal interphalangeal joints, metacarpal phalangeal joints, and wrist joints with flexion contractures of the fingers. (See color insert.)

may limp or refuse to use the affected limbs. Younger children often do not complain of pain and may present only with a limp or a regression in gross or fine motor skills. Anorexia, weight loss, and growth failure may also be seen, particularly in systemic or polyarticular-onset disease. Other extra-articular manifestations include:

- Rash
- Lymphadenopathy
- Hepatosplenomegaly
- Serositis (pleuritis, pericarditis)
- Chronic uveitis
- Delayed development of secondary sexual characteristics

Pauciarticular-Onset Juvenile Rheumatoid Arthritis

JRA with a pauciarticular onset accounts for approximately 40% to 50% of cases of JRA. Four or fewer joints are involved in the first 6 months of disease. The most common pattern is asymmetric involvement of the large joints of the lower extremities. About half of these children have monoarticular arthritis, mainly of the knee.

The onset of most cases of pauciarticular JRA is in early childhood. Children usually present between 1 and 4 years of age. Girls are more often affected than boys. The knees and ankles are typically involved. *Hip involvement at the onset of pauciarticular JRA is very rare.* Although the joints are swollen and warm, children often have very little pain and function well.

In nearly one third of cases, an *asymptomatic chronic anterior uveitis* may develop. *Girls between 1 and 3 years of age with a positive ANA are at particularly high risk for developing uveitis.* Chronic uveitis leads to significant visual impairment in up to 30% of patients; thus, prevention of permanent eye damage caused by uveitis is essential. Other common complications include the development of cataract, glaucoma, and

band keratopathy. Therefore, a routine *ophthalmologic slit-lamp examination* should be performed in all patients with JRA according to the schedule recommended by the American Academy of Pediatrics and the American College of Rheumatology. Young girls with pauciarticular JRA and positive ANA need an ophthalmologic examination every 3 to 4 months for the first 5 to 7 years of their disease.

Local complications of pauciarticular JRA include the development of *flexion contractures, muscle atrophy,* and *leg length discrepancies.* In younger children the affected limb is usually longer than the healthy limb, whereas in older children (>9 years) arthritis may lead to an early closing of the growth plate and a shorter limb. Thirty-three percent to 50% of children with pauciarticular JRA progress to develop a polyarticular course. Often, the outcome of uveitis and development of complications (glaucoma, cataract, visual defects) are the determinants of the long-term prognosis of pauciarticular JRA.

Polyarticular-Onset Juvenile Rheumatoid Arthritis

Approximately 35% of cases of JRA have a polyarticular onset. Five or more joints are involved in the first 6 months of disease. Characteristically, the arthritis is symmetric and affects both large and small joints. Hip, shoulder, and temporomandibular joint involvement are common. The cervical spine can also be involved and is associated with a risk for *atlantoaxial subluxation.* Many children in this subgroup have constitutional symptoms, including low-grade fever, malaise, anemia of chronic disease, mild hepatosplenomegaly, and weight loss or growth delay.

There are two types of polyarticular-onset JRA. The more common type is RF negative polyarticular JRA. The onset is usually early in childhood (2–5 years old), and commonly affects large joints prior to small joints. Girls are affected more often than boys. Children respond well to treatment and have good functional outcomes, although the disease in most children persists to adulthood. Approximately 5% to 10% of these children develop chronic uveitis.

Only approximately *5% to 10%* of children with polyarticular-onset JRA are positive for RF. Many of these children also have antibodies to CCP. The pattern of this disease resembles that of adult-onset rheumatoid arthritis. Girls, mainly adolescent, are affected more often than boys. *Rheumatoid nodules* or *Felty syndrome* (splenomegaly and leukopenia) may develop. The disease progresses rapidly, with *joint erosions* often evident within 6 to 12 months of onset of symptoms. Patients with HLA-DR4 typically have a worse prognosis. These patients should be treated aggressively early in the disease course.

Systemic-Onset Juvenile Rheumatoid Arthritis

Systemic-onset JRA is seen in 10% to 20% patients with JRA and can present at any age. This is the only type of JRA without a definite gender predilection. The arthritis of systemic-onset JRA can be either pauciarticular or polyarticular, affecting both large and small joints. Children with a polyarticular course often have severe disease with a poor outcome.

The arthritis is usually preceded by systemic manifestations for as long as even 6 months. Therefore, children often present with *fever of unknown origin* and undergo extensive evaluations, especially for infection and malignancy (leukemia, neuroblastoma), before other diagnoses are excluded. *Fevers* are intermittent, typically occurring in the evening or with two daily peaks. The *rash* of systemic-onset JRA is transient, occurring more frequently during febrile periods, and is described as an erythematous or *salmon-pink* macular rash. This rash can often be elucidated by minor local trauma *(Koebner phenomena)* or can be seen after a warm bath (Fig. 52.2). *Lymphadenopathy* and *hepatosplenomegaly* are seen in more than two thirds of these children. *Pleuritis* or *pericarditis* is present in approximately 20% to 35% of patients. Rarely, pericarditis may be severe. There are no specific laboratory tests in systemic-onset JRA. Laboratory results reflect an inflammatory state with a markedly increased sedimentation rate and C-reactive protein. Characteristic blood count findings include an elevated white blood cell count with a left shift, severe anemia, and thrombocytosis. Ferritin levels are often markedly increased. Serologic markers (ANA and RF) are usually absent. Uveitis is rarely found in this type of JRA.

Spondyloarthropathies (Enthesitis-Related Arthritis)

This class of arthritis usually presents in males (>80%) older than 8 years, with painful, asymmetric arthritis of the lower extremities (knees, ankles, tarsal joints, and hips) and

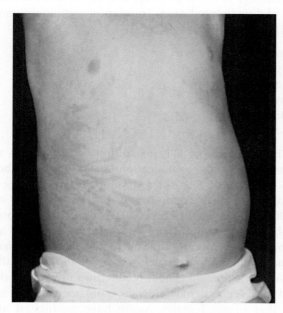

Figure 52.2 Macular, salmon-pink rash of systemic-onset juvenile rheumatoid arthritis. The rash can be elucidated by scratching (Koebner phenomena). This rash is more evident during febrile periods. (See color insert.)

often includes inflammation of the enthesis. Commonly affected enthesis are in the calcaneus, patella, and trochanter regions. An association with HLA-B27 is seen in most cases. Many of these children develop *sacroiliitis* or *ankylosing spondylitis* in adolescence or adulthood. A strong family history is often reported. Fifteen percent to 25% of these children develop *acute* uveitis, which unlike the uveitis of JRA, is associated with *pain, erythema,* and *photophobia.* Other forms of spondyloarthropathies include inflammatory bowel disease–related arthritis (both ulcerative colitis and Crohn disease) and postinfectious reactive arthritis (see subsequent section on Reactive Arthritis).

Psoriatic Arthritis

Fifteen percent to 20% of adults with psoriasis develop arthritis. Although uncommon, psoriatic arthritis is occasionally seen in children (approximately 5% of cases of chronic childhood arthritis). Psoriasis can occur simultaneously with arthritis, precede the development of arthritis by many years, or occur years after the beginning of arthritis. Several clues to the possibility of psoriatic arthritis in children include *a family history of psoriasis* in a first-degree relative, *nail abnormalities* (pitting, onycholysis), or *tenosynovitis* near small joints often in the pattern of *dactylitis* (*sausage* digit). Children with psoriatic arthritis can develop a pauciarticular, polyarticular, or spondyloarthropathy pattern of arthritis.

Diagnosis

The diagnosis of JRA is primarily based on the clinical findings and exclusion of other causes of arthritis. No specific diagnostic laboratory tests for JRA are available, although most patients with pauciarticular (50%–75%) and many patients with polyarticular JRA (40%–50%) have a positive ANA. The erythrocyte sedimentation rate and level of C-reactive protein may be elevated during active disease, but normal acute phase reactants do not rule out JRA. Approximately 5% to 10% of children with JRA are RF and anti-CCP antibody positive. Radiographs of the affected joints in the early stage of disease may show soft tissue swelling, regional osteoporosis, and demineralization. Later signs include bony overgrowth, joint space narrowing, erosions, subluxation, ankylosis, or joint destruction. In questionable cases, magnetic resonance imaging (MRI) (with gadolinium enhancement) may be helpful in the diagnosis of synovitis and the detection of joint damage even before conventional radiographs are done.

Treatment

The goals of therapy for JRA are to decrease the inflammatory process so as to minimize pain and joint damage, improve the function, and decrease the long-term disability. Nonsteroidal anti-inflammatory drugs are considered first-line therapy but mainly affect pain and stiffness, although not significantly affecting the disease process. Therefore, disease-modifying antirheumatic drugs such as methotrexate are used early in the course of the disease, especially in polyarticular and systemic JRA. Intra-articular long-acting corticosteroid injections are used with increasing frequency to treat pauciarticular JRA and prevent flexion contractions and leg length discrepancies. Systemic corticosteroids are reserved for patients with severe systemic features of JRA or as a bridging medication until disease-modifying drugs are effective. In recent years, *biologic-modifying* medications acting on specific molecules in the inflammatory process have been developed for treating arthritis. Etanercept, a soluble receptor of tumor necrosis factor, has been approved for the treatment of polyarticular JRA not responsive to methotrexate. Adalimumab, a humanized tumor necrosis antibody has also been approved for use in polyarticular JRA. Infliximab, a mouse-based tumor necrosis antibody, may be effective for those patients with uveitis not responsive to methotrexate. Abatacept, a T-cell co-stimulator inhibitor was also approved for treatment of polyarticular arthritis. Anti-interleukin 1 and anti-interleukin 6 biologic medications may be effective, especially for patients with systemic JRA.

Physical and occupational therapy is also very important in maintaining joint range of motion and function. Physicians from other specialities participate in the treatment of JRA including ophthalmologists, orthodontists, and orthopedists. It is hopeful that with modern medical therapy less orthopedic intervention, particularly joint replacement surgery, will be necessary.

Prognosis

The prognosis varies with the subtype of JRA. Unfortunately, previously quoted statistics that as many as 80% of children will enter remission before adulthood are incorrect and are not supported by current data. Recent studies have shown that most children with polyarticular JRA and systemic or pauciarticular JRA with a polyarticular course will continue to have active disease as adults. Less than one third achieve long-term remission. Children having systemic-onset JRA with a persistent fever, high platelet count, and a polyarticular course and children with RF-positive JRA will have a particularly poor prognosis, with severe joint erosions and disability. These children require more aggressive therapy.

REACTIVE ARTHRITIS

Reactive arthritis is a nonspecific arthritis associated with particular enteric and genital infections. In early childhood most cases are postgastroenteritis, usually caused by *Shigella, Salmonella, Campylobacter,* or *Yersinia*. Sexually active adolescents may develop posturogenital infectious arthritis, often caused by *Chlamydia*. The triad of postinfectious *arthritis, conjunctivitis,* and *urethritis* is now called

reactive arthritis. (The old term of *Reiter syndrome* was discontinued because of the Nazi activities of Dr. Reiter.) Most children with reactive arthritis are positive for HLA-B27. Rheumatic fever or poststreptococcal reactive arthritis is another form of reactive arthritis.

The arthritis is usually an asymmetric oligoarthritis that primarily involves the lower extremities. Although most children experience an isolated episode of monoarthritis, the clinical course and severity may vary. Symptoms typically last several weeks to 3 to 6 months. The disease may go into remission, or episodes of disease activity may recur for years. Some patients later develop a full-blown spondyloarthropathy. Many cases of reactive arthritis are self-limiting and can be managed effectively with nonsteroidal anti-inflammatory drugs. Therapy with glucocorticoids (including intra-articular) or sulfasalazine may also be effective for severe or disabling polyarthritis.

SYSTEMIC LUPUS ERYTHEMATOSUS

Systemic lupus erythematosus (SLE) is defined as an episodic, multisystem, autoimmune disease characterized by widespread inflammation of blood vessels and other tissues and the presence of autoantibodies, especially ANA. However, the presence of ANA is not sufficient to diagnose SLE. In fact, full development of the disease may be preceded by several years of the involvement of only a few systems.

Etiology and Epidemiology

The etiology of SLE is currently unknown, with the exception of drug-induced cases. Those most commonly associated are as follows:

- Anticonvulsant agents
- Hydralazine
- Isoniazid
- Procainamide
- Minocycline
- α-Methyldopa

The incidence of SLE in children <15 years in the United States is 0.5 to 0.6 cases/100,000 per year. About 15% to 20% of SLE cases develop before the age of 20 years. Prevalence data suggest that between 5000 and 10,000 children in the United States have SLE. The onset can be at any age but is rare before the age of 5 years and becomes more common during adolescence. The female-to-male ratio is approximately 4 to 5:1 in those older than 10 years (there is no gender predilection in younger children). SLE is prevalent worldwide; estimates of disease suggest that among females, Asians have the highest incidence, followed by Afro-Caribbeans, Hispanics, and whites. However, in the United States the highest prevalence is among African-American females.

Pathophysiology

Research suggests that a number of factors, including immune dysregulation, hormonal influences, infection, and genetic predisposition may play a role in the development of the disease. Twin studies have suggested an increased concordance in monozygotic versus dizygotic twins. In addition, the risk of developing SLE or other connective tissue disorders is 10- to 20-fold greater in the siblings of a patient with SLE than in the general population. Several HLA haplotypes, immune regulatory genes, and complement deficiencies have been implicated in the increased susceptibility to SLE. The strongest prevalence (80%) and the most severe disease have been found in patients deficient in either C1 complex or C4 molecules. Environmental factors such as ultraviolet B irradiation (sun exposure), viral infection, drugs, and chemicals also contribute to the development of SLE.

Clinical Presentation

The presentation of SLE can be insidious, rapidly progressive, or anything in between. Because many systems are involved in this disorder, disease of multiple organs is the rule rather than the exception. Constitutional symptoms consisting of fever, anorexia, weight loss, and malaise are very common at the onset of disease and during flares. Most patients present with rash, arthralgia, and/or myalgia. Other common modes of SLE presentation include immune thrombocytopenia (ITP) with a positive ANA, hypertension and/or nephrotic syndrome, seizures, and psychosis or other unusual neurologic syndromes.

Rash occurs in one third to one half of children at the onset of disease and during flares. Described as a *butterfly* rash, it is symmetric over the bridge of the nose, both upper cheeks *(malar)*, and sometimes the forehead with sparing of the nasolabial areas. The rash is often photosensitive. It should be noted that this type of rash may present in other syndromes and is not specific to SLE. Other skin manifestations of SLE include:

- Vasculitic purpura and petechiae (often on the hands)
- Periungual erythema
- Alopecia
- Discoid lesions
- Ulcerations
- Mucosal ulceration
- Raynaud phenomena

Arthritis and arthralgias are common (up to 75% of cases) in children with SLE. Small joints, particularly in the hands, as well as elbows, shoulders, wrists, knees, and ankles, are usually affected. The arthritis is generally mild and rarely causes permanent deformity. Patients with SLE are at risk for avascular necrosis of bone, especially when treated with corticosteroids for an extended period of time.

Renal disease is very common and possibly present in nearly all children with SLE; it is clinically evident in at least 75%. The most common presentation is microscopic hematuria (80%), followed by proteinuria (55%) and hypertension (40%). Serious renal disease typically occurs within 2 years of the onset of SLE but may present much later. Renal disease, the leading cause of morbidity and mortality in these patients, is more frequent and more severe in children with SLE as compared with adults.

Neurologic involvement occurs in most cases, often later in the disease course. Approximately 50% will have some evidence of central nervous system (CNS) disease at onset. Progressive academic difficulty, social problems, and depression are most frequently noted in these patients. Less often, they may have seizures, psychosis, stroke, and chorea; the latter two are thought to be related mainly to antiphospholipid antibodies. Other manifestations include intractable migraine headaches, aseptic meningitis, and transverse myelitis. In all cases of new neurologic symptoms, *infectious* and *metabolic* causes need to be excluded. CNS disease is the second leading disease-related cause of morbidity and mortality in patients with SLE.

Pulmonary disease is also common, occurring in up to 75% of patients. Manifestations include subclinical disease (60%), pleural effusion and pleuritis, pneumonitis (*shrunken-lung* syndrome), infections, and rarely (often fatal) pulmonary hemorrhage.

Cardiac involvement occurs in approximately 30% of cases and most often presents as pericarditis. Myocarditis, myocardial infarction, and valvulitis (classic Libman-Sacks endocarditis lesion) are less common. Pericarditis may be clinically silent but commonly presents with chest pain that is made worse by deep breathing or lying down. Many patients develop *accelerated atherosclerosis*. Atherosclerosis develops later in the course of disease and has multiple causes, including abnormal levels of plasma lipids and the adverse effects of long-term steroid therapy. Atherosclerosis is now considered the major cause of *late* mortality and morbidity in SLE.

Hematologic manifestations include hemolytic anemia, anemia of chronic disease, thrombocytopenia, and leukopenia (mainly lymphopenia). The hemolytic anemia is usually Coombs test positive. In addition, patients may have antiphospholipid antibodies, which are associated with prolonged clotting time, thrombocytopenia, stroke, and thrombosis in all vascular beds (antiphospholipid syndrome). Vasculitis of the small blood vessels is often manifested by Raynaud phenomenon (sequential white, blue, and red color changes in the distal extremities, usually in response to exposure to cold weather). Lupus crisis, the sudden onset of overwhelming systemic disease, is the result of widespread acute vasculitis and thrombosis and can be fatal (rare).

In addition, SLE can affect all other body systems, including the gastrointestinal (GI) tract (hepatitis, pancreatitis), eyes (retinal vasculitis), lymphatic tissues, and thyroid gland.

Systemic Lupus Erythematosus Nephritis: Clinical and Pathologic Correlation

The renal pathology in SLE is relevant to the treatment and outcome. The World Health Organization has defined six classes on the basis of pathologic findings. Class I is defined as *normal or minimal change* by electron microscopy. Class II is *mesangial nephritis*, found in 10% to 20% of patients. Patients with this lesion may have proteinuria and hematuria along with minimal decreases of serum complement, but they usually do not progress to renal insufficiency. Class III, *focal segmental proliferative glomerulonephritis*, occurs in a similar number of patients but is more serious than mesangial nephritis. Proteinuria, hematuria, hypertension, and minimally elevated levels of creatinine may be associated with this renal lesion. Progressive renal disease, however, appears to be uncommon when a small number (<25%) of the glomeruli are affected. Class IV, *diffuse proliferative glomerulonephritis*, is the most severe finding. Proteinuria and hematuria are seen in all such cases, and nephrotic syndrome and renal insufficiency occur in 60%. These *patients have low levels of complement and elevated levels of antibody to double-stranded DNA* (anti-dsDNA). Aggressive therapy (cyclophosphamide) is usually required to stop progression to end-stage renal disease. However, even with treatment, a late decline in renal function may occur. Class V, *membranous glomerulonephritis*, develops in 10% to 20% of patients, who may present without low complement or elevated anti-dsDNA levels. Patients usually have nephrotic syndrome. One third of patients have hypertension. Renal function may be preserved for long periods of time with remission achieved in only 30%; however, in cases of severe nephrotic syndrome, immunosuppressive therapy is warranted. Class VI, *glomerular sclerosis*, represents an end-stage lesion; it usually does not respond to therapy and leads to a slow decline in renal function.

Renal lesions of many patients (as many as 35%) may evolve from one type to the next, often when disease is prolonged.

Diagnosis

The diagnosis of SLE in children is similar to that in adults. Four or more of the 1997 revised classification criteria of the American College of Rheumatology (ACR) must be present either simultaneously or serially during the course of the disease. The criteria include the following:

- Malar rash
- Discoid rash
- Photosensitivity
- Oral ulcers
- Arthritis
- Pericarditis/pleuritis
- Hematologic abnormalities (anemia, leukopenia)
- Nephritis
- Seizures/psychosis
- Elevated levels of ANA
- Other immunologic findings, including positivity for antiphospholipid antibodies, anti-dsDNA antibody, or antibodies to extractable nuclear antigens (ENA), including Sm, SS-A/Ro, SS-B/La, RNP antibodies

ANA is almost always present in children with SLE. *Anti-dsDNA is often present, mainly in active renal disease, and is virtually pathognomonic for SLE.* Antibody to single-stranded DNA (anti-ssDNA) is often present but is often seen in other autoimmune conditions. Anti-Ro (SS-A) and anti-La (SS-B) are seen in neonatal lupus but also in Sjögren syndrome. Patients with these antibodies are at higher risk of photosensitivity reactions. Anti-Sm antibodies are specific for SLE and may be related to CNS disease as are ribosomal antibodies. Antiribonucleoprotein (Anti-RNP) antibodies, when present in high titers and in the absence of other ENA antibodies, are diagnostic for mixed connective tissue disease. Histone antibodies are seen in nearly all patients with drug-induced lupus. Many patients have antibodies to thyroid antigens as well. Titers of these antibodies are not useful, however, for following the course of the disease.

It is important to measure the complement levels in patients who have or are suspected of having SLE. *In most patients with active nephritis, the total hemolytic complement (CH_{50}) is abnormally low. In addition, the levels of the third and fourth components of complement (C3 and C4) are also often depressed, although C3 is less frequently low than C4 or CH_{50}.* Congenitally low levels of C4 complements (*null gene polymorphism*) may be a predisposing cause in the development of SLE.

Many patients with SLE have antiphospholipid antibodies, such as to anticardiolipin or β_2-glycoprotein, which may interfere with the normal process of clotting and cause thrombosis, stroke, thrombocytopenia, chorea, livedo reticularis, and recurrent spontaneous abortions. RF is sometimes present in children with SLE (10%–30%) but is not specific and may raise the possibility of overlap with other rheumatologic diseases.

Urinalysis is important to elucidate the presence of renal disease. Hematuria and red cell casts (seen best on a fresh specimen) are the most important markers of glomerulonephritis. Proteinuria is the most common finding and may persist for long periods even during disease remission. A new finding of proteinuria >500 mg/day is indicative of active renal disease and needs further evaluation. Patients may have nephrotic syndrome and lose a large quantity of protein molecules such as immunoglobulin M (IgM) and IgG. The presence or resolution of these urinalysis findings can be used to determine the treatment and follow the course of the disease.

Treatment

Early diagnosis and aggressive treatment are essential for halting the disease progression. However, because the disease most often occurs in adolescents, patients must be closely monitored for side effects of treatment, such as an altered appearance (which results from steroid use), and adjustment problems such as depression.

Nonsteroidal anti-inflammatory drugs are often used to treat musculoskeletal manifestations, such as arthritis/myalgias and pleuritis/pericarditis. Ibuprofen should be avoided in the treatment of SLE because it has been associated with the development of aseptic meningitis.

Glucocorticoids are the first-line drugs for the treatment of most patients with SLE. The steroid dose will depend on the severity of disease. Patients with moderate to severe disease will likely require therapy with initial high doses of glucocorticoid to gain control of the disease. Once the acute aspects of the disease are controlled, the dose is slowly tapered to a maintenance level. The clinical response, hematologic indices, anti-dsDNA antibodies, C3, C4, or CH_{50} levels, and urinalysis findings are followed up closely to ensure an adequate drug response. If high-dose steroids fail to elicit an adequate response, cannot be weaned, or the side effects of steroids are too prominent, then the adjunctive therapies described in the subsequent text are considered.

Antimalarials such as hydroxychloroquine are often used as adjunctive agents for skin and joint disease and may make it possible to lower the glucocorticoid dose. Antimalarials (especially hydroxychloroquine) are used in nearly all patients with SLE, because some studies have found that they may be beneficial in preventing severe flares and even decrease mortality. They also have cholesterol-lowering potential (important for patients using steroids) and inhibit platelet aggregation. It is important to watch out for the rare adverse effect of ocular toxicity, which can occur especially in the presence of renal insufficiency. Ophthalmology examinations are recommended every 12 months.

Azathioprine has been used as a second-line agent in addition to glucocorticoids. It has been shown to allow a reduction in the dose of glucocorticoids in patients whose disease is poorly controlled by high doses of steroids alone.

Cyclophosphamide is given for treatment of severe lupus nephritis (Class IV) or severe neurologic disease. It is used together with corticosteroids, especially in intravenous pulse regimens. This combination appears to decrease the progression of renal disease. The toxicity of cyclophosphamide, however, is significant and includes hemorrhagic cystitis, infection, gonadal failure, and secondary malignancies.

Recent studies have shown that *mycophenolate mofetil* may be as effective as cyclophosphamide in the treatment of lupus nephritis with a better toxicity profile. However, other studies, including with long-term follow-up are necessary to validate those findings.

Other drugs, including methotrexate, cyclosporine, and Rituximab (an anti–CD-20 mature B-cell antibody), are being investigated for a potential role in the treatment of SLE. Although their efficacy has not yet been conclusively proven, promising results, especially of Rituximab, suggest that these drugs may be of benefit. Other *biologic* drugs targeting specific immune or inflammatory processes in SLE are in the various stages of development and investigation.

Supportive therapy is crucial. Sun protection, prevention and treatment of osteoporosis, treatment of hypertension, hypercholesterolemia, early detection and treatment of infections, and adequate immunizations are crucial in preventing disease flares, mortality, and morbidity related to disease activity, and treatment complications.

Prognosis

The outcome of children with SLE has improved significantly with a marked decrease in mortality. The 10-year survival rate in children is nearly 90%. Several factors have made an impact on the prognosis, including earlier diagnosis of SLE, aggressive therapy (cyclophosphamide for renal disease), and improved supportive treatment. However, there is still considerable morbidity related to damage from disease activity (renal, CNS) or treatment (infection, atherosclerosis, osteoporosis, aseptic necrosis of bone, cataract, infertility). Poor outcomes may be associated with poor compliance, infections (sepsis is now the overall leading cause of death, replacing renal failure), neurologic complications, and severe renal disease (particularly diffuse proliferative glomerulonephritis). Cardiovascular disease, occurring in early adulthood in many patients, is a great concern and the topic of much research in recent years.

Neonatal Lupus

Neonates are thought to acquire SLE by receiving passively transferred auto antibodies, anti-Ro (SS-A) and anti-La (SS-B), from the maternal circulation. *Neonatal lupus develops in approximately 5% of neonates born to mothers affected by SLE or to mothers who have these antibodies without the symptoms of SLE.* However, because the syndrome does not develop in all neonates born to mothers with these antibodies, other undetermined factors may also play a role.

In most babies, neonatal lupus is a mild syndrome consisting of a transient rash that develops after exposure to sunlight or significant light exposure (i.e., phototherapy for hyperbilirubinemia). The rash is usually located in the scalp and periorbital areas. In addition, some infants (1%–2%) born to mothers with SLE may manifest *complete heart block. This is the most common cause of neonatal complete heart block.* The condition is often diagnosed in utero by the finding of bradycardia (or hydrops, if more severe). Infants usually tolerate the block well, if the heart rate is faster than 60 beats/minute, until delivery, when they may become symptomatic. In addition to complete block, other cardiac anomalies include second-degree block, right bundle branch block, prolonged QT interval, and several structural defects, such as coarctation, tetralogy of Fallot, atrial septal defect, and ventricular septal defect. Thrombocytopenia and liver enzyme abnormalities may also be seen.

Treatment in the prenatal period consists of corticosteroids, which rarely may reverse incomplete heart block and also decrease the incidence of fetal hydrops associated with poor cardiac output. A cardiac pacemaker is placed in newborns with congenital heart block to ensure stable rhythm and cardiac output. Rash, caused by maternal antibodies, is transient and usually disappears by the age of 6 months. No treatment is usually needed for noncardiac manifestations of neonatal lupus. The likelihood of the development of a connective tissue disorder in these children is not thought to exceed that of unaffected children of mothers with SLE.

HENOCH-SCHöNLEIN PURPURA

Etiology and Epidemiology

Henoch-Schönlein purpura (HSP), also known as *anaphylactic purpura*, is the most common vasculitic disorder seen in children. It can affect multiple systems, including the skin, GI tract, joints, and kidneys (Table 52.2). Although the true cause is not known, HSP is thought to be an IgA-mediated immune response to many infectious agents, especially *β-hemolytic Streptococcus*. At least 50% of children with HSP have had a *preceding upper respiratory tract infection*. Children with C2 complement deficiency or familial Mediterranean fever are at risk of developing recurrent episodes of HSP.

HSP is seen more commonly in winter or early spring. The male-to-female ratio is approximately 1.5:1. Recent reports indicate an annual incidence of 22.1 cases/100,000. Seventy-five percent of children with HSP are <10 years, and the peak incidence is between 4 and 7 years.

Pathophysiology

Immune complexes become trapped following an inciting event and their deposition in blood vessel walls initiate local complement activation and neutrophil and macrophage

TABLE 52.2

CLINICAL FEATURES OF HENOCH-SCHÖNLEIN PURPURA

Purpura
Arthralgia/arthritis/periarthritis
Abdominal pain
GI bleeding
Renal involvement
Subcutaneous edema
Encephalopathy
Orchitis

GI, gastrointestinal.

adhesion to endothelial cells. Enzymes, leukotrienes, nitric oxide, and reactive oxygen molecules are subsequently released and damage the blood vessel walls. Biopsy of skin lesions reveals a *leukocytoclastic vasculitis with deposits of IgA*. Similar inflammation of the small vessels is seen in joints, the GI tract, and kidneys. In patients in whom nephritis develops, the pathology is similar to that seen in IgA nephropathy (i.e., *proliferative mesangial glomerulonephritis with IgA, C3, fibrin, and fibrinogen deposition seen on renal biopsy*).

Clinical Presentation

Although a rash develops in all patients with HSP, it is the presenting symptom in only 50% of cases. Initially, the rash may appear urticarial or maculopapular. The rash then progresses to the characteristic *palpable purpura and petechiae*, usually on the *buttocks and lower extremities* (Fig. 52.3), or points of pressure.

Abdominal complaints occur in more than two thirds of children and are caused by inflammation of the GI tract. This GI involvement can precede the rash in 15% to 35% of cases. Patients often describe *colicky abdominal pain*. Vomiting and heme-positive or grossly bloody stools may develop. These children are at risk for the development of *intussusception* (1%–5%). It is important to note that the intussusception in HSP is most often *ileoileal rather than the ileocecal* form seen in younger children.

Approximately 50% to 80% of children experience *arthritis, periarthritis, and arthralgias*. Arthritis is the presenting symptom in 25% of cases. The large joints, including the knees and ankles, are more commonly involved. The arthritis is usually self-limiting, lasting several days.

Nephritis develops in 20% to 35% of cases. Symptoms range from microscopic hematuria to rapidly progressive glomerulonephritis and include the development of nephritis or nephrotic syndrome. There is an increased risk

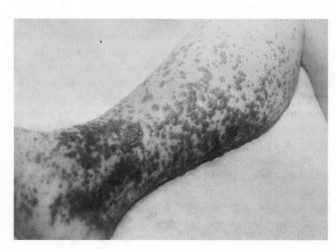

Figure 52.3 Petechial rash and palpable purpura of Henoch-Schönlein purpura. (See color insert.)

of renal disease in those children who present after the age of 7 years, have persistent purpuric lesions, severe abdominal symptoms with GI bleeding, and/or low factor XIII activity. Typical renal disease tends to occur within the first 3 months of the disease onset. One percent to 3% of those with renal involvement progress to renal failure.

Other symptoms include low-grade fever, malaise, non-pitting edema, and headache. Scrotal pain, swelling, and tenderness (orchitis) may also be seen.

Diagnosis

The diagnosis of HSP is based primarily on the history and physical examination findings. No laboratory studies are diagnostic for HSP. Elevated sedimentation rates and white blood cell counts are commonly seen. The serum IgA levels may also be elevated in 50% of patients. The platelet counts are typically normal, as are the results of coagulation studies. Urinalysis may show red blood cells, casts, or protein. The serum is usually negative for ANA, RF, or anti-cytoplasmic neutrophilic antibodies. Although usually unnecessary, punch biopsy of skin lesions will demonstrate a leukocytoclastic vasculitis with IgA and C3 deposition. Ultrasonography may be useful in diagnosing intussusception and orchitis.

Treatment

The goal of HSP management is to provide good supportive care. Physicians should ensure adequate hydration and nutrition. Children should also be monitored for potential complications, including renal involvement and intussusception. Repeat urinalysis should be performed in all children with HSP for at least 3 to 6 months after diagnosis.

The use of steroids for treating HSP is controversial. *Corticosteroids in children who are experiencing abdominal pain or GI bleeding may reduce the severity and duration of symptoms.* There is no evidence that corticosteroid use reduces the rate of intussusception or of the development of renal disease. Steroids are also beneficial in reducing severe edema, especially of the scrotum. However, once started, corticosteroids should be weaned slowly over several weeks because of the risk of a rebound if weaned too rapidly.

Severe renal disease is treated with one of the various experimental immunosuppressive regimens.

Prognosis

Most children with HSP have an *excellent prognosis.* Although the average duration of HSP is 4 weeks, it can range from 3 days to 2 years. Patients may experience several "waves" during the course of the disease; subsequent "waves" are usually milder than the initial presentation. The syndrome may recur in 40% of children.

Early morbidity of HSP is caused mainly by GI involvement. Late morbidity is most often caused by renal

involvement. Older patients or those with early nephrotic syndrome or with a significant proportion of crescents found on performing renal biopsy have a worse renal prognosis. Of those patients in whom nephritic or nephrotic syndrome develops, approximately 44% have long-term renal impairment, with 1% to 3% of these children progressing to end-stage renal failure. HSP is one of the major causes of acquired chronic renal failure in childhood (10%).

The mortality rate of HSP is <1%.

DERMATOMYOSITIS

Juvenile dermatomyositis (JDM) is defined as a multisystem disease characterized by acute and chronic inflammation of skin, GI tract, and striated muscle, resulting from small blood vessel vasculopathy (Table 52.3).

Etiology and Epidemiology

The etiology of JDM is unknown. Several possible pathogenic mechanisms have been suggested, with immunologic mechanisms thought to be involved. Evidence has been gathered that certain genetic polymorphisms, abnormalities of cell-mediated immunity, and infectious agents may be associated with the development of JDM. However, these studies are far from conclusive. Patients with immunodeficiencies, especially B-cell–related or combined variable immunodeficiency, are at higher risk of developing a form of JDM associated with echovirus infection.

The incidence of JDM in children has been estimated to be in the range of 0.5 cases/100,000 per year. The disease occurs more commonly in girls than boys, with an estimated 2:1 ratio overall. The peak onset is between the ages of 4 and 10 years, with a mean of 7 years, although a bimodal incidence includes a second peak in adolescence.

TABLE 52.3

CLINICAL FEATURES OF JUVENILE DERMATOMYOSITIS

Easy fatigue
Progressive proximal muscle weakness
Classic rash
Calcinosis (late)
Fever
Muscle pain or tenderness
Lymphadenopathy
Arthralgia/arthritis
Hepatosplenomegaly
Nonspecific rash
Raynaud phenomena
Dyspnea
Dysphagia
Abdominal pain

The geographic distribution of the disease is widespread. In the United States the disease is seen more among whites than Hispanics and African Americans.

Pathology

Vasculopathy (not vasculitis!) that affects arterioles, venules, and capillaries is noted in the muscles, skin, and GI system. Muscle fibers are often atrophic or necrotic, with signs of fiber regeneration. Fibers of various sizes and increased fat deposition may be present. These findings are not uniformly present throughout the muscle (*skipped* lesions) and can be missed while performing a "blind" biopsy. Skin changes may involve atrophy or hyperplasia of the epidermis with cellular infiltrates. The GI tract is affected by the vasculopathy, and ulceration or perforation may develop. In late disease, calcium deposition may be found in the skin, fascia, and muscles.

Clinical Presentation

JDM is often a difficult disease to recognize and diagnose. Although *classic* cutaneous manifestations have been described, they are often not present at the time of onset. JDM presents initially with constitutional signs and symptoms consisting of low-grade fever, fatigue, anorexia, weight loss, and malaise. These are usually followed by the onset of rash and the gradual development of an objective weakness. Nearly one third of patients have an acute onset of weakness with some developing rhabdomyolysis at the onset.

Rash is found in >75% of patients. The three most common skin manifestations include:

- Heliotrope rash
- Gottron papules (Fig. 52.4)
- Periungual erythema and telangiectasia

The heliotrope rash is a violaceous, reddish eruption over the upper eyelids, often accompanied by swelling.

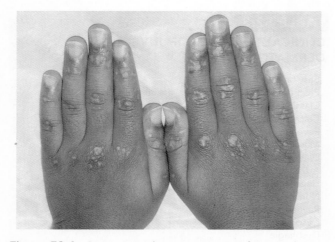

Figure 52.4 Gottron papules on extensor surfaces, pathognomonic for juvenile dermatomyositis. (See color insert.)

Frequently, a malar rash similar to that seen in lupus is also present. Gottron papules are symmetric changes over the dorsal aspect of the fingers, most commonly the proximal interphalangeal joints. Less commonly, the knees, elbows, extensor surfaces of the arms and legs, and entire trunk may be affected. The lesions tend to be shiny-pink to red-scaly plaques and often mimic the changes of psoriasis. Both these eruptions are aggravated by sun exposure. *Gottron papules are considered the most specific manifestation of JDM.* Nail bed changes, such as subungual erythema, telangiectasia, and other abnormalities, may be present in 50% or more of children. Patients with severe disease will develop ulceration. Raynaud phenomenon is commonly seen, with typical periungual capillary abnormalities seen under the microscope.

Muscle weakness is primarily proximal and symmetric. It is usually insidious in onset and gradually worsens over time. Functional difficulties, such as with climbing stairs, arising from a prone position, combing hair, or lifting weights are often present. The *Gower sign* is common, with children having to "climb up" their own body to bring themselves to a standing position. In severely affected patients, difficulty in swallowing and speaking, drooling, and possibly aspiration may be noted. Many patients (30%–80%) have muscle pain and edema. Thirty percent of patients develop arthritis, usually nonerosive. Heart muscle may be involved with the development of myocarditis and conduction abnormalities. Many patients develop a restrictive lung disease related to muscle weakness. Furthermore, an increased risk of aspiration along with disease-related factors may result in interstitial lung disease.

Calcinosis usually has a later onset and may be related to the severity of disease and with a delay in diagnosis and therapy. It develops in approximately 40% of patients. Calcinosis may present as superficial plaques or nodules that do not interfere with function, as deep muscular deposits that may affect movement (especially if near the joints) and break through the skin, or as lesions along myofascial planes that may limit motion and become painful. These calcified deposits may slowly resolve with time.

Less commonly, a symptomatic vasculopathy of the GI tract may occur and is associated with a poorer prognosis. Affected patients may present with abdominal pain and are at risk for GI perforation and hemorrhage. Most early mortality in JDM is caused by GI disease.

Diagnosis

The diagnosis of JDM can often be made on the basis of clinical findings, but in patients without the characteristic rash, certain laboratory, electromyographic, and pathologic findings provide additional evidence. Levels of muscle enzymes, including creatine kinase (CPK), lactate dehydrogenase (LDH), aldolase, aspartate aminotransferase (AST), and alanine aminotransferase (ALT) may be elevated. Most patients (≥90%) have abnormal levels of at least one of these enzymes but may have normal levels of the others. Enzyme levels may be totally normal, especially late in the disease course, in part because of widespread muscle atrophy. Upper GI series are used to evaluate the swallowing mechanism, esophageal peristalsis, and the presence of gastroesophageal reflux. Chest radiographs, computed tomography scan, and pulmonary function tests are used to evaluate the presence of lung involvement.

Results of autoantibody studies are variable and usually not specific for JDM. ANA is present in approximately 60% of patients, whereas RF is usually absent. There are specific myositis-related antibodies. For example, Jo-1 is associated with interstitial lung disease, Pm-Scl with myositis-scleroderma overlap disease, and Mi-2 with a specific rash pattern, malar erythema, and Gottron papules. Increased levels of inflammatory markers, such as erythrocyte sedimentation rate and C-reactive protein, when present, correlate with the degree of clinical inflammation and are useful to differentiate JDM from noninflammatory causes of muscle disorders. However, many patients with JDM do not have increased levels of inflammatory markers. Electromyography can show changes characteristic of myopathy. These changes include decreased amplitude, sharp waves, and fibrillations. It is important to note that these changes are not specific to JDM, and that the electromyogram may appear normal in some children with active disease. *Muscle biopsy is the definitive test in establishing the diagnosis of JDM.* Open biopsy is preferred, and the specimen should be taken from an affected muscle group not previously tested by electromyography. The use of MRI to detect muscle edema on T2 and short inversion time inversion-recovery (STIR) images can be useful in identifying a location for muscle biopsy and following the course of disease and the response to treatment. For the most part, MRI has replaced electromyography in the diagnostic evaluation of JDM.

Treatment

Corticosteroids, usually prednisone, are the initial line of treatment in children with JDM. The exact dose and preferred method of administering prednisone and the use of adjunctive medications, however, vary. Patients with significant disease are typically initially treated with high-dose (usually intravenous in the first few days) prednisone. Monitoring of systemic signs of disease, measurements of muscle strength, serial measurements of muscle enzymes, and occasionally imaging studies (MRI) are used to assess the response to treatment. The clinical response to prednisone may be variable. Fever usually resolves in 1 to 2 days, muscle enzymes decrease in 1 to 2 weeks, and it may take as long as several months before muscle strength is restored. Patients on high doses or prolonged courses of corticosteroids are likely to experience side effects, including osteopenia, aseptic necrosis, growth suppression, and rarely steroid myopathy. Methotrexate is often used as a steroid sparing medication early in the treatment regimen.

Hydroxychloroquine may be used as an adjuvant for the treatment of the skin manifestations of JDM. Intravenous immunoglobulins are often effective as a steroid-sparing agent. Cyclophosphamide is used for critical muscle and GI disease and for interstitial lung disease. Cyclosporin and tacrolimus may be effective in some patients. No therapies have been found to be consistently effective for the treatment of calcinosis. Supportive therapy similar to those mentioned in SLE is crucial in preventing complications. Meticulous skin care is necessary to treat patients with ulcers and calcinosis. Nasogastric feedings, thickened food, and oral suction may be needed for patients with swallowing difficulties and aspiration. In the early stages of disease, oxygen or other respiratory support may be needed. Strenuous physical activity should be avoided during active muscle disease.

Prognosis

The course of JDM may be variable, and the response to therapy is unpredictable. In 30% to 40% of patients, JDM manifests as a single episode that responds well to treatment and never recurs (monophasic). In 10% to 30% of patients, the disease has a polyphasic course with a good overall outcome. In 30% to 50%, JDM has a chronic course. Many of the latter patients develop calcinosis and other disabilities related to damage from disease or treatment. Early diagnosis and adequate treatment strongly influence the overall outcome; patients in whom the institution of treatment is delayed have a higher incidence of severe calcinosis and functional limitation. In the era before steroids, the mortality of JDM approached 40%; however, the mortality is now <10%, with death caused by infection, intestinal perforation, or respiratory failure. Patients who develop early ulcerations and a GI course have a poor prognosis.

REVIEW EXERCISES

QUESTIONS

1. A 15-year-old girl is admitted to your practice with hypertension, proteinuria, and microscopic hematuria. On examination, you notice a rash across the bridge of her nose and upper cheeks. Her family history is positive for autoimmune diseases, including lupus in a maternal aunt. You suspect she has glomerulonephritis secondary to underlying SLE. Of the following, the laboratory test result that would *most* support your diagnosis is:

a) Elevated erythrocyte sedimentation rate
b) Positive RF
c) Decreased levels of C3, C4
d) Elevated platelet count
e) Positive antibodies to single-stranded DNA

Answer

The answer is c. Nephritis associated with lupus most often presents with microscopic hematuria and sometimes also with hypertension and proteinuria. Most patients with lupus have renal involvement at some point in the course of the disease, and the histologic type may correlate with eventual outcome. In many patients, one type of renal disease evolves to another. Patients with renal disease usually have a decreased CH_{50} in addition to low levels of C3 and C4 and the presence of anti–double-stranded DNA antibodies. The erythrocyte sedimentation rate may be elevated, and RFs may be found, but these findings are not specific to lupus. ANA is nearly always present and characteristically the platelet count may be decreased. Antibodies to double-stranded DNA, but not single-stranded DNA, are specific for SLE.

2. A woman with previously diagnosed SLE has just delivered a term newborn. She had excellent prenatal care, and no fetal problems were noted during her pregnancy. The *most* common finding on examination of her newborn is:

a) Complete heart block
b) Rash on the face and scalp that appears to be photosensitive
c) Hematuria
d) Enlarged spleen
e) No pathologic findings

Answer

The answer is e. Most infants born to mothers with SLE *do not* develop neonatal lupus. Complete heart block is the most common *cardiac* finding in babies with neonatal lupus. A transient photosensitive rash is found in most cases of infants *with* neonatal lupus. Usually the rash develops after a significant light exposure, often during phototherapy for hyperbilirubinemia. Because the rash is thought to be related to transferred maternal IgG antibodies (SS-A and SS-B), it is self-limited and almost always resolves by 6 to 8 months of age. Complete atrioventricular (AV) block is usually detected in the second trimester of pregnancy. Therefore, infants who have had excellent prenatal care and no fetal problems will not develop an AV block. This block is permanent and requires the insertion of a pacemaker. Other features of neonatal lupus include transient thrombocytopenia and liver enzyme abnormalities.

3. A 5-year-old boy has a persistent fever of 4 weeks duration. The temperatures are high ($39°C–40°C$ [$102.2°F–104°F$]) and occur each evening. He has a maculopapular erythematous rash that is especially prominent during the febrile periods. He has also had swelling and pain in his knees and ankles for the past week. The liver and spleen tips are palpable. Laboratory

studies reveal a white blood cell count of $20,000/mm^3$, hemoglobin level of 9.0 g/dL, and platelet count of $650,000/mm^3$. Which of the following is a *true* statement?

a) The patient is likely to be positive for RF.
b) Pericarditis is a complication.
c) *Yersinia* is likely to be found on stool culture.
d) Slit-lamp examination of the eyes will commonly reveal uveitis.
e) The patient is likely to be positive for ANA.

Answer

The answer is b. Although the child described has not yet had arthritis for 6 weeks, his symptoms are consistent with systemic-onset JRA. Pericarditis may develop in up to 50% of children with systemic-onset JRA. In most cases, the pericarditis is mild. Patients with systemic-onset JRA are most likely to be negative for RF and ANA. Infectious gastroenteritis caused by *Yersinia* is associated with reactive arthritis. Uveitis is rarely seen in systemic-onset JRA, unlike other subtypes of JRA.

4. A 5-year-old boy has had low-grade fever, abdominal pain, vomiting, and diarrhea for the last 5 days. A palpable, nonblanching rash has now appeared on his lower extremities. On further questioning, you discover he had symptoms of an upper respiratory infection 1 week ago. The *most* likely diagnosis is:

a) Kawasaki disease
b) JRA
c) HSP
d) Meningococcemia
e) ITP

Answer

The answer is c. Up to 15% of children with HSP may have abdominal pain (and even "dysentery") preceding the rash. The characteristic rash of HSP is primarily on the lower extremities or gravity-dependent areas and consists of palpable purpura or petechiae. Many children with HSP have had an upper respiratory infection or strep throat in the weeks preceding HSP. The rash described in the preceding text is not typical of JRA. Kawasaki disease includes high fevers, as well as conjunctivitis, mucous membrane changes, cervical lymphadenopathy, and edema of the extremities. The purpura of ITP is usually not palpable and has a different distribution, although, ITP may also follow a viral illness.

5. The following are associated with the disorder explained in question 4 *except*:

a) Nephritis
b) Testicular swelling
c) Intussusception
d) Periarticular edema
e) Coronary aneurysm

Answer

The answer is e. Nephritis, testicular swelling, and arthritis (with periarthritis from edema) are frequently seen in children with HSP. Three fourths of children with HSP experience some GI involvement, and intussusception develops in 1% to 5%. Children with Kawasaki disease are at risk for the development of coronary aneurysms.

6. A 7-year-old girl is brought in by her mother because she is unable to run and play as she used to. On questioning, the mother states that she does not play tag with her friends anymore and that she seems to have trouble climbing the stairs at home. In addition, she has not been eating well and complains of being tired all the time. The examination reveals that to rise from a seated position on the floor, she must "climb up" her body with her arms. In addition, she is noted to have an erythematous rash over her eyelids and scaly red skin over her knuckles. Of the following, the test that is *most* likely to yield a diagnosis is:

a) Erythrocyte sedimentation rate
b) ANA
c) Creatinine kinase levels
d) An MRI of the brain and spine
e) Decreased complement levels

Answer

The answer is c. This girl has many features consistent with JDM, including fatigue, poor appetite, and proximal muscle weakness. In addition, she has a heliotrope rash and Gottron papules over her knuckles. Of the choices provided, increased creatinine kinase level provides a probable diagnosis. Other muscle enzymes that may be elevated include AST, ALT, LDH, and aldolase. RF is usually negative. ANA is frequently present in patients with JDM but is not specific to this disease. Decreased complement levels are characteristic for SLE.

A brain and spine MRI would be the wrong diagnostic choice for the child with this constellation of symptoms and signs. A muscle MRI on the other hand, would be a very useful test in detecting muscle edema and finding a location likely to yield a positive finding on muscle biopsy. Other diagnostic options include the use of electromyography, although it is usually not necessary in the presence of a classic presentation like the patient in this vignette.

SUGGESTED READINGS

1. Ballinger S. Henoch-Schönlein purpura. *Curr Opin Rheumatol* 2003;15:591–594.
2. Benselar SM, Silverman ED. Systemic lupus erythematosus. *Pediatr Clin North Am* 2005;52:443–467.
3. Cassidy JT, Laxer RM. Systemic lupus erythematosus. In: Cassidy JT, Petty RE, Laxer RM, Lindsley CB, eds. *Textbook of pediatric rheumatology.* Philadelphia: Elsevier Saunders, 2005:342–391.
4. Cassidy JT, Lindsley CB. Juvenile dermatomyositis. In: Cassidy JT, Petty RE, Laxer RM, Lindsley CB, eds. *Textbook of pediatric rheumatology.* Philadelphia: Elsevier Saunders, 2005:407–441.
5. Cassidy JT, Petty RE. Chronic arthritis. In: Cassidy JT, Petty RE, Laxer RM, Lindsley CB, eds. *Textbook of pediatric rheumatology.* Philadelphia: Elsevier Saunders, 2005:184–341.
6. Cassidy JT, Petty RE. Leukocytoclastic vasculitis. In: Cassidy JT, Petty RE, Laxer RM, Lindsley CB, eds. *Textbook of pediatric rheumatology.* Philadelphia: Elsevier Saunders, 2005:496–511.
7. Compeyrot-Lacassagne S, Feldman BM. Inflammatory myopathies in children. *Pediatr Clin North Am* 2005;52:493–520.
8. Hashkes PJ, Laxer RM. Medical treatment of juvenile idiopathic arthritis. *JAMA* 2005;294:1671–1684.
9. Lanzkowsky S, Lanzkowsky L, Lanzkowsky P. Henoch–Schönlein purpura. *Pediatr Rev* 1992;13:130–137.
10. Pachman LM. Juvenile dermatomyositis: a clinical overview. *Pediatr Rev* 1990;12:117–125.
11. Ravelli A, Martini A. Juvenile idiopathic arthritis. *Lancet* 2007;369:767–778.
12. Schneider R, Passo MH. Juvenile rheumatoid arthritis. *Rheum Dis Clin North Am* 2002;28:503–530.
13. Silverman ED, Spence D, Hamilton RM. Neonatal lupus erythematosus. In: Cassidy JT, Petty RE, Laxer RM, Lindsley CB, eds. *Textbook of pediatric rheumatology.* Philadelphia: Elsevier Saunders, 2005:392–405.

Chapter 53

BOARD SIMULATION: Pediatric Rheumatology

Steven Spalding

QUESTIONS

1. You are seeing a 3-year-old white male, who has recently moved to your city, for fever. Going through his chart, you notice that he has been seen about every 4 weeks for fevers for the last 6 months. During the history, his mother reports that he has fever every 26 to 27 days "like clockwork" and that these fevers are associated with sore throat, swollen glands, and abdominal pain. His fevers remain in the 102°F to 103°F range for 4 to 5 days and are minimally responsive to acetaminophen and ibuprofen. He is completely healthy between febrile episodes. On examination, his growth parameters are normal. He is febrile at 39.6°C and is ill-appearing. There is oropharyngeal erythema, tonsillar hypertrophy, posterior pharyngeal ulcers, anterior cervical lymphadenopathy, and abdominal tenderness to palpation. Of the following, which is the most likely laboratory finding in this patient?
a) Tumor necrosis factor receptor super family 1A gene mutation
b) Elevated erythrocyte sedimentation rate (ESR) and C-reactive protein (CRP)
c) Elevated ferritin
d) Mevalonate kinase gene mutation
e) Mediterranean fever gene mutation

Answer
The answer is b. Periodic fever, aphthous stomatitis, pharyngitis, and adenopathy, or PFAPA syndrome is a relatively common cause of recurrent fever in children, but its true prevalence is unknown. Although the exact cause has yet to be determined, this syndrome results in stereotypic attacks of fever lasting 4 to 5 days recurring on a fairly regular interval of approximately 4 to 5 weeks. Although not contained in the acronym, abdominal pain accompanies febrile episodes in up to 60% of patients. Children with PFAPA are completely healthy between attacks and display normal growth and development. During attacks, inflammatory markers such as the ESR and CRP are typically elevated, but return to normal between attacks. Children who remain ill between febrile episodes, have atypical growth and/or development, or persistently elevated inflammatory markers are more likely to have a more serious cause of their recurrent fevers. In general, the prognosis of children with PFAPA is good with nearly 40% either entering spontaneous remission or reduction in frequency and severity of attacks within 2 to 5 years of symptom onset.

2. Which therapeutic option has shown the greatest efficacy in treatment of the condition for the patient in question 1?
a) Adenotonsillectomy
b) Prednisone 1 mg/kg by mouth at onset of symptoms
c) Cimetidine 10 mg/kg by mouth four times a day
d) Infliximab 5 mg/kg every 4 weeks
e) Methotrexate 15 mg/m^2 subcutaneously every week

Answer
The answer is a. There are several treatment options for PFAPA. A single dose of oral prednisone or prednisolone (0.5–2 mg/kg) has been shown to abort attacks if given at the first sign of fever in >90% of PFAPA patients. However, almost 20% of patients who use prednisone to manage their attacks suffer an increase in the frequency and severity of attacks. Cimetidine and colchicine have also been used to prevent PFAPA episodes with success in 33% of patients. The medication must be given every day and missing a single dose can result in an attack. Adenotonsillectomy has been gaining popularity in the management of this condition. To date, close to 100 patients with PFAPA have undergone tonsillectomy reported in the literature, which has resulted in complete cessation of attacks in virtually 100% patients within 12 months after the procedure. There have been no

reported adverse events. Infliximab and methotrexate have not been used for treatment of PFAPA.

3. A 16-year-old white female presents for evaluation of fatigue. For the last 4 months, she has been experiencing intermittent muscle and joint pain, in addition to chronic daily headaches. The pain wakes her from sleep and she often feels tired upon waking. She has not been to school in 2 weeks and takes a 3-hour nap every day. Her examination is normal except for tenderness over her trapezii, second ribs, medial tibial tuberosities, and gluteus medius. What treatment is most likely to result in long-term improvement in this patient?
a) Pregabalin (Lyrica) 50 mg three times a day
b) Referral to pain medicine
c) Physical therapy with cognitive behavioral therapy
d) Oral prednisone at 1 mg/kg per day for 5 days followed by a 2-week taper
e) Oral naproxen at 10 mg/kg twice a day

Answer
The answer is c. Juvenile fibromyalgia syndrome (jFMS) is an increasingly recognized condition. Patients with jFMS complain of a combination of the following six symptoms: fatigue, disordered and nonrestorative sleep, chronic headaches, nonspecific gastrointestinal complaints, widespread musculoskeletal pain above and below the waist, and chronic anxiety or tension. In addition to these somatic complaints, these patients have exquisite tenderness at characteristic musculoskeletal tender points on physical examination. Several medications have recently been marketed as treatment for adult fibromyalgia, including pregabalin and duloxetine. At the time of publication, there have been no prospective studies examining the safety or efficacy of these medications in the treatment of jFMS. Experts in jFMS recommend a multidisciplinary treatment plan including intensive physical therapy, cognitive behavioral therapy, and improved sleep hygiene. Adjunctive use of amitriptyline (<75 mg) in combination with a multidisciplinary care plan may also be beneficial. Longitudinal studies on patients with jFMS are few so prognosis cannot be stated with accuracy. However, successful participation in and completion of a multidisciplinary care plan usually results in sustained return of function but pain may persist for years.

4. A 15-year-old female presents to your office for evaluation of fatigue, low-grade fevers, headaches, abdominal pain after eating, and pain in her left arm with exercise. On examination she is obese and mildly hypertensive (132/89 mm Hg), but your nurse also notes a 15 mm Hg difference in systolic blood pressure between arms. The remainder of your exam is normal. What is the next most appropriate step in your evaluation?
a) Magnetic resonance angiography of aorta and great vessels

b) Referral to physical therapy
c) Referral to neurology
d) Initiate amitriptyline at 25 mg by mouth before bed
e) Initiate enalapril 10 mg once a day

Answer
The answer is a. This patient's signs and symptoms are suggestive of vasculitis, specifically Takayasu's arteritis (TA). TA is a large-vessel vasculitis causing stenotic and rarely aneurismal changes in the aorta and its branches. The thoracic aorta and its branches are commonly involved but the abdominal aorta and renal arteries may be more frequently affected in children. Children with TA may present with constitutional symptoms such as fatigue and malaise or hypertension. In addition, children are less likely than adults to complain of carotidynia (pain over course of internal carotid arteries) and claudication. Recently proposed classification criteria for childhood TA require demonstration of angiographic abnormalities of the aorta or its primary branches using magnetic resonance, computed tomography, or conventional angiography plus at least one of the four following features:

- Hypertension
- Decreased peripheral artery pulses and/or claudication of extremities
- Blood pressure difference of >10 mm HG
- Bruits over aorta and/or it major branches

Typically, these children have elevated acute phase reactants (ESR, CRP, elevated platelets, anemia) on laboratory examination. The mainstay of treatment for children with TA includes high-dose oral prednisone tapered over several months. Approximately 50% of patients treated with prednisone alone achieve good control of their disease. For the patients who are unable to wean from their prednisone, a steroid-sparing immunosuppressing agent such as methotrexate or cyclophosphamide should be initiated.

5. An 8-year-old white female is being seen for a rash. Her mother noted a linear band of violet skin on the left outer thigh, which has become larger and "thicker" over the last several months. On examination, there is an 11-cm × 3-cm plaque with violaceous borders extending from the groin to the knee on the left medial thigh. What information can you offer to this mother about the prognosis of this condition?
a) There is an 80% chance of interstitial lung disease.
b) Many children with this condition develop Raynaud's phenomenon.
c) More than 20% children have extracutaneous manifestations.
d) The rash will get smaller and fade away completely.
e) About 10% develop pulmonary hypertension.

Answer
The answer is c. Linear scleroderma (LS) is an autoimmune condition that results in thickening and

inflammation of the skin and the underlying tissues. It is the most common form of localized scleroderma in childhood. The exact etiology of LS is unknown, but evidence points to disordered fibrogenesis. Females are much more commonly affected than males. In LS, lesions usually occur on the extremities and may extend in proximal and distal directions. If these lesions cross joints, they may result in arthritis and eventual loss of mobility in that joint. The lesions may also extend to the deeper tissues, including the muscle and rarely bone. More than 20% of children with localized scleroderma have extracutaneous manifestations, including arthritis, neurologic symptoms, or other autoimmune conditions. It is extremely rare for localized sclerodermas such as LS or circumscribed morphea to be associated with systemic sclerosis where one commonly sees Raynaud's phenomenon, pulmonary hypertension, and interstitial lung disease. Laboratory examination may reveal elevated acute phase reactants, eosinophilia, and a positive ANA in nearly 50% of patients. Treatment for LS involves topical and systemic steroids in addition to methotrexate. If left untreated, these lesions can result in significant cosmetic damage and functional disability.

6. You are seeing a 16-year-old white female for a routine annual visit. She had been cared for by your partner until his recent retirement. In reviewing her chart, you notice that she has been treated four times in the last year for sinusitis and three times for culture-negative urinary tract infections. On examination, her blood pressure is mildly elevated at 139/88 mm Hg. Inspection of her nasal mucosa demonstrates very edematous and friable mucosa. Her lungs are clear. Her urinalysis today demonstrated 2+ blood, 2+ protein, and 1+ leukocyte esterase. Which of following are her labs most likely to demonstrate?

a) (+)Antineutrophil cytoplasmic antibody, cytoplasmic pattern, anti-myeloperoxidase(+)
b) (+)Antineutrophil cytoplasmic antibody, cytoplasmic pattern, anti-Proteinase 3(+)
c) (+)Antineutrophil cytoplasmic antibody, perinuclear pattern, anti-myeloperoxidase(+)
d) Antinuclear antibody(+), anti–double-stranded DNA(+)
e) Antinuclear antibody(+), anti-Smith(+)

Answer
The answer is b. Wegener's granulomatosis (WG) is a necrotizing vasculitis of the medium and small blood vessels. Females are affected more commonly than males and children most frequently develop symptoms in their second decade of life. Clinically, children may present with the classic triad of:

■ Sinusitis
■ Hemoptysis
■ Glomerulonephritis manifested as hematuria

In addition, constitutional symptoms including fatigue, weight loss, and fevers are very common. WG is considered one of the pulmonary-renal syndromes along with Goodpasture syndrome, microscopic polyangiitis (MPA), and systemic lupus erythematosus. The formation of anti-neutrophil cytoplasmic antibodies (ANCA) is very specific to both WG and MPA, but the conditions can be differentiated by their immunofluorescence patterns as well as antigen specificity. Approximately 80% of children with WG have cytoplasmic staining pattern and presence of anti–proteinase-3 IgG antibodies, whereas almost 90% of all pediatric patients with MPA have presence of ANCA with perinuclear staining on immunofluorescence and IgG antibodies specific for the enzyme myeloperoxidase.

7. Which of the following findings indicate an underlying rheumatologic condition as a cause of Raynaud's phenomenon?

a) Positive antinuclear antibody testing and fatigue
b) Positive antinuclear antibody testing and joint pain with activity
c) Positive antinuclear antibody testing and abnormal nailfold capillaries
d) Positive antinuclear antibody testing and family history of lupus
e) Positive antinuclear antibody testing and hypermobility

Answer
The answer is c. Raynaud's phenomenon (RP) is characterized by episodic color changes in the digits resulting from intermittent vasospasm of the digital arteries because of vasculopathy and/or vascular hyperreactivity. Classically, these color changes are triphasic begin as a stark white discoloration that begins at the tip of the digit and end abruptly at one of the joints. The white color slowly changes to blue then finally to red as perfusion is restored. However, most children with RP experience only monophasic or biphasic color changes. Triggers for RP include cold, stress, and exercise. Females are more often affected than males and onset is usually in the second decade of life. Children may have primary RP, which is unrelated to an underlying autoimmune disease. Children with primary RP are usually adolescent females with a low body mass index. In addition, a recent publication has documented the frequent occurrence of RP in children with attention deficit disorder treated with stimulants. In contrast, children with RP related to a rheumatologic condition, typically SLE, mixed connective tissue disease, juvenile dermatomyositis, or juvenile systemic sclerosis, frequently have a positive antinuclear antibody (ANA) and abnormalities of their nailfold capillaries, including dropout and tortuosity.

8. A 15-year-old African-American male presents for evaluation of shortness of breath. He also reports that his vision has become "blurry" recently and that he has painful "dark red bumps" over his shins. On examination, you note keratic precipitates, tender, erythematous nodules over the shins, and soft crackles in the lower lung fields bilaterally. Pulmonary function tests in your office demonstrate his forced vital capacity (FVC) and forced expiratory volume in 1 second (FEV1) are 60% of predicted and a chest radiograph demonstrates hilar lymphadenopathy. Which of the following tests demonstrates the highest specificity in this condition?

a) Angiotensin converting enzyme
b) Antinuclear antibody
c) Antineutrophil cytoplasmic antibody
d) Inflammatory bowel disease series-7 panel
e) Lymph node biopsy demonstrating noncaseating granulomas

Answer

The answer is e. Sarcoidosis is a rare systemic granulomatous disorder that can affect any organ system. In the United States, African Americans are three times more likely to develop sarcoidosis than whites. Children with sarcoidosis frequently have constitutional symptoms in addition to respiratory symptoms, including cough, chest pain, and shortness of breath. Skin rashes, such as erythema nodosum, and musculoskeletal complaints, including polyarticular arthritis, are also common. Children with sarcoid may present with posterior uveitis, abnormalities of the central nervous system, or nephritis as well. Angiotensin-converting enzyme (ACE) produced by sarcoid granulomas may be elevated in up to 60% of children with sarcoidosis. However, false-positives are frequent, especially in African Americans. Most children with sarcoidosis will have hilar lymphadenopathy on plain radiography and may also demonstrate signs of interstitial lung disease on CT scan or pulmonary function testing. In addition, peripheral adenopathy is a very common finding in childhood sarcoidosis, which may be amenable to biopsy. These nodes demonstrate the classic noncaseating granulomas characteristic for sarcoidosis. However, since similar pathology may be seen in various conditions, great care must be taken to perform a thorough evaluation for other, especially infectious, etiologies.

9. An 8-year-old white male presents for evaluation of recurrent fevers. For the last 9 months, he has had fevers every 5 to 6 weeks that last 3 days and are associated with intense abdominal pain. Several relatives in Italy have had similar symptoms and passed away from renal failure. Which medication will prevent fevers and improve this patient's prognosis?

a) Daily oral prednisone
b) Daily oral colchicine
c) Daily oral aspirin
d) Weekly subcutaneous etanercept
e) Monthly intravenous infliximab

Answer

The answer is b. Although currently rare in the United States, familial Mediterranean fever (FMF) is one of the most common causes of recurrent fevers globally. Patients with FMF can usually trace their heritage to countries surrounding the Mediterranean Sea. (Up to 20% of patients with FMF have their first attack of symptoms before age 10 years, and 80% experience their first attack by age 20 years.) These attacks are usually short-lived, lasting only 2 to 3 days, are characterized by fever, abdominal pain, and arthritis and may occur 8 to 12 times a year. Mutations in the Mediterranean fever (MEFV) gene result in a dysfunctional form of the protein pyrin, which plays a central role in regulating the production of the potent proinflammatory cytokine interleukin-1, thus leading to FMF attacks. The resulting persistent inflammation can result in amyloidosis and renal failure. Daily oral colchicine has been shown to dramatically reduce the frequency and severity of febrile attack in FMF in up to 90% of patients and, most importantly, reduce the risk of amyloidosis from 37% to 5%.

SUGGESTED READINGS

1. Akikusa JD, Schneider R, Harvey EA, et al. Clinical features and outcome of pediatric Wegener's granulomatosis. *Arthritis Rheum* 2007;57(5):837–844.
2. Anthony KK, Schanberg LE. Pediatric pain syndromes and management of pain in children and adolescents with rheumatic disease. *Rheum Dis Clin North Am* 2007;33(3):625–660.
3. Goldman W, Seltzer R, Reuman P. Association between treatment with central nervous system stimulants and Raynaud's syndrome in children: a retrospective case-control study of rheumatology patients. *Arthritis Rheum* 2008;58(2):563–566.
4. Hoffmann AL, Milman N, Byg KE. Childhood sarcoidosis in Denmark 1979–1994: incidence, clinical features and laboratory results at presentation in 48 children. *Acta Paediatr* 2004;93(1): 30–36.
5. Licameli G, Jeffrey J, Luz J, et al. Effect of adenotonsillectomy in PFAPA syndrome. *Arch Otolaryngol Head Neck Surg* 2008;134(2): 136–140.
6. Miller ML, Pachman LM. Vasculitis syndromes. In: Behrman RE, Kliegman RM, and Jenson HB, eds. *Nelson textbook of pediatrics*, 18th ed. Philadelphia: Saunders, 2007.
7. Nigrovic PA, Fuhlbrigge RC, Sundel RP. Raynaud's phenomenon in children: a retrospective review of 123 patients. *Pediatrics* 2003; 111(4 Pt 1):715–721.
8. Ozen S, Ruperto N, Dillon MJ, et al. Ann. EULAR/PReS endorsed consensus criteria for the classification of childhood vasculitides. *Rheum Dis* 2006;65(7):936–941. Epub 2005 Dec 1.
9. Padeh S, Berkun Y. Auto-inflammatory fever syndromes. *Rheum Dis Clin North Am* 2007;33(3):585–623.
10. Renko M, Salo E, Putto-Laurila A, et al. A randomized, controlled trial of tonsillectomy in periodic fever, aphthous stomatitis, pharyngitis, and adenitis syndrome. *J Pediatr* 2007;151(3):289–292. Epub 2007 Jun 14.
11. Tasher D, Somekh E, Dalal I. PFAPA syndrome: new clinical aspects disclosed. *Arch Dis Child* 2006;91(12):981–984.
12. Thomas KT, Feder HM Jr, Lawton AR, et al. Periodic fever syndrome in children. *J Pediatr* 1999;135(1):15–21.
13. Zulian F. Systemic sclerosis and localized scleroderma in childhood. *Rheum Dis Clin North Am* 2008;34(1):239–255.

Chapter 54

Anemia: An Approach to Evaluation

Jawhar Rawwas and L. Kate Gowans

Anemia may be defined as a reduction in red blood cell (RBC) mass or blood hemoglobin concentration. The commonly used measures of anemia are hemoglobin and hematocrit. The hematocrit is the fractional volume of a whole blood sample occupied by RBCs. It is expressed as a percentage. Hemoglobin is a measure of the concentration of the RBC pigment hemoglobin in whole blood, expressed as grams per 100 mL (dL) of whole blood. Hemoglobin value is a direct measurement and is therefore more reliable than hematocrit, which is a calculated value. The overall clinical picture is important in the investigation for the causes of anemia. On the basis of the methods used to determine the normal range for hemoglobin and hematocrit values, it is expected that 2.5% of the healthy population will have apparently low hemoglobin and hematocrit, which may be incorrectly interpreted as anemia. On the other hand, hemoglobin and hematocrit values may be normal in a child with a chronic cardiac or pulmonary disorder, but below the level required to provide adequate tissue oxygenation, resulting in a *functional anemia*.

In general, there is considerable variation in hemoglobin and hematocrit values in pediatric patients. Therefore, it is important to use age- and sex-adjusted norms when evaluating a pediatric patient for anemia.

AGE-DEPENDENT VARIATION

Erythropoiesis is active during intrauterine life. The hemoglobin value at birth of a full term newborn (as seen in cord blood) is approximately 16.6 g/dL, and the lowest acceptable value is 13.8 g/dL (Table 54.1). The mean corpuscular volume (MCV) of RBCs is also increased in the newborn, so that values <96 μ^3 indicate microcytosis. On exposure to increased oxygen after birth, RBC production decreases during the first few days, reaches a minimum during the second week, and subsequently rises to high values at approximately

3 months. This variation in erythropoiesis results in hemoglobin and hematocrit nadirs at 6 to 9 weeks of age (the lowest level is 9 g/dL in a full-term infant), called the *physiologic anemia of infancy*. Erythropoietin levels correspond with these findings, and in term infants these levels are lowest at 1 month and highest at 2 months of age. Anemia in preterm infants may be more pronounced because of inadequate iron stores and because of the shorter lifespan of preterm RBCs. The mean half-life of RBCs in term infants is approximately 23 days, as opposed to 17 days in preterm infants and up to 35 days in adults. The physiologic anemia in a preterm infant may therefore be seen sooner and last longer than observed in a full-term infant.

Infants with inherited RBC membrane abnormalities, such as hereditary spherocytosis, may present with exaggerated anemia in the neonatal period because of the concomitant decrease in erythropoiesis and the increase in splenic RBC destruction that occurs after birth.

During late infancy and childhood, the hemoglobin concentration progressively increases (Table 54.2). With the onset of puberty, differences between the hemoglobin concentration in the sexes become apparent; values for boys are higher by approximately 1 to 1.5 g/dL. African-American children may have hemoglobin levels lower than those of Asian or white children by approximately 0.5 g/dL.

CLASSIFICATION OF ANEMIA

Anemias are commonly classified on the basis of:

- Morphology. The anemia is microcytic, normocytic, or macrocytic. The most reliable laboratory indicator of morphology is the MCV.
- Physiology. The anemia is caused by either decreased production or increased loss or destruction of RBCs or both. The most reliable indicator of physiology is the reticulocyte count.

TABLE 54.1

CORD BLOOD VALUES

	Mean	±2 SD
Hemoglobin	16 g/dL	13.8–20.0 g/dL
Mean corpuscular volume	106 μ^3	96–116 μ^3
Reticulocytes	4%	3%–7%

Values are compiled from various sources.
SD, standard deviation.

It is important to use both systems of classification simultaneously as one proceeds with the investigation for the cause of anemia (Tables 54.3 and 54.4).

HISTORY AND PHYSICAL EXAMINATION

A thorough history and physical examination are critical in the investigation of anemia (Table 54.5).

History

The age and sex of the patient and the duration of the anemia/symptoms are helpful in elucidating the etiology of anemia (Table 54.6). The most frequent causes of anemia in the newborn are hemolysis and blood loss. Primary nutritional iron deficiency anemia occurs more frequently during early toddlerhood and in adolescent girls. Clinical manifestations of the more common hemoglobinopathies are unusual in the neonatal period. The clinical manifestations of anemia (Tables 54.7 and 54.8) depend on age and duration of the anemia and include lethargy, tachycardia, and pallor. Anemic infants may present with irritability and poor oral intake. Patients with chronic anemia may be well compensated and may not have significant complaints. Cardiovascular decompensation is related to the acuity and the severity of the anemia, and neurologic changes become apparent only with the worsening of anemia.

Important historical clues signifying hemolytic episodes include change in urine color, scleral icterus, or jaundice.

TABLE 54.2

HEMOGLOBIN VALUES INDICATING ANEMIA IN DIFFERENT AGE GROUPS

	Age	Hb (g/dL)
Infancy	2–3 Months	9.0 (Term)
		8.5 (Low birth weight)
	3–6 Months	9.5
	6–12 Months	10.0
Childhood	12–24 Months	10.5
	>24 Months	11.5
Adolescence	>13 Years	12.0 (Female)
		13.5 (Male)

TABLE 54.3

MORPHOLOGIC CLASSIFICATION OF ANEMIA

Normocytic (normochromic): normal MCV
Aplastic (hypoplastic) anemia
Anemia secondary to bone marrow infiltration (i.e., leukemia, neuroblastoma)
Secondary anemias
  Hypothyroidism
  Renal disease
  Chronic illness
Transient erythroblastopenia of childhood
Microcytic (hypochromic): decreased MCV, decreased MCH
Iron deficiency anemia
Thalassemia syndromes
Sideroblastic anemia
  Congenital
  Acquired
    Lead intoxication
    Isoniazid toxicity
Anemia of chronic disease (anemia of inflammation)
Rare anemias
  Congenital absence of transferrin
  Copper deficiency
  Lymphoid hamartoma syndrome (Castleman disease)
Hemoglobin E
Macrocytic: increased MCV
Nutritional (primary or secondary): folic acid or B_{12} deficiency
  Malabsorption syndromes
  Juvenile pernicious anemia
  Phenytoin therapy
  Transcobalamin II deficiency
  Congenital folic acid malabsorption
  Congenital B_{12} malabsorption
  Blind loop syndrome
  Surgical resection
Hypothyroidism
Down syndrome
Drug-induced (chemotherapy)
Congenital dyserythropoietic anemias
Primary bone marrow disorders
  Myeloproliferative disorders
  Aplastic anemia (congenital or acquired)
  Diamond-Blackfan anemia
  Pearson syndrome

MCV, mean corpuscular volume; MCH, mean corpuscular hemoglobin.

A history of blood loss is essential and should include:

- Gastrointestinal blood loss, which can manifest as any change in stool color or presence of blood in the stools.
- Vaginal blood loss. Teenaged girls may have excessive menstrual loss, which is not evident to them; therefore, information regarding the menstrual history including duration of periods, flow, quantitation and saturation of tampons or pads, should be obtained.
- Excessive nose bleeds.

Prior anemic episodes, duration, etiology, and resolution, as well as all prior therapy for anemia should be reviewed. A prior complete blood count (CBC) for

TABLE 54.4

FUNCTIONAL (PATHOPHYSIOLOGIC) CLASSIFICATION

Inadequate production (decreased reticulocytes)
Erythroid hypoplasia (decreased red blood cell precursors in the
  bone marrow)
  Aplastic (hypoplastic) anemia
    Congenital
      Fanconi anemia and variants
    Acquired
      Posthepatitis
      Idiopathic
      Paroxysmal nocturnal hemoglobinuria
  Red blood cell aplasia (hypoplasia)
    Congenital
      Diamond-Blackfan anemia
    Acquired
      Transient erythroblastopenia of childhood
      Parvovirus B19 infection
  Tumor infiltration
  Leukemia
  Neuroblastoma
Erythroid hyperplasia (increased red blood cell precursors in the
  bone marrow)
  Iron deficiency
  Vitamin B_{12} deficiency
  Folic acid deficiency
  Sideroblastic anemias
  Thalassemia syndromes
  Dyserythropoietic anemias
Increased destruction or loss (increased reticulocytes)
Blood loss anemia
  Acute (normocytic)
  Chronic (microcytic)
Hemolysis
  Extracorpuscular defect
    Alloimmune
    Autoimmune
    Hypersplenism
    Microangiopathic hemolytic anemia

    Disseminated intravascular coagulation syndromes
    Hemolytic uremic syndrome
    Thrombotic thrombocytopenic purpura
    Macroangiopathic (cardiac) hemolytic anemia
  Intracorpuscular defect
    Membranopathy
      Spherocytosis
      Elliptocytosis
      Stomatocytosis
      Pyropoikilocytosis
      Cation transport
      Paroxysmal nocturnal hemoglobinuria
    Enzymopathy
      Energy-producing (glycolytic) pathway
      Pyruvate kinase deficiency
    Antioxidant (redox) pathway
      Glucose-6-phosphate dehydrogenase deficiency
    Hemoglobinopathy
      Hemoglobinopathies
      Sickle cell disease (SS, SC, S/β thalassemia)
      Thalassemia syndromes
      Unstable hemoglobins
**Decreased production and increased destruction
(ineffective erythropoiesis)**
B_{12} deficiency
Thalassemia major
Folic acid deficiency
Congenital dyserythropoietic anemias

TABLE 54.5

DIAGNOSTIC CLUES TO ANEMIA

Historical Feature	Suggests
Excessive milk intake	Iron deficiency
Pagophagia	Iron deficiency
Pica	Iron deficiency
Neonatal jaundice	Hemolysis
Splenectomy/cholecystectomy	Hemolysis
Abdominal surgery (ileal resection)	Vitamin B_{12} deficiency
Physical examination feature[a]	Suggests
Jaundice	Hemolysis
Splenomegaly	Hemolysis
Maxillary hyperplasia	Hemolysis
Frontal *bossing*	Hemolysis
Koilonychia (spooning of nails)	Iron deficiency
Glossitis	Vitamin B_{12} deficiency
Hepatosplenomegaly	Bone marrow infiltrative disorders

[a]See Tables 54.1, 54.2, and 54.7.

TABLE 54.6

COMMON CAUSES OF ANEMIA IN DIFFERENT AGE GROUPS

Age Groups	Common Causes
Neonatal period	Hemolysis
	Blood loss
Early infancy	Hemolysis
	Blood loss (cow milk protein intolerance)
	Diamond-Blackfan anemia
Late infancy/ Childhood	Iron deficiency
	Secondary anemia (marrow infiltration, blood loss)
	Transient erythroblastopenia of childhood
	Diamond-Blackfan anemia
Adolescence	Iron deficiency
	Secondary anemia (marrow infiltration, blood loss [inflammatory bowel disease])
	Sports anemia

TABLE 54.7

GENERAL CLINICAL MANIFESTATIONS OF ANEMIA

Degree of Anemia	Skin/Mucosae	Cardiovascular System	Central Nervous System
Mild	Normal	No change	No change
Moderate	Pallor	Tachycardia/murmur	Headache
Severe	Marked pallor	Tachycardia/murmur	Fainting
		Heart failure	Syncope/seizure

comparison is helpful. In pediatrics, a frequently seen diagnostic error is when a patient with thalassemia trait is treated with iron supplements because of microcytic anemia. In addition to a complete past medical and surgical history, a careful review of symptoms should be made to elucidate chronic underlying infectious or inflammatory conditions that may result in anemia.

A careful birth history and neonatal course should be obtained, including the blood type of the infant and mother, to ascertain any history of ABO or Rh incompatibility. Any history of exchange or intrauterine transfusion and a history of anemia in the early neonatal period should be obtained. Gestational age at birth is important, as premature infants may have iron deficiency resulting in anemia. The presence of jaundice or need for phototherapy may signify the presence of an inherited hemolytic anemia.

The workup of anemia must include a family history. A family history of anemia, as well as jaundice, gallstones, or splenomegaly should be elicited. A history of family members who have undergone cholecystectomy or splenectomy, particularly at an early age, is important and may aid in the identification of additional individuals with inherited hemolytic anemias. Hemolytic episodes that occur only in male family members may indicate the presence of a sex-linked disorder, such as glucose-6-phosphate dehydrogenase deficiency. Race and ethnic background are helpful in guiding the workup for hemoglobinopathies and enzymopathies. For example, thalassemia syndromes are more common in individuals of Mediterranean and Southeast Asian descent; hemoglobins S and C are most commonly seen in African-American populations.

TABLE 54.8

CLINICAL MANIFESTATIONS OF SOME TYPES OF ANEMIA

Type of Anemia	Clinical Finding
Blood loss	Bleeding site(s)
	Blood in stools
Hemolysis/ dyserythropoiesis	Splenomegaly
	Jaundice
	Frontal or maxillary hyperplasia
Hypoproliferative	See Table 54.9

A history of travel to and from areas of endemic infection (i.e., malaria, hepatitis, and tuberculosis) should be noted and possible infectious etiologies for the anemia should be questioned. It is not unusual to see a mild anemia in the setting of an infection.

Medications and environmental toxin exposure, including the use of well water that contains nitrates and nitrites, should be reviewed. Any history of oxidant-induced hemolysis should be obtained. A history of homeopathic or herbal medications should be elicited, because some of these preparations may contain lead and other toxins. In addition, when evaluating a child with microcytic anemia, specific questions regarding the environment, housing, paint exposure, and cooking materials should be asked, to evaluate for possible lead exposure.

A complete dietary history is critical, to estimate its iron content. The type of diet, type of formula (if iron fortified), and age of the infant at the time of discontinuation of the formula or breast milk should be documented. The quantity and type of milk the infant is drinking should be determined, as *cow milk intake of >900 mL/day in a toddler is associated with iron deficiency.* Goat milk ingestion is associated with folate deficiency. Specific questions as to whether the child has pica may aid in the diagnosis of lead toxicity and/or iron deficiency.

A detailed developmental history is important; loss of milestones or developmental delay in infants with megaloblastic anemia may signify abnormalities in the cobalamin pathway.

Physical Examination

- Skin: Pallor where the capillary beds are visible through the mucosa (e.g., conjunctivae, palms, and nail beds) usually indicates the presence of severe anemia. Hypopigmentation or hyperpigmentation (seen with Fanconi anemia) should be assessed. Jaundice may indicate hemolysis or occasionally ineffective erythropoiesis.
- Nails: Koilonychia (spooning of nails) is associated with iron deficiency.
- Eyes: Pallor and jaundice should be sought. Mild degrees of hyperbilirubinemia are not evident on physical examination. Microphthalmia can be associated with Fanconi anemia.

TABLE 54.9

CONGENITAL SYNDROMES OF BONE MARROW HYPOPLASIA

Type of Anemia	Skin/Mucosae	Other
Fanconi anemia	Skin hyperpigmented/ hypopigmented	Thumb or radius anomalies Short stature Horseshoe kidney Microphthalmia
Diamond-Blackfan anemia	Pallor	Cathie facies (see text) Thumb anomalies Short stature
Dyskeratosis congenita	Dystrophic nails Skin and mucosal lesions	Pathologic fractures
Pearson syndrome	Pallor	Lactic acidemia Pancreatic dysfunction Failure to thrive

- Mouth: Pale oral mucosa and erosion of papillae on the tongue are seen with iron deficiency.
- Facies: Frontal bossing and maxillary hyperplasia can be associated with chronic hemolysis and reactive bone marrow hyperplasia (hemoglobinopathies). Cathie facies (snub nose, thick upper lip, wide-set eyes with an intelligent expression) is associated with congenital hypoplastic (Diamond-Blackfan) anemia (Table 54.9).
- Heart: Abnormal heart sounds or murmurs should be noted.
- Hands: Thumb anomalies are associated with Fanconi anemia and Diamond-Blackfan anemia (Table 54.9).
- Skeletal: Radius abnormalities and short stature are associated with Fanconi anemia.
- Abdomen: Splenomegaly may suggest a hemolytic process.

LABORATORY EVALUATION

The laboratory evaluation should include a CBC comprising RBC indices, a reticulocyte count, and a review of the peripheral blood smear (Table 54.10).

Important facets of individual components of the CBC in the evaluation of anemia include:

- White blood cell (WBC) count: If the WBC count is low, factors such as drugs, viruses, and leukemia, that are suppressing the bone marrow's ability to produce hematopoietic elements, should be considered. A reticulocyte count is helpful in this circumstance. If the WBC count is elevated, morphologically normal white cells are more indicative of stress or infection, whereas morphologically abnormal white cells may be indicative of leukemia.
- RBC count: A normal or elevated RBC count in the setting of a low MCV, is consistent with thalassemia, whereas iron deficiency anemia is associated with a low RBC count.

- Hemoglobin: This is the most reliable measure of anemia because it is a directly measured value (as opposed to hematocrit, which is calculated).
- Hematocrit: A heel stick test on a newborn with poor peripheral perfusion may result in a falsely elevated hematocrit. Hematocrit may be low because of overhydration or dilution with intravenously administered fluids, or it may be high secondary to dehydration.
- MCV: This is a reliable value that is least likely to vary over short periods. Normal values for MCV vary with age. MCV is usually elevated in newborns. Also, because reticulocytes have a greater MCV than mature RBCs, patients with significant degrees of reticulocytosis may have elevated MCV in the face of otherwise normocytic RBCs. An elevated MCV without reticulocytosis or folate/vitamin B_{12} deficiency can be a sign of a primary bone marrow disorder, such as aplastic anemia or myelodysplasia (preleukemia).
- Mean corpuscular hemoglobin (MCH): A low MCH is most useful in the diagnosis of iron deficiency anemia.
- Mean corpuscular hemoglobin concentration (MCHC): This is a calculated value (hemoglobin/hematocrit [Hb/Hct]), which reflects the concentration of hemoglobin in RBCs; this value is usually *decreased in iron deficiency anemia* and increased in cases of loss of intracellular fluid (dehydration or in case of loss of part of the cell membrane). It is most useful in the diagnosis of *hereditary spherocytosis, in which the MCHC is increased* because of a decrease in the surface area of the RBC in an attempt to contain as much hemoglobin as possible.
- Red blood cell distribution width (RDW): This is a quantitative measure of anisocytosis or the degree of variation in the diameter of the RBCs. *RDW is especially helpful in differentiating iron deficiency from thalassemia in the pediatric patient with microcytic anemia. Patients with iron deficiency usually have elevated RDW, whereas patients with thalassemia have cells of homogeneous size and therefore, normal RDW.*

TABLE 54.10

LABORATORY EVALUATION OF ANEMIA

Laboratory Test	Rationale
Peripheral blood smear	Morphologic classification (also evaluates white blood cell count and platelets)
Hemoglobin (Hb)[a]	Documents and quantifies anemia
Hematocrit (Hct)	
Red blood cell count (RBC)	
Red blood cell indices	Confirms morphologic classification
Mean corpuscular volume (MCV) (Hct/RBC)	
Mean corpuscular hemoglobin (MCH) (Hb/RBC)	
Mean corpuscular hemoglobin concentration (MCHC) (Hb/Hct)	
Red blood cell distribution width (RDW)	
Reticulocyte count[b,c]	Pathophysiologic classification (bone marrow activity)
Platelet count	Marrow disorder
	Other associated disorders
White blood cell count	Marrow disorder
	Infection
	Systemic disease

[a]Most blood cell counters quantify RBC, Hb, and MCV and calculate Hct, MCH, MCHC, and RDW.
[b]May be "corrected by the ratio of patient's hematocrit level to normal hematocrit level," or the absolute reticulocyte count can be calculated from the RBC.
[c]The Technicon H$_3$ series blood cell counter provides a reticulocyte hemoglobin content measurement, which may be the first parameter altered in iron-deficient erythropoiesis.

■ Platelet count and mean platelet volume: A low platelet count often indicates a process that is suppressing the bone marrow's production of platelets, or an immune process that is causing the breakdown of both RBCs and platelets. The mean platelet volume may be increased because of freshly produced platelets, which are larger, as seen in immune thrombocytopenia.

■ Reticulocyte count: Reticulocytes are the youngest RBCs in the circulation. They are quantitated by staining with vital dyes, and are reported as a percentage. After the first few months of life, the mean reticulocyte percentage is the same as that of an adult, approximately 1% to 1.5%. The reticulocyte count is an indication of bone marrow erythropoiesis. Anemia with an elevated reticulocyte count suggests bone marrow response to hemolysis or acute blood loss. On the other hand, anemia with a low reticulocyte count indicates a suboptimal bone marrow response and is suggestive of marrow aplasia, infiltration with malignant cells, depression caused by infection or other toxic agents, severe nutritional deficiency, or suboptimal production of erythropoietin. It is important to note that the reticulocyte count may vary during the period of follow-up. One example of this is the increase in reticulocyte count observed after successful therapy for iron deficiency. Another example is patients with transient erythroblastopenia of childhood (TEC), who are usually diagnosed when their reticulocyte count has started to increase after a prolonged period of reticulocytopenia. If, in the setting of anemia, the reticulocyte count is low or reticulocytes are absent and if other ancillary tests fail to indicate the origin of the anemia, a bone marrow examination may be diagnostic. Reticulocytosis absent in the face of anemia is suggestive of:

■ TEC
■ Diamond-Blackfan syndrome
■ Parvovirus B19 infection

■ Blood smear: A review of the peripheral smear is an essential part of any anemia evaluation. A normal RBC is approximately the size of a small lymphocyte; therefore, cell size (MCV) can be estimated visually. The normal mature RBC is a biconcave disc with a central halo. *Increased central pallor indicates hypochromic cells, which most often are seen in iron deficiency and thalassemia. Absence of central pallor is usually seen in spherocytes and reticulocytes.* The peripheral smear is essential in determining the presence of fragmented RBCs, which would indicate a microangiopathic process. Circulating nucleated RBCs usually indicate rapid bone marrow turnover and are seen with hemolytic processes. The peripheral smear is also essential in the evaluation of malignancy (leukemia).

The interpretation of RBC parameters may be complicated by the fact that different etiologies for the anemia can coexist. For example, a patient with leukemia and blood loss secondary to thrombocytopenia can have reticulocytosis even in the setting of partial marrow replacement with leukemia. Another example is concomitant iron and folate deficiency, which can result in normal MCV.

Other studies helpful in differentiating the causes of microcytic, hypochromic anemia include the serum iron level, total iron-binding capacity (TIBC), and serum ferritin level. Children with iron deficiency anemia resulting from either dietary factors or bleeding characteristically have:

- Low serum iron levels (normal range, 22–184 µg/dL)
- High TIBC values (normal range, 100–400 µg/dL)
- Low ferritin levels (normal range, 7–140 ng/mL for children >6 months)

Children with a microcytic, hypochromic anemia secondary to chronic illness or chronic inflammation have iron in storage, but are unable to transport it to erythroblasts. Therefore, these children have:

- Low serum iron levels
- Low TIBC values
- High ferritin levels

An additional source of available laboratory information is a cord blood hemoglobinopathy screening test. In addition to providing an early diagnosis of sickle cell anemia and other hemoglobin variants, it may be especially useful if α-thalassemia is suspected because hemoglobin Bart can be detected in the newborn and can be diagnostic of α-thalassemia. Additional studies useful in specific clinical settings are listed in Table 54.11.

An important principle in the evaluation of anemia is that since erythropoiesis is a dynamic process, a single laboratory determination may not be as accurate as sequential laboratory values. This concept is commonly illustrated in the *therapeutic trial* of iron for children with suspected primary nutritional iron deficiency. In the setting of a microcytic, hypochromic anemia with an elevated RDW and a dietary history suggestive of iron deficiency, a therapeutic trial of iron is indicated. The response to iron therapy is an initial increase in the reticulocyte count, followed by an increase in hemoglobin, and normalization of the RBC indices. These sequential changes not only chronicle the response to iron therapy, but also confirm the diagnostic impression.

TABLE 54.11

ADDITIONAL TESTING IN THE EVALUATION OF ANEMIA

Laboratory Test	Rationale
Occult blood	Suspected gastrointestinal blood loss
Urinalysis	Hemoglobinuria, hematuria
Bilirubin	Suspected hemolysis
Ferritin	To evaluate iron stores
Serum iron, total iron-binding capacity	To assess iron deficiency
Free erythrocyte	To evaluate iron-deficient erythropoiesis
Zinc protoporphyrin	To evaluate protoporphyrin
Transferrin receptor assay	To evaluate iron deficiency

REVIEW EXERCISES

QUESTIONS

1. A 4-year-old boy has short stature, no thumbs, microphthalmia, and horseshoe kidney. Laboratory analysis reveals the following values:

- Hemoglobin = 7.0 g/dL
- Reticulocyte count = 0.3%
- WBC count = 2000/mm^3
- Platelet count = 37,000/mm^3

The *most* likely diagnosis is:
a) Iron deficiency anemia
b) Fanconi anemia
c) Diamond-Blackfan anemia
d) Dyskeratosis congenita
e) None of the above

Answer

The answer is b. Fanconi anemia is a congenital disorder of DNA repair associated with the anomalies outlined in the question. It is also associated with a pancytopenia that is not present frequently at birth or during infancy but develops during childhood. The risk for the development of malignancy is increased. The association of congenital malformations, short stature, and pancytopenia is suggestive of Fanconi anemia. Iron deficiency anemia is not associated with pancytopenia. Diamond-Blackfan anemia can be associated with congenital anomalies, especially developmental abnormalities of the thumb. It is typically an isolated anemia, although later in the course, neutropenia may develop. Dyskeratosis congenita is a very rare condition associated with pancytopenia that typically develops in the second decade of life. Dystrophic nails and premalignant lesions in the mouth are other features.

2. Anorexia gradually develops in a previously healthy 19-month-old boy, and he becomes less active. Laboratory analysis reveals the following values:

- Hemoglobin = 5.1 g/dL
- Reticulocyte count = <0.1%
- WBC count = 4500/mm^3
- Platelet count = 440,000/mm^3
- MCV = 80 µ^3

The *most* likely diagnosis is:
a) Iron deficiency anemia
b) Leukemia
c) TEC
d) Diamond-Blackfan anemia
e) None of the above

Answer

The answer is c. In iron deficiency (a microcytic, hypochromic anemia), the MCV would be expected to be lower for the hemoglobin level presented in the question. In leukemia, which typically involves all the cell lines in the bone marrow, the platelet count would not be in the high range when the hemoglobin level is 5.1 g/dL. It would be distinctly unusual for a child with leukemia to present with isolated anemia and symptoms referable only to the anemia. In Diamond-Blackfan anemia, as in TEC, an isolated anemia is associated with a low reticulocyte count. However, the MCV is elevated in Diamond-Blackfan anemia and is normal in TEC. Most children with Diamond-Blackfan anemia present in the first 6 months of life, and the vast majority by 1 year of age. The gradual and insidious onset of a normocytic anemia with reticulocytopenia in a toddler is very suggestive of TEC.

Questions 3–6
In moderate to severe iron deficiency anemia, the following alterations are noted:

3. The MCV is decreased.
a) True
b) False

Answer
The answer is a. Iron deficiency anemia is a microcytic anemia characterized by small RBCs that results in a low MCV.

4. The RDW is increased.
a) True
b) False

Answer
The answer is a. Iron deficiency anemia is characterized by cells of varying size (anisocytosis). Early changes in iron-deficient RBCs are manifested as an increase in the RDW. In some laboratory reports, this is referred to as the *coefficient of variation of the MCV.*

5. The RBC count is increased.
a) True
b) False

Answer
The answer is b. In iron deficiency anemia, the RBC count is typically decreased, although exceptions are found. This is the basis for the Mentzer index (MCV/RBC). In thalassemia minor, the RBC count is usually normal or increased.

6. The free erythrocyte protoporphyrin (FEPP) or zinc protoporphyrin (ZnPP) level is decreased.
a) True
b) False

Answer
The answer is b. In iron-deficient erythropoiesis, the synthesis of porphyrins is adequate. However, because

of a deficiency of available iron, the FEPP molecules bind to zinc, so that the level of ZnPP is increased. Lead poisoning also results in increased levels of ZnPP.

7. A 2-year-old girl who had neonatal jaundice is found to have a palpable "spleen tip" and the following laboratory data:

■ Hemoglobin = 10.0 g/dL
■ Reticulocyte count = 5.6%
■ WBC count = 6000/mm^3
■ Platelet count = 320,000/mm^3
■ MCHC = 37 g/dL
■ MCH = 28 pg
■ MCV = 82 μ^3
■ RDW = 19

Which of the following will help in the diagnosis?
a) Determination of osmotic fragility
b) Review of the peripheral blood smear
c) Careful family history
d) Review of peripheral blood smear of parents
e) All of the above

Answer
The answer is e. The question describes a clinical picture suggestive of hemolysis:

■ Neonatal jaundice
■ Splenomegaly
■ Anemia with reticulocytosis

The RDW is increased, possibly because of the reticulocytosis. Notably, the MCHC is elevated. This finding suggests dense cells and can be observed in spherocytosis or sickle cell syndromes. The osmotic fragility test confirms the presence of spherocytes, as does a careful examination of the peripheral blood smear. The family history may be revealing because the disorder is commonly inherited as an autosomal dominant trait. Affected family members may have had a splenectomy or a cholecystectomy (for bilirubin gallstones). Spherocytes in the blood smear of the parents also suggest a familial pattern.

8. TEC is characterized by each of the following *except:*
a) Low hemoglobin level
b) Low reticulocyte count
c) Increased MCV
d) Spontaneous resolution
e) Mild neutropenia, occasionally

Answer
The answer is c. An increased MCV is a simple but significant differential feature of Diamond-Blackfan anemia. TEC is characterized by anemia with reticulocytopenia that resolves spontaneously. Occasionally, mild neutropenia may occur (particularly if the TEC was preceded

by a viral infection). In TEC, the MCV is normal, and in Diamond-Blackfan anemia (which is congenital and does not resolve spontaneously), the MCV is increased. (During the recovery phase of TEC, the MCV may be increased.)

9. An increase in the hemoglobin level from 10.0 to 12.5 g/dL after treatment with elemental iron 6 mg/kg per day indicates iron deficiency anemia.
a) True
b) False

Answer

The answer is a. An increase in hemoglobin associated with iron therapy is diagnostic of iron deficiency. Only iron deficiency anemia responds to iron therapy. However, the limitation of a therapeutic trial of iron is that it does not explain what caused the iron deficiency.

10. Iron deficiency anemia in an 8-year-old boy suggests nutritional iron deficiency.
a) True
b) False

Answer

The answer is b. Primary nutritional iron deficiency occurs most frequently during periods of rapid growth: infancy and adolescence (especially in menstruating girls). If iron deficiency is identified during the middle childhood years, other causes must be considered. Gastrointestinal bleeding is frequently suspected.

11. Parvovirus B19 is a leading cause of acquired hemolytic anemia.
a) True
b) False

Answer

The answer is b. Parvovirus B19 infection is associated with neonatal anemia as a complication of intrauterine infection. In children with an underlying chronic hemolytic anemia, such as sickle cell anemia or spherocytosis, it can lead to an aplastic episode associated with a marked decrease in both the hemoglobin level and the reticulocyte count. A similar process of longer duration may occur in children receiving chronic immunosuppressive therapy following solid organ transplantation. Parvovirus B19 infection is not associated with TEC or acquired hemolytic anemia.

12. A reticulocyte count should always be included in an evaluation of anemia.
a) True
b) False

Answer

The answer is a. A reticulocyte count offers a "window" to the bone marrow. It is a measure of effective erythroid activity in the bone marrow and aids in the differential diagnosis of anemia. A bone marrow examination is usually not necessary to evaluate an anemia associated with reticulocytosis. A diagnosis of anemia can be confirmed by measurement of the hemoglobin level or hematocrit or by an RBC count. However, to evaluate the cause of anemia properly, a reticulocyte count is necessary. It is also recommended as part of therapeutic trials with iron.

SUGGESTED READINGS

1. Christensen RD. *Hematologic problems of the neonate.* Philadelphia: Saunders, 2000:117–137.
2. Erslev AJ, Gabuzda TG. *Pathophysiology of blood,* 3rd ed. Philadelphia: Saunders, 1985:28–51.
3. Isbisten JP, Pittiglio HP. *Clinical hematology: a problem-oriented approach.* Baltimore: Williams &Wilkins, 1988:35–80.
4. Miller D. *Blood diseases of infancy and childhood.* St. Louis: Mosby, 1989:26–47.
5. Nathan DG, Oski SH. *Hematology of infancy and childhood,* 5th ed. Philadelphia: Saunders, 1998:237–338, 373–470.
6. Young NS. *Bone marrow failure syndromes.* Philadelphia: Saunders, 2000:47–68.

Chapter 55

Hemoglobinopathies

David J. Slomiany and Michael Levien

Hemoglobin (Hb) is a complex tetrameric protein composed of four polypeptide (globin) chains with prosthetic oxygen-binding heme groups. Normal Hbs in the red blood cell (RBC) are Hb A, Hb A_2, and Hb F. Hb A (the major Hb) is composed of two α-globin chains and two β-globin chains. α-Chains are encoded on chromosome 16. β-Chains are encoded on chromosome 11. During embryonic and fetal development, several distinct globin chains are produced and combine in tetramers to form embryonic and fetal Hb. Mutations in the globin genes can yield:

- Abnormal globin chains and subsequently abnormal Hb molecules (e.g., Hb S in sickle syndromes)
- Abnormal synthesis of globin chains and subsequently decreased amounts of normal Hb (e.g., thalassemias)

The Hbs in an individual's RBCs are characterized by electrophoresis (ELP). The screening of all newborn infants for disorders has led to early diagnosis. Early medical intervention and education have decreased morbidity and mortality in infants with sickling disorders (Table 55.1).

SICKLE CELL DISEASE

Etiology

Sickle cell diseases are a group of genetic disorders with various clinical manifestations; the common feature is that the affected individuals have at least one gene for Hb S. The disorders include homozygous Hb SS disease and disease states in which Hb S is associated with other variant Hbs (e.g., Hb SC, Hb SD, Hb S/β thalassemia) that enhance or promote the sickling phenomenon (Table 55.2). Sickle cell disease is identified in most cases by newborn screening. Confirmation of the diagnosis is by Hb ELP.

The cause of sickle cell disease is a mutation in the *β-globin* gene. An adenine-to-thymine substitution in codon 6 of the *β-globin* gene specifies the insertion of valine for glutamic acid at the sixth position of the β-globin chain to produce Hb S. Hb S occurs frequently among population in areas previously exposed to falciparum malaria, including western coastal Africa, central Africa, India, Saudi Arabia, and the Mediterranean countries. Hb S in these patients provides protection against intraerythrocytic growth of malaria.

Pathophysiology

Hb S crystallizes and polymerizes on deoxygenation, thereby distorting the RBC. Polymerization and distortion lead to destruction of the RBC membrane, decreased RBC deformability, and increased RBC adhesion to vascular endothelium. Sickling of erythrocytes is facilitated by fevers, dehydration, and acidosis.

The clinical problems associated with sickle cell disease are a consequence of hypoxia and acidosis, which are caused by tissue ischemia resulting from vaso-occlusion by irreversibly sickled RBCs. The clinical manifestations include severe hemolytic anemia, an increased frequency and severity of certain infections, tissue infarction with subsequent organ damage and failure, and recurrent episodes of pain. The clinical manifestations are acute and chronic.

Clinical Presentations and Treatments

Sickle cell disease is a chronic condition in which acute events of variable severity occur intermittently. Patients require care in specialized centers. Routine health maintenance is important, with an emphasis on nutrition, education of families, infection prophylaxis, and anticipatory guidance regarding the avoidance of extremes of temperature, dehydration, and physical activity (Table 55.3).

The clinical consequences of sickle cell disease can be broadly grouped into three categories:

- Vaso-occlusive events
- Hemolytic events
- Infectious events

The damage inflicted by sickle cell disease can be acute or chronic in nature.

TABLE 55.1

TABLE 55.1

HEMOGLOBIN PATTERNS ON NEWBORN SCREENING

Newborn Screening Hemoglobin Pattern	Interpretation	Recommended Action
FAS	Hb S trait	Hb ELP 9–12 months
FS	Homozygous sickle cell disease or Hb S trait with other variants (e.g., Hb S/β thalassemia)	Hb ELP plus CBC at initial visit, repeat Hb ELP at 9–12 months, plus CBC
FSC or FSD	Potentially serious sickling disorder	Hb ELP plus CBC at initial visit, repeat Hb ELP at 9–12 months, plus CBC
FAE	Hb E trait	Hb ELP, 9–12 months, plus CBC
FA Bart's	α Thalassemia	Hb ELP, 9–12 months, plus CBC
FE	Homozygous Hb E or hemoglobin E/β thalassemia	Hb ELP, 9 months, plus CBC at 4–6 months. Family studies helpful

A, normal adult hemoglobin; C, hemoglobin C variant; CBC, complete blood cell count; D, D hemoglobin variant; E, hemoglobin E variant; ELP, electrophoresis; F, normal fetal hemoglobin; Hb, hemoglobin; S, sickle hemoglobin variant.

Vaso-occlusive Crisis

Vaso-occlusive crisis occurs when poor RBC deformability, increased viscosity, and adherence of the "sickled" RBCs to endothelial cells cause ischemia/infarction. Vaso-occlusive crisis is also known as *pain crisis*. It most commonly affects bone, lung, liver, spleen, brain, and penis.

Bone infarction or ischemia of the periarticular tissues is the most common form of acute vaso-occlusive pain crisis. The pain is usually diffuse. Localized tenderness, swelling, and limited range of motion are common. Redness and warmth occur but are not prominent. Low-grade fevers usually develop. The severity and frequency of pain crisis increase with age. Initially, pain crisis is usually *dactylitis (hand-foot syndrome)*, most common in children <2 years and involving the metacarpals, metatarsals, and phalanges of one or more extremities. Long bones, spine, clavicles, ribs, and sternum are also frequently affected by pain

TABLE 55.2

CLINICALLY IMPORTANT SICKLING DISORDERS

Hb SS	Majority (60%–70%) of the cases of sickle cell disease in the United States. Second most common form of sickle cell disease in the United States (~20%); moderate chronic hemolytic anemia, less severe than Hb SS
Hb SD	Clinically similar to Hb SS
Hb SO Arab	Clinically similar to Hb SS
Hb S β thalassemia	Heterogeneous clinical disorders with symptoms and severity that depend on the severity of thalassemia component

crisis. Treatment is supportive, with aggressive hydration, narcotic analgesics, and nonsteroidal anti-inflammatory agents. Oxygen is of little value and may actually exacerbate anemia. Infection should be sought out and treated.

Cerebrovascular Events

Two major central nervous system (CNS) complications of Hb SS disease are occlusion in large vessels and aneurysms in small vessels. Stroke occurs in up to 15% of patients with Hb SS, and the reported mortality is 15% to 20%. It is the second leading cause of death in patients with Hb SS. The risk of stroke is four times higher in patients with Hb SS disease compared with patients with Hb SC disease. Stroke is usually the result of infarction, although hemorrhagic strokes do occur. Sickling of RBCs in the vas vasorum of the large vessels leads to infarcts in the blood vessel walls causing stenosis, aneurysms, and occlusion. The distribution is typically the middle cerebral artery and watershed areas, and the stroke may be preceded by a transient ischemic attack.

The presentation is with seizures, paresis, or aphasia. Various findings are noted on magnetic resonance imaging (MRI), computed tomography (CT) scan and arteriography. The recurrence rate without treatment is 70% within 3 years.

Treatment involves reducing the concentration of Hb S to 30% to 50%; this usually requires exchange transfusion but can sometimes be accomplished by a simple transfusion. Erythrocytapheresis is the preferred treatment in an acute event to rapidly reduce the concentration of Hb S. *Chronic transfusion* of RBCs by hypertransfusion or erythrocytapheresis is mandatory to decrease or prevent the recurrence of stroke. Recovery varies, although children recover more fully than adults. A recent study by the National Institutes of Health has concluded that it is not safe to stop

TABLE 55.3

HEALTH CARE MAINTENANCE

Well-child immunizations	Routine childhood immunizations required
	Conjugate 7-valent pneumococcal vaccine: 4 doses prior to age 2 years followed by 23-valent polysaccharide pneumococcal vaccine at ages 2 and 5 years
	Yearly influenza vaccine
Initial evaluation	Physical examination, CBC with RBC indices
	Reticulocyte count
	Confirmatory Hb ELP
	Genetic counseling
	Anticipatory guidance regarding fever, hydration, pain, and acute splenic sequestration (demonstrate and teach parents how to palpate spleen)
	Prophylactic penicillin from 1 month to 5 years of age
	Start folic acid at 6 months (optional)
Newborn–2 years	Every 2–3 months for physical examination
	CBC, reticulocyte count every visit
	G6PD at 6 months
	Confirmatory Hb ELP at 9–12 months
	Anticipatory guidance
	Blood chemistries at 12 months, as needed
	Iron and lead studies
2–6 years	Every 6 months for physical examination, if clinically well
	CBC, reticulocyte count every visit
	Blood chemistries yearly, p.r.n
	Transcranial Doppler ultrasonography every 6 months to 1 year
	Ophthalmology exam yearly
	Urinalysis yearly
	ECHO/ECG at 3–5 years
	Anticipatory guidance
6–18 years	Every 6 months for physical examination, if clinically well
	CBC, reticulocyte count every visit
	Blood chemistries yearly, p.r.n
	Transcranial Doppler ultrasonography every 6 months
	Ophthalmology exam yearly
	Urinalysis yearly
	ECHO/ECG every 3–5 years
	Pulmonary functions age 10, p.r.n or with history of acute chest syndrome
	Hip/shoulder x-rays age 10–14 years
	Anticipatory guidance

CBC, complete blood cell; ECHO/ECG, echocardiography/electrocardiography; ELP, electrophoresis; G6PD, glucose-6-phosphate dehydrogenase; Hb, hemoglobin; p.r.n, as needed; RBC, red blood cell.

RBC transfusions even after 5 years in this patient population due to the risk of stroke recurrence.

It is important to note that 30% of asymptomatic patients with Hb SS disease have "silent" infarcts on MRI surveillance. These patients have never had clinical evidence of stroke. Children with Hb SS disease should have transcranial Doppler (TCD) ultrasonography every 6 months or at least once a year starting at the age of 2 years. TCD measures the velocity of blood flow through the internal carotid and middle cerebral arteries. More frequent studies should be done on patients with borderline high velocities (180–199 cm/second). If the velocity is ≥200 cm/second on two separate occasions 1 to 2 months apart, magnetic resonance arteriography and venography should be done to assess the patient's risk for stroke. If the patient has tortuous vessels with or without stenosis, moyamoya disease

(basal arterial occlusion with telangiectasia), and/or "silent" infarct(s), then commencing a chronic RBC transfusion program is strongly recommended.

The long-term consequences of chronic transfusion program are the result of iron overload and alloimmunization. Iron chelation therapy should be administered in children 3 years and older when the serum ferritin is >1000 ng/mL (although serum ferritin alone is not a reliable measure of total body iron burden). *Deferoxamine* is currently the standard chelating agent. Partial RBC exchange transfusions are another approach to reducing iron overload.

Acute Chest Syndrome

Patients present with chest pain, tachypnea, shortness of breath, cough, fever, leukocytosis, unilateral or bilateral infiltrates, and possibly hypoxemia. Bony tenderness over the ribs, sternum, or spine may occur. Bloody or purulent cough is not prevalent. Increased incidence of acute chest syndrome occurs in patients with low fetal hemoglobin, high steady-state hemoglobin (increased blood viscosity), high white blood cell counts, and in the winter months when the frequency of respiratory infections are increased. Acute chest syndrome may develop after vaso-occlusive pain crisis, which is a consequence of infarcts in long bones creating pulmonary fat emboli. The Hb level can be significantly decreased from baseline at presentation. The respiratory status can quickly deteriorate as hypoxia and acidosis further promote sickling.

Causes of acute chest syndrome include infection, bone infarction, and the formation of fat emboli secondary to bone marrow necrosis. The fatality rate is 10% to 20%; acute chest syndrome is reported to be the leading cause of death in patients with Hb SS disease who are >10 years. It is the most common complication of anesthesia. Repeated episodes can lead to chronic restrictive pulmonary disease, pulmonary hypertension, and cor pulmonale. Early recognition is important. Treatment includes:

- Correction of the hypoxemia with oxygen
- Administration of antibiotics and analgesics
- Transfusion (simple or exchange)
- Incentive spirometry to prevent hypoventilation

Priority should be given to administering RBC transfusions to rapidly decrease Hb S. Intravenous fluids should not exceed maintenance rate. A rapidly deteriorating patient should have exchange transfusion (erythrocytapheresis). These patients can progress to respiratory failure and require tracheal intubation and ventilator support. A multicenter acute chest syndrome trial conducted by the National Institutes of Health accrued 538 patients with 671 episodes of acute chest syndrome. Analysis of bronchial alveolar lavage samples from these patients revealed the following:

- 30%: negative for viral, bacterial, and fungal infection
- 16%: positive for lipid-laden macrophages (pulmonary fat emboli)
- 54%: positive for infection (*Chlamydia* 13%), (*Mycoplasma* 12%), (viruses 12%), (*Staphylococci*, *Streptococci*, and *Haemophilus* 8%)

Empiric intravenous antibiotic therapy should include a 3rd generation cephalosporin, such as ceftriaxone or cefotaxime *and* a macrolide.

Priapism
Priapism is a painful and persistent erection secondary to sickling in the corpora cavernosa, causing vaso-occlusion, which obstructs the venous drainage of the penis. It is more prevalent in teenagers and adults but is likely to be highly underreported in children. The incidence is 42%, and the median age is 21 years; nearly 50% of affected patients are left with sexual dysfunction.

Treatment includes aggressive hydration, analgesia, transfusion if the erection persists >2 hours, and surgical intervention (corporal aspiration and irrigation, saphenous-corporal shunts) if medical measures are unsuccessful within 4 to 6 hours. Recurrent episodes of priapism can result in fibrosis and impotence, even when adequate treatment is provided.

Hematologic Crisis
Hemolytic anemia is generally tolerated but does lead to premature gallstones. Anemia can be life-threatening, especially in the first few years of life. Thirty percent of patients who are chronically transfused will become alloimmunized to minor RBC antigens that are less common in the African-American population. Care should be taken to determine the correct RBC phenotype on all patients with sickle cell anemia and cross matched appropriately to prevent antibody formation, which can result in hyperhemolytic episodes that can be difficult to treat.

Acute Sequestration Crisis
Acute sequestration crisis (ASC) is the acute pooling of the blood volume within the spleen with a resultant precipitous drop in the Hb level, hypovolemia, and cardiovascular collapse. Most initial episodes occur in patients with Hb SS disease between the ages of 3 months and 5 years, with the greatest risk between the ages of 6 months and 2 years. ASC also occurs in patients with other sickling disorders (Hb SC, Hb S/β thalassemia), but at a later age. The mean age in patients with Hb SC disease is 9 years. Signs and symptoms include weakness, lethargy, pallor, dyspnea, tachypnea, tachycardia, abdominal distension, left-sided abdominal pain, emesis, and shock. The recurrence rate is 50% within 2 to 3 months. The mortality rate for the first episode is 12%, for the second episode is 20%, and occurs most commonly in patients with HbSS.

The priority in management is to restore effective circulating blood volume, which is accomplished with emergent RBC transfusion. Caution should be taken not to over transfuse, because when the episode resolves, the spleen will release the trapped RBCs and auto transfuse the patient. Early parental education in spleen palpation and recognizing the signs of acute progressive anemia has decreased the mortality rate. Splenectomy should be considered. Chronic transfusion will delay and may prevent recurrence in some patients. Hepatic sequestration crisis can also occur; it presents with liver enlargement, liver tenderness, hyperbilirubinemia, progressive anemia, and reticulocytosis. Care should be taken not to over transfuse these patients as well, because they will undergo auto transfusion when the crisis resolves.

Aplastic Crisis

Aplastic crisis is the temporary suppression, during viral or bacterial infection, of the markedly increased production of reticulocytes in the marrow. It results in a rapid drop in the Hb level within a few days. RBC survival in patients with sickle cell disease is markedly decreased, so the RBC production must be increased to maintain the Hb level at steady state. *Human parvovirus B19 has a predilection for RBC precursors in the marrow.* Symptoms of severe anemia with a decreased Hb level and little or no compensatory reticulocytosis are diagnostic. Spontaneous recovery is usually accompanied by a markedly elevated peripheral nucleated RBC count, followed by a brisk reticulocytosis. Management consists of transfusion support as necessary.

Infectious Crisis

The spleen functions in phagocytosis and in antibody and opsonin production. It is predisposed to infarction by a vast microcirculation and hypoxic environment. Beginning at approximately 6 months of age, repeated episodes of splenic congestion and infarction produce a fibrotic, nonfunctioning spleen. Autoinfarction of the spleen is complete in most patients with Hb SS disease by the age of 5 years. Patients with splenic dysfunction are at increased risk for infection, especially by encapsulated organisms. These include *Streptococcus pneumoniae, Haemophilus influenzae, Klebsiella,* and *Salmonella.* The increased risk for infection is greatest in children.

Patients with sickle cell disease who have fever require prompt medical attention. Blood cultures and empiric parenteral antibiotics are necessary to avoid potentially fatal septicemia. However, not all febrile patients with sickle cell disease require hospitalization. Prophylactic penicillin has significantly reduced early childhood mortality in these patients (although resistance to antibiotics is becoming problematic). Routine childhood immunizations and pneumococcal vaccine should be given to all patients with sickle cell disease.

Chronic Complications of Sickle Cell Disease

Persistent ischemic damage resulting from overt or occult vaso-occlusion secondary to intravascular sickling can lead to chronic organ dysfunction and subsequent medical problems, including the following:

- Restrictive pulmonary disease with a low vital capacity and reduced total lung capacity
- CNS complications that occur in approximately 25% of patients, cognitive deficits seen in patients with or without overt neurologic damage, possibly secondary to "silent stroke"
- Left ventricular hypertrophy, cardiomegaly, myocardial hemosiderosis, cardiac murmur, pulmonary hypertension, and cor pulmonale

- Infarction of the renal medulla, hyposthenuria, hematuria, and nephrotic syndrome, the common renal abnormalities
- Thrombosis, infarction, and necrosis of bone, especially in the epiphyseal ossification centers of the long bones
- Retinal detachment; tears, holes and vitreous hemorrhages, the common complications in patients with Hb SC disease occur because of retinal arteriolar vascular occlusion, leading to infarction and neovascularization (proliferative retinopathy); retinal detachment occurs from mechanical traction created by chronic, enlarging fibrovascular retinal membranes, occurring as early as 20 months of age, but most commonly at 15 to 30 years.
- Cholelithiasis resulting from chronic hemolysis, can occur as early as 2 to 4 years of age, 30% of patients develop cholelithiasis by 18 years of age, gallbladder sludge may be a consequence of ceftriaxone therapy.
- Decreased growth (height and weight)
- Delayed puberty
- Increased infertility in female patients

Chronic RBC transfusions and the administration of *hydroxyurea* are the more common methods used to influence the sickling phenomenon and decrease the potential long-term complications of sickle cell disease. Hydroxyurea increases fetal hemoglobin in most patients. Increased fetal hemoglobin provides a protective effect against sickling. Hydroxyurea does not prevent strokes. In most patients, it can reduce vaso-occlusive pain crises by 50%. *Bone marrow transplantation* is curative and should arrest the development of further damage. This should only be considered in high-risk patients as bone marrow transplants can cause significant morbidity in some patients. Nonmyeloablative stem cell transplants offer another choice to help arrest the progression of disease with reduction in morbidity. Successful nonmyeloablative transplants can create mixed bone marrow chimeras, creating a patient with "sickle cell trait." The use of cord blood may decrease the risk of graft versus host disease.

Prognosis

Survival is influenced by environmental, social, and economic factors as follows:

- Overall mortality rate is approximately 3%
- Peak incidence of death between the ages of 6 months and 3 years
- Gradual increase in mortality starts in late adolescence
- Survival of 85% of patients with Hb SS disease, beyond the age of 20 years
- The median age of death for affected men: 42 years for patients with Hb SS and 60 years for patients with Hb SC
- The median age of death for women: 48 years for patients with Hb SS and 68 years for patients with Hb SC

THALASSEMIA

Etiology

The thalassemias are a diverse group of genetic blood diseases characterized by an absent or decreased production of normal Hb, which results in a microcytic, hypochromic anemia of varying severity. Mutations affect either the *α-globin* or *β-globin* genes. The result is an impaired production of the corresponding globin molecule and an abnormal ratio of *α-globin* to non–α-globin. The proportion of globin molecules produced in normal amounts becomes excessive; these molecules then form aggregates in the RBCs, are oxidized, and damage the RBC membrane. Hemolysis, ineffective erythropoiesis, or both, occur. The clinical and biochemical manifestations of each type of thalassemia are characteristic.

The distribution of the thalassemias corresponds to areas where *Plasmodium falciparum* infection is common. α Thalassemia is common in southeastern Asia, Malaysia, and southern China. β Thalassemia is common in the areas surrounding the Mediterranean Sea, Africa, and southeastern Asia.

α Thalassemia

Pathophysiology

Normally, four genes control the production of the α-globin molecules; therefore, the loss (deletion) of one to four genes is possible and results in distinct clinical conditions. In α thalassemia, excess amounts of β-globins lead to the formation of β-globin tetramers (β_4), called *Hb H*.

α Thalassemias are difficult to diagnose and identify with certainty because no characteristic elevations in Hb S, Hb A_2, or Hb F occur. However, with the use of molecular diagnostic techniques, the deletions responsible for the common α thalassemias are readily detectable.

Clinical Presentations and Treatment

Silent Carrier

One of the α-genes is lost, and three functional α-genes remain. The patient has no clinically detectable problems and is hematologically normal. A small amount (<5%) of Hb Bart's (γ_4) may be seen on the newborn screening. The patient is a carrier for α-thalassemia minor. The condition is frequent in the population of southeast Asia. Twenty-five percent of African Americans are silent carriers.

α Thalassemia Trait (Minor)

Two α-genes are lost, and two functional α-genes remain. The diagnosis is one of exclusion. The condition produces a mild microcytic, hypochromic anemia and is frequently confused with iron deficiency anemia. No additional clinical problems develop. No therapy is required, and iron replacement is not needed. Hb Bart's is detected on newborn screening in 3% to 10% of total Hb. In Asians, the *cis* type of mutation is most common—that is, the two α-genes are deleted from the same chromosome. The offspring of affected individuals are at risk for severe thalassemia.

α Thalassemia/Hemoglobin Constant Spring

Hb Constant Spring is a minor Hb in which an elongated **α**-chain results from a mutation in a termination codon.

■ It is found mostly in Asians.
■ No hematologic abnormality occurs in the heterozygous state.
■ The homozygous state yields a mild microcytic anemia; 2% to 8% Hb Constant Spring is detected on Hb ELP.
■ It is found in some patients with Hb H disease.

Hemoglobin H Disease

Three α-genes are lost, and one functional α-gene remains. The condition produces a moderate or severe microcytic, hypochromic anemia and can be life threatening. A high percentage (>10%) of Hb Bart's is detected on the newborn screen. The severe imbalance between α- and β-globin production results in an accumulation of β-globin in the RBCs. The formation of β-globin tetramers produces an abnormal Hb, termed *Hb H*. Hb H does not carry oxygen properly and precipitates as the RBC ages. Clinical manifestations are chronic hemolysis with jaundice, cholelithiasis, skin ulceration, bony abnormalities, hepatosplenomegaly, growth retardation, and hemolytic exacerbations. Supportive treatment with transfusions is usually necessary.

Hemoglobin H/Constant Spring

■ Severe, microcytic, hypochromic anemia
■ Steady-state Hb level of 5 to 8 g/dL
■ Patient usually transfusion dependent
■ Moderate or massive splenomegaly
■ Postsplenectomy thrombocytosis with hypercoagulability possible

α Thalassemia Major

The loss of all four α-genes results in hydrops fetalis, which is usually *fatal* in utero. The fetus experiences significant hypoxia with cardiac failure and pulmonary edema. It may survive with intrauterine transfusions. If the fetus is alive at birth, significant Hb Bart's is detected on screening the newborn. Embryonic forms of Hb (e.g., Hb Portland, $\zeta_2\gamma_2$) may also be seen. The condition manifests as severe anemia with marked microcytosis, hypochromasia, and anisopoikilocytosis. The clinical features are massive hepatosplenomegaly, anasarca, and pleural and pericardial effusions. Supportive transfusions and bone marrow transplantation are the only therapeutic options.

β Thalassemia

Pathophysiology

Two genes control β-globin production. Numerous mutations affect the genes and thereby all aspects of β-globin production and stability. In α thalassemia, *α-globin* genes are deleted, whereas in β thalassemia, *β-globin* genes are present but fail to produce adequate globin chains. As a result, an excess of α-globins (α_4) accumulates and precipitates in the RBCs, because of which ineffective erythropoiesis and anemia result. The severity of the thalassemia depends on the amount of β-globin chains produced by the defective genes. The diagnosis is by Hb ELP, which usually shows an increase in Hb A_2 and Hb F. β Thalassemia has been divided into three general categories.

Clinical Presentations and Treatment

β Thalassemia Minor

One β-gene is affected. The condition is usually clinically benign, with a mild microcytic, hypochromic anemia, mild reticulocytosis, and minimal splenomegaly. The blood smear shows target cells, elliptocytes, and basophilic stippling. β Thalassemia minor can be mistaken for iron deficiency anemia. The diagnosis is established by the demonstration of increased amounts of Hb A_2 (approximately two times normal) on Hb ELP. Racial differences in hematologic severity have been noted. Generally, no therapy is required.

β Thalassemia Intermedia

Two β-genes are incompletely affected, therefore the β-globin production is less than in β thalassemia minor but does not fail completely, as in β thalassemia major. This is a descriptive clinical condition, not a pathologic or genetic condition. The clinical presentation is variable and can resemble that of β thalassemia minor or β thalassemia major. Continual evaluations are required because the clinical status may change. A moderate microcytic, hypochromic anemia with moderate splenomegaly is the usual clinical presentation. Bony abnormalities may be seen. Delayed puberty, cardiomegaly, osteoporosis, arthritis, and pathologic fractures are other possible features. The patient may require periodic RBC transfusions; however, if regular transfusions are needed, the patient is considered to have β thalassemia major.

TABLE 55.4

HEMOGLOBIN E

Second most common hemoglobin variant
Point mutation in β-gene producing a truncated β-chain
Common in Cambodia, Thailand, Laos
Heterozygous Hb E: asymptomatic, mild microcytosis, normal hemoglobin, target cells on peripheral smear
Homozygous Hb E: mild microcytic, hemolytic anemia
Can combine with severe β thalassemia to produce transfusion-dependent hemolytic anemia

---

TABLE 55.5

HEINZ BODY HEMOLYTIC ANEMIA

Multiple mutations causing hemoglobin molecular instability and intracorpuscular precipitation (Heinz body)
Precipitated hemoglobin causes red blood cell membrane damage
Broad range of hemolysis ranging from mild to severe microcytic anemia
Variable polychromatophilia, schistocytes, spherocytes, and basophilic stippling on peripheral smear
Aplastic crisis or cholelithiasis may occur
No specific therapy required
Splenectomy may be beneficial

β Thalassemia Major

Two β-genes are identically affected (homozygous mutations), so that little or no β-globin molecules are produced. The clinical presentation consists of severe microcytic, hypochromic anemia with ineffective erythropoiesis, enhanced RBC clearance, hepatosplenomegaly, and bony malformations. Complications include pallor, jaundice, osteoporosis, cholelithiasis, cardiomegaly, cardiac dysfunction, endocrine dysfunction, and immune dysfunction. The blood smear shows target cells, fragmented cells, and nucleated RBCs. Untreated patients usually die in the first decade of life.

Long-term survival requires regularly scheduled transfusions. Transfused patients are highly susceptible to iron overload toxicity, and chelation therapy is required for survival into adulthood. Bone marrow transplantation is curative.

VARIANT HEMOGLOBINOPATHIES

Any Hb with a mutation is a variant Hb. Many variant Hbs exist worldwide. The mutations may or may not cause clinical conditions. Some, such as Hb E, are significant in that they may be inherited together with thalassemia trait to produce a clinical disease that requires treatment (Table 55.4). Mutations may result in the formation of unstable Hbs, as in Heinz body hemolytic anemia (Table 55.5), Hbs with an abnormal oxygen affinity, such as Hb M (Table 55.6), or Hbs with structural abnormalities that are clinically silent.

TABLE 55.6

HEMOGLOBIN M

Mutation in α-gene causes a single amino acid substitution
Decreased oxygen binding
Blood appears brown
Affected patients are cyanotic but clinically asymptomatic
No specific therapy indicated
No lifestyle restrictions
Important to differentiate hemoglobin M from other causes of neonatal cyanosis to avoid unnecessary invasive diagnostic procedures

REVIEW EXERCISES

QUESTIONS

For each numbered item, select the one lettered answer that is best.

1. All of the following are sickling syndromes *except*:
a) Hemoglobin SC
b) Hemoglobin SD
c) Hemoglobin AS
d) Hemoglobin S/β thalassemia
e) Hemoglobin SO Arab

Answer

The answer is c. Many structural variants of Hb exist, most of which have no clinical significance; however, a few are associated with major clinical symptoms. Hb C is an abnormal Hb in which the glutamic acid at position 6 of the β-chain is replaced by lysine. Hb C is less soluble than Hb A. When it is paired with Hb S, usually in a 1:1 ratio, the RBC becomes dehydrated and more rigid because of higher intracellular concentrations of Hb. As a result, the rate of Hb S polymerization is accelerated.

Hb D results from a substitution at position 121 of the β-chain; the most common is a glutamine substitution for glutamic acid in Hb D Punjab. Hb D copolymerizes with Hb S to cause a clinical syndrome similar to that associated with Hb SS.

Hemoglobin O Arab is another β-chain variant involving position 121, a contact point with Hb S. Hb O Arab also copolymerizes with Hb S to produce a clinical condition similar to that associated with Hb SS. The Hb S/β thalassemia syndromes are of variable severity depending on the severity of the thalassemia component. The β+ thalassemias, in which Hb A is present in the RBC, are associated with a milder clinical disease than Hb S/β0 thalassemia, in which no Hb A is present in the RBC.

Hb AS is sickle cell trait. The RBC contains both Hb A and Hb S, but Hb A is always the more prevalent component. Hb A and Hb S in the proportions found in sickle cell trait do not polymerize under physiologic conditions.

2. Newborn screening identifies Hb F and Hb S in an infant. The diagnosis could be:
a) Homozygous sickle cell disease
b) Homozygous sickle cell disease with persistence of Hb F
c) Sickle cell/β thalassemia
d) Any of the above
e) None of the above

Answer

The answer is d. Hb undergoes significant changes during fetal and early infant growth and development. Hb Gower-1, Hb Go-wer-2, and Hb Portland predominate the first 8 weeks of embryonic development. By week 10 of gestation, Hb F is the major Hb in the RBC of the fetus. The production of Hb F decreases as delivery approaches, and the production of Hb A begins. At birth, the RBCs of the neonate contain 70% to 90% Hb F, with Hb A comprising the remainder. During the infant's first 6 months of life, Hb F levels continue to decrease and Hb A levels increase. The level of Hb F in healthy adults usually does not exceed 1%. In patients with Hb SS, the newborn screening Hb ELP pattern is Hb F and Hb S. The ELP patterns of patients with Hb S/β thalassemia are identical to those of patients with Hb SS.

3. Appropriate follow-up for the infant described in question 2 includes all of the following *except*:
a) Penicillin prophylaxis
b) RBC transfusion
c) Well-child immunizations
d) Anticipatory guidance to the family regarding fever, pain, and hydration
e) Plan to administer pneumococcal vaccine

Answer

The answer is b. RBC transfusions are an integral part of the treatment of patients with sickle cell disease. Transfusions can be either acute or chronic, simple or exchange. However, the indications for RBC transfusions are specific. In general, they are used to increase oxygen-carrying capacity or improve microvascular blood flow in an attempt to prevent or treat sickle-related vascular events. Specific indications for RBC transfusions include CNS infarction, acute chest syndrome, sequestration crisis, aplastic crisis, and cardiac or multiple organ failure. Transfusions are also given preoperatively. Chronic RBC transfusions are utilized in CNS infarction, recurrent chest syndrome, debilitating vaso-occlusive pain crisis, chronic organ failure, and recurrent priapism. All infants with Hb SS and Hb S/β0 thalassemia require penicillin prophylaxis beginning at the age of 2 to 3 months and continuing until at least the age of 5 years. Patients with sickling disorders should receive all routine well-child immunizations, including conjugated pneumococcal vaccine. The 23-valent pneumococcal vaccine should be given to patients with sickle cell disease at the ages of 2 and 5 years. Some hematologists also give this vaccination at the age of 10 to 12 years, along with meningococcal vaccine. Appropriate educational information must be provided in verbal and written format. Discussions should include an explanation of the genetics and pathophysiology of sickle cell disease, the importance of routine visits, the need for antibiotic prophylaxis, and the need to seek prompt medical attention in specific instances.

4. A 1-year-old boy with homozygous Hb S is brought to the emergency department with a temperature of

39.5°C (103.1°F). He is irritable when awake and moderately anorexic, and he appears ill. All of the following are appropriate steps in managing this infant *except:*

a) Blood cultures
b) Complete blood cell count with reticulocyte count
c) Intravenous fluids at twice maintenance
d) Empiric parenteral antibiotics (e.g., ceftriaxone)
e) Follow-up in clinic in 24 hours
f) Admission to the hospital for continued evaluation and treatment

Answer
The answer is e. Bacterial sepsis is the leading cause of death in children <3 years with sickle cell disease. The nearly 20% mortality rate of patients in this age group with bacterial sepsis underscores the importance of early evaluation and treatment of young children with sickle cell disease. Fever often indicates bacteremia, and temperatures more than 39°C (102°F) in young children with sickle cell disease are usually associated with sepsis. Other physical findings in patients with sickle cell disease are also associated with a high risk for septicemia. These include hypotension, organ hypoperfusion, severe pain, irritability, a white cell count <5000/mm^3 or >30,000/mm^3, and an age <1 year. Any child with fever and sickle cell disease requires a prompt evaluation that includes a physical examination, blood cultures and laboratory studies, intravenous fluid resuscitation, and the prompt administration of broad-spectrum antibiotics. Chest radiography, urine culture, throat culture, and lumbar puncture may also be required depending on the child's physical examination findings. Admission to the hospital for continued treatment is appropriate in this case given the child's age and physical findings.

5. A 10-year-old girl with homozygous Hb S is brought to your clinic with a 3-day history of increasing back and leg pain. She has been taking acetaminophen with codeine at home once or twice a day. Appropriate steps in managing this patient include all of the following *except:*

a) Admission to the hospital
b) Intravenous fluids at twice maintenance
c) Anti-inflammatory medications
d) Intravenous narcotics, regularly scheduled or through a patient-controlled analgesic device
e) Intravenous narcotics as needed

Answer
The answer is e. Painful events are thought to occur when tissue ischemia is caused by a reduction in blood flow. Tissue hypoxia develops and further exacerbates RBC sickling, which further leads to ischemia and increased pain. Painful events usually last approximately 1 week, but the frequency and severity of painful crises vary. In general, the treatment of a vaso-occlusive pain

crisis is based on three components. First, verify and treat the precipitating events. Second, provide adequate hydration. Third, provide quick and effective pain relief. This patient has attempted outpatient therapy and failed; the pain is escalating. Hospitalization with close monitoring and evaluation is indicated. Intravenous hydration to correct fluid imbalance should be initiated. Intravenous analgesics administered according to a fixed schedule with appropriate dosing intervals or through a patient-controlled analgesic device to provide quick, effective pain control are necessary. Nonsteroidal anti-inflammatory drugs are effective adjuvant agents in managing painful crisis.

6. Screening of a newborn has detected a hemoglobinopathy with Hb Bart's. All of the following statements are true *except:*

a) The infant may have a α thalassemia trait.
b) The infant may be a silent carrier of α thalassemia.
c) The infant may have microcytosis and anemia.
d) The infant may have β thalassemia.
e) The infant may be hematologically normal.

Answer
The answer is d. Hb Bart's is a tetramer of γ-globin chains (γ_4) that forms because of an excess of γ-globins. The γ-globin excess is the consequence of a decrease in α-globin synthesis. The synthesis of α-globin chains is inadequate in α thalassemia. α Thalassemia is difficult to diagnose because no characteristic elevations in Hb A_2 or Hb F are present. Four α-genes are involved in α-globin production. Silent carrier α thalassemia is characterized by the loss of one α-gene. The level of Hb Bart's is low on newborn screening. No hematologic manifestations develop in silent carrier α thalassemia. α Thalassemia trait is characterized by the loss of two α-genes. The level of Hb Bart's is high on newborn screening. Thalassemia trait is clinically characterized by mild microcytosis and mild hypochromic anemia. Hb Bart's (>15%–20%) is also seen in thalassemia with three α-gene deletions and thalassemia with four α-gene deletions if the newborn survives. β Thalassemia is a failure of adequate synthesis of β-globins and is characterized by increased levels of Hb A2 ($\alpha_2\delta_2$) and Hb F ($\alpha_2\gamma_2$).

7. Chronic RBC transfusions for the treatment of thalassemia are associated with:

a) Cirrhosis
b) Congestive heart failure
c) Cardiac arrhythmias
d) Diabetes mellitus
e) All of the above

Answer
The answer is e. Patients with thalassemia major require regularly scheduled RBC transfusions to maintain nearly normal Hb levels. Transfusions are given

in an attempt to prevent chronic anemia and hypoxemia and to suppress extramedullary hematopoiesis while "normal growth and development" can take place. However, the repeated administration of RBC transfusions is not without significant complications. These include alloimmunization, hyperviscosity, the transmission of infectious agents, and iron overload. The ability of the body to excrete iron is limited. Iron overload develops when the intake of iron is increased over time, either by chronic RBC transfusions or an increased absorption of iron from the gastrointestinal tract, both of which occur in thalassemia. Transfusion circumvents the intestinal barriers, and unless the Hb level of a patient with thalassemia is kept nearly normal, the gastrointestinal absorption of iron is increased. Iron overload can cause cardiac, liver, and endocrine problems that lead to premature morbidity and mortality. Cardiac complications include arrhythmias, pericarditis, and heart failure. Liver disease, including cirrhosis, develops over time. Growth retardation, delayed pubertal development, hypothyroidism, hypoparathyroidism, and diabetes mellitus are also common complications.

SUGGESTED READINGS

1. Cao A, Gabutti V, Galanello R, et al. *Management protocol for the treatment of thalassemia patients,* Flushing, NY: Printed and distributed by Cooley's Anemia Foundation, Inc., 1997.
2. Cao A, Saba L, Galanello R, et al. Molecular diagnosis and carrier screening for β-thalassemia. *JAMA* 1997;278:1273–1277.
3. Dover GJ, Platt OS. Sickle cell disease. In: Nathan DG, Orkin SH, eds. *Hematology of infancy and children,* 5th ed. Philadelphia: Saunders, 1998.
4. Huisman THJ. Human hemoglobin. In: Miller Dr, Baehner RL, eds. *Blood diseases of infancy and childhood,* 7th ed. St. Louis, MO: Mosby, 1995.
5. Leiken SL, Gallagher D, Kinney TR, et al. Mortality in children and adolescents with sickle cell disease. *Pediatrics* 1989;84:500–508.
6. Olivieri NF, Weatherall DJ. Thalassemias. In: Lilleyman J, Harn I, Blanchette V, eds. *Pediatric hematology,* 2nd ed. New York: Harcourt Brace, 1999.
7. Orkin SH, Nathan DG. The thalassemias. In: Nathan DG, Orkin SH, eds. *Hematology of infancy and children,* 5th ed. Philadelphia: Saunders, 1998.
8. Pass KA, Lane PA, Fernhoff PM, et al. U.S. newborn screening system guidelines II: follow-up of children, diagnosis, management, and evaluation. Statement of the Council of Regional Networks for Genetic Services (CORN). *J Pediatr* 2000;137(Suppl):4.
9. Reid CD, Charache S, Lubin B, eds. *Management and therapy of sickle cell disease,* 3rd ed. U.S. Department of Health and Human Services, Public Health Service, National Institutes of Health, NIH Publication No. 92-2117, Bethesda, MD, Reprinted 1995; (Suppl):4.
10. Serjeant GR, Serjeant BE. *Sickle cell disease,* 3rd ed. New York: Oxford University Press, 2001.

Chapter 56

Clinical Signs and Prognostic Factors in Common Pediatric Malignancies

Michael Levien and L. Kate Gowans

Cancer as a diagnosis in pediatrics is rare. When the worldwide occurrence of cancer is considered, cases diagnosed within the pediatric and adolescent age groups represent a small proportion of the cancer burden. In the Western industrialized nations, the percentage of cancers occurring within the pediatric age range is approximately 2%. In the United States, approximately 12,400 new cases of cancer in children and in adolescents <20 years are diagnosed annually. In contrast, 150,000 new cases of colon cancer and 150,000 new cases of lung cancer are diagnosed yearly in adults. Pediatricians might see only one to three cases in their entire professional lifetime.

The purpose of this chapter is to review the clinical presentations of common pediatric malignancies and provide an understanding of the prognostic features of each cancer at the time of diagnosis.

The distribution of cancer diagnoses is different for the 0 to 14 year age group and the 15 to 19 year age group. The approximate distribution (%) of cancer diagnoses in these groups is shown in Table 56.1.

COMMON CLINICAL SIGNS AND SYMPTOMS OF PEDIATRIC MALIGNANCY

Lymphadenopathy

Persistent adenopathy is common in children. At least 70% of pediatric patients <7 years have enlarged anterior or posterior cervical nodes, or both.

Size and location are important in assessing children with lymphadenopathy. Lymph nodes are considered enlarged if their greatest diameter is >10 mm. The exception is that epitrochlear nodes are considered enlarged if the diameter is >5 mm. Inguinal nodes are not abnormal unless the diameter is >15 mm. In most children, the cervical, axillary, and inguinal nodes are palpable and small. *Posterior auricular, epitrochlear, and supraclavicular adenopathy all warrant further investigation.* Pathologic cervical adenopathy is usually indicated by a diameter of >15 to 20 mm. Enlargement of lymph nodes to a pathologic size (e.g., >2 cm in the head and neck), followed by a decrease to a nonpathologic or even imperceptible size, probably represents a reactive adenopathy. However, if the same nodes continue to increase and decrease in size over time, especially in a pathologic (e.g., supraclavicular) area, an investigation for malignancy should be undertaken. Within 2 to 3 weeks, most noncancerous nodes should return to normal size.

Infection is the most common cause of acute cervical adenopathy. In cases of localized cervical adenitis with moderate inflammation and fever, the child can be treated with an oral antibiotic empirically. The therapy should include both antistaphylococcal and antistreptococcal coverages, and also anaerobic coverage if a dental source is suspected. When a child does not respond to antibiotic therapy in 7 days, or has a node that is fluctuant or >2 cm, a more extensive workup is necessary. This includes chest radiography, a complete blood cell count, metabolic studies (lactate dehydrogenase, uric acid, phosphorus, calcium and other electrolytes, blood urea nitrogen, creatinine,

TABLE 56.1

DISTRIBUTION (%) OF PEDIATRIC CANCERS

Type	Age 0–14 Years	Age 15–19 Years
Leukemia	30	10
Central nervous system tumors	22	10
Lymphoma	10	25
Neuroblastoma	8	0
Soft-tissue sarcoma	7	7
Wilms tumor	6	0
Osteosarcoma/Ewing sarcoma of bone	5	7
Germ cell tumor	3	12
Retinoblastoma	3	0
Hepatoblastoma	1	0
Thyroid cancer	1	7
Melanoma	1	8

bilirubin, and liver enzymes), measurement of the sedimentation rate, and a tuberculin skin test. Viral, bacterial, and fungal serologies should be obtained only if indicated by the history and physical examination findings. Bone marrow biopsy and aspiration may be indicated if the blood cell counts are abnormal or a mediastinal mass or hepatosplenomegaly is detected.

In chronic lymphadenopathy of the head and neck, malignancy becomes a consideration. Lymph nodes with malignant involvement are usually *firm, rubbery, and matted*. They are generally *nontender*, and when observed over time, they increase in size.

The following malignancies are associated with *generalized adenopathy:*

- Acute lymphocytic leukemia (ALL)
- Acute myeloid leukemia (AML)
- Lymphoma (non-Hodgkin and Hodgkin)
- Neuroblastoma

Patients with these conditions usually have other evidence of systemic disease, such as fever, night sweats, bone pain, arthralgias, easy bruising, petechiae, and peripheral blood changes. A mediastinal mass (see subsequent section) can be found in ALL (usually T-cell ALL) and the lymphomas (Hodgkin and non-Hodgkin).

A lymph node biopsy is suggested for any of the following:

- Enlarging nodes, or nodes that remain enlarged after 2 weeks
- Nodes that are not enlarging but have not decreased in size after 5 to 6 weeks or do not return to normal size after 10 to 12 weeks, especially if unexplained fever, weight loss, or hepatosplenomegaly is present; a biopsy should be performed earlier for enlarged supraclavicular or lower cervical nodes
- Mediastinal mass
- Pathologically enlarged lymph nodes in less common locations (e.g., supraclavicular, epitrochlear, and posterior auricular)

Mediastinal Mass

A number of benign and malignant tumors are found in the thorax. The mediastinum is the site of most intrathoracic masses in children. The location of a mass in one of the three anatomic areas of the mediastinum is a clue to the diagnosis (Table 56.2).

Patients with mediastinal tumors can be asymptomatic; however, with close questioning, more than half are found to have unreported symptoms, such as cough, dyspnea, orthopnea, or stridor caused by the compression or erosion of adjacent structures, such as the respiratory tract or superior vena cava. These patients can present with superior mediastinal syndrome, the most common symptom of which is shortness of breath or dyspnea that develops when the patient is in a supine position. It should be considered a medical emergency, and a workup should be undertaken immediately in the hospital.

Frequently, a mass is discovered on routine chest radiography, leading to computed tomography (CT) scan as the next diagnostic maneuver, which frequently requires

TABLE 56.2

ETIOLOGY OF MEDIASTINAL MASSES IN CHILDREN ACCORDING TO LOCATION

Anterior Mediastinum	Middle Mediastinum	Posterior Mediastinum
Hodgkin disease	Angiomas	Neuroblastoma
Non-Hodgkin lymphoma	Pericardial cysts	Other neurogenic tumors
ALL (usually T cell)	Lymph node lesions	Bronchogenic cysts
Bronchogenic Cysts	Bronchogenic cysts	Enterogenous cysts
Thyroid tumors	Teratomas	Thoracic meningocele
Lipomas	Esophageal lesions	Ewing sarcoma
Aneurysms	Hernia (foramen of Morgagni)	Lymphoma
		Rhabdomyosarcoma

ALL, acute lymphocytic leukemia.

sedation in children. *It is imperative to note that children with a mediastinal mass resulting in orthopnea or tracheal caliber <50% of normal cannot tolerate sedation or general anesthesia.* Specialists in pediatric anesthesia, oncology, and surgery should be consulted together immediately to plan a safe evaluation, which will involve unsedated scans and biopsies.

The most common histologic diagnosis of a mediastinal tumor in children is a "small, blue, round cell tumor," which is one of the following: lymphoma, leukemia (lymphoid), neuroblastoma, rhabdomyosarcoma, or primitive neuroectodermal tumor (PNET/Ewing sarcoma family). *An anterior mediastinal mass is leukemia (usually T-cell ALL) or lymphoma (Hodgkin or non-Hodgkin) until proved otherwise. A posterior mediastinal mass is a neurogenic tumor such as neuroblastoma or PNET until proved otherwise.* If a posterior mediastinal mass is present, magnetic resonance imaging (MRI) of the thoracic spine should be performed, ideally before surgery, to rule out extension of tumor into the spinal canal, which can cause spinal cord compression.

Headache

Headache is one of the most common symptoms seen in pediatric practice. Although very few headaches are associated with an intracranial tumor, it is important to consider this diagnosis when a patient has recurrent headaches.

Brain tumors are the solid tumors most frequently encountered in pediatrics. The diagnosis of brain tumor is initially suspected on the basis of a symptom complex that most often depends on the site of the tumor. Because most brain tumors are so situated that they interfere with the circulation of cerebrospinal fluid, increased intracranial pressure (ICP) is a common problem. Early symptoms may be non-localizing. Supratentorial lesions typically present with signs of high ICP (headache and vomiting) and focal neurologic deficits; infants may have an enlarging head size. Infratentorial lesions tend to present with ataxia or other gait disturbances, signs of high ICP if there is aqueduct compression, and cranial nerve abnormalities if the brain stem is involved. Spinal tumors present with back pain and signs of cord compression (weakness of extremities, and loss of bladder and bowel function).

MRI or CT scan of the brain is indicated in patients who have:

- Recurrent morning headaches or headaches that interrupt sleep
- Recurrent morning headaches that are usually incapacitating, that change in quality, frequency, and pattern, and that are often associated with vomiting
- Headache with vomiting in the absence of a family history of migraine
- Headaches that are associated with abnormal findings on neurologic examination such as seizure or confusion (95% of patients with brain tumors have abnormal findings)

- Ocular findings, such as papilledema, decreased visual acuity, or loss of vision
- Short stature or deceleration of linear growth
- Diabetes insipidus
- Neurofibromatosis
- Past history of cranial irradiation
- Headache and age <3 years

Bone Pain

Most of the pain associated with cancer is the consequence of bone, nerve, or hollow viscus involvement. Childhood cancers rarely present with pain except for bone cancers and leukemia. The differential diagnosis includes malignancy if pain awakens the child from sleep, function is compromised in the absence of trauma, no cause for the pain is apparent within 2 weeks, or there is an associated mass with or without fracture. The pain associated with bone cancer (Ewing sarcoma and osteosarcoma) tends to be intermittent at first and increases in severity with time. In both Ewing sarcoma and osteosarcoma, the time between the onset of symptoms and the diagnosis can be as long as 6 to 12 months.

Bone pain as a presenting complaint or resulting in a limp (or refusal to bear weight or walk in toddlers) has been reported in 27% to 33% of cases of acute leukemia. This is more common in ALL than in acute myeloid leukemia (AML). Patients who are being evaluated for acute rheumatoid arthritis may need to undergo a bone marrow examination to rule out acute leukemia, as leukemic arthritis may be mistaken for various rheumatic diseases.

Bone pain may also be a presenting complaint in children with neuroblastoma. Some children who present with abnormal blood cell counts and bone pain and who are evaluated for leukemia may have stage 4 neuroblastoma. If neuroblastoma is suspected, abdominal ultrasonography should be performed to search for an adrenal mass. If an abdominal mass is present, abdominal CT scan may reveal a *calcified mass consistent with neuroblastoma.* Further workup would include urine collection for catecholamine metabolites (vanillylmandelic and homovanillic acids) and bone marrow examination.

Rarely, children present with metastatic lesions to the bone from other types of tumors, such as rhabdomyosarcoma, other soft-tissue sarcomas, lymphoma, brain tumors (e.g., PNET, or medulloblastoma), and liver cancer (hepatocellular carcinoma).

If a child has persistent or chronic intermittent pain of bone/extremity, a plain film should be obtained and bone scan/MRI considered, especially if the pain is associated with a swelling, mass, or limited motion. If a destructive lesion is seen or the periosteum is disrupted, further workup is indicated. Patients who have persistent bone pain associated with fever should be evaluated for infection, such as osteomyelitis, in addition to malignancy.

Before biopsy, simultaneous input from pediatric oncology and orthopaedic oncology is essential.

Abdominal Masses

A palpable abdominal mass is the most common sign that should suggest a malignant solid tumor, although the mass is more likely to be benign or pseudotumor (e.g., feces, the abdominal aorta, a distended bladder, or hydronephrotic kidneys). Age is important when the differential diagnosis is considered (Table 56.3).

When the history is obtained and the physical examination performed, the presence of generalized adenopathy, pallor, bruising, petechiae, cachexia, gastrointestinal symptoms, genitourinary (GU) symptoms, jaundice, chest pain, dyspnea, shoulder pain, and pain on palpation of the mass should be noted.

Abdominal ultrasonography is the most common initial radiologic study performed to characterize an abdominal mass. CT scan of the chest, abdomen, and pelvis may also be indicated. If a renal mass is present, ultrasonography of the inferior vena cava and the heart is also indicated to rule out a tumor thrombus extending into the inferior vena cava and possibly into the heart. If a neuroblastoma is suspected, a scan with metaiodobenzylguanidine (MIBG) should be performed because this radioactively labeled compound is taken up by catecholaminergic cells, which are found in most neuroblastomas. In cases of neuroblastoma and paraspinal PNET, MRI of the spine should be performed to rule out an extension of the tumor into the spinal canal.

Pancytopenia

Anemia, leukopenia, or thrombocytopenia frequently occur alone as a presenting sign of acute leukemia, or all

TABLE 56.3

TUMORS PRESENTING AS ABDOMINAL MASSES ACCORDING TO AGE GROUP

Age Group	Tumor
Newborn	Neuroblastoma (most common solid tumor in infants)
	Mesoblastic nephroma
	Hepatoblastoma
	Wilms tumor
	Yolk sac tumor of testis
1–11 years	Neuroblastoma
	Wilms tumor
	Hepatoblastoma (usually 0–3 years of age)
	Hepatoma (over 3 years of age)
	Rhabdomyosarcoma
	Leukemia/lymphoma (liver/spleen involvement)
12–19 years	Lymphoma
	Hepatocellular carcinoma
	Soft-tissue sarcoma
	Dysgerminoma

three may develop. Pancytopenia is primarily a consequence of replacement of the bone marrow by tumor cells. Anemia is also associated with malignancy for other reasons. Anemia of chronic disease or hemolytic anemia can develop as a paraneoplastic manifestation of lymphomas (autoimmune hemolytic anemia). Except when the marrow is involved, leukopenia is rarely a manifestation of extramedullary malignancies. The same is true of thrombocytopenia, except for the rare association of immune thrombocytopenic purpura with Hodgkin lymphoma or thrombocytopenia with disseminated intravascular coagulation (DIC), which may occur in widely disseminated tumors such as AML, rhabdomyosarcoma, and neuroblastoma. Any other malignancy that involves the bone marrow can also produce a pancytopenia or depression of any of the cell lines. Pediatric solid tumors that can involve the bone marrow include neuroblastoma, lymphoma, rhabdomyosarcoma, Ewing sarcoma, and retinoblastoma.

Leukocytosis

An elevated white blood cell count is common in acute leukemia. A peripheral white blood cell count >100,000/mm^3 is almost always a manifestation of acute or chronic leukemia. Leukemoid reactions with white blood cell count >50,000/mm^3 are seen in children with septicemia. Lymphoid leukemoid reactions have been seen in infectious lymphocytosis, mumps, varicella, pertussis, and infections with adenovirus and cytomegalovirus. Myeloid leukemoid reactions with cell count >100,000/mm^3 have been reported in premature infants whose mothers received corticosteroids during pregnancy.

Approximately 10% of neonates with Down syndrome may develop a transient leukemia or myeloproliferative syndrome characterized by high leukocyte counts, blast cells in their peripheral blood, and associated anemia, thrombocytopenia, and hepatosplenomegaly. This usually resolves spontaneously within days to weeks after onset, although some very ill children (respiratory compromise caused by massive organomegaly) require a short course of chemotherapy. These infants require close follow-up, as 20% to 30% develop leukemia by age 3 years (median age: 16 months). The most common type of leukemia following TMD (transient myeloproliferative disorder) in a child with Down syndrome is acute megakaryocytic leukemia. TMD may occur in infants who do not have phenotypic features of Down syndrome. Blasts from these patients may show trisomy 21, suggesting a mosaic state. GATA1 mutations (a transcription factor that controls megakaryopoiesis) are present in the blasts from patients with Down syndrome who have TMD and also in those with leukemia.

Leukocytosis secondary to an exaggerated eosinophilia with white blood cell counts in the range of 20,000 to 100,000/mm^3 is often seen in parasitic infections, especially visceral larval migrans. Other causes of eosinophilia include hypereosinophilic syndrome, periarteritis nodosa, and allergic and hypersensitivity reactions. The malignant causes of eosinophilia are eosinophilic leukemia, Hodgkin lymphoma (20% of patients), and acute lymphoid leukemia. Eosinophilia is also seen in sarcoidosis. The absolute eosinophil count is used to quantitate eosinophilia. Many diseases are associated with moderate (1500–5000 cells/μL) or severe ($>$5000 cells/μL) eosinophilia. Patients with sustained blood eosinophilia may develop organ damage, especially cardiac, as found in HES (hypereosinophilic syndrome). These patients need to be monitored closely for evidence of cardiac disease. Eosinophilia is observed in many patients with primary immunodeficiency syndromes, especially hyper IgE syndrome and Wiskott-Aldrich syndrome. Eosinophilia is also seen in syndromes of thrombocytopenia with absent radii (TAR syndrome) and familial reticuloendotheliosis with eosinophilia. Wiskott-Aldrich syndrome may evolve into leukemia or lymphoma. Reticuloendotheliosis, class III, is associated with acute monocytic leukemia and true malignant histiocytosis.

Bleeding

Bleeding is an uncommon initial sign of malignancy in children. When it occurs, it is usually related to thrombocytopenia secondary to primary bone marrow involvement of leukemia or infiltrative marrow disease (e.g., lymphoma, rhabdomyosarcoma). It can represent a systemic consumptive process: disseminated intravascular coagulopathy (DIC) secondary to leukemia. In newly diagnosed acute leukemia, bleeding can also be related to the use of nonsteroidal anti-inflammatory drugs, such as ibuprofen. The use of aspirin in the treatment of bone pain can induce bleeding. High doses of antibiotics such as penicillin and ticarcillin can cause bleeding. This bleeding caused by nonsteroidal anti-inflammatory medications, aspirin, and penicillin is caused by platelet dysfunction. Coagulation abnormalities are also seen in disseminated malignancies. They rarely give rise to signs or symptoms unless DIC develops or there is significant bone marrow involvement causing thrombocytopenia. *DIC is a prominent feature of acute promyelocytic leukemia (APL)*, especially after the institution of chemotherapy. DIC can occur in any type of leukemia presenting with hyperleukocytosis (WBC $>$100,000). DIC also occurs in sepsis syndromes, such as gram-negative sepsis. These infections can be the presenting features in severely neutropenic or immunocompromised patients with undiagnosed acute leukemia and lymphomas.

SUMMARY OF PRESENTING SIGNS AND PROGNOSTIC FEATURES FOR INDIVIDUAL MALIGNANCIES

Brain Tumors

Brain tumors are the second most common cancer, and the most common solid tumor seen in pediatrics.

Presenting Signs

The most common presenting features of brain tumors in children are as follows: recurrent morning headaches that are usually associated with vomiting, coordination problems, ataxia, head tilt, and visual problems. *Patients with neurofibromatosis are at risk for the development of peripheral and central nervous system (CNS) tumors.*

Prognostic Features

Primary brain tumors are a diverse group of diseases that are classified according to histology, whereas tumor location and extent of spread are important factors that affect treatment and prognosis. Immunohistochemical analysis, cytogenetic and molecular genetic findings, and measures of mitotic activity (all elements of *grade*) along with the *stage* (extent of spread) are essential in tumor diagnosis. These evaluations determine the prognosis and subsequent treatment.

Approximately 70% of brain tumors in children are infratentorial, with three fourths of these located in the cerebellum or fourth ventricle. Common infratentorial (posterior fossa) tumors include the following:

- Cerebellar astrocytoma (usually pilocytic [low grade] but occasionally invasive or high grade)
- Medulloblastoma, the most common malignant brain tumor in children
- Ependymoma
- Brainstem glioma (often diagnosed neuroradiographically without biopsy; may be high or low grade)

Juvenile pilocytic cerebellar astrocytomas (JPA) and early stage (M0) medulloblastomas carry the best prognosis. JPA can be treated exclusively with surgery if these tumors are not invasive. Early stage medulloblastoma has a cure rate of 75% with surgery, chemotherapy, and radiation. Current clinical trials are evaluating lower-dose radiation in an attempt to decrease long-term sequelae.

Supratentorial tumors occur in the sellar or suprasellar region and other areas of the cerebrum. Sellar and suprasellar tumors comprise approximately 20% of childhood brain tumors and include the following:

- Craniopharyngioma
- Diencephalic (chiasmatic, hypothalamic, or thalamic) glioma (astrocytoma) of various grades
- Germinoma

The prognosis of these tumors depends on histologic grade and location.

Leukemias and Lymphomas

When leukemia or lymphoma becomes part of any differential diagnosis in a child, posteroanterior and lateral chest radiography should be performed. A mediastinal mass may be present, and airway patency must be fully assessed before these patients undergo any sedation.

Leukemias

ALL is the most common childhood malignancy. The cure rate for childhood ALL is >80%, and most children no longer receive cranial radiation. AML is less common but more aggressive, with the cure rate remaining at approximately 40% to 50%.

Presenting Signs and Symptoms

The most common presenting features include:

- Pancytopenia
- Selective anemia, thrombocytopenia, or leukopenia
- Leukocytosis
- Generalized lymphadenopathy
- Hepatosplenomegaly
- Fever of unknown origin
- Bone pain
- Arthralgias
- Petechiae
- Easy bruising
- Bleeding (the APL form of AML is strongly associated with DIC)
- Pallor and fatigue

Prognostic Features of Acute Lymphocytic Leukemia

In children with ALL, the initial white blood cell count and age are the two most important prognostic variables. "Standard-risk" ALL (prognosis 80%–90%) patients are aged from 1 to 10 years, *and* have a white blood cell count of <50,000/mm^3 at diagnosis. "High-risk" ALL (prognosis 70%) patients are 10 years or older, with any presenting white blood cell count, *or* children of any age with initial white blood cell count >50,000/mm^3. Children <1 year and those with certain molecular or cytogenetic characteristics have a distinctly poor prognosis, some now being classified as "very high-risk" (Table 56.4).

The immunophenotype of the leukemia cell is important prognostically; this predictor is evolving with changing therapy.

- Pre-B ALL (immature B-cell lymphoblast): best prognosis

TABLE 56.4

POOR PROGNOSTIC FEATURES OF ACUTE LYMPHOCYTIC LEUKEMIA

Age at onset is <1 year or >10 years
White blood cell count at diagnosis of >50,000/mm^3
T-cell immunophenotype
Presence of Philadelphia chromosome (translocation 9;22)
Presence of 11q23 rearrangement (MLL)
Presence of cytogenetic extreme hypodiploidy (<44 chromosomes)
Failure of induction chemotherapy (no remission documented by 6 weeks)
MLL, mixed-lineage leukemia.

- B cell (mature B-cell lymphoblast, Burkitt cell): worst prognosis
- T-cell ALL: intermediate to poor prognosis

Cytogenetic abnormalities and chromosome number are also of prognostic significance. Patients with hyperdiploidy (an overall increase in chromosome number) have a favorable prognosis, whereas patients with hypodiploidy, pseudodiploidy, and tetraploidy have a poor prognosis. Those with a nearly haploid number have the worst prognosis. Certain chromosomal translocations, such as t(8;14) (Burkitt's leukemia), and t(9;22) (Philadelphia chromosome), are associated with a particularly poor prognosis, whereas some others are associated with an excellent outcome (t(12;21), known as the TEL-AML translocation, and trisomies of chromosomes 4, 10 and 17, known as triple trisomy).

Treatment outcomes for cancer in older adolescents (age 15–19 years) are worse than for those 14 years and younger. Although true in many childhood cancers, the difference is most dramatic in ALL, where outcomes are 25% to 30% worse in 15- to 19-year-olds. The reasons for this difference are being investigated and appear to be caused in part by better outcomes if teens are treated on pediatric regimens (higher drug intensity and frequency).

Prognostic Factors in Acute Myeloid Leukemia and Chronic Leukemia

In AML, the long-term survival with conventional chemotherapy therapy is 30% at 3 years but is as high as 50% with bone marrow transplant in first remission from a human leukocyte antigens (HLA)–identical sibling. The intensity of the treatment required, as well as the severe immune suppression, makes infection a major cause of morbidity and mortality in AML.

APL leukemia carries the best prognosis. Acute myelocytic leukemia, acute myelomonocytic leukemia, and acute monoblastic leukemia all have a poor prognosis. Acute megakaryocytic leukemia and erythroleukemia have the worst prognosis of the AMLs. Of note, children with Down syndrome and AML have an overall survival that is dramatically superior to non–Down syndrome children with AML.

Chronic myeloid leukemias (juvenile and adult forms), rare in childhood, have a very poor prognosis.

Non-Hodgkin Lymphoma

Non-Hodgkin lymphoma (NHL) is the third most common childhood malignancy, accounting for approximately 6% of cancers in individuals <20 years. Although no sharp age peak is noted, NHL occurs most commonly in the second decade of life and is unusual in children <3 years. NHL is the most frequent malignancy in children with acquired immunodeficiency syndrome (AIDS).

The histopathology of childhood NHL falls into three broad categories:

- Lymphoblastic
- Small noncleaved cell (Burkitt and non-Burkitt)
- Large cell (histiocytic)

The lymphoblastic type is predominantly a T-cell lymphoma and accounts for 30% of cases of childhood NHL. Most of the patients with this histopathologic type have an anterior mediastinal mass and may present with tumor lysis syndrome and/or superior vena cava/superior mediastinal syndrome. The small noncleaved cell type of lymphoma accounts for 40% to 50% of cases of childhood NHL. Most of these tumors are intra-abdominal. Other sites of involvement include the lymphoid tissue of Waldeyer's ring, nasal sinuses, bones, peripheral lymph nodes, skin, bone marrow, CNS, and testes. The large cell lymphomas are a heterogeneous group of tumors accounting for 20% to 25% of cases of childhood NHL.

Presenting Signs and Symptoms
- Lymphadenopathy (focal or diffuse) without fever or weight loss (most common)
- Fever
- Weight loss
- Bone pain (a small percentage have primary cortical bone involvement, some have bone pain and fever secondary to bone marrow involvement and leukemic transformation)
- Pancytopenia or selective blood cell depression secondary to bone marrow involvement
- Headaches and vomiting secondary to CNS involvement
- Cough, dyspnea, pneumonia, dysphagia secondary to anterior mediastinal involvement
- Superior vena cava syndrome (common in T-cell or lymphoblastic lymphoma)
- Abdominal mass, signs of intestinal obstruction (typical of Burkitt or B-cell lymphoma), usually ileocecal involvement
- Patients with advanced-stage lymphoma at presentation, especially NHL with high proliferative cell index (Burkitt lymphoma and T-cell lymphoma), may have signs and symptoms of renal failure because of *tumor lysis syndrome (high potassium, phosphorus, and uric acid, low calcium)*.

Prognostic Features
The most important prognostic determinant, given optimal therapy, is the extent of disease at diagnosis as determined by pretreatment staging. More than 60% of children with NHL survive 5 years on current chemotherapy protocols. Patients with a single extra-abdominal or extrathoracic tumor and those with totally resectable intra-abdominal tumors have an excellent prognosis (5-year survival >90% regardless of histology). Patients with extensive intrathoracic disease and patients with bone marrow or CNS disease have a poorer prognosis.

Hodgkin Lymphoma
Presenting Signs and Symptoms
Painless lymph node enlargement, most often in the cervical or supraclavicular chains, is the most common presentation of Hodgkin lymphoma. The onset is usually subacute and prolonged, whereas it is rapid in NHL. Approximately 30% of patients with Hodgkin disease present with systemic symptoms at the time of diagnosis, which include the following:

- Fever
- Pruritus
- Weight loss
- Night sweats

Specifically, the "B" symptoms of Hodgkin lymphoma, which portend a worsening of prognosis, are fever (38°C [100.4°F] for 3 consecutive days), night sweats, and unexplained weight loss (10% or more of body weight in the preceding 6 months). Two thirds of patients have an anterior mediastinal mass, and therefore may have cough, dyspnea, or orthopnea, but are often asymptomatic. Laboratory findings may include a high sedimentation rate, elevated ferritin and eosinophilia; none of these are prognostic.

In Hodgkin lymphoma, the primary area of involvement is usually *above the diaphragm*, and disease can progress to any lymph node chain above or below the diaphragm. Patients may also present with stage IV disease involving bone, bone marrow, lung, or liver. Although the peak age for Hodgkin lymphoma is during adolescence, this cancer has been diagnosed in children as young as 3 years. It is also important to note that the presenting manifestation of primary disease can uncommonly be below the diaphragm (e.g., inguinal nodes).

Prognostic Features
The prognosis is based on the stage and histopathology. The 5-year survival rate is approximately 75% for patients with stage IV disease, whereas patients with stage I disease have a 95% survival rate. Generally, the lymphocyte-predominant and nodular sclerosing types carry the best prognosis. The mixed cellularity type has an intermediate prognosis, and the lymphocyte-depleted type has the worst prognosis, although with current therapy the prognosis remains good. Current clinical trials seek to find a balance between chemotherapy and radiation that decreases the incidence of second malignancy, which is a significant concern in these survivors.

Neuroblastoma

Presenting Signs and Symptoms
Primary tumors involving the adrenal medulla present with abdominal mass or pain. The mass is firm, irregular, and nontender. Anorexia, vomiting, and change in bowel habits are common.

Signs and symptoms of a neuroblastoma presenting outside the adrenal gland correlate with the site of involvement.

- Cervical ganglia: Horner syndrome, heterochromia
- Thoracic: dysphagia, dyspnea, infections, chronic cough
- Pelvic: difficulty with defecation or urination
- Paraspinal: back pain, paraplegia, retention of stool and urine

Signs and symptoms of metastases include:

- Pain, pancytopenia (bone marrow)
- Pain in long bones, periorbital ecchymosis, proptosis (bone)
- Hepatomegaly (liver)
- Dyspnea (lung)
- Left supraclavicular, cervical, inguinal lymphadenopathy
- Multiple subcutaneous bluish nodules (skin)

Signs and symptoms of paraneoplastic syndromes include:

- Hypertension (stretching of the renal artery): angiotensin effect
- Flushing, hypertension: catecholamine effect
- Watery diarrhea, abdominal distension: vasoactive intestinal peptide effect
- Opsoclonus-myoclonus syndrome: myoclonic jerks, chaotic, conjugate, jerking eye movements (opsoclonus)
- Progressive cerebellar ataxia: also a feature of the opsoclonus-myoclonus syndrome

Neuroblastoma is the most common malignant tumor in infancy, accounting for over half of cancers in the newborn period. It is the most common solid tumor in pediatrics outside of the central nervous system.

Prognostic Features

Poor prognostic indicators include the following.

- Stage III or IV disease
  - Exception: stage IVS—Special category reserved for infants <1 year of age with resectable primary tumors and metastases that are limited to the liver, skin, and bone marrow. Those with metastasis to the cortical bone are excluded. Overall survival for stage IVS is 85%.
- Age >1 year. Overall survival at 5 years from NCI SEER program data are 83%, 55%, and 40% for children <1 year, 1 to 4 years, and 5 to 9 years, respectively. Recent clinical trial data suggest that patients up to 18 months of age with stage IV disease who have biologically favorable characteristics (nonamplification of N-myc oncogene and favorable Shimada histology) demonstrated an 86% 6-year survival.
- Pathologic risk classification. Tumors are classified as Shimada favorable or unfavorable based on the degree of neuroblast differentiation, Schwannian stroma content, frequency of cell division (the mitosis-karyorrhexis

index), and age at diagnosis. A high Shimada rating is unfavorable.

- Cytogenetics and molecular genetics. Although no pathognomonic genetic or chromosomal alteration has been identified, certain molecular and cytogenetic characteristics correlate with poor prognosis. High N-myc amplification (also called MYCN oncogene) or alterations in the total DNA content of the tumor (DNA index or ploidy), which presumably result from mitotic dysfunction, are both associated with worse prognosis and are often found in stage 4 tumors. Tumors associated with a higher DNA content (hyperdiploid with a DNA index of >1) are associated with lower stage, better response to initial therapy, and overall better prognosis than diploid tumors. Gain or loss of certain chromosomes is also reported; loss of heterozygosity (LOH) of chromosome 1p is associated with a poorer prognosis; gain of 17 q (trisomy 17q) occurs in one half of neuroblastomas and is associated with a very aggressive phenotype.

Wilms Tumor

Presenting Signs and Symptoms

The major presenting features of Wilms tumor include:

- An *asymptomatic abdominal mass*, usually in the flank, in a well-appearing child
- Abdominal pain, anorexia, vomiting, listlessness, or a combination of these (one third of patients). Pain is likely related to subcapsular hemorrhage.
- Hematuria (caused by bleeding into the urinary tract)
- Hypertension (caused by distortion of renal vasculature, present in 25% of patients)
- Anemia (caused by bleeding within the tumor)

Although most Wilms tumors have no identifiable genetic abnormality, some of them appear to result from changes in one or more of several genes; accordingly, there are syndromes associated with a higher risk of developing Wilms tumor. Specific germ-line mutations in one of these genes (*WT1*) are associated with the rare Denys-Drash syndrome (pseudohermaphroditism, glomerulopathy, renal failure, and 95% chance of developing Wilms tumor). A gene that causes *aniridia* is located near the *WT1* gene on chromosome 11p13, and deletions encompassing the *WT1* and aniridia genes may explain the association between aniridia and Wilms tumor. WAGR (W-Wilms tumor, A-Aniridia, G-Genital, and/or urinary tract abnormalities, R-mental retardation) syndrome is also associated with WT1 mutation.

A second Wilms tumor gene *(WT2)* appears to be located at or near the Beckwith-Wiedemann gene locus on chromosome 11p15. *Children with Beckwith-Wiedemann syndrome* (macroglossia, *hemihypertrophy*, visceromegaly, mild microcephaly, omphalocele, facial nevus flammeus, characteristic earlobe crease, and renal medullary dyslalia) *are at increased risk (5% incidence) for the development of Wilms tumor* (and hepatoblastoma and adrenocortical carcinoma) and should be screened with ultrasonography *every 3 months* until they are 7 years old. *Patients with aniridia or hemihypertrophy should be screened with renal ultrasonography every 3 months until they are 6 years old.*

Despite the number of genes that appear to be involved in the development of Wilms tumor, hereditary Wilms tumor (either bilateral tumors or a family history of the neoplasm) is uncommon, with 4% to 5% of patients having bilateral tumors and 1% to 2% of patients having a family history positive for Wilms tumor. The risk for Wilms tumor among the offspring of individuals who have had unilateral (i.e., sporadic) tumors is quite low (<2%).

Prognostic Features

Wilms tumor is a curable disease in most of the affected children. More than 90% of patients survive for 4 years after diagnosis. The prognosis is related to:

- Stage of the disease
- Histopathologic features. The most important *poor* prognostic factor is diffuse anaplastic tumor histology, defined as the presence of multipolar polypoid mitotic figures and marked nuclear enlargement with hyperchromia. Although diffuse anaplasia is detected in only 10% to 14% of patients, those with diffuse anaplastic tumors account for >60% of the deaths.
- Patient age. Children <2 years historically have carried a better prognosis; however, with improved therapeutic interventions, the effect of age as a prognostic factor has been reduced.
- Tumor size (tumor weight <250 g carries a better prognosis)
- Biologic markers. Current research suggests that several markers appear to be predictive of outcome. The most promising of these is the loss of heterozygosity (LOH) at chromosomes 16q and 1p. In a recent study from NWTSG (National Wilms Tumor Study Group) of 232 patients, patients with tumor specific LOH at 16q had a relapse rate that was 3.3 times higher and a mortality rate 12 times higher than patients without this marker. In a more recent study from the same group, tumor specific LOH at 16q *and* 1p was independently associated with a higher risk of relapse and death in a subset of patients with favorable histology (nonanaplastic). The current NWTS treatment for stages 1 and 2 with favorable histology evaluates newly diagnosed specimens for the presence of tumor specific LOH of 16q and 1p. Those patients whose tumors show LOH for 16q and 1p have a third chemotherapy agent added to their treatment. Stage 3 and 4 favorable histology patients already have this third drug in their treatment plans. Finally, an increase in gene copy number (aneuploidy) in tumor cells is another biologic marker that appears to be associated with poor outcome.

Rhabdomyosarcoma

Rhabdomyosarcoma is a soft-tissue malignant tumor of skeletal muscle origin that can involve any skeletal muscle of the body.

Presenting Signs and Symptoms

The most common clinical presentation is a painless, enlarging mass or symptoms related to obstruction/transplantation of organs.

The most common sites of involvement include:

- Head, neck, or orbit (35%)
- Extremities (24%)
- GU tract (18%)
- Trunk (11%)

In the head, the sinuses are very common sites of involvement, with potential extension of the tumor into the parameningeal area and brain. The tumor can present in the middle ear and mastoid area, with the same potential for extension into the CNS. Other less common sites include the intrathoracic region, gastrointestinal tract (including the liver and biliary tract), and perianal and anal regions.

Most cases of rhabdomyosarcoma appear to be sporadic, but the disease has been associated with familial syndromes, such as neurofibromatosis, Li-Fraumeni syndrome, Beckwith-Wiedemann syndrome, and Costello syndrome. Li-Fraumeni syndrome (LFS) is characterized by members of affected families who are predisposed to a spectrum of cancers resulting from the inactivation of the p53 tumor suppressor gene. Studies have shown a clear association with inactivation of p53 and rhabdomyosarcoma in children <3 years of age. Beckwith-Wiedemann syndrome is a fetal overgrowth condition that is associated with an increased incidence of solid tumors of childhood, including rhabdomyosarcoma, Wilms tumor, hepatoblastoma, and adrenocortical carcinoma. In Costello syndrome, or faciocutaneoskeletal syndrome (FCS syndrome), there is a predisposition to developing malignancies, including rhabdomyosarcoma.

Prognostic Features

The prognosis is based on the stage, extent of surgical resection, and histopathology. Treatment includes a combination of chemotherapy and surgery and/or radiation, so initial *multidisciplinary referral and evaluation are imperative.* Patients with smaller tumors (<5 cm) have better survival than patients with larger tumors. Patients with metastatic disease at diagnosis have a very poor prognosis, with <30% of patients achieving 5-year survival. For rhabdomyosarcoma, the alveolar histopathologic type (usually in the extremities) is associated with a poorer outcome, whereas the embryonal type is associated with a better prognosis. The vaginal botryoid sarcoma has the best prognosis. Although rhabdomyosarcoma is a very aggressive tumor, current intensive chemotherapy protocols coupled with radiation and surgery have improved the overall survival for all of these patients.

Bone Cancer

Presenting Signs

Bone pain, usually localized to one area, is the most common presenting sign of bone cancer. The history of pain may go back as far as 3 to 6 months, or even longer. The patient may or may not have an associated soft-tissue mass in the area. The distal femur and proximal tibia are the most common sites, followed in decreasing frequency by the proximal humerus and middle and proximal femur.

Bone cancer is usually osteosarcoma or Ewing sarcoma. Ewing sarcoma is one of the "small round blue cell tumors," a categorization that also includes neuroblastoma, lymphoma, leukemia, and rhabdomyosarcoma.

Prognostic Features of Osteosarcoma

The site of the tumor is a significant prognostic factor in localized disease. In children, distal tumors have been associated with a more favorable prognosis, whereas primary tumors of the axial skeleton have a poor prognosis. Proximal humeral tumors have a poor prognosis.

Resectability of the tumor is an important prognostic feature because osteosarcoma is relatively resistant to radiotherapy. Patients with primary tumors of the mandible, iliac crest, pubis, and shoulder blade have a good survival rate with aggressive surgery and intensive multimodal therapy. After initial chemotherapy and at the time of definitive resection, the amount of tumor necrosis seen histologically (expressed as a percentage), remains a prognostic indicator as well; >90% is desirable.

The most important prognostic factor remains the stage (extent of spread). Twenty percent of patients have *metastatic lung disease* at diagnosis. In the era of adjuvant (preoperative) chemotherapy in the frontline treatment of osteosarcoma, the survival of patients with clinically nonmetastatic disease is 70%; the outlook for children with metastatic disease remains poor with an overall survival of <30%.

Prognostic Features of Ewing Sarcoma

The site of the primary tumor and whether it has metastasized are the two most important prognostic features. Presence or absence of metastases at diagnosis appears to be of greater importance. Patients with metastatic disease in lung and *bone at diagnosis fare significantly worse than those with bony mets alone; of metastatic disease that is present in only one location, isolated bony disease is worse than isolated lung disease.* Patients with axial primaries (i.e., pelvis, rib, scapula, skull, clavicle, and sternum) tend to have a worse prognosis than those with extremity lesions. The size of the primary tumor and the histologic response to up-front chemotherapy are prognostic as well. Fever, anemia, and elevated serum LDH at diagnosis all correlate with a greater volume of disease and a poorer prognosis. Molecular genetic analysis of Ewing sarcoma in the last decade has shown that those with a type 1 fusion of the EWS-FLI1 translocation fare better than those with the less common fusion transcript types. This type 1 fusion transcript in which EWS (Ewing sarcoma) exon 7 is fused to FLI1 exon 6 is present in 60% of cases compared with other fusion types. It is associated with a threefold reduction in the risk of developing metastatic disease as compared to non–type 1 transcripts. At least 18 different possibilities for gene fusions have been reported in the Ewing sarcoma family of tumors. Biologic and molecular genetic studies and their potential prognostic significance are ongoing in current and future clinical trials.

Retinoblastoma

Presenting Signs

Leukocoria of one or both eyes, termed "white reflex," but described by parents as an unusual appearance of the eye, is the most frequent presenting sign, present in more than half of children with retinoblastoma. Leukocoria is manifested when the tumor is fairly large or has caused a total retinal detachment, resulting in a retrolental mass that is visible through the pupil. Strabismus is the next most common sign (25%). This occurs when the tumor arises in the macula, causing a loss of central vision and followed by a loss of fusional reflex such that the eye may drift, resulting in esotropia or exotropia. Vision loss is not a symptom because young children are unaware of unilaterally decreased vision. Intraocular tumors are not painful unless secondary glaucoma or inflammation is present. Newly diagnosed cases of retinoblastoma are bilateral 20% to 30% of the time. The median age of onset is 2 years, but bilateral, hereditary cases usually present before the age of 1 year. Bilateral disease is multifocal, with several tumors in each eye.

Prognostic Features

Children with retinoblastoma have an excellent prognosis, with 5-year survival rates >90%. The prognosis is based on stage and therapy. If the tumor is unilateral at presentation and does not extend beyond the cribriform plate in the optic nerve, the cerebrospinal fluid and bone marrow are not involved (bone marrow involvement is rare), and the child is <2 years, the prognosis is excellent. Patients with bilateral disease have a worse prognosis because of the *high incidence of second malignant neoplasms (most frequently osteosarcoma). Soft tissue sarcomas and malignant melanomas are not uncommon in these patients, irrespective of whether they receive radiation as part of their treatment.* This is, however, why radiation should be avoided whenever possible. The incidence of second malignancies in these patients increases with age such that by age 50, there is a 50% chance of developing a new cancer. Children with RB1 mutations are at significant risk for the development of second malignancies.

Patients with bilateral disease should have MRI of the brain to evaluate their pineal gland. Some patients with bilateral retinoblastoma will present with PNET of the pineal gland at diagnosis *(trilateral retinoblastoma)*. This would impart a significantly poorer prognosis.

How would therapy affect the prognosis of patients with retinoblastoma? Since the early 1990s, the use of chemoreduction therapy instead of EBRT (external beam radiation therapy) has become the standard of care. The use of vincristine, etoposide (VP-16), and carboplatin, in most cases, causes significant reduction in the size of these tumors such that the ophthalmologist can apply local therapies (laser photocoagulation, cryotherapy, or brachytherapy). Avoiding the use of EBRT reduces the risk of second malignancies that can occur in the irradiated areas.

Liver Cancer

Liver cancer in children is rare. The two important types of cancers are hepatoblastoma and hepatocellular carcinoma. Hepatoblastoma occurs in very young children; nearly 70% are diagnosed by age 2, 90% by age 5. *Hepatoblastoma is associated with Beckwith-Wiedemann syndrome and familial adenomatous polyposis; it occurs with increased frequency in children with a history of low birth weight (<1000 g).*

Hepatocellular carcinoma occurs primarily in the 12- to 15-year age group, but can be seen in children from birth to 4 years of age. It is associated with *hepatitis B and hepatitis C*, especially in children with perinatally acquired infection.

Presenting Signs

Most tumors of the liver present as a painless abdominal mass palpated by the family or examining physician. In advanced disease, symptoms may include nausea, vomiting, anorexia, weight loss, or abdominal pain. Hepatoblastoma may be associated with anemia and thrombocytosis. A child with the rare hemangioepithelioma may present with signs and symptoms compatible with congestive heart failure.

Prognostic Features

The overall survival rate for children with hepatoblastoma is 75%; it is 25% for those with hepatocellular carcinoma. If the tumor is completely resectable with no metastases at presentation, the survival rate is high. If a hepatoblastoma is completely resected and pulmonary metastases develop, and if the lung metastases are completely excised, patients have an excellent prognosis. Most patients with these tumors have *elevated levels of α-fetoprotein* that usually parallel disease activity. The absence of α-fetoprotein when hepatoblastoma is diagnosed is probably a poor prognostic sign. It is associated with a small cell anaplastic histologic variant that responds poorly to therapy.

Adverse Effects of Chemotherapy

Chemotherapy has adverse effects that are common or rare, and acute or chronic. Many agents cause nausea and myelosuppression. The following is a list of the most frequently encountered adverse effects unique to some of the most commonly used chemotherapeutic agents:

- Alkylating agents (cyclophosphamide, ifosfamide): decreased fertility
- Anthracyclines: cardiomyopathy
- Asparaginase: pancreatitis, coagulation abnormalities, anaphylactic reaction
- Bleomycin: pulmonary fibrosis
- Cisplatin: ototoxicity, renal toxicity
- Cyclophosphamide: bladder irritation, syndrome of inappropriate antidiuretic hormone secretion (SIADH)
- Etoposide: secondary leukemia (AML)
- Ifosfamide: Fanconi renal tubular acidosis, bladder irritation
- Vincristine/vinblastine: neurotoxicity (peripheral neuropathy), constipation

REVIEW EXERCISES

QUESTIONS

1. Bone pain is a common presenting problem in which of the following tumors?
a) Acute leukemia, hepatoblastoma, Ewing sarcoma
b) Osteosarcoma, retinoblastoma, acute leukemia
c) Wilms tumor, acute leukemia, neuroblastoma
d) Osteosarcoma, acute leukemia, Ewing sarcoma
e) Acute leukemia, neuroblastoma, osteosarcoma

Answer
The answer is d. Bone pain is a universal presenting complaint in primary destructive lesions of the bone. This symptom is the reason patients with osteosarcoma and primary bone Ewing (not extraosseous Ewing) sarcoma or primary bone PNET seek a physician's evaluation. A simple radiograph usually reveals a destructive lesion of the bone with or without periosteal elevation. If the radiographic results are questionable and the patient has persistent pain, an MRI can confirm the existence of the lesion. Bone pain and arthralgias are common symptoms in acute leukemia. The bone pain is probably caused by intramedullary expansion of the bones secondary to the proliferation of leukemia cells in the bone marrow. Arthralgias *(leukemic arthritis)* represent referred and inflammatory pain. Stage IV neuroblastoma usually causes bone marrow and lytic bone pain and can mimic acute leukemia clinically. Hepatoblastoma, retinoblastoma, and Wilms tumor rarely present with bony metastatic disease. These tumors are usually diagnosed early enough by virtue of

their common presenting features (abdominal masses in hepatoblastoma and Wilms tumor, leukocoria in retinoblastoma) that it would be unlikely to find osseous metastases.

2. Which of the following are the two *most* important prognostic indicators in children in whom ALL is diagnosed?
a) Age and immunophenotype
b) Sex and white blood cell count
c) Platelet count and immunophenotype
d) Immunophenotype and white blood cell count
e) Age and white blood cell count
f) Race and hemoglobin level

Answer
The answer is e. The initial leukocyte count is probably the most significant prognostic factor in ALL. Patients with an initial white blood cell count >50,000/mm³ have a poorer prognosis (approximately 20% of children with ALL). This usually reflects a higher proliferative index of lymphoblasts. It most certainly represents a greater tumor burden at diagnosis, which is usually manifested by the presence of significant hepatosplenomegaly and lymphadenopathy in any form of ALL and carries a poorer prognosis. Age is also a major prognostic factor. Children <1 year and >10 years at diagnosis have a poorer prognosis than do children in the "standard-risk" age group (1–9.99 years). Infants <1 year have the worst prognosis. Girls fare better than boys (approximately 10% advantage), although male gender is no longer considered an adverse prognostic indicator. Other factors, such as an adverse immunophenotype (T-cell, mature B-cell) and adverse leukemia molecular and cytogenetic features, are usually associated with a high white blood cell count and carry a less favorable prognosis. A low hemoglobin level at the time of diagnosis usually reflects a primary bone marrow disease rather than lymphoma-leukemia syndrome, the latter having a poorer prognosis. The initial platelet count and race are insignificant factors. An initial platelet count >100,000/mm³ may reflect an early primary bone marrow process or leukemic transformation of lymphoma.

3. On a physical examination of a newborn infant, an abdominal mass is discovered. The *most* likely tumor diagnosis is:
a) Lymphoma
b) Wilms tumor
c) Hepatoblastoma
d) Neuroblastoma
e) Retinoblastoma
f) None of the above

Answer
The answer is d. Neuroblastoma is the most common tumor in infancy and accounts for >50% of cancers of

the newborn. Lymphoma is not likely in a patient of this age. Although a hepatoblastoma or Wilms tumor would present with an abdominal mass, presentation in the newborn period is unusual. Although possible but unlikely in a newborn infant, retinoblastoma would not present with an abdominal mass.

4. A chest radiograph reveals a posterior mediastinal mass. The *most* likely tumor diagnosis is:
a) Hodgkin disease
b) Rhabdomyosarcoma
c) Neuroblastoma
d) Non-rhabdomyosarcoma soft tissue sarcoma
e) Lymphocytic lymphoma

Answer
The answer is c. Neurogenic tumors account for 20% of all mediastinal tumors. Posterior mediastinal masses are neurogenic tumors until proved otherwise. These are usually neuroblastomas of all degrees of maturity (neuroblastoma, ganglioneuroblastoma, ganglioneuroma, or composites of all three). Primitive neuroectodermal tumor (Ewing variant) may also present in the posterior mediastinum, which is also a site for neurofibromas. The posterior mediastinum is a possible but much less likely location for lymphomas and sarcomas not of the Ewing type. Lymphomas are more typically located in the anterior mediastinum and are likely to be of the Hodgkin type. Benign entities such as bronchogenic and enterogenous cysts and meningoceles are also included in the differential diagnosis.

5. On a routine health maintenance examination of an apparently healthy 2-year-old girl, you notice leukocoria. Which physician(s) should become involved as possible?
a) Urologist
b) Gynecologist
c) Oncologist and nephrologist
d) Dermatologist
e) Psychiatrist
f) Ophthalmologist and oncologist
g) No one at this time; would observe patient

Answer
The answer is f. Leukocoria, also known as *"white reflex"* is a white-appearing reflex of a large retrolental mass. It occurs when the retinoblastoma is large or has caused a total retinal detachment. The mass is visible through the pupil. Leukocoria is the most common presenting sign of retinoblastoma. Such children should be co-managed by a pediatric ophthalmologist and oncologist.

Case for Questions 6 and 7
A teenage boy has a 3-month history of a 10-kg weight loss, intermittent fevers, and night sweats.

6. Which of the following clinical features would you expect to find on examination and evaluation?

a) Petechiae, tender joints with severe limitation of motion

b) Right lower quadrant abdominal mass; ecchymoses on legs, back, and trunk

c) Horner syndrome, cerebellar ataxia

d) Large tender mass in the right knee, decreased breath sounds in the base of the right lung

e) Significant hepatosplenomegaly, leukocoria

f) Diffuse lymphadenopathy, large anterior mediastinal mass

Answer

The answer is f.

7. The *most* likely tumor diagnosis in question 6 is:

a) Hodgkin lymphoma

b) Neuroblastoma

c) Rhabdomyosarcoma

d) Hepatocellular carcinoma

e) Burkitt lymphoma

Answer

The answer is a. Weight loss, night sweats, and fever are the most common systemic manifestations of Hodgkin lymphoma, in which an "A" or "B" is assigned to the stage. "A" patients are free of the presenting "B" signs and symptoms, whereas patients with the "B" symptoms have systemic manifestations of illness. (Pruritus can be seen, but has been removed from the "B" list of symptoms.) Other non-Hodgkin lymphomas and the leukemias *can* present with fever and weight loss; a Burkitt's lymphoma is less likely to present with constitutional symptoms.

SUGGESTED READINGS

1. Albritton K, Bleyer WA. The management of cancer in the older adolescent. *Eur J Cancer* 2003;39:2584–2599.

2. Breneman JC, Lyden E, Pappo AS, et al. Prognostic factors and clinical outcomes in children and adolescents with metastatic rhabdomyosarcoma: a report from the Intergroup Rhabdomyosarcoma study IV. *J Clin Oncol* 2003;21:78–84.

3. Chantada G, Fandino A, Davila MT, et al. Results of a prospective study for the treatment of retinoblastoma. *Cancer* 2004;100:834.

4. Crist WM, Anderson JR, Meza JL, et al. Intergroup Rhabdomyosarcoma Study IV: results for patients with non-metastatic disease. *J Clin Oncol* 2001;19:3091–3102.

5. D'Angio GJ. Pre- or post-operative treatment for Wilms tumor? who, what, when, where, how, why, and which. *Med Pediatr Oncol* 2003;41:545–549.

6. Demirci H, Shields CL, Meadows AT, Shields JA. Long-term visual outcome following chemoreduction for retinoblastoma. *Arch Ophthalmol* 2005;123:1525–1530.

7. Dome J, Coppes M Recent advances in Wilms tumor genetics. *Curr Opin Pediatr* 2002;14:5–11.

8. Gamis A. Acute myeloid leukemia and Down syndrome evolution of modern therapy: state of the art review. *Pediatr Blood Cancer* 2005;44:13–20.

9. Ganjavi H, Malkin D. Genetics of childhood cancer. *Clin Orthop* 2002;401:75–87.

10. Golden CB, Feusner JH. Malignant abdominal masses in children: quick guide to evaluation and diagnosis. *Ped Clin NA* 2002;49:1369–1392.

11. Gururangan S, Friedman HS. Recent advances in the treatment of pediatric brain tumors. *Oncology* 2004;18:1649–1661.

12. Gurney JG, Bondy ML. Epidemiology of Childhood Cancer. In: Pizzo PA, Poplack DG, eds. *Principles and Practice of Pediatric Oncology, 5th ed.* Philadelphia: Lippincott, 2006:1–13.

13. Grundy PE, Breslow NE, Li S, et al. Loss of heterozygosity for chromosomes 1p and 16q is an adverse prognostic factor in favorable histology Wilms tumor: a report from the National Wilms Tumor Study group. *J Clin Oncol* 2005;23:7312–7321.

14. Hosalkar HS, Dormans JP. Limb sparing surgery for pediatric musculoskeletal tumors. *Pediatr Blood Cancer* 2004;42:295–310.

15. Kalapurakal JA, Dome JS, Perlman EJ, et al. Management of Wilms tumour: current practice and future goals. *Lancet Oncol* 2004;5:37–46.

16. Katzenstein HM, Krailo MD, Malogolowkin MH, et al. Fibrolamellar hepatocellular carcinoma in children and adolescents. *Cancer* 2003;15:2006–2012.

17. Kennedy JG, Frelinhuysen P, Hoang BH. Ewing sarcoma: current concepts in diagnosis and treatment. *Curr Opin Pediatr* 2003;151:53–57.

18. Kleinerman RQA, Tucker MA, Tarone RE, et al. Risk of new cancers after radiotherapy in long-term survivors of retinoblastoma: an extended follow-up. *J Clin Oncol* 2005;23:2272–2279.

19. Mackie AM, Watson CB. Anesthesia and mediastinal masses. *Anesthesia* 1984;39:899–903.

20. Malogolowkin MH, Quinn JJ, Steuber CP, Siegel SE. Clinical assessment and differential diagnosis of the child with suspected cancer. In: Pizzo PA, Poplack DG, eds. *Principles and Practice of Pediatric Oncology*, 5th ed. Philadelphia: Lippincott, 2006:145–159.

21. Meyer WH, Spunt SL. Soft tissue sarcomas of childhood. *Cancer Treat Rev* 2004;30:269–280.

22. Meza JL, Anderson J, Pappo AS, Meyer WH. Analysis of prognostic factors in patients with nonmetastatic rhabdomyosarcoma treated on intergroup rhabdomyosarcoma studies III and IV: The Children's Oncology Group. *J Clin Oncol* 2006;24:3844–3851.

23. Oberlin O, Rey A, Lyden E, et al. Prognostic factors in metastatic rhabdomyosarcoma: results from pooled analysis from United States and European cooperative groups. *J Clin Oncol* 2008;26:2384–2389.

24. Punyko JA, Mertens AC, Baker KS, et al. Long- term survival probabilities for childhood rhabdomyosarcoma. *Cancer* 2005;103:1475–1483.

25. Rodriguez-Galindo C, Wilson MW, Haik BG, et al. Treatment of intraocular retinoblastoma with vincristine and carboplatinum. *J Clin Oncol* 2003;21:2019–2025.

26. Schnater JM, Kohler SE, Lamers WH, et al. Where do we stand with hepatoblastoma? *Cancer* 2003; 98:668–678.

27. Schouten-van Meeteren AY, Moll AC, Imhof SM, et al. Chemotherapy for retinoblastoma: an expanding area of clinical research. *Med Pediatr Oncol* 2002;38:428–438.

28. Stiller CA. Epidemiology and genetics of childhood cancer. *Oncogene* 2004;23:6429–6444.

29. Velez MC. Lymphomas. *Pediatr Rev* 2003;24:380–386.

30. Weinstein JL, Katzenstein HW, Cohn SL. Advances in the diagnosis and treatment of neuroblastoma. *Oncologist* 2003;8:278–292.

31. Young G, Toretsky JA, Campbell AB, et al. Recognition of common childhood malignancies. *Am Fam Physician* 2000;61:2144–2154.

Chapter 57

Bleeding Disorders

Gregory E. Plautz

The evaluation of a child or an adolescent for a bleeding disorder rests on an assessment of whether the bleeding or bruising is abnormal or is within the range of normal. It is typical for toddlers to have small bruises on extensor surfaces and for children to have several episodes of epistaxis. Likewise, menarche frequently raises concerns about irregular bleeding of variable amounts that can lead both parents and patients to evaluation by the pediatrician. As with all evaluations, history, family history, physical examination, and the judicious use of a limited number of key laboratory tests are usually sufficient to diagnose most pediatric bleeding disorders.

This chapter discusses the common pediatric abnormalities in the three components of the coagulation system:

- Platelet disorders
- Coagulopathies
- Thrombophilia

Discussion of platelet abnormalities includes both quantitative defects and functional defects. Similar to many pediatric diseases, there are congenital defects that usually present early in infancy and acquired defects that can present at any age. Most patients harboring abnormalities in plasma components have either von Willebrand disease (vWD) or hemophilia. Finally, inherited disorders that cause thrombophilia, an abnormal propensity to blood clot formation, are briefly described.

NORMAL COAGULATION CASCADE AND LABORATORY SCREENING TESTS

It is helpful to overview briefly the process of coagulation and its relation to the most commonly ordered coagulation tests (Fig. 57.1). The coagulation factors are enzymes that normally exist in an inactive form in plasma. Upon enzymatic cleavage of a portion of the molecule, there is a change in its conformation that activates its proteolytic function. The activated coagulation factors then interact with the next downstream substrate, thereby forming a cas-

cade that amplifies the response and ultimately generates a fibrin plug. It is important to realize that coagulation normally occurs on a negatively charged phospholipid surface provided by the platelet or endothelial plasma membrane.

When a blood vessel is injured, the endothelial surface is disrupted, causing two arms of the coagulation system to become activated. First, platelets are exposed to subendothelial collagen, activating surface glycoproteins and von Willebrand factor (vWF). Second, tissue factor (TF) in the subendothelial space comes in contact with the small amounts of plasma factor VII that exist in an activated form (designated VIIa). The activated platelets clump to form a physical obstruction. In addition, platelets degranulate, releasing substances that cause vasoconstriction, and thereby staunching the blood flow. Exposure of factor VIIa to TF on a phospholipid surface causes cleavage and activation of factor X (designated Xa). Factor Xa, factor VIIa, calcium, and phospholipids combine to form the prothrombinase complex. *The most important step is the conversion of prothrombin (factor II) to thrombin.* Thrombin acts on fibrinogen, which is a relatively abundant substrate in plasma, to generate fibrin monomers. These fibrin monomers are subsequently cross-linked by factor XIII to form a stable clot.

The *prothrombin time (PT)* is performed by adding recombinant TF, a phospholipid complex, and calcium to anticoagulated (citrated) plasma. TF reacts with the small amount of factor VIIa to initiate the "extrinsic" pathway. It is called "extrinsic" because it relies on TF, which is normally extrinsic to the vasculature. *The PT is dependent on factors VII, X, V, II (prothrombin), and fibrinogen.* Several of these factors (II, VII, and X) are vitamin K dependent, and the PT is often used to monitor warfarin therapy. The International Normalized Ratio (INR) is an adjusted PT that was developed to compensate for variability in different batches of reagents to warfarin inhibition, and it represents patient PT/control PT. The INR shows much less interlaboratory variability for patients on warfarin therapy.

The *activated partial thromboplastin time (aPTT)* is performed by adding phospholipids, calcium, and a particulate substance to citrated plasma. This serves to activate the

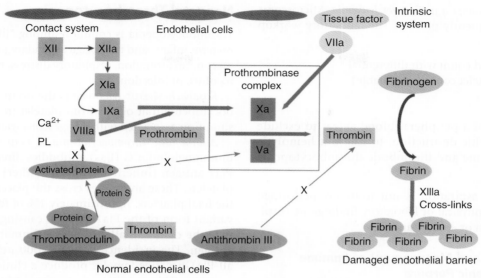

Figure 57.1 Components of the coagulation system. PL, phospholipid.

"intrinsic" pathway because all of the factors are intrinsic to plasma. The earliest step in the cascade involves interaction between the phospholipid surface and "contact" factors, including the following: factor XII, high-molecular-weight kininogen (HMWK), prekallikrein, and factor XI. The initiating factors then cleave to factor IX, thereby activating it (factor IXa). The phospholipid surface also serves as a platform on which factors IXa and VIII combine to activate factor X. Activated factor X (Xa) then combines with factor Va to generate the prothrombinase complex as described in the preceding text.

Feedback Inhibition of the Coagulation Cascade

It is physiologically important to restrict clot formation to the immediate vicinity of the endothelial damage. Consequently, there is feedback through an elaborate antithrombotic system to balance the coagulation cascade. When thrombin is generated, it binds to thrombomodulin and together with protein S enzymatically activates protein C. Activated protein C inactivates factors VIIIa and Va. There is a second system that is maintained in a highly activated state. It consists of the protein antithrombin III, which is bound to heparin sulfate on the surface of intact endothelium. When factors Xa and thrombin drift into a zone of intact endothelium, they are degraded rapidly by antithrombin III. This prevents clot propagation beyond the area of damaged endothelium.

PLATELET DISORDERS

The first step in the evaluation of thrombocytopenia involves determination of whether the platelet count is abnormal. There is a wide range of normal, from 150,000 to 450,000 mm³, but no age-dependent variation in normal level. The platelet count determines the level of severity: A platelet count >50,000/mm³ is mild thrombocytopenia with minimal bleeding risk in the absence of major trauma or surgery. A platelet count 20,000 to 50,000/mm³ is moderately severe with risk of bleeding from contact sports. A platelet count of <20,000/mm³ is considered severe thrombocytopenia and carries an increased risk of spontaneous bleeding. An enlarged spleen can sequester platelets, but it normally does not cause the platelet count to drop <50,000/mm³. The next step is to determine whether there is decreased production or increased destruction of platelets. The normal platelet survival time is approximately 7 days. Similar to red blood cells in anemia, recently produced platelets have an increased volume (mean platelet volume [MPV]) and have residual mRNA. Some laboratories can provide a "reticulated platelet" count, which if low implies a production defect, and if high implies destruction.

Immune Thrombocytopenic Purpura

Immune thrombocytopenic purpura (ITP) is caused by autoantibodies binding to platelets with subsequent clearance by the spleen. In children, the peak incidence is from 2 to 5 years of age. The clinical onset is acute, but often there is a subclinical viral prodrome 1 to 3 weeks prior to the onset of clinical findings. The history is notable for a *lack of previous bleeding or bruising tendency*. Physical signs include bruising in locations other than extensor surfaces and petechiae (1- to 3-mm nonblanching nontender bright red-purple skin lesions). Occasionally, mucous membrane petechiae (wet purpura) are present. *Hepatosplenomegaly and/or diffuse lymphadenopathy are not associated with ITP and if present should prompt a workup for leukemia.* Microscopic hematuria is frequently present. The laboratory workup should include:

■ Complete blood count with differential
■ Reticulated platelet count (if available)
■ Type and screen
■ Coombs test
■ Examination of a peripheral blood smear to exclude microangiopathic destruction, to rule out hemolytic uremic syndrome and thrombotic thrombocytopenic purpura

A bone marrow aspiration is not routinely performed unless particular physical or laboratory findings are suspicious for leukemia or aplastic anemia.

Clinical Course and Management of Immune Thrombocytopenic Purpura

ITP is usually a self-limited disease with 90% of cases resolving within 6 months. The goal of therapy is to prevent life-threatening hemorrhage, which occurs in 0.5% to 2% of cases. Platelet transfusions are not routinely performed because the antibodies are usually directed against common antigens. However, platelet transfusions and emergency splenectomy have been performed for life-threatening bleeding. Patients with platelet count $<10,000/mm^3$ should be hospitalized.

Patients with ITP who are Rh-positive may be treated with anti-Rh globulin, (WinRho 50–75 μg/kg intravenously for one dose). It may be necessary to repeat the dose in 3 to 4 weeks. The anti-Rh globulin binds to red blood cells and overwhelms binding sites in the reticuloendothelial system, thereby decreasing the removal of platelets. Anticipate a drop in the hemoglobin concentrations by 1 to 2 g/dL. Anti-Rh should be used with caution if the baseline hemoglobin concentration is <8 g/dL.

Patients who are Rh negative may be treated with intravenous immune globulin; the recommended dose is 0.8 g/kg. Again, this dose may need to be repeated depending on the response.

Alternative therapies for ITP include a high-dose of methylprednisolone 30 mg/kg per day for 3 days or prednisone 2 mg/kg per day for 2 weeks with subsequent slow taper.

Chronic Immune Thrombocytopenic Purpura

Chronic ITP is defined as ITP lasting for >6 months. There is a 3:1 female to male preponderance, and the typical patient is an adolescent girl. Chronic ITP is often associated with a positive antinuclear antibody and may be the initial manifestation of systemic lupus erythematosus or other connective tissue disorder. Splenectomy is effective in 75% of cases. Rituximab (anti-CD20 mAb) can be used for severe chronic ITP but can cause immunosuppression because of depletion of B lymphocytes.

Neonatal Thrombocytopenia

Thrombocytopenia is common among "ill" neonates and preterm infants and may occur secondary to birth asphyxia, meconium aspiration, respiratory distress, necrotizing enterocolitis, or infection.

Kasabach-Merritt syndrome is the occurrence of thrombocytopenia that occurs from platelet trapping and consumption associated with a *large hemangioma.*

Alloimmune thrombocytopenia is caused by maternal immunoglobulin G (IgG) antibodies directed against the Pla1 antigen (inherited from the father) on the infant's platelets. These antibodies cross the placenta and destroy the fetal platelets. Approximately 1% of females express a variant form of the Pla1 antigen, causing them to recognize the common allele (99% of humans) as a foreign antigen. The incidence is 1 per 5000 newborns, so not all Pla1-negative females produce a clinically significant response. This condition may arise during the first pregnancy, but the severity of disease increases with subsequent affected infants. Intracranial hemorrhage, which may occur prenatally, is the most feared complication of this condition. Management of the infant includes transfusion of *maternal* platelets, which will have normal survival. The platelet count normalizes over 1 to 2 weeks as maternal antibody is adsorbed.

Neonatal thrombocytopenia can also occur in the setting of *maternal ITP.* In this case, the infant can be treated with intravenous immune globulin because transfused platelets will be destroyed. The threshold for treatment of an infant with thrombocytopenia should be lower than that for older children.

Congenital Quantitative Platelet Disorders (Rare)

These are rare disorders that include:

■ Thrombocytopenia-absent radii (TAR). This syndrome presents with hemorrhagic manifestations at birth with thrombocytopenia and aplasia of radii
■ Congenital amegakaryocytic thrombocytopenia
■ Marrow infiltration, such as congenital leukemia, myelofibrosis, and osteopetrosis
■ Fanconi anemia is an autosomal-recessive disorder leading to progressive pancytopenia usually manifesting between 5 and 10 years of age.

Congenital Qualitative Platelet Disorders (Rare)

Bernard-Soulier syndrome is an autosomal-recessive disorder, caused by the absence of glycoprotein Ib/IX/V, which is the receptor for vWF. Although the platelet count is normal, very large platelets are present. The clinical presentation includes easy bruising and severe hemorrhage with trauma or surgery. Adolescent girls with this disorder may present at menarche.

Glanzmann thrombasthenia is an autosomal-recessive disorder, caused by absence of glycoprotein IIb and IIIa, which is the receptor for fibrinogen. The platelet count is normal. Clinical manifestations include bruising and bleeding.

Wiskott-Aldrich syndrome is an X-linked recessive disorder caused by a defect in a protein (Wiskott-Aldrich syndrome protein [WASP]) involved in cytoskeletal reorganization. The platelet count is low, and platelets are small and defective. Other manifestations include severe immune deficiency and eczema.

Drug-Related Platelet Disorders

Heparin-induced thrombocytopenia is a relatively uncommon condition in pediatric patients as compared with adults. This entity results when heparin-dependent antibodies bind to platelet factor 4, causing adherence and clearance from the circulation.

Aspirin inhibits the function of the cyclooxygenase enzymes within the platelet, causing an irreversible reduction of prostaglandin synthesis and inhibition of platelet aggregation for the platelet lifespan (7–10 days).

Indomethacin causes a reversible inhibition (12–24 hours) of platelet aggregation.

DISORDERS OF PLASMA FACTORS

Hemophilia A and B

Hemophilia is a genetic disorder resulting from a deficiency in circulating levels of plasma factors VIII and IX. Deficiency of these factors causes hemorrhage resulting from delayed and abnormally friable clot formation. Hemophilia A (classic hemophilia) is a deficiency of factor VIII, affecting 1 per 5000 males, and accounts for 85% of cases of hemophilia. Hemophilia B (Christmas disease) is a deficiency of factor IX, affecting 1 per 50,000 males, and accounts for 15% of cases of hemophilia. These disorders have an X-linked pattern of inheritance (genes are on the long arm of the X-chromosome), although *one-third of cases are new mutations occurring without a previous family history.* The most common mutation, occurring in 45% of cases, is caused by a gene inversion, which provides a basis for genetic screening. A severe deficiency is defined by the presence of <1% of the normal factor activity level, a moderate deficiency is defined by the presence of 1% to 5% of the normal factor activity level, and a mild deficiency is defined by the presence of >5% of the normal factor activity level.

Clinical Presentation of Hemophilia

The manifestations of hemophilia A and B are similar because both factors VIII and IX function to activate factor X. Patients with severe deficiency have frequent episodes of spontaneous bleeding into joints and deep-tissue spaces after minimal or unknown trauma. Patients with moderate deficiency have occasional bleeding into joint spaces. Mild hemophiliacs may go undiagnosed for

years until significant trauma or surgery. Approximately 30% of affected males present with profuse bleeding after circumcision. The most typical presentation occurs after 6 months of age, at which time easy bruising, oral bleeding, hemarthrosis, and intramuscular bleeding become evident.

Management of Hemophilia

Desmopressin acetate (0.3 µg/kg) can be used for mild to moderate hemophilia A because it causes release of factor VIII from storage pools and a transient increase in level. *The mainstay of therapy, however, is factor replacement.* One U/kg activity will raise the plasma levels by 2 U/kg for factor VIII or 1 U/kg for factor IX. For example, to obtain 100% factor VIII replacement for a 10-kg child, one would give 500 U. To do this for factor IX, one would give 1000 U.

Bleeding is managed on the basis of the location and severity. In general, for minor bleeding episodes, the recommendation is to achieve and maintain the factor levels at 50% to 60%. For severe bleeding, the goal is to achieve and maintain factor levels at 100%.

Home-based therapy for minor bleeding episodes using implanted vascular access devices is now the norm. Prophylactic factor replacement several times per week is recommended for patients with recurrent hemarthrosis to prevent permanent joint damage. Comprehensive hemophilia clinics are utilized to address orthopaedic, social, and hematologic issues.

von Willebrand Disease

vWD is relatively common, affecting 0.5% to 1% of the population and males and females equally. This disease has an autosomal-dominant pattern of inheritance with variable penetrance. There are many different mutations resulting in highly variable severity; however, within a family, the degree of severity is similar. Easy bruising, postoperative bleeding, epistaxis, and menorrhagia are the most common presenting features; hemarthrosis is not typical.

vWF is a glycoprotein that binds to glycoproteins on the platelet surface, which stimulates platelet adhesion and aggregation at the site of vessel wall injury. This factor also is a carrier of factor VIII, and is crucial for its stabilization in the circulation.

vWD is classified into three types. Type 1 disease is the most common, accounting for 70% to 80% of the cases and represents a quantitative deficiency in vWF. Patients with this form of disease present with mild bleeding symptoms. Type 2A (10% of vWD) is a qualitative deficiency of vWF, resulting in defective platelet adhesion. In type 2B (4% of vWD) disease, there is increased affinity of vWF binding to platelets with enhanced platelet function. There may also be associated thrombocytopenia in this form. In type 3 disease, there is complete absence or minimal amount of vWF. Unlike the other types of vWD, this type is inherited in an autosomal-recessive pattern. The clinical illness of type 3 disease is similar to hemophilia because vWF is the carrier protein for factor VIII.

Patients with vWF generally have a normal PT, abnormal platelet function screening test, and prolonged partial thromboplastin time (PTT). Analysis of vWD activity and multimer analysis can determine the presence of vWD and the specific subtypes.

Management of von Willebrand disease

vWF is stored in platelets and endothelial cells. These storage pools can be released by desmopressin acetate, given intravenously or intranasally, to increase the level of vWF and factor VIII. In type 1 vWD, there is normally a very good response to desmopressin therapy, whereas in type 2A vWD, the response is variable. Desmopressin is contraindicated in type 2B vWD because it can exacerbate thrombocytopenia. Type 3 disease does not respond to desmopressin. Therefore, it is important to determine the type of vWD. Patients with vWD who are at risk for surgical bleeding, are treated with plasma-purified factor VIII-vWF concentrate. It is important to remember that recombinant DNA-produced factor VIII products do not contain vWF protein.

Disseminated Intravascular Coagulation

Disseminated intravascular coagulation (DIC) is a life-threatening clinical diagnosis that includes:

- Bleeding
- Thrombosis
- Progressive organ dysfunction

DIC is caused by an underlying process, which causes tissue destruction and release of TF. The subsequent activation of factor VII by TF leads to a *consumption* of platelets and clotting factors. Laboratory findings include:

- Elevated INR
- Elevated aPTT
- Positive fibrin degradation products (FDP)
- Decreased platelet count

The most common cause of DIC is bacterial or viral infection. Other causes include near drowning, trauma, crush injuries, central nervous system injuries, burns, hemolytic transfusion reaction, ischemia-reperfusion injuries, and snakebites.

Management of DIC involves:

- Treating the underlying cause (i.e., draining abscesses, resecting necrotic tissue).
- Supporting perfusion and correcting the acidosis.
- Infusing fresh frozen plasma (FFP) to replace fibrinogen to 50 mg/dL and platelets to >50,000/mm³.

Vascular Purpura

Purpura fulminans, which manifests with widespread thrombosis and skin necrosis, is caused by the development of autoantibodies to protein C. This entity may accompany or follow infections such as varicella, congenital rubella, meningococcemia, and other bacterial infections.

In Henoch-Schönlein purpura, injury to endothelial cells from vasculitis causes release of vWF and thrombosis with simultaneous dysfunction of renal endothelium. In this disorder, laboratory markers of bleeding, such as platelet count, PT, PTT are normal.

THROMBOPHILIA

A genetic susceptibility to venous thrombosis is called thrombophilia.

Common predisposing mutations and disorders resulting in thrombophilia include:

- Factor V Leiden: confers resistance to activated protein C, a natural anticoagulant
- Prothrombin mutation (G20210A): associated with increased plasma prothrombin
- Deficiency of protein C, protein S, or antithrombin III

Laboratory testing for hypercoagulability states should include an activated protein C resistance ratio (indicating factor V Leiden mutation if abnormal), prothrombin 20210A mutation, protein C, protein S and antithrombin activity, as well as anti-phospholipid antibody panel. The management of these disorders depends on the exact genotype, laboratory values, family history, and clinical situation.

REVIEW EXERCISES

QUESTIONS

1. A 3-year-old child was noted at bath time to have several bruises on her back. The following morning, she had numerous tiny red spots on the trunk and abdomen. Examination reveals multiple petechiae on the skin and several on the soft palate but is otherwise normal. The *most* likely diagnosis is:
a) Acute lymphoblastic leukemia (ALL)
b) Nonaccidental trauma
c) Disseminated intravascular coagulation (DIC)
d) Immune thrombocytopenic purpura (ITP)
e) Salicylate ingestion

Answer
The answer is d. The acute onset and otherwise normal examination excludes acute lymphoblastic leukemia. Bruising secondary to nonaccidental trauma typically occurs in linear patterns or on nonextensor surfaces rather than as petechiae, and does not present with soft palate petechiae. DIC is associated with an acute but severe illness and salicylate ingestion presents with other symptoms of intoxication.

2. You are called to the newborn nursery to evaluate a term newborn male, product of uncomplicated pregnancy to a G3P2 healthy mother. The exam is positive for multiple bruises and facial petechiae. The platelet count is 8K, the Hgb is 13 g/dL and WBC is 12K with normal differential. The mother's CBC is normal. What is the most likely cause of the thrombocytopenia?

a) Maternal ITP (Immune thrombocytopenic purpura)
b) TAR syndrome (Thrombocytopenia, absent radii)
c) Neonatal alloimmune thrombocytopenia
d) Hemophilia A
e) Glanzmann's thrombasthenia

Answer

The answer is c. This scenario describes a case of neonatal alloimmune thrombocytopenia in which the immune response is directed against a platelet antigen present on the baby's platelets. The mother's platelet count would be low if this were maternal ITP. Thrombocytopenia absent radii (TAR) has physical abnormalities of the forearms. Hemophilia does not cause low platelet counts and the platelet count is normal in Glanzmann's thrombasthenia, which is a disorder of platelet function.

3. A 15-month-old previously healthy boy who has been walking for 4 months began limping after learning how to jump off the couch. He refuses to bear weight. Examination shows an irritable afebrile infant with unilateral warmth and swelling of the left knee. Which of the following does *not* fit with a presumed diagnosis of hemophilia A?

a) His mother would be expected to have severe bruising and menorrhagia.
b) His PT/INR is normal.
c) His platelet count is normal.
d) The PTT is 70 seconds and corrects to normal after 1:1 mixing with control plasma.

Answer

The answer is a. This scenario describes an infant with hemophilia. The mother and perhaps the sister would be carriers (with 50% levels), but would *not* have bleeding manifestations. The PT is not dependent on Factor VIII activity and therefore is not prolonged. Likewise, the platelet count is normal in hemophilia A. The PTT is prolonged in the presence of very low levels of factor VIII or IX but replacement to 50% of normal levels by 1:1 mixing with normal plasma is sufficient to correct the PTT.

4. An 11-year-old girl has anemia (Hb 7.5 mg/dL) and menorrhagia with onset of menses. She has a history of easy bruising and frequent epistaxis. Her father and paternal uncle have a history of easy bruising and epistaxis. Her platelet count and INR are normal but PTT is prolonged and factor VIII is 40% of normal. Which of the following statements is correct advice?

a) She is a carrier for hemophilia and will have a 50% chance of giving birth to affected sons.
b) Menorrhagia is common and she should return if it persists longer than 6 months.

c) You suspect this is von Willebrand disease and will need to perform additional tests to determine which type.
d) Her younger sister will have a 1:4 chance of developing the same symptoms.

Answer

The answer is c. The presentation with bruising and menorrhagia suggests vWD; hemophilia carriers do not have a bleeding tendency. Inheritance for a bleeding tendency through the paternal lineage is also consistent with vWD, which has an autosomal-dominant mode of inheritance with a 1:2 risk for siblings. It is important to determine the particular type of vWD because desmopressin therapy is contraindicated for one type (type 2B).

5. A 15-year-old boy with acute onset of fever to 40.5°C (104.9°F), hypotension, and severe headache and meningismus develops oozing from his intravenous catheter site and has dusky discoloration of his right foot, which is also cold to touch. Which of the following support a diagnosis of DIC?

a) Elevated PT and aPTT
b) Decreased platelet count
c) Elevated FDP and D-dimer
d) Positive meningococcal culture in the blood
e) All of the above

Answer

The answer is e. This scenario describes DIC associated with presumed meningococcemia. DIC is a clinical diagnosis and is associated with consumption of coagulation factors and platelets, and thrombolysis producing D-dimer.

6. A 6-year-old girl presents with abdominal pain and hepatosplenomegaly 3 days following a viral gastroenteritis and a severe dehydration episode. An abdominal ultrasound demonstrates a thrombus in the portal vein with minimal flow. Predisposing factors to the thrombus might include which of the following?

a) Protein C heterozygosity
b) Factor V Leiden heterozygosity
c) Prothrombin gene mutation
d) Dehydration
e) All of the above

Answer

The answer is e. This patient has thrombophilia. Each of the three listed mutations in coagulation proteins can contribute to an increased risk of venous thrombosis. Dehydration is an independent acquired predisposing factor.

SUGGESTED READINGS

1. Kitchens CS, Alving BM, Kessler CM, eds. *Consultative hemostasis and thrombosis.* WB Saunders, 2002.
2. Nathan DG, Orkin SH, Ginsburg D, et al. *Nathan and Oski's hematology of infancy and childhood.* Philadelphia: Saunders, 2003.

Chapter 58

BOARD SIMULATION:
Hematology-Oncology

Michael Levien and L. Kate Gowans

QUESTIONS

1. The two *most* important prognostic indicators in neuroblastoma are as follows:
a) Age of the patient and stage of disease
b) Stage of disease and histopathology
c) Sex of the patient and catecholamine levels in a 24-hour urine collection
d) Presence of cerebellar ataxia and stage of disease
e) N-*myc* copies and age of the patient
f) None of the above

Answer

The answer is a. The prognosis in neuroblastoma, as in other childhood malignancies, is directly proportional to the extent of disease at presentation. In early (stage I or II) disease, the tumor burden is much smaller than in stage III or IV disease, and the patient can be more easily treated with chemotherapy and surgical excision. The biology of neuroblastoma is highly unusual, with some early stage disease cured with surgery alone or surgery plus 2 to 4 months of chemotherapy. This is in comparison with higher-stage disease that requires surgery, intensive chemotherapy, autologous stem cell transplant, radiation therapy, and possibly biologic therapy. *A unique feature of neuroblastoma is that it is an age-dependent prognosis. Children under the age of 1 year have a much better prognosis in all stages than do children past that age.* This finding is thought to be related to a temporal loss of older infants' ability to differentiate embryonic tissue. In a series of autopsies performed on 4-month-old fetuses, approximately 32% of the adrenal glands had neuroblastoma cells. These tissues differentiate or mature in most cases as the fetus reaches term. Histopathology (favorable vs. unfavorable) and number of N-*myc* oncogene copies are prognostic variables used in tailoring therapy, but outcome is correlated more strongly with age and stage. Gender, presence of ataxia, and 24-hour urine catecholamine levels are not significant predictors of prognosis, although patients presenting with ataxia tend to have lower stage disease at diagnosis.

Neuroblastoma is an excellent example of a childhood cancer with risk-directed or stratified therapy based on cell biology and risk factors present at diagnosis. Long-term survival along this spectrum of disease ranges from >95% to <25%.

2. In which of the following tumors is long-term control *most* likely to be achieved with currently available treatments?
a) Stage IV neuroblastoma in a 3-year-old
b) Stage IV rhabdomyosarcoma in a 2-year-old
c) Stage IV Hodgkin disease, nodular sclerosing type, in a 15-year-old
d) Stage IV osteosarcoma
e) Acute lymphoblastic leukemia in a 17-year-old adolescent

Answer

The answer is c. Stage IV disease (metastases to viscera, such as the lungs) is a poor prognostic indicator in most malignancies of childhood. However, the treatment of Hodgkin disease has been very successful since the introduction of MOPP (nitrogen mustard, vincristine, procarbazine, and prednisone) and ABVD (Adriamycin, bleomycin, vinblastine, and dacarbazine) therapy in the 1960s and 1970s. This is also an exquisitely radiosensitive tumor. The judicious use of radiation therapy and chemotherapy has resulted in event-free survival exceeding 80% in patients with stage IV Hodgkin disease. Hodgkin disease therapy is evolving rapidly, as attempts are being made to decrease the intensity of chemotherapy and eliminate radiation therapy in patients with early complete response to chemotherapy. This aims to decrease the incidence of late effects and second malignancies in these survivors. All other stage IV malignancies have a much lower chance for cure. (A patient with ALL would have the best survival rate at approximately 70%.)

3. Generalized lymphadenopathy is a common presenting sign in which of the following groups of childhood malignancies?

a) Neuroblastoma, acute lymphoblastic leukemia, rhabdomyosarcoma
b) Osteosarcoma, Ewing sarcoma, Wilms tumor
c) Acute lymphoblastic leukemia, neuroblastoma, non-Hodgkin lymphoma
d) Acute nonlymphocytic leukemia, neuroblastoma, hepatoblastoma
e) Acute leukemia, Wilms tumor, retinoblastoma

Answer

The answer is c. Wilms tumor, retinoblastoma, osteosarcoma, and Ewing sarcoma are usually brought to the attention of a physician early in their course because of the presenting features. Wilms tumor and hepatoblastoma present with an abdominal mass. Retinoblastoma presents with leukocoria and other visual problems. Ewing sarcoma and osteosarcoma present with progressive bone pain or palpable mass; rhabdomyosarcoma usually presents with a palpable mass. Peripheral adenopathy can be associated with these tumors in progressive, late-stage, widely metastatic disease. Neuroblastoma often presents in early stages, but when the presentation is in stage IV, the patient may have widespread lymphadenopathy, and the presentation may be very similar to that of acute leukemia (i.e., generalized lymphadenopathy, bone pain, hepatosplenomegaly, petechiae, fever, easy bruising). All forms of lymphoma may present with significant lymphadenopathy.

4. A 4-year-old African-American boy is taking trimethoprim/sulfamethoxazole for acute sinusitis. He develops fatigue, dark urine, and pallor. The *most* likely diagnosis is:

a) Hereditary spherocytosis (HS)
b) Glucose-6-phosphate dehydrogenase deficiency
c) Hepatitis A
d) Autoimmune hemolytic anemia

Answer

The answer is b. This boy's symptoms are consistent with a hemolytic process. Of the choices listed that are hemolytic anemias, glucose-6-phosphate dehydrogenase deficiency is most consistent with this patient's clinical presentation. Glucose-6-phosphate dehydrogenase deficiency is an X-linked disorder characterized by hemolytic anemia. The incidence of this disorder is high in African Americans, Italians, Greeks, and individuals of Middle Eastern ancestry. The most likely inducers of hemolysis in individuals with glucose-6-phosphate dehydrogenase deficiency include:

- Fava beans
- Sulfonamides
- Trimethoprim
- Nitrofurantoin
- Chloramphenicol
- Primaquine
- Chloroquine
- Quinacrine
- Naphthalene

HS is more likely in a white patient and hemolysis tends not to be associated with drugs but rather with viral illnesses. Similarly, autoimmune hemolytic anemia usually develops spontaneously or following a viral illness.

5. Over a 3-day period, petechiae develop over the trunk and extremities of a previously healthy 5-year old. The parents state that he has been bruising easily for the past week. He has been afebrile. A complete blood cell count reveals the following values: white blood cell (WBC) count, 10,500/mm³ with 75% neutrophils and 20% lymphocytes; hemoglobin, 13 g/dL; mean corpuscular volume (MCV), 87 μ³; platelet count, 10,000/mm³. The *most* likely diagnosis is:

a) Henoch-Schönlein purpura
b) Immune thrombocytopenic purpura (ITP)
c) Meningococcemia
d) Rocky Mountain spotted fever
e) Acute lymphocytic leukemia (ALL)

Answer

The answer is b. This child presents with isolated thrombocytopenia but no fever or other clinical manifestations. Therefore, ITP is most likely. This often occurs after an antecedent viral infection (70% of cases) and is characterized by a deficiency of circulating platelets despite adequate numbers of megakaryocytes in the bone marrow. It is likely an immune-mediated process whereby the patient's immune system mistakes a platelet antigen as foreign. The clinical picture is generally one of an acute onset 1 to 4 weeks after a viral illness. A generalized petechial rash and excessive bruising are common, and mucous membrane hemorrhage can be prominent. The children generally appear well, without lymphadenopathy or hepatosplenomegaly to suggest malignancy. Isolated thrombocytopenia (often dramatic, but usually between 10,000–50,000/mm³), with a normal WBC count and hemoglobin level, is the rule. Examination of the bone marrow, although not necessary for diagnosis, reveals normal granulocytic and erythrocytic series, with normal or increased numbers of megakaryocytes. The prognosis is excellent; 80% to 90% of patients will recover in weeks to a few months, with or without treatment. If ITP lasts greater than 6 months, it is termed chronic ITP and can be quite difficult to manage.

6. A 3-year-old girl was noted to have a hemoglobin level of 9.8 g/dL when she presented to the clinic 3 months ago. The MCV was 68 μ³, the mean corpuscular hemoglobin (MCH) 20.6 pg, and the red blood cell distribution width (RDW) 11%. She was placed on ferrous sulfate (elemental iron 6 mg/kg per day). On the return visit 8 weeks later, the reticulocyte count is 1.8%, and the indices are unchanged. The peripheral smear is normal except for small hypochromic red blood cells (RBCs). These data are consistent with:

a) Thalassemia
b) Sickle cell trait
c) Sickle cell disease
d) Folate deficiency

Answer

The answer is a. This child has a microcytic, hypochromic anemia with a low-to-normal RDW. Despite iron therapy, her reticulocyte count is low, and the peripheral smear shows small, hypochromic RBCs. These findings are most consistent with thalassemia. The causes of a microcytic, homogeneous anemia (low MCV, normal RDW) include thalassemia and anemia of chronic disease. Sickle cell disease causes a normocytic, heterogeneous anemia (increased RDW resulting from the presence of reticulocytes). Folate and vitamin B_{12} deficiencies cause a macrocytic anemia and are very unusual in children in developed countries. It is noteworthy that noncompliance with iron treatment should always be a consideration. Serum iron levels can be helpful in distinguishing thalassemia and iron deficiency, but they may coexist. The Mentzer index (MCV/RBC) can also be useful: <11 suggests thalassemia; >11 suggests iron deficiency.

7. Jaundice develops in a healthy white 7-year-old girl. The physical examination reveals splenomegaly. A complete blood cell count reveals the following values: WBC 7400/mm^3, platelets 235,000/mm^3, hemoglobin 9 g/dL; MCV 85 μ^3; reticulocyte count 6%. The *most* likely diagnosis is:

a) ALL
b) Pyruvate kinase deficiency
c) Glucose-6-phosphate dehydrogenase deficiency
d) HS

Answer

The answer is d. Jaundice and splenomegaly, along with a normocytic anemia and reticulocytosis, are characteristic of a hemolytic anemia. In a previously healthy 7-year-old white child, HS would be the most likely diagnosis. HS is transmitted as an autosomal-dominant disorder, but the rate of new mutations is high. It is the most common congenital abnormality of the RBC membrane. Hemolytic disease in children is quite variable (baseline hemoglobin ranging from 9–11 g/dL); it can manifest early in life with severe hemolysis or may not manifest until late in life. Prolonged neonatal jaundice is a common historical finding, and splenomegaly and gallstones are common clinical features. Spherocytes (often microspherocytes) and reticulocytes on the blood smear are characteristic (causing increased mean corpuscular hemoglobin concentration [MCHC] and RDW), and the

findings of splenomegaly, reticulocytosis, and spherocytosis are often diagnostic. The osmotic fragility test confirms the presence of spherocytes in the blood. This test incubates patient RBCs with varying concentrations of saline, and the patient's cells will burst quickly, not withstanding osmotic stress as would a normal biconcave RBC. Splenectomy eliminates most of the hemolysis associated with this disorder.

8. Which of the following sets of labs is consistent with tumor lysis syndrome?

a) ↑ K, ↑ PO$_4$, ↑ Ca, ↑ uric acid
b) ↓ K, ↑ PO$_4$, ↓ Ca, ↑ uric acid
c) ↑ K, ↑ PO$_4$, ↓ Ca, ↓ uric acid
d) ↑ K, ↑ PO$_4$, ↓ Ca, ↑ uric acid
e) None of the above

Answer

The answer is d. Tumor lysis syndrome is an acute metabolic derangement caused by the rapid turnover of dying cancer cells. This can happen spontaneously or as a result of initiation of chemotherapy. As intracellular contents are released, the resulting classic laboratory abnormalities are *elevated potassium, phosphorus, and uric acid, and decreased calcium*. Renal function may deteriorate quickly, necessitating dialysis if electrolytes are not managed aggressively. Management includes frequent monitoring of laboratory values, aggressive intravenous hydration that does not include potassium, and allopurinol (xanthine-oxidase inhibitor), which lowers the production of uric acid. Calcium should be replaced quickly, and many measures can be used to decrease a rising potassium (Lasix, glucose plus insulin, potassium binders). A nephrologist and pediatric intensivist should be notified of any patient who presents at high risk for tumor lysis syndrome. *Burkitt lymphoma* is the pediatric diagnosis most closely associated with this *oncologic emergency*. Acute leukemias that present with a high tumor burden (high WBC count with or without massive organomegaly) are also at risk. Solid tumors do not carry significant risk of tumor lysis syndrome.

9. A 4-year-old boy presents to your office with a 3-day history of fever to 38.33° to 38.88°C (101° to 102°F), decreased oral intake and complaints of abdominal pain. Physical examination reveals scattered cervical adenopathy, a few bruises, and a palpable spleen tip. Which of the following is the *least* likely diagnosis?

a) Infectious mononucleosis
b) ITP
c) Streptococcal pharyngitis
d) Acute lymphoblastic leukemia

Answer

The answer is c. Streptococcal pharyngitis could account for fever, decreased oral intake, abdominal pain, and adenopathy, but it should not be accompanied by any palpable organomegaly. The presence of fever, adenopathy, and palpable organomegaly should lead one to suspect infectious mononucleosis or acute leukemia. The presence of bruises could indicate possible ITP, and mild splenomegaly would not exclude this diagnosis. Fever and adenopathy make ITP somewhat less likely.

10. On the preceding patient, labs reveal WBC 1200/mm^3 with 18% neutrophils, Hgb 9.9 g/dL with normal MCV, and platelets 76,000/mm^3. The *most* likely diagnosis is
a) Infectious mononucleosis
b) ITP
c) Streptococcal pharyngitis
d) Acute lymphoblastic leukemia

Answer

The answer is d. This patient who has presented with fever and malaise has pancytopenia with an abnormally low percentage of circulating neutrophils. This is strongly suggestive of an infiltrative process in the marrow, and a diagnosis of acute lymphoblastic leukemia should be at the top of the list of possibilities. Infection with Epstein-Barr virus can cause pancytopenia and a physical examination similar to this child's. A bone marrow examination would be necessary to make the diagnosis. ITP is not the diagnosis because the WBC count and hemoglobin are both abnormal.

11. Hemihypertrophy and aniridia are associated with:
a) Neuroblastoma
b) Retinoblastoma
c) Hodgkin disease
d) Wilms tumor
e) None of the above

Answer

The answer is d. Wilms tumor appears to result from changes in one or several genes. Specific germ-line mutations of band 13 of the short arm of chromosome 11 (11p13) cause aniridia. The deletions encompassing the Wilms tumor gene 1 *(WT1)* on chromosome 11p13 may explain the association between aniridia and Wilms tumor. Wilms tumor and aniridia combined with genitourinary abnormalities and mental retardation is a well-described entity known as WAGR (*W*-Wilms tumor, *A*-Aniridia, *G*-Genital and/or urinary tract abnormalities, *R*-mental retardation) syndrome. Hemihypertrophy is also associated with Wilms tumor, either as an isolated finding or in conjunction with Beckwith-Wiedemann syndrome (macroglossia, large size, visceromegaly, omphalocele, facial nevus flammeus, characteristic earlobe crease [see Fig. 20.4], and renal medullary dysplasia). The locus of the latter gene is on chromosome 11p 15. Patients with aniridia or hemihypertrophy should be evaluated with abdominal ultrasonography every 3 months until the age of 6 years. Patients with Beckwith-Wiedemann syndrome should undergo abdominal ultrasonography every 3 months until they are 7 years old.

12. Beckwith-Wiedemann syndrome is associated with which of the following malignancies in children:
a) Wilms tumor and hepatoblastoma
b) Retinoblastoma and Ewing sarcoma
c) Hodgkin disease and adrenal tumors
d) Acute leukemia and osteosarcoma
e) Both a and c

Answer

The answer is a. Children with Beckwith-Wiedemann syndrome are at increased risk for the development of Wilms tumor, hepatoblastoma, and adrenal cortical carcinoma.

13. A 23-month-old boy presents with a 2-week history of progressive cerebellar ataxia. The results of magnetic resonance imaging (MRI) of the brain are normal. What other type of malignancy should be sought?
a) Hepatoblastoma
b) Burkitt lymphoma
c) Hodgkin disease
d) Primitive neuroectodermal tumor (Ewing sarcoma) of the spinal cord
e) Neuroblastoma

Answer

The answer is e. Ataxia that is not associated with a cerebellar tumor or primary neurologic disorder can be caused by a neuroblastoma. Because ataxia occurs early in the disease process, and the patient is brought to the attention of a physician, the prognosis is excellent for patients with stage I or II tumors. The tumors are usually very small, and meticulous scanning with metaiodobenzylguanidine (MIBG) may be required to locate them. The ataxia is thought to be the result of an immunologic reaction against the neuroblastoma antigens. The antineuroblastoma antibodies cross-react with cerebellar tissue and cause ataxia.

14. Proptosis as a presenting sign is more commonly seen in which of the following pediatric tumors:
a) Hodgkin disease
b) Retinoblastoma
c) Ewing sarcoma
d) Rhabdomyosarcoma
e) T-cell acute lymphoblastic leukemia
f) Primitive neuroectodermal tumor

Answer

The answer is d. Orbital rhabdomyosarcoma (ocular muscle involvement) may present with proptosis and facial swelling medial or lateral to the orbit. Stage IV neuroblastoma may present with proptosis associated with retrobulbar and orbital infiltration by tumor. These are children who present with the classic "raccoon eye" appearance, often without proptosis. Retinoblastoma is an intraocular, retrolental mass that is usually detected early enough that no outward anatomic distortion of the orbit has occurred. Primary or metastatic involvement of orbital or retroorbital bones with Hodgkin disease, Ewing sarcoma, primitive neuroectodermal tumor or ALL is rare.

15. Coordination difficulties can be a presenting sign in which one of the following tumors:
a) Osteosarcoma
b) Hodgkin disease
c) Primary involvement of the temporal bone with Ewing sarcoma
d) Central nervous system (CNS) leukemia at diagnosis
e) Supratentorial brain tumor
f) Infratentorial brain tumor

Answer

The answer is f. Brain tumors are the most commonly diagnosed solid tumor in children. The most common type is astrocytoma (often requiring only surgery), followed by medulloblastoma (surgery, radiation, intense chemotherapy). The diagnosis of a brain tumor is often initially suspected by a history of headaches and early morning vomiting that are progressive. As most pediatric brain tumors are infratentorial, they often interfere with the normal flow of cerebrospinal fluid; the resulting obstructive hydrocephalus increases the intracranial pressure and causes headaches and vomiting. Tumors tend to involve the fourth ventricle/posterior fossa and infiltrate the cerebellum, thereby causing ataxia and coordination difficulties. Ninety-five percent of patients presenting with a brain tumor have abnormal neurologic examination findings. Older adolescents are more likely to have supratentorial tumors that present with headache, focal neurologic signs, or seizure. In general, seizure as a presenting symptom of CNS tumor in a child is very unusual. Osteosarcoma and Ewing sarcoma are unlikely to present with neurologic findings, even if the skull is involved. Acute leukemia involving the CNS is usually an incidental finding with diagnostic lumbar puncture. Most patients with CNS leukemia are asymptomatic, or they may present with an isolated cranial nerve palsy.

16. A 15-year-old boy has difficulty breathing when lying flat in his bed. When he sits up, he has no trouble breathing. What would you expect to find on his physical examination?
a) Rales at both lung bases
b) Diffuse inspiratory and expiratory wheezing
c) Large goiter
d) Lower cervical and supraclavicular adenopathy
e) Lungs clear to auscultation with no adenopathy detectable
f) Croup-like cough with inspiratory stridor

Answer

The answer is d. This patient's complaint suggests airway compression when lying flat. Such patients usually have lower cervical and supraclavicular adenopathy associated with a mediastinal mass compressing a main

bronchus. Chest radiography will reveal a mediastinal mass (anterior, superior). Chest CT will reveal compression of the airway. This should be treated as a medical emergency. A careful evaluation should be performed before anesthesia. If the airway is compromised, biopsy of a palpable lymph node should be performed under local anesthesia and should provide the diagnosis.

17. The patient described in the preceding question would *most* likely have:
a) Hodgkin disease
b) ALL, pre-B immunophenotype
c) Wilms tumor metastasis
d) Neuroblastoma metastasis
e) Sarcoidosis

Answer

The answer is a. The most likely diagnosis in an adolescent boy with an anterior, superior mediastinal mass causing airway compression is Hodgkin lymphoma. Non-Hodgkin lymphoma and acute lymphoblastic leukemia (usually T-cell immunophenotype) can present in the same way and cause a potentially life-threatening clinical situation. Wilms tumor can metastasize to the mediastinal nodes, usually in stage IV or late-stage disease, but is usually diagnosed in children 2 to 6 years of age. Most children with Wilms tumor who present with stage IV disease and pulmonary involvement have asymptomatic pulmonary parenchymal metastases, not mediastinal disease. Neuroblastoma outside the abdomen usually presents in the posterior mediastinum and would be highly unusual in a patient of this age. Although neuroblastoma is the most common pediatric solid tumor outside the CNS, it is rarely diagnosed in older children. Sarcoidosis can involve the mediastinal nodes, and the presentation can be similar to that of Hodgkin lymphoma. However, this is extremely rare and therefore not high on the list of differential diagnoses.

18. A 10-year-old African-American boy is admitted to the hospital with bilateral leg pain. He has no fever. His hemoglobin is 8.1 g/dL with decreased MCV, bilirubin is 2.6 mg/dL, reticulocyte count 8.4%. Which of the following would be *unlikely* on his blood smear?
a) Target cells
b) Howell-Jolly bodies
c) Spherocytes
d) Sickled cells
e) Microcytes

Answer

The answer is c. This patient likely has sickle cell anemia and is having a vaso-occlusive episode. Target cells are commonly seen in patients who have any hemoglobin S, C, D, E, or thalassemia. Howell-Jolly bodies are an indicator of splenic dysfunction, and are often seen on smears of sickle cell patients. On the basis of the information given that this patient's MCV is decreased, one would expect to see some microcytes, normally shaped but small RBCs (the decreased MCV is also resulting from the sickled cells). Spherocytes are not a typical feature of a sickle cell patient's smear.

19. Which of the following therapies would be *least* important in the preceding patient's hospital management?
a) Anti-inflammatory medications
b) Antibiotics
c) Narcotic analgesia
d) Packed RBC transfusion
e) Intravenous fluids

Answer
The answer is b. This patient has been admitted for a vaso-occlusive episode. The standard of care for these patients includes intravenous hydration, attempting to reverse the ongoing sickling that is caused by dehydration in the RBC, aggressive analgesia (morphine is the drug of choice), anti-inflammatory agents such as ketorolac, and packed RBC transfusion, depending on the patient's hemoglobin compared with baseline and how brisk their reticulocytosis is. It is often difficult to manage these situations without at least one transfusion because intravenous hydration will naturally dilute the patient's hemoglobin value. These patients often require the use of a patient-controlled analgesia pump for continuous analgesia. Their pain rating should be assessed frequently, in addition to vital signs with close attention to respiratory status. (Overuse of narcotics will cause respiratory depression, and too much intravenous fluid can lead to respiratory distress and possibly acute chest syndrome in a patient who already has chest pain, cough, and/or infiltrate on chest radiography.) Hospitalization will last until pain is gone or is well controlled with oral analgesics. Although some patients who are admitted with pain are febrile and require blood culture and intravenous antibiotics, this patient is afebrile and so antibiotics are not indicated.

20. A well-appearing, well-nourished, asymptomatic 2-year boy presents to your office with a large abdominal mass. Which of the following radiographic studies is *not* indicated?
a) Computed tomography (CT) scan of the chest, abdomen, and pelvis
b) MRI of the thoracic, lumbar, and sacral spine
c) Ultrasonography of the inferior vena cava and heart
d) Chest radiography

Answer
The answer is b. The most probable diagnosis in a 2-year-old child who presents with an abdominal mass, who is otherwise healthy, well nourished and playful (not irritable), and has no bone pain, fever or other clinical problems is a Wilms tumor. Children with neu-

roblastoma who present with large abdominal masses usually have significant disease with metastases to the bone marrow and bones, and are generally quite ill in appearance, with irritability and pain. The exceptions are infants with stage IVS disease, who have abdominal masses and disease in the liver, skin, and bone marrow only (not cortical bone) and therefore do not have bone pain. CT scan is the choice of imaging for initial evaluation of an abdominal mass. Ultrasonography is used to rule out extension of a Wilms into the inferior vena cava or right heart. Baseline chest radiography is used to evaluate visible metastatic disease. If a paraspinous mass were suspected, MRI would be the imaging of choice.

21. A 5-year-old girl with neurofibromatosis is being evaluated for progressive visual difficulties and headaches. She should be evaluated for which of the following tumors?
a) Retinoblastoma
b) Orbital rhabdomyosarcoma
c) Optic glioma
d) Medulloblastoma

Answer
The answer is c. Patients with neurofibromatosis 1 are at increased risk for the development of peripheral and CNS tumors. A patient with neurofibromatosis 1 who has visual problems with or without headaches and vomiting should be evaluated for a glioma involving the optic nerve or optic chiasm. These low-grade glial tumors can cause significant visual and hypothalamic problems as they grow. They are usually sensitive to chemotherapy and radiation therapy. Such patients are also at increased risk for the development of tumors of the eighth cranial nerve (acoustic neuromas). They usually present with tinnitus, nerve deafness, loss of the corneal reflex, vertigo, ataxia, and signs of increased intracranial pressure.

22. A patient has been diagnosed with ITP. Which of the following are the *most* common *initial* treatments used?
a) Corticosteroids
b) Splenectomy
c) Anti-D immune globulin
d) Intravenous immune globulin
e) All of the above
f) a, c, and d

Answer
The answer is f. First-line therapy for an Rh-positive patient with new onset ITP is anti-D immune globulin (WinRho, RhoGAM). It works by causing a mild hemolytic anemia, attempting to preoccupy the spleen so that it will ignore passing antibody-coated platelets. In an Rh-negative patient, intravenous immune globulin is the treatment of choice. It will saturate the Fc receptors inside the spleen so that there are fewer receptors

available to capture antibody-coated platelets. Corticosteroids are a reliable treatment for acute (if above measures fail) and chronic ITP; however, the side effects can be limiting. Steroids work by decreasing antibody production and by down-regulating Fc receptor expression in the spleen. Splenectomy is reserved for patients with refractory chronic ITP and is effective approximately 80% to 90% of the time. Those patients who do not respond to splenectomy are presumed to be destroying their platelets in the reticuloendothelial system of the liver.

Questions 23–28

For each of the toxicities listed in the subsequent text, match the chemotherapeutic agent *most* likely to produce the adverse effect.

a) Cisplatin
b) Vincristine
c) Bleomycin
d) Asparaginase
e) Cyclophosphamide
f) Doxorubicin

23. Pancreatitis

Answer

The answer is d. Asparaginase is a chemotherapeutic agent that inhibits protein synthesis. Its major side effects include allergic reactions, anaphylaxis, and pancreatitis, which may be a dose-related and potentially irreversible long-term adverse effect. Coagulopathy (decreased fibrinogen and protein C) is also expected, and these patients are at risk for acute thrombosis.

24. Cardiomyopathy

Answer

The answer is f. Myocardial damage is a late sequela of therapy with the anthracycline chemotherapeutic agents, which include doxorubicin (Adriamycin) and daunorubicin (daunomycin). These agents can cause a severe, dose-dependent cardiomyopathy, which occurs in one third of patients treated with higher doses. Early changes in cardiac function and rhythm can be detected in these patients with the use of serial echocardiography and electrocardiogram.

25. Hemorrhagic cystitis

Answer

The answer is e. Cyclophosphamide is an alkylating chemotherapeutic agent; its major side effects include myelosuppression, mucosal ulceration, and hemorrhagic cystitis. It may also cause infertility later in life. A uroprotective agent (Mesna) is given with this chemotherapy.

26. Neurotoxicity

Answer

The answer is b. Vincristine and vinblastine are microtubule inhibitors, both neurotoxic chemotherapeutic agents. Constipation, cranial nerve palsies, loss of deep tendon reflexes, and foot drop are manifestations of such toxicity. Side effects are usually reversible when therapy is discontinued. Vincristine is lethal if in error given intrathecally. Vinblastine is the more myelosuppressive of the two agents.

27. Pulmonary fibrosis

Answer

The answer is c. Bleomycin can cause irreversible, dose-related pulmonary fibrosis. Patients who receive this drug (Hodgkin lymphoma, germ cell tumors) are screened and followed up with formal pulmonary function testing.

28. Ototoxicity

Answer

The answer is a. Cisplatin is an alkylating agent. A long-term adverse effect, which may be dose related and irreversible, is high-frequency hearing loss. The drug also causes bone marrow suppression and renal tubular toxicity with wasting of electrolytes, particularly potassium, phosphorus, and magnesium.

SUGGESTED READINGS

1. Arndt CAS, Crist WM. Common musculoskeletal tumors of childhood and adolescence. *NEJM* 1999;341:342–352.
2. Beckwith JB. New developments in the pathology of Wilms tumor. *CancerInvest* 1997;15:153–162.
3. Cines DB, Blanchette VS. Immune thrombocytopenic purpura. *NEJM* 2002;346:995–1008.
4. Fischer DS, Knobf MT, Durivage HJ. *The cancer chemotherapy handbook,* 5th ed. Philadelphia: Mosby, 1997.
5. Friebert S, Shurin S. ALL: diagnosis and outlook. *Contemp Pediatr* 1998;15:39–54, 118–136.
6. Griffin IJ, Abrams SA. Iron and breast-feeding. *Pediatr Clin North Am* 2001;48:401–413.
7. Gururangan S, Friedman HS. Recent advances in the treatment of pediatric brain tumors. *Oncology* 2004;18:1649–1661.
8. Haase GM, Perez C, Atkinson JB. Current aspects of biology, risk assessment, and treatment of neuroblastoma. *Sem Surg Oncol* 1999;16:91–104.
9. Lange B, O'Neill JA, Goldwein JW, et al. Oncologic emergencies. In: *Pizzo and Poplack's principles and practice of pediatric oncology,* 4th ed. Philadelphia: Lippincott Williams & Wilkins, 2002:1177–1203.
10. Oski FA, Brugnara C, Nathan DG. A diagnostic approach to the anemic patient. *Nathan and Oski's hematology of infancy and childhood,* 5th ed. Philadelphia: Saunders, 1998:375–384.
11. Raney RB. Hodgkin's disease in childhood: a review. *J Pediatr Hematol Oncol* 1997;19:502–509.
12. Sackey K. Hemolytic anemia: part 1. *Pediatr Rev* 1999;20:152–159.
13. Sackey K. Hemolytic anemia: part 2. *Pediatr Rev* 1999;20:204–208.
14. Segel GB, Hirsh MG, Feig SA. Managing anemia in pediatric office practice. *Pediatr Rev* 2002;23:75–84.
15. Steinberg MH. Management of sickle cell disease. *NEJM* 1999;340:1021–1030.

Chapter 59

Ingestions and Poisonings

Steve Davis

The management of poisonings in pediatric patients is based on an understanding of the basic supportive measures required for most ingestions. The epidemiology of pediatric ingestions is significantly different from that of adult ingestions. Because most are accidental and unwitnessed, the ability to manage ingestions of unknown substances before the results of specific testing are available is critical.

EPIDEMIOLOGY

The epidemiology of pediatric poisonings can be elicited by examining telephone calls made to poison control centers throughout the United States. More than 70% of calls to poison centers involve children under the age of 18 years. Data collected from these centers reveal that:

- Of all pediatric poisonings, 85% involve children <5 years.
- Most of these are unintentional and involve common household products and over-the-counter medications.
- The mortality rate for children with ingestions is exceedingly low.

Adolescent ingestions are more like adult ingestions:

- The majority are intentional and involve either a *suicide attempt* or *drug experimentation*.
- Because they are intentional, involve illicit drugs, or are an attempt at suicide, the rate of severe complications is much higher, and the *associated mortality rate is 15 times that of younger children*.

The most commonly ingested substances in young children in decreasing order of frequency include:

- Cosmetics/hygiene products
- Cleaning products
- Analgesics
- Plants
- Cough and cold medications
- Pesticides
- Vitamins
- Hydrocarbons

Fatalities from ingestion in children are extremely rare. Data from Poison Centers from 2003 revealed that of the approximate 2.5 million calls to these centers, there were 34 reported fatalities. In children <6 years of age, 12 deaths were associated with over-the-counter products, nine were unintentional, *eight were therapeutic errors*, seven were environmental exposures, and two were homicides. In adolescents, approximately 40% involved drug experimentation and 33% were suicides.

Plant exposures account for up to 10% of calls to poison centers. The vast majority do not involve more than minimal symptoms. However, because of the large number of these exposures, fatalities can occur. It is therefore useful to know which types of exposures have the potential to cause severe morbidity or mortality. These include:

- *Jimsonweed:* a plant frequently ingested by adolescents for its hallucinogenic properties
- Hemlock
- Philodendron
- Pokeweed
- Holly
- Castor beans
- Mistletoe
- Leaves and pits of several fruit trees can release cyanide

ROLE OF HISTORY AND PHYSICAL EXAMINATION

The history and physical examination are pivotal in the appropriate management of a child who presents after having ingested an unknown substance. Despite rapid advances in technology, a basic knowledge of the presenting features of the major categories of poisonings is critical to appropriate management because management decisions are routinely made before the results of laboratory tests become available. Most pediatric ingestions are unintentional, and in many cases, the poison is an unknown substance, so that it becomes necessary to elicit a thorough history from the parents. A standard history should be obtained, including what agent was ingested, how much, when, why, and under what circumstances. The location of the ingestion may also be helpful. For example, potential agents ingested in the kitchen may be different than those in the bathroom. It is often helpful to have the parents or caregiver bring in the substance. Many cleaning and household products contain multiple potential toxins, and reviewing the label may be useful. In cases of ingestion involving unknown products,

TABLE 59.1

COMMONLY ENCOUNTERED TOXIDROMES

Category of Toxin (Example of Agent)	Manifestations
Anticholinergic agents (antihistamines, phenothiazines, tricyclic antidepressants, antispasmodics)	Agitation Hallucinations Dilated pupils Red color Dry skin Fever
Sympathomimetic agents (amphetamines, cocaine)	Sweating Tremulousness Hyperactivity Dysrhythmia Dilated pupils
Organophosphate agents (pesticides)	Salivation Lacrimation Urination Diaphoresis Miosis Pulmonary congestion
Hallucinogens (phencyclidine, lysergic acid diethylamide)	Visual hallucinations Sensory distortions Depersonalization
Tricyclic antidepressant agents (imipramine)	Coma Convulsions Cardiac dysrhythmia (prolonged QRS)
Salicylate agents	Vomiting Hyperpnea Fever
Phenothiazine agents (antipsychotics, antinauseants)	Torsion of the head and neck Oculogyric crisis Ataxia
Opioids (narcotics such as morphine and heroin)	Respiratory failure Miosis Coma
Selective serotonin reuptake inhibitors	Hyper-reflexia Myoclonus Hyperthermia Autonomic instability

TABLE 59.2

CHARACTERISTIC ODORS THAT MAY SERVE AS CLUES TO AN UNKNOWN INGESTION

Odor	Substance/Toxin
Garlic	Arsenic Organophosphates
Mothball	Camphor
Rotten eggs	Hydrogen sulfide
Wintergreen	Methyl salicylate
Bitter almond	Cyanide
Acetone	Salicylates Isopropyl alcohol

the parents, with guidance, can often identify a list of potential toxins and medications in the home. A review of the activities of the past 24 hours can often provide a sense of when the ingestion took place, information that helps to determine the severity of exposure, and whether aggressive therapy is needed. It has been estimated that history is the most important factor in identifying unknown ingestions in up to 90% of cases. Information provided by an adolescent who has had an intentional ingestion is often unreliable. Use of illicit drugs is typically underreported. A family history of drug use in an older sibling or parent may often lead to unintentional ingestions in young children.

Unfortunately, the history does not always identify the offending agent, especially in adolescents in whom the ingestion frequently is intentional and unwitnessed. In these situations, the physical examination and a knowledge of *toxidromes* is crucial because treatment often must be instituted before the results of any laboratory testing are known. Toxidromes can identify the ingested toxin or class of ingested agent in more than 80% of cases of ingestion of unknown toxins. The most commonly encountered toxidromes are summarized in Table 59.1.

Certain substances can be rapidly identified during the physical examination by characteristic odors (Table 59.2) or specific examination findings (Table 59.3). Frequent

TABLE 59.3

GENERAL FINDINGS ON PHYSICAL EXAMINATION THAT MAY AID IN DETECTING AN UNKNOWN POISON

Physical Examination Finding	Substance/Toxin
Needle tracts	Drug abuse, particularly with narcotic agents
Gray cyanosis	Agents causing methemoglobinemia
Chocolate blood	Agents causing methemoglobinemia
Cherry-red mucous membranes	Carbon monoxide

physical examinations may provide critical information about the evolution of poisoning and the need for aggressive interventions.

ROLE OF LABORATORY TESTING

Screening laboratory tests are helpful in the management of ingestions because of their easy access and rapid turn-around times. The goal is often to identify the metabolic effects of the poison. However, few are specific.

In most cases, it is easy to calculate an *anion gap* from the electrolyte values in the emergency setting. The anion gap is calculated with the following formula:

- Serum sodium − (serum chloride + serum bicarbonate)

Normal values are <16. An elevated anion gap represents an accumulation of organic acids, such as lactate or formate, which neutralize bicarbonate. However, a normal anion gap does not rule out the presence of organic acids.

An elevated anion gap can be caused by the ingestion of:

- Alcohol
- Toluene
- Methanol
- Paraldehyde
- Ethylene glycol
- Salicylates

Uremia, diabetic ketoacidosis, and lactic acidosis also can cause an elevated anion gap.

An *osmolar gap* can also be calculated easily from the laboratory values for electrolytes and renal function. An osmolar gap indicates the presence of low-molecular-weight toxins, although the absence of an osmolar gap does not rule out the presence of these toxins. The following formula is utilized to calculate an osmolar gap:

- Measured osmolality ([2 × sodium] + [glucose/18] + [blood urea nitrogen/2.8]) = osmolar gap

If the osmolality calculated with this formula is less than the measured serum osmolality, then an osmolar gap is present.

Substances that may cause an osmolar gap include:

- Methanol
- Ethanol
- Diuretics
- Isopropyl alcohol
- Ethylene glycol

Arterial blood gas measurements are useful in significant ingestions. They provide rapid information about acid-base status, as well as oxygenation and ventilation. Urinalysis may indicate the presence of myoglobin from rhabdomyolysis. The presence of calcium oxalate crystals in the urine may indicate an ethylene glycol ingestion.

OTHER TESTS

An electrocardiogram can be useful in the management of poisonings, particularly in patients with abnormal findings on cardiac monitoring. The presence of bradycardia is consistent with the ingestion of:

- Narcotics
- β-Blockers
- Clonidine
- Calcium channel blockers

Agents that can prolong the QT or QRS interval include:

- Anticholinergics (tricyclic antidepressants and phenothiazine agents, carbamazepine)
- Lithium
- Organophosphates
- Ethylene glycol

Radiographs are seldom helpful in the evaluation of poisonings. Very few agents are radiodense or are ingested in large enough quantities to be visible on abdominal films. Substances that may be apparent on radiographs include chloral hydrate, heavy metals, iodine, phenothiazine agents, and enteric-coated tablets. Multivitamins with iron are rarely visible.

Toxicology screens have a role in the management of serious ingestions. However, it is important to realize that treatment must often be instituted before the results of toxicology screens are known. Several types of toxicology screens are available, and knowledge of the types of screens available locally and the agents routinely tested for are important. Examples of agents that may be overlooked on standard toxicology screens include antibiotics, diuretics, ethylene glycol, lithium, aromatic hydrocarbons, and cyanide. The American Association of Clinical Chemists routinely monitors proficiency tests for laboratories conducting toxicology screens. On average, false-negative results are obtained in 10% to 30% of cases, whereas false-positive results are obtained in up to 10% of cases.

The clinical utility of toxicology screens is limited by the fact that:

- Decisions frequently must be made before the results are known.
- Few specific antidotes/interventions are available.
- Morbidity is low if standard decontamination measures are implemented.
- The agent or class of agent is frequently obvious on presentation.

In certain circumstances, toxicology screens are useful or necessary. These include but are not limited to:

- Overdoses in which a quantitative determination is required to predict severity and outcome
- The presence of significant symptoms in the face of an unclear cause

- Situations in which proof of intoxication is of medicolegal importance
- Suspicion of Munchausen by proxy

MANAGEMENT

The management of ingestions is based on basic supportive therapy. The components of management include:

- Resuscitation and stabilization
- Preventing further drug absorption
- Decontaminating the gastrointestinal tract
- Hastening the elimination of already absorbed substances
- Specific management (antidotes) in serious or life threatening ingestions

Resuscitation and stabilization involve the basic principles of attending to the airway, breathing, and circulation.

Gastric-Emptying Strategies

Gastric emptying, which has long been a mainstay of therapy, and charcoal therapy are means of preventing further drug absorption.

Ipecac and gastric lavage are commonly used to empty the stomach. Unfortunately, both are only marginally effective in reducing the amount of drug absorbed, and they are not without risk. In clinical studies, both techniques removed up to approximately 30% of ingested drug when applied within 1 hour of an ingestion. Lavage has been felt to offer several advantages over induced emesis, including the fact that it can be performed without delay, followed by the administration of charcoal through the gastric tube. However, despite these theoretic advantages, the effectiveness of lavage in clinical trials was only equivalent, not superior, to that of induced emesis.

Contraindications to the use of gastric-emptying strategies are rare, but include the following:

- The patient has ingested an alkaline or hydrocarbon substance, so that the risk for further injury as the substance is refluxed into the esophagus during emesis negates any benefit.
- The patient has previously sustained an esophageal injury.
- The ingestion is likely to cause only mild symptoms, and the risk for aspiration is not warranted.
- The patient's airway is compromised.
- The time since ingestion exceeds 1 hour, so that the benefit of gastric emptying may be limited.

The use of activated charcoal to prevent further absorption and to decontaminate the gastrointestinal tract has become the standard of care for most ingestions that are more than minor. Several clinical trials have shown no advantage to adding either induced emesis or lavage to activated charcoal alone. Charcoal can be administered in multiple doses to produce a *gastrointestinal dialysis* and can be used with a cathartic, such as sorbitol, to increase elimination from the gastrointestinal tract. *Sorbitol or other cathartics should be given only with the first dose of charcoal because of a real risk for dehydration and electrolyte abnormalities with repeated administration.*

Activated charcoal should be administered after any ingestion with the potential to produce moderate to severe adverse effects when the toxin ingested is known to be absorbed by charcoal. Charcoal also should be utilized in serious ingestions to enhance the elimination of drugs that can be removed by *gastrointestinal dialysis* (e.g., theophylline, phenobarbital) or drugs that are known to be substantially eliminated through the bile.

Contraindications to charcoal administration include:

- Airway compromise until after endotracheal intubation
- Ingestions of *caustic agents*

Complications of charcoal therapy are rare but can include:

- Vomiting and endotracheal aspiration
- Charcoal inspissation after repeated administration
- Excessive fluid loss after repeated use with a cathartic

Various types of substances are not absorbed by charcoal. These include:

- Simple ions (e.g., iron, lithium, cyanide)
- Simple alcohols (e.g., ethanol, methanol)
- Strong acids or bases (e.g., hydrogen chloride, sodium hydroxide)

Whole-bowel irrigation may be useful for serious ingestions. This labor-intensive and time-consuming procedure involves the administration of a very large volume of an electrolyte solution into the stomach to irrigate the bowel. Whole-bowel irrigation may decrease the bioavailability of ingested substances more rapidly and fully than the use of activated charcoal. The fluid solution is administered until the rectal effluent is clear. This technique is *strongly recommended for serious ingestions involving iron, lithium, and sustained-release agents* and should be also considered for ingestions of heavy metals, lead salts, zinc salts, and packets of illicit drugs.

Methods of hastening the elimination of substances are usually reserved for the most serious ingestions. These methods include:

- Forced diuresis, with or without alteration of pH
- Dialysis
- Hemoperfusion

Alkaline diuresis is contraindicated in patients with cerebral or pulmonary edema and in patients who are in renal failure.

Antidotes

Antidote administration should be considered when a specific antidote is available, the patient has had a significant

TABLE 59.4
ANTIDOTES FOR PEDIATRIC INGESTIONS

Antidote	Toxin
Atropine	Organophosphates
Deferoxamine	Iron
Ethanol	Methanol
	Ethylene glycol
Oxygen	Carbon monoxide
Methylene blue	Agents causing methemoglobinemia
N-Acetylcysteine	Acetaminophen
Naloxone	Narcotics
Physostigmine	Anticholinergic agents

ingestion, and the potential risks of using the antidote are outweighed by the benefits of its use. Antidotes are rarely utilized for pediatric ingestions.

Although the poison control index lists more than 300 specific antidotes for ingestions, only about 15 of these are used with any regularity. Naloxone, administered to treat narcotic ingestions, is by far the most commonly utilized antidote. Other important antidotes are listed in Table 59.4. Even when they are available for a specific ingestion, antidotes should be used as an adjuvant, and are not a replacement for meticulous supportive care.

SPECIFIC INGESTIONS

Acetaminophen

Acetaminophen is present in many over-the-counter medications, either alone or in combination with other substances. Acetaminophen is frequently ingested in large quantities by toddlers because it tastes good, and adolescents ingest it in suicide attempts.

The clinical manifestations typically occur in phases. Patients are asymptomatic or complain of nausea and vomiting in the first 24 hours after the ingestion. The gastrointestinal symptoms typically resolve during the next 24 hours. Evidence of liver injury develops at 72 hours and beyond, if a toxic amount was ingested. Depending on the amount ingested, elevated transaminase levels may be apparent within 24 hours of ingestion.

The minimum toxic dose is considered to be >140 mg/kg. Hepatic toxicity is predicted according to the serum acetaminophen levels plotted on a Rumack nomogram. A serum acetaminophen level obtained at a specified time after the ingestion (usually 4–12 hours afterward) that falls above the nomogram line is associated with hepatic damage, whereas levels falling below the nomogram line are not associated with significant hepatic toxicity. The acetaminophen nomogram does not work for chronic or acute superimposed on chronic ingestion.

The management of minor ingestions consists of supportive care only. For potentially severe ingestions, a spe-

cific antidote, N-acetylcysteine, should be administered. This agent is effective in decreasing hepatic toxicity, if given within 24 hours of the ingestion. If it is not clear how serious the ingestion is, or if it is not possible to determine the acetaminophen level, N–acetylcysteine should be administered pending further information.

Anticholinergic Agents

Anticholinergic agents are included in many over-the-counter cold remedies. Examples of these are antihistamines, phenothiazines, tricyclic antidepressants, and antispasmodics.

The clinical manifestations can be remembered by the saying, "mad as a hatter, dry as a bone, red as a beet, blind as a bat, and hot as a hare." Both central (confusion, memory loss, agitation, hallucinations, and seizures) and peripheral (tachycardia, fever, hypertension, dry mouth, urinary retention) symptoms are present.

Management begins with supportive care as outlined in the preceding text. In patients with significant symptoms, treatment with physostigmine, a cholinesterase inhibitor, counteracts both central and peripheral symptoms.

Salicylates

Salicylates are available as single agents (aspirin) or in combination with other products. As in acetaminophen overdose, a nomogram (Done nomogram) can be used to predict the amount of toxicity based on the serum level at a specified time after the ingestion. This nomogram is accurate only in acute ingestions.

Clinical manifestations are variable and include fever, nausea, vomiting, coagulopathy, hyperpnea, tinnitus, seizures, and coma. Respiratory depression, coma, hepatotoxicity, and renal failure can occur with severe ingestions.

Laboratory findings include metabolic acidosis, respiratory alkalosis, hypokalemia, hypocalcemia, hyperglycemia or hypoglycemia, and hypernatremia or hyponatremia.

Management consists of meticulous supportive measures, including correcting dehydration, treating acidosis, and administering vitamin K for coagulopathy. Alkaline diuresis may also be considered. In severe cases, hemodialysis may be necessary.

Iron

Iron typically is an ingestion of toddlers. The severity is related to the amount ingested.

The clinical manifestations generally occur in stages. The initial stage consists of gastric irritation, manifested by nausea, vomiting, abdominal pain, and bloody diarrhea. This stage is usually followed by a 6- to 12-hour period in which the symptoms resolve. However, the resolution is often only temporary, and the patient progresses to shock. Hyperglycemia, metabolic acidosis, bleeding diathesis, and coma ensue. If the child survives this stage, the final stage is one of hepatic toxicity with jaundice, hypoglycemia, and intestinal scarring and stenosis.

Supportive care and gastrointestinal decontamination are the mainstay of therapy. Chelation therapy with deferoxamine is reserved for symptomatic patients and those with serum iron levels >350 μg/dL.

Tricyclic Antidepressants

Tricyclic antidepressants are most commonly ingested by adolescents attempting to commit suicide. These agents can produce both central and peripheral anticholinergic effects, as noted in the preceding text. They also decrease the reuptake of norepinephrine and so enhance adrenergic stimulation.

The clinical manifestations of ingestion include drowsiness and lethargy progressing to coma. Important myocardial effects include quinidine-like myocardial depression, tachyarrhythmias, second- and third-degree heart block, and a prolonged QRS complex. Peripheral anticholinergic effects, such as blurred vision and dry mucous membranes, may also be seen.

Management consists of supportive care, including vigilant observation of the airway status, and the repeated administration of charcoal to reduce enterohepatic circulation. Alkalinization of the urine, either with hyperventilation or bicarbonate therapy, is recommended. For patients with hypotension, norepinephrine, or epinephrine may be required to increase blood pressure and perfusion.

Opioids

Opioids are commonly ingested by adolescents, but also can be ingested accidentally by toddlers.

The clinical manifestations are usually easily recognized by the toxidrome of miosis, respiratory depression, and coma. Seizures are also possible.

Routine supportive care is paramount. Naloxone is a specific opiate receptor antagonist. A dose of 0.01 mg/kg can be administered initially and repeated up to 10 times if necessary. It is important to remember that the half-life of naloxone is less than that of most opioids, so that either repeated doses or a continuous infusion may be necessary.

The clinical symptoms of patients who have ingested barbiturates closely resemble those of patients with opioid ingestions. In the case of an unknown barbiturate ingestion, a failure to respond to naloxone may be diagnostic.

Selective Serotonin Reuptake Inhibitors

Selective serotonin reuptake inhibitors are now commonly used to treat depression, anxiety and obsessive ruminations. In general, these agents are well tolerated and overdoses typically result in less serious complications that with other antidepressant overdoses. However, in combination

with other drugs, such as monoamine oxidase inhibitors or St. Johns Wort, ingestion of these agents can be fatal.

These agents can rarely produce *serotonin syndrome*, which is caused by overstimulation of central and peripheral serotonin receptors. The clinical manifestations include nausea, vomiting, and diaphoresis in mild cases. More serious ingestions may lead to hyper-reflexia, hyperthermia, myoclonus, muscular rigidity, and autonomic instability. The diagnosis is made clinically. Most cases are mild and require only routine supportive care. If hyperthermia and rigidity are present, cooling measures should be instituted. For severe cases, benzodiazepines and cyproheptadine can be used. *Cyproheptadine is an antihistamine which is a serotonin receptor antagonist.* The need for intubation and paralysis is only rarely necessary in the management of this syndrome.

REVIEW EXERCISES

QUESTIONS

1. A toddler is brought to the emergency department after having ingested unknown quantities of an unknown drug. The clinical manifestations include vomiting, hyperpnea, and fever. Which of the following is a *true* statement?
a) This child likely has a metabolic alkalosis.
b) Bleeding may occur.
c) Metabolic derangements are uncommon with this ingestion.
d) A specific antidote for this ingestion is available.

Answer
The answer is b. Vomiting, hyperpnea, and fever are features of salicylate poisoning. Metabolic derangements are common following salicylate ingestions and include metabolic acidosis, hypoglycemia, and hyponatremia. Bleeding may result from hypothrombinemia and platelet dysfunction, and the administration of vitamin K may be required.

2. Agitation, hallucination, mydriasis, dry skin, and fever are characteristic features of ingestion with which of the following group of agents?
a) Anticholinergics
b) Sympathomimetics
c) Organophosphates
d) Opioids

Answer
The answer is a. The toxidrome of agitation, hallucination, mydriasis, dry skin, and fever suggests anticholinergic poisoning. The toxidromes for the other agents listed as choices can be found in Table 59.1.

3. A 15-year-old girl is brought to the emergency department in a coma. Her pupils are constricted, and she is noted to have severe respiratory depression. Ingestion of

which of the following is *most* likely responsible for her findings?
a) Cocaine
b) Phencyclidine
c) Heroin
d) A tricyclic antidepressant

Answer
The answer is c. The triad of coma, respiratory depression, and miosis is characteristic of opioid ingestion. Heroin and morphine are examples of opioids.

4. A 17-year-old boy presents with profuse sweating and agitation. He is noted to have dilated pupils and tachycardia. Ingestion of which of the following substances is *most* likely responsible for his symptoms?
a) Cocaine
b) Thorazine
c) Heroin
d) Phencyclidine

Answer
The answer is a. The clinical manifestations of sympathomimetic ingestions include sweating, tremulousness, hyperactivity, mydriasis, and dysrhythmias, especially tachycardia.

5. Which of the following is *not* a feature of organophosphate toxicity?
a) Mydriasis
b) Salivation
c) Lacrimation
d) Pulmonary edema

Answer
The answer is a. Miosis, not mydriasis, is a feature of organophosphate toxicity. Other features include salivation, lacrimation, urination, defecation, and pulmonary edema.

6. Which of the following is a feature of serotonin syndrome that may result from a serious ingestion of selective serotonin reuptake inhibitors?
a) Hyporeflexia
b) Rigidity
c) Hypothermia
d) Hypotonia

Answer
The answer is b. The features of serotonin syndrome include hyperreflexia, hyperthermia, rigidity, myoclonus, and autonomic instability. These features occur with severe ingestions of the selective serotonin reuptake inhibitors.

SUGGESTED READINGS

1. Alander SW, Dowd MD, Bratton SL, et al. Pediatric acetaminophen overdose: risk factors associated with hepatocellular injury. *Arch Pediatr Adolesc Med* 2000;154:346–350.
2. Henretig F, Shannon M. Toxicological emergencies. In: Fleisher GR, Ludwig S, eds. *Textbook of pediatric emergency medicine.* Baltimore: Williams & Wilkins, 1993.
3. McGuigan ME. Poisoning potpourri. *Pediatr Rev* 2001;22:295–301.
4. Watson WA, Litovitz TL, Rodgers GC Jr, et al. 2002 Annual report of the American Association of Poison Control Centers Toxic Exposure Surveillance System. *Am J Emerg Med* 2003;21:353.
5. Woolf AD. Poisoning and the critically ill child. In: Rogers MC, ed. *Textbook of pediatric intensive care.* Baltimore: Williams & Wilkins, 1996.

Chapter 60

Musculoskeletal Emergencies

Martin G. Hellman

As a primary care provider, a pediatrician should have a fundamental knowledge of musculoskeletal injuries and fractures in children. Of all childhood injuries, 10% to 15% are musculoskeletal. An understanding of the unique nature of pediatric fractures and their acute care is important to every pediatrician. Recognizing fractures secondary to possible child abuse is critical.

PHYSIOLOGIC HIGHLIGHTS OF CHILDREN'S BONES

Several key points concerning the anatomy of children's bones must be emphasized.

The growth plate (physis) is susceptible to injury because of its relative weakness. The physis, located at the end of long bones, is under compressive forces, and is radiolucent. Ligaments at joints are stronger than the physis until it closes at puberty; therefore, true sprains are rare or nonexistent. An apophysis is a bony prominence to which muscles or tendons are attached. It is joined to the bone by a radiolucent physis that is under traction forces.

Blood is supplied to the epiphysis by penetrating vessels from the joint capsule, whereas the metaphysis and diaphysis of the bone receive blood from nutrient and periosteal vessels. The physeal blood supply is from epiphyseal, metaphyseal, and perichondrial vessels. Fractures to the growth area can cause vascular compromise and subsequent growth problems. The periosteum of children's bones is thicker, stronger, and more vascular, but less attached than that of adult bones. Because of these properties, callus forms more quickly in children, and limits the amount of displacement associated with fractures.

Children's bones are different biomechanically from those of adults; these differences have a direct impact on injuries. The bone is less dense and more porous, especially the metaphysis, which is the area where the bone structure changes most rapidly. For this reason, children's

bones are more "bendable" than those of adults. Because children's bones are less dense, they fail with both compressive forces and tension forces. Some of the unique features of fractures seen in children are directly attributable to these characteristics.

EVALUATION OF THE PATIENT

A cardinal rule in pediatrics is to heed parents when they say that their child is "not acting right." This is particularly true in the evaluation of an injured child. Optimally, a reliable witness or the patient can clarify the mechanism of injury. It is important to note whether longitudinal or rotational forces were applied to the bones. It is also important to keep the normal developmental milestones of childhood in mind when the nature of an accident and the possibility of child abuse are being assessed.

The movements and position of an infant's extremities should be observed while the child is sitting in the guardian's lap. The physician should first examine the unaffected extremity and then other areas of the affected extremity. This may allay the child's fears before the likely injured spot is examined. The examiner should "tune in" for an increase in a small child's crying or screaming when the fracture site is palpated. Preschoolers and older children usually wince and elevate their shoulders when the exact fracture spot is located.

Proper radiographs (x-rays) are crucial in making a diagnosis. A minimum of two perpendicular views is mandatory, but oblique views are often helpful. The lateral radiographic view is often the best one for detecting subtle buckle fractures and growth plate disruptions. The clinician should obtain views of the specific tender area whenever possible so that subtle fractures are more evident as the x-ray beam is aimed directly at the area in question.

Routine comparison views of an extremity are usually not necessary. However, they can be useful in the evaluation of an elbow with its six ossification centers, or when the status of a physis is doubtful. Bone scans are rarely needed to clarify fractures in children, but they can assist in detecting occult fractures.

FRACTURE TYPES SPECIFIC TO CHILDREN

Five types of fractures occur in children's bones:

- Buckle
- Plastic deformation or bowing
- Greenstick
- Complete
- Growth plate

Each type demonstrates unique features related to the anatomy and physiology of growing bone.

Buckle Fractures

Buckle fractures are also known as *torus fractures* in reference to the prominence around the base of an architectural column. They occur in the metaphysis where the bone is more porous and when compressive forces are directed in the longitudinal plane. The physical examination reveals an absence of swelling or ecchymosis at the fracture site. Tenderness can be elicited by direct palpation of the spot. The radiograph shows a bulging of the cortex or an acute angulation of the cortical margin that is best seen on the lateral view. The clinician should always remember that long bones flare out smoothly and any sudden sharp angulation may indicate a torus fracture. Buckle fractures are stable and do not displace acutely. Short-term immobilization is primarily for pain relief while the fracture heals.

Bowing or Bend Fractures

Bowing fractures occur when longitudinal stress causes a microscopic failure in compression on the concave side of a bone with tension on the convex side. If the fracture on the tension side does not continue, then plastic deformation develops when the forces subside. A true fracture of the cortex does not occur, and hemorrhage is absent. Swelling may be limited, and no ecchymosis or callus formation is seen. Comparison radiographs may be the only way to confirm or refute the diagnosis, with the lateral view again being the most informative. The most commonly involved bones in bow fractures are the ulna and fibula, but such fractures can be seen in the radius and rarely in the tibia. Reduction may be necessary in children >4 years.

Greenstick Fractures

Greenstick fractures occur when the tension side of a bone fails and starts to fracture. The compression side

bends, and the fracture does not completely traverse the bone. Completion of the fracture and correction of any angulation may be necessary depending on the degree of angulation, its distance from the physis, and the age of the child.

Complete Fractures

Fractures through both sides of a bone can occur in children as they do in adults. Comminution is rare in children because of the bones' porosity and the relatively strong periosteum. Spiral fractures caused by rotational forces fall in this category. Although they can be accidental, such fractures are often the result of child abuse, especially in the humerus of a child <15 months.

Growth Plate Fractures

Because approximately 15% of pediatric fractures are growth plate fractures, they should always be considered when pain and swelling are noted at a joint. Growth areas are weaker than strong ligaments before puberty, so that sprains in children are very rare. Growth plate injuries have been classified in several ways, but the classification described by Salter and Harris is the one most commonly acknowledged. All types may or may not be displaced.

- A type I fracture (Fig. 60.1) involves the physis itself. Local pain and swelling at the physis result from tearing or avulsion stresses. The radiographic findings may be normal, or physeal widening may be apparent. Stress

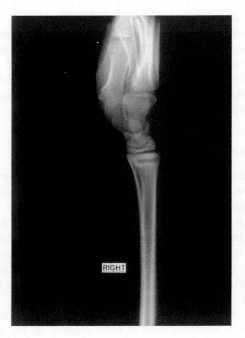

Figure 60.1 Lateral view of the right wrist demonstrates a growth plate injury. Note that the physis is not even across its entire width; it is wider at the dorsal aspect and narrower on the ventral side. This pattern signifies a Salter-Harris type I fracture.

views may accentuate the physeal widening. Some authors believe that type I fractures are really type II fractures without evidence of the metaphyseal chip.

- Type II fractures are the most common (80%–85%) type of growth plate fracture. The fracture extends through the physis and into the porous metaphysis.
- A type III fracture involves the physis and extends into the epiphysis.
- Type IV fractures are very uncommon as they extend through both the epiphysis and metaphysis.
- A type V fracture was originally described as a physis crush injury, but most authors now refute its existence.

Avulsion Fractures

Avulsion fractures, although not characteristic of children, occur when a fragment is pulled off a bone by an attached tendon or muscle. A common site is at the base of the fingers' phalanges or at the pelvic iliac crest. They are best seen on the lateral radiographic view.

COMMON CLINICAL ENTITIES

Clavicle Fractures

Fractures of the clavicle occur when a child lands directly on the lateral aspect of a shoulder, and the force is transmitted medially. Greenstick fractures predominate in the middle third of the clavicle, but fractures can occur at the distal end. They are best treated with reassurance and measures for comfort. Slings can be used for older children to avoid painful arm dangling. Local ice and oral analgesics are also indicated. Figure-of-eight wraps are not useful and may cause harm when they impinge on the axillary area. Neonates can present with a healing callus of the clavicle in the first month of life after a difficult delivery and shoulder dystocia. Radiographic confirmation is necessary only to allay parental fears.

Nursemaid's Elbow

"Nursemaid's elbow," or more accurately *dislocation or tearing of the annular ligament from the radial head,* is a common entity in children between 4 months and 8 years of age; the peak incidence is from 15 to 30 months. Dislocation or subluxation of the elbow does not occur; the articular cartilages remain in direct proximity. This injury is more common in girls than boys and more common in the left than the right arm. Although a variety of histories can be elicited, a "pulling" theme is evident in all cases.

The child typically does not use the affected limb, and sometimes holds the wrist to avoid supination. The physical examination reveals no swelling or ecchymosis at the elbow, and direct palpation of the three most common sites of fracture in the upper limb (middle of the clavicle, distal

humerus, and distal radius) elicits no painful response. The child dislikes even minimal supination of the arm.

When the history and physical examination findings are consistent with a diagnosis of nursemaid's elbow, the clinician should feel comfortable dealing with the problem *without* radiographic guidance. The parent should first be apprised of the situation and informed that a small snap or click may be heard during the procedure. Different techniques can be used, but the easiest way to reduce it is to fully supinate the arm and then completely flex it. The examiner should feel a click or a thud when the procedure is successful. An alternative to that technique is to hyperpronate the arm and then flex it at the elbow. It may take the child a few moments to use the arm effectively, but eliciting the child's now-normal parachute reflex will demonstrate that all is well. The parent should be warned about possible recurrence.

Elbow Fractures

Elbow fractures usually occur when a child falls on an outstretched arm while the elbow is hyperextended, but they can also result from a flexion injury. The supracondylar area is most commonly involved. Localized pain and swelling are usually prominent. The presence or absence of a fat pad sign on the true lateral radiograph is important. Normally, the anterior fat pad should hug the humeral rim, and the posterior fat pad should not be visible. Displacement of either indicates an effusion of blood into the joint, signifying a fracture (Fig. 60.2). Comparison radiographs may be needed to distinguish the six ossification centers in the elbow. The radial shaft should always be in line with the capitellum. A fracture in

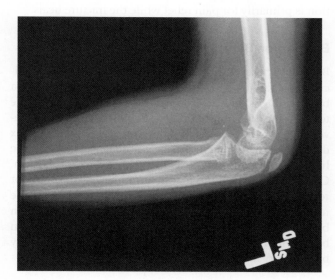

Figure 60.2 Lateral view of an elbow clearly shows abnormal fat pads, implying an intra-articular effusion from a fracture. The anterior pad is pushed superiorly and anteriorly away from the humeral rim. Note the radial head has an irregularity, indicating a fracture at this site.

the ulna midshaft with dislocation of the radius is called a *Monteggia fracture.*

The clinician should always be aware of possible compartment syndromes with supracondylar fractures and keep the five *Ps* (pain, pallor, pulselessness, paresthesia, and paralysis) in mind. Urgent orthopaedic consultation is mandatory in the case of any of these early findings. Most elbow fractures in which displacement is absent or minimal can be splinted with a posterior mold or "sugar tongs" and the patient discharged with appropriate follow-up and instructions. Fractures of the radial head, especially of the buckle type, are also seen occasionally.

Wrist Fractures

Buckle fractures and Salter type II fractures predominate in the distal radius. Sprains are rare before puberty because until then the ligaments are stronger than the porous metaphysis and relatively weak physis. Carpal fractures are rare in preadolescents, but the clinician should be on guard for navicular fractures once the physis begins to close. Volar wrist splints usually suffice to alleviate discomfort, but if supination or pronation causes pain, immobilization should include the elbow.

Hand Fractures

The clinician should be aware of the normal pseudoepiphysis seen occasionally on the distal portion of the thumb metacarpal and not mistake it for a fracture. This is a normal indentation where the metaphyseal ossification is enlarged. The lateral and oblique views of the fingers and hand are usually the most helpful in identifying tiny buckle fractures or avulsions. The position of function should be maintained when the fingers or hand is splinted.

Pelvic Fractures

Pelvic ring fractures are rare in children except in victims of a multiple trauma. Avulsion fractures of the iliac spines may occur in adolescents, usually those who participate in athletic endeavors such as basketball, hurdling, and sprinting. They are treated with bed rest and analgesics.

Fractures of the Femur and Tibia

A spiral or "toddler's" fracture typically occurs between the ages of 10 months and 6 years because of a rotary torque force. The extent of the fracture is usually seen best on the lateral view. The clinician should always consider the possibility of child abuse if the history is suggestive. Nutrient artery canals in the diaphysis can be mistaken for fractures. To differentiate between the two, the physician should palpate the area for tenderness and note the configuration, uniform lucency, and location of the radiographic finding.

A comparison view demonstrating similar findings will alleviate any doubts.

Small metaphyseal chips at the ends of long bones, especially at the knee, may indicate rapid, forceful leg twisting as a form of child abuse. These fractures are often referred to as *corner* or *bucket handle fractures.*

Knee Problems

Before adolescence, fractures of the epiphysis and physis are immensely more common than ligamentous injuries. Patellar fractures are uncommon because direct blows from falls usually result in simple contusions. Bipartite patellae are more common in males, and comparison views should help distinguish them from fractures. Patellar dislocations are more common in female adolescents, and acutely they almost always displace laterally. To relocate them, flex the hip and extend the knee while applying medial pressure to the patella. An osteochondral fracture of the lateral femoral condyle or the medial pole of the patella can result from a dislocation.

Chondromalacia patellae or patellofemoral stress syndrome, are more common in female patients. Chronic pain results from damage to the articular cartilage and is worse after rest and sudden flexion. Exercises to strengthen the quadriceps reduce stress and pain.

Ankle Fractures

Localized pain and swelling over the distal fibular physis imply a growth plate injury and not a sprain until the physis closes in adolescence. It should be splinted with a posterior mold, and follow-up should be arranged. The os trigonum is the normal lateral tubercle of the talus and is sometimes separate, so that it has the appearance of a fracture.

Foot Fractures

The fifth metatarsal apophysis normally runs parallel to the longitudinal plane of the bone. Fractures occurring here from forceful foot twisting appear either oblique or perpendicular to the long axis of the metatarsal. Treatment with a hard-soled shoe usually suffices, but a short-leg walking cast may be necessary. Buckle fractures can occur at the first metatarsal base after a fall and present with localized pain of the foot's dorsum. Calcaneal fractures are rare because tremendous forces are needed to fracture this very hard bone. A pseudoepiphysis analogous to the thumb is often seen in the large toe.

SPLINTING AND MANAGEMENT

The site of an injury or fracture should always be placed in a splint that includes the joint above and the one below the area in question. Anteroposterior splints or posterior molds usually serve this purpose well. The clinician should always be alert for compartment syndromes with any acute supracondylar, midshaft forearm, or tibial fracture. Any increase in pain in an extremity or change in its vascular status after casting or splinting may indicate a compartment syndrome. In this instance, appropriate measures to decrease the pressure should be instituted immediately. A child <9 or 10 years of age may not be safe with crutches unless specialized instructions are available.

CHILD ABUSE AND MUSCULOSKELETAL TRAUMA

It has been estimated that 10% to 70% of abused children sustain some type of skeletal trauma. Half of these cases occur in children <2 years, and a third are in infants <1 year. A variety of fracture patterns can be seen:

- Corner or bucket handle fractures at long bones' ends
- Rib fractures
- Unexplained diaphyseal spiral fractures, especially in the humerus
- Concurrent multiple fracture sites
- Skull fractures

The clinician should consider a skeletal survey whenever child abuse is suspected, especially for children <5 years. Unexpected periosteal new bone formation may be seen as evidence of old fractures.

REVIEW EXERCISES

QUESTIONS

1. Which of the following fractures is *not* a "typical" pediatric fracture but is more commonly seen in adults?
a) Buckle fracture of the wrist
b) Spiral fracture of the tibia
c) Bend fracture of the ulna
d) Comminuted fracture of the radius
e) Greenstick fracture of the clavicle

Answer
The answer is d. Comminuted fractures rarely occur in children.

2. What is the *most* common type of growth plate injury?
a) Salter type I
b) Salter type II
c) Salter type III
d) Salter type IV
e) Salter type V

Answer
The answer is b. Salter type II fractures account for 85% to 90% of growth plate injuries.

3. A 2-year-old girl was playing and she rolled down the hill. She got up crying and is not using her left arm. No swelling is noted. What would you do next?
a) Order an x-ray film of the entire upper extremity
b) Order an x-ray film of the elbow
c) Fully supinate and flex the arm
d) Fully supinate and extend the arm
e) Fully supinate the arm

Answer
The answer is c. One way to reduce a nursemaid's elbow is to fully supinate, then flex the arm.

4. All of the following statements about buckle fractures are true *except*:
a) They occur when longitudinal forces are applied.
b) They are most common in the diaphyses of bones.
c) They are stable fractures.
d) They are often seen best on the lateral view.
e) They are often diagnosed when a bone forms a sudden sharp angle.

Answer
The answer is b. Buckle fractures are most commonly seen in the metaphyses of bones.

5. An isolated ulnar fracture with a displaced radial head is a:
a) Galeazzi fracture
b) Monteggia fracture
c) Biplane fracture
d) Colles fracture
e) Smith fracture

Answer
The answer is b. This is a description of a Monteggia fracture.

6. A pseudoepiphysis can be seen in the:
a) Great toe
b) Distal radius of a newborn
c) Distal ulna of a newborn
d) Small toe of a toddler
e) Proximal phalanx of the thumb

Answer
The answer is a. A pseudoepiphysis can be seen in the great toe and in the metacarpal of the thumb.

7. A 6-month-old boy is admitted for a swollen knee. According to his father, he was rolling around on a bed unattended and fell onto the floor. He has no other injuries except the swollen knee. Physical examination reveals a well-developed, well-nourished, clean child in no acute distress. He is afebrile with a pulse rate of 110/minute, respiratory rate of 28/minute, and good perfusion status. He is playful until his left leg is moved. The examination findings other than for the left knee are completely normal. The left knee is swollen in comparison

with the right, but no ecchymosis, erythema, or perceived warmth is present. Roentgenography of the left knee shows a tiny metaphyseal chip on the medial aspect of the distal femur. Appropriate management includes all the following *except:*
a) Notifying child protective services
b) Immobilizing the leg from the ankle to the thigh
c) Obtaining an orthopaedic consult
d) Obtaining a bone scan

Answer
The answer is d. A posterior mold from the ankle to the thigh would keep the joint immobile until an orthopaedic evaluation is performed. This type of corner fracture is not caused by a direct blow or fall. It is the result of violent shearing forces applied to the lower extremity by an adult. Protective services should be notified.

8. A 6-year-old girl is on a swing, and as she gets off, her foot becomes stuck in the loose dirt. She suddenly twists her ankle and falls down. She is unable to walk. She is brought in by emergency medical services for evaluation. Physical examination reveals a pleasant and cooperative girl until you examine her right ankle. Her blood pressure is 100/66 mm Hg; the pulse rate is 92/minute, and the respiratory rate is 24/minute. She is afebrile. All her physical examination findings except for the right ankle are normal. Examination of the ankle shows swelling over the distal lateral fibula. She is most tender approximately 1 cm superior to the edge of the distal fibula, not anteriorly or posteriorly. She begins to cry when the spot is palpated directly. Roentgenography reveals considerable soft-tissue swelling over the lateral distal fibula, without fracture noted. Which of the following is a *true* statement concerning this case?

a) The lack of an obvious fracture on the x-ray film does not preclude the possibility of a growth plate injury.
b) The girl most likely has a sprain of the ankle.
c) Osteomyelitis must be ruled out.

Answer
The answer is a. The physical examination demonstrates pinpoint pain and swelling at the physis of the distal fibula and not over the anterior talofibular or posterior talofibular ligament. The lack of an obvious fracture on the x-ray film does not preclude the possibility of a growth plate injury, and the child should be splinted and treated for a possible fracture. Osteomyelitis is not a consideration, given the history and physical examination findings.

SUGGESTED READINGS

1. Chacon D, Kissoon N, Brown T, et al. Use of comparison radiographs in the diagnosis of traumatic injuries of the elbow. *Ann Emerg Med* 1992;21:895–898.
2. Cramer K. Orthopedic aspects of child abuse. *Pediatr Clin North Am* 1996;43:1035–1050.
3. Green NE, Swiontkowski MF. *Skeletal trauma in children,* vol 3. Philadelphia: Saunders, 1994.
4. Hilton SW, Edwards DK, Hilton JW. *Practical pediatric radiology.* Philadelphia: Saunders, 1984.
5. Jackman KV. Acute pediatric orthopedic conditions. *Pediatr Ann* 1994;23:240–249.
6. MacEwen GD, Kasser JR, Heinrich SD. *Pediatric fractures.* Baltimore: Williams & Wilkins, 1993.
7. Rang MR. *Children's fractures,* 2nd ed. Philadelphia: Lippincott, 1983.
8. Rockwood CA, Wilkins KE, King RE. *Fractures in children.* Philadelphia: Lippincott, 1984.
9. Strait R, Siegel RM, Shapiro RA, et al. Humeral fractures without obvious etiologies in children less than 3 years of age: when is it abuse? *Pediatrics* 1995;96:667–671.
10. Thomas S, Rosenfield NS, Leventhal JM, et al. Long bone fractures in young children: distinguishing accidental injuries from child abuse. *Pediatrics* 1991;88:471–476.

Chapter 61

Pediatric Trauma

Michelle Walsh

The management of traumatic injuries in children is unique to the field of pediatric emergency medicine. It is an important topic to understand because of the vast number of children presenting for medical care secondary to an injurious event. Trauma is the most common cause of morbidity and mortality in children. There are more than 500,000 pediatric trauma admissions in the United States, and trauma is the leading cause of death in children >1 year of age. There have been many advances in the management of the trauma patient and in the prevention of trauma in the past decade. However, despite the advances, there are >20,000 pediatric deaths each year secondary to trauma.

EPIDEMIOLOGY

Blunt trauma is the mechanism in 80% to 90% of cases of pediatric trauma. Although the number of children being injured by penetrating forces is lower, the mortality rate of penetrating trauma, which would include injuries from knives and firearms, is much higher. The ratio of blunt to penetrating injuries has been changing over the past decade with the rates of penetrating trauma slowly increasing steadily, especially in urban areas. The ease of obtaining firearms and the prevalence of gang violence are two factors contributing to the recent changes.

The age and development of the child play important roles in determining injury patterns. In nonambulating infants, abuse is the leading cause of trauma. The advancing gross motor skills and curiosity of the surrounding world in toddlers make falls the most common cause of injury in this age group. Pedestrian injuries and bicycle accidents are the leading cause of trauma in school-age children. Adolescents have increasing independence in the world, but not always good judgment, making motor vehicle accidents, with or without alcohol use, the most common cause of trauma in this age group.

INITIAL ASSESSMENT AND RESUSCITIATION OF TRAUMA PATIENT

Trauma management is a very systematic process. It begins with the primary survey with simultaneous initial resuscitation. The primary survey is often referred to as the ABCDEs and consists of the following steps:

- Airway control with cervical spine stabilization
- Breathing and ventilation
- Circulation and hemorrhage control
- Disability (neurological screen)
- Exposure

The evaluation begins with the assessment of the airway and proceeds down the list. If serious alterations in one of the body systems is encountered, resuscitative care is performed prior to moving to the next step. For example, an airway would need to be established in a patient with stridor and breathing difficulty before managing a bleeding wound. Once stabilized, a secondary survey is performed. The secondary survey is a focused and detailed evaluation of each body area, proceeding from head to toe. The secondary survey helps to find more subtle injuries that may not be life threatening, but may increase the potential morbidity.

HEAD TRAUMA

Head trauma is the leading cause of morbidity and mortality in children. Children are more prone to head injuries than adults because of their relatively large occiputs as compared with body habitus, weaker neck musculature, and immature cognitive development. Falls are the most common cause of head injuries in children, followed by motor vehicle accidents, bicycle accidents, and assaults. Eighty percent of children who die from trauma have significant head injuries.

Brain injury may be classified as primary or secondary. Primary brain injury refers to the injury that occurs at the time of impact. This injury is very rarely influenced by initial medical interventions. This type of injury includes skull fractures and intracranial hemorrhages. Secondary brain injury occurs after the time of impact and refers to the neuronal injury and neuronal death resulting from hypoxia, ischemia, and mechanical distortion of the neurons. An example of secondary injury is diffuse cerebral edema and herniation after diffuse axonal injury. The goal in the management of the head injured patient is to provide interventions that limit secondary brain injury.

The final common pathway in the development of secondary brain injury is increased intracranial pressure (ICP) and/or decreased cerebral perfusion pressure (CPP). The CPP is influenced by two factors, the ICP and the mean arterial pressure (MAP). The equation CPP = MAP − ICP illustrates the relationship. The goal is to maintain the CPP within normal limits. Maintaining an adequate MAP and limiting elevations of the ICP help to achieve this goal.

The intracranial volume is a fixed and is comprised of three components: CSF volume, blood volume, and brain volume. Changes in one component will directly affect the other two components. Once compliance of the intracranial volume is exceeded, any small changes in any component will lead to large increases in the intracranial pressure. Early symptoms of increased ICP include:

- Headache
- Vomiting
- Altered mental status, or
- Abnormal posturing

The management of increased intracranial pressure includes:

- Intubation
- Mild hyperventilation
- Sedation
- Neuromuscular blockade
- Mannitol

In the evaluation of a child with head trauma, a decision needs to be made concerning potential radiographic studies. One option is to obtain skull films, which can help determine if there are any bony abnormalities, but will not demonstrate any intracranial lesions. A negative skull film does not rule out intracranial injury. The availability of computed tomography (CT) scanning has been increasing significantly over the past decades, and is becoming the study of choice given the ease of access and rapidity of the study. The decision, however, to obtain a CT scan is not always clear. One must weigh the risks of potential radiation exposure and the potential need of sedation when considering the study. The *absolute* indications for a head CT in the evaluation head trauma are:

- Penetrating injury to the head
- Focal neurologic deficits

- Post-traumatic seizures
- Extensive facial injury
- Signs of basilar skull fracture

Relative indications for obtaining a head CT in the management of an injured child include:

- A history of a change in level of consciousness
- Alcohol or drug intoxication
- Suspected child abuse
- Unreliable or inadequate history
- Age <2 years
- Postconcussive amnesia
- Severe headaches

Magnetic resonance imaging (MRI) has no role in the initial evaluation of the head-injured patient.

Skull Fractures

There are several types of skull fracture in children, including linear, depressed, and basilar fractures.

- *Linear* skull fractures are the most common type of skull fracture in children. Isolated linear fractures without intracranial hemorrhage usually result in minimal symptoms except for focal scalp swelling. Management includes symptomatic care with follow-up CT or skull radiographs to determine resolution.
- *Depressed* skull fractures typically occur after a large force strikes a small area (e.g., hammer), causing the bone fragment to be depressed under the inner table of the skull. These can be associated with brain injury. Management includes neurosurgical evaluation with possible elevation of the bone fragment.
- *Basilar* skull fractures are those extending through the basal portion of the skull. They are characterized by periorbital hematomas, periauricular hematomas, cerebrospinal fluid (CSF) rhinorrhea, and hemotympanum, otorrhea, and cranial nerve palsies. Management includes mandatory neurosurgical evaluation. Ninety-five percent of basilar skull fractures heal with bed rest and elevating the head of the bed. Complications of basilar skull fractures include meningitis, CSF fistula, and facial nerve palsies.

Intracranial Hemorrhages

There are several types of intracranial hemorrhages that may occur after head trauma:

- Intracerebral hematoma
- Subdural hematoma
- Epidural hematoma

Each of these injuries has the potential to cause significant brain damage and requires mandatory neurosurgical consultation.

Intracerebral hemorrhages, or cerebral contusions, are bruises of the cerebral cortex. They occur as the brain moves about in the skull. A *coup* injury occurs at the site of the impact, whereas a *contrecoup* injury occurs at the side opposite the impact. Cerebral contusions are characterized by focal parenchyma swelling and small areas of hemorrhage within the brain tissue itself. This type of injury may be associated with other types of intracranial injury.

Subdural hematomas are secondary to tearing of bridging veins and lead to blood accumulating between the dura and arachnoid membrane. Subdural hematomas occur more commonly in infants and young children as compared with older children and adults. The most common mechanism causing subdual hematomas are forces with rapid acceleration and decelerations, such as with shaken impact syndrome. Children often present with signs of increased ICP. Infants with open fontanelles may have delayed symptoms. A crescent shaped density compressing the brain will be noted on CT scan. Mortality rates range from 10% to 20%. Neurologic sequelae are common.

Epidural hematomas occur from the tearing of a meningeal artery, typically the middle meningeal artery. *The classic presentation is a child who sustains a head injury, followed by a lucid interval, and then develops deterioration.* The most common mechanism in children is a fall onto a hard surface from a height or motor vehicle accidents. The majority of epidural hematomas have associated skull fractures. A lens-shaped density is seen on CT scan. Shift of the ventricles across midline with potential herniation can occur with large hemorrhages. The prognosis for a favorable neurologic outcome is good with prompt neurosurgical intervention.

CHEST TRAUMA

Falls, motor vehicle accidents, and sports are the most common mechanisms for chest trauma in children. Penetrating trauma is a less common cause, but is increasing in adolescents. Chest trauma is much less frequent than head trauma in children, but is the second leading cause of mortality from trauma in children. Its presence often signifies potential severe multisystem trauma. Children are more at risk for significant cardiothoracic injuries because of a very compliant chest wall. The bony structures are much more flexible and withstand much larger amounts of force before breaking as compared with adults. This generation of forces may cause intrathoracic damage without evidence of external trauma. Because of the increased chest wall compliance, rib fractures are not prevalent in children. The presence of rib fractures is a risk factor for more severe injury. The earliest symptoms of intrathoracic trauma are tachypnea or hypoxia. Other symptoms include chest pain, noisy breathing, respiratory distress, or failure and bloody sputum.

Pulmonary contusions are the most common intrathoracic injury in children and are caused by blunt forces to the chest. External findings are often missing. These are caused by small areas of bleeding within the lung parenchyma. Symptoms may include chest pain or difficulty breathing. Some children may have only mild symptoms. Chest x-ray shows patchy density in the area of the contusion. Management is typically symptomatic unless there is significant respiratory distress. Patients with pulmonary contusions should be admitted to the hospital for further observation.

Simple pneumothorax is the second most common intrathoracic injury in children. Air accumulates in the pleural cavity secondary to injury to the lung tissue, penetrating injury to the chest, or disruption of the tracheobronchial tree. Patients may complain of difficulty breathing or chest pain. Diagnosis is made by chest x-ray. Treatment consists of chest tube placement, supplemental oxygen, and hospital admission.

Myocardial contusions are caused by blunt force to the chest and are rare in children. Patients often complain of chest pain and localized chest wall tenderness. Tachycardia is often present on examination. Diagnostic studies include obtaining an ECG and echocardiography. Controversy exists regarding the use of cardiac enzymes in the diagnosis of cardiac contusion. Dysrhythmias are a complication. *Commotio cordis* is a rare phenomenon occurring after a forceful direct blow to the chest. The impact causes ventricular fibrillation. This entity is immediately life-threatening and requires defibrillation.

ABDOMINAL TRAUMA

Blunt trauma is the most common cause of abdominal injuries; falls, sports, and motor vehicle accidents are the most common mechanisms. Children are more at risk for intra-abdominal injuries because of their more exposed organs and less overlying fat. Signs and symptoms of children presenting with potential abdominal trauma include abdominal pain and tenderness, abdominal distension, abdominal wall contusions, and vomiting. The spleen and the liver are the most frequently injured intra-abdominal organs.

The spleen is the most commonly injured intraabdominal organ after blunt trauma to the abdomen. Patient may present with *left upper quadrant pain or left shoulder pain.* Because of potential blood loss, hypotension, and tachycardia are also presenting signs. The diagnosis is made by CT scan. The majority of splenic injuries are small lacerations or subcapsular hematomas. Most of these injuries are managed nonoperatively with volume resuscitation.

The liver is the second most commonly injured organ after abdominal trauma. Liver injury should be suspected when there are symptoms of right upper quadrant tenderness. Hypotension and tachycardia may also be present because of the potential volume of blood loss. The diagnosis is made by CT scan of the abdomen. Liver enzymes are often elevated. The majority of liver lacerations in children are managed nonoperatively with observation and fluid resuscitation. Delayed bleeding is more common with liver injuries as compared with splenic injuries.

EYE INJURIES

Eye injuries are a common presenting complaint in children and are important because of the potential loss of vision. Trauma to the eye is the leading cause of monocular blindness in children. The most common mechanisms for eye injuries are blunt trauma to the eye, penetrating trauma and chemical exposure. Common complaints after an eye injury are pain, photophobia, diplopia, and loss of vision in an eye. It is important to note the use of contacts, corrective lenses, any history of systemic disease, and medication use. The ocular exam should include an assessment of visual acuity, extraocular muscle function, papillary reactions, an external exam of the lids, and direct ophthalmoscopy. Common eye injuries presenting for evaluation include corneal injuries, post-traumatic iritic and hyphenate.

Corneal injuries are extremely common in all age groups. Accidental self-inflicted injuries (e.g., fingers) are common as are chemical injuries, contact lens injuries, and foreign bodies. Symptoms may include pain, photophobia, excessive tearing, and a foreign body sensation. On exam, blepharospasm and a red eye may be present. To facilitate evaluation, the use of a topical anesthetic may be warranted. The diagnosis is made by the uptake of fluorescein dye in the area of the abrasion. The management includes cycloplegics to alleviate ciliary spasm. Topical antibiotics are used prophylactically to prevent infection. The use of topical steroids is contraindicated. Patching the eye is controversial; its use is being questioned because it impairs binocular visions and potentially traps infection. There has been no evidence to show that corneal injuries heal faster when a patch was used. Close follow-up with ophthalmology is recommended in order to ensure healing. If there are any concerns about potential embedded foreign body, CT scan is the study of choice, and ophthalmology consultation is recommended.

Post-traumatic iritis usually present 1 to 2 days after blunt trauma to the eye with resultant ciliary spasm. The patient may complain of photophobia, pain, and excessive tearing. There is miosis, marked blepharospasm on exam, and pain with accommodation. A slit-lamp exam will reveal flare and cells in the anterior chamber. Treatment consists of cycloplegics to relax the ciliary muscle and analgesics. Ophthalmology follow-up is recommended because a potential complication is acute glaucoma.

A *hyphema* is the layering of blood in the anterior chamber of the eye between the cornea and the iris. This injury is usually caused by blunt or penetrating trauma to the globe with subsequent bleeding of the vessels supplying the anterior chamber. Post-traumatic glaucoma is a potential complication because of impaired drainage of blood in the

anterior chamber with resultant increased intraocular pressure. Patients are also at risk for potential re-bleeding into the anterior chamber 3 to 5 days after the initial injury. Patients with hemoglobinopathies are at a significantly increased risk for re-bleeding. Management of hyphema includes bed rest with elevation of the head of the bed. Nonsteroidal analgesic and aspirin should be avoided. Because of the high risk complications, ophthalmology consultation is mandatory.

BURNS

There are more than 100,000 children injured because of burns each year in the United States. The majority of burns in children are scald burns, flame burns, or electrical injuries. There are different injury patterns based on age groups. The most common burn in toddlers and preschoolers is scald injuries from hot liquids. Directly touching hot objects, such as a space heater, is also a common mechanism. Unfortunately, young children also suffer from abusive burn injuries when the caretaker burns the child as a form of punishment. School-aged children and teenagers suffer more flame-related burns. In school-aged children, these injuries usually occur after playing with matches or lighters. Risky behaviors such as lighting fireworks or playing with flammable liquids cause burns in many teenagers. House fires also account for a percentage of burns in children despite the increasing use of smoke alarms.

Burns are classified according to the depth of the burn. A common classification system used divides the burns into first-, second-, third-, and fourth-degree burns. Newer classification systems have evolved to more accurately characterize the depth of the burn. The terms superficial, superficial partial thickness, full thickness, and deep full thickness (subdermal) are becoming more frequent in their usage in describing burns.

Superficial burns, previously called first-degree burns, are those burns isolated to the outer layer of the epidermis. These burns are erythematous and painful because of exposure to the superficial nerve endings. Blisters are not present. Typically these burns heal within 1 week without scarring. The treatment includes oral analgesics and topical moisturizers.

Superficial partial thickness burns, previously called second-degree burns, extend through the epidermis and into the top layer of the dermis. These burns are erythematous, moist, and painful because of nerve-ending damage and exposure. Blister formation is present. Treatment includes debridement of any loose necrotic material. Controversy exists as to whether or not intact blisters should be unroofed. Many experts leave the blisters intact and use them as a biological dressing, unless there is interference with joint mobility. Topical antibiotics, dressings, and oral analgesics are also part of the management plan. Scarring is uncommon. Close follow-up is recommended to ensure proper healing.

Deep partial thickness burns, previously third-degree burns, extend through the epidermis into the lower layers of the dermis. Sweat glands, hair follicles, and other adnexal structures are involved because of the depth of the burn giving the burns a dried pale appearance. Often these burns are not painful secondary to damaged and destroyed nerve endings. Scarring is common. The treatment plan includes debridement of devitalized tissue, topical antibiotics, and potential skin grafting. Treatment by a burn specialist is recommended.

Full thickness or subdermal burns, previously considered fourth-degree burns, extend completely through the epidermis and dermis, ending in the deeper subdermal layers, such as muscles and bones. The burn may be white, yellow, brown, or black with eschar formation. No blisters are apparent. The burn is minimally painful. The treatment, which may take months, needs to take place in a burn center, and involve skin grafting. Scarring will always be present.

The management of a patient with burns starts with assessing the "ABCs" and providing intravenous fluids as needed. Patients with extensive burns lose large amounts of fluids secondary to third spacing and capillary leakage. After stabilization, the extent and depths of the burns needs to be assessed. When calculating the percentage of body surface area (BSA) burned, burns affecting only the epidermis (first-degree) are excluded from the calculation. There are several different methods to calculate what percentage of the body surface area is burned. One must be aware that some methods are less accurate in young children because of differences in body habitus between young children and adults (e.g., the rule of nines). After determining the extent of the burn, the burn should be irrigated with sterile saline, devitalized tissue should be removed, topical antibiotics applied (silver sulfadiazine or bacitracin), and the burn covered with a sterile dressing. Tetanus prophylaxis should be updated, if necessary, at this time. Oral antibiotics are not a part of the initial management.

Indications for treatment at a regional burn center include:

- Burns accompanied by respiratory injuries or major trauma
- Major chemical or electrical burns
- Partial thickness burns >20% BSA
- Full thickness burns >2% BSA
- Any full thickness burns of the face, hands, feet, or perineum

One should always be aware of the potential for abusive burns. Examples of abusive burns are:

- Contact burns in recognizable patterns, such as the stocking–glove distribution on feet and hands
- Burns to the buttocks and perineum of young children
- Burns consistent with an object (e.g., hot iron) and circular cigarette burns

REVIEW EXERCISES

QUESTIONS

1. A 5-year-old boy is injured in an unwitnessed bicycle accident. He was not wearing a helmet at the time of injury. It is not known whether he sustained a loss of consciousness. A neighbor saw him lying on the ground, but the patient started moving soon after the fall and slowly walked home. He did not complain of headache or vomiting. A lump on side of head was noted by his mother. His mother called for an emergency squad 4 hours after the event when she found him unresponsive in his bedroom. On arrival to the emergency department, his heart rate was 100/min, BP 140/90, and respiratory rate at 10/minute. He was unresponsive to a sternal rub. He had a hematoma in the left temporal area. His left pupil was 6 mm and nonreactive, right pupil 3 mm and sluggishly reactive. The most likely cause of his clinical findings is:
a) Parenchymal contusion
b) Subdural hematoma
c) Basilar skull fracture
d) Epidural hematoma
e) Concussion

Answer
The answer is d. This is a classic history for epidural hematoma, in which a period of lucidity after the trauma occurs, followed by a significant change in mental status.

2. A 3-year-old male presents to your office after falling and hitting his forehead on furniture at home. He cried immediately. Has had no vomiting. He seems quieter than usual per mother, but fell asleep in the car. On exam, he is active and has a 2-cm hematoma over his mid-forehead. He is able to perform simple tasks. The remainder of exam is unremarkable. The next step in the management plan is to:
a) Obtain skull x-rays.
b) Discharge the child home with instructions.
c) Admit to the hospital for observation.
d) Obtain an MRI of the brain.
e) Obtain a head CT.

Answer
The answer is b. Given that he did not sustain loss of consciousness, has normal mental status, and no focal findings, imaging of the brain is not indicated. The child can be discharged home with instructions to return if he develops disorientation or unusual behavior, unusual drowsiness and sleepiness, inability to wake from sleep, increasing headache, seizure activity, or vomiting more than two times.

3. An 11-year-old boy presents with abdominal pain after being tackled while playing football at home.

His vital signs are normal. He has left upper and lower quadrant tenderness on exam. He also states his left shoulder is hurting. The most likely cause of his symptoms is:

a) Pancreatic injury
b) Duodenal hematoma
c) Renal contusion
d) Bladder rupture
e) Splenic laceration

Answer

The answer is e. The symptoms of left upper quadrant and left shoulder pain are most characteristic of splenic injury following blunt trauma.

4. A 14-month-old female is brought to the emergency department after grabbing and spilling her mother's coffee cup onto her 1 hour ago. On exam, she has edema, erythema and blistering over her right neck and upper chest, tapering toward her abdomen. The burn is very tender to palpation. The appropriate management plan would include the following *except*:

a) Referral to a burn center of plastic surgery
b) Systemic antibiotics
c) Debridement of open lesions
d) Topical antibiotics
e) Application of sterile dressings

Answer

The answer is b. All of the answers are indicated except systemic antibiotics. Immediate management of burns should include stabilization of the ABCs, obtaining intravenous access, and beginning fluid resuscitation, as needed. Assessment of the extent and depth is also important. The wound should be irrigated with sterile saline, devitalized tissue removed, topical antibiotics applied to partial thickness burns, and sterile dressings should be applied. Tetanus prophylaxis should be updated as needed. Systemic antibiotics are not part of the initial management of burns.

SUGGESTED READINGS

1. Baren JM, Rothrock SG, Brennan JA, Brown L, eds. *Pediatric emergency medicine,* 1st ed. Philadelphia: Saunders, 2008.
2. Bord SP, Linden J. Trauma to the globe and orbit. *Emerg Med Clin North Am* 2008;26(1):97–123.
3. Enrione MA. Current concepts in the acute management of severe pediatric head trauma. *Clin Pediatr Emerg Med* 2001;2:28–40.
4. Greenes D. Neurotrauma. In: Fleisher GR, Ludwig S, Henretig FM, eds. *Textbook of pediatric emergency medicine,* 5th ed. Philadelphia: Lippincott Williams & Wilkins, 2006:1361–1387.
5. Mlcak R, Cortiella J, Desai HH, Herndon DN. Emergency management of pediatric burn victims. *Pediatr Emerg Care* 1998;14(1):51–54.
6. Wegner S, Coletti JE, Van Wie D. Pediatric blunt abdominal trauma. *Pediatr Clin North Am* 2006;53(2):243–256.

Chapter 62

BOARD SIMULATION:
Pediatric Critical Care

Michael McHugh

In this chapter, a board simulation format is utilized to review a variety of pediatric emergencies.

QUESTIONS

Case 1

A 4-year-old boy was brought to your office because it was difficult to arouse him this morning. The parents recall no trauma. There are no medications at home that might have caused this. The family does not keep alcohol in the house. On your examination, the child is not moving, and does not rouse with stimulation. You note some diffuse swelling over the right parietal region. You palpate a fracture line of the parietal bone. The left pupil is 8 mm; the right pupil is 3 mm. There are no bruises noted. The rest of the examination is negative.

1. What is the *most* likely clinical diagnosis?
a) Toxic ingestion
b) Benign head trauma
c) Left focal seizure
d) Increased intracranial pressure (ICP) with impending herniation

Answer

The answer is d. The presence of mental status changes makes this scenario most consistent with nonbenign head trauma. The CT scan demonstrated that this child had a left parietal skull fracture with an expanding epidural hematoma. Most simple linear skull fractures in children are not surgical emergencies and require no treatment. In this case, however, the patient had an epidural hematoma with increased ICP and impending uncal herniation. Epidural hematomas often develop secondary to laceration of the underlying middle meningeal artery, and the palpable skull fracture overlying the course for this artery provides a clue to the diagnosis. The new onset of a unilateral dilated pupil indicates that the uncus of the temporal lobe is being displaced medially.

Toxic ingestions usually provide symmetric, nonlocalizing, neurologic signs. There is nothing in the history to suggest the onset of a seizure disorder.

Clinical signs and symptoms of increased ICP in infants and children include:

- Altered mental status
- Vomiting
- Cranial nerve III and VI palsies
- Altered vital signs (increased blood pressure, bradycardia or tachycardia, decreased or irregular respirations)
- Papilledema
- Full fontanelle (infants)
- Separated sutures (infants)
- Decerebrate or decorticate posturing

No single treatment for increased ICP exists. Supportive measures include respiratory and circulatory resuscitation, elevation of the head to 30 degrees, seizure and fever control, and maintenance of an adequate blood volume. Medical management of acutely elevated ICP may include:

- Airway protection using ICP protective strategies (full sedation, lidocaine, and paralysis)
- Controlled hyperventilation (brief)
- Mannitol and furosemide
- Hypertonic saline (3% saline) and control of serum osmolality
- Monitoring of ICP
- Mild to moderate hypothermia
- Dexamethasone
- Induced barbiturate coma
- Glycerol

Case 2 for Questions 2–4

An 18-month-old boy has had profuse watery diarrhea for 2 days. He has had poor oral intake and a low-grade fever. He is producing small amounts of dark urine. His parents report he is hard to arouse. His eyes appear sunken. He has no localizing signs.

2. Which acid-base state is the child *most* likely to have?
a) Metabolic acidosis
b) Metabolic alkalosis
c) Respiratory alkalosis
d) Mixed metabolic alkalosis and respiratory acidosis

Answer

The answer is a. Metabolic acidosis is the most common acid-base problem in pediatric emergencies. It results from a loss of bicarbonate ions or from a gain of hydrogen ions. This baby is hypovolemic and has lost large amounts of bicarbonate in his stool. Poor tissue perfusion and loss of base make metabolic acidosis the most likely acid-base state. Hypovolemia is the most common cause of shock in infants and children. Causes of hypovolemic shock include gastrointestinal hemorrhage, traumatic hemorrhage, fluid and electrolyte losses from gastrointestinal losses, and endocrinologic diseases such as diabetic ketoacidosis.

If electrolytes are checked, this child is most likely to have a normal anion gap acidosis (normal anion gap for a child <2 years is 16 ± 4). A bicarbonate level <12 has correlated with the need for hospitalization.

3. When lab values are drawn, his blood urea nitrogen (BUN) is 35 mg/dL and his creatinine is 1.0 mg/dL. What diagnosis *best* fits these lab values in this situation?
a) Prerenal azotemia
b) Henoch-Schönlein purpura
c) Hemolytic uremic syndrome
d) Acute tubular necrosis

Answer

The answer is a. Azotemia and oliguria may be caused by renal, prerenal, or postrenal etiologies. Prerenal causes of azotemia include decreased cardiac output (as in cardiogenic shock) and decreased intravascular volume (as in hemorrhage, dehydration, and "third-spacing" situations). Prerenal azotemia and hypovolemia cause the kidneys to preserve plasma volume. A BUN: creatinine ratio >20 suggests a prerenal state. If treated promptly, prerenal and postrenal etiologies are usually reversible. Untreated, this child could progress to acute tubular necrosis.

Henoch-Schönlein purpura is a vasculitic process mediated by the deposition of immunoglobulin A (IgA) containing immune complexes that typically present with the classic triad of a purpuric rash, crampy abdominal pain, and joint symptoms. Typically, the child is older than the one presented; the most common age distribution is from 3 to 10 years. There is frequently a history of a precedent upper respiratory infection. The clinical presentation of the child in question does not fit this diagnosis.

Hemolytic uremic syndrome is a syndrome of microangiopathic hemolytic uremia, thrombocytopenia,

and acute renal failure occurring typically in children <3 years. The typical form of the disease follows a diarrheal infection with toxin-producing *Escherichia coli*. This disease is more common in the summer months. It has been associated with contact with animals carrying the toxin-producing bacteria.

4. You decide that the child in case 2 requires volume resuscitation. Which is the *best* fluid to prescribe?
a) 20 cc/kg 5% dextrose water with lactated Ringer solution (D5W/LR)
b) 10 cc/kg 5% albumin
c) 10 cc/kg 0.9% sodium chloride (NS)
d) 20 cc/kg 0.9% NS

Answer

The answer is d. Isotonic crystalloids are the fluids of choice for volume resuscitation. The correct dose for most children is 20 cc/kg given as rapidly as possible. Using D5W/lactated Ringer solution will result in hyperglycemia. Lactated Ringer solution alone is an acceptable resuscitation fluid. Five percent albumin is an acceptable but expensive resuscitation fluid. Sufficient volumes of isotonic crystalloids, titrated to the adequacy of perfusion, are readily available and equally efficacious as resuscitation fluids. Unless there is a prior history of heart disease or a suggestion in the history of possible heart disease, the initial dose of fluid should be 20 mL/kg, given as quickly as possible (<15–20 minutes).

Case 3 for Questions 5–6
A 5-year-old girl darted into the street and was hit by a truck. She is conscious and well oriented, but complains of abdominal pain. Her abdomen is tense and tender. Vital signs reveal a pulse of 160/minute, respiratory rate of 25/minute, blood pressure of 140/90 mm Hg, and oxygen saturation of 98%. En route to the emergency department, she receives two boluses each of 20 cc/kg of 0.9% normal saline.

5. Why is she hypertensive?
a) Over-resuscitation (excessive fluid administration)
b) Traumatic avulsion of one kidney
c) Increased systemic vascular resistance
d) Increased ICP

Answer

The answer is c. The most likely cause is increased systemic vascular resistance. The sympathetic nervous system is rapidly engaged in response to trauma and blood loss. It helps to maintain perfusion of vital organs. Even if blood loss is not excessive, pain will similarly increase sympathetic tone and cause higher blood pressures.

It is highly unlikely that 40 mL/kg of normal saline would be excessive fluid resuscitation in this scenario. Traumatic avulsion of the kidney is possible, but is not as likely a cause of hypertension. Increased ICP is not likely in someone who is alert and oriented.

6. Which is the *best* vascular access for rapid volume resuscitation of this patient?
a) 20-gauge peripheral intravenous (IV) catheter
b) 4 F 15 cm double lumen central venous catheter
c) Intraosseous needle
d) 24-gauge peripheral IV catheter

Answer

The answer is a. A shorter, larger-bore IV line allows for rapid vascular access and rapid resuscitation. Therefore, a 20-gauge IV is preferable to a 4 F, 15-cm central venous line. The length of the catheter dramatically increases resistance to flow and decreases the rapidity of resuscitation. An intraosseous needle is usually used in pediatric patients with circulatory collapse or cardiac arrest and might be used if a peripheral catheter cannot be inserted.

Case 4 for Questions 7–9

A 4-year-old boy had an appendectomy. He was on a morphine infusion at 100 µg/kg/hour. He was found barely breathing by his nurse on rounds. His cardiac rhythm is sinus bradycardia (40 beats/minute).

7. Which is the *most* important drug for treating this child?
a) Naloxone
b) Atropine
c) Epinephrine
d) None of the above

Answer

The answer is a. The findings of coma, respiratory depression, and pinpoint pupils suggest opiate poisoning. Respiratory depression induced by the morphine infusion has likely caused hypoxia. The most common cause of cardiac arrest in children is respiratory failure. Following the mnemonic A (airway), B (breathing), C (circulation), this child first needs oxygen and positive-pressure ventilation. Opening the airway and providing rescue breaths may increase the heart rate. Administration of naloxone may reverse the situation and preclude the need for endotracheal intubation. Epinephrine is the first drug to use for bradycardia unresponsive to basic life support measures of airway opening, rescue breathing, and chest compressions.

Naloxone blocks the action of narcotics. It is rapidly effective, has a very short half-life and very few side effects. Administration of naloxone may reverse respiratory depression and preclude the need for endotracheal intubation. Repeat doses or a continuous infusion of naloxone maybe necessary to maintain the patient's respiratory drive.

8. What size endotracheal tube would you choose for this child?
a) Same size as his thumb
b) 5-0 uncuffed tube
c) 4-0 uncuffed tube
d) 4-0 cuffed tube

Answer

The answer is b. The appropriate-sized tube may be estimated by:

- The size of the patient's little finger
- By the formula $(16 + \text{age in years})/4$

Although these are two methods for estimating endotracheal tube size, it is important to also have the next larger and smaller sized tubes available. Uncuffed endotracheal tubes are typically used for children <7 to 8 years of age. Cuffed endotracheal tubes are used in those situations such as severe pneumonia or adult respiratory distress syndrome (ARDS) where very poor lung compliance is expected.

9. How does epinephrine primarily "work" in an arrest?
a) Decreased systemic vascular resistance
b) Improved coronary perfusion
c) Increased contractility
d) "Jump-starts" the heart

Answer

The answer is b. The *primary* effect of epinephrine is due to its α-adrenergic properties of peripheral vasoconstriction and resultant increase in systemic vascular resistance. This causes diastolic coronary perfusion to improve. Other important β-adrenergic effects do include increased contractility and heart rate.

Case 4 for Questions 10–12

A 12-year-old girl has known severe asthma. She presents with a wheezing episode. Her respiratory rate is 40/minute. She has intercostal and suprasternal retractions. She speaks in one-word responses, answering most questions with nods. She has diffuse bilateral wheezes.

10. Which blood gas is *most* reassuring?
a) pH 7.45; P_{CO_2} 35; P_{O_2} 60
b) pH 7.4; P_{CO_2} 40; P_{O_2} 60
c) pH 7.35; P_{CO_2} 45; P_{O_2} 60

Answer

The answer is a. In the early phase of respiratory distress with obstruction and hypoxemia, the asthmatic child usually responds with hyperventilation and a resultant decrease in P_{CO_2}. Stable asthmatics have metabolic reserve evidenced by a respiratory alkalosis. Therefore, the blood gas will reveal a low P_{CO_2} and an alkalotic pH. A "normal" or acidotic pH in a distressed asthmatic is worrisome, indicating retention of CO_2 and imminent respiratory failure. This patient demands aggressive therapy, follow-up examination and repeat blood gas analysis.

11. Many asthmatics are hypovolemic. Which of the following does *not* contribute to this problem?
a) Poor oral intake
b) Increased insensible losses
c) Syndrome of inappropriate antidiuretic hormone (SIADH) production

Answer

The answer is c. Asthmatics may be too distressed to drink and may have post-tussive emesis. Their rapid respiratory rates increase their insensible water losses. Although SIADH can occur in patients with asthma who have profound hypoxemia, this would result in fluid retention and overload rather than in hypovolemia.

12. Which of the following is an absolute indication for endotracheal intubation in asthma?
a) 85% oxygen saturations on 10 L/minute of oxygen through a nonrebreather mask
b) Depressed mental status
c) Severe wheezing
d) Respiratory acidosis on blood gas

Answer

The answer is b. All of these findings are worrisome and demand very aggressive medical management. Because gas trapping and air leak phenomenon are significant problems for asthmatics who receive mechanical ventilation, every effort is made to avoid intubation. A mental status change with an inability to protect the airway is the only absolute indication for intubation in this population.

Case 5 for Questions 13–16

A 15-year-old boy races mountain bikes. He crashes on a downhill and complains of severe chest pain. He is transported to the emergency department. You hear muffled heart sounds. His vitals are as follows:

- Pulse = 150/minute
- Respiratory rate = 18/minute
- Blood pressure = 90/60 mm Hg
- His oxygen saturations are 100% on room air.

13. What do you think is the *most* likely diagnosis?
a) Myocardial infarction
b) Fractured sternum
c) Pulmonary contusion
d) Cardiac tamponade

Answer

The answer is d. Muffled heart sounds and pulsus paradoxus are features of pericardial tamponade. This occurs when the amount of pericardial fluid reaches a level that compromises on cardiac function. A myocardial infarction is very unlikely. A fractured sternum should not result in muffled heart sounds. The features of pulmonary contusion from blunt injury to the chest include respiratory distress and hypoxia.

Other injuries that can result from blunt trauma to the chest include:

- Open pneumothorax
- Flail chest—resulting from multiple rib fractures
- Hemothorax—resulting from injuries to the aortic arch and systemic vessels
- Tension pneumothorax

- Tracheobronchial rupture
- Myocardial contusion
- Esophageal perforation

14. What should you *not* expect to find on physical examination?
a) Hepatomegaly
b) Abnormally bounding pulses
c) Jugular venous distension
d) Pulsus paradoxus

Answer

The answer is b. Cardiac tamponade compresses the atria, interferes with cardiac filling by decreasing venous return to the heart, and limits cardiac output. If the cardiac dysfunction induced by the tamponade has been present for an adequate period of time, hepatomegaly may be present. Therefore, the physical examination findings include muffled heart sounds, tachycardia, neck vein distension, hepatomegaly, and an increased pulses paradoxus. Tamponade results in weak, rather than in bounding pulses.

Pulses paradoxus is caused by the normal slight decrease in systolic arterial pressure during inspiration. With cardiac tamponade, this normal phenomenon is exaggerated; a pulsus paradoxus of >20 mm Hg is a reliable indicator of cardiac tamponade.

15. Which diagnostic study is indicated first in this patient?
a) 12-lead electrocardiogram (EKG)
b) Spiral computed tomograph (CT) scan of the chest and abdomen
c) Echocardiogram
d) Plain film of the chest

Answer

The answer is d. Plain film of the chest will easily show an enlarged cardiac silhouette in the setting of cardiac tamponade. This inexpensive, easily obtained study provides ample other information as well.

16. As you are looking at the chest x-ray (big heart), the patient has a falling blood pressure (50/30 mm Hg) and complains of being light-headed. What should you do next?
a) Pericardiocentesis
b) Fluid bolus
c) Intubate

Answer

The answer is b. Atrial compression caused by cardiac tamponade may temporarily be reversed with a 20 cc/kg fluid bolus. This allows the pericardiocentesis to be performed on a more stable patient. If pericardiocentesis can be performed, the clinical response is usually very rapid. Attention to the ABCs of advanced life support should be maintained while fluid resuscitation is ongoing. Equipment and personnel should be marshaled for possible additional interventions.

SUGGESTED READINGS

1. Bordley WC, Travers D, Scanlon P, et al. Office preparedness for pediatric emergencies: a randomized, controlled trial of an office-based training program. *Pediatrics* 2003;112:291–295.
2. Committee on Drugs. Drugs for pediatric emergencies. *Pediatrics* 1998;101:e13.
3. Guilli MF. Asthma update: epidemiology and pathophysiology. *Pediatr Rev* 2004;24:299–305.
4. Guilli MF. Asthma update: clinical aspects and management. *Pediatr Rev* 2004;24:335–343.
5. Heath BW, Coffey JS, Malone P, et al. Pediatric office emergencies and emergency preparedness in a small rural state. *Pediatrics* 2000;106:1391–1396.
6. Roberts JS, Bratton SL, Brogan TV. Acute severe asthma: differences in therapies and outcomes among pediatric intensive care units. *Crit Care Med* 2002;30:581–585.
7. Seidel JS, Knapp JF, eds. *Childhood emergencies in the office, hospital and community,* Evanston, IL: American Academy of Pediatrics, 2000.
8. Sartorelli KH, Vane DW. The diagnosis and management of children with blunt injury of the chest. *Semin Pediatr Surg* 2004;13(2):98–105.
9. Schwaderer AL, Schwartz GJ. Acidosis and alkalosis. *Pediatr Rev* 2004;25:350–356.
10. Wetzel R. Multiple trauma in children: a critical overview. *Crit Care Med* 2002;30:S468–S477.

Chapter 63

BOARD SIMULATION: Common Problems in Pediatric Surgery

Anthony Stallion

This chapter is an attempt to highlight common pediatric surgical problems that a pediatric practitioner will likely encounter in practice. This is not meant to be an inclusive or exhaustive summary of pediatric surgery. For more details on the topics covered in this chapter or other pediatric surgical problems please utilize the references given at the end of the chapter. The cases chosen as examples of each problem are representative of cases that you may encounter regardless if your practice is community or hospital based, and topics that are likely to be represented on board examinations. The discussion of each is an attempt to give you the answers as practiced by a significant number of pediatric surgeons. A board simulation format will be utilized for this chapter.

QUESTIONS

Case 1

1. The most appropriate treatment of an umbilical defect in a 4-year-old child is:
a) Expectant treatment
b) Immediate urgent repair
c) To have the child return in 1 year
d) Elective repair
e) Tape silver dollar on umbilicus

Answer

The answer is d. Umbilical hernias occur in about 7% to 8% of the population, with an equal male:female ratio. There is a marked preponderance in the African-American population. The defect results from incomplete closure of the umbilical ring. This natural process normally occurs shortly before or at the time of birth. Children in whom the umbilical ring does not close completely, will be left with an umbilical bulge. In 80% of these children, the defect will close spontaneously by the time they are 3 to 4 years of age. Thus, waiting until that time to see if the defect will close is the best practice. There are no manipulation maneuvers of the defect, such as daily reduction, use of a compressive patch, placement of a constricting coin or truss type of apparatus that will cause it to close spontaneously; either the defect will close or it will not. *If the defect has not closed by the time the child is of preschool age, the recommendation is to perform elective closure of the defect.* The choice of nontreatment will result only in persistence of the hernia, which will usually worsen as the patient gets older. Females will have a significant issue with protrusion, enlargement, and often pain once they begin childbearing.

For those patients that have at baseline a significantly increased intra-abdominal pressure, from entities such as ventriculoperitoneal shunt, ascites or peritoneal dialysis, the defect often will not close and may result with a progressive increase in size. There is also a higher incidence of recurrence if repaired. Under normal circumstances, <1% of patients experience recurrence. However patients with risk factors for increased intra-abdominal pressure have a higher incidence of recurrence after repair.

Patients who experience incarceration or develop recurrent episodes of localized periumbilical abdominal pain secondary to the defect, should undergo repair of the defect regardless of age. Giant defects (>4 cm), will not close spontaneously and often will show some signs of enlargement as the child is getting older. Skin breakdown may occur with larger defects because of constant irritation of the thin umbilical skin and may lead to early repair. If the large defects are uncomplicated, one can explain to the parents that these defects will not close spontaneously but undergo elective repair once the patients are 18 to 24 months of age. If they are repaired prior to that, they have a higher incidence of recurrence. Incarceration is unlikely in these giant, easily reducible umbilical hernias.

Case 2

A 9-year-old male just returned from a Florida vacation with an 8-day history of emesis that had turned bilious. He has a temperature of 101.5°F, acute abdominal pain and abdominal distension with 48 hours of urgency and watery diarrhea. His white blood cell count is 3.5/mm³ with 35% segmented neutrophils and 15% band forms. Urinalysis is positive for white blood cells and negative for leukocyte esterase. Physical examination demonstrates diffuse abdominal tenderness and dehydration. An abdominal radiograph reveals diffuse bowel gas with dilated loops, consistent with an ileus versus an early partial small bowel obstruction.

2. Of the following, the most likely cause of abdominal symptoms in this child is:
a) Gastroenteritis
b) Parasitic infection
c) Inflammatory bowel disease
d) Appendicitis
e) Malrotation

Answer
The answer is d. About 7% of the population will develop appendicitis at some point during their lifetime. The peak incidence is between 14 to 20 years of age. Fifty percent of patients <7 to 10 years of age will present with perforation of the appendix.

The diagnosis of appendicitis is usually made with a combination of history and physical examination findings. Most often, the physical examination tends to be the most reliable, especially with younger patients. Right lower quadrant tenderness is the most consistent feature. Younger patients often demonstrate atypical symptoms or quite often have a very rapid progression of their symptoms, during which they may perforate within 24 to 48 hours of the onset of the symptoms. It is unclear if this is because of a difference in the progression of the disease or because the patient may be less communicative and unable to really voice concerns until he or she becomes very ill. Thus, the abdominal tenderness and often right lower quadrant tenderness may be the only significant and consistent physical finding.

Ultrasonography, which is a reliable tool for experienced radiologist, can be used to assist in making the diagnosis of appendicitis. Those individuals who are comfortable using compressive grading for diagnosis of appendicitis with ultrasound tend to be quite accurate. However, consistent experience with this modality is mandatory for it to be helpful. It is the gold standard for ruling out ovarian pathology, which lends itself to being very complimentary to other modalities and the physical examination in the female patient. Computed tomography (CT) scanning is very reliable in making the diagnosis of appendicitis for all age groups; it is >90% to 95% accurate. The use of CT for the diagnosis of appendicitis is usually performed with oral, rectal, and intravenous contrast.

Once the diagnosis of appendicitis is made, an appendectomy is performed through an open versus a laparoscopic appendectomy. If the diagnosis is certain, the vast majority of the pediatric population at this point has their appendix removed laparoscopically. This has been the progressive trend over the last decade. At one time the decision was based on body habitus; the larger children doing best with a laparoscopic appendectomy versus the very thin, small child having the appendix to be removed through a small, right lower quadrant incision. Now parents actually request and expect that the procedure will be done laparoscopically. Data demonstrate that there is a slight improvement in recovery as well as decreased hospital length of stay for those who undergo laparoscopic appendectomy.

Patients who present with perforation and significant intra-abdominal soiling with gross peritonitis often require an exploratory laparotomy to control the intra-abdominal infection. There are patients who present with a localized phlegmon and/or abscess that can be treated conservatively with antibiotics, plus or minus percutaneous drainage. If successfully treated, they return in 8 to 12 weeks for an interval appendectomy. There are studies that state that the interval appendectomy may not be necessary and that the risk of recurrence of appendicitis is no higher than appendicitis for the general population once they have been adequately treated conservatively. The author recommends and takes all patients for interval appendectomies if the parents agree.

3. The most classic symptoms of appendicitis are:
a) Anorexia
b) Fever
c) Leukocytosis
d) Right lower quadrant tenderness
e) b, c and d

Answer
The answer is e. *The classic triad for appendicitis is right lower quadrant tenderness, fever, and leukocytosis.* However, of all patients who have appendicitis, only 30% present with that classic triad; thus, the majority of patients do not present with the typical or classic symptoms of appendicitis. This is especially true in the younger population.

Case 3
A 2-year-old female presents to your office with poor oral intake and excessive sleeping. Two days ago, she had a night of "trick or treating" and the next morning began having intermittent, severe abdominal pain lasting for 5 to 20 minutes between episodes. She did not have a documented fever. There was one episode of nonbilious emesis the morning of presentation. She had a recent upper respiratory infection 2 weeks ago. Exam demonstrates an afebrile girl with a benign abdomen but the patient is lethargic appearing. Abdominal radiograph demonstrates a nonspecific gas pattern. The white blood cell count is 9.5/mm^3. Urinalysis is negative.

4. Of the following, the most likely cause of these symptoms in a 2-year-old child is:
a) Gastroenteritis
b) Food poisoning
c) Intussusception
d) Appendicitis
e) Malrotation

Answer
The answer is c. The incidence of intussusception is 1 to 4 cases per 1000 live births. The peak incidence occurs between 6 to 18 months of age. The most common type is ileal colic intussusception. The lead point is most

often enlarged mesenteric lymph nodes, which is why there tends to have been a subclinical or clinical prodrome of a viral illness at some point in the recent past. A polyp, a Meckel's diverticulum, or a tumor can be the lead point, but these are much less common. The clinical presentation is the most important factor in making the diagnosis: crampy, debilitating intermittent abdominal pain with intervening periods of normalcy.

In the words of the senior pediatric surgeon Michael Klein, "Intussusception is a diagnosis made with the ears (i.e., by history) versus appendicitis, which is a diagnosis made with your hands (i.e., on physical examination-RLQ tenderness)." The crampy intermittent abdominal pain should increase the suspicion of intussusception. Quite often, the physical examination is unremarkable, as are plain abdominal films. Thus, having a negative x-ray or exam does not rule out intussusception. Other findings, such as the presence of a right upper quadrant mass or currant jelly stools, may be a part of the classic presentation but usually begin to occur when the intussusception has been ongoing for an extended period. Lethargy is part of the presentation in about 10% of cases.

Both diagnosis and treatment are achieved with a contrast enema. Air contrast enema is most commonly used today in place of radiopaque material. This is the case because of a decreased risk of significant intra-abdominal contamination in case of perforation. Quite often, many patients undergo a screening ultrasound, which, in experienced hands, can determine the presence of an intussusception by demonstrating the presence of a "target sign." If the ultrasound is negative, then the patient can be treated expectantly. If the ultrasound is positive, then they can move on to some type of enema. Gaining in popularity is the use of saline enemas under ultrasound guidance to determine reduction of the intussusception. This obviously avoids the use of any x-ray, thus avoiding the child's exposure to radiation.

These methods of reduction are somewhere between 85% and 95% successful. If they are unsuccessful in demonstrating complete reduction, the patient will require operative intervention and a manual reduction of the intussusception. This can be performed via open versus laparoscopic reduction. A small percentage of patients with intussusception that are not able to be reduced require resection of the ileum and cecum with a primary anastomosis as definitive treatment. This is also potentially performed in patients who have had multiple recurrences. There has been some description of the use of delayed enema studies once the patients has had an attempted reduction but cannot demonstrate reflux into the terminal ileum. In this situation, the patient is admitted to the hospital if he or she is clinically stable and returned to the radiology suite 8 to 12 hours after some of the edema has had a chance to resolve. The contrast enema is repeated to demonstrate reflux into the terminal ileum.

Case 4

A 5-week-old male presents with a 7-day history of increasing emesis that was initially described as "spit up," but then has become projectile in nature and consists of formula only. On physical examination, the infant is lethargic, and has depressed fontanels and a benign abdominal exam.

5. The most likely diagnosis in this 5-week-old infant is:
a) Gastroenteritis
b) Dehydration
c) Pyloric stenosis
d) a and b
e) b and c

Answer

The answer is e. Hypertrophic pyloric stenosis, which leads to persistent vomiting, dehydration, and electrolyte abnormalities, is a medical emergency. *The classic presentation is a patient who has a hypochloremic, hypokalemic, contraction, and metabolic alkalosis with paradoxical aciduria.* This electrolyte defect comes from significant emesis with the loss of potassium and hydrogen ions. The patient also becomes profoundly dehydrated. The renal tubules conserve sodium with the exchange of potassium for sodium so that intravascular hydration status can be maintained with conservation of fluids. Once the potassium has been depleted, another positive ion is required for exchange for the sodium. Thus, the body chooses volume status over acid-base status and then begins to release hydrogen ions in exchange for the sodium ions. Although the patient is already alkalotic, acid will be released, resulting in acidic urine in the presence of metabolic alkalosis (i.e., paradoxical aciduria).

The presence of a very low chloride and high bicarbonate levels leads to the potential for a depressed respiratory drive. For those infants that have a severe alkalosis, they may actually present with apnea. The other potential side effect of the electrolyte abnormality is the ability to breath spontaneously will be significantly impaired after completion of the procedure under general anesthesia. Thus, correcting the dehydration and electrolyte abnormalities are the most important issues that need to be addressed. During the course of the diagnostic workup, consideration should be given to other diagnoses such as gastroenteritis, intussusception, malrotation and gastroesophageal reflux. *Ultrasonography*, which can demonstrate the presence of the thickened pylorus as well as the narrowed pyloric channel and the lack of fluid emptying from the stomach, *is the gold standard for making the diagnosis.*
Once the diagnosis is made and the patient has had adequate resuscitation with correction of the electrolytes, he or she can undergo operative pyloromyotomy. This can be done by an open technique with the standard right upper quadrant muscle splitting incision or through a supraumbilical incision. Most recently, this procedure is done laparoscopically. Once the pyloromyotomy had been completed, by whatever method, care is taken intraoperatively to ensure that there is no perforation of the mucosa of the bowel. Patients can begin feeding in the immediate postoperative period, and they are progressed to regular feeds over the next 18 to 24 hours.

Case 5

An 18-month-old male presents with an 8-hour history of increasing irritability and emesis that was initially formula. The emesis has become green by the mother's history. Exam demonstrates a lethargic child with mild abdominal distension without a palpable mass.

6. The best course of treatment for this toddler with emesis and lethargy is:
a) Pedialyte and discharge home
b) Admit for IV hydration and observation
c) Immediate exploration
d) Upper GI and barium enema
e) CT scan of the abdomen

Answer

The answer is d. Given the child's age and this history, the immediate concern has to be malrotation and/or intussusception. Note that in the discussion of this case the most important point is that *bilious emesis is a surgical emergency until proved otherwise.* The history of bilious emesis has to raise significant concern that the patient has malrotation with midgut volvulus. This places the patient at potential risk for severe ischemic intestinal injury. With this patient's presenting symptoms, the differential diagnoses are:

- Gastroenteritis
- Intussusception
- Malrotation
- Potentially perforated appendicitis

The most life threatening is malrotation and this must be ruled out immediately. Malrotation is best described as no or incomplete rotation of the midgut (ligament of Treitz to the mid transverse colon). It occurs because of a failed completion of the normal rotation of the bowel after returning to the abdomen from the yolk sac. The bowel migrates through the umbilical ring at approximately 5 to 10 weeks gestation and elongates in the yolk sac. The mid gut return to the abdomen by the 10th to 11th week and undergoes a 270 degree, counterclockwise rotation with fixation to the retroperitoneum with the ileocecal junction in the right lower quadrant and the duodenal junction in the left upper quadrant to the left of the midline. This broad fixation prevents small bowel volvulus around the main blood supply (superior mesenteric artery). If the bowel does not undergo complete rotation, that allows for a narrow pedicle based upon the superior mesenteric artery and puts the patient at risk for a mid gut volvulus. In addition, the bands that usually reabsorbed with the fixation of the bowel to the retroperitoneum (Ladd's bands) remain and can cause obstruction, mainly at the level of the duodenum.

Unfortunately, the diagnosis can be somewhat difficult to make. Often the plain films are not helpful or they will show signs of bowel obstruction. The diagnosis is best made by an upper GI study, which will demonstrate the position of the ligament of Treitz, which should be left of the midline and up to the level of the pylorus. Often, it is beneficial in an infant this size, to obtain a "limited upper GI" in which just enough contrast will be used to confirm the position of the ligament. This requires an experienced pediatric radiologist. If it is normal, then the patient will have the contrast evacuated via a nasogastric tube and a barium enema can be performed to evaluate further the etiology of the vomiting and obstruction.

In this particular scenario with an acute onset of symptoms and when malrotation is diagnosed, the need for exploration is emergent. This is critical in order to avoid a potentially catastrophic situation with loss of all of the midgut, which occurs secondary to ischemic injury from a volvulus.

Case 6

A 2400-g female newborn born at 34-week gestational age presented with choking at delivery that resolved. APGAR scores were 6 and 10. The infant is now found to have increased secretions as well as choking and spit ups with formula feeds, and difficulty passing a nasogastric tube. The patient is afebrile with a white blood cell count of 15.5/mm^3. The total bilirubin level is 4.5 mg/dL. Exam is unremarkable. The x-ray demonstrates a right lower quadrant atelectasis and normal bowel gas pattern.

7. The most likely diagnosis is:
a) Formula intolerance
b) Gastroesophageal reflux disease (GERD)
c) Esophageal atresia
d) Esophageal atresia/tracheoesophageal fistula (TEF)
e) Prematurity

Answer

The answer is d. The incidence of esophageal atresia/ tracheal esophageal fistula (EA/TEF) is approximately 1 in 3000 live births. The clinical presentation is dependent upon the type of esophageal atresia and/or tracheoesophageal fistula that is present. These patients will often have polyhydramnios. Ultrasound may demonstrate the absence of the gastric bubble that potentially points to a pure esophageal atresia. *There are often associated anomalies, most frequently cardiac defects.* The other common constellation of abnormalities are: *"VACTERL" syndrome, which constitutes vertebral, anal/rectal, congenital heart disease, tracheoesophageal fistula, renal and limb anomalies.*

The most common type EA/TEF is the proximal esophageal atresia with a distal fistula of the esophagus

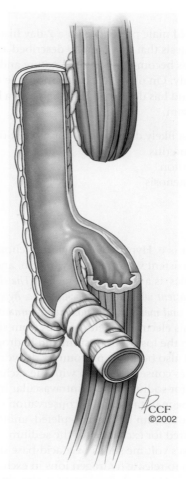

Figure 63.1 Schematic illustration of the most common type of tracheoesophageal fistula in which the lower esophagus is connected to the trachea by a fistula and the proximal esophagus ends blindly.

to the trachea (Fig. 63.1). This accounts for approximately 87% of cases. The next most common is a pure esophageal atresia in which no fistula is present (Fig. 63.2), followed by what is considered an "H type" fistula in which the esophagus is in continuity with a primary fistula between the trachea and the esophagus. The two least common are a proximal fistula with a distal blind pouch and a proximal and distal fistula, both of which account for well <1% of all cases.

The clinical features are secondary to excessive secretions. Infants may choke with attempts at feeding. There is an inability to pass a nasogastric tube. The upper esophagus and pouch can be outlined with air or the curling of the NG tube, which can be demonstrated by x-ray. No further studies are needed. Actually, an upper GI would be contraindicated because of the risk of aspiration. If there is distal fistula, the patients may demonstrate abdominal distension, especially if they are intubated. With positive pressure ventilation there is the potential for significant escape of the ventilated

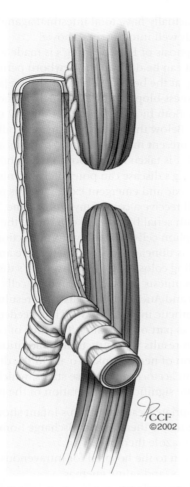

Figure 63.2 Schematic illustration of the second most common type of esophageal atresia in which no fistula is present.

breath through the path of least resistance, which often will be the tracheoesophageal fistula. Depending on its size, this may cause significant abdominal distension and may precipitate the need for emergent operative intervention with gastric decompression and/or ligation of the fistula.

The use of bronchoscopy to evaluate the fistula is important, as this can demonstrate its location. A search for other associated anomalies, such as the VACTERL syndrome, should always be undertaken. The treatment is usually primary repair in most of the cases, depending on the status of the patient, which includes gestational age, size, respiratory status, and other comorbidities. A staged repair may be undertaken if there is any question as to the ability of the patient to tolerate and obtain an adequate outcome with a complete primary repair. This may mean ligation of the fistula if present and the placement of a gastrostomy tube for feeding followed by the treatment of the other underlying issues. Repair of the esophageal atresia and/or fistula can then be accomplished at a later time.

Case 7

A 1-day-old female infant demonstrates intolerance of feeds with emesis that has turned bilious. The patient passed meconium after birth. On exam, she is lethargic but does not have abdominal distension and her abdomen is soft and nontender. She is afebrile. Her white blood cell count is 12.5/mm^3. X-ray reveals a double gas bubble; otherwise, a gasless abdomen.

8. The most likely diagnosis is:
a) Esophageal atresia
b) Duodenal atresia
c) Ileal atresia
d) Malrotation
e) None of the above

Answer

The answer is b. The presentation of duodenal atresia in the newborn is bilious emesis, signifying a high bowel obstruction. *The classic radiographic finding is the "double bubble" gas pattern on plain film of the abdomen* (Fig. 63.3). The etiology is unknown, but at the time of repair, an anterior pancreas or an anterior portal vein is sometimes found. The diagnosis can be made prenatally by demonstrating a gastric bubble and a separate upper intestinal bubble with no other significant bowel gas. However, this entity is often diagnosed postnatally by recognizing the sign of a bowel obstruction with a "double bubble" radiographic sign. *In 30% of cases there are associated anomalies, most commonly cardiac anomalies and/or trisomy 21.* This entity must be distinguished from acute malrotation with midgut volvulus. The treatment is direct primary repair that may require a bypass type anastomosis if there is an annular pancreas or anterior portal vein, since division should not be done in order to relieve the obstruction. The repair is well tolerated and patients begin feeding by

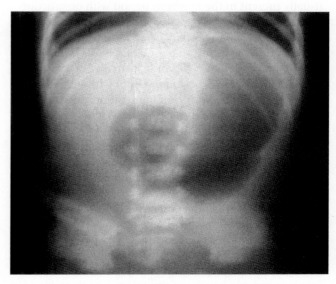

Figure 63.3 Abdominal radiograph illustrating the *double bubble*, characteristic of duodenal atresia.

the 7th to 10th postoperative day with progression of the feeds and without long-term sequelae.

9. The best next step in management of this infant is:
a) NG placement
b) Barium enema
c) Abdominal ultrasound
d) Upper GI
e) Attempt at refeed

Answer

The answer is d. Although the diagnosis is most likely duodenal atresia, given this history, an acute malrotation with acute volvulus must be ruled out, given that this patient did not have a prenatal diagnosis. It is unlikely that this neonate has an ileal atresia, which would result in multiple loops of gas filled of bowel. Thus, an upper GI would be appropriate with this acute onset of symptoms with no prior history.

Case 8

A 1-week-old male has had difficulty passing bowel movements since birth. He had passed a smear of meconium at 24 hours of life. He has had an increase in irritability, emesis, and abdominal distension with associated fever. Exam demonstrates a lethargic child with severe abdominal distension and diffuse abdominal tenderness. The white blood cell count is 22.5/mm^3 with 70% segmented neutrophils and 20% band forms.

10. The most likely diagnosis is:
a) Malrotation
b) Intestinal atresia
c) Hirschsprung's disease
d) Constipation
e) b and d

Answer

The answer is c. Infants with Hirschsprung's disease usually present in the newborn period with obstruction and possibly systemic toxicity. They may also have bilious emesis. A small percentage of patients will not be diagnosed in the newborn period and make it into the toddler years; there will be a much smaller percentage that will actually make it to preschool without a diagnosis. At that point, a significant higher index of suspension is required in order to make the diagnosis. Classically, patients with Hirschsprung's will have significant abdominal distension. A barium enema will demonstrate significant narrowing of the rectum with the rectal sigmoid index demonstrating that the most dilated area of the bowel is the sigmoid colon. Under normal situations the opposite should be the case, with the rectum distending to the greatest diameter of any part of the colon with the enema. Eighty percent of the disease occurs in the rectal sigmoid area. A smaller percentage have long segment Hirschsprung's disease which involves variable lengths of the colon. Less than 5% of patients will have total colonic Hirschsprung's disease

and <1% actually have total intestinal aganglionosis that extends well into the small bowel.

The diagnosis of Hirschsprung's is made with a rectal biopsy that can be done in the newborn period as a suction biopsy at the bedside. This can also be performed as a full-thickness biopsy, which is usually done under anesthesia. Both biopsies should be taken 2 cm from the anal verge. Below this level, there are generally no ganglion cells present in both diseased patients and normal controls. If it is taken much above that, a short segment Hirschsprung's disease can potentially be missed. If the patient is toxic and emergent exploration is required, the patient will receive a colostomy at that time. There is an attempt with serial biopsies to determine the level at which ganglion cells present by frozen section. The colostomy is done at the level where there are ganglion cells (leveling colostomy). Hirschsprung's disease histologically manifests as a lack of ganglion cells in the Meissner's and Auerbach's plexus. This results in lack of parasympathetic innervation which is needed for bowel relaxation as part of peristalsis. This area of constant contraction results in obstruction. In addition, there is proliferation of nerve trunks. To aid in the diagnosis one can perform acetocholinesterase stains, which will also demonstrate significant proliferation of the nerve trunks.

11. Appropriate treatment of this infant should include:
a) Oral Pedialyte therapy and discharge home with oral metronidazole therapy
b) Admission to the hospital for intravenous hydration, antibiotics, and saline enemas
c) Immediate exploration
d) Barium enema
e) b and d

Answer

The answer is e. Given this patient's presentation, the most likely the diagnosis is Hirschsprung's disease. This clinical picture, given the infant's toxic appearance, is very unlikely to be caused by constipation. Thus, intravenous hydration, antibiotics, and a saline enema are necessary in cases of suspected Hirschsprung's disease to relieve the obstruction of stool, the colonic distension, and the systemic toxicity that accompanies the obstruction. A barium enema is obtained to begin the evaluation for the presence of Hirschsprung's disease, but this can be performed once the patient has been stabilized and there is assuredness that the colitis has resolved.

Once the diagnosis has been made the determination as to how to proceed is based upon the clinical status of the patient. Patients who are toxic, with significant obstruction that is not relieved by enemas, require a leveling colostomy. Patients who are able to tolerate enemas and evacuate the colon without any episodes of colitis can then potentially be treated in the newborn period with a primary single stage pull-through. This can either be done openly or laparoscopically.

Case 9

A 1-hour-old infant girl has a protrusion of the abdominal wall containing the liver, small bowel, and stomach. There is a history of meconium-stained amnionic fluid, but the APGARS were 7 and 9, and on exam the infant's color is pink and she has a systolic murmur and large covered abdominal wall defect.

12. An appropriate treatment plan for this patient should include:

a) Intravenous fluids and antibiotics
b) Gastric decompression
c) Cardiac echocardiogram
d) Renal ultrasound
e) All of the above

Answer

The answer is e. Abdominal defects (Table 63.1) were described as early as the 1500s. They occur in 1 of 2000 live births. They are associated with advanced maternal age, and there are multiple modalities for treatment depending on the severity of the defect. They are often associated with malrotation caused by lack of the bowel returning from the yolk sac and undergoing complete fixation because of the abdominal wall defect. There are often associated congenital anomalies. The chromosomal abnormalities and congenital anomalies tend to be associated with omphalocele, rather than gastroschisis. The overall general prognosis tends to be quite good, especially for those patients with the smaller defects.

It is not uncommon for the defects to be diagnosed in utero by ultrasound, which has 75% sensitivity for omphalocele. The first diagnosis is made at 18 plus or minus 6 weeks of gestation. The sensitivity of prenatal ultrasound is 85% sensitivity in detecting gastroschisis, which is usually first diagnosed at 20 weeks ±7 weeks of gestation. There often is an elevated amnionic fluid (polyhydramnios) and serum alpha-fetoprotein (AFP); the acetylcholinesterase (ACHE) is usually 4 to 10 times greater than normal in the second trimester.

The embryology of the *omphalocele* is a true failure of development, migration and closure of the four embryonic folds (two lateral folds, a cranial fold, and a caudal fold) at the midline at the level of the central abdomen or epigastrium. These occur in 1 to 2 per 5000 live births. *The omphalocele is quite often associated with other midline defects such as cardiac, diaphragmatic, pericardial, diaphragmatic, genital urinary, and anal/rectal defects.* The defect is usually >4 cm in size and covered with a sac, unless it has ruptured in utero or during delivery and involves the umbilicus. Quite often, it will contain midgut, liver, and frequently the gonads or the spleen. Also, there may be abnormal insertion of the rectus muscles.

The embryology of *gastroschisis* possibly involves the failure of the umbilical celom to develop or weakening of the abdominal wall associated with the absorption of the right umbilical and abdominal wall vessels resulting in lateral abdominal wall rupture, usually to the right of the umbilicus. The defects are usually <4 cm. There is no sac present. It is often associated with prematurity and respiratory distress. It occurs in 2 to 3 per 5000 live births. The most common associated anomaly is a mid gut atresia. There are not often any other associated anomalies.

There is also a defect that is often called an *umbilical cord hernia*, which is <4 cm with an intact sac and/or is often epithelialized at birth. Associated anomalies are uncommon with this entity and once again the outcome is usually quite good.

There has been discussion regarding the most desired form of delivery with abdominal wall defects (vaginal versus elective C-section). There have been some data demonstrating that immediate repair will lead to better short-term outcome avoiding the development of congestion of the abdominal viscera, which will often delay repair. Long term, there has been no demonstration of any benefit to vaginal versus an elective C-section.

The initial management of abdominal wall defects comprises of gastric decompression, protection of the exposed bowel, thermal regulation, immediate and continual fluid resuscitation, and antibiotics to prevent infection. These patients often require ventilatory support. For patients with a murmur or omphalocele an echocardiogram is done as well as abdominal ultrasound to evaluate the kidneys and a chest x-ray to determine if there is any degree of hypoplastic lungs.

Operative treatment requires placement of a central venous catheter. Often these patients are delayed in their

TABLE 63.1

CHARACTERISTICS OF THE VARIOUS TYPES OF ABDOMINAL WALL DEFECTS

Type	Site	Presence of a Sac	Contents of the Defect	Associated Features	Outcome
Omphalocele	Umbilicus	Yes	Liver, intestine, gonads, spleen	Chromosomal anomalies; cardiac anomalies; midline defects	Fair–good
Gastroschisis	Right of the umbilicus	No	Intestine	Prematurity; respiratory distress; Mid-gut atresia	Good
Umbilical cord hernia	Umbilicus	Yes/No	Intestine	Uncommon	Good

ability to begin feeding and require total parenteral nutrition. A primary closure is preferred as long as the intra-abdominal pressure does not exceed 20 mm of mercury, which can be measured either via gastric or a bladder catheter. If the pressure is elevated after closure, a determination is made whether a patch will be placed versus delayed closure or placement of a silo. The staged repair with a silo can utilize a spring-loaded silo put into place at the bedside or one hand sewn into the fascia followed by serial reduction daily as the edema resolves. Eventual closure occurs at approximately 7 to 10 days after the placement of the silo prior to the onset of infection and sepsis.

The postoperative treatment after primary stage repair is measurement of intra-abdominal pressure to insure that there is no ischemic damage to the mid gut. Continued fluid resuscitation may cause some decreased pulmonary function and may require continuous ventilatory support. At this point gut profusion should take precedence over respiratory status. Intravascular blood pressure must be maintained to insure adequate intestinal perfusion. The use of sedation, rather than paralysis, is recommended for these patients, to avoid the increased third spacing associated with constant paralysis. Often, these patients will have a prolonged ileus requiring parenteral nutrition support until gastrointestinal function returns. Return of gastrointestinal function can be highly variable but loosely correlates with the degree of bowel edema, inflammatory peal, and amount of viscera that requires reduction. It can take up to 3 to 4 weeks before return of bowel function.

CONCLUSION

The cases discussed in this chapter are representative of common problems in pediatric surgery but by no means is it all-inclusive. You are encouraged to utilize the resources provided to gain more insight into what is covered in this chapter and learn more about the areas not discussed. Primary care providers will likely initially encounter these surgical issues. It is imperative pediatric practitioners have a working knowledge of surgical problems so that they can be readily recognized and referred. Remember that "no one wakes up in the morning saying that they need to see a surgeon."

SUGGESTED READINGS

1. Albanese CT, Sylvester KG. Pediatric Surgery. In: Doherty GM, Way LW, eds. *Current surgical diagnosis and treatment*, 12th ed. New York: McGraw-Hill, 2005.
2. O'Neill JA Jr., ed. *Pediatric surgery*, 5th ed. Philadelphia: Mosby, 1998.
3. O'Neill JA Jr., Grosfeld J, Fonkalsrud E, et al. *Principles of pediatric surgery*, 2nd ed. Philadelphia: Mosby, 2003.

Chapter 64

Orthopaedics for the Pediatrician

Thomas E. Kuivila

Orthopaedic problems, conditions, and abnormalities are presenting complaints frequently encountered by pediatricians and other primary care physicians who treat children. The intent of this chapter is to familiarize the practitioner with the common and some of the less common orthopaedic conditions of the neonate, toddler, child, and adolescent.

Orthopaedic congenital abnormalities can be categorized as:

- Structural
- Developmental
- Secondary to intrauterine molding
- Traumatic

Structural problems that represent abnormal intrauterine development are typically caused by an event, teratogenic influence, or genetic abnormality and are manifested in the first trimester of pregnancy. Orthopaedic conditions that fall into this category are frequently associated with visceral abnormalities, most often of the heart and genitourinary tract, because of the temporal proximity of events in development. So-called developmental abnormalities *(fetal arrest)* typically appear later in pregnancy and may be thought of as development that has stopped before completion. These conditions may affect the axial or appendicular skeleton. When an abnormality is in a lateral location, it is not infrequent for it to be manifested bilaterally. Packaging or molding abnormalities are a result of intrauterine forces and are therefore most common in cases of significant "tight packaging." Scenarios contributing to this phenomenon include the primigravida uterus, multiple fetuses, oligohydramnios, and other uterine abnormalities, such as significant fibrosis or a bicornuate uterus.

ABNORMALITIES OF THE NECK

The most common abnormality noted in children at birth is *congenital muscular torticollis,* which results from a sternocleidomastoid contracture. The sternocleidomastoid attaches to the mastoid process, and heads originate from both the sternum and the clavicle. When the muscle is tight or contracted, the head tilts toward and rotates away from the affected side. The condition is more common following prolonged labor and in first-born and high-birth-weight infants. It is associated with other packaging abnormalities, especially developmental dysplasia of the hip and metatarsus adductus.

Torticollis is thought to be caused either by prolonged intrauterine packaging in the noted position or possibly by an ischemic event within the substance of the sternocleidomastoid during a long labor process.

Treatment typically addresses the contracture. If the contracture has not resolved by the age of 12 months, surgical lengthening may be indicated. Persistent sternocleidomastoid contractures can result in long-term skull asymmetry and vision problems.

Klippel-Feil syndrome is a congenital synostosis of the cervical vertebrae. On radiography, the vertebral bodies appear to be fused. The condition results in diminished motion and increased stress across the vertebral segments that are not fused. Long-term instability of the neck and degenerative change can develop. Because this is a structural problem manifested in the first trimester, abnormalities of the genitourinary tract, cardiopulmonary system, and central nervous system are frequently associated with it. The congenital synostoses often cause the neck to appear short, and the hairline may appear low posteriorly.

525

Sprengel deformity is a failure of complete descent of a scapula. This is typically a unilateral condition. When it is severe, surgical intervention may be necessary to bring the scapula further caudal on the dorsal surface. Occasionally, an omovertebral bone may be present. This is a bony or cartilaginous band originating from the superomedial corner of the scapula that attaches to the spinous process.

Cleidocranial dysostosis is bilateral absence of the clavicles, which can result in problems of shoulder instability. However, the orthopaedic manifestations are typically not profound.

Congenital pseudoarthrosis of the clavicle is a condition in which an area of fibrous tissue is interposed in the right clavicle at the midshaft. A prominence in the midshaft of the clavicle is typically seen as early as 1 year. The etiology is unclear, but the condition is thought to be caused by underlying vascular structures on the right. The only reported case of congenital pseudoarthrosis of the left clavicle was associated with situs inversus.

The most common clavicular abnormality noted at birth or at any other time during childhood is a *clavicle fracture*. Birth fractures are typically caused by shoulder dystocia and paradoxically are good. In high-birth-weight infants, shoulder dystocia can stretch the brachial plexus and lead to lifelong debilitating problems. Fracture of the clavicle generally allows the shoulder to pass through the birth canal without nerve stretch. Clavicle fractures at birth and throughout childhood typically heal promptly without long-term sequelae.

DISORDERS OF THE UPPER EXTREMITY

Radial-ulnar synostosis is a congenital condition in which the radius and ulna are connected by a dense fibrous bridge or more commonly a bony bridge at the elbow. This prevents pronation and supination. When the condition is unilateral, typically no treatment is required because sufficient compensation develops. When it is bilateral and the hands are in an abnormal position, surgery is typically indicated to place the dominant hand in mild pronation and the nondominant hand in mild supination.

Another not uncommon finding in the forearm is a *congenitally dislocated radial head*. This condition, which limits pronation and supination in the upper extremity, although not to the same degree as radial-ulnar synostosis, is frequently noted incidentally on radiography performed to evaluate trauma to an upper extremity. It can be mistaken for an acute injury, but the radial head demonstrates classic signs of long-term dislocation, including a typical abnormal shape. Congenital dislocations of the radial head should be left alone because attempts to reduce the abnormality are fraught with complications.

Abnormalities of the hands include failure of formation of the digits with transverse or longitudinal deficiencies. *Duplicated digits* are not uncommon and frequently present as a "duplicate" thumb or sixth digit. These are typically excised early on for cosmesis and function. *Syndactyly*, a congenital connection between the digits, may be simple or complex, complete or incomplete. *Complete* or *incomplete* refers to the length of the digit that is attached to its neighbor. *Simple* or *complex* refers to radiographic appearance and whether or not the bones are similarly conjoined.

TORSIONAL AND ANGULAR ABNORMALITIES OF THE LOWER EXTREMITY

One of the most common reasons for referral to a pediatric surgeon is a malalignment syndrome of the lower extremity. To appreciate what is normal and abnormal, one must understand the etiology and natural history of lower extremity alignment.

Malalignment may be the result of a persistence of intrauterine positioning or part of the natural sequence of development. Children may exhibit deformities of the feet, tibiae, or femora. Although most of these are benign in nature and spontaneously resolve without treatment, some require manipulation, casting, or bracing, and some do eventually require surgery.

Important definitions are listed in Table 64.1.

Internal Tibial Torsion

Tibial torsion, or medial rotation of the tibiae relative to the knee axis, is commonly a result of intrauterine posturing and is frequently associated with metatarsus adductus. Within the uterus, the feet of the fetus are usually internally rotated; this position results in an internal or medial spin of the tibiae. The condition is most commonly noted at about the age a child begins to walk, and the parents bring the child for medical evaluation with concerns about in-toeing and frequent falling.

The natural history of this condition is spontaneous resolution in 95% of cases. Typically, 12 to 18 months after the child starts walking the tibiae are able to rotate to the normal final position of 10 to 15 degrees of external rotation relative to the axis of the knee.

Many braces and devices have been used in the past in an attempt to speed up this resolution. Excellent studies documenting their utility are entirely lacking, and most pediatric orthopaedists prescribe devices such as the Denis Browne bar, but usually only under significant parental pressure. Properly applied the Denis Browne bar does no harm, but it is uncertain whether it truly affects the natural history. Typically, the derotational process does not resolve spontaneously beyond the age of 4 years; therefore, if significant internal tibial torsion persists at this age, a surgical derotational osteotomy can be considered.

TABLE 64.1

IMPORTANT DEFINITIONS

Genu varum: commonly referred to as *bowlegs*.

Genu valgum: commonly known as *knock-knees*.

Genu recurvatum: commonly known as back *kneeing* or *hyperextension of the knees*.

Version: normal rotation present in many long bones with respect to plane of the joint motion axis.

Femoral version: angle between the transcondylar (knee) and transcervical (femoral neck) axes. Normal femoral version is 10 to 15 degrees—that is, a 10- to 15-degree angle is present between the two axes. If the transcondylar axis is aligned with the coronal plane, the transcervical axis is angled *forward* of the coronal plane.

Tibial version: angle between the axis of the knee and the transmalleolar axis. Normal tibial rotation is 5 to 10 degrees of lateral or external rotation.

Torsion: from the Latin *torsio,* "to twist." Pathologic rotational values are those that are two standard deviations from the mean.

Simple rotational deformity: involves one level.

Complex rotational deformity: two levels of involvement. They may compensate or accentuate each other.

Foot progression angle: angle between the longitudinal axis of the foot and the line of travel in gait. By definition, the value is negative in-toeing and positive in out-toeing.

In-toeing: medial or "inward" pointing of toes relative to the line of travel in stance or gait.

Out-toeing: lateral or "outward" pointing of toes relative to the line of travel in stance or gait.

Thigh–foot angle: angle between the long axis of the foot and the femur with the knee flexed 90 degrees.

Tibial–femoral angle: angle on frontal view (with knees fully extended) between the long axis of the tibia and the femur.

Femoral Anteversion

Anteversion of the femur refers to the fact that the plane of the femoral neck is rotated anteriorly to the plane of the knee. The normal adult value of anteversion is 10 to 15 degrees. The average value of hip anteversion at birth is 30 to 45 degrees. One does not typically see medial femoral rotation from anteversion early in life (the first 2 years) because the short external rotators of the hip (piriformis, gemelli, and obturator) are somewhat short and take 1 to 2 years to lengthen slowly. Once these muscles have achieved a normal length, greater internal rotation of the lower extremity is possible, and the consequence of persistent femoral anteversion becomes apparent. The hip is typically held in a position roughly halfway between the two extremes of motion (internal and external rotation). In cases of significant femoral anteversion, the hip is typically held internally rotated halfway between the limits of internal and external rotation.

Genu Varum and Genu Valgum

Most cases of genu varum and genu valgum seen in children are physiologic, not pathologic, in nature. Most children at birth are in 15 degrees or so of varus (bowleggedness). The varus angulation typically improves, and by the age of 18 to 24 months, the legs are straight on an average. The legs continue toward valgus alignment (knock-knees), reaching a nadir of 10 to 15 degrees of valgus at the age of 3 to 4 years. From this point, a gradual drift toward the average adult value occurs and is typically achieved by the age of 7 to 9 years—5 to 7 degrees of valgus in boys and 7 to 9 degrees of valgus in girls. Of course, values within a standard deviation constitute clinical normalcy. Individuals outside this range may have an underlying pathologic condition.

General management principles include the following:

- Avoid predicting the outcome; 95% of cases improve, but it is often impossible to identify the 5% that will not.
- Document the initial baseline values and those noted at subsequent examinations at 3- to 6-month intervals.
- Avoid shoe wedges, certain night braces, and other expensive orthotic devices, which have no scientific documented value.
- Reassure the family. This is important. Most cases improve. Surgery is rarely necessary, but it *can* correct deformities that do not improve.

The features of specific entities causing genu varum and genu valgum are summarized in the following.

Physiologic Bowlegs

- Lateral bowing: birth to 1 year of age, confined to *tibia,* no treatment required
- Physiologic bowing: 1 to 2 years of age, tibia *and* femur, no treatment required
- No bracing required

Physiologic Knock-Knees

- Peak: 3 to 4 years of age
- More pronounced in girls and obese children
- Progression documented by intramalleolar distance (upper limit of 10 cm)
- Resolution in most cases
- Osteotomy/hemiepiphysiodesis if deformity persists

TABLE 64.2

TWO CLINICAL PATTERNS OF TIBIA VARA

Age	1–3 Years	6–18 Years
Bilateral	Yes	No
Symmetric	Yes	Variable
Physeal bridge	No	Sometimes
Anisomelia	Slight	Significant
Resolution	Sometimes	No
Treatment	Brace early; osteotomy if progressive	Physeal bridge resection plus osteotomy

Tibia Vara (Blount Disease)

- Disordered growth of proximal medial physis and metaphysis
- Secondary to osteochondrosis caused by mechanical stress
- Frequently associated with medial tibial torsion
- Increased incidence in African American and obese children
- Two clinical patterns (Table 64.2)
- Radiography
    - Localized deformity at level of proximal tibia, medial metaphyseal lesion
    - Lateral translation of tibia relative to femur
- Treatment
    - Long leg bracing (begin with night bracing)
    - Osteotomy (before age of 4 years if possible)
    - Osteotomy/resection of physeal bar

Rickets

See also Chapter 18.

- Genu varum may be a clinical presentation of vitamin D–resistant rickets.
- It should be suspected in a child:
    - With increasing varus deformity
    - With a positive family history
    - Below the fifth percentile of height for age
- The diagnosis is confirmed by low levels of calcium and phosphorus, and a high level of alkaline phosphatase.
- Full-length anteroposterior (AP) film of lower extremity is required because deformity is *generalized.*
- Treatment:
    - Optimize medical management
    - Efficacy of bracing is controversial
    - Delay surgical correction until end of growth stage

Chronic Juvenile Arthritis

- Valgus deformity, overgrowth secondary to chronic synovitis
- Leg length discrepancy corrected with unilateral physeal sampling

SCOLIOSIS

The management of idiopathic scoliosis continues to advance at a remarkable rate. Although our understanding of its underlying etiology has advanced little in the last few years, the details of its treatment have changed dramatically.

Etiology

The etiology of idiopathic scoliosis is unknown. Abnormalities of vestibular function have been documented in many patients with scoliosis, but how they may cause or affect scoliosis is unclear. Similarly, changes in vibratory sensation (a posterior column function) have been documented, and therefore these may also be a factor. A related finding is that proprioceptive abilities have been noted to be less acute in some patients with scoliosis. One of the driving forces behind the development of the rotation-correcting instrumentation systems has been the belief that scoliosis, particularly in the thoracic spine, begins as an apical lordosis (or relative lordosis). It is postulated that this causes a rotational instability of the spine around which a curve develops. How and why this occurs is presently unknown, but the central nervous system dysfunctions noted in the preceding text may be a factor. It is clear, however, that derotation/translation of the scoliotic curve results in markedly improved alignment in both the coronal *and* sagittal planes.

The one etiologic factor not in dispute is the genetic nature of the disorder. Ruth Wynn-Davies has suggested a multifactorial inheritance pattern based on the prevalence of the disorder among first-, second-, and third-degree relatives. Cowell feels that the condition is more likely to be sex-linked dominant with variable expression and incomplete penetrance.

Natural History

An understanding of the natural history of idiopathic scoliosis is important in a discussion of treatment options, especially the option of observation with patients and their families. Several excellent studies have helped elucidate the natural history of idiopathic scoliosis. Lonstein and Carlson obtained abundant information from 727 patients with curves ranging from 5 to 29 degrees, whom they followed up to maturity or progression. Of this group, 23% overall showed progression, and *only* 18% required treatment. Patients with curves that required treatment tended to progress at a rate of 0.8 degrees/month, whereas those with curves that progressed at a rate of 0.3 degrees/month ultimately did not require treatment. The risk for progression is highest in patients with relatively severe curves noted early and in young and skeletally immature patients (Table 64.3).

TABLE 64.3

RELATIONSHIP BETWEEN INCIDENCE OF SCOLIOSIS PROGRESSION, MAGNITUDE OF CURVE, AND PATIENT AGE AT FIRST EXAMINATION

| Age First Seen (Years) | Percentage of Curves That Progressed | |
	Curves Measuring 5–19 Degrees (%)	Curves Measuring 20–29 Degrees (%)
<10	45	100
11–12	23	61
13–14	8	37
≥15	4	18

From Lonstein JE, Carlson MC. Prediction of curve progression in untreated idiopathic scoliosis during growth. *J Bone Joint Surg Am* 1984;66A:1061–1071, with permission.

Observation

Most curves do not progress to an extent that surgery or bracing is required. Approximately 2% to 3% of the population at the age of 16 years have a curve >10 degrees, but only 0.1% to 0.3% have curves >30 degrees. Observation is the treatment of choice for all idiopathic curves <25 degrees in skeletally immature patients. Curves <40 degrees in mature individuals can also be observed.

Brace Treatment

Bracing has progressed significantly from the Milwaukee brace, the first brace shown to alter the natural history of curve progression. The Milwaukee brace is and will likely continue to be the gold standard by which other bracing systems and protocols are judged. In most cases, however, the Milwaukee brace has been replaced by the lower-profile underarm thoracic lumbar sacral orthosis (TLSO), which has been shown to work well in preventing curve progression. The compliance issue has always markedly influenced the issue of bracing. It is difficult to get anyone, let alone a teenager, to embark on a treatment that creates an appearance "different" from the norm. It is for this reason that patients and their families have accepted shorter bracing periods, even if it is slightly less efficacious. Most orthopaedic surgeons now allow patients being treated with a TLSO to be out of the brace for 6 to 8 hours a day.

Another concept in bracing, the nighttime bending brace, has shown much promise and is far better tolerated than traditional day braces. The first of these was the Charleston bending brace; it was most useful for single thoracic curves and slightly less useful in controlling primary lumbar curves, and least effective in the management of double major curves. Far more popular now is the Providence brace.

The idea behind the night time braces is that the patient is fitted for a brace while bending nearly maximally out of the curve. The brace then holds this position during the hours of sleep, and no other bracing is necessary.

Surgical Management

Posterior spinal fusion remains the most commonly performed surgery for idiopathic scoliosis. Surgical intervention is generally indicated for curves >40 degrees in the skeletally immature and >50 degrees in skeletally mature adolescents.

Anterior release before posterior spinal fusion for rigid curves >60 degrees and all curves >80 degrees is a common rule of thumb. Thoracoscopic release with rib resection is an increasingly commonly used adjunct to posterior spinal fusion that will likely improve curve correction and cosmesis.

Thoracolumbar or lumbar curves with thoracic components <35 degrees are well suited for limited lumbar anterior spinal fusion. The screw-rod constructs available today are markedly better than the Dwyer or Zielke systems of the last decade in correcting scoliosis and restoring lordotic balance. The advantage of limited fusion is that preservation of motion segments may result in a superior correction.

COMMON DISORDERS OF THE HIP

Developmental Dysplasia of the Hip

The term *developmental dysplasia of the hip* has replaced the term *congenital dislocation of the hip* because this name more accurately reflects the fact that not all hip dysplasia in infancy is truly congenital in nature. However, *most cases of hip instability are noted at birth.*

The incidence of frank dislocation of the hip at birth is 1 per 1000 live births. Girls are affected more than boys by a ratio of 4.5:1. The incidence of mild hip instability at birth (i.e., a hip amenable to dislocation or subluxation) is 1 per 100 live births.

The incidence of hip instability in children with frank breech presentation is nearly one in five.

Early developmental dysplasia of the hip is best diagnosed in the newborn nursery or during the first few days of life. Careful examination of the infant is mandatory, and the child must be calm, relaxed, and not crying or fighting the examination. The presence of the *Ortolani sign* is pathognomonic for a *dislocated* hip. The absence of the sign, however, does not mean that the hip is normal. A positive Ortolani sign is reduction of a dislocated hip. The hip is gently abducted and lifted to achieve reduction. The "clunk" of the Ortolani examination is heard when the femoral head returns to the acetabulum. The *Barlow test* is a provocative maneuver in which gentle anterior-to-posterior compression is used to push a hip amenable to subluxation or dislocation partly or completely out of the acetabulum. After the age of 3 months, a dislocated hip is not easily reduced frequently. At this stage, the most common physical finding is asymmetry of abduction. Other physical findings include significant asymmetry of the posterior thigh fat folds and a positive Galeazzi or Allis test result.

Treatment before the age of 6 months is typically with a Pavlik harness. This holds the hips flexed and prevents complete adduction of the hip. If reduction of the dislocated hip is maintained, the capsular structures will tighten and provide normal hip stability 95% of the time. Further management is required when the Pavlik harness protocol fails.

When a hip is fully reduced early, the chance that it will be entirely normal at the age of 2 years and therefore in adulthood is excellent.

Legg-Calvé-Perthes Disease

Legg-Calvé-Perthes disease is a disorder of the growing hip, most frequently noted in children between the ages of 4 and 8 years (range, 2–12 years). It affects approximately two to five of 10,000 growing children; the male:female ratio is 4:1. It is bilateral 10% to 15% of the time, but both hips are rarely affected simultaneously. No evidence of an inheritance factor has been found.

Clinically, the child presents with a gluteus medius limp of insidious onset that is typically intermittent. Mild pain frequently radiates to the anterior thigh or knee. The referral of pain to the anterior medial aspect of the knee is typical in children with hip disease and is a consequence of the distal cutaneous distribution of the anterior branch of the obturator nerve, which also innervates the hip capsule. Internal rotation at the hip is typically limited, and mild muscle atrophy is present.

The radiographic findings initially are normal; later, an increased density of the capital femoral epiphysis is followed by absorption and subsequent reossification. The cause is unclear but is thought to be related to vascular embarrassment of the femoral head. The degree of vascular compromise determines the degree of involvement of the head. The prognosis is better when less than the full femoral head is involved. The prognosis is also typically better in younger than in older patients and better in boys than in girls overall.

The differential diagnosis of Legg-Calvé-Perthes disease includes:

- Toxic synovitis
- Sickle cell disease
- Hypothyroidism
- Idiopathic avascular necrosis
- Gaucher disease
- Hemophilia
- Juvenile rheumatoid arthritis

- Lymphoma
- Neoplasm

In true Perthes disease, the blood supply to the head returns, and the absorbed bone reappears. It is important to maintain containment during the course of the disease to keep the head as spherical as possible. The management for well-contained hips is observation. Hips that are not fully contained in a neutral position are often treated with an abduction brace or with a femoral or pelvic osteotomy.

The incidence of osteoarthritis of the hip is higher in individuals who have had childhood Perthes disease.

Slipped Capital Femoral Epiphysis

Capital femoral epiphyseal slip represents a dehiscence of the capital femoral growth plate. An association with thyroid dysfunction has been noted, but it is felt that a significant mechanical contribution is present in most slips.

The femoral head remains in the acetabulum, and the proximal femoral neck migrates anteriorly and laterally. The severity of the slip is based on how far the neck has moved relative to the femoral head.

As in other hip disorders of children and adolescents, the examiner must have a high index of suspicion to make the diagnosis because the early slip frequently presents as knee pain secondary to the referred pain mechanism. Typically, internal rotation is limited, and the child walks with a limp. In rare instances, the child may not be able to bear weight on the hip if the slip is significantly unstable.

The management of a slipped capital femoral epiphysis is surgical. The current standard management is placement of a single screw from the femoral neck through the growth plate into the femoral head to achieve stability. Significantly unstable slips are frequently fixed with two screws. Although the growth plate is shut down by screw fixation, this arrangement generally does not cause a significant growth discrepancy because the condition typically occurs in adolescents nearing the end of skeletal growth.

Complications of a slipped capital femoral epiphysis include *avascular necrosis* of the femoral head and a condition known as *chondrolysis*.

FOOT DISORDERS

Metatarsus Adductus

Metatarsus adductus (Table 64.4), also known as *metatarsus varus*, is commonly the result of an intrauterine position in which the midfoot is medially deviated because the lateral border of the foot is molded by the uterine wall. Metatarsus adductus is therefore considered a molding phenomenon and is associated with:

- High birth weights
- First births

TABLE 64.4
FEATURES OF METATARSUS ADDUCTUS

Demographics
  In 1000 live births
  Male:female ratio 1:1
  56% of cases bilateral
  10%–15% incidence of hip dysplasia; check for congenital
    dislocation of hip!
  Intrauterine molding vs. muscular imbalance
Natural history
  Prognosis depends on severity and rigidity
  90% nearly normal in 7 years
Treatment
  Nonoperative
    At 1–2 months cast for 1–2 months
    Casting improves results significantly when started at less
      than 8 months
  If flexible
    Mild or moderate
      Before 6 months—observation with or without passive
        stretching
      At 6 months if no improvement—serial casting
    Severe—serial casting
  If rigid—serial casting

■ Multiple births
■ Other conditions of fetal crowding, including oligohydramnios

An association with developmental dysplasia of the hip is noted in 10% to 15% of cases. Therefore, children with metatarsus adductus require a particularly careful hip examination.

Metatarsus adductus can be categorized in a number of ways. A useful classification system is based not so much on the appearance of the foot as on the degree of stiffness. Accordingly, a foot with mild metatarsus adductus would be passively correctable to past neutral, a moderately adducted foot would be correctable to neutral, and a severely adducted foot would be correctable to short of neutral.

In most children (90%) with metatarsus adductus, the condition spontaneously resolves without treatment. Interestingly, a correlation between the initial degree of stiffness and the likelihood of spontaneous resolution has not been found. However, in the United States, most patients who have severe (rigid) metatarsus adductus are treated with serial casting for a period of time. The process of serial casting begins with gentle manipulation of the foot and then placement into a holding cast for a short period of time, followed by further manipulation and casting. It should be noted that the cast itself does not correct the condition but maintains the correction achieved through gentle manipulation. Reverse-last or straight-last shoes are commonly used in the management of metatarsus adductus, although excellent studies demonstrating their efficacy are lacking. Reverse-last shoes are most often used after a period of casting or for feet that are correctable just to neutral. Feet that are passively correctable beyond neutral do not require treatment.

Clubfoot

Unlike metatarsus adductus, which is the persistence of an intrauterine position, structural talipes equinovarus, or clubfoot, is a true congenital deformity involving all bones of the foot. Clubfoot is found in approximately 1 in 1000 live births (incidence is higher in stillbirths). Boys represent 65% of cases (male:female ratio, 2.5:1), and 30% to 40% of cases are bilateral.

The highest incidence of talipes equinovarus is in individuals of Polynesian descent (6.8/1000); the incidence in African Americans is 3.5/1000, and in whites it is 1.2/1000. The lowest incidence is in Asians (0.57/1000). Many genetic diseases have clubfoot as part of the spectrum of problems. These include:

■ Autosomal dominant
  ■ Craniocarpotarsal syndrome
■ Autosomal recessive
  ■ Larsen syndrome
  ■ Diastrophic dwarfism
■ X-linked
  ■ Pierre Robin syndrome
■ Chromosomal abnormalities
  ■ Translocation of chromosomes 6 and 11
■ Neuromuscular
  ■ Increased in myelodysplasia, polio, muscular dystrophy
    and tethered cord

Foot problems are often bundled with other problems; 15% of patients have other congenital anomalies, and the rate of neurologic/congenital developmental dysplasia of the hip with vertical talus is high.

In neonates, the treatment for clubfoot consists of Ponseti casting. Extensive soft tissue releases have dramatically fallen out of favor in the management of idiopathic clubfoot as Ponseti casting typically results in superior correction and long-term improved flexibility. Minor soft tissue procedures may still be required. Bony work is typically reserved for older children and adolescents.

OVERUSE SYNDROMES

Overuse syndromes, perhaps more correctly termed chronic repetitive stress injuries, have become increasingly frequent in the pediatric and adolescent population over the last decade. The reason for this is severalfold. Some of these injuries are a result of poor conditioning, others are a result of inattention to proper warm up and stretching prior to an activity, some are related to increased intensity of activity, others are related to a lack of cross-training, and finally, some are caused by "over intensity." As the philosophical considerations regarding sports participation and parental/coaching involvement are beyond the scope of this chapter, we will focus on the conditions, their pathophysiology, and treatment.

The Inflammatory Osteochondroses

This group of disorders primarily involves inflammation at the tendon–apophyseal (the point on a bone where a tendon inserts) interface. The most commonly encountered condition in this category is *Osgood-Schlatter's disease*, which is an inflammation at the tibial tubercle as a result of repetitive strain on this junction. Tension occurs with each quadriceps contraction, which is more frequent in the jumping and sprinting athlete. With longstanding pull on the tibial tubercle, enlargement of the tubercle secondary to new bone formation can occur. A bony ossicle can actually form within the infrapatellar tendon itself and, in rare cases, a tibial tubercle avulsion can occur. This is a benign self-limiting condition, which improves with maturation and is eliminated with skeletal maturity. A prominent tibial tubercle, if present in adolescence, will persist throughout life. The prominence rarely causes any functional problem. Treatment of this condition is directed at relieving stresses across the tibial tubercle through good stretching of quadriceps and/or activity modification. Additionally, local anti-inflammatory control such as frequent application of ice and the use of an oral anti-inflammatory medication approved for use in children is beneficial. In cases of recalcitrant symptoms, significant activity modification is imperative. In rare instances, short-term immobilization may be necessary to control the discomfort. A thorough explanation of the condition and reassurances relative to the self-limiting nature are useful for the apprehensive teenager.

The calcaneal corollary to Osgood-Schlatter's disease is *Sever's calcaneal apophysitis*. The pain with this condition is located not within the Achilles tendon, nor within the plantar fascia, but rather at the insertion of the Achilles tendon into the posterior aspect of the calcaneus. Squeezing the calcaneus medially and laterally typically results in pain in these patients. Treatment of this condition is similar to that of Osgood-Schlatter in that Achilles tendon stretching, application of ice, and anti-inflammatory medications are useful. In addition, a silicone heal pad or a soft heal cup is a useful adjunct to the other management tools.

Lateral/Medial Epicondylitis

Lateral epicondylitis (tennis elbow) and medial epicondylitis (little league elbow) are common overuse phenomena involving the elbow. Typically, these are dominant extremity disorders and respond nicely, as do the other inflammatory syndromes, to rest, ice application, and anti-inflammatory medications. Little league elbow may have radiographic manifestations with overgrowth of the medial epicondyle. The overgrowth occurs

as a result of the repetitive valgus stress sustained with throwing. As the common flexor origin of the forearm attaches to the medial epicondyle and then to the distal humerus through a physis, elongation and enlargement of the medial epicondyle can occur along with distraction through the physis itself. The development of little league elbow and osteochondritis of the capitellum (see subsequent text) are reasons for limiting the growing athlete's pitch count *and* the number of hard and/or long throws the growing athlete performs on a daily basis. The distractive forces on the medial side of the elbow that result in medial epicondylitis have a corollary in compressive stresses across the lateral aspect of the elbow (radiocapitellar joint), which have greater long-term negative consequences. These compressive forces can result in articular surface injury, osteochondritis dissecans, which can develop into a life-long disability. The practitioner dealing with throwing athletes (baseball and softball) should focus on both medial and lateral aspects of the elbow when faced with a patient with elbow pain. X-ray and magnetic resonance imaging of the elbow are useful in evaluating the radiocapitellar joint.

Tendonitis

Tendonitis, once primarily a disorder of the adult, is for reasons cited earlier seen with increasing frequency in the adolescent population. Tendonitis is inflammation within the substance of the tendon itself and/or within the synovial-lined tendon sheath. Tendons themselves are not elastic, but a stretching of the associated muscle group is useful in diminishing tendon tension and stress. The most useful treatment of tendonitis, however, is rest and ice application. Nonsteroidal anti-inflammatory medications also have a role, but should not be used to supplant the rest program itself. Occasionally, recalcitrant tendonitis requires a splint or cast immobilization for an effective remediation of symptoms.

Ligament Injuries

Ligament injuries about the knee are among the most common ligament injuries in the child and adolescent athlete. The medial collateral ligament (MCL) is torn typically secondary to a valgus or rotational stress to the knee with the foot planted on the ground. Injuries to the anterior cruciate ligament (ACL) may occur in concert with the MCL or may be isolated. The typical mechanism of injury for the ACL is rotatory in nature. *When both MCL and ACL are injured, there is a high likelihood of an associated medial meniscal injury (terrible triad of O'Donoghue) and this should be carefully investigated.* Suspected ligament and/or meniscal injuries should be referred to a pediatric sports medicine specialist for definitive treatment, which may include meniscal and ACL repair. Depending on the patient's age at the time of an ACL rupture, definitive surgical treatment, if indicated, may be deferred until later in adolescence. Contrary to previous widely held dogma, the patient with open tibial and femoral growth plates may undergo an intra-articular ACL reconstruction without adverse results. An ACL injury seen with much greater frequency in the growing athlete than in adults is avulsion of the ACL from the tibial spine. These injuries require prompt treatment for optimal healing. When the fragment reduces well with knee extension, conservative management (casting) is appropriate. For those avulsions that do not spontaneously reduce, surgical intervention is required to reduce the bony fragment and, therefore, reestablish ACL insertional anatomy.

The most common sprain (ligament tear) in the skeletally mature population is in the anterior talofibular ligament of the ankle. Anterior talofibular injuries are rare in young children because the weak link is the physis (growth plate) of the distal fibula. As the physis begins its maturation, the ligament itself becomes a weak link and inversion injuries of the ankle are more likely to result in an anterior talofibular ligament sprain than a Salter-Harris I fracture of the distal fibula. When examining a patient with a ligament injury to the ankle, it is important to fully assess the circumferential ligamentous complex medially, laterally, anteriorly, and posteriorly. Radiography of the ankle (AP, lateral, and Mortise views) is the standard of care in the management of ankle injuries. Ankle sprains require 4 to 6 weeks of protection to achieve optimal healing. Reinjuries of the ligament during the healing phase can result in chronic ligamentous laxity and the tendon problems associated with joint instability. Mild to moderate ankle sprains typically do well with a removable, commercially available, medial–lateral well-padded plastic splint. More severe ankle sprains may require full-time cast immobilization for a short period, to be followed by medial–lateral splinting and subsequent rehabilitation. The value of formal rehabilitation to include range of motion, proprioception, and strength cannot be overemphasized in the management of ankle injuries.

REVIEW EXERCISES

QUESTIONS

1. The greatest risk factor for developmental dysplasia of the hip is:
a) Male sex
b) High birth weight
c) Breech positioning
d) Cesarian section

Answer
The answer is c.

2. Scoliosis >20 degrees in the skeletally immature
a) Should be followed up
b) Should be braced

c) Cannot progress
d) Will always progress
e) Usually requires surgery

Answer
The answer is a.

3. The *most* important function of shoes is to:
a) Provide ankle stability
b) Create an arch to prevent *pes planus*
c) Protect the foot
d) Create a fashion statement

Answer
The answer is c.

4. Metatarsus adductus is found in association with:
a) Tight packaging/high birth weight
b) Developmental dysplasia of the hip
c) Increased tibial torsion
d) All of the above

Answer
The answer is d.

5. A mother brings in her 3-year-old boy because she is worried about his knock-knees. The mother states that the boy was bowlegged at his first birthday; his legs then straightened, but he now has knock-knees. What would you tell the mother? What would you tell her if the knock-knees were significantly asymmetric?

Answer
Most children are born with about 15 degrees of bow-leggedness; the condition improves by 18 months of age, then progresses to moderate valgus before returning to mild valgus positioning. You should tell the mother that symmetric knock-knees are normal at this age. If the deformity is asymmetric, radiography is mandatory.

6. An obese 14-year-old boy presents to your office for evaluation of low-grade, diffuse knee pain. When you examine the patient, what else other than the knee should you examine?

Answer
This is the classic scenario for a slipped capital femoral epiphysis. A careful examination of the hip, with a search for asymmetry, should be performed. Radiography of the hips is also mandatory, including both AP and lateral views of the hip.

7. Significant injuries to the adolescent knee can result in injury to:
a) The ACL
b) The MCL
c) The menisci
d) All of the above and more

Answer
The answer is d.

8. Which factors may be to blame in the development of sports overuse injuries?

a) Inadequate conditioning

b) Bad coaching

c) Insufficient warm up

d) Zealot parents

e) All of the above

Answer

The answer is e.

SUGGESTED READINGS

1. Cowell HR, Hall JN, MacEwen GD. Genetic aspects of idiopathic scoliosis. *Clin Orthop* 1972;86:121–131.
2. Duthie RB, Houghton GR. Constitutional aspects of the osteochondroses. *Clin Orthop* 1981;158:19–27.
3. Guille JT, Pizzutillo PD, MacEwan GD. Developmental dysplasia of the hip from birth to six months. *J Amer Acad Orth Surg* 2000; 8(4):232–242.
4. Herring JA. Legg-Calvé-Perthes disease: a review of current knowledge. In: Barr JS Jr, ed. *American Academy of Orthopaedic Surgeons instructional course lectures, XXXVIII*, Park Ridge, IL: American Academy of Orthopaedic Surgeons, 1989:309–315.
5. Kobayashi K, Burton KJ, Rodner C, et al. Lateral compression injuries in the pediatric elbow: Panner's disease and osteochondritis dissecans of the capitellum. *J Amer Acad Orth Surg* 2004;12(4): 246–254.
6. Lonstein JE, Carlson JM. The prediction of curve progression in untreated idiopathic scoliosis during growth. *J Bone Joint Surg Am* 1984;66A:1061–1071.
7. Lovell WW, Winter RB. In: Morrissy RT, Weinstein SL, ed. *Pediatric orthopaedics*, 6th ed. Philadelphia: Lippincott Williams & Wilkins, 2006.
8. Pritchett JW, Perdue KD. Mechanical factors in slipped capital femoral epiphysis. *J Pediatr Orthop* 1988;8:385–388.
9. Resnick D. Osteochondroses. In: *Bone and joint imaging,* 2nd ed. Philadelphia: Saunders, 1996:960–977.
10. Riddick M, Price C. Time modified brace-wear, an effective alternative treatment regimen. *Presented at the 19th annual meeting of the Scoliosis Research Society, Orlando, FL: September, 1984.*
11. Riseborough EJ, Wynne-Davies R. A genetic survey of idiopathic scoliosis in Boston, Massachusetts. *J Bone Joint Surg Am* 1983;65A: 447–455.
12. Skaggs DL, Tolo VT. Legg-Calvé-Perthes disease. *J Amer Acad Orth Surg* 1996;4(1):9–16.
13. Herring JA, ed. *Tachdjian's Pediatric Orthopaedics*, 4th ed. Philadelphia: Saunders, 2008.
14. Teitz CC, Hu SS, Arendt EA. The female athlete: evaluation and treatment of sports-related problems. *J Amer Acad Orth Surg* 1997; 5(2):87–96.
15. Vitale MG, Skaggs DL. Developmental dysplasia of the hip from six months to four years of age. *J Amer Acad Orth Surg* 2001;9(6): 401–411.
16. Weinstein SL, Ponseti IV. Curve progression in idiopathic scoliosis. *J Bone Joint Surg Am* 1983;65A:447–455.
17. Weinstein SL, Zavala DC, Ponseti IV. Idiopathic scoliosis: long-term follow-up and prognosis in untreated patients. *J Bone Joint Surg Am* 1981;63A:702–712.

Chapter 65

Urology for the Pediatrician

Jonathan H. Ross

HYDRONEPHROSIS IN THE NEWBORN

Etiology and Epidemiology

The widespread use of prenatal ultrasonography has raised new questions regarding the evaluation and management of neonatal hydronephrosis. Before the use of prenatal ultrasonography, most newborn patients with hydronephrosis presented with an abdominal mass or urosepsis. *Indeed, the most common cause of an abdominal mass in the newborn is a multicystic dysplastic kidney and a close second cause is an obstruction at the ureteropelvic junction.* However, most cases of hydronephrosis are now being detected prenatally. Following the introduction of prenatal ultrasonography, approximately 90% of cases of ureteropelvic junction obstruction and 80% of cases of obstructed megaureter seen at the Boston Children's Hospital between 1979 and 1985 were detected prenatally. The postnatal detection rate was not significantly different from that of the era before ultrasonography. These numbers imply that the overall detection rate in infancy for such lesions is five to ten times higher than previous rates.

Pathophysiology

The ultrasonographic appearance of the kidneys changes during gestation. The output of urine begins at approximately 12 weeks of gestation. The bladder and kidneys are first visible at 14 to 16 weeks. By 16 weeks, urine is contributing significantly to the amniotic fluid volume, and the output of urine increases. Because of these changes in urine flow and renal growth, the significance of pyelectasis in utero depends on its degree in relation to gestational age. Prenatal ultrasonography is also able to detect some cases of renal dysplasia.

Diagnosis

Despite improving technology and technique, prenatal ultrasonography cannot be relied on for a definitive diagnosis. The accuracy of prenatal ultrasonography is operator-dependent, and it is generally easier to determine that an abnormality is present than to establish a specific diagnosis. Fortunately, the need to rely on prenatal ultrasonographic findings is very limited because prenatal intervention is rarely indicated.

Because a specific diagnosis cannot be made reliably with prenatal ultrasonography, the postnatal evaluation is crucial and is guided by the spectrum of anomalies seen in patients with prenatal hydronephrosis. Most kidneys prove to be normal postnatally. The frequency of this finding depends on the criteria used to define prenatal hydronephrosis. For those with persistent hydronephrosis postnatally, the differential diagnosis includes:

- Ureteropelvic junction obstruction (the most common cause)
- Obstructed megaureter
- Duplication with an obstructed upper pole moiety (secondary to ureterocele or ectopic ureter)
- Posterior urethral valves
- Prune belly syndrome
- Vesicoureteral reflux (may be the primary cause of hydronephrosis or associated with any of the preceding)

Treatment

Ultrasonography is usually performed in the first few days of life to detect any lesions that may require prompt intervention. These include severe bilateral obstruction or posterior urethral valves. In patients with purely unilateral prenatal hydronephrosis, the initial ultrasonography can be deferred. All infants with prenatal hydronephrosis are placed on antibiotic prophylaxis at birth. Amoxicillin can be used for the first month, and trimethoprim/sulfamethoxazole or nitrofurantoin thereafter. Antibiotics are continued at least until the nature of the lesion is defined. A second ultrasonogram is obtained some time during the first month. This follow-up study is important, even if the findings on the neonatal ultrasonogram are normal. Urine output can be very low in the first days of life and may be inadequate to cause urinary tract dilatation proximal to a significant obstruction. Careful ultrasonography can reliably detect the presence and level of obstruction. It should also detect duplication anomalies, particularly if the degree of pyelectasis differs in the two moieties. A voiding cystourethrogram (VCUG) is also obtained to rule out vesicoureteral reflux. Further management depends on the specific entity that is diagnosed.

Obstruction of the Ureteropelvic Junction

At the first month evaluation, most patients have an obstruction of the ureteropelvic junction. The next step in the management is a diuretic renal flow scan with DTPA (diethylenetriamine penta-acetic acid) or MAG-3 (^{99m}Tc-mercaptoacetyl triglycerine) to determine the degree of obstruction and relative function of the obstructed kidney. The renal flow scan can also distinguish a multicystic kidney, which does not function and appears as a photopenic region on the scan. Unobstructed or equivocal kidneys should be followed up with frequent ultrasonography during the first year of life (roughly every 3 months). In many cases, the hydronephrosis resolves. If it persists, another diuretic renal scan is obtained at 1 year. If the hydronephrosis increases during the period of observation, then the renal scan is repeated sooner than 1 year.

The appropriate management of the unequivocally obstructed kidney (defined by markedly prolonged clearance on the diuretic renal scan) is controversial. If there is decreased ipsilateral function on the renal scan, then surgical intervention is usually recommended. If there is normal ipsilateral renal function despite the obstruction, then close observation or surgical management may be undertaken.

Megaureter

Megaureter is the second most common cause of prenatal hydronephrosis. Evaluation usually consists of a renal/bladder ultrasound and voiding cystourethrography. Typical ultrasound findings are of hydroureteronephrosis with the hydroureter usually being more impressive than the intrarenal distension. Reflux should be absent on the VCUG, though, occasionally faint reflux into an obstructed ureter is seen. The use of diuretic renography is not established in evaluating washout from dilated ureters, although the analog images may be evaluated for a subjective impression of the degree of obstruction. The renal scan does offer a quantitative measurement of relative renal function. Many cases of megaureter resolve spontaneously. Surgical intervention is undertaken if hydronephrosis progresses, renal function

deteriorates, or symptoms such as pain or urinary tract infection develop.

Upper Pole Hydronephrosis in a Duplicated System

Upper pole dilatation in a duplicated system is generally secondary to an ectopic ureter or ureterocele. Lower pole distension may be a consequence of secondary obstruction by an upper pole ureterocele or of vesicoureteral reflux into the lower pole moiety. These lesions can usually be well characterized by a combination of ultrasonography, renal scan, and voiding cystourethrography. In difficult cases, a magnetic resonance urogram or cystoscopy may clarify the anatomy. Surgical intervention is usually indicated, the type of surgery depending on the specifics of the individual anatomy.

Posterior Urethral Valves

Posterior urethral valves are an uncommon cause of antenatal hydronephrosis and represent one of the few entities for which prenatal intervention is occasionally indicated. The diagnosis must be considered in any male neonate with bilateral hydronephrosis. All such patients should undergo postnatal ultrasonography and voiding cystourethrography in the first few days of life. If valves are present in a term infant, they can be treated with primary valve ablation. In a preterm or ill infant, vesicostomy can be performed, with valve ablation deferred until later in life. If renal function remains poor, with persistent hydronephrosis after successful valve ablation or vesicostomy, then higher diversion by cutaneous ureterostomy or pyelostomy is considered.

Multicystic Dysplastic Kidney

The options for managing a multicystic dysplastic kidney are to remove it, follow it, or ignore it. Surgical excision is supported by reports of hypertension and malignancy (both Wilms tumor and renal cell carcinoma) in patients with multicystic kidneys. However, the number of reported cases is small, and the total number of multicystic kidneys, although unknown, is undoubtedly large. Therefore, the risk for any given patient is probably extremely small and may not justify the surgical risk of excision. Most pediatric urologists recommend following up multicystic kidneys with periodic ultrasonography and blood pressure monitoring. Obviously, any patient in whom hypertension or a renal mass developed would undergo nephrectomy.

UNDESCENDED TESTIS

Etiology and Epidemiology

Undescended testis is one of the most common congenital genitourinary anomalies. The incidence of undescended testis is 3% in term infants. Many undescended testes descend spontaneously in the first months of life, and the incidence at 1 year of age is 0.8%. Boys with undescended testes are at increased risk for the development of tumors after puberty, and the testes do not produce sperm if left in an undescended location. When the descent of a testis through the normal pathway is arrested, the testis is said to be undescended. In contrast, the rarer ectopic testis has deviated from the normal pathway of descent. Possible locations for undescended testes include:

- Abdomen
- Inguinal canal (most common)
- Superficial inguinal pouch
- Pubic tubercle
- High scrotum

Ectopic testes may be found in the:

- Femoral canal
- Perineum
- Prepubic space
- Contralateral scrotum

Diagnosis

Because most undescended testes are located in the inguinal canal, they can be evaluated during a clinical examination. Impalpable testes present a more challenging problem and require a more extensive evaluation. When a child presents with an undescended testis, as with any congenital anomaly, a thorough history of the pregnancy and infancy is important. The parents should also be questioned as to whether anyone has ever felt the testis. Was the undescended testis noted at birth? This is particularly important in older children, who may have a retractile testis. A prior normal location of a testis, noted either during examination by the primary care physician or by the parents, suggests that the testis is retractile. Obviously, any previous inguinal surgery is important as a possible cause of secondary testicular ascent or atrophy. Although clinical hernias are uncommon in children with an undescended testis, most have a patent processus vaginalis, and it is important to inquire about a history of hernia.

The physical examination of a child with an undescended testis is a crucial part of the evaluation. A general physical examination is performed to assess surgical risk, and anomalies such as hypospadias, mental retardation, and other central nervous system anomalies, which are sometimes associated with undescended testis, should be sought. It is essential that the child be relaxed and warm during the examination. A cold room or a child's nervousness will exaggerate a retractile testis. Before the child is touched, the genitalia and inguinal region should be visually examined. Because the first touch may stimulate a cremasteric reflex, the best opportunity to see the testis in the scrotum is on initial inspection. A true undescended testis is often associated with a poorly developed hemiscrotum on the ipsilateral side. Placing the child in the frog leg position and gently milking from the inguinal canal to the scrotum often brings a high retractile testis down. If the

testis in question can be brought down in this way and remains in the hemiscrotum without tension, then the diagnosis of retractile testis is made. Applying a small dab of liquid soap to the examining hand can reduce friction and improve sensitivity in detecting an inguinal testis. Continuous age-appropriate conversation with the patient during the examination helps keep the child relaxed and improves the likelihood of detecting a palpable testis. Ectopic sites should also be palpated if no testis is felt in the inguinal region or scrotum.

The physical examination makes it possible to distinguish between an impalpable testis, a palpable undescended testis, and a retractile testis. In equivocal cases, reexamination at a later date often clarifies the diagnosis. When serial examinations leave the question of a retractile testis versus an undescended testis uncertain, a human chorionic gonadotropin (HCG) stimulation test can be performed. A variety of regimens are used. We administer 500 to 2000 IU (depending on body size) every other day for a total of five doses. It is generally agreed that a retractile testis will "descend" in response to HCG stimulation. Some truly undescended testes may also descend in response to HCG, although the actual success rate is controversial. Reported success rates range from 6% to 70%. Most retractile testes ultimately assume a normal scrotal position. However, occasionally a retractile testis will ascend with growth. Therefore, boys with a significantly retractile testis should undergo genital exams on an annual basis.

In the case of a palpable undescended testis, no further evaluation is necessary unless other genital anomalies are present. The most important genital anomaly is hypospadias, which occurs in 5% to 10% of boys with an undescended testis. Hypospadias in association with even one undescended testis raises the possibility of intersexuality. Patients with a unilateral undescended testis and hypospadias may have mixed gonadal dysgenesis and generally exhibit a mosaic karyotype of 45,XO/46,XY. Therefore, patients with an undescended testis and hypospadias should undergo karyotyping. If both testes are undescended, particularly if they are impalpable, then congenital adrenal hyperplasia (CAH) or other less common forms of intersexuality should be considered. CAH should definitely be considered in a newborn with bilateral impalpable testes and hypospadias because it is the most common cause of ambiguous genitalia. However, it should also be considered in the absence of a hypospadias because androgenization can be severe in this disorder. The initial steps in the evaluation are karyotyping and determination of the serum 17-hydroxyprogesterone level. These can rule out the two most common causes of ambiguous genitalia—CAH and mixed gonadal dysgenesis. Rarer causes of ambiguous genitalia, such as true hermaphroditism and male pseudohermaphroditism, must be considered if the child has a normal male karyotype. However, if the only genital abnormality is bilateral cryptorchidism, then a normal male karyotype is sufficient to rule out intersexuality.

In a boy with bilateral impalpable testes, the question arises whether the testes are intra-abdominal or absent. Bilateral anorchia can be diagnosed biochemically with an HCG stimulation test. Three 1500-IU doses of HCG are administered on alternate days. If the serum testosterone level does not rise and the baseline gonadotropin levels are elevated, then the child has anorchia, and no further evaluation is necessary. If the testosterone level rises after the administration of HCG, then the child has at least one functioning testis—presumably intra-abdominal. An HCG stimulation test may be avoided in a newborn by checking a serum testosterone level, which is normally elevated in the first weeks of life. If significant levels are detected, then at least one testis must be present and an HCG stimulation test is not required.

When a boy has a unilateral impalpable testis, an HCG stimulation test is obviously of no value. For such boys, and for boys with bilateral impalpable testes and a positive HCG stimulation test result, further evaluation is indicated. Several radiologic tests are available to identify an intra-abdominal testis. Ultrasonography, computed tomography, and magnetic resonance imaging (MRI) have all been used. The overall accuracy of these tests in localizing an undescended testis is 80% to 90%. However, most testes in reported series are inguinal. The accuracy of these imaging studies for localizing an intra-abdominal testis is <25%. Gonadal venography is more accurate and is able to locate or confirm the absence of an intra-abdominal testis in 75% of cases. However, this modality requires heavy sedation or anesthesia in children, and it is invasive and technically difficult to perform in patients <6 years old.

Because the readily available tests are insensitive for detecting an intra-abdominal testis, they are of little benefit. In the few cases in which a radiologic study identifies an intra-abdominal testis, an operation to bring the testis down is required. However, the failure of any of these tests to identify a testis does not mean the testis is absent; the false-negative rate of each test is significant. Therefore, a negative study result also mandates an operation to locate an intra-abdominal testis or prove definitively that it is absent. Because the results of radiologic tests do not alter management, they are of little value. A possible exception is the child whose body habitus makes physical examination of the inguinal region difficult. If ultrasonography can identify an inguinal testis in such a child, then the child can be spared laparoscopy.

Treatment

The standard treatment of a palpable undescended testis is an orchidopexy. Treatment should be undertaken by 1 year of age to maximize sperm-producing potential. Orchidopexy also places the testis in a palpable location for tumor detection, although it does not reduce the risk of tumor formation. An impalpable testis presents more of a challenge. In approximately 50% of boys with a unilateral impalpable testis, the testis is in fact absent on that side.

Because of the inability of radiologic studies to identify an intra-abdominal testis reliably, an operation is required to determine the presence or absence of an impalpable testis. The addition of laparoscopy to the surgical armamentarium has reduced the morbidity of these explorations. Prior to a formal surgical incision, laparoscopy is performed through a supraumbilical or infraumbilical incision. If an intra-abdominal testis is identified, then an orchidopexy is performed, which can be done laparoscopically. If blind-ending vessels are identified in the abdomen, then the procedure is terminated. If vessels are seen entering the inguinal canal, then inguinal exploration is undertaken. If a testicular remnant is identified, it is removed. If a viable testis is found, an orchidopexy is performed.

ACUTE SCROTAL SWELLING

The differential diagnosis of acute scrotal swelling in children includes:

- Testicular torsion (torsion of the spermatic cord)
- Torsion of the appendix testis
- Epididymoorchitis
- Hernia/hydrocele
- Testis tumor

The last two conditions do not usually present acutely, although they may do so on occasion. Findings suggestive of testicular torsion are an extremely tender high-riding testis, an absent cremasteric reflex, a cord that is thick or difficult to distinguish, and no relief of pain with elevation of the testis (as may occur in epididymitis). Although these findings are typical or suggestive of testicular torsion, their absence does not exclude the possibility. A urinalysis should always be performed because the presence of pyuria is very suggestive of epididymoorchitis.

TESTICULAR TORSION

Diagnosis

Radionuclide testicular scan and color flow Doppler ultrasonography have been employed to assist in the diagnosis of testicular torsion. Doppler ultrasonography is more commonly used and demonstrates an absence of blood flow to the testis in cases of testicular torsion. However, because the intratesticular vessels are small, reliable detection may be difficult and occasional false-negative and -positive results will occur.

Treatment

Surgical exploration is the definitive way to diagnose testicular torsion. Because time is essential, immediate exploration is indicated in any patient suspected of having testicular torsion. Most testes explored within 6 hours of the onset of symptoms are salvaged. Most of those explored after 24 hours are not. Waiting for a nuclear scan or ultrasonography to confirm the diagnosis is inappropriate. Radiographic studies should be reserved for patients in whom the likelihood of testicular torsion is felt to be low. As in appendicitis, occasional negative explorations are to be expected but are far better than a delayed exploration in a boy with torsion. At surgery, the testis is untwisted, and orchidopexy or orchiectomy is performed depending on its viability. Scrotal orchidopexy is also performed on the contralateral testis because the incidence of metachronous contralateral torsion is significant.

Testicular torsion also occurs in the neonatal period and should be considered in a neonate with a hard scrotal mass. Although the mechanism in neonates is different from that in older children, urgent urologic evaluation should be obtained.

TORSION OF THE APPENDIX TESTIS

Torsion of the appendix testis also presents as an acute scrotum. The appendix testis is a small, nonfunctional piece of tissue attached to the upper pole of the testis. It is often attached by a narrow stalk and is prone to torsion. Torsion of the appendix testis tends to develop in prepubertal children, who present with increasing pain and swelling for 1 to 3 days. The pain is usually not as dramatic as in testicular torsion. Often, appendiceal torsion can be diagnosed during the physical examination. A twisted appendix testis has a bluish hue when viewed through the scrotal skin, and a "blue dot" seen at the upper pole of the testis confirms the diagnosis. In the absence of a blue dot and other findings suggesting torsion of the spermatic cord, the diagnosis can still be made if scrotal tenderness is isolated to a hard nodule at the upper pole of the testis. However, by the time these patients present, the inflammatory response has sometimes spread throughout the hemiscrotum and a reactive hydrocele has formed, so that the diagnosis is difficult to make. Doppler ultrasonography can be helpful in ruling out testicular torsion by demonstrating normal blood flow to the testis, but occasionally the diagnosis can be made only by surgical exploration. When diagnosed clinically, appendiceal torsion is treated with nonsteroidal anti-inflammatory drugs, and the pain usually resolves within 7 to 10 days.

EPIDIDYMOORCHITIS

Epididymoorchitis is usually a bacterial infection in adolescents caused by enteric flora or sexually transmitted organisms. Before puberty, the inflammation may be bacterial or chemical. If voiding symptoms or pyuria are present, then epididymoorchitis is the presumptive diagnosis. Doppler ultrasonography confirms good blood flow, which excludes testicular torsion in equivocal cases. Treatment is usually with antibiotics against enteric organisms, although a sexually transmitted pathogen should be sought and treated in sexually active boys.

HYDROCELE AND HERNIA

Hydroceles and hernias may present as an acute scrotal mass. Hydroceles are nontender and transilluminate. A normal testis should be palpable. In equivocal cases, ultrasonography is diagnostic. Most infant hydroceles resolve by 1 year of age. Persistent hydroceles should be repaired to prevent the development of a hernia. Hernias do not transilluminate and can usually be palpated up to the inguinal ring. Bowel may be palpable in the inguinal canal. Again, ultrasonography is helpful in equivocal cases. Hernias should be corrected when diagnosed.

TESTIS TUMOR

Testis tumors usually present as a scrotal mass. They are generally painless and subacute. However, pain may develop in cases of a hemorrhage into the tumor. This should be suspected when acute scrotal swelling occurs after apparently minor trauma.

PENIS PROBLEMS

Phimosis, balanoposthitis, or paraphimosis may develop in uncircumcised boys. *Phimosis* is a progressive scarring of the prepuce that is usually caused by recurrent inflammation. The normal adhesion of the foreskin to the glans penis, and the normal inability to retract the foreskin in young children, should not be confused with pathologic phimosis. Evolution of the potential space between the glans and prepuce is a developmental phenomenon that occurs slowly after birth. Although the foreskin is rarely retractable in newborns, it is retractable by 1 year of age in 50% of cases and by 5 years of age in at least 90%. Virtually all foreskins become retractable during puberty. Therefore, "phimosis" is not a pathologic condition in young children unless it is associated with scarring, balanitis or, rarely, urinary retention. Failure of physicians and parents to appreciate this normal process has led to an overdiagnosis of phimosis. When truly present, phimosis may be treated with steroid cream or surgically by circumcision or preputiotomy (incision of the scar).

Balanoposthitis refers to inflammation of the prepuce and glans penis. Most cases resolve spontaneously, though topical or enteral antibiotics may be employed in more severe cases.

Paraphimosis occurs when the foreskin is retracted and not replaced over the glans penis. As a result, edema of the glans develops, with subsequent tightening of the prepuce. A vicious cycle ensues that may have to be corrected surgically. The problem is often iatrogenic and may be confused with balanitis.

Many penile problems can be avoided in uncircumcised boys if parents are properly educated in the care of the uncircumcised penis. The penis should be washed like any other part of the body, and the foreskin should not be retracted such that pain or preputial bleeding occurs. Forceful retraction is painful and may result in secondary phimosis. Keratin that collects under the prepuce is harmless and does not have to be removed from under the unretractable foreskin. In older boys, the foreskin is easily retracted, and the entire glans and preputial skin may be washed daily.

The most common complication of circumcision is meatitis, which can result in *meatal stenosis*. Many boys have a small urethral meatus. A small meatus is not a stenotic meatus. Meatal stenosis should be diagnosed only if the meatus is obviously scarred or if the observed urinary stream is thin or deflected. Meatal stenosis is easily treated with an office meatotomy after the application of topical anesthetic cream.

Hypospadias is a condition in which the urethral meatus is located on the underside (ventrum) of the penis. In most patients, the foreskin is incomplete ventrally, although not in approximately 5% of cases. Most patients with hypospadias also have *chordee* (ventral curvature of the penis). Chordee may also occur without hypospadias. *Hypospadias and chordee are contraindications to neonatal circumcision and should be repaired at 6 to 12 months of age.*

BLADDER INSTABILITY OF CHILDHOOD

Presentation and Pathophysiology

The most frequent cause of incontinence in children is bladder instability. Such children present with urge incontinence and squatting behavior or "potty dancing." Most have been wet since toilet training, although a dry period of several months after toilet training is not uncommon. Bladder instability represents a normal stage in the development of bladder control. In infants, a normal coordinated bladder contraction occurs with bladder filling. Once toilet trained, most children initially prevent wetting by activating the external sphincter when a bladder contraction is reflexively initiated by bladder filling. Most children quickly progress to direct central inhibition of bladder contractions with filling until they have an appropriate opportunity to void. A delay in the ability to inhibit bladder contractions centrally leads to the typical symptoms of bladder instability. These resolve spontaneously but may persist for many years in some children.

Diagnosis

Young children with typical bladder instability do not require a radiographic evaluation. Boys with severe symptoms or any child with symptoms that are not improving should undergo screening ultrasonography of the kidneys and bladder. A VCUG is obtained in any child with evidence of bladder wall thickening or hydronephrosis (to rule out reflux, neurogenic bladder, and posterior urethral valves). Urodynamic studies are unnecessary in children with typical bladder instability because they predictably reveal normal bladder compliance with uninhibited bladder contractions.

Treatment

Indications to treat the problem include associated urinary tract infections or vesicoureteral reflux. In the absence of these indications, treatment is initiated if the problem is causing enough psychosocial stress that the parents or child desire therapy. Conservative measures include timed voiding and treating any constipation that may be present because constipation is a common cause of bladder instability. If conservative measures fail, then medical management is initiated with oxybutynin chloride 0.5 mg/kg per day in three divided doses. Parents should be warned about the possible side effects of dry mouth, facial flushing, heat intolerance, blurred vision, and constipation. Fewer side effects may occur with more bladder-specific anticholinergic agents, such as tolterodine, which are available for children who can swallow tablets. Patients with associated recurrent urinary tract infections are also placed on antibiotic prophylaxis with trimethoprim/sulfamethoxazole 0.25 to 0.5 cc/kg once daily or nitrofurantoin 1 to 2 mg/kg once daily. Medical therapy is discontinued every 6 to 12 months to determine whether it is still required.

NOCTURNAL ENURESIS

Diagnosis

Most children with bedwetting have primary nocturnal enuresis. These are children who have been bedwetting since birth (although a dry interval of several months following toilet training is not unusual). The diagnosis is made in the absence of any daytime symptoms or history of urinary tract infections. The physical examination and urinalysis findings should be normal. A positive family history supports the diagnosis. In older children, screening renal and bladder ultrasonography may be performed, but this is generally unnecessary.

Treatment

Virtually all bedwetting resolves spontaneously sometime before adulthood. No treatment is necessary unless the problem is distressing to the child. Treatment is discouraged in children <6 years of age. Treatment options include:

- Enuresis (bedwetting) alarm
- Desmopressin
- Imipramine

The safest, most effective, least expensive treatment is a bedwetting alarm. However, the child and family must be committed to using the alarm for several weeks before results are obtained. Medications are reserved for those who fail to respond to an alarm. Two medical treatments are widely used. Oral desmopressin acetate is an expensive but relatively safe form of therapy. Treatment should be titrated to response from one to three tablets at bedtime until the lowest effective dose is determined. Treatment should be discontinued every 6 months to see if it is still required. Imipramine is an older medical treatment that is effective in many patients. Treatment is initiated at a dose of 25 mg every evening before bed. The dose can be increased to 50 mg, and in older children to 75 mg, as needed. It takes several weeks before an optimal effect is reached. Anticholinergic effects, altered sleep patterns, and behavioral changes may occur. Parents should be warned about the risk for accidental death by overdose in patients or younger siblings.

VARICOCELE

Varicocele is a varicose dilatation of the spermatic veins in the scrotum. It is recognized clinically as a "bag of worms," usually in the left hemiscrotum. Varicoceles are associated with infertility in adult men. Approximately 15% of adolescent boys and men have varicocele. Only 20% of adolescent boys and men with varicocele are infertile. Because adolescents have not had a chance to test their fertility and can rarely give a reliable semen sample, selecting which varicocele to correct is problematic. The most common indication for considering pre-emptive intervention is ipsilateral testicular hypotrophy, which occurs in approximately 50% of adolescents with varicocele. Correction is with outpatient surgery or transvenous embolization by interventional radiology.

REVIEW EXERCISES

QUESTIONS

Case 1
A term male infant was noted prenatally to have unilateral hydronephrosis.

1. What is the *most* likely diagnosis?
a) Ureteropelvic junction obstruction
b) Obstructed megaureter
c) Ectopic ureter
d) Ureterocele
e) Posterior urethral valves

Answer
The answer is a. Obstruction of the ureteropelvic junction is the most common cause of prenatally detected hydronephrosis.

2. If the bladder is also thickened, what is the next step?
a) Follow-up ultrasonography in 2 to 4 weeks
b) VCUG as soon as possible
c) VCUG in 2 to 4 weeks
d) Renal flow scan
e) Intravenous pyelography

Answer
The answer is b. With a thickened bladder, one must be concerned about the possibility of posterior urethral valves. It is not unusual for these patients to have unilateral hydronephrosis, so the absence of contralateral hydronephrosis does not rule out the possibility of bladder outlet obstruction. Valves should be treated in the first few days of life, so a VCUG to evaluate the bladder and urethra should be obtained as soon as possible.

Case 2
A newborn boy has a midshaft hypospadias and a right impalpable testis. The left gonad is in the scrotum.

3. Which of the following is *not* a diagnostic consideration?
a) Coincidental hypospadias and undescended intra-abdominal testis
b) Hypospadias and absent right testis
c) A girl with CAH
d) Mixed gonadal dysgenesis
e) True hermaphroditism

Answer
The answer is c. Any patient with hypospadias and an undescended testicle should be evaluated for an intersex condition. The most common cause of ambiguous genitalia is CAH in a girl. However, such patients have ovaries; therefore, both gonads would be impalpable. A scrotal gonad is virtually always a testicle, so this patient cannot be a girl with CAH. The impalpable gonad could be a streak gonad, reflecting a diagnosis of mixed gonadal dysgenesis (defined as the presence of a testicle on one side and a streak gonad on the other), or much less likely an ovary or ovotestis if the patient has true hermaphroditism (defined as the presence of both testicular and ovarian tissue). Although intersexuality is possible in this patient, the most likely scenario is not intersexuality but simply hypospadias and an absent or intra-abdominal testicle.

4. The *most* definitive way to distinguish between these possibilities is:
a) Karyotyping
b) Laparoscopy
c) Determination of the 17-hydroxyprogesterone level
d) HCG stimulation test
e) MRI

Answer
The answer is b. Laparoscopy allows a definitive identification of the impalpable gonad, which is necessary to

make a diagnosis. A karyotype would be very helpful because virtually all patients with mixed gonadal dysgenesis have a mosaic 46,XY/45,XO karyotype and most true hermaphrodites have a 46,XX or 46,XX/46,XY karyotype. However, occasionally patients with either condition have a 46,XY karyotype and the only certain way to make the diagnosis is to identify the impalpable gonad. 17-Hydroxyprogesterone levels are measured to confirm the diagnosis of 21α-hydroxylase deficiency (the most common form of CAH), which is not a possibility in this patient. HCG stimulation is used to determine whether testicular tissue is present. This patient has a testicle on one side, so the test result will be normal regardless of the character of the other gonad. Finally, MRI can identify the location of some impalpable gonads, but it cannot characterize them and does not visualize some gonads that are present. Because the patient will require laparoscopy in any case, MRI is not helpful.

5. If intersexuality is ruled out and an undescended testis is confirmed, at what age should the orchidopexy and hypospadias repairs be performed?
a) 3 months
b) 6 to 12 months
c) 2 years
d) 5 years
e) Puberty

Answer

The answer is b. The appropriate age for an orchidopexy is 6 to 12 months. Many undescended testes descend during the first year of life, most by 6 months of age. However, circumstantial evidence suggests that testicular function is best if an orchidopexy is performed at as young an age as possible. Therefore, once the boy is 6 to 12 months old (at which point the testicles will not descend spontaneously) an orchidopexy should be performed. Hypospadias repair should also be undertaken at 6 to 12 months of age. Waiting beyond that point offers no advantage, and ideally, all genital surgery should be completed by 18 to 24 months of age, at which point a child's genital awareness introduces increasingly problematic psychologic issues regarding genital surgery. Because a few patients require a second operation for complications 6 months after the initial repair, the original surgery should be completed by 1 year of age.

Case 3

An 8-year-old boy presents with acute scrotal swelling of 3-day duration. He has no associated voiding symptoms and rates the pain as 6 on a scale of 10. Physical examination reveals a reactive hydrocele on the right side with associated erythema and tenderness. The testis itself cannot be evaluated because of the hydrocele.

6. On the basis of the history, the *most* likely diagnosis is:
a) Testicular torsion
b) Torsion of the appendix testis
c) Epididymoorchitis
d) Communicating hydrocele
e) Testicular tumor

Answer

The answer is b. The history is typical of torsion of the appendix testis. The child is prepubertal, and the pain is moderate and has been present for a couple of days. Testicular torsion usually occurs in pubertal boys and the pain is more severe such that the presentation is more prompt. However, the historical factors are not definitive. Prepubertal boys can certainly suffer testicular torsion, and pain levels vary. This case is unlikely to be epididymoorchitis given the absence of voiding symptoms and the patient's age. Communicating hydroceles and testis tumors rarely present with acute pain. Acute inflammation within the scrotum secondary to testicular torsion, torsion of the appendix testis, or infection can result in a *reactive* hydrocele, as is seen in this patient.

7. Doppler ultrasonography reveals good flow to the testicles with an edematous mass at the upper pole of the right testis, separate from the testicle. You recommend:
a) Nuclear scan
b) Surgical exploration
c) Nonsteroidal anti-inflammatory drugs as needed
d) Antibiotics

Answer

The answer is c. The normal flow on the Doppler ultrasonogram combined with the history essentially eliminates torsion as a significant consideration. Therefore, neither a nuclear scan nor surgical exploration is needed. The edematous structure is likely a twisted appendix testis, which confirms the suspected diagnosis based on the patient's history. Torsion of the appendix testis is a self-limited disorder; the pain resolves spontaneously during 1 to 2 weeks. Nonsteroidal anti-inflammatory drugs are an adequate treatment of the pain while it lasts.

SUGGESTED READINGS

1. Cendron M, Huff D, Keating MA, et al. Anatomical, morphological, and volumetric analysis: a review of 759 cases of testicular maldescent. *J Urol* 1993;149:570–573.
2. Kass EJ, Stone KT, Cacciarelli AA, et al. Do all children with an acute scrotum require exploration? *J Urol* 1993;150:667–669.
3. Monda JM, Husmann DA. Primary nocturnal enuresis: a comparison among observation, imipramine, desmopressin acetate, and bed-wetting alarm systems. *J Urol* 1995;154:745–748.
4. Ransley PG, Dhillon HK, Gordon I, et al. The postnatal management of hydronephrosis diagnosed by prenatal ultrasound. *J Urol* 1990;144:584.
5. Diamond D. Adolescent varicocele. *Curr Opin Urol* 2007;17: 263–267.

Chapter 66

Ophthalmology Overview

Elias I. Traboulsi

The pediatrician plays an essential role in detecting visual and ocular abnormalities in children. Careful screening of vision by trained and patient assistants and personal examination of the pupils, ocular alignment, red light reflex, and optic nerve head by the pediatrician make it possible to identify such pathologic conditions as major malformations, strabismus, cataracts, and other causes of a white pupil. The child is then referred to the pediatric ophthalmologist for further evaluation and management. Some common ocular problems are easily managed by the pediatrician and referrals are only needed in case of non-resolution. These include nasolacrimal duct obstruction and conjunctivitis. The differentiation of allergic from viral or bacterial conjunctivitis allows the institution of appropriate therapy. In the following brief overview, the basic types of strabismus are covered, and the clinical features, differential diagnosis, and management of some of the common and less common ophthalmic conditions that pediatricians encounter in clinical practice are discussed.

STRABISMUS AND AMBLYOPIA

Ocular misalignment in an infant or child is suspected either because of parental reporting or through direct observation in the office. *Pseudostrabismus* is the false impression of ocular misalignment as a result of a prominence of epicanthal folds or variations in orbital alignment in a young child. Pseudostrabismus may simulate esotropia (inward deviation of an eye) or, less frequently, exotropia (outward deviation of an eye). *Symmetric and centered corneal light reflexes in both eyes and normal fixation patterns are usually sufficient to rule out true strabismus.* Parents can be reassured that epicanthal folds will decrease as the child grows and the nasal bridge becomes more prominent, pulling the skin away from the globe and uncovering more of the nasal sclera. A positive family history of strabismus should raise suspicion of true strabismus, in which case a detailed ophthalmologic assessment is always mandatory.

Amblyopia is the loss of vision caused not by an organic ocular or visual pathway lesion, but rather by disuse of one eye and predominant use of the other. The mechanism of vision loss is of visual cortical system origin. This is a reversible process in younger children; in addition to restoring good ocular alignment and binocular vision, one major aim of the treatment of strabismus is the prevention or reversal of amblyopia. Amblyopia therapy consists of penalizing the better-seeing eye to allow stimulation of the central visual centers from the deviated eye. This could be done either by using a patch or by blurring near vision in the better-seeing eye through cycloplegia with atropine drops. Atropine drops are generally not used in very young children. The younger the child, the faster and more dramatic is the response to short periods of occlusion therapy. Longer periods of patching or atropine penalization are required in older children. The upper limit of age at which amblyopia is still reversible is the subject of some debate; it may be approximately 10 years, however some older children may benefit from a trial of penalization.

Congenital or infantile esotropia may not present at birth but is diagnosed in the first 6 months of life. The angle of ocular deviation is usually large, and refractive error is minimal. Associated conditions include overacting inferior oblique muscles and dissociated vertical deviations, which may manifest later in childhood despite initial surgical therapy and good ocular alignment. Surgery should ideally be performed before the age of 1 year, preferably around 6 months, if binocular vision is to be achieved. A positive family history for this likely autosomal-recessive disease with high gene frequency is often elicited.

Accommodative esotropia is one of the most common types of strabismus and becomes evident in the first few

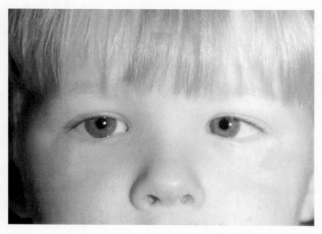

Figure 66.1 Child with left esotropia. Note location of the corneal light reflex at the temporal edge of the pupil. The child also has wide nasal bridge, which accentuates the appearance of esotropia.

years of life (Fig. 66.1). It is the consequence of accommodative efforts made in response to a relatively large degree of hypermetropia. The dysregulated convergence leads to ocular misalignment and the favoring of one eye with rapid development of amblyopia. Patients should be referred promptly. Therapy consists of the use of corrective glasses and surgery for any residual deviation.

Intermittent exotropia is an intermittent outward deviation of either eye that may become evident when the affected child is tired or ill. Exotropic patients often squint in the sunlight. Treatment consists of the correction of any error of refraction and close follow-up. There is no associated amblyopia. Surgery is indicated if binocular fusion breaks down and the ocular deviation is poorly controlled and is present >50% of the time.

Möbius syndrome is characterized by unilateral or bilateral sixth and seventh nerve palsies. Affected children usually demonstrate esotropia and an expressionless face. Babies with this condition have difficulty breast-feeding and sucking their bottles. Associated anomalies include the Poland anomaly (absence of the pectoralis muscle and radial defects) and terminal limb defects.

Extraocular muscle palsies in children result in incomitant strabismus (different magnitude of the deviation in different directions of gaze), with the largest deviation in the field of action of the affected muscle. Children with acquired palsies may not verbalize a complaint of diplopia, but they may squint, cover one eye with a hand, or assume a compensatory head posture to avoid diplopia.

Third nerve palsies are most commonly caused by trauma or increased intracranial pressure, and they may be complete or incomplete. Other causes include inflammation, infectious and parainfectious processes, vascular lesions, tumors, and degenerative and demyelinating disease involving the nerve. Diabetes is not a cause of third nerve palsy in children. Associated neurologic defects are good clues to the location of the lesion causing the nerve palsy.

Like third nerve palsies, *fourth nerve palsies* are commonly caused by trauma or tumor, but many are idiopathic and present at birth. An examination of old photographs reveals the characteristic head tilt and provides a good clue to the chronic and benign nature of congenital fourth nerve palsies. Surgery is indicated to relieve torticollis, which may lead to chronic neck pain and possibly back problems.

Sixth nerve palsies may indicate neurologic disease, but many are transitory and benign and follow viral infections. A sixth nerve palsy may be the result of increased intracranial pressure resulting from hydrocephalus, tumor, intracranial hemorrhage, or cerebral edema. It may be caused by trauma, inflammatory conditions such as meningitis, and degenerative or demyelinating conditions. Benign sixth nerve palsy in children develops 1 to 3 weeks after a febrile illness and usually subsides within 6 months. The child with cranial nerve palsy should undergo a complete neurologic evaluation, including computed tomography or magnetic resonance imaging of the head. A history of recent viral disease should be obtained, and the child should receive care from an ophthalmologist and a neurologist. The acute development of nonaccommodative esotropia and weakness of one or both lateral rectus muscles may indicate the presence of a Chiari malformation.

Nystagmus refers to rhythmic oscillations of the eyes that occur independently of normal movements. In pendular nystagmus, the velocity of movement is equal in the two directions. In contrast, jerk nystagmus has slow and fast components. The different kinds of nystagmus are named according to the refixation and the direction in which the nystagmus occurs (e.g., in right-beating jerk nystagmus, the fast refixation component is to the right). In conjugate nystagmus, the binocular oscillations are in phase, whereas disconjugate or dissociated nystagmus can be monocular or binocular with a slow component that is out of phase. Latent nystagmus is elicited by an interruption of binocular vision, such as the occlusion of one eye. Infantile nystagmus is present at birth and may be associated with abnormal head movements and positions. Visual acuity is usually decreased. Albinism is probably the most common cause of nystagmus in childhood. Tyrosinase-positive oculocutaneous albinism may be difficult to diagnose except with the slit-lamp. Retroillumination reveals iris transillumination in patients with any type of albinism. In addition, patients with albinism exhibit foveal hypoplasia and misrouting of optic nerve fibers. There are numerous causes of sensory (resulting from poor vision) nystagmus, mostly related to structural ocular abnormalities such as aniridia or cataracts that lead to poor vision. Central nervous disease can lead to nystagmus through interference with the centers that control eye movement. Nystagmus can be familial and is most commonly inherited in an X-linked fashion.

OBSTRUCTION OF THE NASOLACRIMAL DUCT

Most cases of obstruction of lacrimal drainage in children are developmental; others are caused by infections, trauma, and lid dysfunction. Obstruction of the nasolacrimal duct, most commonly caused by a failure of the distal membranous end of the nasolacrimal duct to open, occurs in approximately 5% of infants and is bilateral in as many as one third of cases. Obstruction of the nasolacrimal duct may be caused by blockage elsewhere in the lacrimal system or by an absence of the puncti or canaliculi, which interferes with the normal drainage of tears. Rarely, lacrimal obstruction occurs as part of the facial clefting syndromes and the Goldenhar syndrome.

Infants with lacrimal obstruction present with a "wet-eyed" appearance, persistent or intermittent tearing, and various degrees of mucopurulent discharge over the medial canthal area and lids. Pressure over the area of the lacrimal sac expresses whitish material from the lacrimal puncti. Superimposed dacryocystitis may be present, and dacryocystoceles or fistulae may develop.

Most obstructions (90%) resolve spontaneously by 18 months, and lid hygiene alone is the indicated treatment in most cases. Fingertip compressions over the area of the lacrimal sac, with massage directed centrally while the upper end of the lacrimal system is blocked, may be tried for a short period of time; this maneuver increases pressure inside the system, possibly causing the distal membrane to rupture into the nose. Long-term antibiotic therapy should be avoided. Some pediatric ophthalmologists prefer early probing after a short trial of conservative management for 2 to 4 weeks; this results in early patency of the system and avoids potential infections and continuous irritation and annoyance. Probing is performed in the operating room with the patient under inhalation anesthesia. The surgery is successful >90% of cases. If it fails, it can be repeated with or without silicone intubation of the lacrimal system. Silicone stents are left in place for 3 to 6 months. If probing and silicone intubation fail to maintain a patent system, a dacryocystorhinostomy is performed. This procedure provides direct drainage of tears from the lacrimal sac into the nose. Dacryocystitis should be treated with systemic antibiotics and may resolve only after nasolacrimal probing.

The differential diagnosis of tearing in the infant includes congenital glaucoma. The latter can be differentiated from nasolacrimal duct obstruction by the presence of an enlarged and hazy cornea, sensitivity to light, and elevated intraocular pressure in congenital glaucoma.

LEUKOCORIA (WHITE PUPIL): DIFFERENTIAL DIAGNOSIS OF RETINOBLASTOMA

The differential diagnosis of a white pupillary reflex (or for that matter an abnormal pupillary light reflex) in an infant is the differential diagnosis of retinoblastoma. Leukocoria, or white pupil (Fig. 66.2), is a white or tan reflex in the normally black pupillary area. The reflex, which may be observed in certain ambient lighting conditions or only in certain directions of gaze, can theoretically result from the opacification or tumefaction of any structure behind the iris (e.g., lens, vitreous, retina, choroid). The exact cause of the white reflex should be determined as soon as possible so that treatment of the underlying disease can be started.

Retinoblastoma occurs in 1 per 13,000 live births. Forty percent of cases are heritable, 5% are familial, and the rest are sporadic and will not be transmitted to the next generation. *Rb* is a recessive suppressor oncogene located at chromosome 13q14. Both copies of the gene must be mutated for tumors to develop. *Second tumors (other than retinoblastoma) develop in 25% to 30% of patients up to 30 or 40 years later.* Most common are *osteosarcomas* (majority) and *cutaneous malignant melanomas* (7% of second tumors). Cure is achieved >98% of cases if the tumor is diagnosed and treated early with enucleation, chemotherapy, radiation, laser, cryotherapy, or a combination thereof.

Patients present with a white or tan reflex from the pupil, often noted by parents when the child looks to the side. Parents often state that the eyes look funny, or that

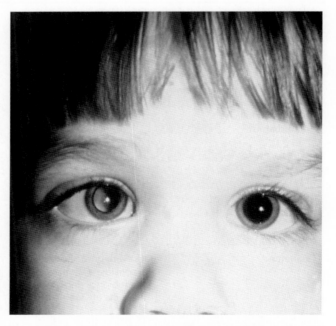

Figure 66.2 Abnormal light reflex from the right eye of a child with retinoblastoma. The pupil can be white (leukocoria), or the reflex may be tan or yellow.

the light reflex in photographs is abnormal. Children can present with strabismus or rarely with nonresolving conjunctivitis or hyphema.

The differential diagnosis of retinoblastoma includes:

- Congenital cataracts
- Retinopathy of prematurity with retinal detachment
- Toxocariasis
- Myelinated nerve fibers
- Coloboma
- Intraocular hemorrhage secondary to child abuse
- Persistent hyperplastic primary vitreous (small eye, cataract, dragged ciliary processes, and peripheral retina into a retrolenticular membrane)
- Coats disease (vascular malformation with leakage of serum and lipids under the retina)

CONJUNCTIVITIS

Three major categories of conjunctivitis are recognized: infectious, allergic, and traumatic or chemical (Table 66.1). Ocular conditions that should be differentiated from simple conjunctivitis include iritis (i.e., inflammation of the iris, a form of anterior uveitis), acute glaucoma, traumatic corneal abrasions, and infectious corneal ulceration.

In *bacterial conjunctivitis*, conjunctival hyperemia is marked, and a moderate to copious purulent discharge is seen. The patient is usually in pain and has a foreign body sensation in the eye. Vision, pupillary reflexes, intraocular pressure, and corneal clarity are all normal. Staphylococcal blepharitis, chronic infection, or inflammation at the lid margins is a common associated finding. Cultures may be obtained, and bilateral antibiotic eye drops or ointment should be started. Broad spectrum antibiotics are useful in shortening the course of the disease to some extent, but bacterial conjunctivitis usually improves within 4 to 5 days irrespective of the treatment.

Viral conjunctivitis may lead to a mild purulent discharge, but tearing and lid swelling, with or without preauricular lymphadenopathy, are the prominent features. Photophobia and blepharospasm with squeezing of the lids, usually in response to light, occur if the cornea is involved. Adenoviruses are common causative agents. Primary herpetic conjunctivitis is not easily recognized unless it is accompanied by herpetic lesions on the lids. The treatment of viral conjunctivitis (except for that caused by herpes simplex virus 1) is symptomatic; mild steroid drops

TABLE 66.1

DIFFERENTIATING FEATURES OF TYPES OF CONJUNCTIVITIS

Viral Etiology	Bacterial	Allergic	Chlamydial
Adenovirus	*Staphylococcus aureus*	Allergic	*Chlamydia trachomatis*
Herpes simplex virus	*Streptococcus pneumoniae*	Atopic	
Herpes zoster virus	*Haemophilus influenzae*	Vernal	
	Neisseria gonorrhea		
Signs and symptoms			
Asymmetric	Symmetric	Itching	Chronic follicular conjunctivitis
Preauricular lymphadenopathy	Purulent discharge	Tearing	Unilateral or bilateral
Clear tears		Stringy discharge	Mucopurulent discharge
Conjunctival follicles		Associated systemic allergies	Giemsa stain
Hemorrhages		Papillae (giant in vernal conjunctivitis)	Immunofluorescence
Corneal irritation		Seasonal	PCR/DNA probe
Treatment			
Cool compresses	Culture if severe or not responding to Rx.	Prevent exposure if allergen is known	Erythromycin 50 mg/kg/day in four doses
Ketorolac	Antibiotics to both eyes	Cool compresses	Topical erythromycin ointment
No steroids	No steroids	Lubricants	
Lasts 2–3 weeks	Lasts up to 1 week	Topical vasoconstrictors/ antihistamines	
Quarantine	If severe or recalcitrant, consider systemic antibiotics depending on results of Gram stain	Cromolyn Na 4%	
		Acular	
		Livostin	
		Alomide	

PCR, polymerase chain reaction.

may be given if inflammation and swelling are severe. Cold compresses and lubricants can be used.

The hallmark of *allergic conjunctivitis* is itching. A stringy mucoid discharge is usually present. Allergic conjunctivitis may be seasonal or associated with hay fever. The patient frequently has a history of allergic disorders. Mild vasoconstrictor, decongestant drops are usually sufficient to improve symptoms in mild cases; mild steroid drops may be necessary in more severe cases. In vernal conjunctivitis, which is a seasonal, and a rather severe allergic ocular condition characterized by large palpebral conjunctival papillae and perilimbal infiltrates, a number of mast cell stabilizing drops have decreased the recurrence rates and shortened the course of the disease if administered frequently and prophylactically. Several agents are available for the treatment of ocular allergy and include the antihistamines olopatadine hydrochloride (Patanol) and levocabastine (Livostin) and the mast cell stabilizer lodoxamide (Alomide).

The classic example of a *chemical conjunctivitis* is the one induced by silver nitrate prophylaxis or a Credé procedure in newborns. Any chemical that reaches the ocular surface is potentially toxic. The most serious of the chemical conjunctivitides are those caused by alkali. Many common household detergents are strong alkalis that can cause serious ocular injuries if they come in contact with the eye. An ophthalmologist should be consulted immediately if an ocular alkali burn is suspected. Pending the ophthalmologist's arrival, topical anesthetic drops should be instilled and the eye copiously irrigated for as long as possible with at least 2 L of normal saline solution or until a litmus paper test reveals a normal pH. Any debris or foreign bodies should be washed out of the conjunctival fornices. Because most of the ocular damage occurs within the first few minutes of exposure, irrigation should be carried out immediately. The ophthalmologist treats the patient for the ocular surface, cornea, and lid problems that are caused by these potentially severe injuries.

OPHTHALMIA NEONATORUM

Conjunctivitis is the most common neonatal ocular disease, occurring in 1.6% to 12% of newborns. The cause and incidence of neonatal conjunctivitis have been altered by the routine use of antibiotic prophylaxis. Erythromycin ointment (0.5%) and tetracycline ointment (1%) are considered equally effective for preventing ocular gonorrheal infection. The efficacy of erythromycin and tetracycline ointments in preventing chlamydial ophthalmia is less clear. Direct immunofluorescent monoclonal antibody staining has proved useful in the diagnosis of neonatal chlamydial conjunctivitis. Of the 100 neonates with conjunctivitis in one study, 43 were found to have chlamydial disease. Rates as high as 73% have been reported. In addition to *Chlamydia trachomatis* and *Neisseria gonorrhoeae*, other causal agents in ophthalmia neonatorum include

Staphylococcus aureus, nontypable *Haemophilus influenzae*, *Streptococcus pneumoniae*, gram-negative aerobic organisms, *Moraxella catarrhalis*, viridans streptococci, and herpes simplex virus.

The external appearance of the eye is generally the same regardless of the causative agent. In addition to swelling of the lids and conjunctivae, a profuse and sometimes bloody discharge is seen, especially if pseudomembranes are formed. *The timing of the infection in relation to birth is helpful, although not diagnostic, in determining the causative agent.* Chemical conjunctivitis and mechanical conjunctivitis occur in the first day of life and are caused by birth trauma and manipulation or silver nitrate prophylaxis itself, if this is used. Gonococcal conjunctivitis, which is acquired in the birth canal, usually manifests between days 2 and 4. The remaining organisms cause conjunctivitis at various time intervals after birth.

An infant suspected of having conjunctivitis should be placed in strict contact isolation. Conjunctival scrapings for Gram and Giemsa staining and for direct immunofluorescent monoclonal antibody staining for *Chlamydia* should be obtained. Aerobic, anaerobic, and chlamydial cultures should all be performed. Therapy is initiated on the basis of the results of the staining, with definitive culture pending.

Patients suspected of having chlamydial disease should be given oral erythromycin (50 mg/kg per day in four divided doses) for 14 days. If gonococcal conjunctivitis is suspected or confirmed, the infant should be hospitalized and treated with one dose of ceftriaxone (25–50 mg/kg intravenously or intramuscularly, not to exceed 125 mg) and saline lavage of the eyes. A search for disseminated gonococcal infection should always be performed. Parents and their sexual partners should be treated for chlamydial and gonococcal infection in the usual manner. Gram-negative bacilli necessitate treatment with one application of gentamicin sulfate ophthalmic ointment four times a day for 1 week. If gram-positive cocci or inflammatory cells without organisms are found, erythromycin ophthalmic ointment should be applied four times a day for 1 week. Pseudomonal conjunctivitis is particularly aggressive and may be complicated by corneal ulceration and blindness. It is acquired in the hospital and should be suspected in infants on mechanical ventilation with other foci of *Pseudomonas* infection.

PEDIATRIC CATARACTS

Cataracts are opacities of the crystalline lens. Cataracts can be categorized according to cause as follows:

- Hereditary cataracts
- Cataracts associated with chromosomal abnormalities
- Cataracts secondary to intrauterine infection
- Cataracts associated with metabolic disorders

- Drug-induced cataracts
- Trauma-induced cataracts
- Cataracts associated with ocular disorders

Hereditary cataracts are not associated with other diseases and are most often transmitted in an autosomal-dominant fashion. More than 20 genes have been identified that cause inherited cataracts.

Chromosomal defects, such as those of trisomy 13, 18, and 21 and Turner syndrome, can be associated with cataracts.

Intrauterine infection with a wide variety of agents can result in the formation of cataracts. Infection with rubella virus is most closely associated with the development of cataracts, but *Toxoplasma*, cytomegalovirus, and herpes simplex virus have also been associated.

Metabolic disorders, especially galactosemia, must be excluded in the infant or child with cataracts. "Classic" infantile galactosemia results from a deficiency of galactose-1-phosphate uridyltransferase and is usually associated with systemic manifestations. Galactokinase deficiency can also result in cataract formation; cataracts are often the sole manifestation in this type of galactosemia and may present later in life.

Long-term *corticosteroid therapy* and other *drug ingestions*, in addition to ocular *trauma*, may lead to the development of cataracts.

Finally, cataracts may be *associated with ocular disorders*, most notably chronic uveitis, retinal detachment, retinopathy of prematurity, aniridia, and microphthalmos.

The evaluation of the infant or child with cataracts includes a full ophthalmologic examination to exclude associated ocular disease and assess visual status. Ocular ultrasonography should be performed in eyes with totally opaque lenses. A family history of congenital cataracts in a parent or grandparent suggests dominant isolated cataracts. Both parents must be examined with a slit-lamp after pupillary dilation for the presence of subclinical lens opacities. The presence of lens opacities in one parent establishes the diagnosis of hereditary cataracts.

Bilateral complete cataracts should be extracted early, and the visual prognosis is generally good if no other ocular disease is present. In the case of unilateral congenital cataracts, surgery is generally performed as early as a few weeks of age to avoid severe sensory amblyopia. Soon after cataract surgery the infant is fitted with a contact lens. In the case of a unilateral cataract, the normal eye is patched for an increasing number of hours each day through middle childhood to treat amblyopia. Frequent refractions and changes of contact lens power are needed, and parents should be aware of the importance of perseverance if good visual results are to be obtained. The conservative management of partial cataracts includes the use of mydriatics if the opacity is central, and patching of the uninvolved eye for the treatment and prevention of amblyopia. During the last few years, intraocular lenses have been increasingly used for the optical correction of aphakia in children of all ages. The current experience with these devices indicates an acceptable level of safety.

ECTOPIA LENTIS

Ectopia lentis is displacement of the lens, which can result from trauma, developmental defects, or ocular disease; it can also be associated with systemic syndromes. Hereditary or simple ectopia lentis is not associated with systemic illness and is usually transmitted as an autosomal-dominant condition. *Marfan syndrome* and *homocystinuria* are two important systemic illnesses associated with ectopia lentis. Ectopia lentis develops in approximately 60% of patients with Marfan syndrome. In most cases of Marfan syndrome, the lens is displaced *superiorly* and temporally, whereas in homocystinuria, the lens is displaced *inferiorly*. The suspicion of a subluxated lens should prompt an extensive workup for Marfan syndrome.

REVIEW EXERCISES

QUESTIONS

1. Nasolacrimal duct obstruction can be differentiated from congenital glaucoma by the:
a) Presence of lacrimation in nasolacrimal duct obstruction but not in glaucoma
b) Occurrence of nasolacrimal duct obstruction in younger and glaucoma in older infants
c) Clouding and enlargement of the cornea in congenital glaucoma but not in nasolacrimal duct obstruction
d) Mode of inheritance

Answer
The answer is c.

2. The differential diagnosis of a white pupillary reflex includes all the following *except*:
a) Retinoblastoma
b) Toxocariasis
c) Congenital cataract
d) Optic nerve glioma
e) Retinopathy of prematurity

Answer
The answer is d.

3. Clues to the diagnosis of allergic conjunctivitis include the presence of itching and tearing and the absence of a mucopurulent discharge.
a) True
b) False

Answer
The answer is a.

4. The use of topical steroids is indicated in mild and moderately severe allergic and viral conjunctivitis.
a) True
b) False

Answer
The answer is b.

5. The first step in the evaluation of children with cataracts is examining the parents for the presence of lens opacities.
a) True
b) False

Answer
The answer is a.

6. Which is a *true* statement concerning the management of infants with gonococcal ophthalmia neonatorum?
a) Intravenous aqueous penicillin G is the treatment of choice.
b) A search for disseminated gonococcal infection need not be performed.
c) One dose of ceftriaxone administered intravenously or intramuscularly, is effective therapy.

d) Ceftriaxone, administered intravenously for 10 days, is the preferred therapy.

Answer
The answer is c.

SUGGESTED READINGS

1. Cassidy L, Taylor D. Congenital cataract and multisystem disorders. *Eye* 1999;13(Pt 3B):464–473.
2. Committee on Practice and Ambulatory Medicine, Section on Ophthalmology, American Association of Certified Orthoptists, American Association for Pediatric Ophthalmology and Strabismus and American Academy of Ophthalmology. Policy statement. Eye examination in infants, children, and young adults by pediatricians. *Pediatrics* 2003;111:902–907, http://aappolicy.aappublications.org/cgi/content/full/pediatrics; 111/4/902.
3. Kiss S, Leiderman YI, Mukai S. Diagnosis, classification, and treatment of retinoblastoma. *Int Ophthalmol Clin* 2008;48:135–147.
4. McLaughlin C, Levin AV. The red reflex. *Pediatr Emerg Care* 2006;22:137–140.
5. Mueller JB, McStay CM. Ocular infection and inflammation. *Emerg Med Clin North Am* 2008;26:57–72.
6. Murphree L. Retinoblastoma. In: Traboulsi EI, ed. *Genetic diseases of the eye*. New York: Oxford University Press, 1999.
7. Reddy MA, Francis PJ, Berry V, et al. Molecular genetic basis of inherited cataract and associated phenotypes. *Surv Ophthalmol* 2004;49:300–315.
8. Wright W, Farzavandi S. *Pediatric ophthalmology for primary care*, 3rd ed. Elk Grove Village, IL: American Academy of Pediatrics, 2008.

Chapter 67

BOARD SIMULATION: Potpourri

Elumalai Appachi

QUESTIONS

1. A 9-month-old infant presents with fever, irritability, and petechial rash for 1 week. He has had multiple ear infections in the past and has a draining right ear. He has seborrhea on his scalp and hepatosplenomegaly on abdominal examination. A radiograph of the skull is shown in Figure 67.1. Radiography of the chest shows multiple pulmonary infiltrates. Which of the following is a *true* statement regarding this infant's condition?
a) A short course of methylprednisolone along with intravenous antibiotics is indicated.
b) A bone scan will be diagnostic.
c) The rash is always caused by thrombocytopenia.

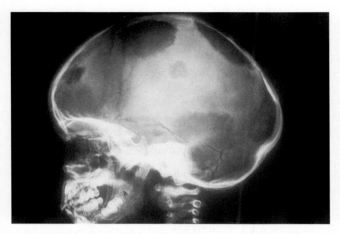

Figure 67.1   Skull radiograph of the patient in question 1. See explanation of question 1 for details.

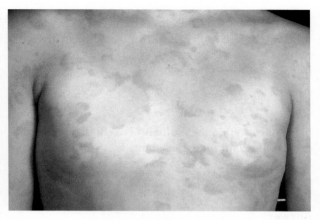

Figure 67.2   Rash in patient in question 2. See explanation of question 2 for details. (See color insert.)

d) The serum sodium level may be elevated.

e) The prognosis is excellent with appropriate therapy.

Answer

The answer is d. Langerhans cell histiocytosis is a multisystem disorder with a variable presentation. The skeleton is the most commonly affected site; osteolytic lesions are most often seen in the skull (Fig. 67.1). Chronically infected, draining ears are a frequent feature and associated with destruction of the mastoids. Skin involvement may be manifested as seborrheic dermatitis of the scalp or diaper area or as a petechial rash, even in the absence of thrombocytopenia. Localized or generalized lymphadenopathy with hepatosplenomegaly is also common. Infants with pulmonary disease and multiple infiltrates present with respiratory distress and progressive respiratory failure. Hypothalamic and pituitary dysfunction may result in growth retardation and diabetes insipidus, which may present as irritability, dehydration, and hypernatremia. Systemic manifestations include fever, weight loss, irritability, and failure to thrive. Skeletal survey, tissue biopsy, chest radiography, a determination of the serum sodium level and urine osmolality, and a detailed evaluation of all organ systems are necessary to establish the diagnosis and plan therapy. Multisystem involvement requires systemic chemotherapy. The prognosis in infants with multisystem disease is poor.

2. An 8-year-old girl presents with a history of fever, joint pain, and rash for 3 days (Fig. 67.2). On examination, she has swollen ankle and knee joints, and a pericardial rub is heard on auscultation. Which of the following is the *most* appropriate next step in the management of this girl?

a) Obtain a throat culture before administering antibiotics.

b) Administer intravenous immunoglobulin therapy.

c) Administer high-dose intravenous methylprednisolone.

d) Perform knee joint aspiration at the bedside and send the aspirates for bacteriologic cultures.

e) Consult a cardiologist for pericardiocentesis.

Answer

The answer is a. Acute rheumatic fever is difficult to diagnose, given that no single test or clinical sign confirms the diagnosis. The Jones criteria are helpful in making the diagnosis. The presence of erythema marginatum (Fig. 67.2), a lesion characterized by a serpiginous appearance and blanching in the middle, is one of the major criteria for the diagnosis of rheumatic fever. It often occurs in patients with carditis. The other major criteria include carditis, migratory polyarthritis, chorea, and subcutaneous nodules. The minor criteria include fever, arthralgia, elevated acute phase reactants (elevated sedimentation rate, increased C-reactive protein), and a prolonged PR interval on the electrocardiogram. The presence of two major criteria or of one major and two minor criteria with evidence of streptococcal infection strongly suggests rheumatic fever. However, when a child presents with unexplained chorea or carditis, the diagnosis of rheumatic fever should be considered, even if the criteria are not met. All patients with acute rheumatic fever should be treated for group A streptococcal infection. Immunoglobulin therapy is not indicated for the child in question. Corticosteroid therapy is indicated for patients with moderate to severe carditis. Pericardiocentesis is indicated if evidence of pericardial effusion and tamponade is present.

3. An 11-year-old boy presents with a history of fever, joint pain, and the rash pictured in **Figure 67.3**. He also has abdominal pain and a swollen scrotum. He had a streptococcal throat infection a week ago. Which of the following is a *true* statement regarding his condition?

a) He has poststreptococcal glomerulonephritis.

b) His platelet count is likely to be normal.

c) A lumbar puncture should be performed and the child should receive broad spectrum antibiotics.

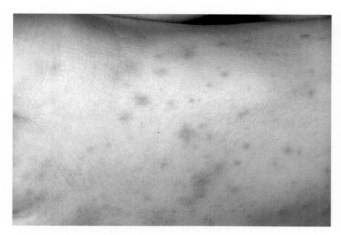

Figure 67.3 Rash in patient in question 3. See explanation of question 3 for details. (See color insert.)

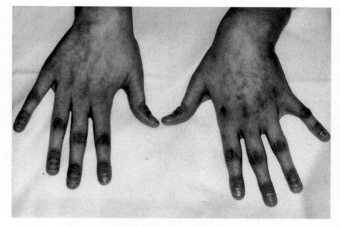

Figure 67.4 Hands of patient in question 4. See explanation of question 4 for details.

d) He has Kawasaki disease.

e) Bone marrow aspirate will be diagnostic.

Answer

The answer is b. Henoch-Schönlein purpura is the most common cause of nonthrombocytopenic purpura in children. The etiology is unknown. Abdominal pain is usually secondary to vasculitis of the gastrointestinal tract and may mimic acute abdomen. Intussusception may occur occasionally. Scrotal edema and tenderness may mimic acute torsion of a testis. Renal involvement, in the form of hematuria, occurs in 25% to 50% of patients. Therapy with IV steroids is usually reserved for life-threatening intestinal and central nervous system complications. The diagnosis is based on the clinical features; routine laboratory tests are not necessary, and bone marrow aspiration is not indicated.

4. A 14-year-old adolescent girl (**Fig. 67.4**) presents with exertional dyspnea and palpitations. Examination reveals a heart murmur. Each of the following statements is appropriate regarding her diagnosis and management *except*:

a) She has a 25% chance of having an offspring with a similar condition.

b) She requires a slit-lamp examination of her eyes and an ophthalmologic evaluation.

c) She requires endocarditis prophylaxis for dental and invasive surgical procedures.

d) Therapy with propranolol is indicated in most cases.

e) A urinary cyanide nitroprusside test is indicated.

Answer

The answer is a. Marfan syndrome is inherited in an autosomal-dominant pattern, but nearly 30% of cases are new mutations. Because the inheritance is autosomal-dominant, the chance that an offspring will be affected is 50%. Slit-lamp examination may reveal lens dislocation and iridodonesis. Morbidity is usually

caused by cardiovascular defects, including aortic root dilatation, and mitral valve prolapse. Propranolol or atenolol may be used therapeutically to reduce cardiovascular morbidity. The cyanide nitroprusside test or specific amino acid assays can be performed to differentiate Marfan syndrome from homocystinuria.

5. A 13-month-old infant is brought to the emergency department with a 5-day history of high fever, bilateral non purulent conjunctivitis, fissured lips, maculopapular rash, joint swelling, and irritability. She received her measles-mumps-rubella vaccine 4 days ago. The next *most* appropriate step is to:

a) Reassure the parents that her symptoms are a reaction to the vaccine.

b) Administer intravenous penicillin and obtain an urgent electrocardiogram.

c) Administer high-dose intravenous methylprednisolone therapy.

d) Admit her and perform a lumbar puncture to rule out meningitis.

e) Consult a pediatric cardiologist for echocardiography.

Answer

The answer is e. Kawasaki disease is an acute febrile vasculitis. Coronary artery dilatation and aneurysms are the most feared complications of this syndrome and occur in approximately 20% of untreated individuals. The diagnosis of Kawasaki disease is made clinically on the basis of diagnostic criteria. Adverse reactions to measles-mumps-rubella vaccine in the form of fever and rash classically develop 10 to 14 days after vaccination. Currently, corticosteroid therapy is not given initially to patients with suspected Kawasaki syndrome. Given the clinical picture, the next logical step is to obtain an echocardiogram to examine the coronary arteries and myocardial function. Depending on the child's appearance, a lumbar puncture may be appropriate. Children

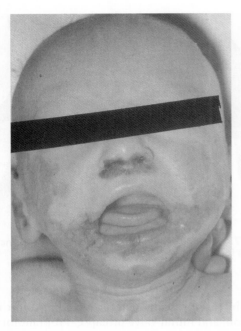

Figure 67.5 Eczematous lesions of patient in question 6. See explanation of question 6 for details.

with Kawasaki syndrome can be so irritable that meningitis cannot be ruled out with confidence. In this instance, a lumbar puncture and empiric antimicrobial therapy are certainly warranted.

6. A 12-month-old infant is admitted for chronic enteritis, failure to thrive, and eczematous lesions over the perioral and perianal areas (Fig. 67.5). Which of the following is *true* regarding her condition?
a) Treatment with high-dose zinc and close monitoring of levels is indicated.
b) She may have an elevated serum alkalinephosphatase level.
c) Therapy with acyclovir is indicated.
d) A gluten free diet should be introduced slowly.
e) The condition may be inherited as an autosomal-dominant pattern.

Answer
The answer is a. Acrodermatitis enteropathica is inherited in an autosomal-recessive pattern, and the symptoms are caused by zinc deficiency secondary to malabsorption. Affected infants usually exhibit cutaneous manifestations in the form of vesiculobullous, dry, eczematous lesions (Fig. 67.5) distributed over perioral, acral, and perianal areas. Chronic enteritis and failure to thrive are other manifestations in affected infants. Similar clinical features can be seen in infants with secondary zinc deficiency, especially those receiving prolonged parenteral nutrition without zinc supplementation. The diagnostic features include low levels of zinc and a low level of alkaline phosphatase in serum.

7. A 16-year-old high school student presents with one week history of abdominal pain, vomiting, and loss of appetite. On examination, she has scleral icterus and mildly dehydrated. Blood work reveals the following values:

    Hemoglobin = 6 g/dL
    Hematocrit = 21 mL/dL
    White cell count = 12,000/mm^3
    Platelets = 260,000/mm^3
    Reticulocytes = 12%

The liver profile shows elevated liver enzymes. The urinalysis indicates glycosuria, aminoaciduria, and phosphaturia. The next *most* appropriate step is to:
a) Inform her that she has infectious hepatitis and arrange for a follow-up visit in 2 weeks.
b) Admit her to the hospital for N-acetylcysteine therapy.
c) Order an urgent abdominal ultrasonographic examination.
d) Perform a slit-lamp examination of her eyes.
e) Perform a bone marrow aspiration and biopsy.

Answer
The answer is d. Wilson disease is an autosomal-recessive condition of abnormal copper metabolism. Multisystem involvement includes hepatic injury, degenerative changes in the brain, renal tubular acidosis, and hemolytic anemia. The accumulation of copper in the corneas causes a pathognomonic feature called Kayser-Fleischer rings (Fig. 67.6), which are detectable on slit-lamp examination of the eyes. The best screening test is measurement of the serum level of ceruloplasmin, which is low in patients with Wilson disease.

8. A 5-year-old child (Fig. 67.7) is brought in for a pre-kindergarten physical examination. His mother is concerned that he does not play much and tires easily.

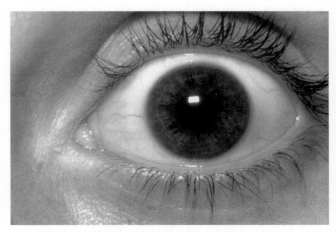

Figure 67.6 A patient with Wilson disease. Note the presence of Kayser-Fleischer rings, indicating an accumulation of copper in the cornea. (See color insert.)

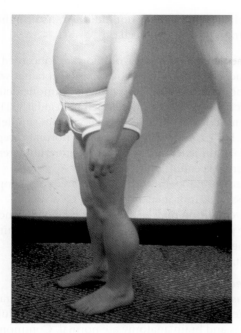

Figure 67.7   Child in question 8. See explanation of question 8 for details.

Further history reveals that he first walked at 22 months of age. The following are all true regarding his condition *except:*

a) Some intellectual impairment will develop in this child.

b) The chance that his son will be affected with the same condition is 50%.

c) He is at risk for heart failure.

d) The mother may not be a carrier of the disease.

e) Further workup, including muscle biopsy, is indicated.

Answer

The answer is b. Duchenne muscular dystrophy is an X-linked recessive disorder; therefore, a father cannot transmit the defective gene to his son. Gross motor skills may be delayed or normal during infancy. All patients have some intellectual impairment, and cardiomyopathy resulting in heart failure is a constant feature. Approximately 30% of cases are the result of new mutations, and the mother is not a carrier. Grossly elevated serum levels of creatine kinase, a myopathic pattern on electromyography, and characteristic features on the muscle biopsy specimen help establish the diagnosis.

9. A 12-year-old boy who has recently immigrated to the United States from Eastern Europe presents with a 1-month history of intermittent fevers and a painful rash on his shins. He has also lost 8 kg in the past month. Which of the following should be obtained/performed as part of the *initial* workup?

a) Cardiology evaluation for rheumatic fever

b) Urinalysis for glycosuria

c) Tuberculin skin test

d) Allergy panel

e) Gastrointestinal contrast studies to search for inflammatory bowel disease

Answer

The answer is c. Erythema nodosum is associated with multiple infectious and inflammatory conditions and is considered a hypersensitivity reaction. The nodules are usually red, shiny, and tender (see Fig. 51.4). The most common infectious cause to be ruled out in an immigrant is tuberculosis. Diabetes and inflammatory bowel disease are included in the differential diagnosis, but in this patient, tuberculosis is more likely the cause.

10. A 16-year-old girl presents to the clinic with fever, headache, and an erythematous malar facial rash. She tires easily and has arthralgia. The *most* appropriate management at this point would be to:

a) Prescribe oral antibiotics and hydrocortisone locally for the rash.

b) Order blood work for antinuclear antibody.

c) Arrange for cranial computed tomography (CT) scan.

d) Start IV acyclovir.

e) Start tetracycline therapy.

Answer

The answer is b. Systemic lupus erythematosus is a rheumatic disease that affects multiple organs and systems, including the central nervous system, kidneys, blood cells, and musculoskeletal system. The disease more often affects girls and women, and an onset of illness before 8 years of age is rare. A photosensitive malar ("butterfly") rash is a characteristic feature of lupus. Antinuclear antibody is often a screening investigation, whereas levels of anti–double-stranded DNA are more specific for lupus. The facial rash does not require treatment with acyclovir, tetracycline, or hydrocortisone. CT scan of the brain is indicated when focal neurologic changes are present.

11. A 12-year-old girl is seen for intractable acne. She has been treated with multiple topical therapies without benefit. Further history reveals that she has a sibling with a seizure disorder. On physical examination, a hypopigmented patch is seen on her trunk. Of the following, the *most* appropriate plan of action for this girl would be to:

a) Administer oral tetracycline therapy.

b) Refer her to a dermatologist.

c) Obtain a renal ultrasonogram.

d) Order karyotyping.

e) Administer anticonvulsant therapy.

Answer

The answer is c. Tuberous sclerosis affects many organs, including the brain, kidneys, heart, bones, and skin. It is inherited as an autosomal-dominant trait and is a heterogenous condition with various presentations. Ash leaf macules and hypopigmented patches (see Fig. 35.5) are common skin manifestations of tuberous sclerosis and provide clues to the diagnosis. Hamartomas or polycystic disease of the kidneys may cause renal insufficiency. Children in whom polycystic kidney disease develops before the age of 10 years should be evaluated for tuberous sclerosis. Adenoma sebaceum (see Fig. 35.6) of the face may resemble acne and is sometimes the only manifestation of the disease. Infantile spasms with a hypsarrhythmic pattern on electroencephalography are common in infancy; myoclonic epilepsy develops at later age.

12. An 11-year-old girl is seen for fever, sore throat, and the rash pictured in **Figure 67.8**. She had a heart transplant 2 years ago for a severe cardiomyopathy. Which of the following is *true* regarding her diagnosis?
a) Treatment with ampicillin might make the rash worse.
b) Household contacts of the child should receive rifampicin prophylaxis.
c) An electrocardiogram and an antistreptolysin O titer should be obtained.
d) High-dose aspirin and immunoglobulin therapy are indicated.
e) None of the above

Answer
The answer is e. Progressive or hemorrhagic varicella is a severe and dreaded complication of infection with the varicella-zoster virus. Severe abdominal pain, hemorrhagic vesicles, and signs of shock are common features at the onset. This condition is more prevalent in children with a deficiency of cell-mediated immunity or malignancy; pregnant women and neonates are also at risk. Systemic manifestations include pneumonia, hepatitis, encephalitis, and disseminated intravascular coagulation. Management consists of meticulous supportive care along with the administration of IV acyclovir. The child in question does not have meningococcal sepsis; hence,

rifampicin prophylaxis is not indicated. Aspirin therapy is contraindicated in varicella.

13. The parents of a 5-year-old boy are concerned about his headache, which does not seem to get better with acetaminophen. The boy has a growth hormone deficiency and receives growth hormone therapy regularly. He is fully immunized and takes regular vitamin supplementation. His examination is essentially normal except for bilateral papilledema. The following are true statements regarding his condition *except:*
a) A lumbar puncture with measurement of the opening pressure is indicated after cranial CT scan.
b) The condition may be caused by hypervitaminosis A.
c) The growth hormone therapy must be discontinued.
d) Repeated lumbar punctures may be required.
e) Acetazolamide therapy may be helpful.

Answer
The answer is c. In pseudotumor cerebri, the intracranial pressure is increased but the cerebrospinal fluid findings and brain anatomy are normal. Common causes include:

■ Prolonged corticosteroid therapy
■ Growth hormone therapy
■ Hypervitaminosis or hypovitaminosis A
■ Obesity
■ Hypoadrenalism
■ Hypoparathyroidism
■ Medications, such as oral contraceptives and tetracycline

The management focuses on treating the underlying cause. Although this is a benign, self-limited disease, prolonged symptoms may cause optic atrophy and visual disturbances. Repeated lumbar punctures may be necessary to reduce the intracranial pressure. An initial lumbar puncture should be performed to determine the opening pressure after cranial CT scan or magnetic resonance imaging has ruled out a structural problem. Acetazolamide, a carbonic anhydrase inhibitor, and corticosteroids have been useful in the management of pseudotumor cerebri.

14. A 4-year-old boy has a history of fever for 4 days and was evaluated at a community emergency department 2 days ago, otitis media was diagnosed, and trimethoprim/sulfamethoxazole was prescribed. Today, he presents with a generalized rash. On physical examination he has cool extremities and altered mental status. The *most* important *initial* step in management should be:
a) Perform a CT scan of the head.
b) Obtain rapid IV access and administer a fluid bolus.
c) Administer IV hydrocortisone or dexamethasone.
d) Perform a lumbar puncture to rule out meningitis.
e) None of the above

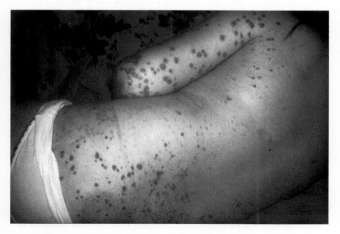

Figure 67.8 Rash of patient in question 12. See explanation of question 12 for details. (See color insert.)

Answer

The answer is b. The rash of Stevens-Johnson syndrome typically consists of erythematous macules initially, which rapidly change into vesicles, bullae, and areas of denudation. The mucosal surfaces are involved in the oropharynx, eyes, gastrointestinal tract, and anogenital region. Pain secondary to mucosal ulceration can be very severe, and multisystem involvement may be manifested as pneumonitis, carditis, hepatitis, enterocolitis, polyarthritis, and acute tubular necrosis. Disseminated bullae and mucosal ulceration may cause extensive fluid loss that leads to hypovolemic shock as in the case described. The management of the overall condition is supportive and symptomatic.

15. An 8-month-old infant is seen with a 3-week history of diarrhea, abdominal distension, rectal prolapse, and poor weight gain. The past medical history is significant for hospitalization for a staphylococcal pneumonia at the age of 3 months. The *most* appropriate plan of action is to:
a) Obtain an urgent surgical evaluation.
b) Obtain serum immunoglobulin levels.
c) Obtain serum antigliadin antibodies.
d) Change her milk formula to a soy-based formula.
e) Perform a sweat chloride test.

Answer

The answer is e. Rectal prolapse is a common clinical feature in infants with cystic fibrosis. It is usually caused by malnutrition, chronic diarrhea, and persistent cough. Any infant with rectal prolapse should be investigated for cystic fibrosis. The prolapsed rectum can be replaced manually in most instances, and surgery is rarely required. The rectal prolapse resolves with overall improvement in the nutritional status and a reduction in steatorrhea following supplementation of pancreatic enzymes.

16. A 5-year-old boy has a history of malaise, fever, headache, nausea, and vomiting for the past 24 hours. A purpuric rash developed an hour ago. Now he is lethargic, confused, and combative. His pulse is 160 beats/minute, and his blood pressure is 70/40 mm Hg. Blood work has been obtained and an IV line placed. The *most* appropriate plan of action is to:
a) Perform a lumbar puncture.
b) Obtain urgent CT scan of the brain
c) Administer a fluid bolus of normal saline solution.
d) Determine the blood levels of ammonia.
e) Administer dopamine infusion

Answer

The answer is c. Meningococcal meningitis is a serious and potentially fatal disease. The causative organism is *Neisseria meningitidis*, a gram-negative diplococcus. Disseminated meningococcal disease is associated with a severe acute inflammatory response. Hemorrhage and intravascular coagulation in multiple organs may lead to tissue necrosis. The spectrum of disease varies, ranging from occult bacteremia (rare) to florid sepsis. Meningococcal septicemia may occur without meningitis and is caused by widespread hematogenous dissemination. Disseminated intravascular coagulation, hypotension, acidosis, adrenal hemorrhage, renal failure, coma, and overall rapid deterioration leading to death characterize septic shock. An altered sensorium is a sign of shock and poor cerebral perfusion. The rash of meningococcal disease can be maculopapular or purpuric, or it can be frank ecchymosis. Because the disease can be rapidly progressive, the management is based on clinical suspicion, and therapy should be initiated without delay. Shock and hypotension should be treated with multiple boluses of fluid and if necessary with inotropic support. Waiting for the results of CT scan and performing a lumbar puncture on an unstable patient with shock are neither necessary nor appropriate. Along with fluid resuscitation, IV antibiotics should be administered as soon as possible. The antibiotic of choice is penicillin once the organism has been identified, but cefotaxime or ceftriaxone should be used initially to treat other potential pathogens.

17. A 3-year-old toddler presents to you for recurrent ear infections and sinusitis. He is recovering from a recent bout of bacterial pneumonia. On examination, prominent blood vessels are noted in the conjunctivae. The mother informs you that he has been unsteady on his feet for the past week. Appropriate management includes all of the following *except:*
a) Measuring serum immunoglobulin levels
b) Measuring serum α-fetoprotein level
c) Performing a sweat chloride test
d) Performing a CT scan of the head
e) Informing the parents that the child is at risk for progressive neurologic impairment at a later age

Answer

The answer is b. The most common features of ataxia-telangiectasia include:

■ Progressive cerebellar ataxia
■ Oculocutaneous telangiectasia
■ Humoral and cellular immunodeficiency causing chronic sinopulmonary disease
■ High incidence of malignancies

The ataxia is progressive, and the child is bound to a wheelchair by the age of 10 to 12 years. Telangiectasia develops around the age of 3 to 6 years. Progressive neurologic dysfunction is common and appears at a later age. Immunoglobulin A is absent, and levels of immunoglobulin E are very low. The thymus is often hypoplastic in association with a defective function of lymphocytes. The cells are unduly sensitive to ionizing radiation, and chromosomal breakage occurs. The genetic defect is in the long arm of chromosome 11. Any child with recurrent sinopulmonary disease should be evaluated for cystic fibrosis.

18. A 2-year-old boy presents with an abdominal mass, which was noticed by the mother while she was bathing him. He has hemihypertrophy and aniridia. Which of the following is *true* regarding the abdominal mass in this child?

a) A laxative or an enema is indicated.
b) Associated hypertension is very rare.
c) Siblings are at increased risk for a similar condition.
d) Surgical management is rarely necessary.
e) All of the above

Answer

The answer is c. Wilms tumor is the most common renal malignancy seen in childhood. It is associated with congenital anomalies, such as genitourinary malformations, hemihypertrophy, and sporadic aniridia. Deletions of chromosome 11 have been associated with Wilms tumor. The most common presenting symptom is an abdominal mass, usually noticed by a parent who is bathing the child. Hypertension is present in approximately 60% of cases of Wilms tumor and is caused by renal ischemia. Wilms tumor should be suspected in any child with an abdominal mass. Abdominal ultrasonography or CT scan will define the tumor. Pulmonary metastasis has occurred in approximately 15% of patients at the time of diagnosis. The treatment of choice is surgical removal of the tumor, even if pulmonary metastasis is present. Radiation therapy or chemotherapy for the residual tumor follows the surgery. Siblings are at increased risk for development of the tumor in comparison with the general population.

19. A 10-year-old young man with sickle cell disease presents with acute abdominal pain, fever, lethargy and cool extremities. All of the following are *true* regarding his diagnosis and management *except*:

a) He may have spontaneous peritonitis.
b) He should receive an isotonic fluid bolus and maintained on IV hydration.
c) His symptoms are caused by acute splenic sequestration.
d) He should receive broad spectrum intravenous antibiotics after appropriate culture specimens are obtained.
e) He should receive an intravenous narcotic analgesic.

Answer

The answer is c. Altered splenic function and deficient opsonins predispose patients with sickle cell disease to infections, such as peritonitis, meningitis, and sepsis. Encapsulated organisms such as pneumococci and *Haemophilus influenzae* and Salmonella are common causes of infection in this patient population. Iron over load causes cardiomegaly/cardiomyopathy and

parenchymal injury to liver and spleen. Progressive impairment in renal function resulting from diffuse glomerular and tubular fibrosis results in hyposthenuria in children >5 years of age. Zinc deficiency is prevalent and contributes to poor growth and maturation. Splenic sequestration is uncommon after 5 years of age.

20. A 2-year-old toddler presents with failure to thrive, diarrhea, irritability and abdominal distension. Which of the following is true regarding celiac disease?

a) A sweat chloride test is diagnostic.
b) A prolonged course of metronidazole is necessary.
c) Children with this entity require a gluten-free diet until the adolescent growth spurt.
d) There is increased risk of developing bowel lymphoma.
e) The majority of children with this condition develop precocious puberty.

Answer

The answer is d. Children with gluten sensitive enteropathy present between 6 months and 2 years of age. Prolonged exposure to gluten, which is present in wheat, rye, and barley, but not in oats, causes the disorder. The immunologic response to gluten results in villous atrophy (short flat villi) and crypt hyperplasia, which results in malabsorption and failure to thrive. Children with celiac disease have growth retardation, diarrhea, vomiting, and muscle wasting. Also they are often clingy, irritable, unhappy, and difficult to comfort. Measurement of serum IgA endomysial antibodies (almost 100% sensitive and specific) and antibody to tissue transglutaminase antigen help to make the diagnosis. Initial small bowel biopsy is probably still needed in spite of available immunologic investigations. The gluten sensitivity is a lifelong condition and treatment requires a lifelong strict gluten-free diet. Longstanding enteropathy from poor compliance with the diet may predispose to bowel lymphomas.

SUGGESTED READINGS

1. American Academy of Pediatrics Committee on Genetics. Health supervision for children with Marfan syndrome. *Pediatrics* 1996; 98:978.
2. Bhatia S, Nesbit ME, Egeler RM, et al. Epidemiologic study of Langerhans cell histiocytosis in children. *J Pediatr* 1997;130:774.
3. Branski D, Lerener A, Lebenthal E. Chronic diarrhea and malabsorption. *Pediatr Clin North Am* 1996;43:307.
4. Bunn HF. Pathogenesis and treatment of sickle cell disease. *NEJM* 1997;337:762.
5. Dajani AS, Ayoub E, Bierman FZ, et al. Guidelines for the diagnosis of rheumatic fever: Jones criteria, update 1993. *Circulation* 1993; 87:302.
6. Feigin RD, McCracken GH, Klein JO. Diagnosis and management of meningitis. *Pediatr Infect Dis J* 1992;11:785.
7. Gershon AA, Mervish N, LaRussa P, et al. Varicella-zoster virus infection in children with underlying human immunodeficiency virus infection. *J Infect Dis* 1997;176:1496.
8. Lehman TJ, McCurdy DK, Bernstein BH, et al. Systemic lupus erythematosus in the first decade of life. *Pediatrics* 1989;83:235.

9. Mattson SN, Riley EP, Gramling L, et al. Heavy prenatal alcohol exposure with or without physical features of fetal alcohol syndrome leads to IQ deficits. *J Pediatr* 1997;131:718.
10. Melish ME. Kawasaki syndrome. *Pediatr Rev* 1996;17:153.
11. Petruzzi MJ, Green DM. Wilms' tumor. *Pediatr Clin North Am* 1997;44:939.
12. Smith GC, Davidson JE, Hughs DA, et al. Complement activation in Henoch-Schönlein purpura. *Pediatr Nephrol* 1997;11:477.
13. Sternlieb I. Perspective on Wilson disease. *Hepatology* 1990;12:1234.
14. Swinson CM, Slavin G, Coles EC, et al. Celiac disease and malignancy. *Lancet* 1983;1:111.
15. Voit T. Congenital muscular dystrophies: 1997 update. *Brain Dev* 1998;20:65.
16. Webb DW, Clarke A, Fryer A, et al. The cutaneous features of tuberous sclerosis: a population study. *Br J Dermatol* 1996;135:1.

Chapter 68

BOARD SIMULATION: Potpourri

Robert J. Cunningham III and Camille Sabella

QUESTIONS

1. Respiratory distress develops in a 10-hour-old term infant. Physical examination reveals tachypnea, diminished breath sounds on the left side of the chest, and a scaphoid abdomen. The *most* likely diagnosis is:
a) Sepsis
b) Transient tachypnea of the newborn
c) Pneumothorax
d) Congenital diaphragmatic hernia
e) Meconium aspiration

Answer

The answer is d. The findings of a scaphoid abdomen and diminished breath sounds in the chest of a newborn infant are characteristic of congenital diaphragmatic hernia. A poster lateral defect (Bochdalek type) is most common, and 75% to 85% of defects occur on the left side; 5% are bilateral. Chest radiography is diagnostic, although the diagnosis can be made prenatally with ultrasonography. A 40% to 50% mortality rate is associated with congenital diaphragmatic hernia; long-term complications, such as growth and developmental delays, gastroesophageal reflux, pectus excavatum, and scoliosis, are common.

2. Bilious vomiting develops in a 1-day-old infant (Fig. 68.1). This infant's condition is *most* closely associated with:
a) Cystic fibrosis
b) Turner syndrome
c) Trisomy 21
d) DiGeorge syndrome
e) Vertebral anomalies

Answer

The answer is c. Bilious vomiting and the appearance of a "double bubble" (Fig. 68.1) in a newborn infant are characteristic of duodenal atresia, which accounts for 25% to 40% of all cases of intestinal atresia. Fifty percent of infants with duodenal atresia are premature, and associated anomalies include:

- Trisomy 21 (20%–30%)
- Malrotation (20%)
- Esophageal atresia (10%–20%)

Bilious vomiting without abdominal distension, maternal polyhydramnios, and the "double bubble" finding on abdominal x-ray film are common features.

3. A 6-month-old boy is brought in for a well-baby visit. On examining the infant, you note a white pupil in his

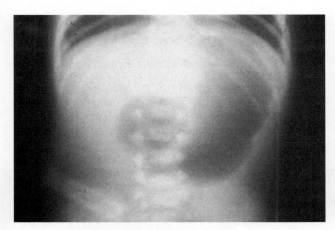

Figure 68.1 Abdominal film of the patient in question 2. See explanation of question 2 for details.

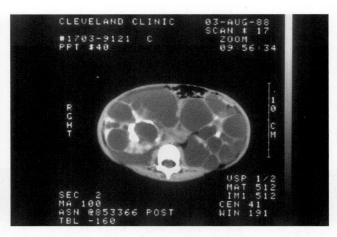

Figure 68.2 Renal ultrasonogram of the patient in questions 4 and 5.

left eye. The infant was born at 33 weeks of gestation with a birth weight of 2000 g. The *least* likely cause of a white pupil in this infant is:
a) Congenital cataract
b) Glaucoma
c) Retinoblastoma
d) Retinopathy of prematurity

Answer

The answer is d. The differential diagnosis of leukocoria includes all of the choices listed in this question. Although retinopathy of prematurity is a cause of leukocoria, it occurs in infants who are born before 33 weeks of gestation, with a birth weight <1500 g. Therefore, the leukocoria of the infant described in the question is *least* likely to be associated with retinopathy of prematurity.

Case for Questions 4–5

A girl who is now 5 years old was taken to her pediatrician at 6 months of age with abdominal masses. At 18 months of age, she had seizures 5 days after vaccination with diphtheria-tetanus-pertussis booster. She is severely developmentally delayed. Her renal ultrasonogram is shown in Figure 68.2.

4. The *most* likely diagnosis is:
a) Infantile polycystic kidney disease
b) Adult polycystic kidney disease
c) Tuberous sclerosis
d) Multicystic kidney disease

Answer

The answer is c. The most likely diagnosis is tuberous sclerosis, which is usually inherited in an autosomal-dominant manner. Tuberous sclerosis is characterized by a seizure disorder, pathognomonic skin lesions (ash leaf lesions and hypopigmented macules; see Fig. 35.5), calcified tubers in the brain, rhabdomyomas of the heart, and hamartomas or polycystic disease in the kidneys.

The clinical manifestations vary widely from patient to patient. The incidence of tuberous sclerosis is high in infants who present with infantile spasms.

5. What is the *best* study to confirm your diagnosis?
a) Urinalysis
b) Ultrasonography of the liver
c) Computed tomography (CT) scan of the brain
d) Cerebral angiography

Answer

The answer is c. Tubers in the brain are diagnostic of tuberous sclerosis. They are typically found in the subependymal region and undergo calcification (Fig. 68.3). The tubers may not be apparent until a patient with tuberous sclerosis is 3 to 4 years of age.

6. A 3-year-old boy is referred to you with a history of increasingly severe headaches. Physical examination reveals skin lesions (Fig. 68.4). The child's father has similar lesions on his trunk and a "lumpy" tumor at

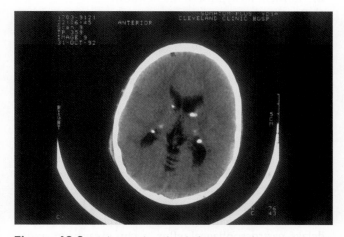

Figure 68.3 Subependymal calcifications of a patient with tuberous sclerosis.

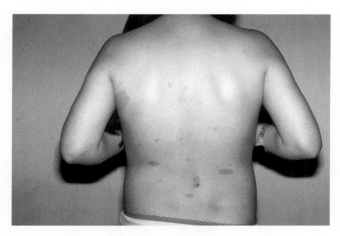

Figure 68.4 Skin lesions in patient in question 6. See explanation of question 6 for details. (See color insert.)

the base of his wrist. The child's blood pressure is 150/110 mm Hg. The *most* likely cause of this child's hypertension is:
a) Coarctation of the aorta
b) Conn syndrome
c) Renal artery stenosis
d) Multicystic kidney disease

Answer

The answer is c. The presence of *café au lait* lesions, which are evident in Figure 68.4, and the family history of similar lesions are consistent with a diagnosis of neurofibromatosis. Patients with neurofibromatosis have an increased incidence of:

■ Renal artery stenosis
■ Pheochromocytoma
■ Optic gliomas
■ Neurofibromas

Renal artery stenosis is common in children with neurofibromatosis, whereas pheochromocytoma is common in adults with neurofibromatosis.

7. A worried mother brings her two sons to your office. They are 5 and 7 years of age. Her concern is that her father's brother has just been started on dialysis and has adult-onset polycystic kidney disease. The mother's father was evaluated and had normal findings on renal ultrasonography. Which of the following studies should be performed to alleviate the mother's concern?
a) Renal ultrasonography
b) Intravenous pyelography
c) Abdominal CT scan with contrast
d) Liver function studies and liver ultrasonography
e) None of the above

Answer

The answer is e. Adult-onset polycystic kidney disease is transmitted in an autosomal-dominant pattern.

Therefore, if the mother's father does not have the disease, the mother is not at risk and her children cannot be affected. Patients with adult-type polycystic kidney disease (autosomal dominant) usually begin to have symptoms at 40 to 60 years of age, although cysts may be present early in life. Approximately 12% of patients have associated berry aneurysms.

8. You are asked to see an expectant mother for prenatal counseling because the fetus has been noted to have two large kidneys, both with numerous large cysts. The mother wants to know whether her child has polycystic kidney disease and if so what problems the infant might have. Which of the following is *true*?
a) The infant will most likely be born with renal failure and will require immediate dialysis.
b) Severe respiratory distress in the early newborn period is likely.
c) The risk that siblings will be affected is 50%.
d) Signs of hepatic fibrosis may develop in older children with infantile polycystic kidney disease.

Answer

The answer is b. The infantile type of polycystic kidney disease is transmitted in an *autosomal-recessive* fashion. Therefore, the risk that subsequent children will have the disease is 25%. The clinical manifestations appear early in infancy; *hypoplastic lungs are commonly associated, so that respiratory distress in the newborn period is likely.* The disease is also associated with congenital hepatic fibrosis.

9. A 13-year-old mentally retarded and institutionalized child with tuberous sclerosis is brought to your office with swelling of both wrists, which appear painful when touched. No erythema or fever is present. Radiographs show widening of the epiphyseal plates and "fraying." Which historical factor is important?
a) History of milk allergy
b) Family history of osteoporosis
c) Seizure disorder controlled with phenytoin (Dilantin)
d) History of stopping multivitamins 3 months earlier
e) History of a fractured rib

Answer

The answer is c. This is a summary of one of the first cases of anticonvulsant-induced rickets. The child was institutionalized and found to have rickets on radiography. The radiographic features of rickets include widened, concave, and frayed epiphyses (Fig. 68.5 and see Fig. 18.2). Although she lived in the United States and her intake of milk was normal, her exposure to sunlight was limited. She was being treated with both phenytoin and phenobarbital, and these agents stimulate the liver enzymatic systems that accelerate the destruction of 1,25-dihydroxycholecalciferol. Anticonvulsant therapy is a rare but important cause of rickets.

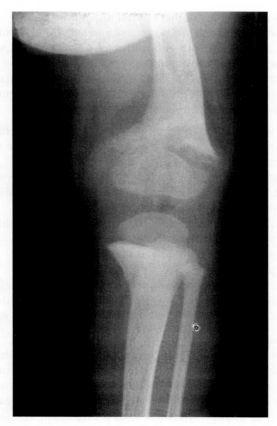

Figure 68.5 Knee radiograph of a patient with vitamin-D deficiency rickets. Note the widened and frayed epiphysis of the femur.

10. You are asked to perform a preoperative evaluation for a patient who is undergoing surgery to correct ptosis. The patient previously had an orchiopexy, is below the fifth percentile for height, and has a webbed neck. Physical examination reveals a midsystolic murmur heard over the entire chest and pronounced over both sides of the back. You conclude that the child has:
a) Holt-Oram syndrome
b) Menkes disease
c) Russell-Silver syndrome
d) Noonan syndrome

Answer

The answer is d. This child likely has Noonan syndrome, a usually sporadic disorder in which the karyotype is normal. The anomalies of Noonan syndrome also occur in girls with Turner syndrome. The most common ones include:

■ Short stature
■ Webbed neck
■ Pectus excavatum or carinatum
■ Congenital heart disease
■ Characteristic facies (hypertelorism, epicanthus, ptosis, micrographic)
■ Moderate mental retardation (25% of cases)

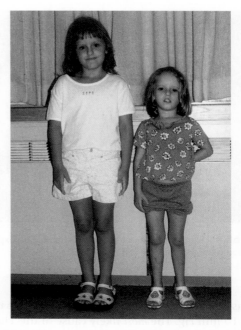

Figure 68.6 The young girl on the right has Russell-Silver syndrome. She is pictured next to her normal twin sister. Note the short stature and small, triangular face of the affected twin and the asymmetry of her lower extremities.

The most common cardiac defects are pulmonic valvular stenosis and atria septal defect. Russell-Silver syndrome (Fig. 68.6) is characterized by:

■ Short stature that becomes apparent even before birth
■ Small, triangular face
■ Asymmetry of the limbs
■ Small, inwardly curved little finger
■ Large, persistent fontanelle

Holt-Oram syndrome is characterized by both skeletal and cardiovascular abnormalities. The common skeletal abnormality is a defect of the upper limb (absent thumb, syndactyly, or an absent radius). This often is asymmetric, with only one side involved, but occasionally involvement is bilateral. The most commonly associated cardiac defects are ostium secundum atrial septal defect and ventricular septal defect.

Menkes disease is an X-linked–recessive defect of copper metabolism. The levels of both ceruloplasmin and copper have been low in all patients studied. The disease is characterized by a profound neurologic deficit that becomes evident by 1 to 2 months of life, and the process is degenerative. Death usually occurs by 3 years of age. The unusual feature of this disease is *kinky hair*. The hair is sparse and lightly pigmented, and twisting and partial breakage are apparent when the hair is viewed through a magnifying glass.

11. A 13-year-old girl is seen for a routine physical examination after having moved to the United States from Egypt. She has had three past episodes of swelling in the middle of her neck associated with redness and exquisite tenderness. Her symptoms have resolved with antibiotic therapy. During the examination, a small mobile mass is noted just above the hyoid bone in the midline of the neck. The mass feels "fluctuant," and it moves up and down when the patient sticks out and retracts her tongue. The *most* likely diagnosis of this mass is:
a) Branchial cleft cyst
b) Follicular carcinoma of the thyroid
c) Early lymphoma
d) Thyroglossal duct cyst

Answer
The answer is d. Thyroglossal duct cysts are defects located in or near the midline of the neck; they may extend to the base of the tongue, and they occasionally contain aberrant thyroid tissue. Branchial cleft cysts are lateral in origin and may open to the skin surface or drain into the pharynx. They may become secondarily infected and require antimicrobial therapy. Thyroid carcinoma and lymphoma are very unlikely given this case history.

12. The State Health Department notifies your office that a newborn screening test has revealed a low thyroxine (T_4) level in an infant now 7 days old. The *best* course of action is to:
a) Repeat measurements of the T_4, thyroid-stimulating hormone (TSH), and free T_4 levels.
b) Obtain a thyroid scan.
c) Begin thyroid replacement therapy now.
d) Obtain a skull film to assess sutures.
e) Answers a and b are correct.
f) Answers a and c are correct.
g) Answers a, b, and c are correct.

Answer
The answer is f. Confirmation of the screening test result is necessary. Therefore, the infant's T_4, TSH, and free T_4 levels should be measured. Once the results are available, therapy with levothyroxine should begin without delay. Therapy is discontinued if the confirmatory test results are negative. A thyroid scan should be performed only if the diagnosis of hypothyroidism is confirmed. Prolonged open sutures are a sign of congenital hypothyroidism, but this sign is not helpful diagnostically.

13. If the laboratory studies in the preceding question confirm the diagnosis of hypothyroidism, which of the following studies will *most* likely reveal the cause?
a) Triiodothyronine (T_3) resin uptake
b) Thyroid scan
c) CT scan of the neck
d) Thyroid-binding globulin determination

Answer
The answer is b. Approximately 60% of patients with congenital hypothyroidism have ectopic thyroid tissue, and another 30% are athyrotic. Measurement of the T_3 resin uptake does not help determine the cause of the hypothyroidism. Ten percent of patients have metabolic defects, determined with studies of ^{131}I uptake. A deficiency of thyroid-binding globulin does not represent true congenital hypothyroidism but rather the absence of a binding protein. Studies in this situation would show a decrease in the total T_4 level but a normal free T_4 level and a normal TSH level.

14. A 17-year-old boy is referred to you for evaluation of a heart murmur noted on his precollege physical examination. He has noted decreased stamina when playing basketball. Physical examination reveals a muscular boy with mild perioral cyanosis and bluish nail beds. A grade 2/6 holosystolic murmur is heard, and his blood pressure is 130/80 mm Hg. The *most* likely diagnosis is:
a) Tetralogy of Fallot
b) Atrial septal defect
c) Ventricular septal defect
d) Truncus arteriosus
e) Wolff-Parkinson-White syndrome

Answer
The answer is a. Tetralogy of Fallot is the most common congenital heart defect that presents in later life with cyanosis. The pulmonary stenosis is relative and along with the ventricular septal defect may finally become severe enough to cause right-to-left shunting.

15. A 3-year-old girl is referred for recurrent skin infection, four episodes of cavitary pneumonia, and numerous episodes of lymphadenitis. The *most* likely diagnosis is:
a) Severe combined immunodeficiency
b) Chronic granulomatous disease
c) X-linked hypogammaglobulinemia
d) Adenosine deaminase deficiency

Answer
The answer is b. Severe combined immunodeficiency and adenosine deaminase deficiency present early in life with overwhelming viral and bacterial infections. Patients with X-linked hypogammaglobulinemia are prone to a wide variety of bacterial infections, most frequently sinopulmonary, ear, and lung infections. The combination of cavitary pneumonia, skin infections, and lymphadenitis is most consistent with a neutrophil function disorder, such as chronic granulomatous disease.

16. A 13-year-old girl presents with a history of swelling of eyelids and feet for the last 2 weeks. Physical examination reveals a blood pressure of 130/100 mm Hg. Mild pretibial edema is present. Urinalysis shows 2+ protein and 2+ hemoglobin, and microscopic examination reveals two red blood cell casts per high-power field. Blood work values are as follows:

Serum creatinine = 1.0 mg/dL
Blood urea nitrogen = 29 mg/dL
C3 (complement) = 35 mg/dL (normal, 70–150)
Hemoglobin = 11.2 g/dL

Possible causes include all of the following *except:*
a) Systemic lupus erythematosus
b) Acute poststreptococcal glomerulonephritis
c) Membranoproliferative glomerulonephritis
d) Immunoglobulin A nephropathy

Answer

The answer is d. Glomerulonephritis with a *low* C3 level nearly always indicates systemic lupus erythematosus, acute poststreptococcal glomerulonephritis, or membranoproliferative glomerulonephritis. Systemic lupus erythematosus and membranoproliferative glomerulonephritis are seen with increased frequency in adolescent girls.

17. An 8-year-old boy is seen in the emergency department following a motor vehicle accident. He was not wearing a seat belt and was in the front passenger seat when the car was struck by another vehicle at the front passenger door. Physical examination reveals a pale boy in moderate distress with rapid shallow respirations. His blood pressure is 130/80 mm Hg; he has a laceration on his right arm, and glass particles are embedded in his right cheek. Chest radiography reveals three fractured ribs on the right side and no pneumothorax. Urinalysis shows 3+ blood and no protein, and microscopic examination shows numerous red blood cells but no casts. The *most* appropriate study to obtain next is:
a) Renal ultrasonography
b) Plain abdominal radiography (kidneys, ureter, and bladder)
c) Intravenous pyelography
d) CT scan of the abdomen

Answer

The answer is d. The presence of blood in the urine signifies severe trauma. The major concern is not the kidney but the other intra-abdominal organs, especially the liver and spleen. The trauma is right-sided, further increasing your concern for liver injury.

18. A 6-month-old infant presents to the emergency department with a sudden onset of tremors, vomiting, and poor responsiveness. He was breast-fed exclusively until recently, is now taking a bottle, and has just begun fruit juices. His blood sugar on admission to the emergency room is 22 mg/dL. The abdominal examination findings are unremarkable. The *most* likely diagnosis is:
a) Galactosemia
b) Hereditary fructose intolerance
c) Nesidioblastosis
d) Glycogen storage disease type I

Answer

The answer is b. Hypoglycemia develops in patients with hereditary fructose intolerance in response to fructose (or sucrose) ingestion. This child has just started fruit juices, which are often fortified with sucrose. Other features of this disorder include:

■ Failure to thrive
■ Hepatomegaly (with long-term ingestion)
■ Aminoaciduria

Galactosemia would present at an earlier date because breast milk contains galactose. Type I glycogen storage disease also would present at an earlier date, likely in association with hepatomegaly. Patients with nesidioblastosis, also known as *neonatal hyperinsulinemic hypoglycemia*, usually presents shortly after birth with severe hypoglycemia. The condition rarely appears after the age of 3 months. It is caused by an abnormality of the islet cells and an imbalance between the cells that produce insulin (β cells) and those that produce somatostatin.

Case for Questions 19–22

You are called by the state laboratory on a Friday afternoon about the positive result of an infant screening study for galactosemia. The infant is now 8 days old and has been fed formula since birth.

19. Of the following, what physical finding are you *least* likely to observe in this infant?
a) Hepatomegaly
b) Cataracts
c) Lethargy
d) Hypotonia
e) Cardiomegaly

Answer

The answer is e. Cardiomegaly is not normally a feature of galactosemia, whereas the other physical findings are associated with this disorder.

20. Which of the following laboratory tests would be *most* helpful in making the diagnosis?
a) Blood glucose determination
b) Liver enzyme determination
c) Prothrombin time and partial thromboplastin time
d) Urinalysis
e) Urine for reducing substances

Answer

The answer is e. The presence of reducing substances would be consistent with the diagnosis of galactosemia.

21. Which of the following formulas would be *best* for this child?
a) Enfamil
b) Isomil
c) SMA
d) Similac
e) Breast milk

Answer
The answer is b. Isomil is a soy-based formula in which the sugar source is sucrose, not lactose (which is glucose and galactose). This is not recommended for long-term treatment.

22. If this child is not treated, the *most* likely long-term outcome will be:
a) Mental retardation
b) Death from liver failure
c) Seizure disorder
d) Death from *Escherichia coli* sepsis

Answer
The answer is d. Infants with galactosemia are susceptible to frequent infections with *E. coli.* These include sepsis and meningitis.

23. Which of the following is *not* a correct statement regarding Waardenburg syndrome?
a) It is inherited in an autosomal-dominant pattern.
b) Patients often exhibit a broad nasal root.
c) Patients have a white forelock.
d) Sensorineural hearing loss occurs in 20% of patients.
e) The incidence of mental retardation is 50%.

Answer
The answer is e. Waardenburg syndrome is characterized by lateral displacement of the medial canthi, partial albinism, and congenital deafness. A broad nasal root is found in approximately 80% of patients, congenital deafness in 20%, and a white forelock in approximately 20%. The condition is inherited in an autosomal-dominant manner. Mental retardation is not usually a feature.

24. A 14-month-old infant was seen in the emergency department for severe abdominal pain and was given a Fleet enema. This was repeated because no result was obtained with the first enema. Thirty minutes after the second enema, the infant had a grand mal seizure. The *most* likely cause of the seizure was:
a) Hypoglycemia
b) Hypertension
c) Hypocalcemia
d) Hypophosphatemia
e) Pyridoxine depletion

Answer
The answer is c. This child likely has hypocalcemia secondary to acute phosphate overload. The Fleet enema contained phosphate, which was absorbed. The resultant fall in the serum calcium level provoked the seizure. Phosphate enemas should be given to infants and young children with great care, or not at all.

25. During the examination of a newborn boy, you note that he is larger on the right side than on the left. The arm, leg, and trunk are all involved. This newborn is at increased risk for all of the following *except:*
a) Wilms tumor
b) Hepatoblastoma

c) Adrenal carcinoma
d) Acute lymphocytic leukemia
e) Adrenal adenoma

Answer
The answer is d. Hemihypertrophy is not associated with an increased risk for acute lymphocytic leukemia. It is associated with an increased risk for the development of adrenal tumors, Wilms tumor, and hepatoblastoma.

26. A 16-month-old boy who had been walking since the age of 12 months is brought to you because his gait is not improving; rather, he is less steady than he was at 13 months of age. You note that his eyes are bloodshot; the parents say the condition is constant and appears to be getting worse. This infant has a disorder characterized by all of the following *except:*
a) Susceptibility to sinopulmonary infections
b) Increased incidence of lymphoma
c) Thymic hypoplasia
d) Progressive jaundice
e) Decreased levels of immunoglobulin A and immunoglobulin E

Answer
The answer is d. Ataxia-telangiectasia is an autosomal-recessive disorder. A defective DNA repair mechanism leads to progressive cerebellar ataxia and the development of multiple telangiectases, which are most obvious in the sclerae. Individuals with this disorder have a deficiency of immunoglobulins A and E and a variable degree of T-cell deficiency. Recurrent sinopulmonary problems and bronchiectasis affect many patients. They are also at risk for the development of neoplasms, most commonly lymphoreticular malignancies. Thymic hypoplasia, which may be severe, is sometimes a feature of this disorder and contributes to the T-cell deficiencies. Progressive jaundice is not a feature of ataxia–telangiectasia, although hepatic abnormalities are present and the level of α-fetoprotein may be increased.

27. A premature infant, born at 35 weeks of gestation, is noted to have macrosomia, a large tongue, and an initial hematocrit of 67%. His birth weight is 4.9 kg. This infant will have all of the following *except:*
a) Very large adrenal glands on CT scan or magnetic resonance imaging
b) A tendency to develop hypoglycemia
c) An increased chance for the development of Wilms tumor
d) A life expectancy of 20 to 25 years

Answer
The answer is d. This infant has Beckwith-Wiedemann syndrome. Such infants are often premature and large and have large tongues; adrenal cortical cytomegaly is a constant feature. The incidence of Wilms tumor is increased (6.5%), especially in those infants who also have hemi-hypertrophy. Omphaloceles are relatively common

in these infants. Affected children who survive infancy are generally healthy. Hypoglycemia in infancy must be recognized and treated aggressively.

28. A 16-year-old previously healthy boy presents with cervical lymphadenopathy. Physical examination reveals a healthy-appearing boy with a left-sided, 2-cm, firm, nontender posterior cervical lymph node and a left-sided, 5-cm, firm, nontender supraclavicular lymph node. The *most* likely diagnosis is:
a) Hodgkin disease
b) *Mycobacteria avium* complex infection
c) Cat scratch disease
d) Reactive lymphadenitis

Answer
The answer is a. The finding of firm, nontender lymph nodes, especially in the supraclavicular area, raises a concern for malignancy. The age of the patient and the fact that he appears healthy are consistent with a presentation of Hodgkin lymphoma. *Mycobacterium avium* complex infection and other mycobacterial infections in addition to tuberculosis may present with firm, nontender cervical adenopathy, but are most commonly seen in children between the ages of 1 and 4 years. The adenitis of cat scratch disease and reactive adenitis are usually tender and rarely involve the supraclavicular areas.

29. A 14-year-old boy is brought to the emergency department after being hit by a car while riding his bicycle. He was not wearing a helmet at the time of the impact. Physical findings include bloody discharge from the right middle ear and an area of ecchymosis in the right post auricular area. Of the following, the *most* likely diagnosis is:
a) Basilar skull fracture
b) Subarachnoid hemorrhage
c) Epidural hematoma
d) Concussion

Answer
The answer is a. The findings of bloody ear drainage, or hemotympanum, along with ecchymosis of the mastoid area (Battle sign) are most consistent with a *basilar skull fracture* involving the temporal bone. Other manifestations of basilar skull fractures, which may involve the frontal, ethmoid, sphenoid, or occipital bones, include:

■ Periorbital ecchymosis (raccoon eyes)
■ Cerebrospinal fluid rhinorrhea or otorrhea
■ Unilateral hearing loss
■ Cranial nerve involvement (VII and VIII)

Basilar skull fractures are difficult to detect radiographically. Epidural hematomas are usually the result of rupture of the middle meningeal artery, which results in an initial loss of consciousness followed by a lucid interval and subsequent neurologic deterioration. Subarachnoid hemorrhage manifests with severe headache and photophobia. CT scan of the head is helpful in diagnosing these entities.

30. The boy in question 29 does well except for persistent clear otorrhea. Several days later, a stiff neck, headache, and fever develop. Lumbar puncture reveals white blood cells 1250/mm³, 90% of which are neutrophils. The cerebrospinal fluid protein level is 90 mg/dL, and the glucose level is 10 mg/dL. Of the following, the *most* likely organism causing this boy's meningitis is:
a) *Staphylococcus aureus*
b) *Neisseria meningitidis*
c) *Streptococcus pneumoniae*
d) *Eikenella corrodens*
e) *Moraxella catarrhalis*

Answer
The answer is c. A cerebrospinal fluid leak, which is a well-known complication of basilar skull fracture, has developed in this child. Cerebrospinal fluid otorrhea and rhinorrhea are the major manifestations of cerebrospinal fluid leaks. The most likely organism associated with such leaks is *S. pneumoniae,* which is often a normal inhabitant of the nasopharynx. Nontypable *Haemophilus influenzae* is another cause of meningitis in this clinical situation. The organisms gain entry into the meninges from the nasopharynx because of the anatomic disruption in the base of the skull.

Case for Questions 31–32
A 13-year-old girl presents with a history of increasingly severe headaches for the past 2 months. The headaches are frontal in location and pounding, and they have awakened her from sleep three times in the past week. Physical examination reveals a blood pressure of 110/70 mm Hg, hyperreflexia without focal findings, and mild hepatomegaly (13 cm).

31. Which of the following is a clue to the cause of the headaches?
a) She was in an automobile accident 4 months ago, after which she underwent CT scan of the brain. Findings were normal.
b) She has grown 10 cm taller in 7 months.
c) Teachers have noted that she is very easily distracted.
d) She became a vegetarian 6 months ago and began taking vitamin supplements.
e) She takes tetracycline once daily.

Answer
The answer is d.

32. Particular attention should be paid to her intake of:
a) Vitamin A
b) Vitamin C
c) Vitamin D
d) Vitamin E
e) Vitamin K

Answer
The answer is a. This girl likely has vitamin A toxicity. Because vitamin A is a fat-soluble vitamin, overdoses can

cause significant toxicity. Signs of vitamin A *toxicity* include:

- Headache
- Pseudotumor cerebri
- Dryness of the mucous membranes
- Hepatomegaly

Signs of vitamin A *deficiency* include:

- Poor night vision
- Xerosis conjunctivae (drying of the conjunctivae)
- Keratomalacia (clouding of the cornea)
- Formation of dry, silver-gray plaques on the bulbar conjunctivae (Bitot spots)
- Apathy
- Anemia
- Mental and physical growth retardation
- Follicular hyperkeratosis

33. Which of the following is an indication for immunotherapy for bee sting prophylaxis?
a) Cardiovascular collapse
b) Large local reaction
c) Generalized hives
d) Joint swelling
e) All of the above

Answer

The answer is a. The indications for immunotherapy include systemic symptoms of anaphylaxis, including cardiovascular collapse and respiratory distress.

34. A 6-year-old girl is referred by her schoolteacher. She often loses concentration for periods of 10 to15 seconds, and then resumes her previous activity. The frequency of these episodes is increasing, and she may have 12 to 15 of them each hour. Her physical examination findings, growth, and development are normal. The patient will *most* likely:
a) Improve with methylphenidate (Ritalin) therapy
b) Require behavior feedback therapy
c) Have a 3/second spike and wave pattern on her electroencephalogram
d) Respond to phenytoin (Dilantin) therapy

Answer

The answer is c. The episodes are most consistent with petit mal seizures. These are characterized by a sudden cessation of motor activity or speech and a blank facial expression. Such seizures are more prevalent in girls than in boys, are never associated with an aura, rarely persist >30 seconds, and are not associated with a postictal state. The seizures can be induced by hyperventilation, and the characteristic electroencephalographic pattern is a 3/second spike and generalized wave discharge. Phenytoin is not effective for petit mal seizures; *ethosuximide and sodium valproate are effective medications.*

Questions 35–39
Match the deficiency states of the following vitamins with the symptom:

35. Vitamin A

36. Vitamin C

37. Vitamin D

38. Vitamin E

39. Vitamin K
a) Growth failure, low serum levels of calcium and phosphate
b) Bleeding in the gastrointestinal tract in a 1-day-old infant
c) Dry eyes
d) Bleeding in the joints and mucous membranes
e) Anemia in a premature infant

Answers

35. The answer is c. Vitamin A deficiency is associated with dry eyes and poor night vision.
36. The answer is d. Vitamin C deficiency is associated with bleeding in the joints and mucous membranes.
37. The answer is a. Vitamin D deficiency results in growth failure and low serum levels of calcium and phosphate.
38. The answer is e. Premature infants may have low levels of vitamin E, and a hemolytic anemia may develop that can be corrected by the administration of vitamin E.
39. The answer is b. Vitamin K deficiency results in a bleeding diathesis in neonates.

Questions 40–43
Match the toxicity state of the following vitamins with the clinical description:

40. Chronic hypervitaminosis A

41. Vitamin D toxicity

42. Vitamin C toxicity

43. Acute vitamin A toxicity
a) Renal stones
b) Anorexia, pruritus, poor weight gain
c) Pseudotumor cerebri
d) Nephrocalcinosis

Answers

40. The answer is b. *Chronic* hypervitaminosis A develops with the ingestion of excessive doses for weeks and months. It manifests with anorexia, pruritus, and poor weight gain. Other features include:

- Increased irritability
- Fissuring at the corners of the mouth
- Increased intracranial pressure
- Hepatomegaly

41. The answer is d. Vitamin D toxicity may result in hypercalcemia and hypercalciuria, which lead to nephrocalcinosis. Other manifestations of vitamin D toxicity include:

- Hypotonia
- Anorexia
- Irritability
- Constipation
- Polydipsia
- Polyuria

42. The answer is a. Vitamin C toxicity can lead to secondary hyperoxaluria, which is associated with the development of renal stones.

43. The answer is c. Acute vitamin A toxicity can result in nausea, vomiting, drowsiness, and increased intracranial pressure. Pseudotumor cerebri, characterized by evidence of increased intracranial pressure, may also occur.

44. A 3-year-old girl returned from vacation and found her bottle of Flintstones vitamins with iron in her suitcase. She ingested the remaining contents of the bottle, which her mother found a few hours later (it had been about half full). Which of the following is likely to develop?
a) Tremors and possible seizures
b) Jaundice
c) Diarrhea
d) Hematuria
e) Headache

Answer
The answer is c. Iron toxicity acutely results in gastrointestinal symptoms, which are caused by the local irritative effects of iron on the gastrointestinal tract. Nausea, vomiting, diarrhea, abdominal pain, hematemesis, and bloody diarrhea can occur. Hypoglycemia and metabolic acidosis may also occur 12 to 24 hours after the ingestion of iron. Severe hepatic necrosis can develop 2 to 4 days after iron poisoning. What prevented a serious overdose in this child was the fact that she ingested children's vitamins with iron, not adult iron medication. For this reason, the ingestion of prenatal vitamins with iron may be life threatening and lead to all the consequences listed in this question.

45. An 18-year-old boy with a recent diagnosis of cystic fibrosis is found to have absent deep tendon reflexes, a positive Romberg sign, mild tremors, and an inability to direct his gaze upward. He *most* likely has:
a) Zinc deficiency
b) Vitamin B deficiency
c) Vitamin C deficiency
d) Vitamin E deficiency
e) Iron deficiency

Answer
The answer is d. Patients with cystic fibrosis do not absorb fat-soluble vitamins. These include vitamins A, D,

K, and E. A degenerative neurologic syndrome may develop in patients with malabsorption and vitamin E deficiency.

46. A 3-year-old child is seen because he is listless and irritable. Approximately 6 months ago, his fingers and toes became pink. Now his hands, feet, and nose are pink, and he complains of pain and itching in his hands and feet. He lives on his grandfather's farm in rural Mississippi. This child *most* likely has which of the following?
a) Linoleic acid deficiency
b) Lead intoxication
c) Zinc deficiency
d) Mercury intoxication
e) Copper deficiency

Answer
The answer is d. The child has mercury intoxication, or acrodynia. This deficiency state was common in the 1940s and 1950s, but is rare today because mercury has been removed from most household products. The skin findings, neurologic symptoms, and painful hands and feet are characteristic.

47. A newborn infant is found to have hypocalcemia following a generalized seizure. Workup reveals that the child has a truncus arteriosus and an absent thymus. Which of the following statements is *true* regarding this child?
a) Only irradiated packed red blood cells should be utilized for blood transfusion during surgical correction of the child's heart disease.
b) The hypocalcemia is likely caused by renal anomalies.
c) Infections with encapsulated organisms are the current problem.
d) The cause of this child's condition is not known.

Answer
The answer is a. This child has DiGeorge syndrome, an inherited disorder resulting from microdeletions in chromosome 22. Manifestations include hypoplasia or aplasia of the thymus and parathyroid glands secondary to dysmorphogenesis of the third and fourth pharyngeal pouches. Hypocalcemia results from parathyroid gland dysfunction. Abnormal T-cell function results from absence or hypoplasia of the thymus gland and predisposes infants to infections with organisms controlled by functioning T cells, such as *Candida* and *Pneumocystis*.

An abnormal facies, characterized by a short philtrum, hypertelorism, mandibular hypoplasia, and low-set, notched ears, may also be present. Truncal anomalies are the most common congenital heart lesions associated with this disorder.

Only irradiated blood products can be given to these infants until their immune status is clarified to avoid severe and fatal graft versus host disease.

48. Which of the following is a *true* statement regarding infants of diabetic mothers?

a. Most of these infants are small for gestational age.
b. The neonatal mortality rate of these infants is similar to that of infants of nondiabetic mothers of similar gestational age and birth weight.
c. Symptomatic hypoglycemia occurs in most of these infants.
d. They have an increased incidence of congenital anomalies.

Answer

The answer is d. Infants of diabetic mothers have a significantly increased risk of congenital anomalies, including the following:

- Lumbosacral agenesis
- Cardiac malformations
  - Ventricular septal defect
  - Atrial septal defect
  - Transposition of the great vessels
  - Truncus arteriosus
  - Coarctation of the aorta
  - Double outlet right ventricle
- Neural tube defects
- Renal anomalies
- Duodenal or anorectal atresia
- Small left colon syndrome
- Holoprosencephaly

These infants may develop small left colon syndrome (Fig. 68.7), caused by a transient delay in development of the left side of the colon; infants with this maturation delay clinically present with abdominal distension.

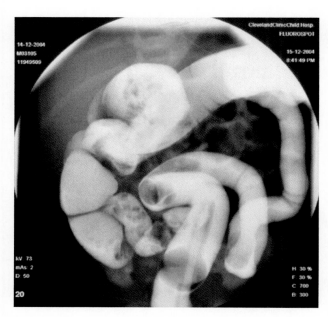

Figure 68.7 A water-soluble contrast study of the colon in an infant of a diabetic mother who presented with abdominal distension. Note that the left side of the colon is smaller in caliber than the more proximal large bowel.

Because of fetal hyperglycemia and hyperinsulinemia, most infants of diabetic mothers are large for their gestational age. The neonatal mortality rate for these infants is significantly greater than that for infants of nondiabetic mothers. Hypoglycemia occurs in 25% to 50% of these infants, although only a small percentage of these infants become symptomatic.

49. Which of the following conditions is *not* an indication for Growth Hormone therapy?
a) Chronic renal failure
b) Small for gestational age infant
c) Cystic fibrosis
d) AIDS wasting

Answer

The answer is c. Growth hormone therapy is approved by the Food and Drug Administration (FDA) for the following indications:

- Growth hormone deficiency
- Chronic renal failure
- AIDS wasting
- Small for gestational age infant
- Height 2.25 SD below the mean (<1 percentile)
- Short gut syndrome
- SHOX defect
- Turner syndrome
- Noonan syndrome
- Prader-Willi syndrome

Growth hormone therapy is not currently indicated for patients with cystic fibrosis.

SUGGESTED READINGS

1. Boxer LA. Neutrophil abnormalities. *Pediatr Rev* 2003;24:52–62.
2. Chen YT. Defects in galactose metabolism. In: Behrman R, Kliegman R, Jenson H, eds. *Nelson textbook of pediatrics*, 17th ed. Philadelphia: Saunders, 2004:475–476.
3. Finberg L. Feeding the healthy child. In: McMillen JA, DeAngelis CD, Feigin RD, Jones RD, eds. *Oski's pediatrics*, 4th ed. Philadelphia: Lippincott Williams & Wilkins, 2006:109–118.
4. Fisher DA. Disorders of the thyroid in the newborn and infant. In: Sperling MA, ed. *Pediatric endocrinology*, 2nd ed. Philadelphia: Saunders, 2002:161–186.
5. Haller JA. Blunt trauma to the abdomen. *Pediatr Rev* 1996;17:29–31.
6. Haslam RHA. Neurocutaneous syndromes. In: Behrman R, Kliegman R, Jenson H, eds. *Nelson textbook of pediatrics*, 17th ed. Philadelphia: Saunders, 2004:2015–2019.
7. Heird WC. Vitamin deficiencies and excesses. In: Behrman R, Kliegman R, Jenson H, eds. *Nelson textbook of pediatrics*, 17th ed. Philadelphia: Saunders, 2004:177–190.
8. Joiner TA, Foster C, Shope T. The many faces of vitamin D deficiency rickets. *Pediatr Rev* 2000;21:296–302.
9. Misra M, Pacaud D, Petryk A, et al. on behalf of the Drug and Therapeutics Committee of the Lawson Wilkins Pediatric Endocrine Society. Vitamin D deficiency in children and its management: review of current knowledge and recommendations. *Pediatrics* 2008;122:398–417.
10. Root AW, Diamond FB II. Calcium metabolism. In: Sperling MA, ed. *Pediatric endocrinology*, 2nd ed. Philadelphia: Saunders, 2002:65–95.

Index

Page numbers in italic refer to figures; those followed by *t* refer to tables.

A

Abdominal distention, 83
Abdominal masses, 470
Abdominal pain, 37–45, 442
  common causes of, 39–41
    carbohydrate intolerance, 40–41
    constipation, 41
    gastritis/peptic ulcer disease, 40
    gastroesophageal reflux, 32,
      39–40, 259
    intestinal parasites, 41
  functional, 37–39
  less common causes of, 41–43
    celiac disease, 43, 78–79
    cholelithiasis, 42
    Crohn disease, 41–42, 46, 49t
    intussusception, 34, 42, 518
    pancreatis, 42–43
  with organic causes, 39–44
  red flags of, 37
  uncommon causes of, 43–44
    acute intermittent porphyria, 43–44
    choledochal cyst, 43
    familial Mediterranean fever, 44, 447
    Henoch-Schönlein purpura, 44,
      438–439, 438t, 551
    uteropelvic junction, 44, 536, 541
Abdominal trauma, 508–509
Abdominal wall defects, 523
Abnormalities of neck, 525–526
Acanthosis nigrans, 106
Accelerated atherosclerosis, 435
ACE. *See* Angiotensin-converting enzyme
Acellular pertussis vaccination, 24
Acetaminophen, 497
Achondroplasia, 332
Acid
  azelaic, 9
  bichloracetic, 364
  disopropyliminodiacetic, 74
  fatty, oxidation, 343
  folic, 306
  hepatic dimethyliminodiacetic, 74
  hydrofluoric, 67
  ingestions, 67
  trichloroacetic, 364
  uric, 488
Acid-base/complex fluid and electrolyte
    problems, 109–116
Acidosis
  gap, 112t
  lactic, 106
  metabolic, 513
  renal tubular, 109, 143
  severe, 110
  worsening central nervous system, 112

Acne, 8–9
Acquired heart disease, 194–200
  acute rheumatic fever, 195–196,
    199, 550
  dilated cardiomyopathy, 197
  hypertrophic cardiomyopathy,
    197–198
  infective endocarditis, 194–195
  Kawasaki disease, 196, 199, 213, 551
  myocarditis, 197
  pericarditis, 196, 199
  preventive cardiology, 198
Acquired hypothyroidism, 131, *132*
Acquired primary adrenal insufficiency,
    124–125
Acrodermatitis enteropathica, 3, 552
ACTH. *See* Adrenocorticotropic hormone
Active immunization, 54
Acute chest syndrome, 459–460
Acute confusional migraines, 261
Acute hepatitis B infection, *55*
Acute intermittent porphyria, 43–44
Acute intestinal obstruction, 411
Acute leukemia, 477
Acute lymphoblastic leukemia, 489
Acute lymphocytic leukemia (ALL), 468,
    472, 563
Acute myeloid leukemia (AML), 469, 472
Acute osteomyelitis, 390t
Acute rheumatic fever, 195–196, 199, 550
Acute scrotal swelling, 538
Acute sequestration crisis (ASC), 460
Acutely ill neonate, 346
Acyclovir, 415
Adenoma sebaceum, 269
Adenotonsillectomy, 444
ADHD. *See* Attention deficit hyperactivity
    disorder
Adolescent development, 350–356
  delayed puberty, 353, 371
  treatment/prognosis, 352–353
Adolescent menstrual cycle, 369
ADPKD. *See* Autosomal-dominant
    polycystic kidney disease
Adrenal androgen, 126, 128
Adrenal cortex, 123–128
Adrenal disorders, 123–129
Adrenal hyperplasia, 343
Adrenal insufficiency, 125
  acquired primary, 124–125
  congenital primary, 123–124
  primary, 123
  secondary, 125
Adrenal medulla, 128
Adrenal steroidogenesis pathway, *124*
Adrenocorticotropic hormone (ACTH), 149

Adrenoleukodystrophy (ALD), 346
Adult respiratory distress syndrome
    (ARDS), 514
Adult-onset polycystic kidney disease,
    559
Afebrile pneumonia syndrome, 426
AFP. *See* Serum alpha-fetoprotein
Age-dependent variation, 448
Aggressive antibiotic therapy, 381
Air flow patterns, 236t
Airway abnormalities, 154
Airway/pulmonary disorders, 233–240
Alagille syndrome, 72
Albinism, 271, 544
Albuterol, 232
ALD. *See* Adrenoleukodystrophy
Alkalosis, 114
ALL. *See* Acute lymphocytic leukemia
Allergic conjunctivitis, 547
Allergic disorders, 214–218
  allergic conjunctivitis, 547
  allergic rhinoconjunctivitis, 214–215
  anaphylaxis, 215–216
  stinging insect allergy, 216
  urticaria, 6, 216–217
Allergic rhinoconjunctivitis, 214–215
Allergies, 241–247
  egg, 19
  food, 34
  latex, 215
  peanut/tree nut, 243
  stinging insect, 216
Alopecia, 129
Alpers-Huttenlocher syndrome, 290
Alport syndrome, 98
Alternative educational placement,
    321–322
Ambiguous genitalia, 178
Amblyopia, 543–545
Amebiasis, 388
Amebic dysentery, 388
Amelioration, 14
Amenorrhea, 368–376
  definition of, 368
  with delayed puberty, 353, 371
  etiology of, 369–370
  evaluation of, 370–374
  with hirsutism/normal pubertal
    development, 374
  menstrual cycle, 368–369
  with normal pubertal development,
    350, 371–373
  principles of treatment, 374
Amino acid metabolism, 341, 343
Aminosalicylates, 50
AML. *See* Acute myeloid leukemia

Ammonia metabolism, 343
Ammonium chloride, 110
Amoxicillin, 195
Amyoplasia, 337
ANA. *See* Antinuclear antibody
Anabolic steroids, 30
Anaphylaxis, 215–216
Androgenic changes, 354
Anemia, 448–456
    additional testing in evaluation of, 454
    age-dependent variation, 448
    classification of, 448–449
    clinical manifestations of some types
        of, 451, 451*t*
    common causes of, in different age
        groups, 450*t*
    diagnostic clues to, 450*t*
    Diamond-Blackfan, 455
    Fanconi, 176, 454
    folate deficiency, 82
    functional/pathophysiologic classifica-
        tion, 448, 450*t*
    general clinical manifestations of, 451*t*
    Heinz body hemolytic, 463*t*
    hemoglobin values indicating, 449*t*
    hemolytic, 71, 435
    history/physical examination, 449–452
    hypochromic, 454, 488
    of infancy, 448
    laboratory evaluation, 452–454, 453*t*
    morphologic classification of, 449*t*
    physical examination of, 451–452
    workup of, 451
Angelman syndrome, 328
Angiokeratomas, 122
Angiotensin-converting enzyme (ACE),
    188, 447
Anhydrotic ectodermal dysplasia, 334
Animal slaughterhouses, 408
Ankle fractures, 503
Anomalous left coronary artery, 192, 194
Anterior cruciate ligament injury, 30–31
Anthrax, 429, 430
Antibiotics, 491
Antibodies
    antineutrophil cytoplasmic, 446
    antinuclear, 431
    heterophil, 420
    perinuclear antineutrophil
        cytoplasmic, 49
    positive antinuclear, 446
Anticholinergic agents, 497
Anticonvulsant therapy, 136, 247–257
Anticyclic citrullinated peptide (CCP),
    431
Antidotes, 496–497
Antiepileptic medications, 251–254
Antifungal therapy, 401
Anti-IgE therapy, 231
Antimalarials, 410, 437
Antimicrobial therapy, 419
Antineutrophil cytoplasmic antibody, 446
Antinuclear antibody (ANA), 431
Antiseptic medication
    adverse effects, 254*t*
    drug–drug interactions, 254
    efficacy of, 251*t*

monitoring, 253–254
    treatment with, 252–253
Antituberculous agents, 404*t*
Aortic arch, 244
Aphthous, 48
Aplastic crisis, 461
Apnea, 173
Appendectomy, 514
Appendicitis, 517, 518
ARDS. *See* Adult respiratory distress
    syndrome
ART. *See* Automated reagin test
Arteries
    anomalous left coronary, 192
    coronary, 211
    mean, pressure, 507
    migraines, 261
    normal coronary, branching pattern,
        191
    transposition of great, 190, 212
Arthritis, 442
    childhood chronic, 431*t*
    juvenile rheumatoid, 430–434
    migratory, 424
    pauciarticular-onset juvenile rheuma-
        toid, 432
    polyarticular-onset juvenile rheuma-
        toid, 432
    psoriatic, 433
    reactive, 385, 434
    septic, 390
    systemic-onset juvenile rheumatoid,
        432–433
ASC. *See* Acute sequestration crisis
Ascaris lumbricoides infections, 411
Ascites, 100
Aseptic meningitis, 392
Ash leaf spot, 269
Asparaginase, 492
Aspergillus species, 244, 402
Aspirin, 32, 199, 210
Asthma, 219–233
    assessing, control, 225*t*, 226*t*
    classifying severity/initiating treatment
        in, 222*t*, 223*t*
    clinical presentation of, 220
    diagnosis of, 220
    differential diagnosis of
        infant/childhood, 221*t*
    environmental control therapy, 231
    environmental factors of, 231*t*
    etiology/epidemiology of, 219
    leukotriene modifiers, 230–231
    management/treatment of, 220–231
    pathophysiology of, 219–220
    pharmacotherapy for, 221–231
        corticosteroids, 222–224
        cromolyn sodium/nedocromil,
            224–227, 232
        long acting β$_2$-Agonists, 227–229
        methylxanthines, 229–230
    prognosis of, 231–232
    stepwise approach for managing, 228*t*,
        229*t*, 230*t*
Asymptomatic abdominal mass, 474
Asymptomatic HIV infection, 18
Ataxia-telangiectasia, 379

Atherosclerosis, 435
Athetoid CP, 304
Athletic training, 213
Atopic dermatitis, 1, 2, 2, 241
Atrial fibrillation, 203
Atrial flutter, 203, 207
Atrial septal defects, 181, 188–189
Atrioventricular canal defects, 189
Attention deficit hyperactivity disorder
        (ADHD), 309–311, 323
    differential diagnosis of, 310
    summary of, 309*t*
    treatment of, 310–311
Atypical absence seizures, 248
Aureus, 396
Autism
    assessment, 321
    clinical presentation, 308
    diagnosis, 308–309
    etiology, 308
    pharmacologic therapy, 309
    summary of, 308*t*
    treatment, 309
Autoimmune thyroiditis, 131
Automated reagin test (ART), 362
Autosomal-dominant dystrophies, 277
Autosomal-dominant polycystic kidney
        disease (ADPKD), 117
Autosomal-recessive dystrophies,
        278–279
Autosomal-recessive fashion, 559
Autovirus infection, 387
Azelaic acid, 9
Azotemia, 513

B
B core antigen, 428
B. pertussis, 419
Babesioses, 411
Bacteremia, 212
Bacterial agents, 10
Bacterial conjunctivitis, 546
Bacterial infections, 383–386, 422
Bacterial meningitis, 396, 425
Bacterial peritonitis, 121
Bacterial pneumonia, 393–394
Bacterial sepsis, 465
Bacterial superinfection, 422
Bacterial vaginosis, 363–364, 366
Balanoposthitis, 539
Barium enema, 522
Barium swallow, 234
Barlow test, 529–530
Bartonella henselae, 392
Basilar artery migraines, 261
Batteries, 65–66
BCA. *See* Bichloracetic acid
Beckwith-Wiedemann syndrome, 328,
        563
Bed wetting, 28
Benign focal epilepsy, 249
Benign myoclonus, 263
    neonatal, 259
Benign paroxysmal vertigo, 261
Benign thyroid replacement, 561
Benzodiazepines, 249
Bernard-Soulier syndrome, 482–483

Bethlem myopathy (BM), 278
Bichloracetic acid (BCA), 364
Bilateral acoustic neuromas, *268*
Biliary atresia, 75
Bilious emesis, 83, 519
Bilious vomiting, 557
Bilirubin, 76
Biochemical components, 156
Biotin metabolism, 343
Biotinidase deficiency, 343
Bladder instability of childhood, 540
Bleeding disorders, 471, 480–485
   disorders of plasma factors, 483–484
   normal coagulation cascade/laboratory
      screening tests, 480–481
   platelet disorders, 481–483
Blood urea nitrogen (BUN), 90
Bloody diarrhea, 48, 383
Bloody ear drainage, 564
Blunt trauma, 508
BM. *See* Bethlem myopathy
Body fluids, 110
Body plethysmography, 236
Bone cancer, 476
Bone marrow hypoplasia, 452*t*
Bone pain, 469–470
Bordetella pertussis, 24, 392, 419
Borrelia burgdorferi, 392, 408
Bowing/bend fractures, 501
Bradycardias, 203–204
Brain abscess, 393
Brain tumors, 471, 490
Breath holding, 206, 213, 258
Broad-spectrum antibiotics, 465
Bronchoconstriction, 219
Bruton's agammaglobulinemia, 378
Buccal cellulitis, *389*
Buckle fractures, 501, 504
Bulbous impetigo, 175, 423
BUN. *See* Blood urea nitrogen
Burkitt lymphoma, 488
Burns, 509–510
   deep partial thickness, 510
   pediatric trauma, 509–510
   superficial, 509
Butterfly rash, 435
Byler disease, 72

C

Café au lait spots, 151, 266, 273, 559
CAH. *See* Congenital adrenal hyperplasia
Calcium/phosphorus metabolism,
   135–140
Caliciviruses, 387
Campylobacter infection, 385–386, 396
Cancers
   bone, 476
   liver, 477
   pediatric, 468*t*
Candida, 401
Carbamazepine, 250, 252
Carbohydrate intolerance, 40–41
Carbohydrate metabolism, 343
Carboplatin, 477
Cardiac anomalies, 521
Cardiac catheterization, 193, 210
Cardiac echocardiogram, 523

Cardiac rate/rhythm
   bradycardias, 203–204
   disorders of, 200–207
   irregular rhythms, 204
   long QT syndrome, 205–206
   syncope, 204–205
   tachycardias, 201–203
   variability in sinus rhythm, 201
Cardiac tamponade, 515
Cardiogenic shock, 185
Cardiology, 208–214
   preventive, 198
Cardiomegaly, 562
Cardiomyopathy, 492
   dilated, 197
   hypertrophic, 197–198
Cardiopulmonary resuscitation (CPR), 203
Cardiorespiratory decompensation, 239
Cardiovascular disorders, 180–187
   cardiogenic shock, 185
   chest pain, 183
   congestive heart failure, 184–185
   heart murmurs, 180–182
   modes of presentation, 183–184
   neonatal cyanosis, 183
   participation screening, 182–183
Cartilaginous matrix, 137
Cat scratch adenitis, 417
Cataracts, 547–548, 548
CATCH 22 Syndrome, 329–330
Caustic ingestions, 62–70
   clinical manifestations, 67
   epidemiology of, 66–67
   long-term complications, 68
   management, 67–68
   mechanism of injury, 67
CCP. *See* Anticyclic citrullinated peptide
CD. *See* Crohn disease
CDC. *See* Center for Disease Control and
   Prevention
Ceftriaxone, 425
Celiac disease, 43, 81
   clinical manifestations, 78
   diagnosis, 78–79
   dietary factors, 78
   epidemiology, 78
   pathogenesis, 78
Cell-mediated immunity, 379–380
Center for Disease Control and
   Prevention (CDC), 359
Central core myopathy, 280
Central nervous system infections,
   390–393
   clinical manifestations, 391
   diagnosis, 391
   prevention, 392
   prognosis/complications, 391
   treatment, 391
Central precocious puberty, 351, 354
Cerebral palsy (CP), 303–305
   athetoid, 304
   clinical presentation of, 303–304
   comorbidities, 305
   diagnosis of, 304–305
   etiology/epidemiology, 303
   summary of, 303*t*
   treatment, 305

Cerebrospinal fluid (CSF), 177, 402, 564
Cerebrovascular events, 458–459
Cervical culture, 427
CGD. *See* Chronic granulomatous disease
Chancroid, 362
CHARGE association, 336
Chemical pneumonitis, 157
Chemotherapy, 477, 486
Chest pain, 183
Chest radiograph (CXR), 234
Chest roentgenogram, *394*, 395
Chest trauma, 508
Chest x-ray film, *63*
Childhood chronic arthritis, 431*t*
Childhood functional abdominal pain,
   38–39
Chlamydia trachomatis, 416, 547
   infection, 359–360
Chlamydophila, 416
   pneumonia infection, 395
Chlorambucil, 96
Chloramphenicol, 425
Chloride ions, 114
Chocolate, 218
Cholecystectomy, 451
Choledochal cyst, 43
Cholelithiasis, 42
Chromosomal abnormalities, 325–330
Chromosomal analysis, 147, 175
Chromosomal breakage studies, 177
Chromosomal defects, 548
Chromosomal disorders
   examples of, 326–330
   incidence of, 326
   indications for, 326
Chronic arthritides, 430–434
Chronic diarrhea, 85
Chronic granulomatous disease (CGD),
   241, 382, 561
Chronic hepatitis B infection, *55*
Chronic hepatitis delta, *57*
Chronic hypervitaminosis, 565
Chronic ITP, 482
Chronic nonspecific diarrhea, 85
Chronic RBC transfusion, 461
Chronic renal disorders, 141
Chronic severe illness, 131
Classic galactosemia (GG), 348
Classic roseola, 399
Classical salt wasting, 126
Clavicle fractures, 502
Cleidocranial dysostosis, 525
Cleft lip/palate, 338
Clindamycin, 9
Clinically important sickling disorders, 458*t*
Clonidine, 495
Clostridium botulinum, 285, 429
Clostridium difficile infection, 386
Clubfoot, 531
Coagulase-negative staphylococci, 429
Coagulation cascade, 481
Coagulation system, 481
Coagulopathies, 480
Coarctation of the aorta, 193
Cocaine, 66, 499
Cognitive delay, 296
Cognitive milestones, 298*t*

Cognitive/social-emotional milestones, 297–298
Colic, 212
Colicky abdominal pain, 438
Comminuted fractures, 504
Common disorders of hip, 529–530
Common mucosal/luminal disorders, 78–82
Common transient neonatal skin conditions, 1
Common variable immune deficiency (CVID), 240, 378
Commonly encountered toxidromes, 494t
Complement deficiency disorders, 380–381
Complete fractures, 501
Complex partial seizures, 248
Compound tomography, 558
Computed tomography (CT), 152, 393, 491
Concomitant eye findings, 4
Congenital adrenal hyperplasia (CAH), 124, 126, 127t, 147, 537
Congenital anomalies, 331, 567
Congenital cataract, 548
Congenital diaphragmatic hernia, 161
Congenital duodenal obstruction, 83
Congenital fiber-type disproportion, 281
Congenital hairy nevus, 6
Congenital heart disease, 182, 184, 185, 187–194, 379
Congenital hypothyroidism, 130–131, 130t, 134, 149
Congenital infections, 163–174, 168t
Congenital intrauterine infections, 167–172
    congenital syphilis, 170–172
    cytomegalovirus infection, 167–169
    rubella, 19, 169, 173, 416
    toxoplasmosis, 169–170, 173
Congenital lactose deficiency, 80
Congenital muscular dystrophies, 278t
Congenital muscular torticollis, 525
Congenital myopathies, 279–281
    central core myopathy, 280
    centronuclear/myotubular myopathy, 280–281
    common forms of, 280t
    minicore myopathy, 280
    nemaline rod myopathy, 280
Congenital nephrotic syndrome, 97, 118
Congenital primary adrenal insufficiency, 123–124
Congenital pseudoarthrosis of the clavicle, 526
Congenital qualitative platelet disorders, 482–483
Congenital syphilis, 170–172
Congestive heart failure, 212
Conjunctival granuloma, 418
Conjunctivitis, 546–547
Constipation, 41
Consumptive coagulopathy, 5
Contact dermatitis, 3
Contaminated farm ponds, 407
Continuous positive airway pressure (CPAP), 238

Coombs-negative hyperbilirubinemia, 71t
Cor pulmonale, 185
Cord blood values, 449t
Corneal injuries, 509
Cornelia de Lange syndrome, 336
Coronary anomalies, 191–192
Coronary artery abnormalities, 211
Cortical hamartomas, 269
Corticosteroids, 222–224
Cortisol, 148
CP. See Cerebral palsy
CPAP. See Continuous positive airway pressure
CPK. See Creatine kinase
CPR. See Cardiopulmonary resuscitation
Cranial nerve involvement, 564
Craniotabes, 31
Creatine kinase (CPK), 440, 443
Creatine phosphokinase, 107
Cri Du Chat Syndrome, 329
Crigler-Najjar syndrome, 71
Crohn disease (CD), 41–42, 46, 47t, 49t
Cromolyn sodium, 224–227, 232
Cryptococcus neoformans, 402
Cryptosporidium, 410
    infection, 387–388
CSF. See Cerebrospinal fluid
CT. See Computed tomography
Cushing syndrome, 144, 148
Cutaneous anthrax, 430
CVID. See Common variable immune deficiency
CXR. See Chest radiograph
Cyanotic heart lesions, 189–192
    coronary anomalies, 191–192
    obstructive left-sided lesions, 191
    tetralogy of Fallot, 189–190, 561
    total anomalous pulmonary venous return, 190–191
    transposition of great arteries, 190, 212
Cyanotic spells, 258–259
Cyclic vomiting, 259
Cyclophosphamide, 95, 437
Cystic fibrosis, 32, 79–80, 238, 567
    evolution of, 80
    gastrointestinal manifestations, 79–80
    pancreatic insufficiency, 79
    pathogenesis, 79
Cysticercosis, 412–413
Cysts
    choledochal, 43
    thyroglossal duct, 561
Cytomegalic inclusion disease, 168
Cytomegalovirus, 167–168
Cytotoxic T lymphocytes, 55

D

Dacryocystitis, 545
Decreased calcium, 488
Deep partial thickness burns, 510
Deeper hemangiomas, 5
Deformation, 331
Dehydration, 90, 91
    isotonic, 35
Delayed puberty, 353, 371
Demerol, 287

Deoxygenated blood, 187
Dermatitis
    atopic, 1, 2, 2, 241
    contact, 3
    rhus, 3
    seborrheic, 1, 2
Dermatomyositis, 439–441
    clinical presentation of, 440
    diagnosis, 440–441
    etiology/epidemiology, 439–440
    pathology of, 440
    prognosis, 441
    treatment, 441
Development, 315–325
Development assessment batteries, 320
Development dysplasia of hip, 529–530
Developmental abnormalities, 154
    cerebral palsy, 303–305
Developmental disabilities, 300–315
    attention deficit hyperactivity disorder, 309–311, 323
    autism/pervasive developmental disorders, 307–309, 321
    fetal alcohol syndrome, 179, 311–312, 337, 337
    language/speech delay, 313
    learning disabilities/educational issues, 312–313
    mental retardation, 300–307
    myelomingocele, 305–307
Dextroamphetamine, 311
Diabetes, 102–108
    insipidus, 114
    type 1, 79
Diamond-Blackfan anemia, 455
Diarrhea, 90, 111, 566
    bloody, 48, 383
    chronic, 85
Diarrheal illness, 385
DIC. See Disseminated intravascular coagulation
DiGeorge syndrome, 243, 381
Digoxin, 184
Dilated cardiomyopathy, 197
Dimorphic pathogenic fungi, 400–401, 401t
Diphtheria vaccine, 15–17
Diplopia, 509
Diseases. See also Acquired heart disease; Inflammatory bowel disease
    ADPKD, 117
    adult-onset polycystic kidney, 559
    Byler, 72
    celiac, 43, 78, 79, 81
    chronic granulomatous, 241, 382, 561
    congenital heart, 182, 184, 185, 187–194, 379
    Crohn, 41–42, 46, 49t
    cytomegalic inclusion, 168
    early disseminated, 408
    familial cardiovascular, 182
    glycogen storage, 73t
    Graves, 132t, 133
    hemoglobin H, 462
    hemorrhagic, cystitis, 492
    hemorrhagic, of newborn, 84
    Hirschsprung's, 522

Hodgkin, 490, 564
interstitial lung, 446
Kawasaki, 196, 199, 213, 551
Legg-Calvé-Perthes, 530
liver, 70–77
lyme, 408–409, 409t
lysosomal storage, 301
maple syrup urine, 347
Menkes, 560
minimal change, 95–96, 117
Moyamoya, 459
mycobacterial, 402–404
neonatal graves, 133
Osgood-Schlatter, 29–30, 532
pelvic inflammatory, 358, 360–361, 361t
peptic ulcer, 40
pneumococcal, 21
representative, 342t
sickle cell, 457–461
slapped cheek, 404
Stage IV Hodgkin, 486
Tay-Sachs, 344
thin basement membrane, 98
thyroid, 129–135
ulcer, 40
von Willebrand, 483–484
Wilson, 289, 552
DISIDA. See Disopropyliminodiacetic acid
Disopropyliminodiacetic acid (DISIDA), 74
Disorders
adrenal, 123–129
airway/pulmonary, 233–240
allergic, 214–218
attention deficit hyperactivity, 309–311, 323
of cardiac rate/rhythm, 200–207
cardiovascular, 180–187
chromosomal, 326–330
chronic renal, 141
clinically important sickling, 458t
common mucosal/luminal, 78–82
complement deficiency, 380–381
congenital qualitative platelet, 482–483
eosinophilic, 80–81
foot, 530–531
gastrointestinal, 259
hypothalamic, 369
inherited immunodeficiency, 377–382
lysosomal storage, 344–345
medication related movement, 263
mitochondrial, 344–345
neuromotor, 293
neuromuscular, 274–282
paroxysmal movement, 261–263
pediatric thyroid, 134t
peroxisomal, 345–346
pervasive developmental, 314
phagocyte, 380
pituitary, 369–370
of plasma factors, 483–484
thrombophilia, 480, 484
von Willebrand disease, 483–484
platelet, 480–483
rare systemic granulomatous, 447

rheumatic, 430–443
trinucleotide repeat, 277
of upper extremity, 526
ureal cycle, 347
urticaria, 6, 216–217
Disruption, 331
Disseminated gonococcal infection, 427
Disseminated intravascular coagulation (DIC), 470, 484
DMD. See Duchenne muscular dystrophy
Dog bites, 31
Dopamine infusion, 147
Double bubble fast pattern, 521
Double-bubble sign, 83
Down syndrome, 79, 302, 326
Drop-like lesions, 4
Duchenne muscular dystrophy (DMD), 275, 289, 553
Duodenal obstruction, 178
Dysentery syndrome, 411
Dyskeratosis congenita, 454
Dyskinetic type, 304
Dysmenorrhea, 358
Dysmorphic syndromes, 331–340
congenital anomalies, 331
examples of, 332–340
Dysmorphology, 331
Dysphagia, 64
Dysplasia, 331
anhydrotic ectodermal, 334
of hip, 529–530
thanatophoric, 334
Dystrophies
autosomal-dominant, 277
autosomal-recessive, 278–279
congenital muscular, 278t
Duchenne muscular, 275, 289, 553
Emery-Dreifuss muscular, 277
facioscapulohumeral muscular, 277–278
Limb-Girdle muscular, 279
muscular, 274–279
myotonic, 152, 277, 281, 284
oculopharyngeal muscular, 278
x-linked, 275–277
Dystrophin-associated glycoproteins, 274
Dystrophin-associated protein complex, 275

E

Early disseminated disease, 408
EBV. See Epstein-Barr virus
Ectopia lentis, 548
Eczematous rashes, 1–3
EE. See Eosinophilic esophagitis
Effective prophylactic therapy, 287
EG. See Eosinophilic gastroenteritis
Egg allergies, 19
Ehlers-Danlos Syndrome, 333
Ehrlichiosis, 407
Elbow fractures, 502–503
Electric cardioversion, 209
Electrocardiography, 199
Electroencephalography, 302
Electrolytes, 513
normalization, 90
Electromyography (EMG), 276

Electrophoresis (ELP), 457
Elevated erythrocyte sedimentation rate (ESR), 444
Elevated potassium, 488
ELISA. See Enzyme-linked immunoadsorbent assay
ELP. See Electrophoresis
Embryogenesis, 129, 270
Emery-Dreifuss muscular dystrophy, 277
EMG. See Electromyography
Encephalitis, 392–393, 420
Encephalopathy, 314
Endocrine neoplasia syndrome, 128
Endocrinologist, 354
Endocrinology, 147–153
End-organ defects, 370
Entamoeba histolytica, 410
Enteric adenovirus infection, 387
Enteric organisms, 427t
Enterobacter, 164
Enterobius vermicularis, 412
Enteropathogenic Escherichia coli, 385
Enteroviruses, 167
Enthesis, 433
Enuresis, 120
Environmental toxin exposure, 451
Enzyme-linked immunoadsorbent assay (ELISA), 58
Eosinophilia, 470
Eosinophilic disorders, 80–81
Eosinophilic esophagitis (EE), 80
Eosinophilic gastroenteritis (EG), 81
Eosinophilic leukemia, 471
Epididymoorchitis, 539
Epidural hematomas, 508, 510
Epiglottis, 237
Epilepsy
benign focal, 249
idiopathic, 248
juvenile myoclonic, 256
temporal lobe, 249
Epilepsy/anticonvulsant therapy, 247–257
classification of seizure, 247–250
etiology of, 247
pregnancy of, 254–255
Epstein-Barr virus (EBV), 415
EPT. See Expatiated partner therapy
Erythema, 433
infectiosum, 9
marginatum, 424
multiforme rash, 422
nodosum, 49, 553
toxicum, 1
Escherichia coli, 164, 385, 563
Esophageal atresia, 520
Esophageal foreign bodies
clinical/radiographic features, 63
management, 64
symptoms, 64
Esophageal injury, 68
ESR. See Elevated erythrocyte sedimentation rate
Ethosuximide, 252
Ethylene glycol, 121, 495
Euthyroid sick syndrome, 131
Ewing sarcoma, 476, 487
Expatiated partner therapy (EPT), 358

Expiratory airflow obstruction, 236
Extracellular volume, 88
Extraocular muscle, 544
Eye injuries, 509
Eye–hand coordination, 293

F

Facial dysmorphism, 244
Faciocutaneoskeletal syndrome, 475
Facioscapulohumeral muscular
        dystrophies, 277–278
Familial cardiovascular disease, 182
Familial hypocalciuric hypercalcemia, 139
Familial Mediterranean fever (FMF),
        44, 447
Family history, 338
Fanconi anemia, 176, 454
Fasting lipids, 376
Fat-soluble vitamin supplementation, 75t
Fatty acid oxidation, 343
Febrile illnesses, 167, 399
Febrile seizures, 250, 399
    clinical features of, 250
    generalized epilepsy with, 250
    treatment, 250
Felbamate, 252
Femoral anteversion, 527
Femoral epiphysis, 530
Femur, 503
FEPP. *See* Free erythrocyte protoporphyrin
Fetal alcohol syndrome, 179, 311–312,
        337, *337*
Fetal Dilantin syndrome, 338
Fetal echocardiography, 208
Fever, 211
    acute rheumatic, 195–196, 199, 550
    FMF, 44, 447
    periodic, 444
    rat bite, 409
    of unknown origin, 433
Fine motor milestones, 293, 296t
Fine reticulogranular pattern, 155
FISH. *See* Fluorescence in situ
        hybridization
Flash-lamp-pumped pulsed dye laser, 176
Floppy infant syndrome, 279
Fluid administration, 93
Fluid bolus, 515
Fluid replacement solutions, 91
Fluid requirements, 90
Fluids/Electrolytes, 88–94
Fluorescence in situ hybridization
        (FISH), 325
FMF. *See* Familial Mediterranean fever
Focal segmental glomerulosclerosis
        (FSGS), 94, 96
Folate deficiency anemia, 82
Folic acid, 306
Food allergy, 34
Foot disorders, 530–531
Forced vital capacity (FVC), 236
Foreign bodies, 62–70
    epidemiology of, 62–63
    esophageal, 63–64
    gastric/small intestinal foreign bodies,
        64–65
    ingestion, gang initiation and, 62

magnets, 66
management of, 65–66
    batteries, 65–66
    cocaine, 66
    impacted meat, 65
sharp/pointed, 66
Fosphenytoin, 255
Fractures
    ankle, 503
    bowing/bend, 501
    buckle, 501, 504
    clavicle, 502
    comminuted, 504
    complete, 501
    elbow, 502–503
    greenstick, 501
    growth plate, 501–502
    pelvic, 503
    skull, 507
    wrist, 503
Fragile X syndrome, 328
Free erythrocyte protoporphyrin
        (FEPP), 455
Free water deficit, 89t
Free water excess, 89t
FSGS. *See* Focal segmental
        glomerulosclerosis
Full thickness, 510
Functional abdominal pain, 37–39
    childhood, 38–39
    functional dyspepsia, 38
    irritable bowel syndrome, 38
Functional anemia, 448, 450t
Functional dyspepsia, 38
Fungal agents, 10
Fungal infections, 400–402
    dimorphic pathogenic fungi causes,
        400–401
    opportunistic fungal infections, 401–402
    of the scalp, 28
Furosemide therapy, 186, 212
Future pregnancies, 175
FVC. *See* Forced vital capacity

G

Gabapentin, 252
Galactosemia, 32, 343, 562
Gap acidosis, 112t
Gastric decompression, 162, 523
Gastric ulceration, 65
Gastric-emptying strategies, 496
Gastritis, 40
Gastroenteritis, 387–388
Gastroenterology, 82–87
Gastroesophageal reflux, 32, 39–40, 259
Gastrointestinal disorders, 259
Gastrointestinal infections, 383–388
Gastrointestinal manifestations, 79–80
Gastroschisis, 523
GBS. *See* Group B streptococcus
General absence seizure, 248
General pediatrics, 27–36
Generalized tonic-clonic seizures, 248
Genetic terms, 339t
Genital ulcers, 361
Genu valgum, 527
Genu varum, 527

GG. *See* Classic galactosemia
GI. *See* Upper gastrointestinal
Giardia lamblia infection, 387
Gilbert syndrome, 86
Gingival hyperplasia, 96
Gitelman syndrome, 122
Glabella, 4
Glanzmann thrombasthenia, 482
Glomerular filtrate, *110*
Glomerular lesion, 100
Glomerulonephritis, 99, 562
Glucocorticoids, 51, 125–126, 437
Glucose-6-phosphate dehydrogenase
        deficiency, 487, 488
Glucuronidase, 71
Gluten sensitive enteropathy, 556
Glycogen storage diseases, 73t
Glycol, 495
Goldenhar syndrome, 335, 545
Gonococcal ophthalmia, 549
Gordon diagnostic text, 310
Gottron papules, *440*
Graves disease, 132t, 133
Greenstick fractures, 501
Gross motor milestones, 292–293, 295t
Group B streptococcus (GBS), 159, 164
Growth failure, 48, 128
Growth hormone
    deficiency, 141, 143–145
    therapy, 145
Growth plate fractures, 501–502

H

Haemophilus ducreyi, 362
Haemophilus influenzae, 14, 19, 164, 389,
        547
Hair loss, 96
Hand-foot syndrome, 458
Hb S polymerization, 464
HCC. *See* Hepatocellular carcinoma
HCG. *See* Human chorionic
        gonadotropin
HCV. *See* Hepatitis C virus
Head banging, 260
Head fractures, 503
Head trauma, 506–507
Headache, 469
Health care maintenance, 459t
Hearing screening, 317, 324
Heart failure, 139
Heinz body hemolytic anemia, 463t
Hemangiomas, 4–5
Hemarthrosis, 31
Hematocrit, 452
Hematologic crisis, 460
Hematology-oncology, 486–492
Hematuria, 98–99
    causes of, 98t, 99
    recommended studies for, 99t
Hemihypertrophy, 489
Hemiscrotum, 537
Hemoglobin
    E, 463
    H disease, 462
    M, 463t
    mean corpuscular, 452
    patterns on newborn screening, 458t

Hemoglobinopathies, 21, 457–466
  sickle cell disease, 457–461
  thalassemia, 462–463
  variant, 463
Hemolytic anemia, 71, 435
Hemolytic uremic syndrome, 385
Hemophilia A/B, 483
Hemorrhages
  intracerebral, 508
  intracranial, 507–508
  intraventricular, 218
  pulmonary, 156
  transplacental, 179
Hemorrhagic disease cystitis, 492
Hemorrhagic disease of newborn, 84
Hemorrhagic varicella, 554
Henoch-Schönlein purpura (HSP),
    44, 551
  clinical features of, 438t
  diagnosis, 439
  etiology/epidemiology, 438
  pathophysiology, 438
  prognosis of, 439
  treatment, 439
Hepatic dimethyliminodiacetic acid
    (HIDA), 74
Hepatic dysfunction, 348
Hepatic failure, 166
Hepatitis A, 53–54
  vaccine, 22, 25
Hepatitis B virus (HBV), 54–57, 121, 428
  serology, 55–57
  vaccines, 19–20, 56
Hepatitis C virus (HCV), 53, 57–59
Hepatitis delta, 57
Hepatitis E, 59
Hepatitis G virus (HGV), 59
Hepatoblastoma, 489
Hepatocellular carcinoma (HCC), 55
Hepatomegaly, 73
Hepatosplenomegaly, 171, 209
Hepatotoxicity, 311
Hereditary cataracts, 548
Hereditary fructose intolerance, 347, 562
Hernias, 549
  congenital diaphragmatic, 161
  left-sided congenital diaphragmatic,
    162
  umbilical, 516
Heroin, 499
Herpangina, 9
Herpes simplex virus, 9, 165–167
  infection, 362–363, 363t
Heterophil antibodies, 420
Heterophil-positive mononucleosis, 420
Heterosexual relations, 358
HGV. See Hepatitis G virus
HHV-6. See Human herpesvirus 6
    infection
HIDA. See Hepatic dimethyliminodiacetic
    acid
Hirschsprung's disease, 522
Hirsutism, 374
Histocompatibility complex (MHC), 56
Histoplasma capsulatum, 244
HIV. See Human immunodeficiency virus
HLA. See Human leukocyte antigen

Hodgkin disease, 490, 564
Holt-Oram syndrome, 334, 560
Homocystinuria, 343
Hookworm, 411
Hormones
  adrenocorticotropic, 149
  growth, 141, 145
  low adrenocorticotrophic, 125
  parathyroid, 152
  secretion of antidiuretic, 115
  short stature/growth, 141–146
  thyroid-stimulating, 561
Hospitalized neonates, 163
HPG. See Hypothalamic pituitary gonadal
HPO. See Hypothalamic-pituitary-ovarian
HPV. See Human parvovirus infection
HSP. See Henoch-Schönlein purpura
Human chorionic gonadotropin
    (HCG), 537
Human herpesvirus 6 infection (HHV-6),
    398–399
Human hypersensitivity, 245
Human immunodeficiency virus
    (HIV), 357
  antiretroviral therapy, 400
  clinical features, 399–400
  diagnosis, 399
  general care of, 400
  infection, 18–19, 399–400
  perinatal transmission, 399
  prevention of opportunistic
    infections, 400
Human leukocyte antigen (HLA), 431
Human papillomavirus
  infection, 364–365
  vaccines, 22–23
Human parvovirus infection (HPV), 398
Hunter syndrome, 345, 345
Hurler syndrome, 150, 345
Hydrocele, 539
Hydrocortisone, 148
Hydrofluoric acid, 67
Hydronephrosis, upper pole, 536
Hydronephrosis in newborn, 535–536
  diagnosis, 535
  etiology/epidemiology, 535
  pathophysiology, 535
  treatment, 535–536
11-Hydroxylase deficiency, 127
21-Hydroxylase deficiency, 126
Hydroxyprogesterone, 542
Hyperammonemia, 343
Hyperbilirubinemia, 70–72, 71t, 76
Hypercholesterolemia, 117
Hypercyanotic spell, 186
Hyperglycemia, 92
Hypergonadotropic hypogonadism, 371
Hyperlipidemia, 102–108, 198t
Hypernatremia, 92
Hypernatremic dehydration, 92
Hyperparathyroidism, 139
Hyperpigmentation, 267
Hyperplasia, 343
  adrenal, 343
  congenital adrenal, 124, 126, 127t,
    147, 537
  gingival, 96

Hypertension, 31, 104, 116, 556
  classification of, by age group, 103t
  definitions of, 103
  diagnostic evaluation, 104–105
  drugs approved for treatment of,
    105t, 106t
  etiology, 103–104
  management and treatment of, 105
  persistent pulmonary, 159
  pulmonary, 157
Hyperthyroidism, 131–133, 132t
Hypertonic dehydration, 91
Hypertrophic cardiomyopathy, 197–198
Hypertrophic pyloric stenosis, 178, 519
Hyphema, 509
Hypoalbuminemia, 117
Hypocalcemia, 92, 291, 563, 566
Hypochondroplasia, 143
Hypochromic anemia, 454, 488
Hypokalemia, 111
Hypomelanosis, 271
Hyponitremia, 115
Hypoparathyroidism, 138–139, 244
Hypoplasia
  bone marrow, 452t
  pulmonary, 158
Hypoplastic left colon syndrome, 83
Hypospadias, 537, 540
Hypotension, 246
Hypothalamic disorders, 369
Hypothalamic hamartoma, 356
Hypothalamic pituitary gonadal
    (HPG), 350
Hypothalamic-pituitary-ovarian
    (HPO), 368
Hypothermia, 120
Hypothyroidism, 79, 343
  acquired, 131, 132
  congenital, 130–131, 130t, 134, 149
  subclinical, 134
Hypoxemia, 466

I

IBD. See Inflammatory bowel disease
Ice cube test, 218
ICP. See Increased intracranial pressure
Idiogenic osmoles, 91
Idiopathic epilepsy, 248
IFSPs. See Individual family service plans
IgG subclass deficiency, 378
Ileum, 518
Immediate swelling, 217
Immune thrombocytopenic purpura
    (ITP), 435, 481–482, 484, 487
Immunizations, 14–26, 75
  active, 15–23, 54
    diphtheria, 15–17
    haemophilus influenzae type b
      vaccines, 19
    hepatitis A vaccine, 22, 25
    hepatitis B vaccines, 19–20, 56
    human papillomavirus vaccine, 22–23
    influenza vaccine, 21–22, 242
    measles vaccine, 18–19
    meningococcal vaccine, 22, 427
    mumps vaccine, 19
    pertussis vaccines, 17

Immunizations (*continued*)
  pneumococcal vaccines, 20–21
  poliovirus vaccines, 17–18
  tetanus vaccine, 15
  varicella, 20
  contraindications to vaccination, 15
  general considerations, 14–15
  recommended, *16*
Immunoglobin, 414
  deficiencies, 377–378
  intravenous, 243
  A nephropathy, 99
  product, 15*t*
  therapy, 554
Immunologic memory, 19
Immunologic reactions, 245
Immunoreactive trypsinogen (IRT), 238
Immunotherapy, 242
Impacted meat, 65
Impetigo, 10
Important language milestones, 297*t*
IN. gonorrhoeae, 366
Inactivated influenza vaccine, 25
Inactivated poliovirus vaccine (IPV), 17
Inadequate caloric intake, 141
Incontinentia pigmenti, 5, 271
Increased intracranial pressure (ICP), 507, 512
Increased systemic vascular resistance, 513
Inderal, 107
Indirect (unconjugated) hyperbilirubine-mia, 70–72
Individual family service plans (IFSPs), 321
Infantile botulism, 285
Infantile esotropia, 543
Infantile spasms, 273
Infections
  acute hepatitis B, *55*
  ascaris lumbricoides, 411
  autovirus, 387
  bacterial, 383–386, 422
  Campylobacter, 385–386, 396
  central nervous system, 390–393
  chlamydia trachomatis, 359–360
  chlamydophila pneumonia, 395
  chronic hepatitis B, *55*
  clostridium difficile, 386
  congenital, 163–174, 168*t*
  cryptosporidium, 387–388
  disseminated gonococcal, 427
  enteric adenovirus, 387
  fungal, 28, 400–402
  gastrointestinal, 383–388
  Giardia lamblia, 387
  herpes simplex virus, 362–363, 363*t*
  HIV, 18–19, 399–400
  human papillomavirus, 364–365
  neisseria gonorrhoea, 360, 360*t*
  neonatal herpes simples virus, 166*t*
  opportunistic fungal, 401–402
  parasitic, 410–413
  parvovirus B19, 456
  rotavirus, 386–387
  salmonella, 383–384, 384*t*
  shigella, 384–385, 384*t*
  skin/soft tissue/bone/joint, 388–390
  streptococcal, 4
    tapeworm, 412–413
    tick-borne/zoonotic, 406–409
    Trichomonas vaginalis, 363
    upper respiratory, 186
    urinary tract, 177
    viral, 220, 398–400
    Yersinia, 386
Infectiosum, 9
Infectious crisis, 461
Infectious diseases, 383–430. *See also*
    Infections
Infective endocarditis, 194–195
Inflammatory bowel disease (IBD), 46, *144*
  Crohn disease, 41–42, 46, 49*t*
  diagnosis, 49
  epidemiology of, 46
  etiologic considerations, 47
  symptoms, 47–49
  therapy for, 50
  treatment, 50–51
  ulcerative colitis, 47, 47*t*
Inflammatory osteochondroses, 532
Influenza vaccine, 21–22, 242
Infratentorial brain tumor, 490
Ingestings/poisonings, 493–499
  characteristics odors, 494*t*
  epidemiology, 493
  general findings on, 494*t*
  history/physical examinations, 493–495
  laboratory testing, 495
  management, 496–497
    antidotes, 496–497
    gastric-emptying strategies, 496
  mercury, 65
  specific ingestion, 497–498
    acetaminophen, 497
    anticholinergic agents, 497
    iron, 456, 497–498
    opioids, 498
    salicylates, 497
    selective serotonin reuptake inhibitors, 498
    tricyclic antidepressants, 498
  tests, 495–496
Inhalation anthrax, 429
Inherited immunodeficiency disorders, 377–382
  b-cell/immunoglobulin deficiencies, 377–378
  complement deficiency disorders, 380–381
  diagnosis/treatment of inherited immunodeficiencies, 381
  phagocyte disorders, 380
  t lymphocytes/cell-mediated immunity, 379–380
Initial leukocyte count, 478
Injuries
  anterior cruciate ligament, 30–31
  corneal, 509
  esophageal, 68
  eye, 509
  ligament, 532–533
Innocent murmurs, 181*t*
Intermittent exotropia, 544
Internal tibial torsion, 526
Interphalangeal joints, 432
    Intersexuality, 542
Interstitial lung disease, 446
Intestinal nematodes
  ascaris lumbricoides infections, 411
  Enterobius vermicularis, 412
  hookworm, 411
  Trichuris trichiura, 411–412
Intestinal parasites, 41
Intoxications
  mercury, 566
  salicylate, 112, 210
Intra-abdominal pressure, 516
Intracerebral hemorrhages, 508
Intracranial hemorrhages, 507–508
Intradermal blisters, 9
Intramuscular penicillin, 199
Intranasal corticosteroid, 242–243
Intraoperative anaphylaxis, 216
Intrauterine growth retardation, 168
Intravenous ampicillin, 195
Intravenous fluids, 523
Intravenous immunoglobin, 243
Intraventricular hemorrhage, 218
Intussusception, 34, 42, 518
Ions
  chloride, 114
  simple, 496
Ipecac, 68
IPV. *See* Inactivated poliovirus vaccine
Iron, 497–498
  therapy, 456
Irradiated packed red blood cells, 566
Irregular rhythms, 204
Irritable bowel syndrome, 38. *See also*
    Inflammatory bowel disease
IRT. *See* Immunoreactive trypsinogen
Isolated clefts, 338*t*
Isoniazid, 425
Isotonic crystalloids, 513
Isotonic dehydration, 35
ITP. *See* Immune thrombocytopenic purpura

J

Jarisch-Herxheimer reaction, 362
JDM. *See* Juvenile dermatomyositis
jFMS. *See* Juvenile fibromyalgia syndrome
Jimsonweed, 493
Jitteriness, 262
Joint effusion, 31
Junctional nevi, 7
Juvenile dermatomyositis (JDM), 439
Juvenile fibromyalgia syndrome (jFMS), 445
Juvenile myoclonic epilepsy, 256
Juvenile rheumatoid arthritis, 430–434
  clinical presentation of, 431–432
  diagnosis of, 433
  epidemiology/etiology, 430–431
  pathology of, 431
  prognosis of, 434
  treatment of, 433–434

K

Kallmann syndrome, 369
Kartagener syndrome, 240
Karyotype determinations, 353

Karyotyping, 325
Kasabach-Merritt syndrome, 5, 482
Kawasaki disease, 196, 199, 213, 551
Klinefelter syndrome, 328
Klippel-Feil anomaly, 337
Klippel-Feil syndrome, 525
Klippel-Trenaunay-Weber syndrome, 270, 271
Knee problems, 503
Koilonychia, 451

L

Laboratory screening tests, 480–481
Lactic acidosis, 106
Lactose intolerance, 80
LAD1. *See* Leukocyte adhesion deficiency
Lamotrigine, 256
Langerhans cell histiocytosis, 550
Language functioning, 320
Laparoscopy, 541
Laryngomalacia, 234, 235
Late epiphyseal closure, 30
Lateral cervical spine, *337*
Lateral epicondylitis, 532
Latex allergy, 215
Latex-fruit syndrome, 244
Learning disabilities, 312–313
    clinical presentation of, 312
    comorbidities, 312–313
    diagnosis of, 312
    etiology/epidemiology, 312
    prognosis, 313
    treatment, 313
Left-sided congenital diaphragmatic hernia, *162*
Legg-Calvé-Perthes disease, 530
Leigh syndrome, 284
Lennox-Gastaut syndrome, 249
Leptospirosis, 407–408
Lesions
    cyanotic heart, 189–192, 212, 561
    drop-like, 4
    glomerular, 100
    microvesicular, *2*
    multiple vesicular, *166*
    noncyanotic heart, 188–189
    obstructive left-sided, 191
    papulosquamous, *4*
    pigmented, 5–8
    vesicular, 9
    vesiculobullous, 170
Less common neurocutaneous syndrome, 271–272
Leukemias, 471–472, 472
    acute, 477, 489
    ALL, 468, 472, 563
    AML, 469, 472
    eosinophilic, 471
    lymphomas, 472
Leukocoria, 476, 545–547
Leukocyte adhesion deficiency (LAD1), 380
Leukocytosis, 470–471
Leukodystrophies, 344
Leukopenia, 96
Leukotriene modifiers, 230–231
Levetiracetam, 252
LFS. *See* Li-Fraumeni syndrome

LGMDs. *See* Limb-Girdle muscular dystrophies
Li-Fraumeni syndrome (LFS), 475
Ligament injuries, 532–533
Limb-Girdle muscular dystrophies (LGMDs), 279
Linear scleroderma (LS), 445
Listeria monocytogenes, 164–165
Liver cancer, 477
Liver disease, 70–77
Liver ultrasonography, 349
Localized phlegmon, 518
Löffler syndrome, 411
Long-acting β_2-Agonists, 227–229, 232–233
Long QT syndrome, 205–206
Low adrenocorticotropic hormone, 125
LS. *See* Linear scleroderma
Lyme disease, 408–409, 409*t*
Lymphadenitis, 382, 405
Lymphadenopathy, 467–468
Lymphogranuloma venereum, 363
Lymphomas, 471–472
    ALL, 468, 472, 563
    AML, 469, 472
    bone cancer, 476
    Burkitt, 488
    Hodgkin, 473
    leukemias, 472
    liver cancer, 477
    neuroblastoma, 473–474, 478, 486, 489
    Non-Hodgkin, 472–473
    pediatric malignancies, 467–472
    presenting signs/symptoms, 473
    prognostic features of, 473
    retinoblastoma, 476–477, 487, 545–547
    rhabdomyosarcoma, 475–476, 489
    Wilms tumor, 474–475, 487, 489
Lysosomal storage disease, 301
Lysosomal storage disorders, 344–345

M

M. pneumoniae. See Mycoplasma pneumonia
Magnetic resonance imaging (MRI), 283, 314, 538
Maintenance electrolyte requirements, 89*t*
Malabsorption syndromes, 136
Malalignment, 526
Malaria, 410–411, 410*t*
Malformation, 331
Malignant melanoma, 7
Mallory-Weiss tear, 36
Malrotation, 519
Mannitol administration, 113
MAP. *See* Mean arterial pressure
Maple syrup urine disease, 347
Marfan syndrome, 332, 548
Marginatum, 424
MAS. *See* Meconium aspiration syndrome
Masturbation, 264
McCune-Albright syndrome, 352
MCH. *See* Mean corpuscular hemoglobin
MCL. *See* Medial collateral ligament
Mean arterial pressure (MAP), 507
Mean corpuscular hemoglobin (MCH), 452

Measles, 416
    vaccine, 18–19
Measured osmolality, 495
Mechanical abnormalities, 154
Mechanical ventilation, 163
Meckel diverticulum, 85
Meconium aspiration syndrome (MAS), 157, 234
Meconium ileus, 179
Meconium stool, 33, 35
Meconium-stained amniotic fluid, 157
MECP2 gene sequencing, 287
Media epicondylitis, 532
Medial collateral ligament (MCL), 532
Medial pharyngeal groove, 154
Mediastinal masses, 468–469, 468*t*
Medication related movement disorder, 263
Medium-Chain Acyl Coenzyme A Dehydrogenase deficiency, 343
Medulla, 123
Megaureter, 536
Membranoproliferative glomerulonephritis (MPGN), 94, 96–97
Membranous glomerulonephritis, 100
Meningitis, 173, 421
    aseptic, 392
    bacterial, 396, 425
    meningococcal, 555
    typical cerebrospinal fluid findings, 391*t*
Meningococcal vaccines, 22, 427
Meningococcemia, 396
Meningoencephalitis, 179, 392
Menkes disease, 560
Menstrual cycle, 368
Mental retardation, 300–307
    clinical presentation of, 301–302
    comorbidities, 302
    diagnosis of, 302
    etiology/epidemiology, 300–301
    prognosis, 302–303
    summary of, 301*t*
Mercury intoxication, 566
Mercury poisoning, 65
Mesalamine preparations, 50
Metabolic acidosis, 513
Metabolism
    amino acid, 341, 343
    ammonia, 343
    biotin, 343
    calcium/phosphorus, 135–140
    carbohydrate, 343
    inborn errors of, 341–349
        dietary management of, 346–347
        examples of, 342*t*
        factors in, 346
        mitochondrial disorders, 344–345
        peroxisomal disorders, 345–346
        principles of nonselective screening of newborns, 341
        selected disease errors, 341–344
    pharmacologic agents for disorders of inborn errors of, 347*t*
Metatarsus adductus, 530–531
Methicillin, 425
Methimazole, 133
Methotrexate, 51

Methylphenidate, 256, 311
Methylxanthines, 229–230
Metoclopramide, 86
MHC. *See* Histocompatibility complex
Microcephaly, 317
Microorganism, 14
Microvesicles, 2
Microvesicular lesions, *2*
Midshaft hypospadias, 541
Migraines
  acute confusional, 261
    basilar artery, 261
    variants, 261
Migratory arthritis, 424
Mild gut volvulus, 519
Mild proteinuria, 100
Miliary tuberculosis, *403*
Mineralocorticoid deficiency, 126
Mineralocorticoid excess, 126
Minicore myopathy, 280
Minimal change disease, 95–96, 117
Miosis, 499
Mites, 10
Mitochondrial disorders, 344–345
Möbius syndrome, 544
Molluscum contagiosum, 9
Monotherapy, 251
Monteggia fracture, 504
Moraxella, 547
Motor assessment, 321
Moyamoya disease, 459
MPGN. *See* Membranoproliferative
    glomerulonephritis
MRI. *See* Magnetic resonance imaging
Mucopolysaccharidoses, 344–345, 345*t*
Mullerian agenesis, 370
Multicystic dysplastic kidney, 536
Multidisciplinary assignment of
    language, 319
Multiforme rash, *422*
Multiple miscarriages, 319
Multiple sclerosis, 318
Multiple vesicular lesions, *166*
Mumps vaccine, 19
Muscle weakness, 440
Muscular dystrophies, 274–279
  autosomal-dominant dystrophies, 277
  classifications of, 276*t*
  Emery-Dreifuss muscular dystrophy, 277
  x-linked dystrophies, 275–277
Musculoskeletal emergencies, 500–505
  avulsion fractures, 502
  child abuse/musculoskeletal trauma, 504
  common clinical entities, 502–503
    ankle fractures, 503
    clavicle fractures, 502
    elbow fractures, 502–503
    femur/tibia, 503
    foot fractures, 503
    head fractures, 503
    knee problems, 503
    nursemaid's elbow, 502
    pelvic fractures, 503
    wrist fractures, 503
  evaluation of patient, 500–501
  fracture types specific to children,
    501–502

bowing/bend fractures, 501
    buckle fractures, 501
    complete fractures, 501
    greenstick fractures, 501
    growth plate fractures, 501–502
  physiologic highlights of children's
      bones, 500
  splinting/management, 503–504
Musculoskeletal trauma, 504
Mycobacterial disease in children,
    402–404
Mycobacterium paratuberculosis, 47
Mycoplasma pneumonia, 395, 416
Mydriasis, 499
Myelomeningocele, 305
  clinical presentation, 306
  diagnosis of, 306
  gastrointestinal concerns, 307
  mobility of, 306–307
  neurologic issues of, 306
  orthopedic problems, 307
  other concerns, 307
  skin breakdown, 307
  spina bifida occulta, 307
  summary of, 305*t*
  treatment of, 306
  urologic problems, 307
Myocardial contusions, 508
Myocarditis, 197
Myoclonic seizures, 248, 256
Myoclonus syndrome, 261
Myotonic dystrophy, 152, 277, 281, 284
Myotubular myopathy, 280–281, 281

N
Naloxone, 514
Narcolepsy/cataplexy, 260–261
Narcotics, 495
Nasal cannula, 155
Nasolacrimal dust, 543, 545
Nedocromil, 224–227
Neisseria gonorrhoea, 547
  infection, 360, 360*t*
Neisseria meningitidis, 22, 390
Nemaline rod myopathy, 280
Neonatal alloimmune thrombocytopenia,
    485
Neonatal bacterial sepsis, 163–165
  prevention, 165
  therapy, 165
Neonatal benign myoclonus, 259
Neonatal cholestasis, 72–75
  causes/frequency of, 72*t*
  clinical presentation, 73–74
  diagnosis, 74
  etiology, 72
  first-line diagnostic studies, 74*t*
  pathophysiology, 72–74
  prognosis, 75–76
  treatment, 74–75
Neonatal cyanosis, 183
Neonatal herpes simples virus infection,
    166*t*
Neonatal hyperinsulinemic hypoglycemia,
    562
Neonatal hypocalcemia, 379
Neonatal intensive care unit (NICU), 153

Neonatal jaundice, 70–77
  clinical presentations, 71
  diagnosis of, 71
  prognosis, 72
  treatment/complications, 72
Neonatal lupus, 442
Neonatal pneumonia, 159
Neonatal sepsis, 163–174
  bacteriology of, 163–164
  diagnosis of, 165
  Escherichia coli, 164, 385, 563
  group B streptococci, 159, 164
Neonatal thrombocytopenia, 482
Neonates, 173
Neonatology, 175–180
Neoplastic transformation, 6
Nephritis, 438, 442
Nephrology, 116–122
A Nephropathy, immunoglobin, 99
Nephrotic singers, 122
Nephrotic syndrome, 95*t*
Neural tube defects, 254, 338
Neuroblastoma, 473–474, 478,
      486, 489
Neurocardiogenic syncope, 207
Neurocutaneous syndromes, 266–273
  more common, 266–268
  pathophysiology, 266
Neurofibromatosis (NF), 7, 116, 151, 352
  type 1, 266, 283
  type 2, 268
Neurologic involvement, 435
Neurologic soft signs, 301
Neurology, 282–291
Neuromotor disorder, 293
Neuromuscular disorders, 274–282
  classification, 274
  muscular dystrophies, 274–279
Neuropathy, 275*t*
Neurotoxicity, 492
Neutropenia, 167
Neutrophils, 1
Nevus sebaceous of Jadassohn, 5
Newborns
  hemorrhagic, diseases, 84
  hydronephrosis in, 535–536
  nonselective screening of, 341
  RDS in, 234
  respiratory diseases of, 153–162
  screening, 458*t*
NF. *See* Neurofibromatosis
NHL. *See* Non-Hodgkin lymphoma
NICU. *See* Neonatal intensive care unit
Night terrors, 27, 260
Nightmares, 27, 260
Nikolsky sign, 175
Nitroblue tetrazolium test, 246
Nitrofurantoin, 118
Nocturnal enuresis, 540–541
Nodosum, 49, 553
Noisy breathing, 235*t*
Nonbalancing rash, *421*
Noncyanotic heart lesions, 188–189
  atrial septal defects, 181, 188–189
  atrioventricular canal defects, 189
  patent ductus arteriosus, 189
  ventricular septal defects, 188, 192

Nonepileptic paroxysmal disorders in children, 258–265
  approaches to, 258
  common events in, 258–259
  gastrointestinal disorders, 259
  migraine variants, 261
  miscellaneous events during wakefulness, 263–264
  paroxysmal movement disorders, 261–263
  sleep-related events, 7, 259–261
Nonepileptic seizures, 264
Nongonococcal urethritis, 359
Non-Hodgkin lymphoma (NHL), 472–473
Nonselective screening of newborns, 341
Nonsteroidal anti-inflammatory drugs, 437, 542
Nontuberculous mycobacteria, 404
Nontyphoidal salmonella, 384t
Noonan syndrome, 336, 560
Normal child growth/development, 292–300
  cognitive/social–emotional milestones, 297–299
  fine motor milestones, 293, 296t
  gross motor milestones, 292–293
  parameters of physical growth, 292
  speech/language milestones, 293–296
Normal coronary artery branching pattern, 191
Normal pubertal development, 350, 371–373
Normal thyroid physiology, 129–130
Nursemaid's elbow, 502
Nutritional therapy, 51

O
Oak tree pollen, 217
Obesity, 102–108
Obstructed total anomalous pulmonary venous return, 193
Obstructive left-sided lesions, 191
Obstructive sleep apnea (OSA), 237
Oculocutaneous albinism, 272
Oculocutaneous telangiectasia, 555
Oculopharyngeal muscular dystrophy, 278
Olfactory hallucinations, 283
Oliguria, 513
Omphalocele, 523
Oocytes, 387
Ophthalmia neonatorum, 547
Ophthalmology
  cataracts, 547–548
  conjunctivitis, 546–547
  ectopia lentis, 548
  leukocoria, 476, 545–547
  nasolacrimal duct, 543, 545
  ophthalmia neonatorum, 547
  overview, 543–549
  strabismus/amblyopia, 543–545
Ophthalmoplegia, 389
Opioids, 498
Opportunistic fungal infections, 401–402
Opsoclonus, 261
Optic glioma, 267, 491
Optimal fluid regimen, 91

Oral antihistamine, 3
Oral aspirin, 199
Oral leukotriene receptor antagonist, 246
Orbital rhabdomyosarcoma, 489
Ornithine transcarbamylase deficiency, 283
Orthopaedics, 525–534
  abnormalities of neck, 525–526
  common disorders of hip, 529–530
  consult, 505
  disorders of upper extremity, 526
  foot disorders, 530–531
  overuse syndrome, 531–533
  scoliosis, 528–529
  torsional/angular abnormalities of lower extremity, 526–528
Orthostatic proteinuria, 98t
OSA. See Obstructive sleep apnea
Osgood-Schlatter disease, 29–30, 532
Osmolar gap, 495
Osmolarity, 114
Osteogenies imperfecta, 333–334
Osteomyelitis, 389–390, 390t
Osteosarcoma, 476, 477, 487
OTC deficiency, 343–344
Ovarian disorders, 370
Overuse syndromes, 531–533
Oxcarbazepine, 252–253
Oxygen, 193, 213

P
P. aeruginosa, 423
PACs. See Premature atrial contractions
Pain, 433
  abdominal, 37–45, 442
  bone, 469–470
  chest, 183
  childhood functional abdominal, 38–39
  colicky abdominal, 438
  crisis, 458
  functional abdominal, 37–39
  vaso-occlusive, 465
Pallid spells, 259
pANCA. See Perinuclear antineutrophil cytoplasmic antibody
Pancreatic insufficiency, 79
Pancreatis, 42–43
Pancytopenia, 470
Panhypopituitarism, 150
Papanicolaou smear, 365t
Papulosquamous lesions, 4
Papulosquamous rashes, 3–4
Paracentesis, 121, 418
Paradoxical aciduria, 519
Parainfluenza viruses, 428
Paraphimosis, 539
Parasitic infections, 410–413
  babesioses, 411
  intestinal nematodes, 411–412
  malaria, 410–411, 410t
  protozoa, 410
Parathyroid hormone (PTH), 152
Parenchyma, 117
Parenchymal conditions, 154
Paroxysmal dyskinesias, 262–263
Paroxysmal infantile torticollis, 262
Paroxysmal movement disorders, 261–263

Parvovirus B19 infection, 456
Passive immunoprophylaxis, 54
Pasteurella multocida, 423
Pastia lines, 10
Patient ductus arteriosus, 189, 211
Patient-delivered partner therapy (PDPT), 358
Pauciarticular-onset juvenile rheumatoid arthritis, 432
PDPT. See Patient-delivered partner therapy
Peanut/tree nut allergies, 243
Pectus excavatum, 557
Pediatric cancers, 468t
Pediatric causes of death, 27
Pediatric critical care, 512–515
Pediatric dermatology, 1–13
Pediatric ingestions. See Foreign bodies
Pediatric malignancies. See also Leukemias; Lymphomas
  abdominal masses, 470
  bleeding, 471
  bone pain, 469–470
  clinical signs/prognostic factors in, 467–479
  common clinical signs of, 467–471
  headache, 469
  leukocytosis, 470–471
  mediastinal mass, 468–469, 468t
  pancytopenia, 470
  presenting signs, 471–477
Pediatric rheumatology, 444–447
Pediatric surgery, 516–524
Pediatric thyroid disorders, 134t
Pediatric trauma, 506–511
  abdominal trauma, 508–509
  burns, 509–510
  chest trauma, 508
  epidemiology, 506
  eye injuries, 509
  head trauma, 506–508
  initial assessment/resuscitation of trauma, 506
  intracranial hemorrhages, 507–508
  skull fractures, 507
Pelvic fractures, 503
Pelvic inflammatory disease (PID), 358, 360–361, 361t
Penicillin, 215
Penis problems, 539–540
Peptic ulcer disease, 40
Pericarditis, 196, 199
Perinuclear antineutrophil cytoplasmic antibody (pANCA), 49
Periodic fever, 444
Periorbital cellulitis, 389
Periorbital ecchymosis, 564
Peripheral blood smear, 407
Peripheral edema, 184
Peripheral precocious puberty, 350, 351
Peritonitis
  bacterial, 121
  primary, 96
Perixosomal disorders, 345–346
Permanent manifestations, 169
Peroxisomal disorders, 345–346
Persistent pulmonary hypertension, 159
Pertussis vaccines, 17

Pervasive developmental disorder, 314
Phagocyte disorders, 380
Phenylketonuria, 341
Phenytoin, 250, 253, 559
Phimosis, 539
Phonophobia, 286
Phosphate, 138
Phosphatidylglycerol, 156
Phosphorus, 138, 488
Photophobia, 286, 509
Physical therapy referrals, 445
Physiologic anemia of infancy, 448
Physiologic bowlegs, 527
Physiologic knock-knees, 527
Physiologic moisturizers, 3
Physiology of menstrual cycle, 368
PID. *See* Pelvic inflammatory disease
PIE. *See* Pulmonary interstitial emphysema
Pigmented hamartomas, *267*
Pigmented lesions, 5–8
Pilosebaceous unit, 1
Pincer grasp, 316
Pituitary disorders, 369–370
Pituitary resistance, 134
Pityriasis rosea, 3, 29
Plague, 409
Plastic mattress encasing, 217
Platelet disorders, 480–483, 483
Pleural cavity, 239
Plexiform neurofibromas, 267
PNE. *See* Primary nocturnal enuresis
Pneumococcal disease, 21
Pneumococcal vaccines, 20–21
Pneumocystosis, 381
Pneumomediastinum, 239
Pneumonia, 173, 393–395
    bacterial, 393–394
    mycoplasma, 395
    neonatal, 160
    viral, 394
Pneumothorax, 160
Poliovirus vaccines, 17–18
Polyarticular-onset juvenile rheumatoid
    arthritis, 432
Polycystic ovary syndrome, 371, 374, 376
Polymicrobial, 393
Poor lung compliance, 161
Poor prognostic factors, 421
Positive antinuclear antibody testing,
    446
Postconcussive syndrome, 285
Posterior embryotoxon, 73
Posterior urethral valves, 536
Poststreptococcal glomerulonephritis
    (PSGN), 119, 550
Post-traumatic iritis, 509
Postural proteinuria, 97
Potassium hydroxide, 28
PPHN. *See* Pulmonary hypertension
Prader-Willi syndrome (PWS), 284, 328
Preauricular lymphadenopathy, 418
Precocious puberty, 151, 351
Pregnancy test, 375
Premature adrenarche, 350
Premature atrial contractions (PACs),
    204
Premature ventricular contractions, *204*

Prematurity, 558
Prenatal history, 338
Prevalence rate, 323
Preventive cardiology, 198
Previous growth data, 355
Priapism, 460
Primary adrenal insufficiency, 123
Primary nocturnal enuresis (PNE), 28
Primary nutritional iron deficiency, 456
Primary peritonitis, 96
Productive cough, 426
Progressive cerebellar ataxia, 555
Progressive gait ataxia, 285
Progressive jaundice, 563
Progressive neurologic deterioration, 150
Progressive renal failure, 118
Progressive varicella, 554
Prominent exocervix, 366
Propylthiouracil, 133
Prostaglandin synthesis, 86
Proteinuria, 94–101, 119
Proteinuria/nephrotic syndrome, 94–98
Proteus syndrome, 272, *272*
Protozoa, 410
Proximal tubular dysfunction, 113
Prune belly syndrome, 177
Pseudohypoparathyroidism, 139
Pseudomotor cerebri, 554
Pseudostrabismus, 543
PSGN. *See* Poststreptococcal
    glomerulonephritis
Psoriasis, 4
Psoriatic arthritis, 433
PTH. *See* Parathyroid hormone
Puberty
    central core precocious, 354
    central precocious, 351
    delayed, 353, 371
Pulmonary air-leak syndromes, 160
Pulmonary branch stenosis, 181
Pulmonary contusions, 508
Pulmonary fibrosis, 492
Pulmonary hemorrhage, 156
Pulmonary hypertension (PPHN), 157
Pulmonary hypoplasia, 158
Pulmonary interstitial emphysema
    (PIE), 160
Pulmonary overcirculation, 188
Pulmonary stenosis, 186
PWS. *See* Prader-Willi syndrome
Pyloric stenosis, 33
Pyoderma gangrenosum, 49
Pyrazinamide, 425
Pyruvate dehydrogenase, 348

R
Rabies vaccines, 23
Radial-ulnar synostosis, 526
Radioactive iodide uptake scan, 134
Rapid destructive phase, 288
Rapid plasma reagin (RPR), 171, 174
Rare systemic granulomatous disorder,
    447
Rat bite fever, 409
Raynaud's phenomenon, 446
RBC. *See* Red blood cell
RDS. *See* Respiratory distress syndrome

Reactive arthritis, 385, 434
Receptor antagonists, 40
Recombinant immunoblot assay
    (RIBA), 58
Recommended immunization schedule, *16*
Rectal prolapse, 411, 413, 555
Recurrent *Neisseria*, 382
Red blood cell (RBC), 448, 464
Regular insulin, 148
Reiter syndrome, 434
Relative efficacy, 287
Reliable skin testing, 218
Renal insufficiency rickets, 138
Renal stones, 100
Renal tubular acidosis (RTA), 109, 143
Renal ultrasonography, 117, 523
Renin, 128
Replenishing, 90
Representative diseases, 342*t*
Resection of ileum, 87
Respiratory diseases of newborn, 153–162
Respiratory distress syndrome (RDS),
    155, 237*t*
    in the newborn, 234
    radiograph showing of, *156*
Resultant hyperoxia, 157
Reticulocyte count, 453
Retinoblastoma, 476–477, 487, 545–547
Retinopathy, 558
Rett syndrome, 287, 336
Reye syndrome, 33
Rhabdomyolysis, 290
Rhabdomyosarcoma, 475–476, 489
Rheumatic disorders, 430–443
    dermatomyositis, 439–441
    reactive arthritis, 385, 434
    systemic lupus erythematosus,
        434–439, 553
Rhonchi, 111
Rhus dermatitis, 3
Rhythm strip, *203*
RIBA. *See* Recombinant immunoblot assay
Rice cereal, 86
Rickets, 31, 137–138, 528*t*
Rifampin, 425
RMSF. *See* Rocky Mountain Spotted Fever
Rocky Mountain Spotted Fever (RMSF),
    406–407
Rotavirus infection, 386–387
RPR. *See* Rapid plasma reagin
RTA. *See* Renal tubular acidosis
Rubella, 19, 169, 173, 416
Russell-silver syndrome, 336

S
S. pneumoniae. See Streptococcus pneumoniae
Sacroiliitis, 433
Salicylate intoxication, 112, 210
Salicylates, 497
Salmon patch, 4
Salmonella infection, 383–384, 384*t*
Salmonella sp., 424
Salter type II, 504
Sarcoidosis, 447
Scabies, 10
Scaphoid abdomen, 557
Scoliosis, 528–529

brace treatment, 529
etiology, 528
natural history, 528–529
observation, 529
progression, 529t
surgical management, 529
Seborrheic dermatitis, 1, 2
Secondary adrenal insufficiency, 125
Secondary syphilis, 3, 29
Secretion of antidiuretic hormone
   (SIADH), 115
Seizures, 139, 247–248, 385
   atypical absence, 248
   complex partial, 248
   febrile, 250, 399
   general absence, 248
   generalized tonic-clonic, 248
   nonepileptic, 264
Selective serotonin reuptake inhibitors, 498
Sensitivity, 322
Separation anxiety, 27
Septic arthritis, 390
Septicemia, 385
Serotonin reuptake inhibitors, 205
Serum alpha-fetoprotein (AFP), 523
Serum osmolarity, 91
Serum RPR, 174
Serum serologic testing, 413
Serum sodium, 495
Severe acidosis, 110
Severe cluneal apophysitis, 532
Severe laboratory abnormalities, 93
Severe wheezing, 515
Sexually transmitted diseases (STDs),
   357–367
   bacterial vaginosis, 363–364, 366
   chancroid, 362
   chlamydia trachomatis infection,
      359–360
   herpes simplex virus infection, 9,
      165–167, 362–363, 363t
   human papillomavirus infection,
      22–23, 364–365
   lymphogranuloma venereum, 363
   neisseria gonorrhoeae infection, 360,
      360t, 547
   newer treatment for, 358–359
   nongonococcal urethritis, 359
   pelvic inflammatory disease, 358,
      360–361, 360t
   screening, 358
   syphilis, 170, 361–362
   trichomonas vaginalis infection, 363
Shagreen patch, 8
Shiga toxin-producing Escherichia coli, 385
Shigella infections, 384–385, 384t
Shin splints, 30
Short stature/growth hormone therapy,
   141–146
   clinical entities associated with normal
      variations in growth, 142
   growth hormone deficiency, 141,
      143–145
   important historical features and, 144t
   initial laboratory tests in, 145t
   pathologic clinical entities causing short
      stature, 142–143

specific physical examination findings
   and, 144t
   typical growth, 142
Shudder attacks, 263
SIADH. See Secretion of antidiuretic
   hormone
Sickle cell disease, 457–461, 461
   clinical presentation/treatments,
      457–461
   etiology, 457
   pathophysiology, 457
Significant motor delay, 318
Silencing, 288
Simple ions, 496
Simple pneumothorax, 508
Simplex polymerase chain reaction, 177
Sinus rhythm, 201
Skeletal maturation, 355
Skin biopsy, 218
Skin/soft tissue/bone/joint infections,
   388–390
Skull fractures, 507
Slapped cheek disease, 404
SLE. See Systemic lupus erythematosus
Sleep-related events, 259–261
   benign neonatal myoclonus, 259, 263
   head banging, 260
   narcolepsy/cataplexy, 260–261
   night terrors, 7, 260
   nightmares, 7, 260
   sleepwalking, 260
Sleepwalking, 260
Slipped capital femoral epiphysis,
   530, 533
Slit lamp examination of cornea, 289
Social/emotional milestones, 298t
Sodium bicarbonate, 112
Spasmus nutans, 263
Spastic quadriplegia, 304
Speech delay, 313
Speech/language milestones, 297t
Spherocytes, 490
Spina bifida, 305–307
Spinal cord involvement, 5
Spine MRI, 314
Splenic laceration, 511
Spondyloarthropathies, 433
Spontaneous pneumothorax, 239
Sporadic vaginal irritation, 29
Sprengel deformity, 526
Stage IV Hodgkin disease, 486
Staphylococcal scalded skin syndrome,
   175, 420
Staphylococcus aureus, 394, 547
Staring spells, 263
Status epilepticus, 255
STDs. See Sexually transmitted diseases
Stenosis, 104, 116, 559
Stereotypes, 262
Steroids
   anabolic, 30
   cortico, 222–224
   intranasal cortico, 242–243
   topical ocular, 215
Stinging insect allergy, 216
Stool-withholding, 263–264
Strabismus, 543–545

Streptobacillus moniliformis, 424
Streptococcal infection, 4
Streptococcal pharyngitis, 488
Streptococcal vulvovaginitis, 29
Streptococcus mitis, 211
Streptococcus pneumoniae, 172, 238,
      393–394, 405, 424–428, 547, 564
Streptococcus pyogenes, 416
Stridor, 234, 235t
Sturge-Weber syndrome, 176, 270
Subacute lymphadenopathy, 417
Subacute thyroiditis, 132, 133
Subclinical hypothyroidism, 134
Subependymal nodules, 269
Suicide attempt, 493
Sulfasalazine, 51
Superficial burns, 509
Superficial hemangioma, 5
Superficial partial thickness burns, 509
Supinate, 504
Supplemental testosterone, 355
Suppurative adenitis, 417
Supraventricular adenopathy, 490
Supraventricular tachycardia (SVT), 201
   reentrant, 208
   treatment of, 202
SVT. See Supraventricular tachycardia
Sweat chloride, 81
Swelling, 100
Swimming, 209
Syncope, 204–205, 264
Syndactyl, 526
Syndromes
   acute chest, 459–460
   adult respiratory distress, 514
   afebrile pneumonia, 426
   Alpers-Huttenlocher, 290
   Alport, 98
   Angelman, 328
   Beckwith-Wiedemann, 328, 563
   Bernard-Soulier, 482–483
   CATCH 22, 329–330
   congenital nephrotic, 97, 118
   Cornelia de Lange, 336
   Cri Du Chat, 329
   Crigler-Najjar, 71
   Cushing, 144, 148
   DiGeorge, 243, 381
   Down, 79, 302, 326
   dysentery, 411
   dysmorphic, 331–340
   Ehlers-Danlos, 333
   endocrine neoplasia, 128
   euthyroid sick, 131
   faciocutaneoskeletal, 475
   fetal alcohol, 179, 311–312, 337, 337
   fetal Dilantin, 338
   floppy infant, 279
   fragile X, 328
   Gilbert, 86
   Gitelman, 122
   Goldenhar, 335, 545
   hand-foot, 458
   hemolytic uremic, 385
   Holt-Oram, 334, 560
   Hunter, 345, 345
   Hurler, 150, 345

Syndromes *(continued)*
  Hypoplastic left colon, 83
  irritable bowel, 38
  juvenile fibromyalgia, 445
  Kallmann, 369
  Kartagener, 240
  Kasabach-Merritt, 5
  Klinefelter, 328
  Klippel-Feil, 525
  Klippel-Trenaunay-Weber, *270*
  latex-fruit, 244
  Leigh, 284
  Lennox-Gastaut, 249
  less common neurocutaneous,
    271–272
  Li-Fraumeni, 475
  Löffler, 411
  Long QT, 205–206
  malabsorption, 136
  Marfan, 332, 548
  McCune-Albright, 352
  meconium aspiration, 157, 234
  Möbius, 544
  myoclonus, 261
  nephrotic, 95*t*
  neurocutaneous, 266–273
  Noonan, 336, 560
  overuse, 531–533
  polycystic ovary, 371, 374, 376
  postconcussive, 285
  Prader-Willi, 284, 328
  proteinuria/nephrotic, 94–98
  proteus, 272, *272*
  prune belly, 177
  pulmonary air-leak, 160
  RDS, 155, *156*, 234, 237*t*
  Reiter, 434
  Rett, 287, 336
  Reye, 33
  Russell-silver, 336
  staphylococcal scalded skin, 175, 420
  Sturge-Weber, 176, 270
  Treacher Collins, 334–335
  triple A, 124
  Turner, 117, 327–328
  Waardenburg, 272, 563
  WAS, 245, 379, 382, 483
  Weil, 408
  Williams, 329
  WPW, 205
  x-linked hyper-IgM, 378
Syphilis, 170, 361–362
Systemic antibiotics, 511
Systemic lupus erythematosus (SLE),
    434–439, 553
  clinical presentation of, 435
  clinical/pathologic, 436
  diagnosis of, 436
  Henoch-Schönlein purpura, 44,
    438–439, 551
  neonatal, 437–438
  prognosis, 437
  treatment, 436–437
Systemic steroid therapy, 245
Systemic-onset juvenile rheumatoid
    arthritis, 432–433
Systolic ejection murmurs, 182

T
T lymphocytes, 379–380
TA. *See* Takayasu's arteritis
Tachycardias, 201–203, *202*, 208–209
Takayasu's arteritis (TA), 445
Tanner staging, 350–356, 351
Tantrums, 316
Tapeworm infections, 412–413
TAR. *See* Thrombocytopenia-absent radii
Tay-Sachs disease, 344
TCA. *See* Trichloroacetic acid
TCD. *See* Transcranial Doppler
TEF. *See* Tracheoesophageal fistula
Telegraphic speech, 296
Temporal lobe epilepsy, 249
Tendonitis, 532
Tension pneumothorax, 239
Testicular torsion, 538–539
Testis tumor, 539
Tetanus vaccine, 15
Tetracycline therapy, 553
Tetralogy of Fallot, 189–190, 561
Thalassemia
  β, 463
  clinical presentations/treatment of, 462
  etiology, 462
  hemoglobin H disease, 462
  major, 462
  pathophysiology, 462
Thanatophoric dysplasia, 334
Theophylline, 229
Therapy
  aggressive antibiotic, 381
  anticonvulsant, 136, 247–257
  antifungal, 401
  anti-IgE, 231
  antimicrobial, 419
  effective prophylactic, 287
  furosemide, 186, 212
  immunoglobin, 554
  inflammatory bowel disease, 50
  neonatal bacterial sepsis, 165
  nutritional, 51
  patient-delivered partner, 358
  short stature/growth hormone,
    141–146
  systemic steroid, 245
  tetracycline, 553
Thin basement membrane disease, 98
Third-degree heart block, 209
Thoracic lumbar sacral orthosis
    (TLSO), 529
Thrombocytopenia, 5, 170, 420
  neonatal, 482
  neonatal alloimmune, 485
Thrombocytopenia-absent radii (TAR),
    482
Thrombocytosis, 419
Thrombophilia, 480, 484
Thumb sucking, 27–28
Thyroglossal duct cyst, 561
Thyroid disease, 129–135
Thyroid function tests, 149
Thyroid nodules, 132–134
Thyroid-stimulating hormone (TSH), 561
Thyrotoxicosis, 149
Tibia, 503, 526, 528*t*

Tick-borne/zoonotic infections,
    406–409
  ehrlichiosis, 407
  leptospirosis, 407–408
  lyme disease, 408–409, 409*t*
  plague, 409
  rat bite fever, 409
  Rocky Mountain Spotted Fever, 406–407
  tularemia, 407
Tics, 262
Tinea capitis, 11, 28
Tinea corporis, 10
Tinea versicolor, 10
Tissue nematodes, 412
Tissue transglutaminase, 79
TLSO. *See* Thoracic lumbar sacral orthosis
TNF. *See* Tumor necrosis factor
Tobacco smoke, 232
Toilet training, 299
Topical adapalene, 8
Topical nasal corticosteroids, 215
Topical ocular steroids, 215
Topiramate, 287
Torsion of appendix testis, 539, 542
Torsional/angular abnormalities of lower
    extremity, 526–528
Total anomalous pulmonary venous
    return, 190–191
Toxicum, 1, 2, 178
Toxidrome of agitation, 498
Toxoplasmosis, 169–170, 173
Tracheoesophageal fistula (TEF), 520
Tracheomalacia, 234
Transcranial Doppler (TCD), 459
Transient hypoglycemia, 150
Transient rashes, 18
Transplacental hemorrhage, 179
Transposition of great arteries, 190, 212
Transverse lucent bands, *171*
Transverse myelitis, 420
Trauma
  abdominal, 508–509
  blunt, 508
  chest, 508
  head, 506–507
  musculoskeletal, 504
  pediatric, 506–511
Treacher Collins syndrome, 334–335
Treponema palladium, 170, 362
Trichinella spiralis, 412
Trichloroacetic acid (TCA), 364
Trichomonas vaginalis infection, 363
Trichophyton tonsurans, 28
Trichotillomania, 10
Trichuris trichiura, 411–412
Tricyclic antidepressants, 498
Trinucleotide repeat disorders, 277
Triple A syndrome, 124
Trisomy 13, 326
Trisomy 18, 326–327
TSH. *See* Thyroid-stimulating hormone
Tubercle apophysitis, 29–30
Tuberculosis, 402–404
  clinical manifestations, 402–403
  diagnosis, 403
  epidemiology, 402
  prophylaxis/treatment, 403–404

Tuberous sclerosis, 8, 268–270, *269*, 288, 553, 558
Tularemia, 407
Tumor necrosis factor (TNF), 51
Tumors
    brain, 471, 490
    testis, 539
    TNF, 51
    Wilms, 474–475, 487, 489
Turner syndrome, 117, 327–328
Type 1 diabetes, 79
Type I Rickets, 137
Type II diabetes, 102–108
Type II Rickets, 137–138

U

UC. *See* Ulcerative colitis
UDPG. *See* Urodine diphosphate glucose
Ulcerative colitis (UC), 47, 47*t*, 49*t*
Ulcers, 361
    disease, 40
Ultrasonography, 349, 517, 519
Umbilical hernias, 516–517
Undescended testis, 536–538
    diagnosis, 537–538
    epidemiology, 536–537
    etiology, 536–537
    treatment, 538
Unilateral hearing loss, 564
Upper gastrointestinal (GI), 84, 519, 522
Upper pole hydronephrosis, 536
Upper respiratory infection, 186
Ureal cycle disorders, 347
Ureteropelvic junction, 44, 536, 541
Uric acid, 488
Urinalysis, 216, 436
Urinary tract infections, 177
Urine osmolarity, 115
Urodine diphosphate glucose (UDPG), 70
Urology for pediatrician, 535–542
    acute scrotal swelling, 538
    bladder instability of childhood, 540
    epididymoorchitis, 539
    hydrocele, 539
    hydronephrosis in newborn, 535–536
    nocturnal enuresis, 540–541
    penis problems, 539–540
    testicular torsion, 538–539
    testis tumor, 539
    torsion of appendix testis, 539, 542
    undescended testis, 536–538
    variocele, 541
Urticaria, 216–217
    pigmentosa, *6*, 216

V

Vaccine Adverse Event Reporting System (VAERS), 14
Vaccine-associated paralytic poliomyelitis (VAPP), 17
Vaccines
    acellular pertussis, 24
    diphtheria, 15–17
    HBV, 19–20, 56
    hepatitis A, 22, 25

human papillomavirus, 22–23
    inactivated influenza, 25
    inactivated poliovirus, 17
    influenza, 21–22, 242
    meningococcal, 22, 427
    mumps, 19
    pertussis, 17
    pneumococcal, 20–21
    poliovirus, 17–18
    rabies, 23
    tetanus, 15
    23-valent polysaccharide pneumococcal, 25
    varicella, 20
VAERS. *See* Vaccine Adverse Event Reporting System
23-valent Polysaccharide pneumococcal vaccine, 25
Valsalva maneuver, 202
VAPP. *See* Vaccine-associated paralytic poliomyelitis
Varicella, 15*t*
    vaccines, 20
Varicella Zoster virus (VZV), 159
Varicella-Zoster Ig, 415
Variocele, 541
Vascular malformations, 4–5
Vascular purpura, 484
Vascular ring, 162
Vascular thromboses, 96
Vaso-occlusive crisis, 458
Vaso-occlusive pain, 465
VATER association, 336
VCD. *See* Vocal cord dysfunction
VCUG. *See* Voiding cystourethrogram
VDRL. *See* Venereal disease research laboratory
Venereal disease research laboratory (VDRL), 171, 362
Venipuncture, 205
Venom immunotherapy, 242
Venous hum, 181
Ventricular arrhythmias, 203
Ventricular septal defects (VSDs), 188, 192
Ventricular tachycardia, *202*, 209
Vermicularis, 35
Vesicular lesion, 9
Vesiculobullous lesions, 170
Viral conjunctivitis, 546
Viral gastroenteritis, 386–387
Viral hepatitis, 53–60
Viral infections, 220, 398–400
Viral pneumonia, 394
Viral sepsis, 165–167
Viral upper respiratory infections, 220
Viruses. *See also* Human immunodeficiency virus
    Epstein-Barr, 415
    hepatitis B, 19–20, 54–57, 121, 428
    hepatitis C, 53, 57–59
    hepatitis G, 59
    herpes simplex, 9, 165–167, 362–363, 363*t*
    parainfluenza, 428
    Varicella Zoster, 159

Visceral hyperalgesia, 37
Visceral larva migrans, 412
Vision screening, 317, 324
Visual-perceptual function, 321
Vitamin A, 564
    deficiency, 565
    toxicity, 565
Vitamin B$_{12}$, 82, 86
Vitamin C, 34
    deficiency, 565
    toxicity, 566
Vitamin D deficiency, 137, 565
    rickets, 136–137
Vitamin D-deficient rickets, 31
Vitamin D-resistance rickets, 136
Vitamin E, 83
Vitamin K deficiency, 565
Vitiligo, *7*
Vocal cord dysfunction (VCD), 239
Voiding cystourethrogram (VCUG), 536
Vomiting
    bilious, 557
    cyclic, 259
von Willebrand disease, 483–484
VSDs. *See* Ventricular septal defects
vulvovaginitis, 29
VZV. *See* Varicella zoster virus

W

Waardenburg syndrome, 272, 563
Warts, 10
WAS. *See* Wiskott-Aldrich syndrome
WBCs. *See* White blood cells
Weil syndrome, 408
Wheezing, 413
White blood cells (WBCs), 118
White reflex, 476
Whole-bowel irrigation, 496
Williams syndrome, 329
Wilms tumor, 474–475, 487, 489
Wilson disease, 289, 552
Wiskott-Aldrich syndrome (WAS), 245, 379, 382, 483
Wolff-Parkinson-White syndrome (WPW), 205
Worsening central nervous system acidosis, 112
WPW. *See* Wolff-Parkinson-White syndrome
Wrist fractures, 503

X

X-linked agammaglobulinemia, 378
X-linked dystrophies, 275–277
X-linked hyper-IgM syndrome, 378

Y

Yellow jackets, 217
Yersinia infection, 386

Z

Zinc, 33, 64
Zona fasciculata, 123
Zona glomerulosa, 123
Zona reticularis, 123
Zonisamide, 253